D0930809

SECOND EDITION

# THE 5-MINUTE ORTHOPAEDIC CONSULT

## Section Editors

Simon C. Mears, MD, PhD
*Arthroplasty*

John T. Campbell, MD
*Foot and Ankle*

Dawn W. LaPorte, MD
*Hand*

Timothy S. Johnson, MD
*History and Physical Examination*

Laura M. Fayad, MD
*Imaging*

Frank J. Frassica, MD
*Oncology*

Paul D. Sponsellar, MD
*Pediatrics*

A. Jay Khanna, MD
*Spine*

John H. Wilckens, MD
*Sports*

Simon C. Mears, MD, PhD
*Trauma*

# THE 5-MINUTE ORTHOPAEDIC CONSULT

SECOND EDITION

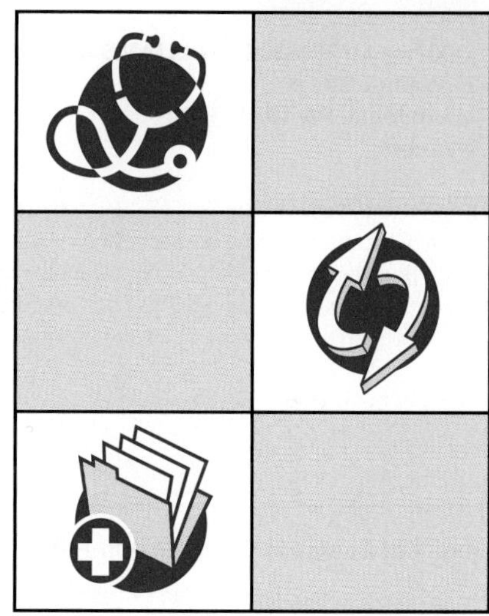

**Frank J. Frassica, MD**
**Paul D. Sponseller, MD**
**John H. Wilckens, MD**

Lippincott Williams & Wilkins
a Wolters Kluwer business
Philadelphia • Baltimore • New York • London
Buenos Aires • Hong Kong • Sydney • Tokyo

*Acquisitions Editor:* Robert Hurley
*Managing Editor:* David Murphy
*Project Manager:* Rosanne Hallowell
*Manufacturing Coordinator:* Kathleen Brown
*Marketing Manager:* Sharon Zinner
*Design Coordinator:* Teresa Mallon
*Cover Designer:* Becky Baxendell
*Production Service:* TechBooks
*Printer:* R. R. Donnelley


**530 Walnut Street**
**Philadelphia, PA 19106 USA**
**LWW.com**



Printed in the USA

---

**Library of Congress Cataloging-in-Publication Data**

The 5-minute orthopaedic consult / [edited by] Frank J. Frassica, Paul D. Sponseller, John H. Wilckens. – 2nd ed.
p. ; cm.
Includes bibliographical references and index.
ISBN-13: 978-0-7817-9971-3 (hardcover : alk. paper)
ISBN-10: 0-7817-9971-6 (hardcover : alk. paper)
1. Orthopedics—Handbooks, manuals, etc. I. Frassica, Frank J. II. Sponseller, Paul D. III. Wilckens, John H. IV. Title: Five minute orthopaedic consult.
[DNLM: 1. Orthopedics—Handbooks. WE 39 Z999 2007]
RD732.5.A16 2007
616.7–dc22 2006032865

---



To purchase additional copies of this book, call our customer service department at (800) 638-3030 or fax orders to (301) 223-2320. International customers should call (301) 223-2300.

Visit Lippincott Williams & Wilkins on the Internet: http://www.LWW.com. Lippincott Williams & Wilkins customer service representatives are available from 8:30 am to 6:00 pm, EST.

10 9 8 7 6 5 4 3 2 1

*We dedicate this book to our wives, Debbie, Amy, and Peggy.*

*We also dedicate this book to the memory of Drs. James F. and Lidia Z. Wenz, who died tragically in a motor vehicle accident on January 20, 2004. James Wenz, an Associate Editor of the first edition of the 5-Minute Orthopaedic Consult, was a superb clinician and innovator, a respected teacher, and a trusted mentor and friend. His thumbprints continue to mark the clinical, educational, and research endeavors of the Johns Hopkins University, including this book. Lidia, his gracious wife and an accomplished child psychiatrist, was a friend and inspiration who will never be forgotten.*

# PREFACE

The *5-Minute Orthopaedic Consult* is designed to provide easy-to-use, subject-specific information. The organization and indexing of topics make this book a reference clinicians can use to help make decisions on the spot while seeing patients in the clinic or in the hospital. The consistent page presentation within each topic enables the user to scan the topic to find specific information or to gain an overview of the topic within minutes by reading it completely. We have included some relevant in-depth information, such as causes and pathogenesis, but in a condensed fashion.

This second edition represents more than an update of useful clinical information in orthopaedics. The authors in this second edition have been specifically charged to provide evidence-based information, clinical material that has met the rigorous process of peer review and is appropriately referenced. These chapters also have been organized a little differently: They all appear in alphabetic order, so that the reader can find the necessary information more quickly, without having to check various sections of the book for the desired topic.

We want this book to be a useful reference. Please take a few minutes to leaf through it and get an idea of its scope and organization. We welcome suggestions for future editions. Please feel free to send us an e-mail at psponse@jhmi.edu.

# ACKNOWLEDGMENTS

The authors would like to express their heartfelt appreciation to Mrs. Elaine P. Henze, BJ, ELS, Senior Medical Editor of the Department of Orthopaedic Surgery at the Johns Hopkins University. She provided not only the rigorous standards but also the professional encouragement to make this project a reality. We also would like to acknowledge Ms. Gwen Walls, MS, our Assistant Editor, who was tireless in verifying and inputting into our reference database all the published material cited in this second edition.

The authors also would like to thank Jenny Kim and Mary Choi, (at Lippincott Williams & Wilkins) and Stephanie Lentz and Jeri Litteral (at TechBooks, York, PA) for helping to bring this new edition to completion. Many of the expert line drawings by Hong Cui, MD, provided for the topics in the first edition, have been retained.

Without the help of these individuals, this second edition would not have been possible!

# CONTRIBUTORS

The following individuals contributed to this book during their residency at the Johns Hopkins University School of Medicine in the Department of Orthopaedics.


**Nicholas Ahn, MD**

**Kris J. Alden, MD, PhD**

**Fariba Asrari, MD**

**Michael S. Bahk, MD**

**Scott Berkenblit, MD, PhD**

**Henry Boateng, MD**

**Michelle Cameron, MD**

**John T. Campbell, MD**

**John J. Carbone, MD**

**Brett M. Cascio, MD**

**Marc D. Chodos, MD**

**Mark Clough, MD**

**David B. Cohen, MD**

**Constantine A. Demetracopoulos, BS**

**Rohit Robert Dhir, BA**

**William J. Didie, MD**

**Damien Doute, MD**

**Adam J. Farber, MD**

**Kevin W. Farmer, MD**

**Laura M. Fayad, MD**

**Deborah A. Frassica, MD**

**Frank J. Frassica, MD**

**Gregory Gebauer, MD, MS**

**Sergio A. Glait, BS**

**Ricardo A. Gonzales, MD**

**Jason W. Hammond, MD**

**Bill Hobbs, MD**

**Emmanuel Hostin, MD**

**Marc W. Hungerford, MD**

**Chris Hutchins, MD**

**John J. Hwang, MD**

**Heather A. Jacene, MD**

**Jamil Jacobs-El, MD**

**Peter R. Jay, MD**

**Clifford L. Jeng, MD**

**Timothy S. Johnson, MD**

**A. Jay Khanna, MD**

**Melanie Kinchen, MD**

**Dennis E. Kramer, MD**

**Dawn M. LaPorte, MD**

**Tung B. Le, MD**

**Andrew P. Manista, MD**

**Theodore T. Manson, MD**

**Sanjog Mathur, MD**

**Lawrence A. McGuigan, PA-C, MMS**

**Simon C. Mears, MD, PhD**

**Daniel L. Miller, BS**

**Misty A. Moore, MSN, FNP**

**Tariq A. Nayfeh, MD, PhD**

**Philip R. Neubauer, MD**

**Derek F. Papp, MD**

**Dhruv B. Pateder, MD**

**Andrew M. Richards, MD**

**William W. Scott, Jr, MD**

**Michael K. Shindle, MD**

**Eric D. Shirley, MD**

**Karl A. Soderlund, BS**

**David Solacoff, MD**

**Paul D. Sponseller, MD**

**Anirudh Sridharan, MD**

**Uma Srikumaran, MD**

**Ryan K. Takenaga, BS**

**Darryl B. Thomas, MD**

**Marc Urquhart, MD**

**Matthew D. Waites, AFRCS (Ed)**

**Barry Waldman, MD**

Jinsong Wang, MD

Kristy L. Weber, MD

James F. Wenz, Sr, MD

Carl Wierks, MD

John H. Wilckens, MD

# CONTENTS

SECOND EDITION

# THE 5-MINUTE ORTHOPAEDIC CONSULT

# ACCESSORY NAVICULAR

*Kris J. Alden, MD, PhD*

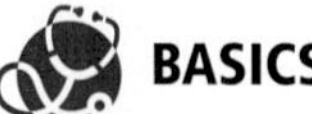

## BASICS

### DESCRIPTION

- This anatomic variant consists of an accessory ossicle located at the medial edge of the navicular (Fig. 1).
- Accessory ossicles are derived from unfused ossification centers.
- Considered an incidental finding on radiographs, but may become symptomatic
- Classification: 3 major types of accessory navicular adjacent to the posteromedial navicular tuberosity (1)
  - Type I: Small, 2–3-mm sesamoid bone in the PTT; referred to as "os tibiale externum"
  - Type II:
    - Larger ossicle than type I
    - Secondary ossification center of the navicular bone
  - Type III: Enlarged navicular tuberosity, considered a fused variant of a type II, often with pointed shape
- Synonyms: Os tibiale; Os tibiale externum; Naviculare secundum

#### *Pediatric Considerations*

Often presents in adolescent patients or young adults, with flatfoot deformity and arch pain

### EPIDEMIOLOGY

#### *Incidence*

- 4–21% incidence; 89% of cases are bilateral (2).
- One of the most common accessory ossicles in the foot
- It is seen over the medial pole of the navicular bone, usually in adolescent patients (3).
- It is most commonly symptomatic in the 2nd decade of life and causes medial foot pain (4).
- <1% of patients become symptomatic.

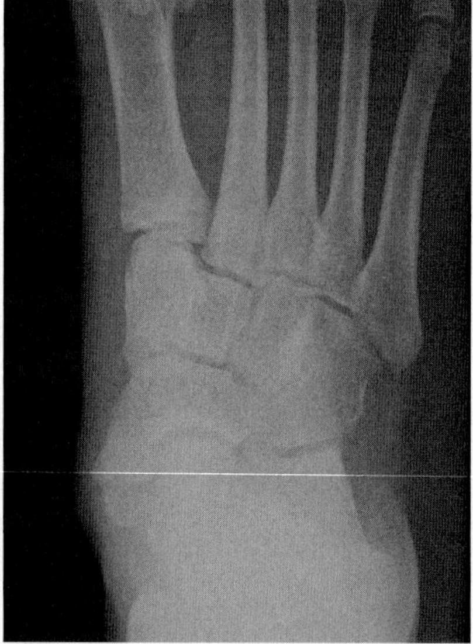

**Fig. 1.** AP radiograph showing an accessory navicular.

- Incidence by classification (1):
  - Type I: ~30% of all accessory navicular bones
  - Type II: ~50%
  - Type III: ~20%

#### *Prevalence*

- Usually affects teens and young adults
- More frequent in females
- May be seen in older adults as incidental finding or, in rare cases, as symptomatic

### ETIOLOGY

- The accessory navicular is a variant of normal anatomy.
- It may become symptomatic from the bony prominence impinging against shoe wear.
- The patient may have diffuse medial and plantar arch pain.
- It may cause problems by destabilizing the insertion and diminishing the pull of the PTT.
- In patients with associated severe flatfoot deformity, lateral pain may occur secondary to impingement of the calcaneus against the fibula.
- A traumatic event can cause injury to the fibrocartilaginous synchondrosis that attaches the ossicle to the main navicular.

### ASSOCIATED CONDITIONS

- Flatfoot deformity
- Secondary Achilles tendon contracture

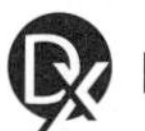

## DIAGNOSIS

### SIGNS AND SYMPTOMS

- Pain may begin after wearing ill-fitting shoes, with weightbearing activities or athletics, or after trauma to the foot.
- Characteristics:
  - Pain and tenderness along the medial aspect of the foot in the region of the accessory navicular
  - Pain or weakness when the patient attempts to rise on toes, run, or jump
  - Often increased prominence over the medial end of the navicular

#### *History*

- The pain is localized to the medial aspect of the navicular.
- Symptomatic accessory tarsal navicular may develop in young athletes (5–7).
- Exacerbated by weightbearing, walking, athletic activity, or the wearing of narrow shoes
- Pain often is relieved by rest.

#### *Physical Exam*

- Tenderness is localized to the medial pole of the navicular.
  - May be exacerbated by abducting and adducting the foot
- Assess the insole of the shoe, which may exacerbate symptoms.
- Assess the strength of the PTT by manual resistance testing against plantarflexion-inversion and by determining the ability to perform multiple single-limb heel rises.
- Assess ankle and subtalar joint motion.
- Identify contracture of the Achilles tendon.

### TESTS

#### *Imaging*

- Obtain routine standing AP, external oblique, and lateral radiographs of the foot.
  - Type-II accessory ossicle has smooth borders, is triangular or heart-shaped, and measures 9 × 12 mm in size.
  - The base is situated 1–2 mm from the medial and posterior aspects of the navicular bone.
  - The accessory ossicle may be best visualized on the internal oblique view.
  - Smooth margins with well-formed cortex differentiate this condition from acute fracture.
- Bone scan:
  - May show increased activity over an accessory navicular
  - May be needed if a navicular stress fracture is suspected in the differential diagnosis
- MRI:
  - Useful when plain films are unremarkable
  - Often, a type-II accessory navicular is attached to the tuberosity by a fibrocartilage or hyaline cartilage layer, and MRI may show soft-tissue edema consistent with a synchondrosis sprain or tear.
  - Shows altered signal intensity and bone marrow edema, suggestive of chronic stress and/or osteonecrosis (8)
  - Also helpful in showing PTT degeneration

#### *Pathological Findings*

- This separate osteocartilaginous fragment is located in place of the normal medial pole of the navicular.
- The PTT inserts on the accessory navicular, navicular body, and cuneiforms.

### DIFFERENTIAL DIAGNOSIS

- Navicular fracture may mimic an acute avulsion fracture of the tuberosity of the navicular.
- Posterior tibial tendinitis
- Stress fracture of navicular

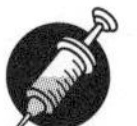

## TREATMENT

### GENERAL MEASURES

- The patient should rest and avoid athletics or aggravating activities.
- Anti-inflammatory medication
- Shoe-wear modification, including use of a softer, wider shoe
- If flatfoot is present, a medial arch support may be useful, but often the patient may not tolerate it because of direct pressure on the ossicle.
- Below-the-knee walking cast or removable fracture boot may be used for 3–6 weeks for persistent symptoms.
- Physical therapy, including strengthening exercises and cryotherapy, may be helpful.

### MEDICATION (DRUGS)

No evidence suggests that one NSAID is superior to another.

### SURGERY

- If pain is progressive or does not remit with nonoperative treatment, surgical excision may be considered.
- In the Kidner procedure, the accessory navicular is excised, and the PTT is rerouted into a more plantar position (9).
- Contemporary surgical treatment:
  - Includes excision of the ossicle and reattachment of the PTT insertion to the navicular, with suture anchors or sutures passed through drill holes
  - Typically provides satisfactory outcome and good pain relief, particularly in adolescents
- Severe flatfoot deformity with lateral impingement symptoms may require concomitant osteotomy of the calcaneus and/or medial column of the foot to improve alignment and decrease mechanical stress of the PTT insertion.

## FOLLOW-UP

### COMPLICATIONS

Weakness, incomplete pain relief, continued deformity

### REFERENCES

1. Sella EJ, Lawson JP, Ogden JA. The accessory navicular synchondrosis. *Clin Orthop Relat Res* 1986;209:280–285.
2. Miller TT. Painful accessory bones of the foot. *Semin Musculoskelet Radiol* 2002;6:153–161.
3. Lawson JP, Ogden JA, Sella E, et al. The painful accessory navicular. *Skeletal Radiol* 1984;12:250–262.
4. Romanowski CAJ, Barrington NA. The accessory navicular—an important cause of medial foot pain. *Clin Radiol* 1992;46:261–264.
5. Mygind HB. The accessory tarsal seaphoid [sic]. Clinical features and treatment. *Acta Orthop Scand* 1953;23:142–151.
6. Ray S, Goldberg VM. Surgical treatment of the accessory navicular. *Clin Orthop Relat Res* 1983;177:61–66.
7. Veitch JM. Evaluation of the Kidner procedure in treatment of symptomatic accessory tarsal scaphoid. *Clin Orthop Relat Res* 1978;131:210–213.
8. Demeyere N, De Maeseneer M, Osteaux M. Quiz case. Symptomatic type II accessory navicular. *Eur J Radiol* 2001;37:60–63.
9. Kidner FC. The prehallux (accessory scaphoid) in its relation to flat-foot. *J Bone Joint Surg* 1929;11:831–837.

### ADDITIONAL READING

- Coughlin MJ. Sesamoids and accessory bones of the foot. In: Coughlin MJ, Mann RA, eds. *Surgery of the Foot and Ankle*, 7th ed. St. Louis: Mosby, 1999:437–499.
- Kidner FC. The prehallux in relation to flatfoot. *JAMA* 1933;101:1539–1542.
- Kopp FJ, Marcus RE. Clinical outcome of surgical treatment of the symptomatic accessory navicular. *Foot Ankle Int* 2004;25:27–30.

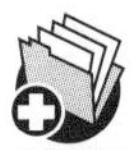

## MISCELLANEOUS

### CODES

#### *ICD9-CM*

- 754.61 Pes planus, congenital
- 755.56 Accessory navicular

### PATIENT TEACHING

- Instruct patients on the typically benign nature of the condition.
- If the condition is secondary to medial pressure from the shoe, suggest a wider, softer shoe.
- Recommend rest from sports with gradual return when symptoms subside.

### FAQ

- Q: What is the most common type of accessory navicular seen radiographically?
  - A: Type-II, with a large accessory ossicle, is the most common.
- Q: What are the standard treatment methods for initial management of a symptomatic accessory navicular?
  - A: Rest, NSAIDs, restriction from sports, immobilization with a boot brace or walking cast, physical therapy, and orthotic arch supports.

# ACHILLES TENDINITIS

*Dennis E. Kramer, MD*

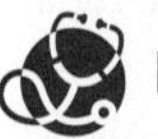

## BASICS

### DESCRIPTION

- Common overuse injury
- Represents a spectrum of disorders involving the Achilles tendon, paratenon, and retrocalcaneal bursa
- Ranges from painful inflammation of the Achilles tendon and its sheath to chronic degenerative tendinosis and tearing
- Definitions:
  - Retrocalcaneal bursitis: Inflammation of the retrocalcaneal bursa, sparing tendon
  - Paratenonitis: Paratenon inflammation
  - Achilles tendinitis: Acute inflammation of the tendon with paratenon inflammation
  - Tendinosis: Intrasubstance degeneration of the tendon
- Location: Noninsertional (several centimeters above attachment to the calcaneus) versus insertional (at insertion point on the posterior calcaneus)

### GENERAL PREVENTION

- Avoid excessive running uphill.
- Avoid training errors, such as overly rapid increase in running mileage.

### EPIDEMIOLOGY

- Occurs particularly in recreational and competitive athletes, especially long-distance runners
- Common in active middle-aged individuals
- The Male:Female predominance approximately parallels the percentage of Male:Female participation in a given athletic activity.
- Degenerative tendinosis also occurs in middle-aged to elderly individuals, regardless of sports participation.

#### *Incidence*

Occurs in 6% of runners (1)

### RISK FACTORS

- Large posterosuperior calcaneal tuberosity (Haglund process)
- Microvascular disease: Diabetes, lupus, rheumatoid disease
- Hemodialysis or peritoneal dialysis: Renal disease
- Connective-tissue disease

### PATHOPHYSIOLOGY

- Achilles tendon anatomy (2):
  - 95% type-I collagen
  - Wavy configuration at rest
  - Surrounded throughout its length by a thin gliding paratenon that functions as an elastic sleeve, permitting free tendon movement
  - Achilles tendon blood supply:
    - Intrinsic vascular system at the musculotendinous and osteotendinous junctions
    - Extrinsic vascular supply via paratenon
    - Zone of hypovascularity 2–6 cm proximal to tendon insertion
  - Paratenonitis/tendinitis: Chronic inflammatory changes (uncommon)
  - Tendinosis: Chronic mucoid degenerative changes with disorganization of collagen fibers (common)

### ETIOLOGY

- Training errors (60–80%): Sudden increase in training regimen (mileage), change in shoe wear or terrain (2,3)
- Rough terrain or uneven surfaces
- Improper shoe wear
- Adverse weather conditions (ice, snow, cold)
- Biomechanical abnormalities of the lower extremity, from lumbar spine to foot (2,3)
  - Hyperpronation
  - Cavus foot
  - Leg-length discrepancy
- Chronically inappropriate, short, or absent warm-up and stretching period

### ASSOCIATED CONDITIONS

Achilles tendon rupture

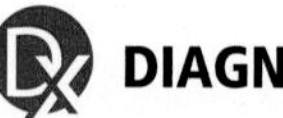

## DIAGNOSIS

### SIGNS AND SYMPTOMS

- A gradual increase in painful swelling and warmth occurs at any point along the tendon substance, from the musculotendinous junction to the bony insertion (os calcis).
- Most pain is 3–5 cm proximal to the insertion onto the calcaneus.
- Microtrauma, such as continued running, or even gross trauma, such as a single leap (in jumpers), exacerbates the symptoms.
- Pain is relieved somewhat by rest.

#### *Physical Exam*

- Check for pain on dorsiflexion of the ankle.
  - Palpate the tendon to localize the pain.
  - In severe cases, the tendon sheath may be swollen and crepitant with ankle motion (Figs. 1 and 2).
- Feel for nodular swelling in the tendon.
- Use the Thompson test to rule out tendon rupture.
- Swelling, warmth, or bogginess immediately anterior to the tendon insertion suggests retrocalcaneal bursitis.
- Test single-limb heel rise.
- Note any intrinsic foot, ankle, or leg deformities: Pes cavus, leg-length discrepancy, scoliosis, equinus deformity

### TESTS

#### *Lab*

- Usually none are indicated.
- Serum chemistry study with glucose is recommended if diabetes is suspected.
- Evaluate for inflammatory arthritis if clinically indicated.

#### *Imaging*

- Standing foot radiographs:
  - AP, lateral, oblique views
  - Assess Haglund prominence.
  - Identify:
    - Insertional spurring of the calcaneus
    - Intratendinous calcification, indicative of chronic tendinosis

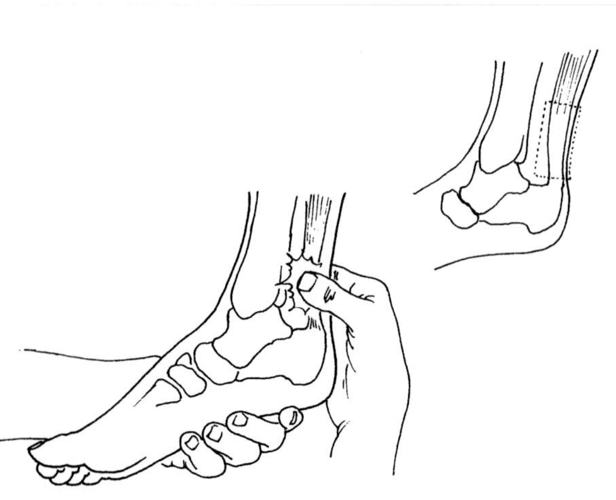

**Fig. 1.** The area of tenderness in Achilles tendinitis is above the heel, over a broad area.

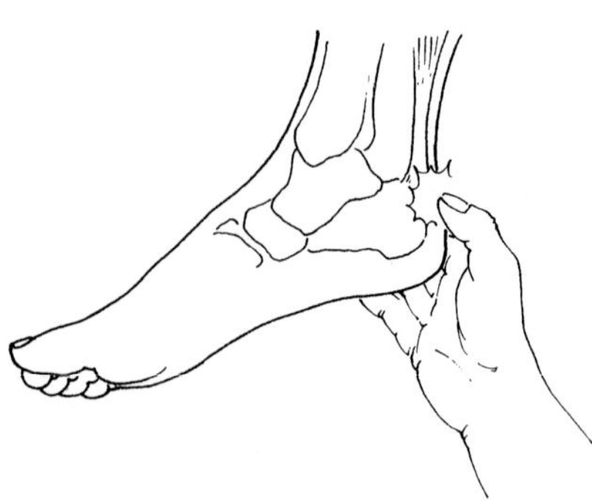

**Fig. 2.** Retrocalcaneal bursitis produces pain in the back of the heel, at the insertion of the Achilles tendon.

- MRI is indicated if the clinical picture suggests tendinosis (4).
  - MRI of a normal Achilles tendon:
    - Homogenous low signal on all sequences
    - Flat or concave anterior margin
    - Crescentic shape
    - Ovoid shape at its insertion onto the calcaneus
    - Normal thickness <8 mm
  - MRI of acute paratenonitis:
    - Loss of sharp interface between tendon and pre-Achilles fat
    - On T2-weighted views, high signal intensity around the tendon and pre-Achilles fat
    - Low signal intensity within tendon itself
  - MRI of chronic Achilles tendinopathy:
    - Thickened >8 mm, enlarged tendon
    - Loss of normal concave margin anteriorly
    - On T1-weighted views, heterogeneous increased signal intensity within tendon
  - MRI of Achilles rupture:
    - Usually occurs 3–5 cm above calcaneal insertion
    - Partial rupture has focal areas of high signal intensity on T2-weighted sequence images within the tendon substance, with preservation of continuity of the tendon.
    - Complete rupture shows loss of continuity with gap formation (high signal area on T2-weighted views).
- Ultrasound:
  - Technique is technician-dependent.
  - Shows fluid around tendon or peritendinous adhesions

### DIFFERENTIAL DIAGNOSIS

- Precalcaneal bursitis
- Retrocalcaneal bursitis
- Peroneal tendinitis or rupture
- Posterior tibialis tendinitis or rupture
- Achilles tendon rupture, partial or complete, may represent terminal stage.
- Inflammatory arthritis

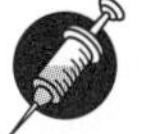

## TREATMENT

### GENERAL MEASURES

- Early, acute phase:
  - NSAIDs, ice, rest, heel lift, foot-wear modification, and orthotic correction of the foot and leg abnormality
  - Modify activities; perform Achilles stretching.
  - Retrocalcaneal bursa injection also may help relieve symptoms and inflammation.
  - For patients unresponsive to the previously-listed treatments, a trial of cast or boot immobilization is appropriate.
  - Corticosteroid injection of the tendon sheath may precipitate rupture and should be avoided.

### SPECIAL THERAPY

#### *Physical Therapy*

- Ultrasound therapy (during proliferative phase healing), phonophoresis, iontophoresis, and short-term heel wedge use (to unload tendon unit)
- Eventually, flexibility, strengthening, and conditioning through *eccentric* exercise to gain maximal benefit

### MEDICATION (DRUGS)

#### *First Line*

- NSAIDs
- Analgesics

### SURGERY

- For patients for whom nonoperative treatment for 3–6 months has failed:
  - Paratenonitis:
    - Treatment involves removal or release of the paratenon through a straight medial incision.
  - Achilles tendinosis:
    - Requires intratendinous débridement, retrocalcaneal bursectomy, and Haglund exostectomy (5,6)
    - May require augmentation or local tendon transfer (e.g., plantaris or flexor hallucis longus) if Achilles tendon has extensive disease (7)

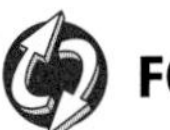

## FOLLOW-UP

### PROGNOSIS

The prognosis is good, but recovery can be prolonged.

### COMPLICATIONS

Tendon degeneration and eventual rupture with loss of function, particularly with a high rate of surgical failure, are possible.

### PATIENT MONITORING

Routine follow-up is indicated until the symptoms have resolved.

### REFERENCES


1. Clement DB, Taunton JE, Smart GW. Achilles tendinitis and peritendinitis: etiology and treatment. *Am J Sports Med* 1984;12:179–184.
2. Paavola M, Kannus P, Jarvinen TAH, et al. Achilles tendinopathy. *J Bone Joint Surg* 2002;84A: 2062–2076.
3. Schepsis AA, Jones H, Haas AL. Achilles tendon disorders in athletes. *Am J Sports Med* 2002;30:287–305.
4. Recht MP, Donley BG. Magnetic Resonance Imaging of the foot and ankle. *J Am Acad Orthop Surg* 2001;9:187–199.
5. McGarvey WC, Palumbo RC, Baxter DE, et al. Insertional Achilles tendinosis: surgical treatment through a central tendon splitting approach. *Foot Ankle Int* 2002;23:19–25.
6. Watson AD, Anderson RB, Davis WH. Comparison of results of retrocalcaneal decompression for retrocalcaneal bursitis and insertional Achilles tendinosis with calcific spur. *Foot Ankle Int* 2000;21:638–642.
7. Martin RL, Manning CM, Carcia CR, et al. An outcome study of chronic Achilles tendinosis after excision of the Achilles tendon and flexor hallucis longus tendon transfer. *Foot Ankle Int* 2005;26:691–697.


### ADDITIONAL READING


- Clain MR, Baxter DE. Achilles tendinitis. *Foot Ankle* 1992;13:482–487.
- Saltzman CL, Tearse DS. Achilles tendon injuries. *J Am Acad Orthop Surg* 1998;6:316–325.


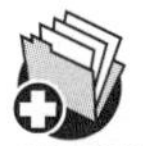

## MISCELLANEOUS

### CODES

#### *ICD9-CM*

- 726.71 Achilles tendinitis
- 727.82 Calcium deposits in tendon and bursa

### PATIENT TEACHING

#### *Activity*

Proper shoe wear and terrain adjustment, with avoidance of steep hills and stairs

#### *Prevention*

Adequate pretraining stretching and warm-up

### FAQ

- Q: What is the most common location for Achilles tendinosis?
  - A: In the zone of avascularity, 2–6 cm proximal to the tendon's insertion onto the calcaneus.
- Q: How long should nonoperative treatment be attempted for Achilles tendinosis before proceeding with surgery?
  - A: At least 6 months of nonoperative treatment are recommended before surgical treatment.
- Q: What are the MRI findings in Achilles tendinopathy?
  - A: On T1-weighted MRI images, a thickened (>8 mm) Achilles tendon with loss of normal concave anterior margin and increased signal intensity within the tendon.

# ACHILLES TENDON RUPTURE

*Marc D. Chodos, MD*

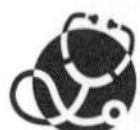

## BASICS

### DESCRIPTION

- The Achilles tendon is the strongest tendon in the body and is subject to loads of 5–7 times body weight.
- Definition: Tendon disruption in its watershed region
- Anatomy (1):
  - The terminal segment of the medial and lateral gastrocnemius and the soleus muscles
  - Is ~15 cm long and inserts on the posterior calcaneal tuberosity
  - Is surrounded by a paratenon, which allows it to glide freely
  - Is composed mainly of type 1 collagen
  - The blood supply to the tendon is poorest in a watershed region from 2–6 cm proximal to the tendon's insertion on the calcaneus.
  - The tendon rotates 90° as it courses distally, concentrating mechanical stress in the watershed area.
- Classification:
  - Acute versus chronic
  - Open versus closed
  - Complete versus incomplete

### GENERAL PREVENTION

Training and stretching result in tendon adaptation, including increased cross-sectional area.

### EPIDEMIOLOGY

- Bimodal distribution (2):
  - Young to middle-aged athletes (30–40 years old)
    - 60–75% occur during sports activity.
    - The most common sports to cause acute Achilles tendon rupture varies from country to country, depending on which sports are most popular in that area.
  - Older nonathletes (~13% of ruptures)

#### *Incidence*

- Unclear, varying from 2–37.3 per 100,000 in several studies (2,3)
- Increasing incidence seen in recent decades

#### *Prevalence*

- It predominantly affects males.
- Left side injury is more common than right (possibly because right-hand dominant athletes push-off with the left leg).
- More common in industrialized countries and among "weekend warriors"

### RISK FACTORS

- In 1 study, previous Achilles tendon rupture was a risk factor for future contralateral tendon rupture in up to 6% of patients (4).
- Several medications are associated with an increased risk of tendon rupture (2,3).
  - Corticosteroids, either oral or injected locally into the Achilles tendon area
  - Anabolic steroids
  - Fluoroquinolone antibiotics
- Multiple systemic diseases have been associated, but not often, with spontaneous ruptures (3,5).
  - Diabetes
  - Rheumatoid arthritis and other inflammatory arthritides
  - Gout

### PATHOPHYSIOLOGY

Histopathology from Achilles tendon ruptures almost always shows evidence of degenerative changes and chronic tendinosis.

### ETIOLOGY

- Most common: Indirect mechanism:
  - Pushing off with weightbearing foot while extending the knee
  - Eccentric contraction of gastrocnemius–soleus complex
- Rarely, direct trauma such as a laceration or gunshot wound can tear the Achilles tendon.

### ASSOCIATED CONDITIONS

- Achilles tendinopathy
  - Insertional: Retrocalcaneal bursitis, insertional tendinopathy
  - Noninsertional: Tendinosis, peritendinitis

## DIAGNOSIS

### SIGNS AND SYMPTOMS

- Usually, a sudden "snap" or "pop" is felt in the back of the ankle.
- Patient may describe a sensation of being kicked in the back of the leg.
- Pain may be severe.
- Local pain, swelling with a palpable gap along the Achilles tendon near its insertion site, and weak active plantarflexion strength all strongly suggest the diagnosis.

#### *History*

In addition to a general foot and ankle history, enquire about previous pain or symptoms of tendinopathy.

#### *Physical Exam*

- Perform general foot and ankle examination, concentrating on the following specific areas:
  - Examine the posterior ankle for tenderness, swelling, or a palpable gap in the tendon.
  - Check muscle strength.
    - Patient still may be able to plantarflex the ankle by compensating with other muscles, but strength will be weak.
    - Single-limb heel rise will not be possible.
  - Knee flexion test:
    - Check resting position of ankle with patient prone and knees flexed 90°.
    - Loss of normal resting gastrocnemius–soleus tension will allow ankle to assume a more dorsiflexed position than that on the uninjured side.
  - Thompson test:
    - Position the patient prone with ankles clear of the table.
    - Squeezing the calf normally produces passive plantarflexion of the ankle.
    - If the Achilles tendon is not in continuity, the ankle will not passively flex with compression of calf muscles.

### TESTS

#### *Lab*

Obtain preoperative laboratory tests only if surgery is planned.

#### *Imaging*

- Plain radiographs to evaluate bony structure
- If evidence is present of a calcaneal tuberosity fracture and Achilles tendon avulsion, CT can help to assess the calcaneus fracture pattern.
- Acute Achilles tendon rupture usually is a diagnosis made clinically.
  - If the diagnosis is in question, MRI or, occasionally, ultrasound can help to make the diagnosis.

### DIFFERENTIAL DIAGNOSIS

- Achilles tendinopathy
- Partial Achilles tendon rupture
- Calcaneus fracture

## TREATMENT

### INITIAL STABILIZATION

- Once the diagnosis is made, the ankle should be splinted in equinus with a well-padded, below-the-knee, nonweightbearing splint.
- Ice and elevation help to control swelling.

### GENERAL MEASURES

- Management can be operative or nonoperative, depending on the patient's age, general health, activity level, and preferences.
  - In general, surgical treatment is preferred in young, active, healthy individuals.
- Surgical and nonsurgical techniques are associated with treatment-specific risks and benefits that both surgeon and patient must consider (3).
- Nonoperative management:
  - Immobilization protocol:
    - Below-the-knee cast with ankle in full equinus is placed initially.
    - During the following 6–10 weeks, the ankle is gradually brought to a plantigrade position with cast changes approximately every 2 weeks.
    - Weightbearing is allowed after 4–6 weeks.
    - After casting, a heel lift usually is worn for several months.
  - Functional bracing protocol:
    - Boot or brace that limits dorsiflexion but allows plantarflexion
    - The dorsiflexion block is gradually relaxed, allowing more ankle motion.

#### *Activity*

With the nonoperative treatment technique, weightbearing usually is not permitted for 4–6 weeks.

### SPECIAL THERAPY

#### *Physical Therapy*

- Many rehabilitation protocols are available.
- Generally, therapy initially involves progressive, active ankle motion and progresses to weightbearing and strengthening.

### SURGERY

- Open technique (6):
  - Surgery is delayed ~1 week to allow for swelling diminution.
  - Prone position: Both legs should be draped into the operative field so that resting ankle position can be approximated to the normal side when sutures are tied.
  - A medial longitudinal incision along Achilles tendon often is used to decrease the risk of sural nerve injury.
  - A running locking technique with 2 suture strands in each segment of tendon produces the strongest repair (7).
  - The paratenon should be preserved and repaired to help prevent adhesions.
    - If present, the plantaris tendon can be unfolded and wrapped around the repair to minimize adhesion formation.
- Percutaneous techniques: Several techniques using special instruments and multiple stab incisions have been described (8–10).
- Surgical management of chronic ruptures:
  - The repair technique depends on the size of the gap and the presence of muscle atrophy.
    - If end-to-end repair is not possible, V–Y lengthening, turndown advancement flap, tendon transfer or augmentation (flexor hallucis longus, flexor digitorum longus), and allograft tendon are options.

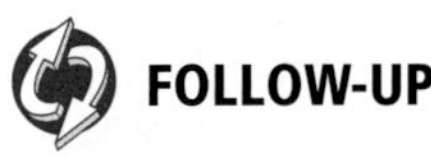

## FOLLOW-UP

### PROGNOSIS

- The prognosis is good for both operatively and nonoperatively managed Achilles tendon tears.
  - In a prospective randomized trial of 112 tears treated operatively or nonoperatively, no differences were noted in return to sports, isokinetic strength, endurance, or ankle motion at 1 year (11).
  - A meta-analysis of 421 patients showed a nonsignificant difference in the proportion of patients who regained normal function after surgical or nonoperative management (71% versus 63%) (12).

### COMPLICATIONS

- Meta-analysis of 356 patients (13):
  - Rerupture rate: 3.5% in the surgical group versus 12.6% in the nonsurgical group
  - Overall incidence of complications in the surgical group: 34.1%
    - 19.7% adhesions
    - 9.8% altered sensation (sural nerve most common)
    - 4% wound infection or dehiscence
  - Overall incidence of complications in the nonsurgical group: 2.7%
    - Adhesions, excessive tendon lengthening, and DVT were the most common.
- Compared with open techniques, percutaneous surgery has been associated with a shorter operative time, lower infection rate, higher rate of rerupture, and higher rate of sural nerve injury (14).
  - These results may improve with newer techniques (14).

### PATIENT MONITORING

- Sutures are removed ~2 weeks after surgery.
- Casting/bracing and progressive therapy are instituted as described earlier.
- Consider prophylaxis for DVT.

### REFERENCES


1. O'Brien M. The anatomy of the Achilles tendon. *Foot Ankle Clin* 2005;10:225–238.
2. Movin T, Ryberg A, McBride DJ, et al. Acute rupture of the Achilles tendon. *Foot Ankle Clin* 2005;10:331–356.
3. Jarvinen TA, Kannus P, Maffulli N, et al. Achilles tendon disorders: etiology and epidemiology. *Foot Ankle Clin* 2005;10:255–266.
4. Aroen A, Helgo D, Granlund OG, et al. Contralateral tendon rupture risk is increased in individuals with a previous Achilles tendon rupture. *Scand J Med Sci Sports* 2004;14:30–33.
5. Kannus P, Jozsa L. Histopathological changes preceding spontaneous rupture of a tendon. A controlled study of 891 patients. *J Bone Joint Surg* 1991;73A:1507–1525.
6. Myerson MS, Mandelbaum B. Disorders of the Achilles tendon and the retrocalcaneal region. In: Myerson MS, ed. *Foot and Ankle Disorders*. Philadelphia: WB Saunders Co., 2000:1367–1398.
7. Watson TW, Jurist KA, Yang KH, et al. The strength of Achilles tendon repair: an *in vitro* study of the biomechanical behavior in human cadaver tendons. *Foot Ankle Int* 1995;16:191–195.
8. Calder JD, Saxby TS. Early, active rehabilitation following mini-open repair of Achilles tendon rupture: a prospective study. *Br J Sports Med* 2005;39:857–859.
9. Lim J, Dalal R, Waseem M. Percutaneous vs. open repair of the ruptured Achilles tendon–a prospective randomized controlled study. *Foot Ankle Int* 2001;22:559–568.
10. Ma GWC, Griffith TG. Percutaneous repair of acute closed ruptured Achilles tendon: a new technique. *Clin Orthop Relat Res* 1977;128:247–255.
11. Moller M, Movin T, Granhed H, et al. Acute rupture of tendon Achillis. A prospective randomised study of comparison between surgical and non-surgical treatment. *J Bone Joint Surg* 2001;83B:843–848.
12. Bhandari M, Guyatt GH, Siddiqui F, et al. Treatment of acute Achilles tendon ruptures: a systematic overview and metaanalysis. *Clin Orthop Relat Res* 2002;400:190–200.
13. Khan RJK, Fick D, Brammar TJ, et al. Interventions for treating acute Achilles tendon ruptures. *Cochrane Database Syst Rev* 2006;3(CD003674):1–37.
14. Young JS, Kumta SM, Maffulli N. Achilles tendon rupture and tendinopathy: management of complications. *Foot Ankle Clin* 2005;10:371–382.


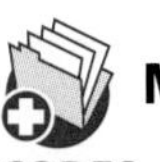

## MISCELLANEOUS

### CODES

#### *ICD9-CM*

- 727.67 Nontraumatic
- 845.09 Traumatic

### PATIENT TEACHING

The patient should be actively involved in the decision-making process, with a clear understanding of the risks and benefits of surgical and nonsurgical treatments.

### FAQ

- Q: Which nerve is at greatest risk for injury during operative treatment of an Achilles tendon rupture?
  - A: The *sural* nerve runs lateral to the Achilles tendon and is at risk.
- Q: In which situation is urgent surgical intervention required for a closed Achilles tendon injury?
  - A: Occasionally, the Achilles tendon will avulse a piece of the calcaneal tuberosity instead of producing an intratendinous tear. Because this area is subcutaneous, the bony fragment can place pressure on the skin, causing necrosis of the area. *Calcaneal tuberosity avulsion fractures should be fixed urgently if the skin is compromised.*
- Q: Can the ankle be plantarflexed if the Achilles tendon is ruptured?
  - A: Yes. Other muscles, including the tibialis posterior, flexor hallucis longus, flexor digitorum longus, and peroneals, pass posterior to the center of rotation for the ankle joint. Compensation using these muscles can plantarflex the ankle, but strength will be markedly diminished.
- Q: What is the main advantage of surgical treatment for an acute Achilles tendon tear?
  - A: The main advantage of operative management is the significantly lower rate of rerupture. In essence, for every 10 patients treated with surgical repair, 1 rerupture will be prevented. However, surgical repair has a higher risk of infection, wound healing problems, and sural nerve injury than nonoperative management (12).

# ACHONDROPLASIA

*Paul D. Sponseller, MD*

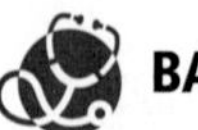

## BASICS

### DESCRIPTION

- Achondroplasia is the most common skeletal dysplasia.
- Characteristics:
  - Patient height <4.5 feet at maturity
  - The greatest shortening occurs in the proximal humerus and femur (1).
  - Hypoplasia of the midface and frontal bossing may be present (Fig. 1).
  - Arthritis is rarely seen, but spinal stenosis is the most serious possible complication.
  - Affects the skeletal and neurologic systems
  - Its features are immediately evident at birth, but life expectancy is not substantially altered in the heterozygote:
    - Skeleton: Ligamentous laxity, undergrowth of long bones
    - Neurologic: Stenosis of the foramen magnum in infancy or the lumbar spine near maturity
    - Skeletal dysplasia: Rhizomelic short stature

### EPIDEMIOLOGY

#### *Incidence*

- The incidence of spinal stenosis and degenerative disc disease increases with age.
- It affects males and females equally.

#### *Prevalence*

1 per 15,000 population (1)

### RISK FACTORS

- Parental age >37 years
- Achondroplastic parent

#### *Genetics*

- Autosomal dominant
- Acquired by most patients (70%) as a new mutation (1,2)
- Homozygous patients (with 2 affected parents) usually die.

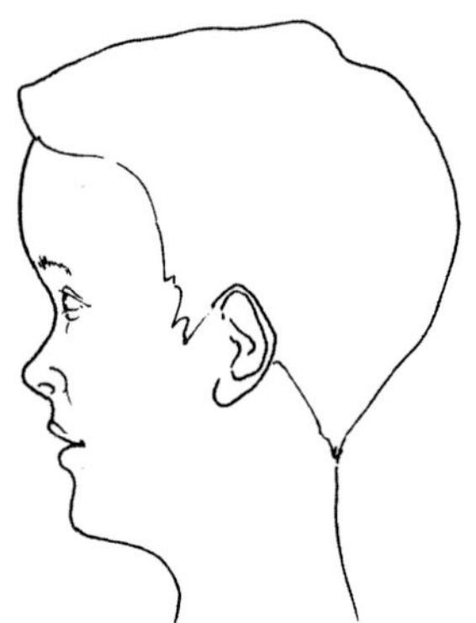

**Fig. 1.** Frontal bossing and midface hypoplasia are seen in achondroplasia.

### PATHOPHYSIOLOGY

- Growth plates show decreased cellular organization and activity, resulting in a defect in endochondral osteogenesis.
- Bones and other tissues are otherwise normal.
- Growth plates are of normal width; microscopically, the normal, orderly arrangement of cartilage cells into columns is defective.
- Membranous bone formation, which accounts for circumferential growth of the shafts of the long bones, proceeds normally.
- Changes can be recognized radiographically as early as 3 months of gestation.

### ETIOLOGY

- Achondroplasia results from a defect in the fibroblast growth factor receptor-3 protein (1).
- The pathologic process begins *in utero*: The epiphyseal cartilage plate growth is slowed and disordered, with a resulting decrease in longitudinal growth.

### ASSOCIATED CONDITIONS

- Spinal stenosis
- ± Hydrocephalus
- Overweight

## DIAGNOSIS

### SIGNS AND SYMPTOMS

- Disproportionately short stature, long trunk, and rhizomelic shortening of the limbs are evident at birth (Fig. 2).
- Large head, with a prominent forehead and parietal bossing
- Midfacial hypoplasia

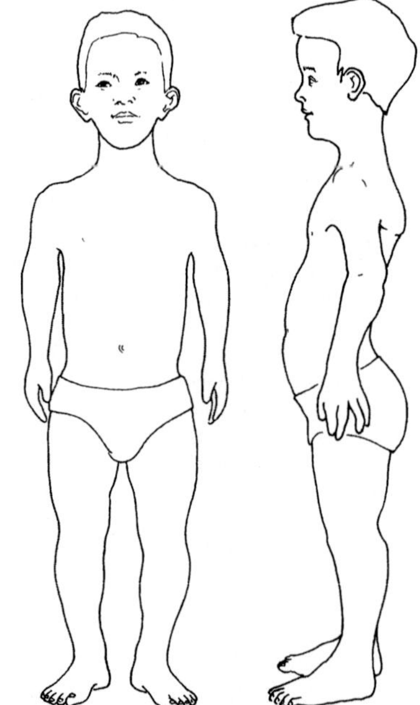

**Fig. 2.** Characteristic features in achondroplasia include rhizomelic shortening (thighs and upper arms most markedly shortened) and increased lumbar lordosis.

- Initially, the legs appear straight, but genu varum may develop with growth.
- Short, broad, and stubby digits (Fig. 3)
- Restricted elbow extension (but little functional importance)
- Excessive lumbar lordosis and anterior pelvic tilt, as well as a waddling gait
- Stenosis of the lumbar spine, prolapse of the intervertebral discs, osteophytes, and deformed vertebral bodies may compress the spinal cord and nerve roots.
- Adult height ranges from 42–56 inches.

#### *History*

- A developmental history should be taken.
  - Although milestones are not met at the usual times, norms are available for this condition.
  - In many cases, stenosis of the foramen magnum resolves spontaneously.

#### *Physical Exam*

- Head: Frontal bossing; midface hypoplasia
- Spine: Exaggerated lumbar lordosis; possible thoracolumbar kyphosis
- Extremities:
  - Short, especially proximally in the humerus and femur
  - Muscular appearance
- Elbow flexion contracture ± dislocated radial head
- Space between long and ring fingers, giving appearance of "trident" hand (3 groups of digits)
- Bowed (varus) knees common; varus–valgus laxity and hyperextension often are seen in childhood.
- Lumbar stenosis in adults, possibly producing motor weakness in ankles, feet, and bladder function
- Cervical or thoracic stenosis, possibly causing hyperreflexia

### TESTS

#### *Lab*

- No characteristic laboratory findings
- DNA testing is not used clinically.

#### *Imaging*

- Radiography:
  - Skull:
    - A shortened skull base, a large cranium with prominent frontal and occipital areas, and superimposition of the spheno-occipital synchondrosis over the mastoid
    - Small foramen magnum

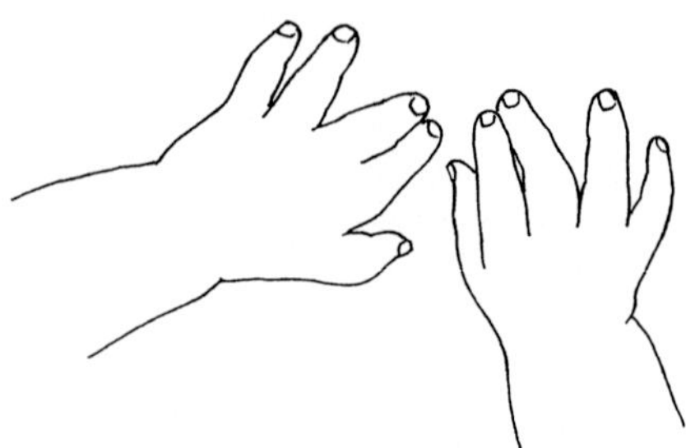

**Fig. 3.** A characteristic separation between the 3rd and 4th fingers leads to the "trident hand" of achondroplasia.

- Lumbar spine:
  - Decreased interpedicular distance, spinal stenosis, and posterior scalloping of the vertebral bodies
  - Thoracolumbar kyphosis, commonly seen in infancy, usually disappears with ambulation and is replaced by an exaggerated lumbar lordosis.
- Pelvis: Broad with wide, "square" iliac wings, small and deep greater sciatic notches, and horizontal superior acetabular margins
- MRI:
  - Obtain of the head and neck if milestones are delayed beyond the achondroplastic norms

### *Diagnostic Procedures/Surgery*
- Sleep studies are possibly indicated for infants with developmental delay.
- Routine genetic testing is not indicated.

### *Pathological Findings*
None

### DIFFERENTIAL DIAGNOSIS
- Pseudoachondroplasia: Normal facial appearance; irregular epiphyses of hips and knees
- Hypochondroplasia: Height usually >54 inches, no spinal stenosis, no caudal approximation of the pedicles

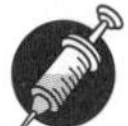

## TREATMENT

### GENERAL MEASURES
- No effective treatment for the cartilage growth difference is available.
- Occasionally, osteotomy is required to correct specific limb deformities (1,2).
- In adults, low back pain may require symptomatic measures.
- Neurologic complications, including hydrocephalus, nerve root compression, spinal stenosis, and paraplegia, may necessitate surgery.
- Foramen magnum decompression is performed for severe infantile stenosis (2).
- Thoracolumbar kyphosis is monitored, and patients are treated with a brace if the condition persists beyond the age of 2–3 years.
- Laminectomy is indicated for severe spinal stenosis and should include fusion for a patient with severe kyphosis or skeletal immaturity.
- Restriction from sports is not usually necessary.
- Custom chairs and automobile hand controls are helpful.
- Close follow-up for any signs of neurologic compromise is important.
- Children with achondroplasia should not be evaluated against normal developmental milestones but, rather, against standards developed for children with the condition.
- Motor skills often are delayed because of the physical difficulties imposed by short limbs and hypotonia.
- Cognitive skills usually are attained at the expected ages.

### SPECIAL THERAPY

### *Physical Therapy*
A therapist may be helpful in adapting a child to the environment or monitoring developmental progress.

### SURGERY
- Tibial valgus-derotation osteotomy:
  - Usually indicated for persistent varus and torsion of the knees; internal tibial torsion usually accompanies the varus.
  - Fibular shortening has not been proven effective in this condition.
- Spinal fusion:
  - Indicated for severe kyphosis of >40° that fails to respond to bracing by the age of 8–10 years (3,4)
- Laminectomy:
  - If indicated for spinal stenosis, it should be extensive: Usually decompression of the entire lumbar spine and sometimes of the lower thoracic spine.
  - Kyphosis may need to be corrected at the same time if it is severe or if the patient is growing.
- Limb lengthening:
  - May produce substantial gains in height
  - May improve lumbar lordosis and stenosis by stretching hamstrings
  - Usually, however, bilateral lengthening of the femur, tibia, and humerus is necessary to achieve acceptable proportions, a treatment program that lasts several years.
- Foramen magnum decompression:
  - Should be done by an experienced neurosurgeon, after multidisciplinary consultation, if patient fails to improve.

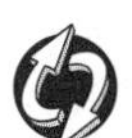

## FOLLOW-UP

### PROGNOSIS
- Good, except for spinal stenosis
- Visceral involvement is absent.
- The rare, homozygous form usually results in death in a few weeks to months.
- Heterozygous individuals have a normal life span.
- Intelligence is normal.
- Patients usually are independent in daily life.

### COMPLICATIONS
- Spinal stenosis
- Nerve root compression
- Knee pain

### PATIENT MONITORING
- Given the high propensity to orthopaedic problems, patients should be seen routinely.
- Periodic examinations of extremity strength and bladder control are warranted.

### REFERENCES

1. Sponseller PD, Ain MC. The skeletal dysplasias. In: Morrissy RT, Weinstein SL, eds. *Lovell and Winter's Pediatric Orthopaedics*, 6th ed. Philadelphia: Lippincott Williams & Wilkins, 2006:205–250.
2. Nicoletti B, Kopits SE, Ascani E, et al. *Human Achondroplasia. A Multidisciplinary Approach*. New York: Plenum Press, 1988.
3. Ain MC, Shirley ED. Spinal fusion for kyphosis in achondroplasia. *J Pediatr Orthop* 2004;24:541–545.
4. Ain MC, Shirley ED, Pirouzmanesh A, et al. Postlaminectomy kyphosis in the skeletally immature achondroplast. *Spine* 2006;31: 197–201.


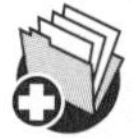

## MISCELLANEOUS

### *ICD9-CM*
259.4 Dwarfism
724.00 (general) Spinal stenosis
756.4 Achondroplasia

### PATIENT TEACHING
- Genetic counseling
- Weight control, which is often a problem and is helped by exercise
- Early detection of spinal stenosis
- Vocational counseling, to avoid physical labor occupations
- Usually no restriction on activity unless spinal stenosis occurs
- Mention Dwarf Amateur Athletic Association, a competitive forum

### *Activity*
- Counsel patient to:
  - Remain physically active on a regular basis
  - Avoid excessive weight gain
  - Avoid hyperextension stress

### *Prevention*
Patients should be told about the signs and symptoms of spinal stenosis so that it can be detected at the earliest possible point.

### FAQ
- Q: How should a patient with achondroplasia be followed?
  - A: Especially in childhood, a geneticist usually has the most knowledge about the entire spectrum of the condition. He or she should see the patient at least yearly and can consult other specialists as needed.
- Q: What are the signs and symptoms of spinal stenosis in achondroplasia?
  - A: Spinal stenosis is heralded by thigh and leg pain that is worse with walking and not localized just to the knee. Physical stamina may become challenged. The need to stoop forward and rest holding the thighs is a characteristic move.

# ACROMIOCLAVICULAR JOINT ARTHRITIS

*Michael S. Bahk, MD*

## BASICS

### DESCRIPTION

- The AC joint can become a source of pain in the shoulder, often because of degenerative osteoarthritis, posttraumatic arthritis, or distal clavicle osteolysis.
- Diagnosing problems of the AC joint:
  - Best diagnosed with pain on palpation, reproduction of pain with cross-body adduction, and diagnostic injections
  - Plain radiographs, especially the Zanca view, or bone scans may help image the AC joint.
- Nonoperative management can be successful, but some patients require operative distal clavicle resection.
- The results of arthroscopic or open distal clavicle resection are good.

### GENERAL PREVENTION

Limitation of exacerbating activities such as bench-presses, dips, push-ups, and overhead activities

### EPIDEMIOLOGY

Patients >50 years old and patients involved in activities that stress the AC joint are at risk.

#### *Incidence*

- Degenerative osteoarthritis is more common with advanced age.
- AC joint arthritis is much less common than hip, knee, or glenohumeral arthritis.
- Posttraumatic arthritis is a more common cause than primary osteoarthritis.
- Distal clavicle osteolysis, an even less-common cause, occurs in certain power athletes (e.g., weight-lifters).

### RISK FACTORS

Advanced age, previous AC injury, weight-lifting

### PATHOPHYSIOLOGY

- The AC joint is a hyaline cartilage joint with a fibrocartilage meniscal disc.
- The disc starts to break down with normal aging and, by early adulthood, is minimal or may be injured with an AC separation or with repetitive activity.

### ETIOLOGY

- Osteoarthritis results from the normal aging process.
- Posttraumatic arthritis is associated with AC separations and distal clavicle fractures, especially intra-articular fractures.
- Distal clavicle osteolysis is associated with repetitive trauma, resulting in resorption of fatigued bone, especially in weight-lifters.

### ASSOCIATED CONDITIONS

Rotator cuff impingement

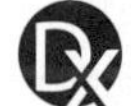

## DIAGNOSIS

### SIGNS AND SYMPTOMS

#### *History*

- Patients usually report pain in the anterior or superior shoulder.
- Activities that load the joint, including reaching across or behind the body, cause pain.
- Activities such as bench-pressing also stress the joint.
- Patients may have night pain, especially when they roll onto the affected side.
- Patients also may complain of trapezoid or neck pain.

#### *Physical Exam*

- Reproduction of pain with palpation is important, and reproduction of pain at the AC joint with cross-body adduction is helpful.
  - The arm is elevated to 90° while the arm is adducted across the body by the examiner.
- Relief of pain with a local anesthetic injection also is helpful in diagnosing AC joint arthritis.

### TESTS

#### *Imaging*

- Radiography:
  - Normal shoulder radiographs may not adequately reveal the AC joint.
  - A Zanca view best exhibits the AC joint.
    - The x-ray beam is aimed cephalad 15° while the voltage is decreased to about 1/2 that of a normal shoulder radiograph.
  - Images reveal sclerosis, subchondral cysts, joint space narrowing, and osteophyte formation.
  - However, radiographs with distal clavicle osteolysis reveal loss of bone at the end of the distal clavicle.
  - Comparison of the affected shoulder with the contralateral AC joint may prove helpful.
- Bone scan:
  - Useful in identifying the AC joint as the source of pain in a patient with unclear radiographs (increased uptake over the joint)

#### *Diagnostic Procedures/Surgery*

Local anesthetic injection into the AC joint with relief of symptoms is a good diagnostic test for AC joint pathology.

#### *Pathological Findings*

- The disc often is degenerated.
- The joint is arthritic with loss of normal hyaline cartilage.

### DIFFERENTIAL DIAGNOSIS

- Rotator cuff impingement is the most common problem in the differential.
  - These diagnoses often are interconnected because AC arthritis may contribute to cuff impingement.
- Other shoulder problems include calcific tendinitis, frozen shoulder, and glenohumeral arthritis.
- Nonshoulder problems include cervical disc disease or cervical arthritis.

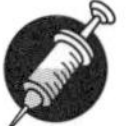

## TREATMENT

### INITIAL STABILIZATION

- Activity modifications, such as temporarily avoiding dips or changing the grip distance for bench presses, may be beneficial.
- NSAIDs and corticosteroid injections can provide relief.

### GENERAL MEASURES

- Nonoperative management is the initial treatment plan.
- Activity modification, NSAIDs, and corticosteroid injections may prove helpful.
- After 6 months of nonoperative management with persistent symptoms, surgery can be considered, but the specific treatment plan should be tailored to the patient, the occupation, and the activity level.

#### *Activity*

Refraining from offending activities may provide relief.

### SPECIAL THERAPY

#### *Physical Therapy*

Minimal role in AC joint arthritis

### MEDICATION (DRUGS)

Analgesics such as NSAIDs for pain relief

### SURGERY

- Can be considered after 6 months of unsuccessful nonoperative interventions
- Distal clavicle resection may produce good results.
  - The painful AC joint is removed.
  - Adequate resection is important to prevent continued bony contact between the clavicle and acromion.
  - The resection may be performed through an open incision or arthroscopically.

## FOLLOW-UP

### PROGNOSIS

- Medical management can be useful but can require a protracted course.
- For open surgical distal clavicle resection, 62–100% have good to excellent results (1).
- For arthroscopic procedures, 90% have good to excellent results (2).
- Both techniques have similar long-term results, with arthroscopic resection potentially allowing an earlier return to activity.

### COMPLICATIONS

- The most common complication of surgical management is incomplete resection and continued pain after surgery.
- Excessive resection of the distal clavicle, which might include the coracoclavicular ligaments, can lead to distal clavicle instability.

### REFERENCES

1. Novak PJ, Bach BR, Jr, Romeo AA, et al. Surgical resection of the distal clavicle. *J Shoulder Elbow Surg* 1995;4:35–40.
2. Snyder SJ, Banas MP, Karzel RP. The arthroscopic Mumford procedure: an analysis of results. *Arthroscopy* 1995;11:157–164.

### ADDITIONAL READING

- Mazzocca AD, Sellards R, Garretson R, et al. Shoulder. Section A: Functional anatomy and biomechanics of the shoulder. Part 1: Injuries to the acromioclavicular joint in adults and children. In: DeLee JC, Drez D, Jr, Miller MD, eds. *DeLee and Drez's Orthopaedic Sports Medicine: Principles and Practice*, 2nd ed. Philadelphia: WB Saunders, 2003:912–934.
- Shaffer BS. Painful conditions of the acromioclavicular joint. *J Am Acad Orthop Surg* 1999;7:176–188.

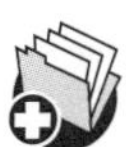

## MISCELLANEOUS

### CODES

#### *ICD9-CM*

715.1 Acromioclavicular joint arthritis

### PATIENT TEACHING

- Patients should understand that the source of pain often is arthritis or degeneration of the joint.
- Patients >50 years old, patients with distal clavicle fractures, and weight-lifters or power athletes are predisposed.
- Nonoperative management is initially pursued with activity modification, NSAIDs, and corticosteroid injections.
- Surgical management (open or arthroscopic) often is successful.

### FAQ

- Q: How can one differentiate the shoulder pain of AC joint arthritis from that of rotator cuff impingement?
  - A: A diagnostic injection of anesthetic into the AC joint will relieve pain associated with AC joint arthritis.
- Q: What radiographs best visualize AC joint arthritis?
  - A: Traditional radiographs of the shoulder are inadequate for visualizing the AC joint. AP and cephalad tilt views of the AC joint are the best for visualizing arthritic changes. Similar views of the contralateral AC joint are helpful for comparison.

# ACROMIOCLAVICULAR JOINT SEPARATION

*Adam J. Farber, MD*

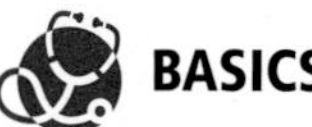

## BASICS

### DESCRIPTION

- AC joint injuries range from a mild sprain of the supporting ligaments to a complete separation of the AC joint.
- The AC joint is a diarthrodial joint formed by the distal clavicle and the medial facet of the acromion.
  - Interposed in the joint is a fibrocartilaginous disc, which helps distribute the forces from the upper extremity to the axial skeleton.
- The AC joint has a thin capsule that is stabilized by anterior, posterior, superior, and inferior AC ligaments.
  - These AC ligaments provide horizontal joint stability to the AC joint.
  - The superior AC ligament is the most important of these 4 ligaments.
- The coracoclavicular (the trapezoid and conoid) ligaments pass from the inferior surface of the clavicle to the base of the coracoid process of the scapula.
  - These strong ligaments provide vertical stability to the AC joint.
- Tossy et al. (1) originally classified AC joint injuries into 3 types; Rockwood et al. (2) later added 3 more types to complete the current classification system based on physical examination findings and radiographs.
  - Type I: Sprain of the AC ligaments only; no displacement of the distal clavicle
  - Type II: Disrupted AC ligaments and joint capsule; intact coracoclavicular ligaments; <10% vertical subluxation of the clavicle
  - Type III: Disrupted AC ligaments, coracoclavicular ligaments, and joint capsule; complete separation of the AC joint with the clavicle displaced superiorly; complete loss of contact between the clavicle and acromion
  - Type IV: Disrupted AC ligaments, coracoclavicular ligaments, and joint capsule; completely displaced AC joint with the clavicle displaced posteriorly into or through the trapezius muscle
  - Type V: Disrupted AC ligaments, coracoclavicular ligaments, and joint capsule; completely displaced AC joint with the clavicle displaced superiorly (>300%); distal clavicle detached from the deltoid and the trapezius.
  - Type VI: Disrupted AC ligaments, coracoclavicular ligaments, and joint capsule; completely displaced AC joint with the clavicle displaced inferiorly to the acromion and coracoid process.

### GENERAL PREVENTION

No effective preventive measures are known.

### EPIDEMIOLOGY

#### *Incidence*

- AC joint injuries represent approximately 40% of shoulder injuries in athletes.
- This injury is especially common in athletes participating in hockey, rugby, football (3), wrestling, and lacrosse.
- Peak incidence is in the second decade of life.
- The injury is rare in skeletally immature patients.
- The injury is 5 times more common in males than in females.
- Type I and type II injuries each occur twice as frequently as the other types.

### ETIOLOGY

- Most of these injuries result from direct trauma; classically, when an individual lands on the point of the shoulder.
- The AC joint is at risk for traumatic injury because of its subcutaneous position on the top of the shoulder.
- The magnitude of the force determines the injury severity and the structures involved.
  - Typically, the force is absorbed initially by the AC ligaments.
  - If the force is great enough, the coracoclavicular ligaments and deltotrapezial fascia are affected.
- Indirect trauma, such as a fall on a flexed elbow or outstretched arm, also may lead to AC joint injury.

### ASSOCIATED CONDITIONS

- Fractures of the distal clavicle or the coracoid
- Brachial plexopathy

## DIAGNOSIS

### SIGNS AND SYMPTOMS

#### *History*

Injury to the AC joint should be suspected in anyone with pain after a traumatic injury to the shoulder region.

#### *Physical Exam*

- Inspection may reveal prominence of the outer end of the clavicle, abrasion, or swelling in the area of the AC joint.
- Palpation reveals local tenderness and swelling.
- A palpable step-off may be felt in type III to VI separations.
- Pain is associated with arm movements.
- Hypermobility of the clavicle is difficult to appreciate in the acute situation because of patient discomfort.
- In type VI injuries, the shoulder has a flat appearance with a prominent acromion.

### TESTS

#### *Imaging*

- Radiographic evaluation should include an AP view of the AC joint and an axillary view of the shoulder.
  - Axillary views are useful for evaluating the position of the distal clavicle with respect to the acromion in the anteroposterior plane, particularly in type IV injuries.
- A 15° cephalic-tilt view (Zanca view) is useful for assessing joint displacement and intra-articular fractures.
- Stress or weighted radiographs are not recommended because of their ineffectiveness and because of patient discomfort.

### DIFFERENTIAL DIAGNOSIS

- Clavicle fracture, in which tenderness usually is located more medially and more swelling is present
- Epiphyseal separation of the clavicle
- Shoulder dislocation

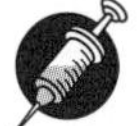

## TREATMENT

### GENERAL MEASURES

- Type I injuries lack evidence of instability and should be treated nonoperatively: A sling (for up to 1 week), analgesic medication to provide comfort, and ice to reduce swelling.
- Type II injuries are treated similarly to type I injuries: A sling (for up to 2 weeks), analgesics, and ice as necessary for patient comfort.
- Treatment of type III injuries remains controversial.
  - Surgical treatment has no proven distinct advantage over nonoperative care, and currently most authors (2) recommend nonoperative treatment except for overhead athletes and heavy manual laborers, open injuries, and patients with brachial plexopathy.
  - Nonoperative treatment is similar to that used for type I and II injuries: A sling (up to 4 weeks) followed by gentle mobilization and strengthening.
- Early surgical treatment is recommended for all type IV, V, and VI injuries.

#### *Activity*

- Type I injuries:
  - Return to sports should not be allowed until the athlete has painless ROM.
  - Most athletes return to competition within 1–2 weeks.
- Type II injuries:
  - Return to athletic activity is predicated on the restoration of painless motion and strength.
  - Most athletes return to competition by 6–8 weeks.
- Type III injuries:
  - Guarded return to sports and work are allowed after a period of sling immobilization, depending on the return of full painless ROM and the stability of the joint.
  - The time to return to sports is controversial, and many high-level athletes never return to their previous levels of function with nonoperative treatment.

## MEDICATION (DRUGS)

### *First Line*

An analgesic of choice is given for 2–4 weeks.

## SURGERY

- Surgical treatment is recommended for:
  - Open injuries
  - Closed type IV, V, and VI injuries
  - Patients who sustain type III injuries but continue to have pain and discomfort despite an adequate trial of nonoperative therapy
- Some clinicians (2,4) also recommend surgery for:
  - Type III injuries in overhead athletes and heavy manual laborers
  - Patients with brachial plexopathy
- Surgical treatment options for type III injuries include:
  - Dynamic muscle transfers
  - Primary AC joint fixation
  - Primary coracoclavicular ligament fixation
  - Distal clavicle excision with or without coracoclavicular ligament reconstruction
- A dynamic muscle transfer may be performed as the tip of the coracoid process and the attached coracobrachialis and short head of the biceps are transferred to the undersurface of the clavicle. This technique:
  - Risks nonunion and musculocutaneous nerve injury
  - Has a high rate of failure with persistent pain
  - Is recommended only for patients with chronic injuries that failed nonoperative treatment
- Primary AC joint transfixion may be performed using wires, pins, plates, or screws. This procedure:
  - Usually is undertaken with repair or reconstruction of the AC or coracoclavicular ligaments
  - Currently is unpopular because of risks of loss of fixation, pin breakage, and pin migration, and the necessity for a 2nd surgical procedure for hardware removal
- Primary coracoclavicular ligament fixation with a coracoclavicular screw may be performed with or without supplemental repair of the coracoclavicular ligaments.
  - This procedure is limited by the necessity for a 2nd surgical procedure for hardware removal.
- The most commonly performed surgical intervention for AC separation is an anatomic reconstruction of the injured ligaments.
  - Reconstruction of the coracoclavicular ligaments is performed by using the coracoacromial ligament as a substitute, and by the placement of a synthetic augmentation device (such as a band made of absorbable braid or ribbon) between the coracoid and clavicle.
  - Distal clavicle excision often is used to supplement this procedure.
- Increasingly popular is reconstruction at the coracoclavicular ligaments with a free tendon graft, which allows anatomic reconstruction and obviates the need for supplemental fixation.
- Surgical treatment options for type IV injuries include:
  - Closed reduction, converting the injury to a type III, and then treating nonoperatively or with open reduction (see "Surgery" outlined earlier)
  - Meticulous closure of the deltotrapezial fascia over the clavicle augments stability
- Type V injuries are treated surgically with one of the procedures described earlier. Again, care is taken to close meticulously the deltotrapezial fascia.
- Type VI injuries are rare.
  - Reduction is rarely achieved in a closed fashion.
  - Distal clavicle excision aids in reduction.

# FOLLOW-UP

## PROGNOSIS

- Excellent results in >90% of all patients (5)
- Excellent results in nearly 100% of patients with type I and type II injuries
- Most patients return to their usual activities in several months.

## COMPLICATIONS

- Complications may occur as a result of the injury or its treatment.
- Complications related to the injury include:
  - Associated fractures of the distal clavicle or the coracoid
  - Propensity toward degenerative arthritis of the AC joint and osteolysis of the distal clavicle
- Complications related to surgical treatment include:
  - Injury to the great vessels
  - Possible mortality related to pin migration
  - Continued pain if resection of the distal clavicle is inadequate, particularly if the joint remains unstable
  - Compromised stability if clavicle resection is excessive
  - Erosion into the clavicle by synthetic augmentation devices
  - Wound infection
  - Osteomyelitis
  - AC arthritis
  - Late fracture
  - Recurrent deformity

## REFERENCES


1. Tossy JD, Mead NC, Sigmond HM. Acromioclavicular separations: useful and practical classification for treatment. *Clin Orthop Relat Res* 1963;28:111–119.
2. Rockwood CA, Jr, Williams GR, Jr, Young DC. Disorders of the acromioclavicular joint. In: Rockwood CA, Jr, Matsen FA, III, eds. *The Shoulder*, 2nd ed. Philadelphia: WB Saunders Co., 1998:483–554.
3. Kaplan LD, Flanigan DC, Norwig J, et al. Prevalence and variance of shoulder injuries in elite collegiate football players. *Am J Sports Med* 2005;33:1142–1146.
4. Lemos MJ. The evaluation and treatment of the injured acromioclavicular joint in athletes. *Am J Sports Med* 1998;26:137–144.
5. Phillips AM, Smart C, Groom AFG. Acromioclavicular dislocation. Conservative or surgical therapy. *Clin Orthop Relat Res* 1998;353:10–17.


## ADDITIONAL READING


- Bannister GC, Wallace WA, Stableforth PG, et al. The management of acute acromioclavicular dislocation. A randomised prospective controlled trial. *J Bone Joint Surg* 1989;71B:848–850.
- Bossart PJ, Joyce SM, Manaster BJ, et al. Lack of efficacy of 'weighted' radiographs in diagnosing acute acromioclavicular separation. *Ann Emerg Med* 1988;17:20–24.
- Nuber GW, Bowen MK. Acromioclavicular joint injuries and distal clavicle fractures. *J Am Acad Orthop Surg* 1997;5:11–18.


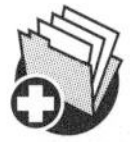

# MISCELLANEOUS

## CODES

### *ICD9-CM*

831.04 Dislocation of the acromioclavicular joint

## PATIENT TEACHING

## FAQ

- Q: Are stress views recommended in the evaluation of AC separations?
  - A: No. They only subject the patient to unnecessary pain, without providing additional useful information.
- Q: What is the role of braces to reduce the joint (such as a Kenny-Howard brace)?
  - A: These braces are no longer widely used because of the risk of pressure sores and because of good results with only a simple sling.
- Q: If an athlete suffers an AC separation, what is the timeframe for return to sports/competition?
  - A: The answer depends on the severity of the injury:
    - Type I: 1–2 weeks for most
    - Type II: 6–8 weeks for most
    - Type III: 3 months or more
    - Types IV, V, and VI: 4–6 months after surgical stabilization

# ANEURYSMAL BONE CYST

*Frank J. Frassica, MD*

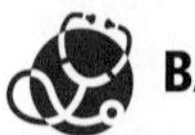

## BASICS

### DESCRIPTION

- Destructive, painful, lytic bone lesions occurring in young patients
- May occur primarily in bone (*de novo*) or develop within another benign bone lesion
- Can be locally aggressive and can cause a bone to "balloon" as a result of aneurysmal cystic expansion
- Occurs most often at the proximal ends of long bones and 2nd most commonly in the vertebral column
- In general, considered benign active or aggressive lesions
- Children with open physes are much more prone to local recurrence (up to 50%) (1,2).

### EPIDEMIOLOGY

- Can occur in any decade of adult life, but nearly 80% occur in the 2nd decade (2).
- Occurs equally in males and females (1)

#### *Incidence*

Rare

### RISK FACTORS

May develop within other benign bone tumors

### PATHOPHYSIOLOGY

- Appears to be hemorrhagic and consists of a combination of "fleshy" tissue and unclotted blood
- Often brown soft tissue because of hemosiderin deposition
- Normally, at the periphery of the lesion is an eggshell-like layer of periosteal bone around the lesion.
- Microscopically, there appear to be cavernous spaces filled with blood.
- The walls of the spaces contain fibroblastic cells, multinucleated giant cells, and strands of bone.

### ETIOLOGY

- No known causes
- However, nearly 1/2 are seen to occur in conjunction with another benign tumor and may represent a breakdown in the body's reaction to the other tumor.

### ASSOCIATED CONDITIONS

- May occur in other benign bone tumors or processes:
  - Giant cell tumor
  - Chondroblastoma
  - Osteoblastoma
  - Fibrous dysplasia
  - NOF

## DIAGNOSIS

### SIGNS AND SYMPTOMS

- Pain (usually mild and intermittent) is the most common symptom.
- The involved area may swell.
  - Swelling will tend to increase until the lesion is treated.
- If the lesion is located in the vertebral column, it may cause signs and symptoms of spinal cord compression (leg weakness, bowel or bladder dysfunction).

#### *Physical Exam*

- Check the affected area for tenderness to palpation and the presence of swelling.
- Quantify ROM.
- Check for neurologic deficits.

### TESTS

#### *Imaging*

- Radiography:
  - Plain radiographs show a "ballooned" expansion of the affected bone.
  - No matrix mineralization is present in the lesion.
  - Lesions most commonly are seen in the metaphyseal regions of the femur and tibia, as well as in the posterior elements of the vertebra.
  - One often can see a sclerotic rim or a fine shell of periosteal bone surrounding the lesion.
- CT:
  - Can be used to assess lesions of the pelvis or vertebral column more precisely than radiography
  - Often allows the physician to assess carefully the presence of the periosteal rim of bone around a lesion
  - Often shows a fluid level in the lesion
- MRI:
  - Allows more accurate assessment than CT or radiography of the extent of an aneurysmal bone cyst
  - Allows quantification of soft-tissue expansion and minor involvement by the lesion that points away from the lesion
  - On T2-weighted images, the lesions have high signal levels, and layering in the blood (fluid-fluid levels) often can be seen.

### DIFFERENTIAL DIAGNOSIS

- Depending on the location of the tumor, a widely varying differential diagnosis is possible, based on symptoms.
- Based on radiographs, the differential diagnosis includes:
  - Unicameral bone cyst
  - Giant cell tumor
  - Osteosarcoma (telangiectatic type)
  - Osteoblastoma
  - Fibrous dysplasia
- Based on histologic features, the differential diagnosis includes:
  - Giant cell tumor
  - Giant cell reparative granuloma
  - Simple bone cyst
  - Telangiectatic osteosarcoma

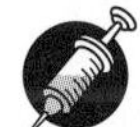

## TREATMENT

### GENERAL MEASURES

- After appropriate evaluation of the lesion with radiologic studies, a needle or open biopsy may be performed, followed by excision, curettage, and bone grafting.
- Once the bony defect is healed, patients return to normal function.
- Lesions can recur locally; the treatment is repeat surgical excision.

#### *Activity*

- Most patients need to limit weightbearing activity on the involved region while bony healing occurs.
- Once the bone has healed, no limitations on activity are necessary.

### SPECIAL THERAPY

#### *Physical Therapy*

Physical therapy may be needed to regain joint motion or to assist in gait training after surgery.

### SURGERY

- Treatment of aneurysmal bone cysts involves excision of the ballooned cortex, curettage with hand and power instruments, chemical cauterization of the cyst walls, and bone grafting (2).
- If the cyst is in an expendable bone (rib or fibula), resection of the lesion may be performed.
- Radiation therapy should be used only when no surgical option exists.
- Embolization may be effective as an adjunct to control bleeding or control the lesion in difficult sites such as the pelvis, sacrum, or vertebral bodies.

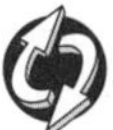

## FOLLOW-UP

Radiotherapy should be reserved for progressing or untreatable lesions.

### PROGNOSIS

- With modern treatment, 95% of patients can be expected to be cured of these lesions (1).
- An aneurysmal bone cyst should not be expected to metastasize unless rare malignant transformation occurs.
- If a patient does have a local recurrence, repeat surgical excision can be performed.

### COMPLICATIONS

- Complications of surgical treatment vary greatly, but the most common problem after appropriate treatment is local recurrence of the tumor.
- Other surgical complications, such as infection and neurologic or vascular injury, occur with a low frequency.

### PATIENT MONITORING

After surgical treatment, regular follow-up is required for several years to evaluate bony healing and to look for local recurrence of the tumor.

### REFERENCES

1. Dorfman HD, Czerniak B. Cystic lesions. In: *Bone Tumors*. St. Louis: Mosby, Inc, 1998:855–912.
2. McCarthy EF, Frassica FJ. Bone cysts. In: *Pathology of Bone and Joint Disorders: With Clinical and Radiographic Correlation*. Philadelphia: WB Saunders, 1998:277–289.

### ADDITIONAL READING

- Bruckner JD, Conrad EU, III. Musculoskeletal neoplasms. In: Kasser JR, ed. *Orthopaedic Knowledge Update 5: Home Study Syllabus*. Rosemont, IL: American Academy of Orthopaedic Surgeons, 1996:133–148.
- Wold LE, McLeod RA, Sim FH, et al. Aneurysmal bone cyst. In: *Atlas of Orthopedic Pathology*. Philadelphia: WB Saunders, 1990:232–237.

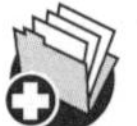

## MISCELLANEOUS

### CODES

#### *ICD9-CM*

213.9 Aneurysmal bone cyst

### PATIENT TEACHING

Patients must be educated to look for signs and symptoms of local recurrence of the tumor, including onset of pain or localized swelling in the area of a previous lesion.

### FAQ

- Q: Can aneurysmal bone cysts be confused with other bone conditions?
  - A: The pathologist must study the histologic specimens carefully to exclude an underlying condition. Telangiectatic osteosarcoma, a highly malignant tumor, can be confused with an aneurysmal bone cyst.
- Q: Is aneurysmal bone cyst a neoplasm?
  - A: Probably not. Most clinicians believe they are benign reactive conditions, occurring in the presence of a disturbance of the vascular system.
- Q: Can patients with aneurysmal bone cysts be observed to see if this bone lesion will resolve?
  - A: Aneurysmal bone cysts can grow quickly and destroy large areas of the bone. Curettage and grafting rather than observation should be the treatment of choice.

# ANKLE ARTHRITIS

*Mark Clough, MD*

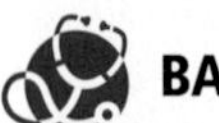

## BASICS

### DESCRIPTION

- The ankle joint is subject to osteoarthritis, but less frequently than other joints, such as the hip and knee (1).
- Trauma and abnormal ankle mechanics are the most common causes of ankle arthritis (2,3).
- Demographically, posttraumatic ankle arthritis presents in a younger age group than does primary osteoarthritis.
- Chronic ankle instability, OCDs, and osteonecrosis also lead to degenerative arthritis.
- Ankle and foot arthritis are common in patients with rheumatoid arthritis and other inflammatory arthropathies.
- Cartilage in the ankle is thinner and more uniform in its matrix than is that in the hip and knee (4).

#### *Geriatric Considerations*

Caution with NSAIDs or COX-2 inhibitors for symptomatic treatment because of potential cardiovascular complications

#### *Pediatric Considerations*

No specific considerations

#### *Pregnancy Considerations*

To avoid bleeding complications, do not treat a symptomatic pregnant patient with NSAIDs.

### GENERAL PREVENTION

- Proper treatment of ankle fractures may decrease the development of posttraumatic arthritis (5).
- Weight loss is helpful in reducing joint loading, which may help to slow or prevent the development of arthritis.

### EPIDEMIOLOGY

#### *Incidence*

Symptomatic ankle arthritis is rare and has been reported to be 9 times less common than symptomatic knee and hip arthritis (6).

### RISK FACTORS

- Ankle trauma
- Ankle instability
- Inflammatory arthritis

### ETIOLOGY

- Trauma:
  - Malleolar fractures
  - Tibial plafond (pilon) fractures
  - Talar fractures
- Ankle instability
- Inflammatory disease (e.g., rheumatoid arthritis)
- Osteonecrosis
- OCD of the talus
- Infection

## DIAGNOSIS

### SIGNS AND SYMPTOMS

- Pain
- Swelling
- Giving way or locking
- Stiffness
- Deformity

#### *History*

- Identify previous trauma and treatment.
- Identify underlying medical problems.

#### *Physical Exam*

- Examine the patient (seated and standing).
- Palpate for ankle joint effusion or warmth.
- Assess ROM and ankle ligament stability.
- Palpate the ankle joint line for tenderness and differentiate it from subtalar pain.
- Assess motor and sensory function to evaluate for neurologic impairment.
- Palpate dorsalis pedis and posterior tibial pulses; check capillary refill.
- Observe gait pattern, identify antalgic pattern, and identify external rotation or circumduction secondary to diminished dorsiflexion

### TESTS

#### *Imaging*

- Radiography:
  - Obtain standard radiographs of the ankle, including AP, lateral, and mortise views.
  - Assess for arthritic changes, including joint space narrowing, subchondral cysts, osteophytes, and sclerosis.
- A CT scan may show the extent of the arthritis, including subtalar involvement.
- Consider MRI if an OCD, osteonecrosis, or tumor is suspected on radiographs, or to evaluate further for soft-tissue and/or tendinous abnormalities.

### DIFFERENTIAL DIAGNOSIS

- Osteochondritis dissecans
- Osteonecrosis/AVN
- Posterior tibial tendinitis
- Subtalar joint arthritis
- Tumor

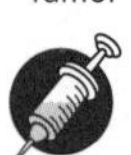

## TREATMENT

### GENERAL MEASURES

- First line treatment is generally nonoperative.
  - NSAIDs
  - Orthotic devices, including ankle-foot orthosis (brace)
  - Footwear modifications (e.g., rocker bottom sole, solid ankle cushion heel)
  - Intra-articular corticosteroid injections
  - Weight loss
- If nonoperative treatment is ineffective after 3–6 months, the patient may be counseled about surgery.

#### *Activity*

- The patient should decrease excessive walking and avoid high-impact activities such as running, jumping, or cutting maneuvers.
- Encourage low-impact exercise, including stationary bicycle and aquatic exercises.
- Consider use of assistive devices such as a cane or crutches.

### SPECIAL THERAPY

#### *Physical Therapy*

Not typically prescribed in primary management but may be useful postoperatively

### MEDICATION (DRUGS)

#### *First Line*

- NSAIDs
- Analgesics

#### *Complementary and Alternative Therapies*

It is unclear if glucosamine is efficacious in the treatment of ankle arthritis.

### SURGERY

- Considered after failure of nonsurgical measures
- Ankle arthroscopy can be used for débridement of impinging osteophytes, loose bodies, and chondral defects.
- Articular distraction arthroplasty of ankle joint with external fixation is an option for mild to moderate stages of arthritis (7).
- Supramalleolar tibial osteotomy for fracture malunion, tibial malalignment, or partial joint arthritic involvement (8)
- Ankle arthrodesis (fusion) via screw fixation is the gold standard of salvage surgery for ankle arthritis (Fig. 1).
  - Fusion has the widest indications, including posttraumatic or degenerative arthritis, postinfection arthritis, large OCDs, rheumatoid or inflammatory arthritis, and talar osteonecrosis (9).

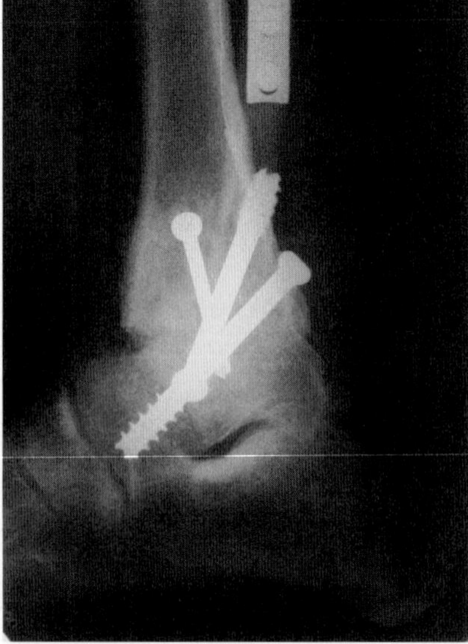

**Fig. 1.** Lateral radiograph of ankle arthrodesis (fusion).

- Patients generally are satisfied with outcomes and pain relief despite limitations in ROM (9).
- Total ankle arthroplasty is becoming more accepted with the introduction of later-generation designs (10) (Fig. 2).
  - Possible advantages compared with fusion: Greater ROM and potential for less hindfoot/midfoot arthritis from altered mechanics
  - Disadvantages compared with fusion: More perioperative complications, finite lifespan of implants, potential for implant failure and bony loss that can complicate future revision surgery

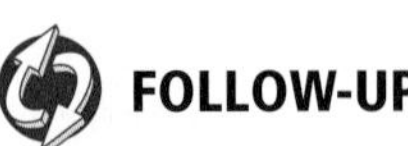

## FOLLOW-UP

### PROGNOSIS
- Prognosis is fair.
- Many patients with severe arthritis ultimately need surgery to control pain.

### COMPLICATIONS
- Nonoperative treatment: Few complications
- Surgical management: Wound-healing problems, malalignment, secondary hindfoot and midfoot arthritis, infection, and damage to local nerves and blood vessels

### PATIENT MONITORING
The patient with ankle arthritis should be followed to monitor symptoms and to discuss treatment options.

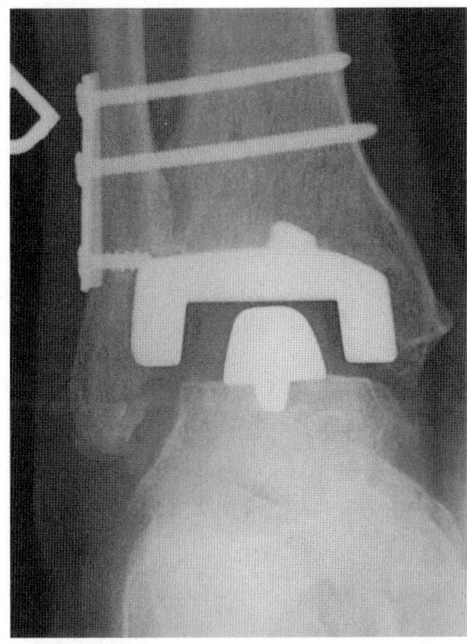

**Fig. 2.** Anteroposterior radiograph of total ankle arthroplasty (replacement).

### REFERENCES

1. Stauffer RN, Chao EYS, Brewster RC. Force and motion analysis of the normal, diseased, and prosthetic ankle joint. *Clin Orthop Relat Res* 1977;127:189–196.
2. Miller RA, DeCoster TA, Mizel MS. What's new in foot and ankle surgery? *J Bone Joint Surg* 2005; 87A:909–917.
3. Demetriades L, Strauss E, Gallina J. Osteoarthritis of the ankle. *Clin Orthop Relat Res* 1998; 349:28–42.
4. Swann AC, Seedhom BB. The stiffness of normal articular cartilage and the predominant acting stress levels: implications for the aetiology of osteoarthrosis. *Br J Rheumatol* 1993;32:16–25.
5. Lindsjo U. Operative treatment of ankle fracture-dislocations. A follow-up study of 306/321 consecutive cases. *Clin Orthop Relat Res* 1985;199:28–38.
6. Cushnaghan J, Dieppe P. Study of 500 patients with limb joint osteoarthritis. I. Analysis by age, sex, and distribution of symptomatic joint sites. *Ann Rheum Dis* 1991;50:8–13.
7. van Valburg AA, van Roermund PM, Lammens J, et al. Can Ilizarov joint distraction delay the need for an arthrodesis of the ankle? A preliminary report. *J Bone Joint Surg* 1995;77B:720–725.
8. Stamatis ED, Cooper PS, Myerson MS. Supramalleolar osteotomy for the treatment of distal tibial angular deformities and arthritis of the ankle joint. *Foot Ankle Int* 2003;24:754–764.
9. Coester LM, Saltzman CL, Leupold J, et al. Long-term results following ankle arthrodesis for post-traumatic arthritis. *J Bone Joint Surg* 2001; 83A:219–228.
10. Knecht SI, Estin M, Callaghan JJ, et al. The Agility total ankle arthroplasty. Seven to sixteen-year follow-up. *J Bone Joint Surg* 2004;86A:1161–1171.


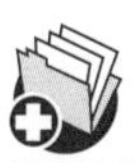

## MISCELLANEOUS

### CODES
#### *ICD9-CM*
716.97 Arthropathy, ankle not otherwise specified

### PATIENT TEACHING
The clinician should thoroughly discuss with the patient the risks and benefits of surgical treatment, as well as alternatives and expected outcomes.

### FAQ
- Q: What is the most common cause of ankle arthritis?
  - A: Trauma.
- Q: How does arthritis of the ankle differ from arthritis of the hip and knee?
  - A: Most cases of ankle arthritis are posttraumatic in nature and present at a younger age than do hip or knee arthritis, which are typically primary osteoarthritis.
- Q: What are potential nonsurgical treatment options?
  - A: Activity modification, medications, corticosteroid injections, brace, shoe modifications, cane.
- Q: What is currently the most common surgical option for severe ankle arthritis?
  - A: Ankle arthrodesis (fusion).

# ANKLE FRACTURE

*Simon C. Mears, MD, PhD*
*Barry Waldman, MD*

## BASICS

### DESCRIPTION

- Fractures of the distal end of the fibula and tibia are termed ankle fractures.
  - Usually caused by the twisting of the body around a planted foot or a misstep that results in overstressing the ankle joint
  - Severe fractures may result in dislocation of the ankle.
- 2 fracture classification systems are used currently: Lauge-Hansen (1) and Weber (2) (or AO); each has disadvantages that prevent its use as a precise guide to treatment (3).
  - Lauge-Hansen system is based on foot position at the time of injury and force applied to it:
    - The 1st word in the classification refers to position and the 2nd is the force applied.
    - The 4 main types are supination-external rotation, supination-adduction, pronation-external rotation, and pronation-abduction.
  - The Weber or AO system is simpler, and based on the level of the fibular fracture:
    - A, below the ankle-joint line
    - B, at the joint line
    - C, above the joint line
- A tibial plafond, or pilon, fracture is a comminuted fracture of the distal end of the tibia that is caused by high-energy trauma (see "Tibial Plafond Fracture").

### EPIDEMIOLOGY

#### *Incidence*

- Ankle fractures are the 2nd or 3rd most common type of fracture (4).
- Fractures in children typically involve the growth plate.
- Fractures in adolescents (Tillaux fractures) can have special patterns because of the partial closure of the growth plates (5).

### RISK FACTORS

Fracture rates are thought to be highest in young adults (6).

### ETIOLOGY

- Most often, ankle fractures result from acute trauma, such as a fall, misstep, or sports injury.
- Rarely caused by a pathologic lesion

### ASSOCIATED CONDITIONS

- Ankle sprain
- PTT sprain

## DIAGNOSIS

### SIGNS AND SYMPTOMS

- Pain in the ankle and inability to bear weight
- Deformity may be present with a fracture/dislocation.
- Swelling and ecchymosis are common.

#### *Physical Exam*

- Palpate the affected area and inspect for any breaks in the skin or tenting.
- Check the dorsalis pedis and posterior tibial pulses and all motor and sensory nerves to the foot.
  - Inversion injury of the ankle can cause peroneal nerve palsy (7).
- Examine for severe swelling and compartment syndrome in the lower leg and foot.

### TESTS

#### *Lab*

Generally, testing is for preoperative evaluation only.

#### *Imaging*

- Radiography:
  - Although a tendency exists to obtain radiographs of the ankle of any patient who complains of pain and swelling, limiting radiography to those ankles with specific indications reduces radiograph usage by 50% without missing any clinically significant fractures (8).
    - These indications are called the Ottawa ankle rules and include gross deformity, instability of the ankle, crepitus, localized bone tenderness, swelling, and inability to bear weight (9).
  - 3 radiographic views of the ankle are obtained: An AP view, a lateral view, and 15° internally rotated oblique view (called a mortise view).
  - Stress views are helpful in evaluating ligamentous injuries and should be obtained in patients with evidence of fibular fracture without medial malleolar fracture (10).
- Patients with severely comminuted intra-articular fractures may benefit from a CT scan.

### DIFFERENTIAL DIAGNOSIS

- Ligamentous injury (sprain) resulting from acute trauma and is not evident on a radiograph
- Stress fractures of the distal fibula
- Osteochondritis dissecans
- Metatarsal fracture

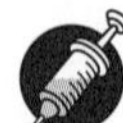

## TREATMENT

### GENERAL MEASURES

- Pain medication and elevation should be prescribed.
- All ankle fractures should be splinted in a neutral position acutely (Fig. 1).
- Isolated fibular fractures or undisplaced fractures of the medial malleolus may be treated in a below-the-knee cast.
- Stable fractures should be treated functionally with an air splint and gradual advancement of weightbearing.
- Congruity of the ankle joint is thought to be important in reducing the incidence of posttraumatic arthritis.
- Dislocations should be reduced with adequate sedation as soon as possible.
- Patients with open fractures should be taken to the operating room for irrigation, débridement, and fixation within 6–8 hours of the injury.
- Patients should be kept nonweightbearing on the affected side until pain has subsided and some signs of fracture healing appear on follow-up radiographs.
- Bimalleolar fractures or fibular fractures with medial ligament injury or syndesmotic injury are treated surgically.

#### *Activity*

- The ankle should be elevated to reduce swelling.
- Early weightbearing and ROM are important to prevent stiffness.

#### *Nursing*

Care should be taken to avoid rubbing on the splint or cast.

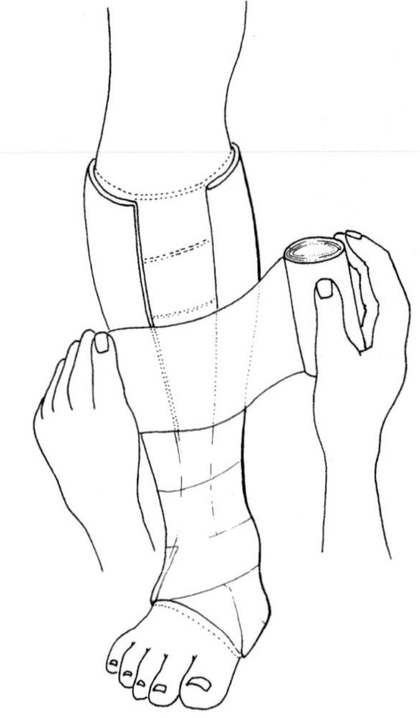

**Fig. 1.** Ankle fractures or other injuries may be splinted by a "sugar tong" method of using a layer of padding, fiberglass, or plaster and an elastic (Ace) bandage.

## SPECIAL THERAPY

### *Physical Therapy*

ROM of the MTP joints and, later, of the ankle and midfoot are important to prevent contractures and to reduce scarring of soft tissues.

## MEDICATION (DRUGS)

### *First Line*

Analgesics

## SURGERY

- Fractures of the ankle that are displaced or unstable generally are treated surgically:
  - Bi- or trimalleolar ankle fractures
  - Distal fibular fractures with medial ligament injury
  - Fibular fractures with syndesmotic injury
  - Medial malleolar fractures
  - Open fractures
- A determination of medial injury should be made with an external rotation stress view of the ankle (11,12).
- The fibular fracture usually is plated through a lateral incision (either a lateral plate or a posterior antiglide plate) (13).
- Medial malleolar fractures are stabilized with compression screws.
  - A buttress plate is used for unstable vertical fractures.
- A syndesmotic injury that is unstable under fluoroscopic testing should be treated with syndesmotic screw fixation.
- Open or unstable fractures may require an external fixator with or without internal fixation.

# FOLLOW-UP

- A patient should have a follow-up visit at 1–2 weeks to check radiographs.
- After the initial splint is removed, patients are placed in a below-the-knee cast or moon boot for 4 weeks.
- Radiographs are obtained and assessed at 6-week intervals until fracture healing.

## DISPOSITION

### *Issues for Referral*

Unstable or displaced fractures should be referred to an orthopaedic surgeon.

## PROGNOSIS

Most ankle fractures heal without incident, and the patient is able to return to normal activities (14).

## COMPLICATIONS

- With severe fractures, blisters may occur and may compromise skin integrity.
- Peroneal tendon lesions can be caused by posterior antiglide plates (15).
- Painful hardware may necessitate its removal after fracture healing.
- Compartment syndrome
- Open fractures may become infected and may require irrigation and débridement.
- Nonunion, often requiring fusion surgery
- Malunion, sometimes requiring corrective osteotomy
- Elderly patients:
  - May have osteoporotic bone, which makes surgery more difficult
  - Are at higher risk for skin or wound breakdown, and special care must be taken to ensure the blood supply (16)
- Posttraumatic arthritis:
  - Occurs in 25% of patients with displaced ankle fractures and may require ankle fusion (17)
  - The number of patients with ankle pain and arthritic changes seems to increase with the length of follow-up after fracture (17).

## PATIENT MONITORING

Radiographs should be taken every 2–6 weeks, depending on the fracture pattern and signs of healing.

## REFERENCES


1. Lauge-Hansen N. Fractures of the ankle. II. Combined experimental-surgical and experimental-roentgenologic investigations. *Arch Surg* 1950;60:957–985.
2. Weber BG. *Die Verletzungen des oberen Sprunggelenkes*. Bern: Verlag Hans Huber, 1966.
3. Whittle AP, Wood GW, II. Fractures of lower extremity. In: Canale ST, ed. *Campbell's Operative Orthopaedics,* 10th ed. St. Louis: Mosby, 2003:2725–2872.
4. van Staa TP, Dennison EM, Leufkens HGM, et al. Epidemiology of fractures in England and Wales. *Bone* 2001;29:517–522.
5. Kay RM, Matthys GA. Pediatric ankle fractures: evaluation and treatment. *J Am Acad Orthop Surg* 2001;9:268–278.
6. Hasselman CT, Vogt MT, Stone KL, et al. Foot and ankle fractures in elderly white women. Incidence and risk factors. *J Bone Joint Surg* 2003;85A:820–824.
7. Redfern DJ, Sauve PS, Sakellariou A. Investigation of incidence of superficial peroneal nerve injury following ankle fracture. *Foot Ankle Int* 2003;24:771–774.
8. Bachmann LM, Kolb E, Koller MT, et al. Accuracy of Ottawa ankle rules to exclude fractures of the ankle and mid-foot: systematic review. *Br Med J* 2003;326:1–7.
9. Stiell IG, Greenberg GH, McKnight RD, et al. Decision rules for the use of radiography in acute ankle injuries. Refinement and prospective validation. *JAMA* 1993;269:1127–1132.
10. Egol KA, Amirtharage M, Tejwani NC, et al. Ankle stress test for predicting the need for surgical fixation of isolated fibular fractures. *J Bone Joint Surg* 2004;86A:2393–2398.
11. Egol KA, Tejwani NC, Walsh MG, et al. Predictors of short-term functional outcome following ankle fracture surgery. *J Bone Joint Surg* 2006;88A:974–979.
12. McConnell T, Creevy W, Tornetta P, III. Stress examination of supination external rotation-type fibular fractures. *J Bone Joint Surg* 2004;86A:2171–2178.
13. Lamontagne J, Blachut PA, Broekhuyse HM, et al. Surgical treatment of a displaced lateral malleolus fracture: the antiglide technique versus lateral plate fixation. *J Orthop Trauma* 2002;16:498–502.
14. Bhandari M, Sprague S, Hanson B, et al. Health-related quality of life following operative treatment of unstable ankle fractures: a prospective observational study. *J Orthop Trauma* 2004;18:338–345.
15. Weber M, Krause F. Peroneal tendon lesions caused by antiglide plates used for fixation of lateral malleolar fractures: the effect of plate and screw position. *Foot Ankle Int* 2005;26:281–285.
16. Kettunen J, Kroger H. Surgical treatment of ankle and foot fractures in the elderly. *Osteoporos Int* 2005;16:S103–S106.
17. Day GA, Swanson CE, Hulcombe BG. Operative treatment of ankle fractures: a minimum ten-year follow-up. *Foot Ankle Int* 2001;22:102–106.


## ADDITIONAL READING


Takao M, Uchio Y, Naito K, et al. Diagnosis and treatment of combined intra-articular disorders in acute distal fibular fractures. *J Trauma* 2004;57:1303–1307.


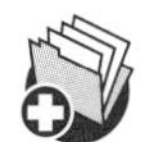

# MISCELLANEOUS

## CODES

### *ICD9-CM*

824.9 Fracture, ankle

## PATIENT TEACHING

Patients should be aware of the potential for posttraumatic arthritis later in life.

### *Prevention*

Avoidance of irregular walking and running surfaces

## FAQ

- Q: How long does it take to recover from an ankle fracture?
  - A: Patients make substantial improvement in function in the first 6 months after injury. Evaluations of patients' driving skills after fracture fixation have shown that the use of car brakes returns to normal at 9 weeks after fracture. Overall recovery continues up to a year and is slower for elderly patients.

# ANKLE INSTABILITY

*Dennis E. Kramer, MD*

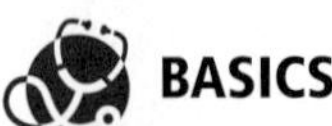

## BASICS

### DESCRIPTION

- Recurrent ankle sprains occurring primarily from an inversion stress on a plantarflexed ankle, which lead to chronic ankle pain and instability
- Divided into 2 types:
  - Functional instability:
    - Pain causes ankle to be unstable.
    - Feeling of ankle "giving way"
    - Neuromuscular deficit
  - True mechanical instability:
    - Frank insufficiency of ligaments
    - Physiologic ROM is exceeded.
    - Positive anterior drawer or talar tilt test

### GENERAL PREVENTION

- Treat initial ankle sprains aggressively using:
  - Activity modification
  - Bracing
  - Functional rehabilitation program

### EPIDEMIOLOGY

#### *Incidence*

- Ankle sprains account for as many as 40% of all athletic injuries (1).
- 27,000 ankle sprains occur each day in the United States (2).
- Symptomatic ankle instability will develop in up to 20% of patients after an inversion sprain of the lateral ankle ligaments (3).

#### *Prevalence*

High in soccer and basketball players

### RISK FACTORS

- History of previous sprain (most common risk factor)
- Connective-tissue disorders
- Cavovarus foot alignment

### ETIOLOGY

- Complex causes of functional instability:
  - Neural: Proprioception, reflexes, muscle reaction time
  - Muscular: Strength, power, endurance
  - Mechanical: Lateral ligamentous laxity
- Ankle sprains cause sequential disruption of:
  - Anterolateral joint capsule
  - ATFL
  - CFL
- Primary static restraints to ankle inversion injury:
  - ATFL:
    - Most commonly injured ankle ligament
    - Primary restraint to inversion with ankle plantarflexed
    - Torn in inversion, plantarflexion, and internal rotation
  - CFL:
    - Stabilizes ankle and subtalar joints
    - Resists inversion with ankle dorsiflexed
    - Tears in inversion and dorsiflexion
- Primary dynamic restraints:
  - Peroneal tendons
- Key anatomy:
  - ATFL:
    - Originates 1 cm proximal to tip of lateral malleolus
    - Inserts into talus 18 mm superior to subtalar joint, coursing anteriorly at a 90° angle to fibula
    - 7 mm wide, 10 mm long
    - Intimately associated with joint capsule
  - CFL:
    - Originates adjacent to the ATFL, 8 mm proximal to tip of fibula
    - Courses at a 130° angle to the fibula, heading posteriorly and distally to insert on the calcaneus 13 mm distal to subtalar joint
    - Extracapsular: Floor of peroneal sheath
  - Posterior talofibular ligament: Rarely injured except with ankle dislocations

### ASSOCIATED CONDITIONS

Connective-tissue disorders: Ehlers-Danlos

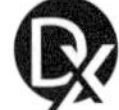

## DIAGNOSIS

- Must differentiate functional from mechanical instability.
- 15–30% of simple ankle sprains result in residual symptoms with peroneal weakness (functional instability) (3,4).

### SIGNS AND SYMPTOMS

Recurrent ankle pain and swelling

#### *History*

- Recurrent sprains with minimal trauma
- Subjective feeling of ankle "giving way"
- Repeated episodes of instability with asymptomatic periods between episodes

#### *Physical Exam*

- Assess hindfoot alignment.
- Evaluate gait.
- Neurovascular examination: Increased superficial peroneal nerve injuries in patients with recurrent ankle sprains
- Palpate peroneal tendons.
- Assess ankle ROM.
  - Crepitus and pain with ROM may be indicative of cartilaginous injury.
- Assess subtalar motion.
  - Rigidity may suggest tarsal coalition.
- Assess subtalar stability.
  - Assess CFL integrity.
  - Dorsiflex ankle and apply inversion force to calcaneus.
  - Medial translation of calcaneus is indicative of subtalar instability.
- Evaluate for mechanical instability.
  - Anterior drawer test:
    - Evaluates ATFL
    - Position ankle in neutral and apply anterolateral force to heel.
    - Positive test: >10 mm of anterior translation on involved side, >3 mm of anterior translation greater than on uninvolved side; confirm with lateral stress radiograph.
  - Talar tilt test:
    - Evaluates CFL
    - Patient seated, ankle neutral
    - Apply inversion force to hindfoot and midfoot as a unit.
    - Do not allow forefoot to rotate medially.
    - Positive test: Talar tilt >9° total, talar tilt 3° more on involved than uninvolved side; confirm on stress mortise radiograph.

### TESTS

#### *Imaging*

- Lateral and mortise radiographs:
  - Posttraumatic changes:
    - Tibial marginal osteophytes
    - Talar exostoses (at ATFL insertion)
    - Osteochondral lesions of talus
    - Os subfibulare
- Mortise and lateral stress radiographs:
  - Anterior translation (assesses ATFL):
    - Measured on lateral stress radiograph
    - Perpendicular distance between posterior edge of tibial articular surface and talus
    - Anterior translation 3–5 mm more than other side or 10 mm absolute is indicative of mechanical instability.
  - Talar tilt (assesses CFL):
    - Measured on mortise stress view
    - Angle between tibial and talar surfaces
    - Talar tilt angle 3–5° more than the other side or 10° absolute is indicative of mechanical instability.

### DIFFERENTIAL DIAGNOSIS

- Ankle pain may be associated with ankle instability.
- Other causes of ankle pain include (2,5):
  - Intra-articular fibrosis/synovitis
  - Talus OCD
  - Peroneal tendon tears
  - Peroneal tendon subluxation
  - Lateral process of talus fracture

## TREATMENT

### GENERAL MEASURES

- Initial treatment for ankle instability is nonoperative.
  - RICE protocol
  - Ankle brace:
    - Moderate to severe sprains may be braced for 6 months to allow return to sports.
  - Functional rehabilitation
  - Residual lateral ankle pain and functional instability most often are secondary to inadequate rehabilitation.

#### *Activity*

- Restrict sports until:
  - Rehabilitation program is completed.
  - Strength and ROM are normal.
  - Patient is able to perform sport-specific tasks (cutting, jumping).
- Functional bracing or taping during return to athletics may help prevent recurrence.
  - Braces do not interfere with performance.

### SPECIAL THERAPY

#### *Physical Therapy*

- Should emphasize:
  - ROM, concentric and eccentric muscle strengthening
  - Endurance training of peroneals
  - Proprioception
  - Tilt-board exercises

### SURGERY

- Indications for surgery:
  - Persistent instability after a functional rehabilitation program
  - Extreme laxity
  - Recurrent sprains with normal activities
  - Instability with sports despite bracing/taping
- Surgical techniques:
  - Anatomic repair:
    - Best results for patients with good-quality soft tissues
    - Benefits: Restores normal anatomy, preserves subtalar motion, preserves peroneals (dynamic stabilizers)
    - Contraindications: Connective-tissue disorder (Ehlers-Danlos), failed previous surgery, severely attenuated tissue (>10 years of instability)
    - Broström repair (6): Direct late repair, torn ends of ATFL shortened and repaired; sometimes CFL imbrication is necessary
    - Gould modification (7): Immobilization and reattachment of inferior extensor retinaculum to fibula after imbrication of ATFL and CFL; provides additional stability
    - Combination of Broström and Gould technique is the gold standard, with 90% success rate (8).
  - Reconstruction (Chrisman-Snook, Evans):
    - Indications: Patient with poor-quality soft tissue (ligaments are attenuated), salvage for a failed Broström procedure, obesity/high-demand patient
    - Benefits: Increased strength of repair
    - Problems: Nonanatomic reconstruction, loss of talocrural and subtalar motion, adjacent peroneal nerve injury
    - Chrisman-Snook reconstruction (9): Split peroneus brevis at its attachment to base of 5th metatarsal; harvest proximal portion of split peroneus brevis and weave it anterior to posterior through a drill hole in fibula; then weave it posterior to anterior through a calcaneal bone tunnel; suture it back to itself.
    - Evans reconstruction (10): Harvest proximal portion of peroneus brevis; weave it anterior to posterior through a fibular drill hole; does not address subtalar instability
  - Realignment procedures: Hindfoot varus—calcaneal osteotomy can be performed in conjunction with repair or reconstruction.

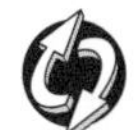

## FOLLOW-UP

- Postoperatively:
  - Cast in eversion for 2–6 weeks
  - Then switch to removable brace
  - Physical therapy for 3 months
  - Protective brace for at least 6 months

### PROGNOSIS

- High success rate regardless of anatomic repair or tenodesis procedure (1)
- Predictors of poor outcome after surgery:
  - $\geq$10 years of symptoms
  - Ankle osteoarthritis
  - Joint hypermobility

### COMPLICATIONS

- Highest percentage occur in nonanatomic reconstruction procedures
  - Loss of subtalar and talocrural motion
  - Peroneal nerve injury
  - Tendon failure: Tendons are stiffer and have less strain to failure than ligaments.

### REFERENCES

1. Colville MR. Surgical treatment of the unstable ankle. *J Am Acad Orthop Surg* 1998;6:368–377.
2. Renstrom PAFH. Persistently painful sprained ankle. *J Am Acad Orthop Surg* 1994;2:270–280.
3. Freeman MAR. Instability of the foot after injuries to the lateral ligament of the ankle. *J Bone Joint Surg* 1965;47B:669–677.
4. Gerber JP, Williams GN, Scoville CR, et al. Persistent disability associated with ankle sprains: a prospective examination of an athletic population. *Foot Ankle Int* 1998;19:653–660.
5. Digiovanni BF, Fraga CJ, Cohen BE, et al. Associated injuries found in chronic lateral ankle instability. *Foot Ankle Int* 2000;21:809–815.
6. Broström L. Sprained ankles. VI. Surgical treatment of "chronic" ligament ruptures. *Acta Chir Scand* 1966;132:551–565.
7. Gould N, Seligson D, Gassman J. Early and late repair of lateral ligament of the ankle. *Foot Ankle* 1980;1:84–89.
8. Bell SJ, Mologne TS, Sitler DF, et al. Twenty-six-year results after Broström procedure for chronic lateral ankle instability. *Am J Sports Med* 2006;34:975–978.
9. Snook GA, Chrisman OD, Wilson TC. Long-term results of the Chrisman-Snook operation for reconstruction of the lateral ligaments of the ankle. *J Bone Joint Surg* 1985;67A:1–7.
10. Evans DL. Recurrent instability of the ankle—a method of surgical treatment. *Proc R Soc Med* 1953;46:343–344.

### ADDITIONAL READING

- Baumhauer JF, O'Brien T. Surgical considerations in the treatment of ankle instability. *J Athletic Training* 2002;37:458–462.
- Girard P, Anderson RB, Davis WH, et al. Clinical evaluation of the modified Broström-Evans procedure to restore ankle stability. *Foot Ankle Int* 1999;20:246–252.
- Povacz P, Unger F, Miller K, et al. A randomized, prospective study of operative and non-operative treatment of injuries of the fibular collateral ligaments of the ankle. *J Bone Joint Surg* 1998;80A:345–351.
- Thacker SB, Stroup DF, Branche CM, et al. The prevention of ankle sprains in sports. A systematic review of the literature. *Am J Sports Med* 1999;27:753–760.

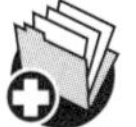

## MISCELLANEOUS

### CODES

#### *ICD9-CM*

718.87 Ankle instability

### PATIENT TEACHING

#### *Activity*

Modify activities until appropriate rehabilitation program is completed.

#### *Prevention*

Brace may prevent recurrence during athletics.

### FAQ

- Q: Does the patient have functional or mechanical instability?
  - A: Check anterior drawer and talar tilt test to document presence or absence of mechanical instability.
- Q: What are the initial treatment recommendations for a patient presenting with functional ankle instability?
  - A: Activity modification, ankle brace, functional rehabilitation program focusing on proprioception and endurance training of peroneals.
- Q: What is the gold standard initial surgery for mechanical ankle instability in a healthy athlete?
  - A: An anatomic repair procedure such as the Broström repair with Gould modification.

# ANKLE PAIN

*Brett M. Cascio, MD*

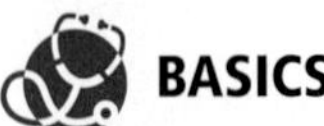

## BASICS

### DESCRIPTION
- Ankle pain can result from a variety of underlying causes, including trauma, arthritis, sports-related conditions, infection, systemic disorders, and neoplastic processes.
- Successful treatment requires a full understanding of ankle anatomy, a proper history, and a thorough physical examination to yield an appropriate differential diagnosis.
- Ankle anatomy:
  - Bones: The ankle joint is comprised of the talus, distal tibia, and distal fibula.
  - Ligaments:
    - Lateral: ATFL, CFL, PTFL
    - Syndesmotic: Anterioinferior tibiofibular ligament, posteroinferior tibiofibular ligament

### EPIDEMIOLOGY
#### *Incidence*
- Extremely common
- More common with increasing age

### ETIOLOGY
- Trauma
- Arthritis: Degenerative, inflammatory
- Stress fracture, overuse
- OCD of talus
- Tendinitis or tendon tear
- Acute ligament sprain or chronic instability
- Infection: Septic arthritis, osteomyelitis
- Neoplasm

#### *Geriatric Considerations*
Common causes of ankle pain include degenerative or inflammatory arthritis, PTT dysfunction, chronic tendinosis, and gout.

#### *Pediatric Considerations*
Ankle pain commonly is secondary to trauma, occult tarsal coalition, or bone or soft-tissue tumor.

#### *Pregnancy Considerations*
Pregnant patients may experience transient ankle pain secondary to lower extremity edema or altered lower extremity mechanics in addition to other adult causes.

### ASSOCIATED CONDITIONS
- Rheumatoid or inflammatory arthritis
- Gout
- Lyme disease
- Tarsal coalition

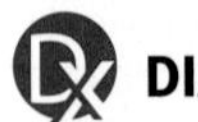

## DIAGNOSIS

### SIGNS AND SYMPTOMS
- Ankle pain that is well localized after a traumatic episode may represent an ankle sprain, fracture, or tendon injury.
- Pain without a history of trauma but with substantial joint swelling, warmth, and extreme pain with passive ROM could indicate a septic joint or an acute gouty attack.
- Chronic symptoms related to activity in adult patients may indicate degenerative arthritis of the ankle, whereas morning pain and stiffness may indicate an inflammatory condition.
- Ankle pain, swelling, and a skin rash after a tick bite may represent Lyme disease.

#### *History*
- Elicit a careful history of factors that caused or exacerbate the pain.
  - History of trauma
  - Activities that exacerbate symptoms
  - Presence of morning pain and stiffness
  - History of gouty involvement of hallux
  - Constitutional symptoms, such as fever, night sweats, weight loss, night or rest pain
  - History of tick bite
  - Athletic history

#### *Physical Exam*
- Localize area of maximum tenderness:
  - Medial and lateral malleoli
  - Tendons: Posterior tibialis, peroneals, Achilles, extensor tendons
  - Ligaments: Deltoid ligament, lateral ligaments, and syndesmotic ligaments
  - Anterior joint line/capsule
- Assess active and passive ROM of the affected ankle and compare with that of the contralateral ankle.
- Assess ligament stability and manual muscle strength.
- Examine the skin about the ankle and assess for focal swelling, warmth, or joint effusion.
- Assess the neurovascular status of the foot.
- Assess the patient's gait.

### TESTS
#### *Lab*
- Order serum laboratory tests based on the level of suspicion for specific clinical entities:
  - Septic arthritis: Complete blood count with differential, erythrocyte sedimentation rate, C-reactive protein
  - Rheumatoid arthritis or other inflammatory arthritis: Rheumatoid screen, rheumatoid factor, antinuclear antibody
  - Gout: Serum uric acid level
  - Lyme disease: Lyme antibody screen

#### *Imaging*
- Radiography:
  - Standing AP, lateral, and mortise views of the ankle are necessary.
  - An oblique radiograph of the foot may be indicated to rule out calcaneonavicular coalition.
- MRI:
  - May be necessary to detect occult processes such as stress fractures, OCD, tendon abnormality, or neoplasm
  - Also can evaluate traumatic injuries and identify OCDs, occult fractures, and tendon tears
- CT:
  - Can help define fracture fragments and intra-articular involvement
  - Can help identify neoplastic processes such as cysts or osteoid osteoma
  - May be indicated to identify tarsal coalition

#### *Diagnostic Procedures/Surgery*
- Arthrocentesis is a useful method for diagnosing septic arthritis or gout.
  - In septic arthritis, findings include positive Gram stain and/or culture, most commonly *Staphylococcus aureus*.
  - In gout and pseudogout, findings include urate or calcium pyrophosphate crystals, respectively.

### DIFFERENTIAL DIAGNOSIS (1)
- Ankle sprain
- Ankle fracture
- Tendon strain or rupture
- Stress fracture
- Tendinitis or degenerative tendinosis
- Osteoarthritis or degenerative arthritis
- Rheumatoid or inflammatory arthritis
- Septic arthritis (2)
- Lyme disease
- Acute gout
- Osteochondritis dissecans of the talar dome
- Bone tumor
- Soft-tissue neoplasm
- Tarsal coalition

# TREATMENT

## GENERAL MEASURES

- Ankle sprains or low-grade trauma can be treated with the RICE protocol and gradual weightbearing as tolerated.
- Patients with ankle fractures should be splinted, instructed to remain nonweightbearing, and referred to an orthopaedist for definitive care.
- Hot, swollen, erythematous ankles may warrant arthrocentesis to rule out a gouty attack or septic arthritis.

### *Activity*

- Patients with ankle sprains and low-grade trauma should begin to bear weight gradually as tolerated.
- Nonweightbearing activity is appropriate in a patient with an ankle fracture, pending evaluation by an orthopaedist.
- Protected weightbearing in a cast or boot brace often is useful for patients with conditions such as tendon strain, tendinitis/tendinosis, stress fracture, OCD of the talus, or symptomatic tarsal coalition.

## SPECIAL THERAPY

### *Physical Therapy*

May be indicated in certain cases once diagnosis and specific treatments are performed

## MEDICATION (DRUGS)

### *First Line*

- NSAIDs are used for tendon injuries, sprains, stress fractures, and arthritis.
- Narcotics are used for fracture pain.
- Gouty attacks may require NSAIDs and colchicine, whereas allopurinol may be needed for suppression of chronic attacks.
- Septic joints require antibiotics and either aspiration or surgical debridement (2).
- Corticosteroid injection is used for arthritis pain.

## SURGERY

- Unstable fractures typically require surgical reduction and fixation.
- Pain from ligament instability, tendon tear, or OCD of the talus may ultimately require surgical treatment.
- Septic arthritis is treated with surgical irrigation and debridement rather than serial aspirations in patients with chronic, Gram-negative or *Staphylococcus* infection; patients who are immunocompromised; or patients for whom antibiotics and aspirations have failed (2).
- Arthritis pain that does not respond to appropriate nonsurgical means may necessitate ankle arthrodesis (fusion) or arthroplasty.
- Bony or soft-tissue neoplasm typically requires appropriate staging workup and biopsy, followed by definitive surgical treatment (e.g., bone grafting of benign cyst, wide resection with limb-sparing surgery, or even amputation).

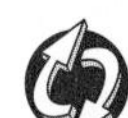

# FOLLOW-UP

## DISPOSITION

### *Issues for Referral*

- Acute fracture should prompt referral to an orthopaedist for definitive management.
- Chronic conditions unresponsive to rest, activity and sports restriction, medications, and immobilization should lead to referral to an orthopaedist for additional evaluation and management.
- Bone or soft-tissue neoplasm should be referred to musculoskeletal oncologist for staging workup and biopsy.

## PROGNOSIS

Depends on underlying cause

## COMPLICATIONS

Many of the causes of ankle pain can lead to progressive pain and stiffness.

## PATIENT MONITORING

Careful short-term follow-up is necessary to monitor ROM and prevent contractures.

## REFERENCES

1. Renstrom PAFH. Persistently painful sprained ankle. *J Am Acad Orthop Surg* 1994;2:270–280.
2. Ross JJ. Septic arthritis. *Infect Dis Clin North Am* 2005;19:799–817.

## ADDITIONAL READING

- Pfeffer GB (ed). *Chronic Ankle Pain in the Athlete.* Rosemont, IL: American Academy of Orthopaedic Surgeons, 2000.
- Richardson EG (ed). *Orthopaedic Knowledge Update: Foot and Ankle 3.* Rosemont, IL: American Academy of Orthopaedic Surgeons, 2004.

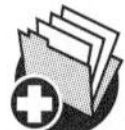

# MISCELLANEOUS

## CODES

### *ICD9-CM*

719.47 Ankle joint pain

## PATIENT TEACHING

### *Activity*

Activity depends on abnormality.

### *Prevention*

Maintenance of strength and flexibility

## FAQ

- Q: What are 7 possible causes of ankle pain?
  - A: Fracture, sprain, tendon injury, tendinitis, arthritis, infection, or neoplasm.
- Q: What structures comprise the medial and lateral ankle ligaments?
  - A: Superficial and deep deltoid, ATFL, PTFL, and CFL.
- Q: What type of condition is suggested by morning stiffness and ankle pain?
  - A: Rheumatoid or inflammatory arthritis.
- Q: What conditions likely require referral to an orthopaedist?
  - A: Acute fracture, neoplasm, and a chronic condition unresponsive to initial nonsurgical treatment attempts.

# ANKLE SPRAIN

*Dennis E. Kramer, MD*

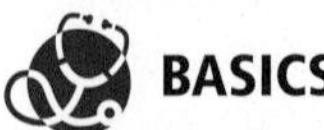

## BASICS

### DESCRIPTION

- Acute sprains of the lateral ligaments about the ankle are the most common injury in sports (1) and also occur commonly in the general population.
- Most commonly a partial tear or complete rupture of the ATFL occurs (2).
  - More severe injuries include the CFL (2).
  - Lateral ankle sprain results from an inversion mechanism.
- Classification (3):
  - Grade I: Partial tear of the ligaments
  - Grade II: Partial to complete tear of the ATFL, partial tear of the CFL
  - Grade III: Complete rupture of the ATFL and CFL
- Ankle sprains cause sequential disruption of:
  - Anterolateral joint capsule
  - ATFL
  - CFL
- Primary static restraints to ankle inversion injury:
  - ATFL:
    - Most commonly injured ankle ligament
    - Primary restraint to inversion with ankle plantarflexed
    - Torn in inversion, plantarflexion, and internal rotation
  - CFL:
    - Stabilizes ankle and subtalar joints
    - Tears in inversion with ankle neutral or dorsiflexed
- Primary dynamic restraints:
  - Peroneal tendons

### EPIDEMIOLOGY

#### *Incidence*

- In the United States, ~27,000 of these injuries occur every day (4).
- Most common athletic injury (1)

### RISK FACTORS

- Athletes
- Dancers
- Children with congenital tarsal coalition
- Cavovarus foot alignment

### ETIOLOGY

The injury results from inversion of the foot with the ankle in varying degrees of plantarflexion when weight is placed on the ankle.

## DIAGNOSIS

### SIGNS AND SYMPTOMS

- Pain, tenderness, and swelling over the lateral aspect of the ankle
- Often difficult to bear weight on extremity

#### *History*

- Mechanism of injury causing sprain:
  - Inversion in plantarflexion: ATFL injury
  - Inversion in dorsiflexion: CFL injury

#### *Physical Exam*

- Tenderness and swelling are noted along the lateral aspect of the ankle inferior and anterior to the tip of the lateral malleolus.
- Perform manual strength testing of muscle groups, including the peroneal tendons.
- Assess the neurovascular status of the limb, including the superficial peroneal nerve that can sustain a stretching injury with inversion sprain.
- Assess the ligament stability of the ankle.
  - Compare with the uninjured ankle.
  - Anterior drawer test:
    - Evaluates ATFL stability
    - Holding the distal tibia firmly with one hand, place the other hand around the heel and displace the hindfoot anteriorly with the ankle in a neutral position.
  - Inversion tilt test:
    - Evaluates CFL stability
    - Position ankle in neutral dorsiflexion.
    - Stabilize distal tibia with 1 hand and apply inversion force to hindfoot with other hand.

### TESTS

#### *Imaging*

- AP, lateral, and mortise radiographic views of the ankle are obtained.
  - Rule out fracture, OCD of talus, or arthritic changes.
- CT is indicated if occult fracture or tarsal coalition is suspected.
- MRI:
  - Rarely needed for acute ankle sprains
  - Can be indicated if concomitant tendon tear is suspected

### DIFFERENTIAL DIAGNOSIS (5)

- Fibular fracture
- Osteochondral fracture of the talar dome
- Peroneal tendon subluxation
- Congenital tarsal coalition
- Talar fracture
- Calcaneal fracture

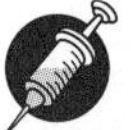

## TREATMENT

### GENERAL MEASURES (1,4)

- RICE protocol
- Partial weightbearing with crutches in the acute phase (first 3–7 days), which is advanced as tolerated to full weightbearing
- Stirrup ankle brace to facilitate early ambulation
- NSAIDs may help with pain.
- Gentle active ROM as tolerated is advised.
- For severe sprains, consider a formal strengthening and proprioception retraining program with physical therapy (4).
- Activity modification (rest, sports restriction) until strength returns

### SPECIAL THERAPY

#### *Physical Therapy*

ROM, strengthening exercises, and proprioceptive retraining are indicated (4).

### MEDICATION (DRUGS)

#### *First Line*

NSAIDs and analgesics can be used for severe sprains, but they usually are not necessary.

### SURGERY

- Surgical repair of acute ankle ligament tear is rarely indicated (4).
  - Primary repair of ATFL and CFL (6)
- Surgery may be indicated for patients with recurrent instability.
  - In such patients, repair of the lateral ankle ligaments or reconstruction with part of the peroneus brevis tendon usually is successful.

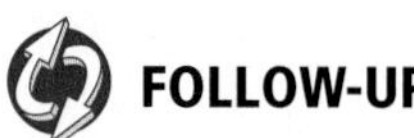

## FOLLOW-UP

### PROGNOSIS

The prognosis, which depends on injury severity, is excellent for most patients.

### COMPLICATIONS

- OCD
- Recurrent sprains

### PATIENT MONITORING

- Patients should show full strength and ROM before returning to sports.
- Functional bracing or taping during return to athletics may help prevent recurrence.

### REFERENCES

1. Clanton TO, Schon LC. Athletic injuries to the soft tissues of the foot and ankle. In: Mann RA, Coughlin MJ, eds. *Surgery of the Foot and Ankle,* 6th ed. St. Louis: Mosby-Year Book Inc, 1993:1095–1224.
2. Brostrom L. Sprained ankles. I. Anatomic lesions in recent sprains. *Acta Chir Scand* 1964;128: 483–495.
3. Leach RE, Schepsis AA. Acute injuries to ligaments of the ankle. In: Evarts CM, ed. *Surgery of the Musculoskeletal System,* 2nd ed. New York:Churchill Livingstone, 1990:3887–3913.
4. Kannus P, Renstrom P. Treatment for acute tears of the lateral ligaments of the ankle. Operation, cast, or early controlled mobilization. *J Bone Joint Surg* 1991;73A:305–312.
5. Renstrom PAFH. Persistently painful sprained ankle. *J Am Acad Orthop Surg* 1994;2:270–280.
6. Brostrom L. Sprained ankles. V. Treatment and prognosis in recent ligament ruptures. *Acta Chir Scand* 1966;132:537–550.

### ADDITIONAL READING

- Chabra A, Katolik LI, Pavlovich R, et al. Sports medicine. Section 3. Leg, foot, and ankle. In: Miller MD, ed. *Review of Orthopaedics*, 4th ed. Philadelphia: WB Saunders Co, 2004:228–231.
- Thacker SB, Stroup DF, Branche CM, et al. The prevention of ankle sprains in sports. A systematic review of the literature. *Am J Sports Med* 1999;27:753–760.

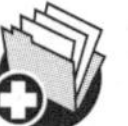

## MISCELLANEOUS

### CODES

#### *ICD9-CM*

845.0 Ankle sprain

### PATIENT TEACHING

#### *Activity*

An appropriate return to activity plan is determined based on the severity of the ankle sprain.

#### *Prevention*

Proprioceptive training has been shown to decrease recurrent sprains.

### FAQ

- Q: Which ligaments are involved and in what sequence in a lateral ankle sprain?
  - A: A lateral ankle sprain injures the following, in order: anterolateral joint capsule, ATFL, and occasionally the CFL.
- Q: What condition must be ruled out in an adolescent patient with a rigid flatfoot and recurrent ankle sprains?
  - A: Tarsal coalition.
- Which ligament provides primary static restraint to inversion injury with the ankle plantarflexed?
  - ATFL.
- What are appropriate initial treatments for acute ankle sprain?
  - RICE protocol, stirrup brace, early ambulation, and ROM exercises.

# ANKYLOSING SPONDYLITIS

*Philip R. Neubauer, MD*

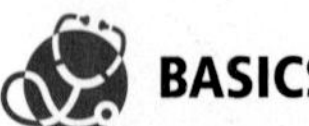

## BASICS

### DESCRIPTION

- AS is a seronegative spondyloarthritis.
- It is an inflammatory oligoarthritis of the spine and peripheral joints.
- Primarily affects the spine, especially the SI joint, as well as the hips and shoulders
- May affect any spinal level
- Affects synovial and fibrous joints, causing chronic synovitis with joint, destruction, erosions, and sclerosis, which eventually leads to joint fibrosis and ankylosis
- Ocular, cardiac, and mucocutaneous manifestations also may be seen.

### EPIDEMIOLOGY

- Primarily affects young males in the 3rd and 4th decades of life.
- Manifestations after age 40 are rare.
- Cause is unknown.
- Associated with the HLA genes of the major histocompatibility complex, in particular HLA-B27.

#### *Incidence*

- The incidence in North America is 0.1–0.3% (1).
- In patients with the HLA-B27 gene, the incidence increases 100-fold (1).
- In 1st-degree relatives of patients with AS, the incidence increases 20-fold (2).

#### *Prevalence*

It should be noted that, although a link exists between AS and HLA-B27, <5% of patients with the HLA-B27 gene develop AS (3).

### RISK FACTORS

- HLA-B27 gene
- Positive family history

#### *Genetics*

- Strong positive family history
- Concordance rate in identical twins is 63% compared with a 23% concordance in fraternal twins (3).
- Associated with several genes of the major histocompatibility complex, including HLA-B27, HLA-DRB1, and HLA-B60
- Other genes implicated include CYP2D6 and IL-1B.

### PATHOPHYSIOLOGY

- Inflammatory arthropathy, affecting the SI joint 100% of the time (1).
- Affects both synovial and fibrous joints of the spine and the periphery
- Inflammation of the tendons and ligaments also are seen.
- The inflammatory process leads to joint destruction and ankylosis.
- Onset usually is insidious, with flares and remissions.
- The disease affects both males and females but is more severe in males.
- Severity also is proportional to age at onset, with early onset showing a more severe course.

### ETIOLOGY

- Exact cause is unknown.
- May be associated with viral or bacterial infection
- *Klebsiella* has been implicated, but studies to investigate the bacterial relationship with AS have been inconclusive (4).
- Some evidence suggests a link between AS and inflammation of the small intestine.

### ASSOCIATED CONDITIONS

- Plantar fasciitis
- Achilles tendinitis
- Inflammatory uveitis
- Aortic insufficiency, cardiomegaly, and conduction defects

## DIAGNOSIS

### SIGNS AND SYMPTOMS

- The diagnosis of AS is made clinically and radiographically, and is suggested by the following signs and symptoms, which should be present for at least 3 months:
  - Pain relieved by exercise, and not made better with rest
  - Morning stiffness
  - Limited spine motion
  - Fatigue
  - Decreased chest expansion
  - Weight loss
  - Chest pain secondary to costosternal involvement
  - Apical fibrosis of the lungs
  - Kyphosis and/or flattening of lumbar spine
  - Upper extremities are rarely involved.

#### *History*

- Insidious onset of discomfort of the lumbosacral spine, buttocks, and hips.
- Onset age <40 years
- Persistence of symptoms for >3 months
- Morning stiffness
- Improvement of pain and stiffness with exercise

#### *Physical Exam*

- Early in the disease, patients may be asymptomatic.
- Careful neuromuscular, pulmonary, and optic examinations are essential.
- Careful examination of the lumbar spine will show loss of motion in flexion and extension.
- Pain with palpation of the SI joint

### TESTS

#### *Lab*

- HLA-B27 gene
- The ESR is elevated in 80% (3).
- Antinuclear antibodies and rheumatoid factor are not useful.

#### *Imaging*

- Radiography:
  - Radiographs may be negative in the early stages of AS.
  - Radiographic changes of the SI joint are pathognomonic for AS.
  - Radiographic findings usually are symmetric.
  - Early signs are erosions and sclerosis of the SI joint, which lead to a blurring of the joint margins and pseudo widening of the SI joint.
  - Late changes are calcification with osseous bridging of the SI joint.
  - *Bamboo spine* is seen in the lumbar spine as a result of inflammation of the annulus fibrosis, with erosion of the corners of the vertebral bodies and subsequent osteophyte bridging of the adjacent bodies.
  - AP, lateral, and oblique radiographs should be studied carefully because fracture lines may be difficult to detect.
- CT scans with 3D reconstructions are sensitive for detecting fractures.
- MRI can be used to detect epidural hematomas.

### DIFFERENTIAL DIAGNOSIS

- The differential diagnosis should include any of the seronegative arthropathies:
  - Reactive arthritis (formerly known as "Reiter syndrome"): Nongonococcal urethritis and arthritis
  - Psoriatic arthritis
  - Crohn disease
  - Ulcerative colitis
  - Infection of the SI joint
  - Osteoarthritis
  - Rheumatoid arthritis
  - Herniated nucleus pulposus

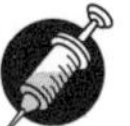

## TREATMENT

### INITIAL STABILIZATION
- The mainstay of treatment is exercise.
- Back exercise and flexibility training reduce pain and improve function.
- NSAIDs

### GENERAL MEASURES
In general, recreational activities and the pursuit of a healthy, active lifestyle should be encouraged.

### SPECIAL THERAPY
#### *Physical Therapy*
- Hyperextension exercises are helpful in preventing kyphosis.
- Flexibility training provides pain relief and improves quality of life.

### MEDICATION (DRUGS)
#### *First Line*
- NSAIDs
- The selection is empiric: No specific drugs, including the COX-2 inhibitors, have shown superiority (3).

#### *Second Line*
- Many other medications have been used:
  - Corticosteroids
  - Sulfasalazine
  - Antibiotics
  - Pamidronate
  - Thalidomide
  - TNF-$\alpha$ blockers

### SURGERY
- The role of surgery for patients with AS is primarily to treat the complications that develop as a result of the disease.
  - Most commonly, total hip arthroplasty
  - Stabilization for vertebral fractures
  - Spinal osteotomy for the correction of the kyphotic deformity (seen in late-stage AS).

## FOLLOW-UP

### PROGNOSIS
- Patients with early-onset disease and inflammation of peripheral joints have a relatively poor prognosis.
- No cure exists for this disorder, but with aggressive preventive measures, much of the disability associated with it can be avoided.

### COMPLICATIONS
- Spinal fractures may occur with minimal trauma because the ossified spine is brittle and is therefore overall less elastic than the normal spine.
  - Epidural hematomas may occur with a cervical spine fracture.
    - If unrecognized, the hematoma may compress the spinal cord and cause irreversible paralysis.
- Spinal fractures should be braced or internally fixed urgently to reduce risk of subsequent paralysis.
- Uveitis develops in 25% of patients and may require topical steroids (5).

### PATIENT MONITORING
- Patients should be seen on a routine basis (every 6 months) to monitor posture, reinforce the importance of exercises, and adjust analgesics.
- Patients should be monitored for uveitis and the development of cardiac and pulmonary problems.

### REFERENCES
1. van der Linden S, van der Heijde D. Ankylosing spondylitis. In: Ruddy S, Harris ED, Jr, Sledge CB, eds. *Kelley's Textbook of Rheumatology,* 6th ed. Philadelphia: W.B. Saunders, 2001:1039–1053.
2. Reveille JD, Arnett FC, Keat A, et al. Seronegative spondyloarthropathies. In: Klippel JH, ed. *Primer on the Rheumatic Diseases,* 12th ed. Atlanta: Arthritis Foundation, 2001:239–258.
3. Reveille JD, Arnett FC. Spondyloarthritis: update on pathogenesis and management. *Am J Med* 2005;118:592–603.
4. Stone MA, Payne U, Schentag C, et al. Comparative immune responses to candidate arthritogenic bacteria do not confirm a dominant role for *Klebsiella* pneumonia in the pathogenesis of familial ankylosing spondylitis. *Rheumatology (Oxford)* 2004;43:148–155.
5. Martin TM, Smith JR, Rosenbaum JT. Anterior uveitis: current concepts of pathogenesis and interactions with the spondyloarthropathies. *Curr Opin Rheumatol* 2002;14:337–341.

### ADDITIONAL READING
- Bono CM, Garfin SR, Tornetta P, et al. *Spine*. Philadelphia, Lippincott Williams & Wilkins, 2004.
- Brashear HR, Jr, Raney RB, Sr. Chronic arthritis. In: *Handbook of Orthopaedic Surgery*, 10th ed. St. Louis: CV Mosby, 1986:140–186.
- Clark CR. Common neck problems. In: Clark CR, Bonfiglio M, eds. *Orthopaedics: Essentials of Diagnosis and Treatment*. New York: Churchill Livingstone, 1994:285–294.

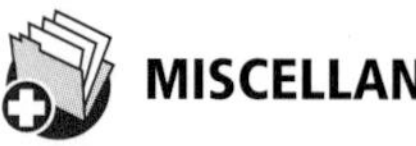

## MISCELLANEOUS

### CODES
#### *ICD9-CM*
720.0 AS

### PATIENT TEACHING
- More information can be found on the following web sites:
  - www.spondylitis.org
  - www.arthritis.org

#### *Activity*
- Activity should not be prohibited, but patients should be told about the increased risk and danger of spine fracture and should avoid situations placing them at risk for this injury.
- Patients should avoid contact sports and other activities such as skydiving and bungee jumping.

#### *Prevention*
- Patients should be discouraged from smoking.
- Patients should be counseled about a 10–20% risk of transmitting the disease to their children.

### FAQ
- Q: What is the cause of AS?
  - A: The exact cause is unknown, but it appears that AS (much like rheumatoid arthritis) is an autoimmune inflammatory disease that affects the spine and other joints in the body.
- Q: What are the treatment options for patients with AS?
  - A: Exercise is the cornerstone of treatment. Physical therapy and anti-inflammatory drugs also are used.
- Q: If a patient with AS presents to the emergency department with neck pain after a fall and evidence of AS but no evidence of a fracture, what should be the next step?
  - A: Advanced imaging with MRI or CT to evaluate for a nondisplaced fracture.

# ANTERIOR CRUCIATE LIGAMENT INJURY

*Adam J. Farber, MD*

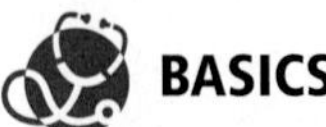

## BASICS

### DESCRIPTION

- The ACL is critical for knee function in athletes who require knee stability in activities such as running, cutting, jumping, and kicking.
- The ACL originates on the posteromedial aspect of the lateral femoral condyle and inserts anterior to and between the intercondylar eminences of the tibia.
- The ACL is composed of 2 bundles—an anteromedial bundle and a posterolateral bundle.
- The ACL functions as the primary restraint to limit anterior tibial translation and as a secondary restraint to internal rotation of the tibia.
- In the skeletally immature patient, injury to the ACL most often occurs at the bone–ligament interface, as an avulsion of the tibial spine.
- In the adult patient, rupture of the midsubstance of the ligament is more common.

### EPIDEMIOLOGY

#### *Incidence*

ACL injuries commonly are associated with sports such as football, hockey, basketball, lacrosse, gymnastics, wrestling, and volleyball.

### RISK FACTORS

ACL injury rate is 4–6 times higher in females than males in competitive sports (1).

### ETIOLOGY

- Etiologic factors include anatomic features, such as an elevated Q angle, notch stenosis, a narrower than normal ACL, and neuromuscular factors (landing with decreased knee flexion and increased knee valgus).
- ACL injuries often are the result of a noncontact injury that occurs while decelerating, changing direction, or landing from a jump.
- Direct contact to the knee with a valgus load and external rotation of the tibia, such as a clipping injury, is another common mechanism.

### ASSOCIATED CONDITIONS

- "Bone bruises" (trabecular microfractures), which occur in >50% of acute ACL injuries, typically are located on the posterior portion of the lateral tibial plateau and near the sulcus terminalis on the lateral femoral condyle.
- Meniscal injuries (>50%) (2):
  - Acutely, lateral meniscal injuries are more common than medial.
  - In patients with chronic ACL deficiency, medial meniscal injuries are more common than lateral.
- Collateral ligamentous injuries in the knee
- Articular cartilage injuries

## DIAGNOSIS

### SIGNS AND SYMPTOMS

#### *History*

- The injury often is associated with immediate pain and an audible "pop."
- Swelling of the knee is noted within a few hours (acute hemarthrosis).
- The patient often states that the knee feels too unstable to continue playing and that weightbearing is difficult.

#### *Physical Exam*

- A careful physical examination can diagnose most ACL injuries.
- The results of the physical examination of the injured knee must be compared with those of the normal knee.
- Inspection usually reveals a moderate to severe effusion.
- Typically, full knee extension is limited secondary to pain, effusion, hamstring spasm, and ACL stump impingement.
- Flexion often is limited by effusion.
- Care should be taken to observe that anterior translation or drawer testing is not reducing a posteriorly sagged tibia (PCL injury) from a subluxated position.
- The Lachman test is the most sensitive examination for acute ACL injuries.
  - The knee is placed in 30° of flexion, the femur is stabilized, and an anteriorly directed force is applied to the proximal calf.
  - The examiner assesses the magnitude of anterior translation and the firmness (firm versus soft) of the endpoint.
  - Differences between the injured and uninjured knees are clinically significant.
- The pivot shift test is used to assess the anterior subluxation of the lateral tibial plateau on the femoral condyle.
  - It is difficult to perform this test in an awake patient in the acute setting, but it is helpful in evaluating an ACL-deficient knee.
  - This test is especially helpful when the patient is anesthetized.
  - Procedure:
    - Patient supine, knee extended
    - With the tibia internally rotated, apply a valgus force to the knee as it is passively flexed.
    - If, at approximately 20–40° of knee flexion, the patient experiences a sudden jerk as the iliotibial band reduces the anteriorly subluxated tibia, the test is considered positive.
- The anterior drawer test is the least reliable test for acute ACL injuries (3).
  - The hip is flexed at 45°, and the knee is flexed to 90°.
  - An anterior force is directed by the examiner to the proximal calf.
  - The examiner assesses the magnitude of anterior translation and the firmness (firm versus soft) of the endpoint.
  - Differences between the injured and uninjured knee are clinically significant.
- Instrumented knee laxity measurements can be performed using a device such as the KT-1000.
  - These devices are useful for quantifying knee laxity objectively, but they are not necessary for diagnosis.
  - A difference of >3 mm of anterior tibial translation between the injured and uninjured knee is considered pathologic.

### TESTS

#### *Imaging*

- Radiography:
  - Evaluation should include AP, lateral, and tunnel views of the knee.
  - Plain radiographic findings suggestive of an ACL injury include a tibial spine avulsion fracture, a Segond fracture (lateral capsule avulsion fracture of the tibial plateau), or a deepened sulcus terminalis.
- MRI is the imaging modality of choice for evaluating the ACL and associated bony contusions and ligamentous or meniscal injuries.
  - MRI has an overall accuracy of 95% in diagnosing ACL injuries (3).
  - On sagittal MRI, an ACL tear is visualized as a discontinuity in the ligament.

### DIFFERENTIAL DIAGNOSIS

- Osteochondral fracture
- Tibial plateau fracture
- Meniscal injury
- Cartilage injury
- MCL or LCL injury
- PCL injury

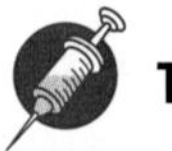

## TREATMENT

### INITIAL STABILIZATION

- The initial treatment of the acutely injured ACL is splinting and the use of crutches for comfort and early active ROM. The goal is to obtain full ROM.
- Ice, elevation, and analgesics are prescribed in the initial postinjury period.

### GENERAL MEASURES

- Treatment decisions should be based on many factors, including patient age, activity level, type of sporting activity (especially jumping, cutting, and pivoting sports), degree of instability, and associated knee pathology.
- Treatment options in the skeletally mature patient include nonoperative interventions and intra-articular ligamentous reconstruction.
- Nonoperative treatment is preferred for elderly patients or those with sedentary lifestyles (see "Physical Therapy" section).
- For the skeletally immature patient with a midsubstance ACL injury:
  - Some clinicians favor nonoperative treatment and rehabilitation measures until skeletal maturity is reached (3).
  - Others favor physeal sparing surgical reconstructive procedures (4).
- Nondisplaced and minimally displaced tibial spine avulsion fractures in skeletally immature individuals are treated with closed reduction.

#### *Activity*

- Patients should be counseled concerning high-risk activities, such as cutting, pivoting, and jumping.
- Regardless of treatment modality, functional knee bracing after ACL injury is controversial.

## SPECIAL THERAPY

### *Physical Therapy*

- Preoperative, postoperative, and nonoperative rehabilitation emphasizes early ROM (especially full extension of the knee) and early weightbearing.
  - For patients treated nonoperatively or surgically, strengthening is achieved by using closed-chain weightbearing exercises.
  - The goal is to return the function of the hamstring and quadriceps muscles to within 90% of that of the contralateral limb.
  - In patients treated surgically, agility and strengthening exercises typically are started 6 weeks after surgery.

## MEDICATION (DRUGS)

### *First Line*

- In the acute period:
  - NSAIDs
  - Acetaminophen
  - Mild narcotic analgesics

## SURGERY

- Before surgery, the patient should undergo physical therapy to regain full ROM and minimize swelling.
- Intra-articular ACL reconstruction currently is favored for:
  - Those with active lifestyles but acute ACL deficiency
  - Those with chronic ACL deficiencies that result in functional instability that endangers the menisci
- Intra-articular ACL reconstruction with grafting can be performed effectively via either open or arthroscopic techniques.
- Graft selection depends on patient factors and surgeon preference.
  - Autograft: Bone–patellar tendon–bone, 4-strand hamstrings, or quadriceps tendon
  - Allograft: Fascia lata and Achilles, quadriceps, patellar, hamstring, and anterior and posterior tibialis tendons
  - Allograft is associated with lessened donor-site morbidity, but it has the potential for viral transmission (5).
- Primary repair is favored for a displaced tibial spine avulsion fracture but is not recommended for a midsubstance ACL rupture.
- In the skeletally immature patient with a midsubstance ACL injury, a variety of reconstructive procedures may be performed based on the maturity of the patient (6).
  - Tanner stage 1 patients: Physeal-sparing procedures
  - Tanner stage 2 patients: Partial transphyseal techniques
  - Tanner stage 3 and above (those approaching skeletal maturity): Complete transphyseal reconstructions

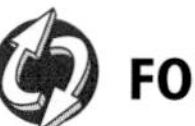

# FOLLOW-UP

## PROGNOSIS

- In the ACL-deficient knee, meniscal tears, cartilage damage, and possibly degenerative arthrosis may ensue.
- Prognosis is excellent for appropriately selected patients who have undergone ACL reconstruction.

## COMPLICATIONS

- Nonoperative-related (i.e., the chronic ACL-deficient knee):
  - Higher incidence of complex meniscal tears than in surgically treated patients
  - Possibly more prone to development of late osteoarthritis (controversial)
- Surgery-related:
  - Graft failure, graft impingement, quadriceps weakness, patellofemoral pain, infection, arthroscopic fluid extravasation and compartment syndrome, deep vein thrombosis, reflex sympathetic dystrophy (<1%), nerve and vascular injuries (<1%), and arthrofibrosis.
  - Harvesting bone–patellar tendon–bone autograft is associated with anterior knee pain, kneeling pain, and (rarely) patellar fracture and patellar tendon rupture (3).

## PATIENT MONITORING

Patients should be followed carefully at 4–6-week intervals to ensure that they regain ROM and strength of the quadriceps and hamstrings.

## REFERENCES


1. Gray J, Taunton JE, McKenzie DC, et al. A survey of injuries to the anterior cruciate ligament of the knee in female basketball players. *Int J Sports Med* 1985;6:314–316.
2. Noyes FR, Barber-Westin SD. A comparison of results in acute and chronic anterior cruciate ligament ruptures of arthroscopically assisted autogenous patellar tendon reconstruction. *Am J Sports Med* 1997;25:460–471.
3. Larson RL, Tailon M. Anterior cruciate ligament insufficiency: principles of treatment. *J Am Acad Orthop Surg* 1994;2:26–35.
4. Stanitski CL. Anterior cruciate ligament injury in the skeletally immature patient: diagnosis and treatment. *J Am Acad Orthop Surg* 1995;3:146–158.
5. Nemzek JA, Arnoczky SP, Swenson CL. Retroviral transmission by the transplantation of connective-tissue allografts. An experimental study. *J Bone Joint Surg* 1994;76A:1036–1041.
6. Tanner JM, Davies PSW. Clinical longitudinal standards for height and height velocity for North American children. *J Pediatr* 1985;107:317–329.


## ADDITIONAL READING


- D'Amato MJ, Bach BR, Jr. Knee. Section J. Anterior cruciate ligament injuries. Part 1: ACL reconstruction in the adult. In: DeLee JC, Drez D Jr, Miller MD, eds. *DeLee & Drez's Orthopaedic Sports Medicine: Principles and Practice,* 2nd ed. Philadelphia: WB Saunders, 2003:2012–2067.
- Linko E, Harilainen A, Malmivaara A, et al. Surgical versus conservative interventions for anterior cruciate ligament ruptures in adults. *Cochrane Database Syst Rev* 2005;CD001356.
- Pigozzi F, DiSalvo V, Parisi A, et al. Isokinetic evaluation of anterior cruciate ligament reconstruction: quadriceps tendon versus patellar tendon. *J Sports Med Phys Fitness* 2004;44:288–293.
- Sloane PA, Brazier H, Murphy AW, et al. Evidence based medicine in clinical practice: how to advise patients on the influence of age on the outcome of surgical anterior cruciate ligament reconstruction: a review of the literature. *Br J Sports Med* 2002;36:200–203.


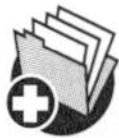

# MISCELLANEOUS

## CODES

### *ICD9-CM*

- 717.83 Old disruption of the anterior cruciate ligament
- 844.2 Acute sprain of cruciate ligament of knee

## PATIENT TEACHING

Most patients do not return to their previous level of activity if they were high-performance athletes, but most patients can return to sports.

## FAQ

- Q: If I choose not to undergo ACL reconstruction, what activity modifications will I have to make?
  - A: Patients permanently should avoid high-impact or cutting motions and contact sports. Straight-away running and closed-chain exercises are excellent for conditioning and strengthening.
- Q: If I undergo ACL reconstruction, how long will I be out of sports?
  - A: In uncomplicated cases and depending on the sport, athletes can expect to return to full sports participation in approximately 6–9 months after ACL reconstruction.
- Q: What is the role of bracing to prevent ACL injuries?
  - A: Although the issue is controversial, use of knee braces during aggressive athletic activity, such as football, has not been shown to decrease incidence of knee injuries and may give the player a false sense of security.

# ARTHROCENTESIS

*Michelle Cameron, MD*
*Timothy S. Johnson, MD*

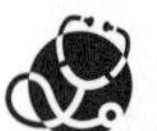

## BASICS

### DESCRIPTION

Aspiration of synovial joints is performed for diagnostic or therapeutic purposes.

### ETIOLOGY

- Causes of joint effusions:
  - Infection
  - Crystalline arthropathies
  - Hemophilia
  - Autoimmune arthropathies
  - Trauma
  - PVNS

## DIAGNOSIS

### SIGNS AND SYMPTOMS

- Synovial joints (Table 1) are aspirated for myriad reasons, the most common of which include:
  - To rule out infection
  - To diagnose arthropathies
  - To relieve pain
- Joints with enough fluid to perform arthrocentesis generally have a palpable effusion.
- Infectious, autoimmune, and crystalline arthropathies often are warm to the touch and may display overlying erythema or cellulitis.

#### *Physical Exam*

- An effusion usually is palpable.
- The patient with infectious and crystalline arthropathies or trauma may have difficulty with ROM of the affected joint.
- There may be outward signs of trauma or inflammation such as abrasions, erythema, or cellulitis.

**Table 1 Best Locations for Aspirating Joint Effusions**

| Joint | Site of Aspiration |
|---|---|
| Elbow | Posterolaterally |
| Shoulder | Anteriorly (ultrasound, CT, fluoroscopy are helpful) |
| Hip | Anteriorly or laterally (CT, fluoroscopy are helpful) |
| Knee | Laterally or medially from suprapatellar pouch |
| Ankle | Anterolaterally |

**Table 2 Joint Fluid Analysis**

| Type | Appearance | White Blood Cell Count | Polymorphonuclear Cells (%) | Comment |
|---|---|---|---|---|
| Noninflammatory | Straw-colored | 200 | 25 | Osteoarthritis: Serum glucose and protein equivalent to aspirate values |
| Inflammatory | Cloudy yellow | 2,000–75,000 | 50 | Gout: Strongly, negatively birefringent crystals<br>Calcium pyrophosphate deposition disease (pseudogout): Weakly, positively birefringent crystals<br>Rheumatic disease: Serum studies help elucidate type. |
| Infection | Purulent/opaque | >80,000 | >75 | +Gram stain and culture<br>Serum glucose >aspirate glucose<br>Serum protein <aspirate protein<br>Polymerase chain reaction: May be helpful for detecting Lyme disease |
| Traumatic | Bloody | Few | <25 | Consider fracture if a fat-fluid separation develops in syringe after a few minutes. |

### TESTS

#### *Imaging*

Radiographs often are helpful to rule out trauma and to evaluate degenerative changes within the joint.

#### *Pathological Findings (Table 2)*

- Crystalline arthropathies show crystals when specimens are examined with polarized light:
  - Gout: Monosodium urate crystals appear sharp (needle-like) by normal light microscopy and are brightly birefringent on compensated polarized microscopy.
  - The calcium pyrophosphate crystals of pseudogout have blunt ends and are not birefringent.
- Aspirates from septic arthritis often have cell counts >100,000 with >80–90% polymorphonuclear cells, and they may have organisms present on Gram staining.
- Crystalline and inflammatory arthropathies also can have high white cell counts in the 50,000/mm$^3$ range.

### DIFFERENTIAL DIAGNOSIS

- Septic arthritis
- Gout
- Pseudogout
- Autoimmune disorders, such as rheumatoid arthritis or systemic lupus erythematosus
- Trauma
- Hemophilia

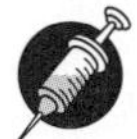

## TREATMENT

### GENERAL MEASURES

- Patients with traumatic effusions should be treated appropriately for their underlying traumatic injury, but arthrocentesis of the affected joint often makes these patients more comfortable.
- Patients with septic arthritis require joint irrigation and débridement; the type of débridement depends on the joint involved.
- Appropriate antibiotics also should be administered after all cultures are obtained.
- Patients with inflammatory and crystalline arthropathies generally respond well to anti-inflammatory medications and should be referred to a rheumatologist for evaluation.

### SURGERY

- Sterile skin preparation is required before aspiration.
- Injection of local anesthetic with a small-gauge needle into the skin may lessen the pain of aspiration (especially if more than 1 attempt is necessary).
- The needle gauge should be large enough to withdraw the viscous joint fluid (usually 18 gauge or larger) (Fig. 1).

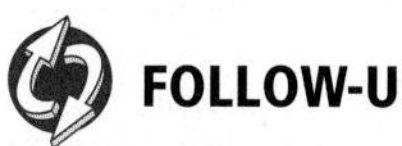

## FOLLOW-UP

### COMPLICATIONS

- Risk of iatrogenic infection:
  - Care should be taken, especially when aspirating a potentially infected joint.
  - If cellulitis is present, care should be taken to aspirate through uninvolved skin to avoid infecting a previously aseptic joint.
- Aspiration may be predisposing in as many as 23% of all cases of septic arthritis (1,2).

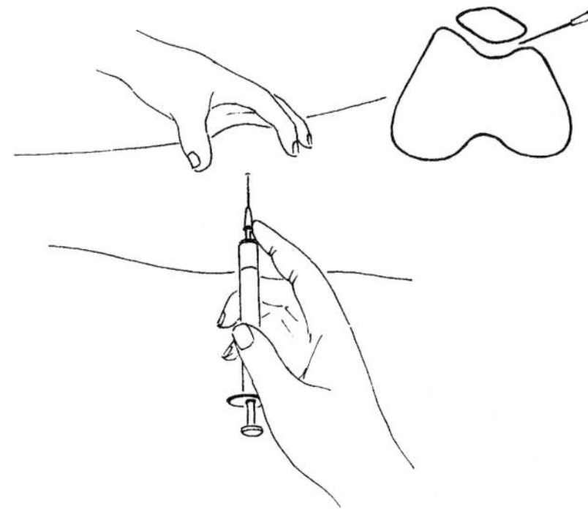

**Fig. 1.** Arthrocentesis of the knee is most easily done from the lateral side, under the patella.

### REFERENCES

1. Esterhai JL, Jr, Gelb I. Adult septic arthritis. *Orthop Clin North Am* 1991;22:503–514.
2. Tsumura H, Ikeda S, Torisu T. Debridement and continuous irrigation for the treatment of pyogenic arthritis caused by the use of intra-articular injection in the osteoarthritic knee: indications and outcomes. *J Orthop Surg (Hong Kong)* 2005;13:52–57.

### ADDITIONAL READING

Park AL, Diabach JA. Infectious arthritis. In: Canale ST, ed. *Campbell's Operative Orthopaedics*, 10th ed. St. Louis: Mosby, 2003:685–711.

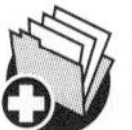

## MISCELLANEOUS

### FAQ

- Q: What is the appearance of the joint aspirate under light microscopy in the setting of gout?
  - A: Sharp, needle-like crystals.
- Q: A joint aspirate with a white blood cell count >100,000 per high-powered field is consistent with which type of arthritis?
  - A: Septic arthritis.

# ARTHROSCOPY

*Marc Urquhart, MD*
*John H. Wilckens, MD*

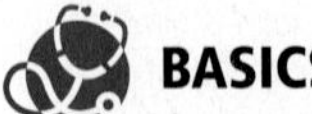

## BASICS

### DESCRIPTION

- Arthroscopy should be performed after a complete history and physical examination and after appropriate imaging studies have been obtained.
- Most procedures can be performed on an outpatient basis.
- Knee:
  - Indications:
    - Meniscal repair or débridement
    - Meniscal cyst
    - Treatment of osteochondral lesions
    - ACL or PCL tear débridement or reconstruction
    - Synovial biopsy or synovectomy
    - Determination of uncertain origin of instability or pain
    - Débridement of degenerative joint disease
  - Procedure:
    - 2 or more portal incisions ~0.5 cm in length allow visualization through the arthroscope and instrument placement through another portal.
    - The articular cartilage can be visualized in the 3 compartments of the knee (patellofemoral, medial, and lateral).
    - The medial and lateral menisci, as well as the ACL and PCL, can be visualized and probed to assess stability and integrity.
    - Meniscal tears often can be treated with débridement or repair.
    - ACL and PCL tears also can be reconstructed with arthroscopic assistance.
  - Rehabilitation:
    - Postoperatively, most patients can resume partial to full weightbearing with crutch assistance.
    - The rehabilitation period after arthroscopy varies, depending on the type of procedure performed.
    - Many patients who have undergone arthroscopy have some physical therapy for strengthening of the core, quadriceps, and hamstrings; the duration and method of rehabilitation are specific to the injury.
- Shoulder:
  - Indications (1):
    - Treatment of instability
    - Biopsy
    - Removal of loose bodies
    - Treatment of impingement
    - Rotator cuff repair
    - Management of SLAP tears
  - Procedure:
    - Involves 2 or more 0.8-cm portals
    - The articular cartilage of the glenoid and humeral head can be visualized for any pathologic process (e.g., osteoarthritis, osteochondral fragments).
    - The soft-tissue stabilizers of the shoulder also can be assessed: Inferior glenohumeral ligament complex, middle glenohumeral ligament complex, superior glenohumeral ligament complex.
    - The integrity of the labrum also can be determined arthroscopically.
    - If the patient has rotator cuff symptoms, arthroscopy includes visualizing the subacromial space and rotator cuff for causes of impingement.
    - Definitive procedures that can be performed arthroscopically: Soft-tissue stabilization procedures for instability of recurrent dislocations (e.g., Bankart capsulorrhaphy), acromioplasty, rotator cuff repair, and SLAP repairs or débridements (encouraged)
  - Rehabilitation:
    - Physical therapy is a necessary modality for anyone who has undergone shoulder arthroscopy.
    - In general, the emphasis is on regaining motion and strengthening the shoulder girdle muscles and dynamic stabilizers of the shoulder.
    - The duration and mode of rehabilitation vary with the type of injury and surgical procedure.
- Hip:
  - Indications (2):
    - Synovial biopsy or synovectomy
    - Loose-body removal
    - Treatment of labral tears
- Ankle:
  - Indications (3):
    - Synovial biopsy or synovectomy
    - Loose-body removal
    - Bone-spur removal
    - Treatment of osteochondral lesions
- Elbow:
  - Indications (4):
    - Synovial biopsy or synovectomy
    - Loose-body removal
    - Débridement of cartilage lesions and osteophytes
- Wrist:
  - Indications (5):
    - Synovial biopsy or synovectomy
    - Loose-body removal
    - Diagnosis or débridement of TFCC injuries

## REFERENCES

1. Ellman H. Shoulder arthroscopy: current indications and techniques. *Orthopaedics* 1988;11:45–51.
2. Byrd JWT. Hip arthroscopy. The supine position. *Clin Sports Med* 2001;20:703–731.
3. Drez D, Jr, Guhl JF, Gollehon DL. Ankle arthroscopy. Technique and indications. *Clin Sports Med* 1982;1:35–45.
4. Poehling GG, Ekman EF. Arthroscopy of the elbow. *J Bone Joint Surg* 1994;76A:1265–1271.
5. Whipple TL. The role of arthroscopy in the treatment of wrist injuries in the athlete. *Clin Sports Med* 1998;17:623–634.


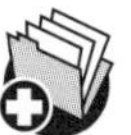

## MISCELLANEOUS

### FAQ

- Q: What is arthroscopy?
  - A: Arthroscopy is a procedure whereby a fiberoptic camera is inserted into a joint via a portal (stab) incision to visualize the articular surfaces and the supporting soft tissues.
- Q: Is arthroscopy only diagnostic, or can it be used operatively to repair, reconstruct, or remove injured structures?
  - A: Arthroscopy has evolved from being just diagnostic to having the ability to address most abnormalities of a joint. Accessory portals allow the introduction of additional instruments.
- Q: Is arthroscopy safer than traditional surgery?
  - A: Arthroscopy, properly performed, results in less morbidity and pain than traditional open surgical incisions and approaches. Arthroscopy has a steep learning curve and requires additional training to become familiar with the arthroscopic anatomy and facile with the arthroscopic equipment. In inexperienced hands, arthroscopy can be less effective and more dangerous than standard open surgical procedures.

# BACK PAIN

*Rohit Robert Dhir, BA*
*Damien Doute, MD*
*A. Jay Khanna, MD*

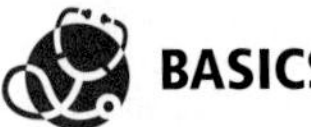

## BASICS

### DESCRIPTION

- Low back pain, the most common musculoskeletal condition, is responsible for the loss of 17 million work days per year in the United States and ~$60 billion of the annual U.S. health care budget (1).
- 70–80% of adults experience severe back pain at some time during their lives (1,2).
- Back pain, which affects the bones, joints, ligaments, and muscles of the back, is a symptom that occurs primarily in middle-aged adults, but it also may occur in children and adolescents.
- Pathologic back pain can originate within the spine (spondylogenic or neurogenic) or outside the spine (viscerogenic, vascular, or psychogenic) (3).
- The clinician must evaluate each patient carefully to determine the nature of the pain.
- Synonyms: Backache; Low back pain
- Classification is organized broadly into traumatic and atraumatic conditions.

### EPIDEMIOLOGY

- Age:
  - Adults: Common
  - Children: Uncommon:
    - Children and adolescents with scoliosis may have mild pain.
    - Severe back pain in children should alert the clinician to look for a potentially serious problem, such as a tumor or infection.
- Gender: Back pain is more common in males than in females because of their higher rates of involvement with manual labor, motor vehicle injuries, and industrial accidents.

#### *Incidence*

The estimated incidence of low back pain is 15–20% in the United States (4).

#### *Prevalence*

- The lifetime prevalence of low back pain ranges from 13.8–31% (2).
  - Low back pain usually appears in the 3rd decade of life, peaks between the ages of 35 and 55 years (1), and decreases thereafter (2).
  - After 6 months, 7% of patients still experience back pain symptoms, but this figure drops to 2% after 1 year (5).

### RISK FACTORS

- Obesity
- Smoking
- Manual labor
- Accidents

#### *Genetics*

No genetic predispositions are known.

### PATHOPHYSIOLOGY

No pathologic findings are applicable.

### ETIOLOGY

- Traumatic:
  - Fractures/microfractures (causes severe immediate back pain) (6)
  - Dislocations
  - Herniated discs
  - Ligament tears
- Atraumatic:
  - Degenerative disc disease
  - Degenerative spinal stenosis
  - Inflammatory arthritis
  - Osteoporosis
  - Spondylolysis and spondylolisthesis
  - Neoplasms
  - Primary or metastatic tumor
  - Infection

### ASSOCIATED CONDITIONS

- AS
- Rheumatoid arthritis
- Sciatica with low back pain
- Cauda equina syndrome

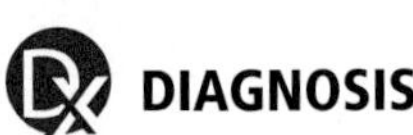

## DIAGNOSIS

### SIGNS AND SYMPTOMS

- Symptoms:
  - Low back discomfort/pain
  - Stiffness
  - Numbness
- Signs:
  - Paravertebral muscle spasm
  - Motor weakness
  - Loss of deep tendon reflexes
  - Loss of sensation
  - Clonus
  - Positive Babinski sign

#### *History*

- Because diagnostic and radiographic studies generally are ineffective, it is essential to obtain a thorough history.
- It is important for the physician to use an objective, history-taking approach to eliminate the subjectivity of the pain experienced by the patient (2).
  - This procedure includes having the patient map out the area of pain instead of merely describing its location (7).

#### *Physical Exam*

- Begin with a general inspection of the spine.
- Note any asymmetry of the ribs, flank, or pelvis, and inspect the natural sagittal curvatures of the patient.
- Assess ROM and determine local tenderness.
- Note flexion, extension, lateral bending, and rotation of the lumbosacral spine.
- Sudden pain accompanying movement is suggestive of a mechanical abnormality (7).
  - Pain with extension is common in patients with facet joint arthritis and spinal stenosis (5).
- Elicit paravertebral muscle spasms and percussion tenderness.
- The neurologic examination is crucial, and the following should be evaluated:
  - Motor testing
  - Strength testing
  - Deep tendon reflexes
  - Sensation
  - Gait examination

### TESTS

#### *Lab*

- No specific laboratory tests
- If one suspects infection, a complete blood count and ESR should be performed.
  - The ESR is more useful, however, and is consistently higher in infection.
- These determinations also are useful in patients >50 years old as a screening test for multiple myeloma.
- In young patients with substantial stiffness, a serum HLA-B27 test can be used to assess for AS.

#### *Imaging*

- Imaging techniques rarely are relevant clinically unless they strongly correlate with the patient's history and physical examination (8).
- Conventional radiographs, CT scans, MRI, and technetium bone scans should be used only to confirm pathology or rule out a specific diagnosis (8).
  - Radiographs are not always necessary for patients with the 1st episode of back pain, especially if it is caused by minor trauma (such as lifting).
  - However, radiographs should be obtained if evidence from the history and physical suggest that a patient might have a substantial structural abnormality, such as AS (8,9).
  - CT and MRI scans (alone or in combination) are useful for detecting and localizing structural abnormalities precisely.
    - CT is useful for detecting bone abnormalities such as fractures or osteoid osteomas.
    - MRI is useful for detecting marrow abnormalities or soft-tissue processes such as metastatic bone disease.
  - Technetium bone scans are useful for detecting early bone infections and localizing metastatic bone lesions.

### DIFFERENTIAL DIAGNOSIS

- The differential diagnosis is extensive and can be broadly outlined based on the age of the patient and whether a traumatic event occurred.
- Adults:
  - Traumatic:
    - Herniated discs
    - Compression fractures
    - Fracture/dislocation
    - Spondylolysis (traumatic)
  - Atraumatic:
    - Degenerative disc disease
    - Spinal stenosis
    - Inflammatory arthritis: Rheumatoid arthritis, AS
    - Spondylolysis and spondylolisthesis
    - Ligament strains
    - Neoplasms: Metastatic bone disease, multiple myeloma
- Children:
  - Traumatic:
    - Herniated disc
    - Fracture
  - Atraumatic:
    - Scoliosis
    - Disc space infection
    - Vertebral osteomyelitis
    - Neoplasms

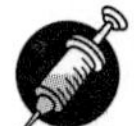

## TREATMENT

### GENERAL MEASURES

- Most patients with low back pain can be treated nonoperatively with short-term bed rest in the supine position, NSAIDs, and physical therapy to improve muscle strength of the lower back.
- Surgical treatment is rare: Only 1–2% of back pain sufferers are candidates (2).
- Prolonged bed rest is not beneficial; the patient may have 2–3 days of bed rest after the incident of back pain (5,10).
- During the initial period of severe spasm and pain (usually 2–7 days), patients may have restricted mobility.
- If plain radiographs are normal, patients should be mobilized progressively with physical therapy and aerobic conditioning.

### SPECIAL THERAPY

#### *Physical Therapy*

- Physical therapy, aimed at increasing endurance and strength, lowers the recurrence rate and shortens the history of back pain (5).
- Effective low back exercises include the Williams flexion program and the McKenzie hyperextension program (10).
- Patients are educated regarding activity modification and injury prevention.
- Patients who are injured on the job often are referred for a work-hardening program.
- Passive modalities of therapy, such as massage, acupuncture, and electrical stimulation, can provide immediate relief, but they do not help in long-term treatment (5,10).

### MEDICATION (DRUGS)

- NSAIDs are the medications of choice for decreasing inflammation.
  - Generally, they are prescribed for an initial 4–6 weeks.
  - If the pain resolves, the medication is discontinued.
- Muscle relaxants do not have a major role, although they can be very helpful in patients with severe spasm and anxiety.
  - They are best used for short-term pain relief rather than for long-term use.
- In the presence of an infection, intravenous antibiotics and rest are required to treat the infection and normalize ESR.

### SURGERY

- The many operative procedures for back pain (the choice of modality depends on the nature of the individual's problem) have several principles in common:
  - Decompression of any nerve root or spinal cord compression
  - Fusion to achieve a stable spine
  - Consideration of realignment and fusion to correct spinal deformities (i.e., scoliosis and spondylolisthesis)
- Instrumentation is important to achieve fusion in a reliable manner, and multiple systems, including pedicle screws, interbody devices, and rods, are available.
- More recently, lumbar disc arthroplasty has been suggested as a surgical method for treating discogenic low back pain that is refractory to nonoperative management.
  - Some controversy exists within the spine community as to whether this modality will become a widely accepted procedure for the treatment of discogenic low back pain.

## FOLLOW-UP

### PROGNOSIS

- The prognosis is good (not always excellent) in patients who do not have major structural abnormalities.
- Patients with major fusions can return to most activities, but they generally do not tolerate heavy work or repetitive loading of the back.

### COMPLICATIONS

- Most complications stem from iatrogenic surgical failure (11) and include infection, neurologic trauma, pseudarthrosis (nonunion), loss of fixation, and chronic unexplained pain.
- Cauda equina syndrome is a devastating complication that occurs when a lesion causes nerve root compression of the cauda equina.
  - Unchecked compression results in permanent neurologic loss, leading to paralysis of the lower extremities and loss of bladder and bowel function.

### PATIENT MONITORING

- Patients are followed at 4–6-week intervals until the pain subsides.
- With rest, activity modification, and NSAIDs, patients should show progressive improvement.
  - If not, suspect a structural problem.

### REFERENCES


1. McCulloch J, Transfeldt E. Epidemiology and natural history of spondylogenic backache. In: *Macnab's Backache,* 3rd ed. Baltimore: Williams & Wilkins, 1997:240–246.
2. Kahanovitz N. Epidemiology. In: *Diagnosis and Treatment of Low Back Pain*. New York: Raven Press, 1991:1–3.
3. McCulloch J, Transfeldt E. Classification of low back pain. In: *Macnab's Backache,* 3rd ed. Baltimore: Williams & Wilkins, 1997:86–89.
4. Borenstein DG, Wiesel SW, Boden SD. Epidemiology of low back pain and sciatica. In: *Low Back Pain: Medical Diagnosis and Comprehensive Management,* 2nd ed. Philadelphia: W. B. Saunders, 1995:22–27.
5. Kahanovitz N. Idiopathic low back pain. In: *Diagnosis and Treatment of Low Back Pain.* New York: Raven Press, 1991:67–75.
6. McCulloch J, Transfeldt E. Spondylogenic back pain: osseous lesions. In: *Macnab's Backache,* 3rd ed. Baltimore: Williams & Wilkins, 1997:90–148.
7. McCulloch J, Transfeldt E. The history. In: *Macnab's Backache,* 3rd ed. Baltimore: Williams & Wilkins, 1997:247–256.
8. Kahanovitz N. Radiographic and laboratory tests. In: *Diagnosis and Treatment of Low Back Pain.* New York: Raven Press, 1991:43–66.
9. McCulloch J, Transfeldt E. The investigation. In: *Macnab's Backache,* 3rd ed. Baltimore: Williams & Wilkins, 1997:277–357.
10. McCulloch J, Transfeldt E. Treatment of lumbar disc disease. In: *Macnab's Backache,* 3rd ed. Baltimore: Williams & Wilkins, 1997:393–413.
11. Kahanovitz N. Postoperative complications and failed back. In: *Diagnosis and Treatment of Low Back Pain*. New York: Raven Press, 1991: 121–126.


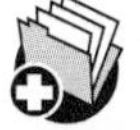

## MISCELLANEOUS

### CODES

#### *ICD9-CM*

847.9 Back sprain

### PATIENT TEACHING

Education is important so that patients understand their condition and the various methods for preventing recurrent injuries.

#### *Prevention*

Prevention is best accomplished through the use of specific back exercises, avoidance of exacerbating activities, and implementation of aerobic conditioning.

### FAQ

- Q: Is lumbar spine surgery a 1st-line treatment for most patients with low back pain?
  - A: No. Most low back pain resolves spontaneously or with nonoperative management. Only a very small percentage of patients with persistent discogenic back pain become candidates for surgical intervention.
- Q: If infection is the suspected cause of an episode of back pain, which laboratory studies should be ordered?
  - A: Complete blood count, ESR, and C-reactive protein in addition to other laboratory studies, as indicated.

# BICEPS TENDON RUPTURE

*Michael S. Bahk, MD*

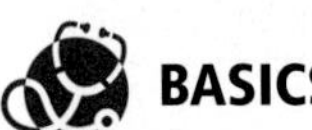

## BASICS

### DESCRIPTION

- The biceps tendon can rupture proximally near the shoulder or distally near the elbow (1).
  - Most ruptures occur proximally.
- Proximally, the biceps helps depress and stabilize the humeral head, whereas distally it is the primary supinator of the forearm and assists in elbow flexion.

### EPIDEMIOLOGY

#### *Incidence*

- Typically occurs in males >40 years old
- These injuries can be seen in young athletes, and anabolic steroid use should be investigated.
- Typically occurs in the dominant extremity

### RISK FACTORS

- >40 years of age
- Rotator cuff impingement
- Anabolic steroids

### PATHOPHYSIOLOGY

- Tendon degeneration, symptomatic and asymptomatic, is thought to be the cause of biceps tendon ruptures (2).
  - Proximally, degeneration from decreased vascularity or from mechanical impingement from the coracoacromial arch
  - Distally, the degenerated tendon usually avulses from the radial tuberosity when a large extension force is applied to a flexed elbow.

### ASSOCIATED CONDITIONS

Rotator cuff disease

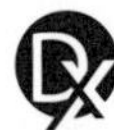

## DIAGNOSIS

### SIGNS AND SYMPTOMS

#### *History*

- Patients may complain of anterior shoulder, arm, or antecubital pain.
- Patients may have antecubital elbow pain with forearm supination or flexion.

#### *Physical Exam (3)*

- Ecchymosis and swelling may be present in the antecubital fossa, arm, or shoulder.
- The retracted biceps muscle belly presents as a large distortion of the arm ("Popeye sign").
  - Muscle retracts away from the tendon tear.
- Some weakness or pain may present with supination or flexion.

### TESTS

#### *Imaging*

MRI is the best diagnostic study for biceps tendon rupture.

### DIFFERENTIAL DIAGNOSIS

- Rotator cuff impingement
- Rotator cuff tear

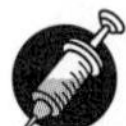

## TREATMENT

### GENERAL MEASURES

- For proximal tears, treatment initially is nonoperative.
  - Patients who sustain these injuries often are >40 years old with minimal functional deficits or weakness.
  - Patients <40 years old or those who are athletes, who are concerned about cosmesis, or who wish an optimal return of function can consider surgery.
- For distal lesions, surgical repair offers the best functional result.
  - Nonoperative treatment may result in activity-related pain and decreased strength in flexion and supination.

#### *Physical Therapy*

- Acutely, rest is recommended until pain and swelling resolve, followed by gentle ROM.
- Advance activity as tolerated.

### MEDICATION (DRUGS)

NSAIDs and acetaminophen are recommended acutely.

### SURGERY

- Proximal tears:
  - For isolated tears, the biceps tendon is tenodesed in the bicipital groove.
  - If associated with rotator cuff disease, acromioplasty is performed in addition to the tenodesis.
- For distal tears, the biceps tendon is reattached to the radial tuberosity through 1 or 2 incisions.

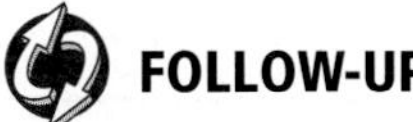

## FOLLOW-UP

### PROGNOSIS
- In general, patients undergoing surgical repair of distal tears can expect a near-full return of strength.
- Patients with proximal lesions treated with tenodesis can expect pain relief.

### COMPLICATIONS
- Without surgery:
  - Some patients may continue to experience activity-related pain.
  - Patients can expect a loss of supination strength.

### REFERENCES

1. Strauch RJ, Michelson H, Rosenwasser MP. Repair of rupture of the distal tendon of the biceps brachii. Review of the literature and report of three cases treated with a single anterior incision and suture anchors. *Am J Orthop* 1997;26:151–156.
2. Yamaguchi K, Bindra R. Disorders of the biceps tendon. In: Iannotti JP, Williams GR, Jr, eds. *Disorders of the Shoulder: Diagnosis and Management*. Philadelphia: Lippincott Williams & Wilkins, 1999:159–190.
3. Curtis AS, Snyder SJ. Evaluation and treatment of biceps tendon pathology. *Orthop Clin North Am* 1993;24:33–43.


### ADDITIONAL READING

- Bennett JB, Mehlhoff TL. Arm. Section A: Soft tissue injury and fractures. Part 1: Soft tissue injury and fractures of the arm in the adult. In: DeLee JC, Drez D, Jr, Miller MD, eds. *DeLee & Drez's Orthopaedic Sports Medicine: Principles and Practice*, 2nd ed. Philadelphia: WB Saunders, 2003:1171–1191.
- Ramsey ML. Distal biceps tendon injuries: diagnosis and management. *J Am Acad Orthop Surg* 1999;7:199–207.


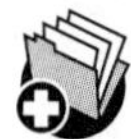

## MISCELLANEOUS

### CODES
#### *ICD9-CM*
727.62 Ruptured biceps tendon

### PATIENT TEACHING
- Patients with proximal biceps tendon tears often have associated rotator cuff or impingement problems.
- The best functional results, especially with distal tears, are obtained with surgery.
- Patients should use caution when lifting heavy objects (e.g., piano, furniture) because they are at risk for a distal biceps tendon tear.

### FAQ
- Q: If I have ruptured my biceps tendon distally, must I have surgery?
  - A: No. However, you may experience weakness in elbow flexion and, more commonly, in forearm supination, and you may have difficulty with simple tasks of daily living such as turning doorknobs or grabbing heavy objects off a shelf. Strength is best restored through primary repair of the tendon.
- Q: If I rupture my biceps tendon proximally, do I need surgery?
  - A: No. Because usually only the long head of the biceps tendon ruptures proximally, strength can still be generated through the short head of the biceps. Because proximal ruptures can be associated with rotator cuff disease, the cuff may require surgery.

# BITE TO THE HAND

*Dawn M. LaPorte, MD*
*Chris Hutchins, MD*

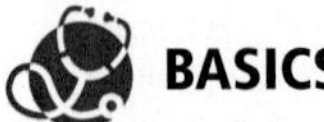

## BASICS

### DESCRIPTION

- Hand bites (direct or indirect) are serious injuries that, if not managed correctly, may result in substantial morbidity to the hand.
- A direct bite to the hand, such as a dog bite or intentional human bite, can occur in any location.
- The more common "clenched-fist" (or indirect) injury occurs over the MCP joint (the knuckle) when a fist strikes an opponent's mouth.
  - This seemingly benign injury is, in fact, treacherous and, unfortunately, common.
  - A tooth may lacerate the extensor tendon, the joint capsule, or the joint itself.
  - As the digit is straightened, the underlying wound is obscured by normal soft tissue.
- Classification:
  - Minor: Small puncture wound
  - Major: Large lacerations and soft-tissue damage (2–5 cm, exposed bone or cartilage, tendon rupture)
- Synonyms: Clenched fist injury; Fight bite; Dog or cat bite

### GENERAL PREVENTION

- Little can be done in terms of prevention for direct or indirect bites except to counsel patients about avoiding unknown animals and fighting, respectively.
- Complications may be minimized by recognizing the human bite wound as a serious injury and treating with early irrigation, débridement, and appropriate antibiotics (1).

### EPIDEMIOLOGY

#### *Incidence*

- Common
- >1 million dog bites reported annually

### RISK FACTORS

- Alcohol abuse
- Fighting

### ETIOLOGY

- Fist fights
- Dog or cat exposure

### ASSOCIATED CONDITIONS

Fractures

## DIAGNOSIS

### SIGNS AND SYMPTOMS

- Signs:
  - Puncture or laceration to the hand is present.
  - Associated swelling and erythema may be present.
  - Cellulitis and lymphangitis are present if an infection occurs.
  - If a tendon has been lacerated, the patient may experience difficulty with finger extension.
- Symptoms:
  - Decreased hand function, such as difficulty with grasping or moving an individual digit
  - Pain

#### *History*

Many combatants are embarrassed or hesitant to admit injury to this region or the mechanism of injury and consequently present late for evaluation and treatment.

#### *Physical Exam*

- Examine the hand closely for any sign of skin puncture, particularly over the 3rd and 4th MCP joints in instances of clenched-fist injuries.
- Assess the motor, sensory, and vascular status of the hand and digits.
- If the injury is of a clenched-fist type, have the patient make a fist, if possible; this procedure may reveal the underlying soft-tissue damage and may facilitate deep wound inspection.
- In clenched-fist injuries, the damage to underlying structures is proximal to the skin wound when the fingers are in the extended, anatomic position (Fig. 1).

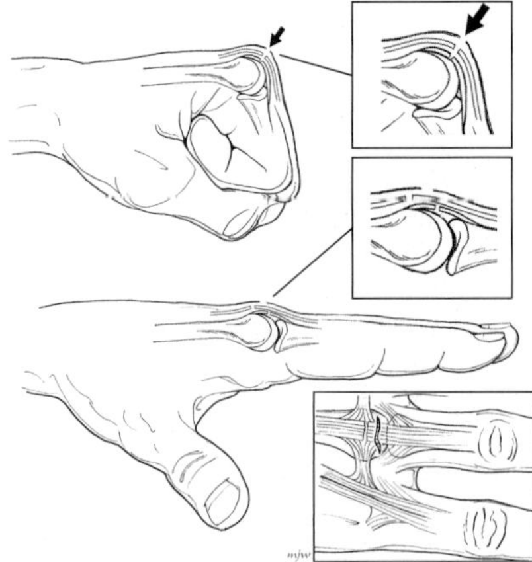

**Fig. 1.** With a bite to the hand, the extensor injury usually is proximal to the skin laceration because the MCP joint is flexed at the time of injury.

### TESTS

#### *Lab*

Cultures in the acute period before surgical débridement are unlikely to be helpful.

#### *Imaging*

- Obtain radiographs of the hand to assess for fracture and tooth fragments.
- In subacute presentations, look for osteomyelitis.

### DIFFERENTIAL DIAGNOSIS

Any puncture wound over the MCP joints must be regarded with great suspicion and treated as a clenched-fist–type bite injury.

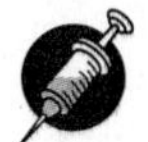

## TREATMENT

### GENERAL MEASURES

- If the patient has not been immunized within the past 10 years, tetanus toxoid should be administered.
- The most important therapeutic interventions are aggressive irrigation and débridement, to remove all devitalized tissue and to irrigate the wound copiously with normal saline solution, povidone-iodine (Betadine), or both.
- The wound may need to be extended surgically to facilitate exposure of the injured tissue.
- In clenched-fist injuries, the skin wound is distal to the zone of deeper injury.
- After irrigation and débridement, the wound should be packed, and the hand should be immobilized and elevated.
- *Do not suture bite wounds.*
- Antibiotics should be commenced (amoxicillin [Augmentin] is a reasonable 1st line agent) and should be continued for 5–7 days in the absence of overt infection.
- At 24 hours, the packing should be removed, the patient should be reexamined, and warm soaks should be started.
- If infection is present, the wound should undergo repeat irrigation and débridement, and the patient should be admitted for parenteral antibiotic therapy.
- For patients presenting late to evaluation and treatment, and for those in whom infection is manifest, urgent irrigation and débridement followed by parenteral antibiotics are essential.
- Immediate referral to a hand specialist should be considered for any patient presenting >24 hours after the initial injury, for those who have infected wounds, and for those who have sustained injury to the tendon, capsule, joint, or bone.

### SPECIAL THERAPY
#### *Physical Therapy*
- Physical therapy is not necessary in the acute period.
- At 1 week after treatment, ROM exercises should be started to prevent stiffness (especially of the MCP joints).

### MEDICATION (DRUGS)
#### *First Line*
- More than 40 bacterial species have been isolated from infected bite wounds.
- The most common organisms are *Eikenella corrodens* and group A *Streptococcus* species in human bite wounds and *Pasteurella multocida*, *S. aureus*, and Bacteroides in animal bite wounds (2–4).
- Augmentin provides satisfactory coverage for all organisms.
- Treat infection empirically with intravenous antibiotics for 48 hours, then adjust based on cultures.

### SURGERY
- Irrigation and débridement consist of cleaning infected tissues and removing devitalized tissues.
- Cultures should be obtained.
- Wounds should be left open and managed with dressing changes.
- Extensor tendon injury should not be repaired until infection resolves.

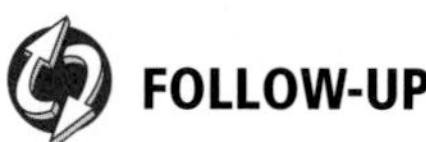

## FOLLOW-UP

### PROGNOSIS
Prognosis usually is good if infection is avoided or treated early.

### COMPLICATIONS
- Infection: Both soft tissue and bone
- Stiffness
- Pain
- Extensor tendon injury

### PATIENT MONITORING
- At 24 hours, the packing should be changed.
- The patient should be followed closely until the wound shows satisfactory healing with no evidence of infection.
- When doubt exists about the stability of the wound, the patient should be followed at 24–48-hour intervals.

### REFERENCES

1. Mennen U, Howells CJ. Human fight-bite injuries of the hand. A study of 100 cases within 18 months. *J Hand Surg* 1991;16B:431–435.
2. Dire DJ. Emergency management of dog and cat bite wounds. *Emerg Med Clin North Am* 1992;10:719–736.
3. Garcia VF. Animal bites and *Pasturella* infections. *Pediatr Rev* 1997;18:127–130.
4. Talan DA, Citron DM, Abrahamian FM, et al. Bacteriologic analysis of infected dog and cat bites. *N Engl J Med* 1999;340:85–92.


### ADDITIONAL READING

- Abrams RA, Botte MJ. Hand infections: treatment recommendations for specific types. *J Am Acad Orthop Surg* 1996;4:219–230.
- Baratz ME, Schmidt CC, Hughes TB. Extensor tendon injuries. In: Green DP, Hotchkiss RN, Pederson WC, et al., eds. *Green's Operative Hand Surgery*, 5th ed. Philadelphia: Elsevier Churchill Livingstone, 2005:187–217.
- Siverhus DJ, Stern PJ. Avoiding complications of human bite injuries. *J Musculoskelet Med* 1996;13:32–36, 43.
- Stevanovic MV, Sharpe F. Acute infections in the hand. In: Green DP, Hotchkiss RN, Pederson WC, et al., eds. *Green's Operative Hand Surgery*, 5th ed. Philadelphia: Elsevier Churchill Livingstone, 2005:55–93.


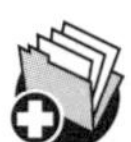

## MISCELLANEOUS

### CODES
#### *ICD9-CM*
882.1 Wound hand complicated

### PATIENT TEACHING
- Patients are instructed in cases of open wounds to watch for signs of infection.
  - Open packing
  - Soaking
  - ROM
  - Redness
  - Pain
  - Fever
  - Drainage
  - Inability to move finger

### FAQ
- Q: What are the most important treatment interventions in a bite to the hand?
  - A: The 1st priority is prevention of infection, which consists of prompt surgical exploration with irrigation and débridement of the joint and treatment with intravenous antibiotics.
- Q: When should an extensor tendon laceration secondary to a bite wound be repaired?
  - A: In this setting, repair of the extensor tendon can be delayed 7–10 days until the infection is resolved.

# BLOUNT DISEASE

*Paul D. Sponseller, MD*

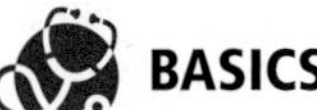

## BASICS

### DESCRIPTION

- Bowing of the legs can be a normal stage of growth for infants and toddlers.
  - This phase is called "physiologic bowing" and resolves spontaneously by approximately 2 years of age.
  - The vast majority of children presenting with bowed legs have this benign physiologic state.
- More rarely, bowed legs may be pathologic.
  - The most common cause of this condition is Blount disease.
  - It is an abnormality of the proximal tibial growth plate secondary to overload.
  - It causes progressive varus alignment of the knees (bowed legs) in children or adolescents (1,2) (Fig. 1).
- Classification:
  - Infantile form: Presents in children 0–4 years old
  - Juvenile form: Presents at >4–9 years of age in obese children
  - Adolescent form: Presents in children >10 years old; has excellent prognosis with surgery
- Synonyms: Infantile tibia vara (0–4 years); Juvenile tibia vara (>4–9 years); Adolescent tibia vara (10–16 years); Pathologic bowlegs

### GENERAL PREVENTION

- Weight control
- Extremely early standing or walking should not be encouraged.
- Early bracing sometimes is effective.

### EPIDEMIOLOGY

#### *Incidence*

- Infantile tibia vara is the most common cause of pathologic bowing in young children and accounts for <1% of all bowed legs (2).
- The juvenile form is much less common: Only 60 reports in the literature in the United States.

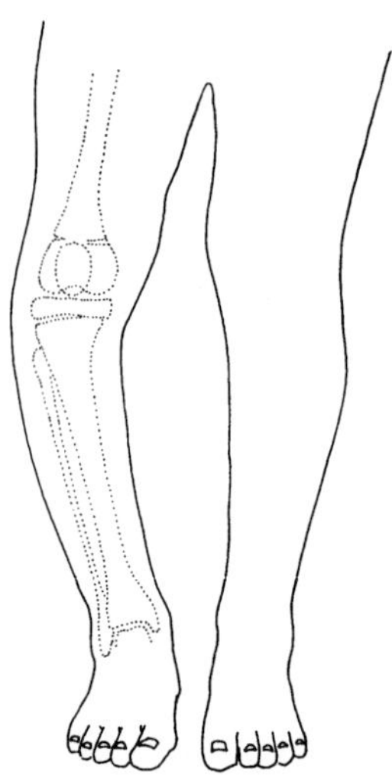

**Fig. 1.** In Blount disease, the varus is focal at the upper tibia.

- The adolescent form is becoming more commonly recognized.

#### *Prevalence (1,2)*

- The infantile form is more common in girls.
- The juvenile or adolescent form is more common in boys.
- The disorder is more common in African American children than those of other races.

### RISK FACTORS

- African American ethnicity
- Obesity
- Early age of walking
- Varus greater on the tibial than the femoral side is a risk factor for infantile and juvenile Blount disease (1).

#### *Genetics*

- No genetic pattern has been proved.
- More likely, patients inherit a body habitus that predisposes them to the disorder.

### PATHOPHYSIOLOGY

- The growth plate shows islands of densely packed cartilage cells with more hypertrophy than normal, islands of almost acellular fibrous cartilage, and abnormal groups of capillaries (2).
- Biopsy is not indicated.

### ETIOLOGY

Decreased growth of the proximal medial tibial growth plate (physis) causes varus angulation (bowing) and internal rotation of the proximal tibia secondary to weight-related overload of this portion of the growth plate.

### ASSOCIATED CONDITIONS

Obesity

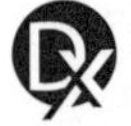

## DIAGNOSIS

### SIGNS AND SYMPTOMS

- Patients with infantile tibia vara usually present between 14 and 40 months of age with increasingly bowed legs (usually bilateral involvement).
- Adolescent presentation also involves progressive varus deformity (bowing), but many of these patients also have medial knee pain and often only 1 leg is affected.
- If untreated, the infantile form may progress to become severe.
- The juvenile and adolescent forms rarely become as severe.
- Some internal tibial torsion usually is present along with the bowing.

#### *Physical Exam*

- Record the patient's height, weight, and percentiles.
- The finding of short stature suggests rickets or a skeletal dysplasia.
- Note the location of any pain.
- Record the gap between the medial sides of the knees and check knee ROM and ligamentous laxity.
- Assess tibial torsion by the thigh–foot angle.
- Perform a routine knee examination, observe gait, and measure the foot progression angle (angle of the feet with the direction of walking).

### TESTS

#### *Lab*

- Testing is indicated if rickets is suspected.
- In Blount disease, calcium, phosphorus, alkaline phosphatase, and renal function tests are all normal (2).

#### *Imaging*

- Radiography:
  - Appropriate radiographs: A long leg AP view of the tibia and femur to evaluate the tibiofemoral angle and mechanical axis (1–5).
  - The radiograph should show the whole limb from the hip to the ankle, and it should be a true AP view of the knee (4).
  - The metaphyseal–diaphyseal angle differentiates Blount disease and physiologic varus:
    - $<11^\circ$ is physiologic varus.
    - $\geq 16^\circ$ indicates Blount disease.
    - Values between $11^\circ$ and $16^\circ$ signify a risk of potential Blount disease.
  - Reveals a medial physeal bar (disappearance of the growth plate with metaphysis–epiphysis fusion) in more advanced disease
- CT or MRI:
  - Can be useful in delineating the physeal damage that later may form a bar.
  - Patients with adolescent Blount disorder (Fig. 2) show less deformation of the epiphysis and rarely form a bar, but they usually have some deformity on the femoral as well as on the tibial side

### DIFFERENTIAL DIAGNOSIS

- Physiologic bowed legs
- Hypophosphatemic rickets
- Trauma to metaphysis or growth plate
- Osteochondroma
- Metaphyseal chondrodysplasia
- Focal fibrocartilaginous dysplasia

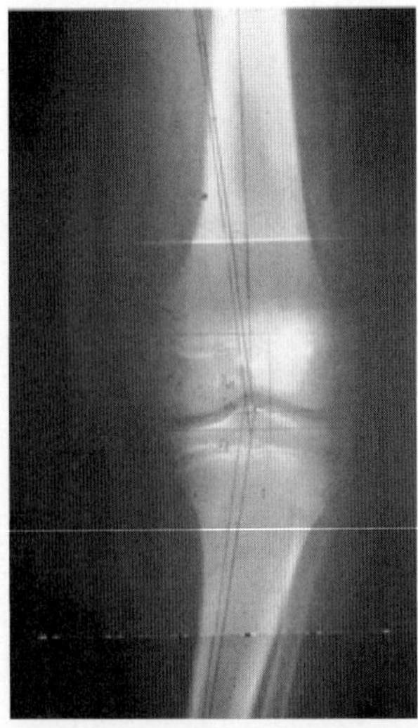

**Fig. 2.** Adolescent Blount disease. Note the physeal widening and relative preservation of the epiphysis of the tibia.

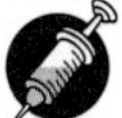

# TREATMENT

## GENERAL MEASURES

- Children <3 years old who present with Blount disease may be braced, preferably with a long brace from the hip to the ankle that is locked at the knee (2).
- Full-time bracing (22 hours a day) puts a corrective valgus stress on the knee (more knock-kneed) and decreases the stress on the medial physis.
  - If bracing is begun when the deformity is mild, this treatment allows the growth plate to "catch up" the growth medially.
- If the patient is being braced, full weightbearing is encouraged.
- If bracing fails to correct the deformity, or if a patient >3 years old presents with moderate to severe deformity, an osteotomy is needed (6,7).
- If osteotomy is performed, the patient is kept nonweightbearing until healing (8–12 weeks) of the osteotomy; then full weightbearing can be resumed.
- Hemiepiphysiodesis is also an alternative in juveniles if the deformity is moderate (6).

### *Activity*

- No activity restriction on unbraced patients
- Bracing restricts participation in sports.

## SPECIAL THERAPY

### *Physical Therapy*

- Does not help improve knee varus
- Crutch training after osteotomy
- Regaining knee ROM after osteotomy

## SURGERY

- Osteotomy (cutting and realigning the proximal tibia) will decrease the stress on the medial physis and can allow healing.
- If a physeal bar has formed:
  - An osteotomy often is combined with completion of the closure of the proximal tibial physis.
  - The whole growth plate should be fused to prevent the lateral portion of the growth plate from causing recurrent varus (5); patients with advanced cases may have a secondary deformity of the distal femur and/or the distal tibia.
- If substantial leg-length inequality develops, it may be treated by lengthening the short limb or by growth plate closure of the longer limb.
- Adolescent Blount disease may be treated with tethering ("stapling") of the lateral sides of the growth plate to allow the bone to correct itself.
- In more advanced cases, osteotomy of the tibia and/or the femur is needed.

# FOLLOW-UP

## PROGNOSIS

- Because the recurrence rate is higher in patients treated after 4 years of age (70–75%) than in patients treated before age 4 (20–30%) (2), early osteotomy (before age 4) should be performed if bracing is not successful.
- Patients with late treatment or incomplete treatment have an increased risk of arthritis of the knee.

## COMPLICATIONS

- Recurrence of deformity leads to abnormal limb alignment and degenerative arthritis.
- Limb-length inequality may result.
- Postosteotomy complications include neurovascular complications and compartment syndrome.

## PATIENT MONITORING

- Patients should be followed until skeletal maturity.
- The interval between visits is determined by the severity of the disease.

## REFERENCES

1. Bowen RE, Dorey FJ, Moseley CF. Relative tibial and femoral varus as a predictor of progression of varus deformities of the lower limbs in young children. *J Pediatr Orthop* 2002;22:105–111.
2. Schoenecker PL, Rich MM. The lower extremity. In: Morrissy RT, Weinstein SL, eds. *Lovell and Winter's Pediatric Orthopaedics,* 6th ed. Philadelphia: Lippincott Williams & Wilkins, 2006:1157–1211.
3. Doyle BS, Volk AG, Smith CF. Infantile Blount disease: long-term follow-up of surgically treated patients at skeletal maturity. *J Pediatr Orthop* 1996;16:469–476.
4. Gordon JE, Heidenreich FP, Carpenter CJ, et al. Comprehensive treatment of late-onset tibia vara. *J Bone Joint Surg* 2005;87A:1561–1570.
5. Stanitski DF, Stanitski CL, Trumble S. Depression of the medial tibial plateau in early-onset Blount disease: myth or reality? *J Pediatr Orthop* 1999;19:265–269.
6. Gordon JE, King DJ, Luhmann SJ, et al. Femoral deformity in tibia vara. *J Bone Joint Surg* 2006;88A:380–386.
7. Henderson RC, Kemp GJ, Jr, Greene WB. Adolescent tibia vara: alternatives for operative treatment. *J Bone Joint Surg* 1992;74A:342–350.

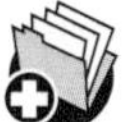

# MISCELLANEOUS

## CODES

### *ICD9-CM*

732.4 Blount's disease

## PATIENT TEACHING

- The patient's family must understand the benefit of regular monitoring and weight reduction.
- If they elect to use bracing in patients with infantile Blount disease, the braces must be worn 22 hours a day to exert their corrective effect on growth.

## FAQ

- Q: How can Blount disease be distinguished from physiologic bowing of the tibia?
  - A: They can be distinguished by the metaphyseal–diaphyseal angle in young children (<3 years old) being >11° and by the shape of the tibial deformation in older children.
- Q: What is the cause of Blount disease?
  - A: The cause is overload of the medial growth plate of the upper tibia.
- Q: Is surgery always necessary?
  - A: Surgery is recommended for all patients who are symptomatic or who have varus of >10°.
- Q: Does adolescent Blount disease develop from infantile Blount disease?
  - A: No, adolescent Blount disease develops spontaneously in older-aged children than does infantile Blount disease.

# BRACHIAL PLEXUS BIRTH PALSY

*Paul D. Sponseller, MD*

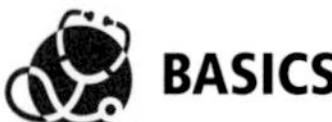

## BASICS

### DESCRIPTION

- Brachial plexus palsy results from stretch during birth that is caused by downward or upward traction on the arm.
- Secondarily, the muscles and bones of the upper extremity become contracted or deformed over time because of the resultant muscle imbalance.
- Although the injury occurs at birth, in mild cases it may not be detected until the baby tries to use the extremity (1–3).
- Classification (3):
  - Type I (Erb palsy): Injury to roots 4–6 of the cervical spine
  - Type II (whole-brachial plexus palsy): C4–T1 involved; also known as "Erb-Duchenne-Klumpke" palsy
  - Type III (Klumpke palsy): C8–T1 involved
- Synonyms: Birth palsy; Obstetric palsy; Erb palsy; Klumpke palsy

### GENERAL PREVENTION

- Sometimes obstetricians will advise a caesarean section if a baby seems extremely large or cephalopelvic disproportion is present.
- Not all cases can be anticipated or prevented.

### EPIDEMIOLOGY

#### *Incidence*

- Currently, the incidence is 0.8 per 1,000 live births (2).
  - This figure is a decline from the rate in 1900, when it was reported twice as often.
  - The change most likely results from improved obstetric care.
- Erb palsy is ~4 times as common as Klumpke palsy.
- No recognized difference exists in incidence between boys and girls.

### RISK FACTORS

- Fetal malposition
- Shoulder dystocia
- Cephalopelvic disproportion
- High birth weight:
  - Maternal diabetes
- Use of forceps in delivery

### PATHOPHYSIOLOGY

- Pathologic findings vary from stretch to disruption of the nerves of the brachial plexus (3).
- The injury may occur at the cervical foramen as the nerves exit the spinal canal (poorer prognosis), or farther down in the neck and shoulder.
- Secondary muscle atrophy and contracture ensues.

### ETIOLOGY

- Erb palsy results from downward traction on the shoulder or arm or lateral traction against the neck.
- Klumpke palsy is secondary to upward traction on the arm.
- Both occur because of the force needed in a difficult extraction.

### ASSOCIATED CONDITIONS

- High birth weight
- Gestational diabetes

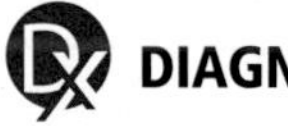

## DIAGNOSIS

### SIGNS AND SYMPTOMS

- Decreased active use of the extremity
- Arm held in internal rotation (2)
- Loss of full active or passive external rotation
- Inability to abduct (raise) the shoulder
- Atrophy of the involved muscles (late) (Fig. 1)
- Elbow flexion contracture
- Possible Horner syndrome in Klumpke palsy
- The condition is not painful.
- A loss of sensation may be noted with complete plexus injuries.

#### *History*

- Decreased infant arm movements sometimes are noted from birth.
- In other cases, more subtle decreases in shoulder movement or presence of arm contracture may not be noted until later.

#### *Physical Exam*

- Physical examination is the primary means of diagnosis.
  - Palpate for tenderness over the clavicle, proximal humerus, and ribs.
  - Test sensation by responses to light touch or pinch.
  - Test the function of all muscles in the shoulder, elbow, and hand by stimulation and observation.
- In patients with Erb palsy, the shoulder is internally rotated and lacks external rotation and abduction.
- In Klumpke palsy, loss of finger and interosseous function occurs.

### TESTS

#### *Imaging*

- Plain radiographs often are indicated at birth to rule out other injuries that may cause decreased movement of the infant's arm (clavicle fracture, proximal humerus fracture); such injuries may coexist with brachial plexus birth palsy.
- At the time of late reconstruction in a child >4 years old who has residual shoulder imbalance, plain radiographs and CT scans are indicated to assess the shape of the glenohumeral joint.

#### *Diagnostic Procedures/Surgery*

- An electromyogram should be obtained if no clinical return of deltoid or biceps function occurs by 3–6 months of age.
  - Lack of reinnervation may be a relative indication for surgery.
- Cervical myelography may be helpful for diagnosing the level of injury.
  - Meningoceles seen at the root levels in the cervical spinal cord indicate that roots were avulsed from the cord, and the prognosis is poor.
  - A finding of meningoceles indicates that different strategies may be needed at surgery.

### DIFFERENTIAL DIAGNOSIS

- Clavicle fracture:
  - Usually painful to palpation
  - Some shoulder motion may be elicited.
- Proximal humeral physeal fracture:
  - Same findings as clavicle fracture, with tenderness over the proximal humerus; the abnormality may not show on radiographs because the proximal humerus is not ossified at birth.
  - Ultrasound or MRI studies may be diagnostic, as are plain films 7–10 days later.
- Septic arthritis of the shoulder:
  - May cause pseudoparalysis
  - Fever in the newborn may not be pronounced.

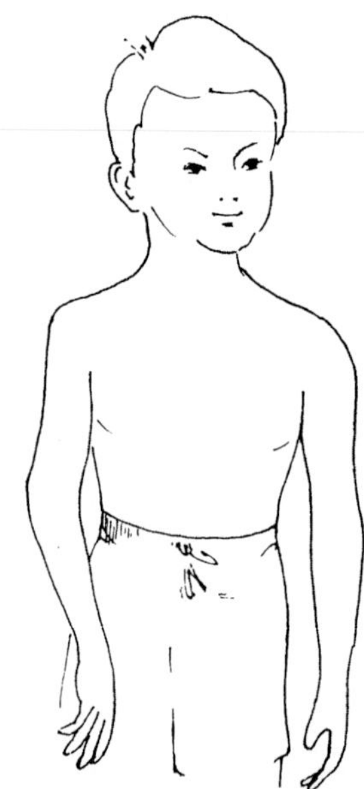

**Fig. 1.** The most typical deformity after infantile brachial plexus palsy is an internally rotated arm that does not abduct fully or flex at the elbow. This deformity results from damage to the C5–C6 roots.

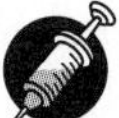

# TREATMENT

## GENERAL MEASURES

- Parents should stretch the infant's arm several times a day as directed by the occupational therapist (1–3).
- The patient should be referred to a specialized pediatric orthopaedic surgeon for monitoring and decision-making.
- Observation and passive ROM are indicated for the newborn; ~80% of patients recover spontaneously by 1 year of age (4).
- Splinting is not necessary, but continued follow-up is needed.
- Surgery is indicated for the remaining 20% of patients, with grafting of the injured nerves (if no meningoceles are present and the elapsed time is not >1–2 years) or with tendon transfers to improve muscle balance (2–5).

### *Activity*

- No restrictions
- Encourage passive ROM.

## SPECIAL THERAPY

### *Physical Therapy*

- An occupational therapist is helpful in teaching the parents how to stretch and what contractures to watch for.
- Splinting is not needed, but stretching and passive ROM are encouraged.

## SURGERY

- Nerve repair/reconstruction:
  - May be performed with an operative microscope with direct repair or grafting of the injured nerves if the patient's function does not return in ~6 months.
  - The exact timing is controversial.
- Tendon transfers may be performed later to restore external rotation to the shoulder.
- Release of the tight internal rotators also may be indicated.
- Humeral osteotomy is another way to restore an externally rotated position.
- Several muscle transfers are available to restore elbow flexion, most notably the latissimus transfer.
- Transfers for finger and wrist function are least commonly needed.

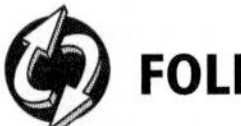

# FOLLOW-UP

## DISPOSITION

### *Issues for Referral*

It is important to refer the baby with brachial birth palsy to an orthopaedic surgeon with an interest in this condition because it is a specialized field.

## PROGNOSIS

- 80% of patients with brachial plexus birth palsy recover spontaneously.
- Surgery may help many of the remainder.

## COMPLICATIONS

- Contracture of shoulder, elbow, or wrist
- Affected extremity smaller in length and girth
- Sensory loss
- Shoulder dislocation

## PATIENT MONITORING

The patient should be seen approximately every 2–3 months to look for return of function and to plan for appropriate diagnostic testing.

## REFERENCES


1. Boome RS, Kaye JC. Obstetric traction injuries of the brachial plexus. Natural history, indications for surgical repair and results. *J Bone Joint Surg* 1988;70B:571–576.
2. Waters PM, Bae DS. Effect of tendon transfers and extra-articular soft-tissue balancing on glenohumeral development in brachial plexus birth palsy. *J Bone Joint Surg* 2005;87A:320–325.
3. Waters PM. Update on management of pediatric brachial plexus palsy. *J Pediatr Orthop* 2005;25:116–126.
4. Smith NC, Rowan P, Benson LJ, et al. Neonatal brachial plexus palsy. Outcome of absent biceps function at three months of age. *J Bone Joint Surg* 2004;86A:2163–2170.
5. Hoffer MM, Wickenden R, Roper B. Brachial plexus birth palsies. Results of tendon transfers to the rotator cuff. *J Bone Joint Surg* 1978;60:691–695.


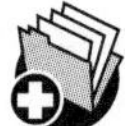

# MISCELLANEOUS

## CODES

### *ICD9-CM*

767.6 Brachial plexus birth palsy

## PATIENT TEACHING

- The prognosis should be outlined to the parents, so they can plan ahead.
- The possibility of contractures should be explained, so the parents will be motivated to continue the stretching exercises.

### *Activity*

No activity restrictions

### *Prevention*

- Management of gestational diabetes
- Caesarean delivery if cephalopelvic disproportion is clinically significant.

## FAQ

- Q: Why is immediate surgical repair of the brachial plexus not indicated at birth?
  - A: Because most lesions are stretch lesions (neurapraxias) that will improve spontaneously. Surgery on these nerves may disrupt intact channels.
- Q: What is the latest age at which nerve repair may be performed?
  - A: It should not be performed much after the age of 12–18 months because reinnervation may not succeed.

# BUNION/HALLUX VALGUS

*Gregory Gebauer, MD, MS*

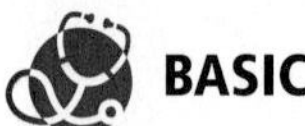

## BASICS

### DESCRIPTION

- A bunion is an enlargement of the medial eminence of the 1st metatarsal with soft tissue and bursal swelling.
- Hallux valgus occurs primarily at the MTP joint and consists of lateral deviation of the great toe with medial deviation of the 1st metatarsal.
- Subluxation of the MTP joint often occurs.

### GENERAL PREVENTION

Avoidance of narrow footwear

### EPIDEMIOLOGY

- Occurs predominantly in middle-aged to elderly women, but can be seen in adolescents and young adults
- Females are affected more than males.
- Occurs almost exclusively in shoe-wearing societies

#### *Prevalence*

Reported to occur in up to 33% of individuals (1)

### RISK FACTORS

- Heredity
- Shoe wear

#### *Genetics*

- May be an unidentified genetic component
- Positive family history in 2/3 of patients
- Hallux valgus also is seen commonly as a component of a hyperlaxity syndrome that is thought to have a genetic component.

### ETIOLOGY

- Shoes with narrow toe boxes and high heels are believed to be related to the development of hallux valgus.
  - Higher incidence in shod versus unshod societies and increasing incidence in populations that adopt more Westernized shoe styles (Fig. 1) (1)
- Pes planus also may be a causative factor: Part of a laxity syndrome and associated with mechanically abnormal pressure on the 1st MTP joint secondary to a pronated gait.

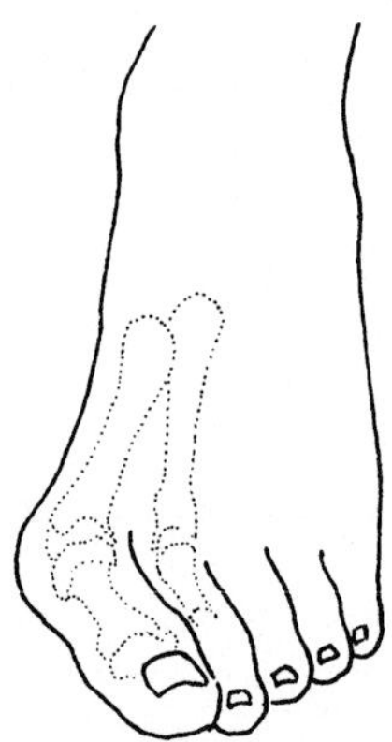

**Fig. 1.** A bunion is produced by an underlying imbalance of the soft tissues and extrinsic pressure.

- Metatarsus primus varus is associated; a strong relationship exists between an increase in the angle between the 1st and 2nd metatarsal joints and the development of hallux valgus.
- Acquired joint laxity (e.g., from rheumatoid arthritis, gout, or trauma) can contribute to the development.
- Other miscellaneous conditions (e.g., amputation of another toe, severe hammering of the toes, Achilles tendon contracture) also may be associated.

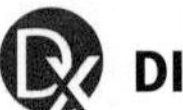

## DIAGNOSIS

### SIGNS AND SYMPTOMS

- The primary symptom is pain over the medial eminence, often caused by shoe wear pressure.
- The patient has lateral deviation of the great toe and prominence of the medial eminence.
- The deformity may be accentuated with weightbearing.
- When the condition is advanced, impingement by the great toe on the 2nd toe can lead to 2nd-toe pain and deformity.
- Can be associated with pain under the 2nd metatarsal head (transfer metatarsalgia), 1st metatarsal joint pain, and arthritis.
- Patients' complaints often are cosmetically based and concern difficulty with shoe wear.

#### *Physical Exam*

- Examine the sitting and standing patient.
- Assess for Achilles tendon and gastrocnemius contracture with the knee flexed and extended (indicated by limited ankle dorsiflexion).
- Check motion at the ankle, subtalar, midfoot, and metatarsal joints.
- Manually assess for increased laxity or instability of the 1st metatarsocuneiform joint with vertical shear or stress.
- Assess the flexibility or rigidity of the hallux valgus deformity by manually reducing the alignment of the toe.
- Pay attention to foot morphology and arch status.
- Perform a complete neurovascular and musculoskeletal examination of the entire lower extremity.

### TESTS

#### *Imaging*

- Obtain standing AP, oblique, lateral, and axial (sesamoid) foot radiographs.
  - Assess for the intermetatarsal angle, hallux valgus angle, hallux IP angle, distal metatarsal articular angle, and the sesamoid incongruence.
  - Evaluate for joint incongruence and arthrosis, which greatly influences the treatment plan.
  - Evaluate lesser toe alignment.

#### *Pathological Findings*

- 2 broad categories of hallux valgus occur, each with different entities and different pathoanatomic features: A noncongruent joint and a congruent joint.
- Incongruent joint:
  - Multiple static and dynamic anatomic components
  - The 1st metatarsal head drifts medially (varus), thus increasing the angle between the 1st and 2nd metatarsals.
  - The sesamoid complex is held in place by the transverse metatarsal ligament and thus becomes relatively laterally positioned as the metatarsal head displaces medially.
  - With progressive deformity, the axis of pull for the adductor hallucis, the flexor hallucis brevis, extensor hallucis longus, and the abductor hallucis become lateralized, which dynamically contributes to the lateral displacement of the great toe.
  - The medial joint capsule and ligaments become attenuated, whereas the lateral joint capsule and ligaments become contracted.
- Congruent joint:
  - A laterally sloped articular surface is present, with no pathologic articulation, so progression of deformity is less likely.

### DIFFERENTIAL DIAGNOSIS

Gout

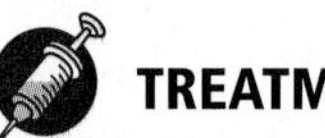

## TREATMENT

### GENERAL MEASURES

- Hallux valgus should be treated initially with nonoperative measures.
- Appropriate shoe wear is essential.
  - Pointed shoes and high heels must be avoided.
  - Lace-up styles have wider forefeet.
  - Soft leather shoes can be stretched to accommodate the bunion.
  - No stitching should be present over the medial eminence.
- Numerous off-the-shelf cushions, pads, or splinting devices may alleviate pressure over the medial bunion.
- Heel cord stretching and custom orthotic arch support may have a role for patients with associated Achilles contracture and pes planus (2).
- Prescription shoes, wide with increased depth, can be ordered if needed.

### SPECIAL THERAPY

#### *Physical Therapy*

Not usually helpful for symptom relief

### MEDICATION (DRUGS)

Analgesic medications may be necessary for symptomatic control.

## SURGERY

- Goals of surgery: Pain relief, correction of the deformity, restoration of normal biomechanics, and maintenance of adequate joint motion
- Indications for surgery:
  - Failed nonsurgical treatments
  - Worsening pain and deformity
  - Decreased function and inability to tolerate shoe wear
- Contraindications for surgery:
  - Cosmetic complaints alone without symptoms
  - Vascular insufficiency
- Options:
  - Multiple surgical procedures exist.
  - A decision tree for appropriate care is based on multiple factors.
    - Age
    - The angle between the 1st and 2nd metatarsal joint ( normal, 9°)
    - The MTP angle (normal, 15°)
    - Congruity or incongruity of the joint
    - In the presence of degenerative joint disease, the options are to fuse or to place a prosthesis; currently, prosthesis technology is associated with high complication and failure rates and is not recommended for active individuals (3).
    - The presence of a rigid joint
- Overview of surgical procedures:
  - Silver procedure:
    - Resection of the medial eminence should be used only for elderly patients.
    - Low complication rate, high recurrence rate
  - Modified McBride procedure (4):
    - Soft-tissue repair with resection of the medial eminence; release of the contracted lateral joint capsule, adductor hallucis tendon, and transverse metatarsal ligament; and imbrication of the medial capsule
    - Corrects hallux valgus angle
    - Can be used for mild deformities
    - More effective when performed with a proximal metatarsal osteotomy
    - Complications include hallux varus (overcorrection) and stiffness.
  - Distal metatarsal chevron osteotomy combined with a medial eminence resection and medial capsule plication (5):
    - The metatarsal head fragment is translated laterally, correcting intermetatarsal angle.
    - Appropriate for mild to moderate deformity (cannot adequately correct more severe deformities)
    - Can be complicated by malunion, osteonecrosis, or hallux varus
  - Metatarsocuneiform arthrodesis and distal soft-tissue correction (Lapidus procedure) (6):
    - For hallux valgus deformities with hypermobility or instability of 1st metatarsocuneiform joint
    - Corrects increased intermetatarsal angle
    - Combined with modified McBride correction at the MTP joint
  - Proximal metatarsal osteotomy and distal soft-tissue correction (4,7):
    - For more severe hallux valgus deformities
    - Corrects increased intermetatarsal angle
    - Numerous configurations of proximal osteotomies have been described, including crescentic, oblique, opening wedge, and proximal chevron osteotomies.
    - Combined with modified McBride correction at the MTP joint.
  - MTP arthrodesis (8):
    - For severe deformities in elderly individuals; hallux valgus with degenerative or inflammatory arthritis, underlying spasticity, or connective tissue disorders, and as salvage for failed surgery
    - Fusion has dependable rates of pain relief and satisfaction but does result in hallux stiffness.
  - Resection arthroplasty (Keller) bunionectomy (9):
    - Involves removal of the medial eminence and base of the proximal phalanx
    - Appropriate only for older, sedentary patients
    - Can be associated with multiple complications, including recurrent valgus, transfer metatarsalgia, and cock-up 1st toe.
  - Akin phalangeal osteotomy procedure (10):
    - A medial closing wedge osteotomy of the proximal phalanx
    - For isolated hallux valgus interphalangeus or in combination with more proximal metatarsal osteotomy or fusion

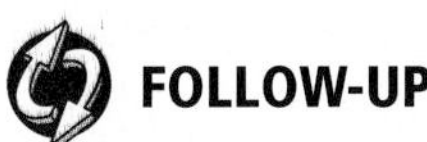

# FOLLOW-UP

## PROGNOSIS

- Mild deformities and congruent deformities have lower rates of progression with nonoperative management than do severe or incongruent deformities.
- Surgical treatment with appropriate indications and decision-making typically results in pain relief and deformity correction in most patients.

## COMPLICATIONS

Surgical complications include wound breakdown and infection, recurrence of the deformity, overcorrection leading to hallux varus, malunion or nonunion of osteotomy or fusion procedures, joint stiffness, neuroma, and transfer metatarsalgia.

## REFERENCES


1. Sim-Fook L, Hodgson AR. A comparison of foot forms among the non-shoe and shoe-wearing Chinese population. *J Bone Joint Surg* 1958;40A:1058–1062.
2. Torkki M, Malmivaara A, Seitsalo S, et al. Surgery vs orthosis vs watchful waiting for hallux valgus: a randomized controlled trial. *JAMA* 2001;285:2474–2480.
3. Shereff MJ, Jahss MH. Complications of silastic implant arthroplasty in the hallux. *Foot Ankle* 1980;1:95–101.
4. Mann RA, Rudicel S, Graves SC. Repair of hallux valgus with a distal soft-tissue procedure and proximal metatarsal osteotomy. A long-term follow-up. *J Bone Joint Surg* 1992;74A:124–129.
5. Trnka HJ, Zembsch A, Easley ME, et al. The chevron osteotomy for correction of hallux valgus: Comparison of findings after two and five years of follow-up. *J Bone Joint Surg* 2000;82A:1373–1378.
6. Sangeorzan BJ, Hansen ST, Jr. Modified Lapidus procedure for hallux valgus. *Foot Ankle* 1989;9:262–266.
7. Chiodo CP, Schon LC, Myerson MS. Clinical results with the Ludloff osteotomy for correction of adult hallux valgus. *Foot Ankle Int* 2004;25:532–536.
8. Coughlin MJ, Grebing BR, Jones CP. Arthrodesis of the first MTP joint for idiopathic hallux valgus: intermediate results. *Foot Ankle Int* 2005;26:783–792.
9. Vallier GT, Petersen SA, LaGrone MO. The Keller resection arthroplasty: a 13-year experience. *Foot Ankle* 1991;11:187–194.
10. Frey C, Jahss M, Kummer FJ. The Akin procedure: an analysis of results. *Foot Ankle* 1991;12:1–6.


## ADDITIONAL READING


Coughlin MJ. Hallux valgus. *J Bone Joint Surg* 1996;78A:932–966.


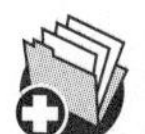

# MISCELLANEOUS

## CODES

### *ICD9-CM*

- 727.1 Bunion
- 735.0 Hallux valgus
- 754.52 Metatarsus primus varus

## PATIENT TEACHING

### *Activity*

Once the patient is no longer in the perioperative period, few limitations are placed on activity.

### *Prevention*

The most important factor in prevention is the use of proper shoe wear and the avoidance of high-heeled shoes with narrow toe boxes.

## FAQ

- Q: When is bunion surgery indicated?
  - A: Bunion surgery is indicated for painful lesions that have not responded to nonoperative therapy, including trials of wide toe-box shoe wear.
- Q: What can be done to prevent recurrence?
  - A: Avoidance of high-heeled, narrow toe-box shoe wear is critical to preventing recurrence.

# BURNERS (STINGERS)

*Michael K. Shindle, MD*
*Marc Urquhart, MD*

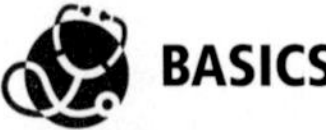

## BASICS

### DESCRIPTION
- Burners (also termed "stingers") are traction injuries that result in a neurapraxia of the brachial plexus.
- Patients typically report pain that radiates into the shoulder and down the arm to the hand, which is usually described as a "dead arm."
- These injuries are common in tackling sports and usually occur in teenagers and young adults.
- One of the most common injuries in football
- Usually associated weakness of shoulder abduction (deltoid), elbow flexion (biceps), and external humeral rotation (spinati) (1)
- The brachial plexus injury typically involves only the upper trunk (2) (Fig. 1).

### EPIDEMIOLOGY
Males are affected more often than are females.

### RISK FACTORS
- High-impact sports
- Motorcycle crashes
- Cervical stenosis may predispose an athlete to a burner syndrome because of concomitant foraminal narrowing with nerve root compression.

### ETIOLOGY
- Typically secondary to ipsilateral shoulder depression with lateral neck deviation to the contralateral side (3) (Fig. 1)
- A direct blow to the supraclavicular area may occur in football and other contact sports, as well as in motorcycle accidents.

### ASSOCIATED CONDITIONS
- Horner syndrome
- Suprascapular nerve compression

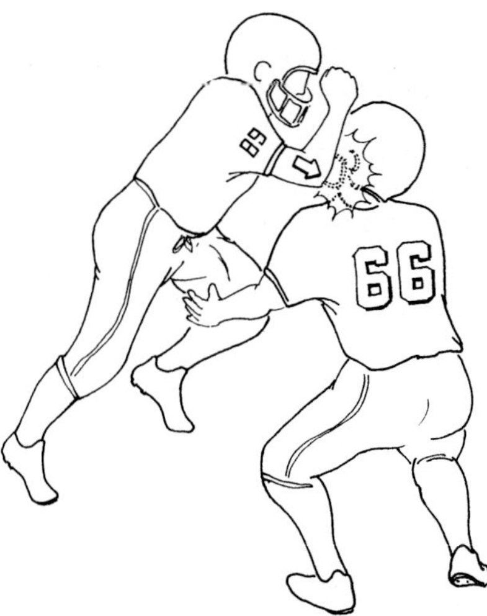


**Fig. 1.** Burners and stingers are produced by a downward blow to the shoulder or by a lateral force to the hand and neck.

## DIAGNOSIS

### SIGNS AND SYMPTOMS
- The distribution of symptoms depends on the level of the brachial plexus injury.
- Transient numbness or tingling may be present.
- Weakness of shoulder abduction (deltoid), elbow flexion (biceps), and external humeral rotation (spinati) may occur.

#### *Physical Exam*
- Sideline evaluation should include:
  - Palpation of the cervical spine for tenderness and cervical ROM testing: Cervical tenderness or painful or limited ROM are red flags for a more serious problem.
  - A complete but brief neurologic examination of all four extremities: Sensation and movement may be checked by having the patient flex and extend each joint; test sensation on anterior and posterior surfaces of each limb segment.
  - Manual muscle testing in the affected upper extremity: Arm weakness with decreased sensation may be present, but athletes usually have a normal examination by the time they reach the sideline (4).
  - Testing for tenderness in the brachial plexus: Tinel sign in the supraclavicular fossa indicates damage to at least 1 nerve root.

### TESTS
#### *Lab*
Electromyographic and nerve conduction velocity studies should be obtained if no recovery of neurologic function occurs in 2–3 weeks (rare).

#### *Imaging*
- Radiography:
  - Plain radiographs of the cervical spine, including active flexion and extension views to look for cervical instability and oblique views to visualize the cervical nerve root foramen (5).
  - Scapular AP and lateral views plus axillary views of the shoulder
- MRI of the cervical spine for patients with recurrent stingers or persistent neurologic deficit

### DIFFERENTIAL DIAGNOSIS
- Cervical spine injury or stenosis
- Thoracic outlet syndrome
- Long thoracic nerve palsy
- Suprascapular nerve compression

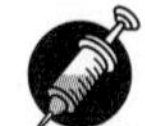

## TREATMENT

### GENERAL MEASURES
- Observation and serial evaluations should be performed.
- Most patients recover within minutes.
- Return to play is allowed when full strength has returned, all neurologic signs and symptoms have resolved, and cervical ROM is pain free.
- Patients with recurrent or prolonged (hours to weeks) burner syndrome mandate additional evaluation, including:
  - AP, lateral, oblique, and odontoid views of the cervical spine for assessment of cervical stenosis (6).
  - If those radiographs are negative, then flexion–extension views to identify ligamentous instability
- The affected extremity may be placed in a sling for comfort, as needed.
- The patient should be restricted from sports until the symptoms have resolved and any needed workup is complete.
- If stingers are recurrent, a change in sport should be considered.

### SPECIAL THERAPY
#### *Physical Therapy*
An aggressive neck and shoulder strengthening program should be initiated.

### MEDICATION (DRUGS)
Analgesics may be taken, if needed.

### SURGERY
In general, surgery is not indicated.

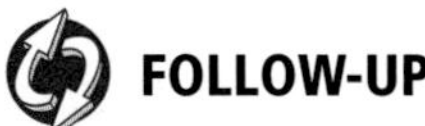

## FOLLOW-UP

### PROGNOSIS
- The prognosis is generally poor for patients with supraclavicular injuries and patients with complete neurologic deficits.
- The prognosis is more favorable for patients with infraclavicular injuries or incomplete neurologic deficits.

### COMPLICATIONS
- Incomplete recovery
- Muscle weakness or wasting
- Pain

### REFERENCES

1. Feinberg JH. Burners and stingers. *Phys Med Rehabil Clin N Am* 2000;11:771–784.
2. Weinberg J, Rokito S, Silber JS. Etiology, treatment, and prevention of athletic "stingers." *Clin Sports Med* 2003;21:493–500.
3. Vaccaro AR, Watkins B, Albert TJ, et al. Cervical spine injuries in athletes: current return-to-play criteria. *Orthopaedics* 2001;24:699–703.
4. Safran MR. Nerve injury about the shoulder in athletes, part 2: long thoracic nerve, spinal accessory nerve, burners/stingers, thoracic outlet syndrome. *Am J Sports Med* 2004;32:1063–1076.
5. Kelly JD, IV, Aliquo D, Sitler MR, et al. Association of burners with cervical canal and foraminal stenosis. *Am J Sports Med* 2000;28:214–217.
6. Levitz CL, Reilly PJ, Torg JS. The pathomechanics of chronic, recurrent cervical nerve root neurapraxia. The chronic burner syndrome. *Am J Sports Med* 1997;25:73–76.


### ADDITIONAL READING

- Fagan KM. Head and neck injuries. In: Andrews JR, Clancy WG, Jr, Whiteside JA, eds. *On-Field Evaluation and Treatment of Common Athletic Injuries*. St. Louis: Mosby, 1997:1–15.
- Torg JS. Cervical spine injuries. In: Garrick JG, ed. *Orthopaedic Knowledge Update: Sports Medicine 3*. Rosemont, IL: American Academy of Orthopaedic Surgeons, 2004:3–18.
- Zarins B, Prodromos CC. Shoulder injuries in sports. In: Rowe CR, ed. *The Shoulder*. New York: Churchill Livingstone, 1988:411–433.


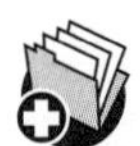

## MISCELLANEOUS

### CODES
#### *ICD9-CM*
767.6 Injury to brachial plexus

### PATIENT TEACHING
- Proper tackling technique should be taught.
- The motion and position that produce brachial plexus stretch should be explained.
- Patients should avoid impact on the top of the shoulder or the side of the neck.

#### *Prevention*
- Physical therapy with emphasis on a neck-strengthening program
- High-profile shoulder pads or a cowboy collar to limit the extent of lateral flexion and extension
- Education about proper blocking and tackling techniques

### FAQ
- Q: In the stinger syndrome, weakness most commonly occurs during strength testing of which muscles?
  - A: In most cases, this injury involves the upper trunk (C5, C6) of the brachial plexus. Thus, weakness may include the deltoid (C5), biceps (C5, C6), supraspinatus (C5, C6), and infraspinatus muscles (C5, C6).
- Q: What criteria should be used to decide if an athlete can return to play?
  - A: Most athletes have full recovery within minutes. If full strength has returned and all neurologic signs and symptoms have resolved, return to play is allowed. More prolonged symptoms and/or 3 or more previous episodes of the stinger/burner syndrome should prohibit return to play until additional evaluation is performed.
- Q: What condition may predispose an athlete to develop the burner/stinger syndrome?
  - A: Cervical stenosis may predispose an athlete to experiencing a burner syndrome because of concomitant foraminal narrowing with nerve root compression.

# CALCANEOVALGUS FOOT

*Paul D. Sponseller, MD*

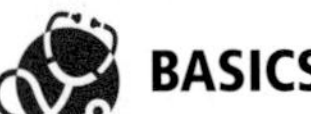

## BASICS

### DESCRIPTION

- Calcaneovalgus foot is a congenital condition thought to result from intrauterine positioning (1).
- The hindfoot is held in valgus and the foot is markedly dorsiflexed, with the dorsum of the foot nearly touching the anterior tibia.

### EPIDEMIOLOGY

- The condition occurs in neonates.
- No gender predominance is noted.
- It is one of the most common congenital foot disorders.

#### *Prevalence*

Present to varying degrees in 5% of all births

### PATHOPHYSIOLOGY

- The Achilles tendon is stretched temporarily, but it recovers spontaneously after birth.
- No bony abnormalities are present.

### ASSOCIATED CONDITIONS

- Infants with a calcaneovalgus foot should be checked for other positioning deformities, such as DDH or torticollis.
- No evidence suggests that this condition may predispose the patient to the development of pes planus (flat feet).

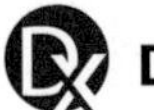

## DIAGNOSIS

### SIGNS AND SYMPTOMS

- This condition, present at birth, has no symptoms.
- The foot is markedly dorsiflexed, with the dorsum of the foot resting against the anterior tibia.
- The hindfoot is held in valgus and, occasionally, a contracture of the anterior muscles (dorsiflexors) is present.
- The deformity usually is supple, and the foot can be passively plantarflexed easily.

#### *Physical Exam*

- The appearance of the foot usually is diagnostic.
- The foot is easily plantarflexed and supinated, but it may not be passively correctable right away (Fig. 1).
- Note the orientation of the calcaneus to rule out convex pes planus (vertical talus).
  - In vertical talus, the hindfoot is in equinus.
  - In calcaneovalgus foot, the hindfoot is dorsiflexed (heel is pointing down)

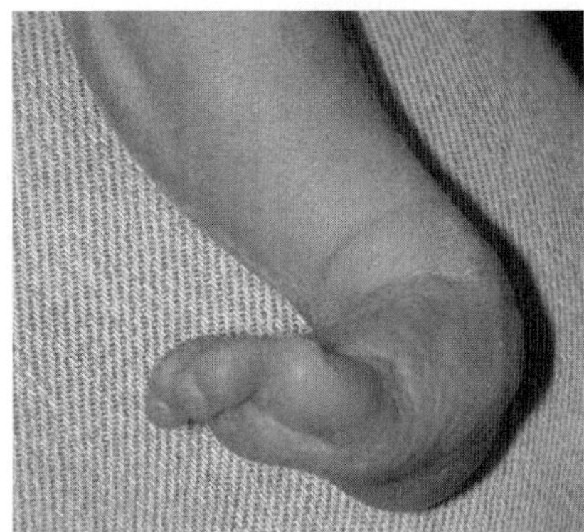

**Fig. 1.** Calcaneovalgus foot in a newborn.

### TESTS

#### *Imaging*

If the physical examination alone is not diagnostic, obtain routine AP and lateral foot and ankle radiographs to rule out bony abnormalities.

### DIFFERENTIAL DIAGNOSIS

- Convex pes valgus (congenital vertical talus) (1):
  - To differentiate the 2 conditions, note the position of the calcaneus.
    - In congenital vertical talus, the calcaneus is fixed in plantarflexion with contracture of the Achilles tendon and dislocation of the navicular on the dorsal neck of the talus (i.e., the heel points upward).
    - In calcaneovalgus foot, the calcaneus is dorsiflexed (i.e., the heel points downward) and is somewhat in valgus.
- Posteromedial bow of the tibia:
  - In this condition, the foot is in the same position as the calcaneovalgus foot (dorsiflexed and everted), but the cause is a bow in the tibia rather than in the joint.
  - The bony abnormality can be palpated.
- L5 paresis, as seen in spina bifida, can produce a fixed dorsiflexed foot because of muscle imbalance.

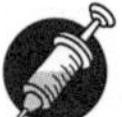

## TREATMENT

### GENERAL MEASURES

- Reassure the patient's parents that the condition self-corrects with time.
  - Treatment often requires repeated counseling to convince the parents that this is not a fixed deformity.
- To maintain the child's foot in a corrected position, the parents may perform gentle stretching maneuvers several times per day.
  - Parents who wish to be actively involved may be taught to plantarflex and supinate the patient's feet passively; however, the deformity corrects on its own.
- Occasionally, serial casting can be used to speed correction.

#### *Activity*

No activity restrictions are indicated because the malposition usually resolves quickly.

### SURGERY

Surgery is never needed for this condition.

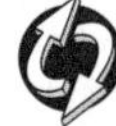

## FOLLOW-UP

### DISPOSITION

#### *Issues for Referral*

Newborns with substantial deformity or possible congenital convex pes valgus should be referred to an orthopaedist for monitoring.

### PROGNOSIS

- This benign condition corrects over time.
- Prognosis is excellent for development of normal shape, strength, and function.
- No definite evidence suggests that the foot is prone to be flat in later life.

### COMPLICATIONS

- On rare occasions, subluxation of the peroneal tendons may occur with this condition.
- This subluxation resolves with serial cast treatment.

### REFERENCE

1. Kasser JR. The foot. In: Morrissy RT, Weinstein SL, eds. *Lovell and Winter's Pediatric Orthopaedics,* 6th ed. Philadelphia: Lippincott Williams & Wilkins, 2006:1257–1328.

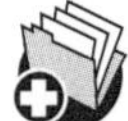

## MISCELLANEOUS

### CODES

#### *ICD9-CM*

754.69 Calcaneovalgus foot

### PATIENT TEACHING

Inform the family about the benign natural history of the condition and the tendency for the foot to correct on its own.

### FAQ

- Q: Will the foot be flat as the baby grows older?
  - A: No evidence suggests that this outcome is more likely than in any other infant.
- Q: Should the baby wear casts or special shoes?
  - A: Such measures are not necessary because the condition should improve on its own.

# CALCANEUS FRACTURE

*Theodore T. Manson, MD*
*Clifford L. Jeng, MD*

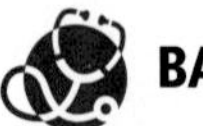

## BASICS

### DESCRIPTION

- Calcaneus fractures affect the calcaneus (heel bone) and the subtalar joint (between the talus and calcaneus).
  - Often high-energy injuries with substantial bony comminution and soft-tissue swelling
  - As such, often very difficult to treat
- Calcaneus fractures may be intra-articular, involving the subtalar joint, or extra-articular.
  - Extra-articular fractures have better outcomes and can be treated nonoperatively.
  - Intra-articular fractures have a worse prognosis and can be associated with severe heel widening, shoe wear problems, gait abnormalities, foot stiffness, and chronic pain.

### EPIDEMIOLOGY

#### *Incidence*

Uncommon, but the calcaneus is the most commonly fractured tarsal bone.

### RISK FACTORS

- Osteoporosis
- Jumping activities
- Work at heights

### PATHOPHYSIOLOGY

- Fracture patterns depend on the following:
  - Force of impact
  - Orientation of the heel
  - Geometry of the calcaneus

### ETIOLOGY

Fall from a height

### ASSOCIATED CONDITIONS

- Spinal fractures
- Ankle fractures
- Foot compartment syndrome

## DIAGNOSIS

### SIGNS AND SYMPTOMS

- Extreme hindfoot pain and tenderness
- Gross heel widening
- Soft-tissue ecchymosis

#### *History*

Patients typically are involved in high-energy trauma, such as a fall from a height or a motor vehicle crash.

#### *Physical Exam*

- Check for the following:
  - Skin integrity
  - Heel ecchymosis
  - Extreme heel tenderness
  - Ankle tenderness
  - Heel widening
  - Soft-tissue swelling about the heel
  - Possible spinous process tenderness in the lower spine (if an associated lower spinal fracture is present)
- Perform a comprehensive neurologic examination, looking for signs and symptoms of compartment syndrome.

### TESTS

#### *Imaging*

- Radiography:
  - AP, lateral, and oblique views of the foot
  - AP, lateral, and mortise views of the ankle
  - A calcaneal axial view (Harris view)
- CT:
  - Useful in determining whether a calcaneal fracture is intra-articular and in classifying intra-articular injuries
  - It is very important that the CT scan be ordered as a "CT scan of the calcaneus."
  - The foot is placed in neutral and the beam is oriented at a 30° oblique angle from the coronal plane.
- The Sanders classification system is used for surgical planning and is based on the CT images of the posterior facet (1).
  - Type 1: Nondisplaced
  - Type 2: 2-part fractures of the posterior facet
  - Type 3: 3-part fractures with 2 fracture lines
  - Type 4: ≥4-part fractures with severe comminution

#### *Diagnostic Procedures/Surgery*

- Patients with extreme swelling or pain may have compartment syndrome.
- Pressure measurement may be necessary to differentiate severe pain from swelling and the injury from that of a compartment syndrome of the hindfoot.

### DIFFERENTIAL DIAGNOSIS

- Subtalar dislocation
- Talar fracture
- Ankle fracture
- Severe ankle sprain

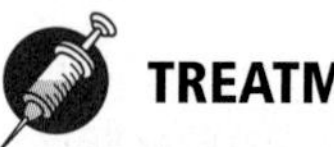

## TREATMENT

### GENERAL MEASURES

- Closed calcaneal fractures can be managed initially in a bulky soft dressing and plaster splint; this dressing *must be well padded* and is fabricated as follows:
  - Several layers of cast padding wrapped around the foot, ankle, and leg
  - Next, a layer of bulky cotton dressing (commonly called "rolled cotton," "Red Cross cotton," or "bulky Jones dressing")
  - Then, a posterior plaster slab and "stirrup" U-shaped plaster slab are placed around the foot and leg and wrapped with an Ace wrap.
- Strict elevation for several days after the fracture reduces swelling.
- Admission to the hospital for pain control and monitoring for compartment syndrome may be indicated for more severe fractures.
- A foot pump may be placed within the dressing to reduce soft-tissue swelling.
- Nondisplaced fractures can be treated with splinting initially, followed by cast immobilization and nonweightbearing.
- Open calcaneal fractures are operative emergencies.
- Compartment syndrome occurs in 10% of calcaneal fractures (2).
  - Monitor patients for severe pain or neurologic deficits, and have a low threshold for foot compartment pressure measurement.
  - Patients with compartment syndrome may require emergent fasciotomy.

### Activity
Activity is nonweightbearing until the fracture has healed (a minimum of 6 weeks).

## SPECIAL THERAPY
### Physical Therapy
- Gait training is indicated for nonweightbearing on the affected side until it is healed.
- After immobilization, therapy should address ankle and foot motion.

## MEDICATION (DRUGS)
### First Line
Narcotic analgesics frequently are required for pain management.

## SURGERY
- The decision to operate is individualized based on the severity of the fracture and the patient profile.
  - Smokers, patients >50 years old, laborers, and those involved in workers compensation claims tend to have poorer outcomes after surgery (3).
  - Diabetic and vasculopathic patients also are poorly served by surgery and may have better results from nonoperative treatment.
  - Conversely, younger patients with good soft-tissue viability and displaced intra-articular fractures usually have better outcomes with surgical treatment.
- Reconstruction of the calcaneus:
  - Performed through a lateral "L" incision
  - The lateral border of the calcaneus is exposed subperiosteally, and a pin is placed in the posterior fragment to improve exposure of the fracture and to facilitate reduction.
  - A plate is placed laterally after the fracture has been reduced, and fixation is provided by placing screws into a stable fragment, commonly the sustentaculum tali.
  - Residual bony defects may require bone grafting.
  - The incision is closed primarily, and the foot is placed into bulky cotton dressing with a posterior splint postoperatively (4,5).
- Open fractures of the calcaneus should be treated with operative débridement.
  - The condition of the soft tissue guides subsequent treatment.
  - Early soft-tissue coverage is important, and a plastic surgeon should be consulted.
  - The soft-tissue coverage drives the ultimate outcome (6).
  - If coverage can be achieved, reduction and fixation may be accomplished.

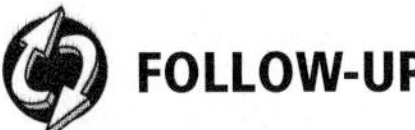

# FOLLOW-UP

## DISPOSITION
### Issues for Referral
- All patients with a calcaneus fractures should be referred to an orthopaedic surgeon.
- All patients who have signs or symptoms of compartment syndrome should be seen in the emergency room by an orthopaedic surgeon.

## PROGNOSIS
- Nondisplaced, extra-articular fractures have an excellent prognosis.
- Patients with displaced intra-articular fractures may develop posttraumatic arthritis.
- Intra-articular fractures are life-changing events, with long-term pain and loss of function (7).

## COMPLICATIONS
- Subtalar arthritis
- Heel widening, preventing normal shoe wear
- Gait difficulties
- Foot stiffness
- Peroneal tendinitis
- Sural nerve irritation
- Loss of soft-tissue viability
- Postoperative wound infection

## PATIENT MONITORING
Serial radiographs are obtained every 6 weeks to monitor healing.

## REFERENCES

1. Sanders R. Intra-articular fractures of the calcaneus: present state of the art. *J Orthop Trauma* 1992;6:252–265.
2. Fulkerson E, Razi A, Tejwani N. Review: acute compartment syndrome of the foot. *Foot Ankle Int* 2003;24:180–187.
3. Folk JW, Starr AJ, Early JS. Early wound complications of operative treatment of calcaneus fractures: analysis of 190 fractures. *J Orthop Trauma* 1999;13:369–372.
4. Bajammal S, Tornetta P, III, Sanders D, et al. Displaced intra-articular calcaneal fractures. *J Orthop Trauma* 2005;19:360–364.
5. Buckley RE, Tough S. Displaced intra-articular calcaneal fractures. *J Am Acad Orthop Surg* 2004;12:172–178.
6. Heier KA, Infante AF, Walling AK, et al. Open fractures of the calcaneus: soft-tissue injury determines outcome. *J Bone Joint Surg* 2003;85A:2276–2282.
7. Westphal T, Piatek S, Halm JP, et al. Outcome of surgically treated intraarticular calcaneus fractures–SF-36 compared with AOFAS and MFS. *Acta Orthop Scand* 2004;75:750–755.


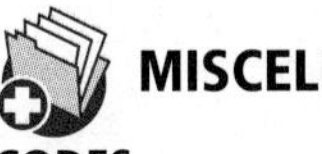

# MISCELLANEOUS

## CODES
### ICD9-CM
- 825.1 Open calcaneus fracture
- 825.2 Closed calcaneus fracture

## PATIENT TEACHING
Intra-articular fractures can lead to subtalar arthritis and the late onset of pain.

### Activity
- The activity level of patients with intra-articular calcaneus fractures usually does not return to normal.
- Patients often have stiffness of the ankle, preventing them from ladder use or heavy loading.
- Patients may require additional surgery to fuse the ankle and subtalar joints.

### Prevention
Prevention involves avoiding falls from height and high-energy trauma.

## FAQ
- Q: Will I return to my job?
  - A: Patients with high-energy calcaneus fractures and extensive intra-articular involvement rarely return to running, jumping, or climbing activities.
- Q: Should I have surgery for my calcaneus fracture?
  - A: Some patients, including those who have diabetes or who smoke, are at high risk for wound infections. Patients with heel widening or articular step-off may benefit from surgery.

# CAMPTODACTYLY

*Dawn M. LaPorte, MD*

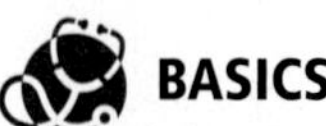

## BASICS

### DESCRIPTION
- A nontraumatic flexion deformity of the PIP joint that may progress gradually (1,2)
- Usually involves the little finger alone, but sometimes also affects adjoining fingers
- May or may not be associated with a syndrome
- 2 recognized types: Early (develops in the 1st year of life) and delayed (or late; onset after age 10)
  - The early form is the more common, and it affects the genders equally.
  - The delayed form affects mostly girls.
  - Although these forms also are called "congenital" and "adolescent," respectively, some clinicians believe the terms early and delayed (or late) should be used, because these manifestations likely represent variations of the same condition.
- The best results occur when treatment is initiated in childhood or adolescence.
- The results of treatment initiated in adulthood are poor.

### EPIDEMIOLOGY
#### *Incidence*
<1% of the population is affected (3).

### RISK FACTORS
Family history

#### *Genetics*
Many cases are sporadic; others have simple autosomal dominance.

### PATHOPHYSIOLOGY
- All structures that could possibly cause flexion deformity at the PIP joint have been considered possible deforming factors.
- Findings may include:
  - Absence, atrophy, or abnormal insertion of the lumbricalis muscle into the lumbrical canal
  - A band of fibrous tissue arising from the A1 pulley and inserting into the flexor superficialis tendon
  - Origination of the flexor superficialis from the palmar fascia in the mid aspect of the palm
  - Anomalous tendons
  - Short flexor digitorum profundus
  - Contracture of the collateral ligaments or the volar plate

### ETIOLOGY
- Camptodactyly is caused by an imbalance between the flexor and extensor mechanisms of the PIP joint.
- Anatomic anomalies occur frequently and include abnormal insertions of the lumbricalis, flexor digitorum superficialis, and retinacular ligaments.

### ASSOCIATED CONDITIONS
- Trisomy 13–15
- Oculodentodigital syndrome
- Orofaciodigital syndrome
- Aarskog syndrome
- Cerebrohepatorenal syndrome
- Mucopolysaccharidosis
- Osteo-onychodysostosis
- Jacob-Downey syndrome

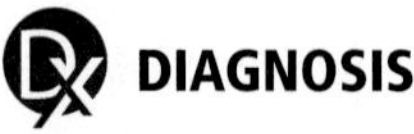

## DIAGNOSIS

### SIGNS AND SYMPTOMS
- A flexion deformity of the PIP joint of the little finger
- Digital angulation in the AP plane is not to be confused with clinodactyly, which describes angulation in the radioulnar plane.
- Occasionally, flexion deformity of the PIP joint of adjoining fingers also occurs.
- ~2/3 of patients show bilateral involvement, with the degree of contracture not necessarily symmetric.
- When only 1 hand is affected, it is usually the right one.
- In children, the deformity usually disappears when the wrist is flexed.
- The MCP joint usually is held in slight hyperextension.
- In severe contractures, with rotatory deformity in the digit, the patient may complain that the finger interferes with tapping or gripping activities.
- Pain and swelling usually are absent, even with severe flexion contracture.

#### *Physical Exam*
- The range of active and passive flexion and extension of the PIP and MCP joints should be quantified, with the wrist in both flexion and extension.
- A flexible deformity should be differentiated from a fixed flexion contracture (Fig. 1).

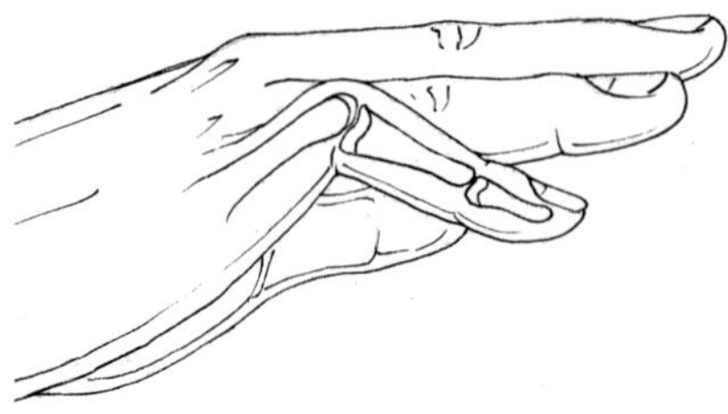

**Fig. 1.** The flexion deformity seen in camptodactyly.

### TESTS
#### *Imaging*
- Plain films of the digit should be obtained.
- Radiographic changes that occur with time and growth include broadening of the base of the middle phalanx, indentation of the neck of the proximal phalanx, a narrowed joint space, and dorsal flattening of the condyle of the proximal phalanx with flattening of the palmar surface.
- These findings bode poorly for chances of correcting the clinodactyly.

### DIFFERENTIAL DIAGNOSIS
- Differentiation is based on a thorough history and physical examination.
  - Clinodactyly, which describes digital angulation in the radioulnar plane
  - Trauma residual
  - Dupuytren contracture
  - Arthrogryposis
  - Absence or hypoplasia of an extensor tendon
  - Marfan syndrome
  - Beal syndrome (contractural arachnodactyly)
  - Pterygium syndrome
  - Symphalangism
  - Boutonniere deformity

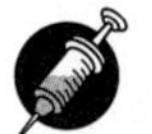

## TREATMENT

### GENERAL MEASURES
- No single successful treatment exists because no single cause of the condition exists.
- Treatment is designed to restore normal flexor–extensor balance.
  - In the early form, normal balance may be achieved best by progressive extension splinting.
  - In the delayed form, surgery often is indicated if splinting fails and the deformity is severe or progressive.
- Best results are obtained with surgical treatment in young patients, but the outcome is not completely predictable.
- Because the results of treatment in adults are poor, corrective operations in adults are no longer recommended.
- For most activities, dysfunction remains so slight that many surgeons discourage surgery because the results of operative treatment are unpredictable.

- A contracture of <30–40° does not interfere with function.
  - The patient and family should be advised to accept the deformity and avoid surgical intervention (4,5).
  - Splinting or serial plaster casting should be tried before surgery.
- Patients with marked contracture may need corrective treatment; the decision should be left up to the patient.
- Medical treatment:
  - Splinting
  - Serial casting

### SPECIAL THERAPY

#### *Physical Therapy*

- Occupational therapy may help those with early (congenital) or late (adolescent) camptodactyly.
- The occupational therapist may supervise stretching and splinting. Static splinting at night is recommended to prevent progression.

### SURGERY

- Surgery is designed to correct the aberrant anatomy through release or transfer of abnormal origins or insertions.
- Unfortunately, the results of these procedures are often disappointing.
- Tendon transfer may be considered for adolescent camptodactyly.
- If radiographs reveal bone and joint changes, corrective extension osteotomy is indicated, rather than procedures designed to increase motion through the joint itself.

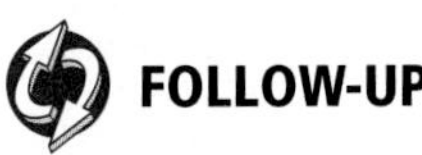

## FOLLOW-UP

### PROGNOSIS

- Left untreated, the condition will worsen progressively in 80% of cases.
- The deformity often worsens during growth spurts.
- The condition usually does not progress after the age of 18–20 years.

### COMPLICATIONS

Surgery in adults may produce increased joint stiffness and pain.

### PATIENT MONITORING

- The deformity may progress with growth spurts.
- Successful treatment is greatest at younger ages; therefore, it is best to treat early and to monitor the patient's progress.

### REFERENCES


1. Flatt AE. Crooked fingers. In: *The Care of Congenital Hand Anomalies*. St. Louis: Quality Medical Publishing, Inc., 1994:196–227.
2. Senrui H. Congenital contractures. In: Buck-Gramcko D, ed. *Congenital Malformations of the Hand and Forearm*. London: Churchill Livingstone, 1998:295–309.
3. Kozin SH, Kay SP. Congenital contracture. Camptodactyly. In: Green DP, Hotchkiss RN, Pederson WC, et al., eds. *Green's Operative Hand Surgery*, 5th ed. Philadelphia: Elsevier Churchill Livingstone, 2005:1512–1521.
4. McCarroll HR. Congenital anomalies: a 25-year overview. *J Hand Surg* 2000;25A:1007–1037.
5. Siegert JJ, Cooney WP, Dobyns JH. Management of simple camptodactyly. *J Hand Surg* 1990;15B:181–189.


### ADDITIONAL READING


- Milford L: Congenital anomalies. In: Crenshaw AH, ed. *Campell's Operative Orthopaedics*, 7th ed. St. Louis: CV Mosby, 1987:419–450.
- Waters PM: Wrist and hand: pediatric aspects. In: Kasser JR, ed. *Orthopaedic Knowledge Update 5: Home Study Syllabus*. Rosemont, IL: American Academy of Orthopaedic Surgeons, 1996:293–309.


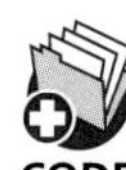

## MISCELLANEOUS

### CODES

#### *ICD9-CM*

755.59 Camptodactyly

### PATIENT TEACHING

- Skin monitoring around splints is important.
- Stretching should be continued after the splinting or casting program to maintain the gain achieved.

#### *Activity*

- Generally, no limitations are placed on activity.
- In severe cases, the deformity may pose a problem in sports or occupations requiring fine work with the hands.

#### *Prevention*

No effective means of prevention exists.

### FAQ

- Q: How often does camptodactyly affect both hands?
  - A: It is bilateral in ~2/3 of cases; the 5th finger is most commonly involved.
- Q: Is surgery recommended to correct the deformity?
  - A: Mild contracture (<30–40°) does not interfere with function and should be treated nonoperatively. Surgical results are not consistent, and surgery usually is reserved for more severe cases that hinder activity.

# CARPAL TUNNEL SYNDROME

Dawn M. LaPorte, MD
Tung B. Le, MD

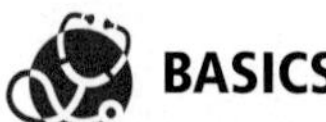

## BASICS

### DESCRIPTION

- CTS is a neuropathy caused by compression of the median nerve within the carpal tunnel.
- The floor of the tunnel is formed by the volar radiocarpal and intercarpal ligaments.
- The transverse carpal ligament forms the roof of the tunnel.
- 9 long flexors of the wrist and fingers and 1 nerve (median) run within this spatially limited and relatively rigid tunnel.
- Thus, any increase in pressure within the tunnel compresses the injury-prone median nerve.
- A decrease in thenar muscle strength occurs, along with a numbness or a decrease in the sensibility of the palmar surface of the radial 3 1/2 digits, especially the middle and index fingers.

#### *Pregnancy Considerations*

- Occurs more frequently in pregnant than in other individuals
- Usually resolves postpartum
- Avoid surgery during pregnancy.
  - Treat with nighttime cockup wrist splint(s) ± corticosteroid injection.

### EPIDEMIOLOGY

#### *Incidence*

- 50% of cases are reported to occur in patients 40–60 years old; average age at carpal tunnel release is 54 years (1).
- CTS occurs predominantly in females (70%), although the number of males with CTS may be underestimated (1).

#### *Prevalence*

- The prevalence of CTS has been reported to vary between 0.6% and 61% in different occupational groups (2).
- It is the most commonly diagnosed site of nerve compression in the upper extremity (2,3).

### RISK FACTORS

- Repetitive hand work
- Endocrine imbalance
- History of neuropathy
- Associated conditions
- Rheumatoid arthritis
- Pregnancy
- Thyroid myxedema
- Acromegaly
- Amyloidosis
- Multiple myeloma
- Diabetes
- Trauma
- Alcoholism
- Gout
- Space-occupying lesions within carpal tunnel

#### *Genetics*

No genetic predisposing factor to CTS has been described.

### PATHOPHYSIOLOGY

- Internal fibrosis of the median nerve
- Epineural scarring and constriction
- Reduced nerve conduction velocity

### ETIOLOGY

- Any factor that increases the pressure within the tunnel compresses the median nerve and leads to CTS.
- The most common causes include flexor tenosynovitis; trauma to the carpal bones; ganglion, fibroma, or lipoma within the tunnel; rheumatoid cyst; gout; and diabetic neuropathy (Fig. 1).

## DIAGNOSIS

- CTS can be diagnosed accurately by careful history and physical examination, inspection for thenar atrophy, and detection of sensory disturbance via light touch or a pinwheel.
- Provocative tests, such as the Phalen test (which consists of placing the affected wrist in hyperflexion in an attempt to reproduce the numbness in the hand) or tapping over the course of the nerve in the tunnel to elicit a Tinel sign, also serve to confirm the diagnosis.

### SIGNS AND SYMPTOMS

- These symptoms can be aggravated with use of the affected hand:
  - Paresthesia in the median nerve distribution in the hand
  - Weakness or clumsiness in the hand
  - Pain in the hand, wrist, or distal forearm
  - Awakening from sleep with pain or numbness in the hand
  - Tinel sign: Tapping the median nerve over the carpal tunnel with resultant paresthesias in the radial $3^1/_2$ fingers
  - Phalen sign: Paresthesias in the median nerve distribution with full flexion for at least 1 minute

#### *Physical Exam*

- The hand should be examined to detect thenar muscle atrophy.
- 2-point discrimination should be checked at the tips of the fingers on the radial and ulnar borders (should be <5–6 mm).
- Provocative tests such as the Phalen and Tinel tests should be performed (Figs. 2 and 3).

### TESTS

- The following basic tests should be ordered to rule out systemic causes of CTS:
  - Sedimentation rate
  - Serum glucose concentration
  - Serum uric acid level
  - Thyroid function test
  - Electromyography/nerve conduction velocity can confirm diagnosis and help determine severity.

#### *Imaging*

- Radiography
  - Plain radiographs of the wrist in patients with previous trauma or in patients with a long history of inflammatory disease should be performed.
  - Cervical spine radiographs also can reveal a cervical rib, if thoracic outlet syndrome is suspected.
- Electromyographic studies can help rule out proximal injury to the median nerve or identify peripheral neuropathy.

### DIFFERENTIAL DIAGNOSIS

- TOS
- Compression of the lower cervical roots by cervical degenerative disc disease or tumors

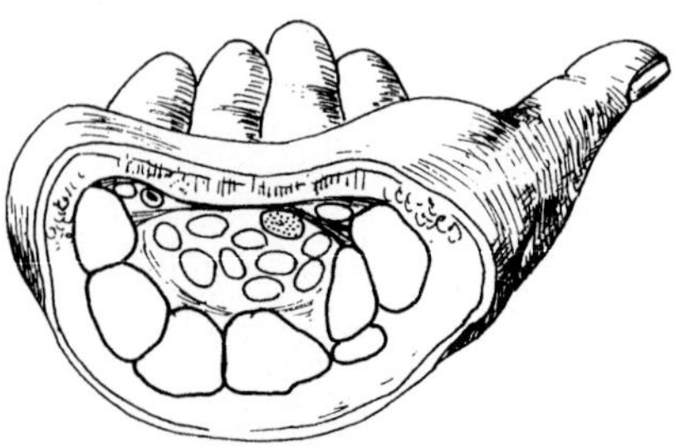

**Fig. 1.** The median nerve is shown in the carpal tunnel with the finger flexor tendons, under the transverse carpal ligament.

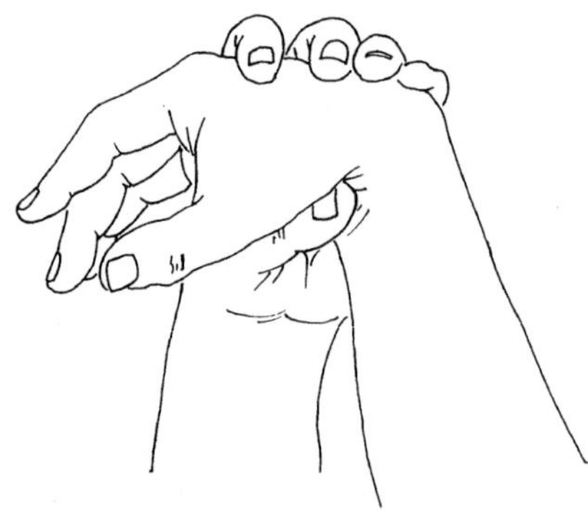

**Fig. 2.** The Phalen test for median nerve compression in the carpal tunnel is performed by holding the wrist flexed 90° for 30 seconds and checking for paresthesias in the fingers.

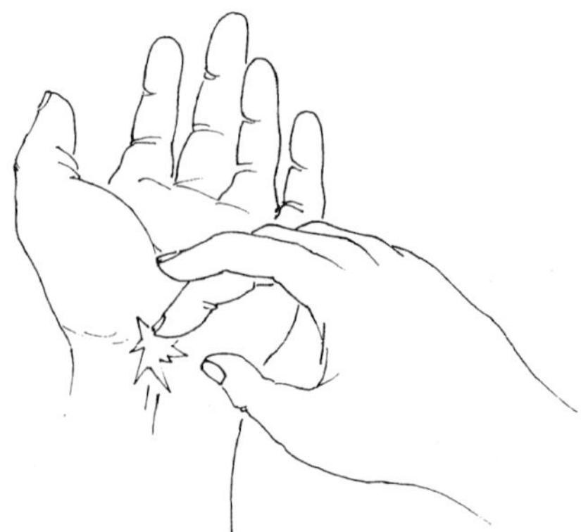

**Fig. 3.** A Tinel sign indicates an irritated median nerve. It refers to radiating pain down the fingers after percussion of the carpal tunnel.

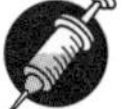

## TREATMENT

### GENERAL MEASURES

- Nonoperative intervention:
  - Modalities: Cockup wrist splinting, NSAIDs (not proven effective), diuretics, and cortisone injections (which must be performed by an experienced physician to avoid direct injury to the median nerve)
  - The patient should wear a wrist splint during sleep (4,5).
- Activity modification in work-related CTS is recommended.
- Surgical release of the transverse carpal ligament is performed when nonoperative measures have failed or in patients with constant numbness, motor weakness, or increased distal median nerve motor latency noted on electromyography.

### SPECIAL THERAPY

#### *Physical Therapy*

- Occupational or physical therapy should be consulted for activity modification teaching or for nerve gliding exercises that might decrease symptoms of nerve compression (6,7).
- Postoperative therapy is aimed at minimizing the development of painful scars and increasing ROM and strength.

### MEDICATION (DRUGS)

- No effective medication specifically to treat CTS has been described.
- Corticosteroid injection into the carpal tunnel is indicated when the median nerve compression is predicted to be temporary, as in pregnancy or when the patient's activity can be modified.
  - Injections must be done with great care to avoid injury to the median nerve.

### SURGERY

- Open carpal tunnel release is made through a longitudinal incision that begins on the distal border of the transverse carpal tunnel ligament and extends proximally to the proximal wrist crease, in line with the ulnar border of the axis of the ring finger.
- The incision then is carried through the palmar fascia to the transverse carpal ligament.
- The ligament then is divided carefully via a combination of scalpel and scissors.
- Care should be taken to avoid the palmar cutaneous branch or the motor branch of the median nerve.
- After division of the ligament, the carpal tunnel and the median nerve should be inspected for any space-occupying lesion or any signs of chronic inflammation requiring neurolysis.
- The skin then is reapproximated with nylon sutures.
- Compared with open carpal tunnel release, endoscopic carpal tunnel release has equivalent results at 1 year after surgery but return to work may be faster.

## FOLLOW-UP

### PROGNOSIS

- Most patients with CTS associated with the repetitive trauma commonly seen in the workplace respond to a combination of splinting, cortisone injection into the carpal tunnel, and activity modification.
- If job modification is not in the patient's nonoperative treatment program, splinting and cortisone injections may provide only temporary relief.
- The maximum return of strength after carpal tunnel release can take 6 months or longer.

### COMPLICATIONS

- Iatrogenic injuries to the median nerve or its branches may occur with open or endoscopic release.
- Painful surgical scars may ruin the results of a successful decompression procedure.
- Flexion tendon bowstringing may occur in a few patients.

### PATIENT MONITORING

- To obtain maximal beneficial results, the splint should be worn full-time for at least 3–4 months, after which time use of the splint can be discontinued gradually.
- If symptoms return with removal of the splint, the patient becomes a surgical candidate.
  - The patient usually experiences immediate pain relief after carpal tunnel release, whereas numbness gradually improves over the next several months.

### REFERENCES


1. Trumble TE. Compressive neuropathies. In: Trumble TE, ed. *Principles of Hand Surgery and Therapy.* Philadelphia: WB Saunders, 2000:324–341.
2. Lo SL, Raskin K, Lester H, et al. Carpal tunnel syndrome: a historical perspective. *Hand Clin* 2002;18:211–217.
3. Amadio PC. The first carpal tunnel release? *J Hand Surg.* 1995;20B:40–41.
4. Celiker R, Arslan S, Inanici F. Corticosteroid injection vs. NSAID and splinting in carpal tunnel syndrome. *Am J Phys Med Rehabil* 2002;81:182–186.
5. Chow JCY. Endoscopic carpal tunnel release. Two-portal technique. *Hand Clin* 1994;10: 637–646.
6. Rozmaryn LM, Dovelle S, Rothman ER, et al. Nerve and tendon gliding exercises and the conservative management of carpal tunnel syndrome. *J Hand Ther* 1998;11:171–179.
7. Seradge H, Parker W, Baer C, et al. Conservative treatment of carpal tunnel syndrome: an outcome study of adjunct exercises. *J Okla State Med Assoc* 2002;95:7–14.


### ADDITIONAL READING


- Hanel DP. Wrist and hand: reconstruction. In: Kasser JR, ed. *Orthopaedic Knowledge Update 5. Home Study Syllabus*. Rosemont, IL: American Academy of Orthopaedic Surgeons, 1996:329–347.
- Lister G. Compression. In: *The Hand, Diagnosis and Indications,* 3rd ed. New York: Churchill Livingstone, 1993:283–322.
- Mackinnon SE, Novak CB. Compression neuropathies. In: Green DP, Hotchkiss RN, Pederson WC, et al., eds. *Green's Operative Hand Surgery,* 5th ed. Philadelphia: Elsevier Churchill Livingstone, 2005;999–1045.

## MISCELLANEOUS

### CODES

#### *ICD9-CM*

354.0 CTS

### PATIENT TEACHING

Activity modification teaching is important to prevent recurrence.

#### *Prevention*

The patient should avoid prolonged and repetitive motions of the wrist.

### FAQ

- Q: If CTS presents during pregnancy, should surgery be considered?
  - A: CTS symptoms presenting during pregnancy often resolve after delivery and therefore treatment should be with nighttime splinting ± corticosteroid injection if indicated. Ideally, surgery should be avoided until postpartum to allow for evaluation of resolution of symptoms after delivery.
- Q: Does CTS recur after surgical release?
  - A: CTS should not recur after surgical release. Persistent or recurrent symptoms after surgery are most likely secondary to incomplete release, but they also can be secondary to incorrect diagnosis or untreated "double crush" syndrome with a more proximal etiology or coexisting peripheral neuropathy.
- Q: What are the symptoms of CTS?
  - A: Patients present with complaints of pain, numbness and tingling, and perhaps difficulty with fine motor tasks. The numbness is typically in the thumb, index finger, middle finger, and radial 1/2 of the ring finger. Weakness, when it is present, is in the abductor pollicis brevis.

# CASTS AND SPLINTS

*Gregory Gebauer, MD, MS*
*Simon C. Mears, MD, PhD*

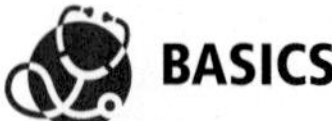

## BASICS

### DESCRIPTION

- Casts and splints are used to immobilize injured bones and joints.
- Because casts are circumferential and do not accommodate postinjury swelling, acute injuries usually should be treated with splints, which have a lower risk of iatrogenic compartment syndrome.
- In the field after an injury, almost anything can be used as splint material, including sticks, slats of wood, a pillow, or cardboard.
- It is important to pad the splint in areas where it contacts the skin to prevent pressure injuries and protect the soft tissues.
- Splints are applied to immobilize not only the fractured bone, but the joint above and below the fracture.
- In a hospital setting, splints and casts are made of 2 substances, plaster and fiberglass.
  - Plaster of Paris:
    - Made of muslin stiffened by dextrose or starch and impregnated with the hemihydrate of calcium sulfate
    - When water is added, the calcium sulfate crystallizes in an exothermic reaction.
    - Plaster solidifies in ~15 minutes.
  - Fiberglass:
    - More modern material made of a fiberglass substrate impregnated with a polyurethane resin that is activated by moisture to polymerize
    - Hardens in ~7 minutes and weighs less than plaster
    - Disadvantages:
      - Sticky and hard-to-remove from exposed skin; latex gloves should be used to protect the hands (1).
      - The fast hardening time can make molding more difficult than with plaster.

### PATHOPHYSIOLOGY

- Injured bones and muscles release inflammatory substances such as interleukin-6.
- Motion of broken bones at a fracture site creates more inflammation and potential muscle injury.
- Immobilization of the limb and fracture limits this motion and leads to pain relief and gradual decrease of inflammation (2).

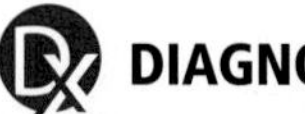

## DIAGNOSIS

### SIGNS AND SYMPTOMS

#### *History*

Patients with fractures after trauma

#### *Physical Exam*

- Examine patients for wounds and open fractures that require urgent surgical débridement.
- Examine joints for signs of dislocation.
- Evaluate neurovascular status thoroughly for nerve or vessel injury.
- Examine patients for swelling and signs of compartment syndrome.

### TESTS

#### *Imaging*

Patients with painful bones or joints should be evaluated with radiographs for fracture or dislocation.

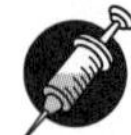

## TREATMENT

### GENERAL MEASURES

- Immobilization in the acute period after an injury is best provided by a splint.
- After swelling of the initial injury has been reduced, a cast may be applied to hold the fracture until healing.
  - Generally, injuries are casted 1 or 2 weeks after the injury.
  - If casts are applied immediately after injury, they should be cut or bivalved and loosely wrapped.
- Before splint or cast application, the extremity must be padded well with cast padding or felt, especially over bony prominences.
- Rings or bracelets must be removed from the affected extremity.
- Limbs should be splinted in the position of function of the joint.
- The joints above and below the fracture should be immobilized.
- Hot water should not be used because it may lead to thermal burns under the splint.
- Indentations from fingers may cause pressure points and should be avoided.
- 3-point fixation and molding should be used to stabilize the fracture.
- Open fractures, which require emergency surgery, should be splinted before surgery.
- Specific consideration should be given by anatomic area.
  - Proximal humerus and humeral shaft fractures:
    - Place plaster over the shoulder and on either side of the arm.
    - Place a sling.
    - Place a removable pad in the armpit so it can be changed and the armpit cleaned.
    - When fractures have begun to heal, a fracture brace may be applied to the humerus.
  - Elbow:
    - Splint the elbow at 90°, with plenty of padding and with a back slab.
    - A side slab can be used for reinforcement.
    - The wrist should be supported by the splint, but the hand should be free.
    - An above-the-elbow cast can be placed after swelling has reduced.
  - Forearm and wrist:
    - A sugar-tong splint extends around the elbow, with the elbow bent at 90°.
    - On either side of the hand, it is important to leave the MCP joints free.
    - Below-the-elbow casts should leave the hand and thumb free to move.
  - Hand and fingers:
    - The "boxer splint" or ulnar gutter splint can be used for 4th and 5th metacarpal fractures (3).
    - Place 4-inch plaster from the tip of the 5th finger to 2 inches from the antecubital fossa, with a gauze pad between the 4th and 5th fingers.
    - The splint is applied to the ulnar side of the hand to create a "gutter."
    - The wrist is positioned at 25–30° of extension and the MCP joint at 90° of flexion.
    - To splint finger fractures, use structural aluminum malleable splints (made of a strip of soft aluminum, coated with polyethylene foam), which can be cut into strips with scissors.

- Femur and hip:
  - Thomas splints are a premade splinting device used to apply traction to a leg.
  - The splint has a ring that measures 2 inches more than the circumference of the proximal thigh and engages the ischial tuberosity for countertraction.
  - A strap is placed anteriorly and attached to the end of the splint with an ankle hitch.
  - This splint can be used temporarily to apply traction to the leg but should not be left in place for >2 hours because the ankle hitch places substantial pressure on the skin and may cause skin necrosis.
- Knee and tibia:
  - Above-the-knee splints extending to the end of the foot should be used; the ankle should be splinted at 90°.
  - Care must be taken to pad the peroneal region around the knee and the ankle.
  - For stable fractures, above-the-knee casts may be used after swelling has subsided.
- Ankle and foot:
  - Below-the-knee splints are applied with a U around the ankle and a back slab.
  - The ankle should be kept at 90° to avoid Achilles contracture.
  - Below-the-knee casts must be padded carefully.
  - Ankle injuries that require less support may be treated with an ankle air splint.

#### *Activity*

Patients should be encouraged to move the joints above and below the splint to prevent joint stiffness; joints that stiffen quickly include the shoulder, elbow, and hand.

#### *Nursing*

- Patients should be evaluated (including a neurovascular check) to make sure that the splint is not too tight.

### MEDICATION (DRUGS)

#### *First Line*

Patients with fractures generally require narcotic pain medicines.

### SURGERY

Fractures that are open, intra-articular, or displaced may require surgical fixation.

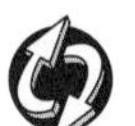

## FOLLOW-UP

### DISPOSITION

#### *Issues for Referral*

- Patients with splinted fractures should be referred to an orthopaedist for management.
- In general, patients should be seen within a week to assess the reduction of the fracture and the need for operative intervention.

### COMPLICATIONS

- Casts or splints may be too tight.
  - Patients complaining of continued pain and tightness should be examined, and the splint or cast should be loosened.
  - If loosening is not effective in reducing pain, the limb should be checked carefully for compartment syndrome.
    - Cut the splint material and assess the limb.
    - Check pressure measurements to evaluate the intracompartmental pressure.
    - If compartment syndrome is diagnosed, urgent fasciotomy is required to preserve limb function (4).
- To prevent skin breakdown, careful attention should be paid to providing adequate padding to boney prominences.

### PATIENT MONITORING

- Patients require monitoring for soft-tissue swelling and compartment syndrome.
- Fracture reduction should be monitored with serial radiographs until healing.

### REFERENCES

1. Bowker P, Powell ES. A clinical evaluation of plaster-of-Paris and eight synthetic fracture splinting materials. *Injury* 1992;23:13–20.
2. Hildebrand F, Giannoudis P, Kretteck C, et al. Damage control: extremities. *Injury* 2004;35:678–689.
3. Zenios M, Kim WY, Sampath J, et al. Functional treatment of acute metatarsal fractures: a prospective randomised comparison of management in a cast versus elasticated support bandage. *Injury* 2005;36:832–835.
4. Walker RW, Draper E, Cable J. Evaluation of pressure beneath a split above elbow plaster cast. *Ann R Coll Surg Engl* 2000;82:307–310.

### ADDITIONAL READING

- Harkess JW, Ramsey WC, Harkess JW. Principles of fractures and dislocations. In: Rockwood CA, Jr, Bucholz RW, Green DP, et al., eds. *Rockwood and Green's Fractures in Adults*, 4th ed. Philadelphia: Lippincott-Raven, 1996:3–120.
- Smith GD, Hart RG, Tsai TM. Fiberglass cast application. *Am J Emerg Med* 2005;23:347–350.

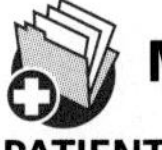

## MISCELLANEOUS

### PATIENT TEACHING

- After application of any splint or cast, the patient should be instructed to:
  - Be aware of the signs and symptoms of compression from swelling within the splint (numbness, tingling, pain).
  - Keep the splint dry.
  - Call the clinician in case of splint problems or symptoms of compression.
  - Make appointment for a follow-up examination.

#### *Activity*

- Comply with weightbearing restrictions.
- Exercise joints not incorporated in the splint.
- Elevate the injured limb above the level of the heart for 2–3 days.

### FAQ

- Q: Can I take the splint off?
  - A: No, the splint must remain in place unless removal is needed for more detailed examination of the extremity or if it is to replaced by another splint or cast. Splints should not be removed for radiographs unless any metal will obscure images, in which case a nonradiodense splint should be applied.
- Q: Why is a cast not applied immediately after the injury?
  - A: Casts are circumferential and do not allow for swelling. Splints apply pressure only on 1 or 2 sides of the extremity, which should allow for swelling. However, if the splint feels too tight, it should be loosened.

# CAVUS FOOT

*Clifford L. Jeng, MD*

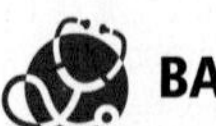

## BASICS

### DESCRIPTION

Cavus foot is defined by an elevation of the medial longitudinal arch, often with an associated deformity of the hindfoot or forefoot (Fig. 1).

### EPIDEMIOLOGY

#### *Incidence*

Cavus feet are common and may be associated with several underlying conditions that affect the muscle balance of the foot.

### RISK FACTORS

- Neuromuscular disorders
- Trauma
- Connective-tissue disorders
- Congenital deformities

#### *Genetics*

- Several of the diseases responsible for the development of cavus feet are hereditary.
- The most common hereditary cause is Charcot-Marie-Tooth disease, which is autosomal dominant.

### PATHOPHYSIOLOGY

Neuromuscular disorders are the etiologic factor for most cavus foot deformities, causing muscle imbalance that leads to atrophy or fibrosis, deformity, and joint contractures.

### ETIOLOGY

- Causes include:
  - Muscle imbalance, such as peroneus longus or posterior tibialis overpull
  - Weakness of the intrinsic muscles of the foot with overpull of the long flexor tendons
  - Connective-tissue disorders, such as Marfan syndrome

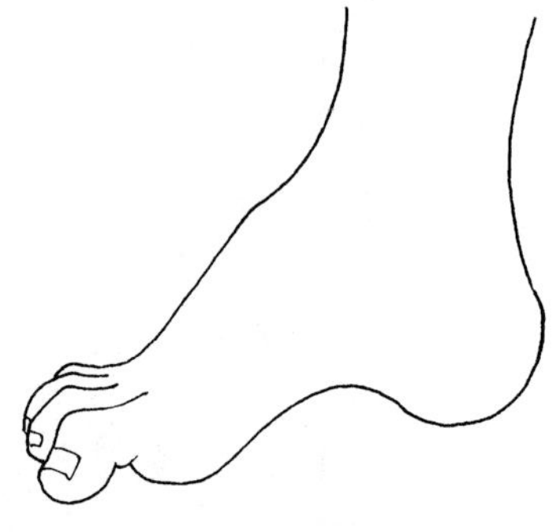

**Fig. 1.** A relatively high arch, which may be flexible or rigid, characterizes a cavus foot.

### ASSOCIATED CONDITIONS

- Charcot-Marie-Tooth disease
- Friedreich ataxia
- Spina bifida, syringomyelia
- Diabetic neuropathy
- Poliomyelitis
- Previous compartment syndrome of the leg or foot
- Partially treated clubfoot
- Idiopathic clubfoot
- Marfan syndrome
- Beal syndrome

## DIAGNOSIS

### SIGNS AND SYMPTOMS

- High arch
- Calluses on forefoot or hindfoot
- Difficulty with shoe wear
- Patient:
  - May have heel varus or plantarflexion of the 1st metatarsal
  - May be asymptomatic
  - May complain of metatarsalgia (pain under metatarsal head region)
  - May develop recurrent ankle instability and/or sprains secondary to severe varus heel malalignment

#### *Physical Exam*

- Measure the motor strength of all muscles crossing the ankle on both legs.
- Look for associated claw-toe deformities.
- Assess for plantar fascia contracture.
- Check reflexes and sensation to light touch.
- Examine the upper extremities, especially for intrinsic wasting.
- Observe the spine for dimples, markings, and scoliosis.

### TESTS

- Coleman block testing determines whether the hindfoot varus is flexible or rigid (1).
  - The patient stands on a block with the first metatarsal and hallux suspended freely in the air.
  - This position eliminates contribution from a relatively plantarflexed 1st metatarsal, which in turn causes varus alignment of hindfoot.
  - In a flexible cavus deformity, Coleman block testing removes forefoot contribution and allows the hindfoot varus to correct.
  - In a rigid deformity, no hindfoot correction occurs.

#### *Lab*

Electromyography and nerve conduction studies are helpful in diagnosing Charcot-Marie-Tooth disease, hereditary motor sensory neuropathies, and lumbar radiculopathy.

#### *Imaging*

- Standing radiographs of the foot should be obtained to evaluate the calcaneal pitch angle (angle between the calcaneus and the floor) and the Meary angle (angle between the talus and the 1st metatarsal).
- As part of the workup for undiagnosed cavus foot deformity, plain radiographs and MRI of the spine may be indicated to identify occult abnormalities.

### DIFFERENTIAL DIAGNOSIS

Muscle atrophy may cause the arch to appear higher.

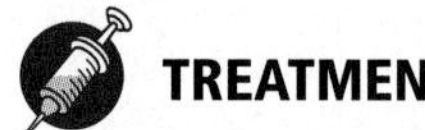

## TREATMENT

### GENERAL MEASURES

- No treatment is indicated if the patient is asymptomatic and the skin is in good condition.
- A padded insole with an arch support and/or metatarsal bar may relieve metatarsalgia.

- A lateral heel wedge may help correct a flexible hindfoot varus deformity.
- A brace may help stabilize a severely weakened cavus foot or concurrent chronic ankle instability.
- Stretching may help prevent worsening deformity and maintain flexibility.
- In general, cavovarus foot is tolerated poorly because of progressive deformity, shoe wear difficulties, ankle instability, and arthritis.

### SPECIAL THERAPY

#### *Physical Therapy*

- Stretching of a tight plantar fascia and of other tight muscles may help slow progression of the condition.
- Muscle strengthening, proprioceptive training, and closed-chain balance exercises may help if the cavovarus deformity has led to ankle instability.

### SURGERY

- Usually, surgery is indicated for progressive deformity, recalcitrant pain, chronic ankle instability, difficulty with shoe wear, or rigid deformity with resultant arthritis.
- Careful examination helps to identify the components of the deformity and the degree of flexibility or rigidity, leading to a customized stepwise surgical plan to address all aspects.
- Flexible deformities can be addressed with soft-tissue rebalancing procedures, whereas rigid deformities require bony osteotomies or arthrodesis (fusion) procedures for correction.
- Plantar fasciotomy may help lower the high arch.
- Midfoot and metatarsal osteotomies are needed for a rigid cavus foot (2).
- A lateral closing-wedge calcaneal osteotomy is performed if the heel varus is rigid (2).
- Tendon lengthening procedures or tendon transfers are necessary to treat muscle imbalance.
- Chronic ankle instability is addressed by ligament reconstruction and often concomitant tenodesis stabilization.
- Triple arthrodesis is reserved mainly as a salvage procedure if other surgical treatments fail or if the patient has painful arthritis.

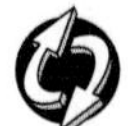

## FOLLOW-UP

- Patients with a cavus foot deformity must be followed regularly by an orthopaedic surgeon for progression of the deformity or muscle weakness.
- Progression may necessitate earlier reconstructive surgery to avoid fusion.

#### *Issues for Referral*

All patients with symptomatic cavus feet should be referred for orthopaedic consultation.

### PROGNOSIS

- Patients with cavus feet secondary to neuropathy usually experience progressive deformity over time.
- Patients with diabetes and Charcot-Marie-Tooth disease may lose protective sensation and develop neuropathic ulcerations that eventually lead to osteomyelitis and amputation.
- Therefore, great care and attention must be paid to appropriate orthoses and shoe wear to prevent abnormal skin pressure from occurring.

### REFERENCES

1. Coleman SS, Chesnut WJ. A simple test for hindfoot flexibility in the cavovarus foot. *Clin Orthop Relat Res* 1977;123:60–62.
2. Sammarco GJ, Taylor R. Cavovarus foot treated with combined calcaneus and metatarsal osteotomies. *Foot Ankle Int* 2001;22:19–30.

### ADDITIONAL READING

- Alexander IJ, Johnson KA. Assessment and management of pes cavus in Charcot-Marie-tooth disease. *Clin Orthop Relat Res* 1989;246:273–281.
- Dwyer FC. The present status of the problem of pes cavus. *Clin Orthop Relat Res* 1975;106:254–275.
- Kirchner JS. Charcot-Marie-Tooth disease and the cavovarus foot. In: Richardson EG, ed. *Orthopaedic Knowledge Update: Foot and Ankle 3*. Rosemont, IL: American Academy of Orthopaedic Surgeons, 2004:135–143.
- Wapner KL. Pes cavus. In: Myerson MS, ed. *Foot and Ankle Disorders*. Philadelphia: WB Saunders Co., 2000:919–941.

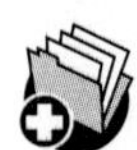

## MISCELLANEOUS

### CODES

#### *ICD9-CM*

- 754.59 Cavovarus foot
- 754.71 Cavus foot

### FAQ

- Q: What is the cause of most cavus feet?
  - A: Neurologic disorders cause many cavus foot deformities secondary to muscle imbalance between plantarflexor-invertors and dorsiflexor-evertors.
- Q: When is surgery indicated for cavus foot deformity?
  - A: Surgery is indicated in symptomatic cavus feet that show progressive deformity, ankle instability, claw toes, and metatarsalgia or failure of shoe wear modifications and orthotic use.

# CEREBRAL PALSY

*Paul D. Sponseller, MD*

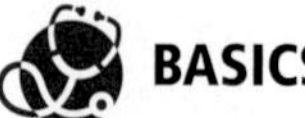

## BASICS

### DESCRIPTION

- Cerebral palsy is a general term covering a wide range of presentations.
  - The common theme is a static neuropathy developing in the first 3 years of life.
  - The cause may vary, and typically only the result is seen, through its effect on the trunk and extremities.
  - Although the neurologic lesion does not change, the functional level may change as the person grows older (1).
- Classification is by anatomic and physiologic types; a patient should be classified according to both parameters.
  - Anatomically: Hemiplegic (ipsilateral arm and leg), diplegic (both legs), and "totally involved"
  - Physiologically: Spastic, athetoid, mixed, and dystonic (1).

### EPIDEMIOLOGY

#### *Incidence*

This disorder affects 1–2% of all children (1).

### RISK FACTORS

- Difficult delivery
- Prematurity
- Postnatal central nervous system injury

### PATHOPHYSIOLOGY

- Peripheral nerves are normal.
- Brain involvement depends on the specific cause.
- Muscles of the affected limb show some degree of fibrosis.
- Typically, no biopsy is indicated.

### ETIOLOGY

- Prenatal brain dysplasia
- Maternal infection
- Fetal hypoxia
- Vascular event
- Encephalitis
- Meningitis
- Trauma
- Kernicterus

### ASSOCIATED CONDITIONS

Associated defects in some patients may include visual or hearing impairment, seizures, osteoporosis, and learning disability (2).

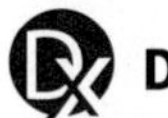

## DIAGNOSIS

### SIGNS AND SYMPTOMS

- Hypotonia followed by spasticity is the most common pattern.
- Milestones may be delayed, and gait is abnormal.
- Deep tendon reflexes are increased after the 1st year of life, and clonus may develop in certain muscles.
- Contractures develop, especially in the Achilles tendon, hamstrings, and adductors.
- Typical findings:
  - Diplegic type: Normal intelligence with equinus or equinovalgus feet
  - Hemiplegic type: Normal intelligence with equinovarus feet and upper extremity spasticity or flexion
  - Totally involved form: Scoliosis, hip dysplasia, and contractures, usually with some cognitive deficit.
  - Athetoid form:
    - Contracture does not develop, and irregular movements occur in the extremities.
    - Normal or mildly impaired intellect (1)

#### *Physical Exam*

- Examine:
  - Upper extremity for deformity, sensation, and use (3)
  - Spine for scoliosis or dysraphism
- Measure limb lengths and document:
  - Contractures at all joints
  - Muscle excursion at all levels, including ankle dorsiflexion, popliteal angle, and hip abduction
- Observe the gait several times, if possible, with and without braces.

### TESTS

#### *Imaging*

- MRI:
  - Indicated if a diagnostic dilemma presents
  - In a patient with spastic diplegia:
    - Typical finding is periventricular leukomalacia, the end result of ventricular hemorrhages.
    - However, the MRI scan may be normal in such patients.
  - In a patient with spastic hemiplegia, typical findings are focal infarct or cyst.
- Radiography:
  - The cervical spine may be imaged with radiographs in some patients with severe diplegia.
  - Routine films of the hip should be obtained for the child with severe diplegia or total involvement (4).
  - If a deformity is apparent, scoliosis films should be obtained for patients with the totally involved variant.

### DIFFERENTIAL DIAGNOSIS

- Brain or upper spinal cord tumor
- Instability of the upper cervical spine
- Neurodegenerative disorder
- Metabolic disorder
- Familial spastic paraparesis
- Early stage of myopathy or neuropathy
- Rett syndrome

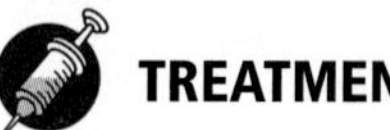

## TREATMENT

### GENERAL MEASURES

- Infant stimulation and encouragement of mobility are the most important measures.
- At-risk muscles (hamstrings, gastrocnemius-soleus) should be stretched if no improvement occurs.
- Intrathecal baclofen may help to decrease peripheral spasticity.
- Diazepam (Valium) has little benefit except in the year of any surgery.
- Physical therapy is best suited to address specific, short-term goals; to monitor changes over time; and to advise on adaptive equipment.

### SPECIAL THERAPY

#### *Physical Therapy*

Physical therapy is useful for gait training, for instruction in stretching to prevent contractures and the use of braces, and for aid in activities of daily living.

### SURGERY

- Foot deformities almost always should be corrected if the patient has limited ambulatory potential.
  - Lengthening contracted muscles decreases their spasticity or triggering during gait.
  - This principle applies especially to the Achilles tendon, hamstrings, and adductors, but the rectus femoris also may be tight.
- Hand muscle tightness or dysfunction rarely benefits from surgery because of the lack of sensory integration (3).

- Before degenerative changes occur, hip subluxation should be treated (4).
  - Adductor muscle lengthening, femoral osteotomy, and possibly an iliac osteotomy
  - Rarely, femoral head removal is indicated if the subluxation has been detected after severe pain develops.
- If the child has trunk imbalance with difficulty in sitting or back pain, scoliosis treatment is indicated.
  - A brace may help the patient to sit more comfortably, but it does not keep the curve from worsening.
  - Surgical correction and fusion are the best choices for those who are having trouble sitting in a stable, comfortable fashion.
- Other surgical treatments for patients with cerebral palsy include rhizotomy and an intrathecal baclofen pump.
  - Dorsal rhizotomy:
    - A procedure to decrease spasticity at the more central level of the spinal cord
    - The dorsal afferent rootlets are checked for the ability to generate a spastic reflex arc, and the most abnormal ones are sectioned.
    - This treatment works for patients $<10$ years old with ambulatory diplegia.
  - Intrathecal baclofen:
    - Interrupts spasticity at the spinal level by pharmacologic means
    - Used mostly for nonambulatory patients

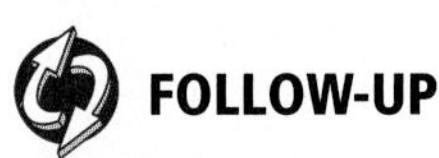

## FOLLOW-UP

### DISPOSITION

#### *Issues for Referral*

- It is best for children with cerebral palsy to be seen on a routine basis at least once a year during growth.
- This monitoring allows detection of deformities and hip dysplasia or scoliosis at a time when they can be treated most effectively.

### PROGNOSIS

- The prognosis depends on the extent of cerebral palsy.
  - Patients with totally involved cerebral palsy have a shortened life expectancy, but those with other types show no decrease in life expectancy (1,3).
  - Most children with cerebral palsy show some decline in walking ability near maturity because, for them, walking demands much energy.

### COMPLICATIONS

- Weight gain is a common problem in both childhood and adulthood and contributes to debility.
- Fractures are common in patients with the totally involved type of cerebral palsy.
- Patients with totally involved cerebral palsy are likely to have respiratory problems.

### PATIENT MONITORING

Children are seen at least once a year to check on ambulatory ability and status of activities of daily living.

### REFERENCES


1. Renshaw TS, Deluca PA. Cerebral palsy. In: Morrissy RT, Weinstein SL, eds. *Lovell and Winter's Pediatric Orthopaedics,* 6th ed. Philadelphia: Lippincott Williams & Wilkins, 2006:552–603.
2. Henderson RC, Lark RK, Kecskemethy HH, et al. Bisphosphonates to treat osteopenia in children with quadriplegic cerebral palsy: a randomized, placebo-controlled clinical trial. *J Pediatr* 2002;141:644–651.
3. Chin TYP, Duncan JA, Johnstone BR, et al. Management of the upper limb in cerebral palsy. *J Pediatr Orthop B* 2005;14:389–404.
4. Presedo A, Oh CW, Dabney KW, et al. Soft-tissue releases to treat spastic hip subluxation in children with cerebral palsy. *J Bone Joint Surg* 2005;87A:832–841.


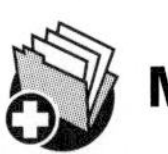

## MISCELLANEOUS

### CODES

#### *ICD9-CM*

343.9 Infantile cerebral palsy, unspecified

### PATIENT TEACHING

- Patients are encouraged to remain as active as possible and to keep their weight down.
- It is ideal if they can be referred to a sports program for special-needs children.
- Patients should understand that the condition cannot be totally cured, and they should beware of any claims that seem too optimistic.
- They should learn that oral medications offer no substantial help for the disease.

#### *Activity*

To be encouraged

#### *Prevention*

Regular follow-up can prevent advanced hip dislocation.

### FAQ

- Q: What is the cause of cerebral palsy?
  - A: A number of different causes exist, but all have in common a 1-time injury to the brain during early childhood.
- Q: How much physical therapy should a child with cerebral palsy have?
  - A: Physical therapy should be individualized. Its main role is to help children adapt to their own motor abilities. Rarely does a child need intensive therapy throughout childhood.

# CERVICAL DISC HERNIATION

*Karl A. Soderlund, BS*
*David B. Cohen, MD*
*A. Jay Khanna, MD*

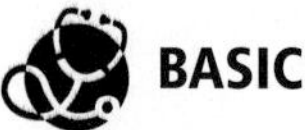

## BASICS

### DESCRIPTION

- Cervical disc herniation is a condition in which retropulsion of disc material occurs, with resulting compression of the neural elements (nerve root[s] and/or spinal cord), resulting in neck pain, radiculopathy, and/or myelopathy.
- Classification
  - Herniation is classified as acute or chronic.
  - The classification of myelopathy is based on physical function.

### GENERAL PREVENTION

- No good evidence exists regarding preventive measures, but smoking cessation may help decrease the chances of neck pain and radiculopathy.
- However, nonsmoking is a predictor of positive outcome after anterior cervical decompression and fusion (1).

### EPIDEMIOLOGY

- Most common in individuals >30 years old, with a mean age of 50 years (2)
- Radiculopathy rarely progresses to myelopathy.

#### *Incidence*

- 107.3 males and 64.5 females per 100,000 population (annual age-adjusted incidence) (3)
- 203 per 100,000 population is the age-specific annual incidence rate for 50–54-year-olds (3).

#### *Prevalence*

- Up to 2/3 of adults will have at least 1 major episode of neck pain in their lifetime (4).
- Radiographic evidence of disc degeneration is seen in nearly 60% of individuals >40 years old (5).

### RISK FACTORS

- Repetitive lifting
- Smoking
- Overhead work

#### *Genetics*

The risk of disc herniation is higher in a person with a positive family history than in a patient without such a history.

### PATHOPHYSIOLOGY

- The mechanical nature of neural element compression is well understood.
- Substance P concentration is elevated in compressed nerve roots.
- Decreased blood flow in a compressed nerve root also may play a role in pain.

### ETIOLOGY

Cervical disc herniations may be traumatic or nontraumatic.

### ASSOCIATED CONDITIONS

- Congenital cervical stenosis
- Ossified posterior longitudinal ligament
- Cervical spine spondylosis

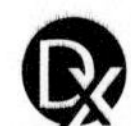

## DIAGNOSIS

### SIGNS AND SYMPTOMS

- Symptoms can develop acutely or insidiously.
- The spectrum of symptoms includes neck pain, occipital pain, shoulder girdle pain, and regional upper extremity symptoms (pain, paresthesias, hypesthesia, or weakness).
- Symptoms often are exacerbated by particular neck motions and positions.
- Nerve root compression at a specific level may cause "classic" findings of motor, sensory, or reflex symptoms.
- The Spurling test (axial loading of the neck while the head is rotated and laterally bent toward the affected side) often recreates the radicular symptoms.
- Cervical myelopathy usually presents insidiously, with a wide variety of symptoms, including:
  - Gait deterioration (unsteadiness and falls)
  - Deterioration of manual dexterity
  - Generalized weakness
  - Bowel and bladder dysfunction
- Patients may complain of losing balance or of "jumpy" legs.
- A Babinski reflex in the lower extremities or a Hoffmann reflex in the upper extremities may be seen.

#### *History*

- Patients may present with pain, paresthesias, and motor weakness.
- Pain in the trapezial and scapular region may accompany radicular pain.
- Sensory abnormalities do not necessarily follow a dermatomal pattern.
- Pain generally worsens when the neck is tilted to the affected side (because of narrowing of the neural foramina).
- Patients with C6 and C7 radiculopathy often complain of breast pain or anginal symptoms.
- Myelopathic patients complain of gait abnormalities, weakness, and motor skills problems.

#### *Physical Exam*

- Neck ROM
- Motor examination to evaluate for weakness
- Sensory examination
- Reflexes
  - C5: Biceps
  - C6: Brachioradialis
  - C7: Triceps
- Evaluate for myelopathy.

### TESTS

- Spurling maneuver
- Babinski: A positive test is indicated by extension of the great toe with noxious stimulation of the plantar surface of the toes.
- Hoffmann reflex: Elicited by pinching the nail of the middle finger.
  - Positive Hoffmann reflex: Reflexive contraction of the thumb and index finger
  - The Hoffmann reflex is absent in a normal patient (6).
- Finger escape sign: Indicated by spontaneous abduction of the small finger secondary to greater involvement of hand intrinsic muscles because of cervical myelopathy.

#### *Lab*

Electrodiagnostics, including electromyography and nerve conduction velocities, can be used as objective diagnostic tools but are recommended only for patients with inconsistencies in history, physical examination, and radiographic studies.

#### *Imaging*

- Conventional radiographs:
  - Allow assessment of skeletal alignment and the presence of degenerative changes in disc spaces.
  - Oblique views visualize the neural foramina.
  - Flexion and extension views can be used to assess stability.
  - However, because almost 50% of all people ≥40 years old show degenerative changes, radiographs should be reserved for patients with acute trauma or for whom nonoperative therapy has failed.
- CT myelography:
  - Allows accurate evaluation of the degree of neural compression from bony and soft tissues
  - Myelography, an invasive procedure, should be reserved as a tool for surgical planning.
- MRI of the cervical spine:
  - Noninvasive
  - Involves no radiation exposure
  - Provides excellent images
  - Should be reserved for patients who do not respond to nonoperative interventions because up to 30% of people ≥40 years old have an asymptomatic disc bulge or foraminal stenosis (5).

#### *Diagnostic Procedures/Surgery*

Selective injections can be used to localize the source of pain in patients with multiple sites of neural compression and unclear findings.

#### *Pathological Findings*

Disc material (nucleus pulposus) herniates through the disc annulus and compresses a nerve root, causing radiculopathy, or compresses the spinal cord, causing myelopathy.

## DIFFERENTIAL DIAGNOSIS

- Intrinsic disease of the shoulder, elbow, or wrist (degenerative joint disease, impingement, rotator cuff disease, or instability)
- Peripheral nerve entrapments (CTS, cubital tunnel, Guyon canal, TOS)
- Neurologic disorders (brachial plexopathy, multiple sclerosis, amyotrophic lateral sclerosis, spinal cord or brain tumors)
- Infectious discitis
- Vertebral osteomyelitis
- Metastatic cancer

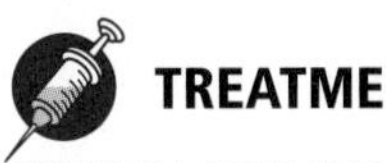

# TREATMENT

## GENERAL MEASURES

- Most patients can be treated nonsurgically with the following:
  - Rest (activity modification)
  - Medication (analgesics, NSAIDs, and muscle relaxants)
  - Intermittent mobilization (soft collar)
  - Physical therapy (exercises or traction)
- Patients for whom a minimum of 6 weeks of nonsurgical care fails, who develop increased symptoms or neurologic deficit, or who present with a myelopathy or a progressive or severe motor deficit should be referred for possible surgical treatment.

## SPECIAL THERAPY

### *Physical Therapy*

- Cervical traction, either in therapy or at home, may help reduce radicular symptoms.
- Initially, passive modalities may help decrease acute pain.
- Subsequent active stretching and exercises may help patients return to normal activities.

## MEDICATION (DRUGS)

No role for maintenance opiates

### *First Line*

- NSAIDs (as long as no gastrointestinal side effects are noted)
- Enteric coated aspirin (fewer gastrointestinal side effects)
- Acetaminophen

### *Second Line*

- COX-2 inhibitors (Be aware of changing side-effect profile.)
- Cervical epidural steroids

## SURGERY

- Anterior cervical discectomy and fusion or posterior laminotomy and foraminotomy can be used to treat a herniated disc that is refractory to nonoperative treatment.
  - A recent study showed that the fusion rates of 1-level anterior cervical decompression and fusion with plate fixation and with bone allograft or autograft are equal (7).
- Anterior cervical decompression and fusion is the preferred surgical treatment for cervical radiculopathy when the herniation is located centrally or when kyphosis or axial neck pain is present (8).
- Posterior laminotomy and foraminotomy may be performed for lateral soft disc herniation with arm pain (8).
- Laminoplasty provides a good alternative to laminectomy or anterior cervical decompression and fusion for multilevel cervical spondylotic radiculopathy (9).

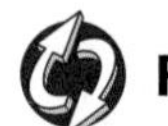

# FOLLOW-UP

## DISPOSITION

### *Issues for Referral*

- Shoulder pathology can present with symptoms similar to those of cervical spine disease.
- Patients with shoulder pathology must be referred to a general orthopaedic surgeon or a shoulder specialist for additional evaluation.

## PROGNOSIS

In a population-based study of cervical radiculopathy, ~90% of patients were treated satisfactorily with surgery or nonoperative procedures (3).

## COMPLICATIONS

- Complications of surgical treatment:
  - Infection
  - Persistence of neurologic deficit
  - New onset neurologic deficit, particularly C5 nerve root palsy
  - Worsening deficit
- Moderate and severely myelopathic patients are likely to remain myelopathic.
- Patients having an anterior cervical discectomy may complain of:
  - Dysphagia (usually improves over 6 months)
  - Pain from pseudarthrosis
  - Late degeneration at an adjacent disc
  - Adjacent level degeneration secondary to anterior plate impingement
  - Hoarseness secondary to injury of the recurrent laryngeal nerve

## PATIENT MONITORING

No regular monitoring is needed.

## REFERENCES


1. Peolsson A, Hedlund R, Vavruch L, et al. Predictive factors for the outcome of anterior cervical decompression and fusion. *Eur Spine J* 2003;12:274–280.
2. Kokubun S, Sakurai M, Tanaka Y. Cartilaginous endplate in cervical disc herniation. *Spine* 1996;21:190–195.
3. Radhakrishnan K, Litchy WJ, O'Fallon WM, et al. Epidemiology of cervical radiculopathy. A population-based study from Rochester, Minnesota, 1976 through 1990. *Brain* 1994;117:325–335.
4. Wolsko PM, Eisenberg DM, Davis RB, et al. Patterns and perceptions of care for treatment of back and neck pain: results of a national survey. *Spine* 2003;28:292–297.
5. Boden SD, McCowin PR, Davis DO, et al. Abnormal magnetic-resonance scans of the cervical spine in asymptomatic subjects. A prospective investigation. *J Bone Joint Surg* 1990;72A:1178–1184.
6. Denno JJ, Meadows GR. Early diagnosis of cervical spondylotic myelopathy. A useful clinical sign. *Spine* 1991;16:1353–1355.
7. Samartzis D, Shen FH, Goldberg EJ, et al. Is autograft the gold standard in achieving radiographic fusion in one-level anterior cervical discectomy and fusion with rigid anterior plate fixation? *Spine* 2005;30:1756–1761.
8. Albert TJ, Murrell SE. Surgical management of cervical radiculopathy. *J Am Acad Orthop Surg* 1999;7:368–376.
9. Herkowitz HN. Cervical laminaplasty: its role in the treatment of cervical radiculopathy. *J Spinal Disord* 1988;1:179–188.


## ADDITIONAL READING


- Garvey TA, Eismont FJ. Diagnosis and treatment of cervical radiculopathy and myelopathy. *Orthop Rev* 1991;20:595–603.
- Levine MJ, Albert TJ, Smith MD. Cervical radiculopathy: diagnosis and nonoperative management. *J Am Acad Orthop Surg* 1996;4:305–316.


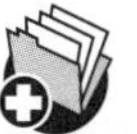

# MISCELLANEOUS

## CODES

### *ICD9-CM*

- 722.0 Displacement, intervertebral disc (with neuritis, pain, or radiculitis)
- 722.71.1 Displacement, intervertebral disc (with myelopathy)

## PATIENT TEACHING

- Patients should be informed that, in the absence of neurologic changes, this condition can be treated nonoperatively with fairly good results.
- For most patients unable to attain pain relief with medications and/or steroids, surgery has excellent results.

## FAQ

- Q: Which provocative physical examination maneuvers can be used to help evaluate for a herniated cervical disc?
  - A: The Spurling test (radiculopathy), Babinski sign (myelopathy), and testing of the Hoffman reflex (myelopathy).
- Q: Which reflexes should be evaluated at C5, C6, and C7?
  - A: C5, biceps; C6, brachioradialis; C7, triceps.

# CERVICAL SPINE ANATOMY AND EXAMINATION

*Sergio A. Glait, BS*
*Sanjog Mathur, MD*
*A. Jay Khanna, MD*

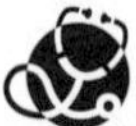

## BASICS

### DESCRIPTION

- Anatomy:
  - The cervical spine contains 7 cervical vertebrae, from which arise 8 nerve roots.
    - The normal cervical spine has a lordotic curvature.
    - Intact functional cervical vertebrae are vital because they protect both the spinal cord and the vertebral artery.
    - Of the 8 nerve roots that arise from the cervical vertebrae, all but 1 (C8) exit above their numbered vertebral body through the vertebral foramina; C8 exits below its numbered vertebral body.
- Vertebral anatomic structures consist of 2 lamina, 2 arches, 2 pedicles, 2 transverse processes, a spinous process, and a body.
- C1 and C2 are unique in that C1 (atlas) lacks a vertebral body and C2 (axis) has a bony protrusion on the superior side of the body called the "odontoid process."
- Most flexion and extension occurs at the atlanto-occipital joint, whereas rotation occurs mostly at the atlantoaxial joint (1).

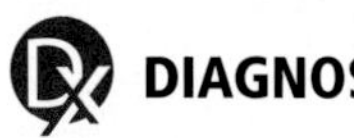

## DIAGNOSIS

### SIGNS AND SYMPTOMS

#### *Physical Exam*

- The cervical spine provides support and stability to the head while allowing for a wide ROM.
- A thorough neck examination should evaluate the soft tissues and bony structures while also testing neurologic function.
- Motor examination:
  - Levator scapulae: Resisted elevation (C3, C4, sometimes C5)
  - Deltoids: Shoulder abduction (C5)
  - Biceps: Arm flexion (C6)
  - Wrist extension (C6)
  - Triceps: Elbow extension (C7)
  - Wrist flexion (C7)
  - Finger extension (C7)
  - Finger flexion and thumb adduction (C8)
- Deep tendon reflexes:
  - An abnormal reflex response may be indicative of spinal stenosis or nerve root compression.
  - Reflex amplification is a symptom of spinal stenosis with myelopathy, whereas diminished reflexes indicate nerve root compression.
    - Biceps (C5)
    - Brachioradialis (C6)
    - Triceps (C7)
- Sensation:
  - When tracing abnormal sensation, patients should be asked to be as specific as possible.
  - C2, C3, and C4 sensation should move from the posterior to the anterior neck.
  - C5–T2 has very specific dermatomes on the arm, wrist, and fingers.
    - C5: Lateral shoulder
    - C6: Radial 2 digits
    - C7: Middle finger
    - C8: Ulnar 2 digits
    - T1: Medial forearm
- Inspection: It is important to evaluate:
  - Posture of the head
  - Posture of the body, motion, gait
  - Pain
  - Scars on the anterior or posterior neck
- Bony palpation: Anterior (2):
  - Note any abnormalities such as tenderness, lumps, asymmetries, or misalignments.
  - May use surface landmarks to localize cervical spine level:
    - Hyoid bone: C3 vertebral body
    - Superior notch of thyroid cartilage: C4 vertebral body
    - 1st cricoid ring: C6 vertebral body (swallowing allows easier palpation.)
    - Carotid tubercle: C6 transverse process (the 2 carotid tubercles of the C6 vertebra should be palpated separately because simultaneous palpation can restrict the flow of both carotid arteries).
    - Trachea: Make sure no deviations are present from the midline and palpate for abnormalities.
- Bony palpation: Posterior (2)
  - Occiput:
    - Inion: The lower, most palpable part of the occiput
  - Spinous processes:
    - C7 and T1 are the most prominent.
    - All the spinous processes should be aligned.
    - Any deviation may be secondary to a unilateral facet dislocation.
    - C3–C5 may be bifid.
  - Facet joints: Approximately 2.5 cm lateral to the spinous processes, the most common joint involved in osteoarthritis is C5–C6 (3).
- Soft-tissue palpation: Anterior:
  - Sternocleidomastoid
  - Parotid gland
  - Lymph nodes
  - Thyroid gland: Symmetric and smooth
  - Carotid pulse
  - Supraclavicular fossa: Palpate for bulges or cervical ribs.
- Soft-tissue palpation: Posterior:
  - Trapezius: Evaluate for lymph nodes, palpable only because of pathologic causes
  - Greater occipital nerves: If palpable, may be secondary to whiplash injury.
  - Ligamentum nuchae: Inion to C7 spinous process
- ROM:
  - Active ROM is a crucial part of the cervical neck examination and includes flexion, extension, lateral bending, and rotation of the neck.
  - Flexion and extension:
    - 50% occurs between the occiput and C1, and the remainder is distributed from C2–C7.
    - Slightly greater motion occurs at the C5–C6 level.
    - Tests sternocleidomastoid muscle (flexor) and paravertebral extensor and trapezius (extensors) (4)
  - Rotation:
    - 50% occurs between C1–C2, and the remainder is evenly distributed in the remainder of the cervical spine.
    - To examine, rotate the chin 60–80° to the right and left.
    - Tests sternocleidomastoid muscle (primary rotator) (4)
  - Lateral bending:
    - Evenly distributed throughout the cervical spine and usually not a pure movement but, rather, functions in conjunction with rotation
    - To examine, touch the ear to the ipsilateral shoulder without moving the shoulder; normal lateral bending is 45°.
    - Tests scalene muscles (4).
- Special maneuvers to help to identify the cause of the cervical spine symptoms:
  - Modified Spurling maneuver (5):
    - Extend the neck and rotate the head to 1 side as axial pressure is applied.
    - A positive test is specific for cervical root compression but with low sensitivity.
  - Distraction test (2):
    - Apply vertical traction to the head in slight flexion and extension.
    - Symptoms of compressed nerve roots may regress temporarily.
  - Lhermitte test (2):
    - Patient flexes head forward.
    - If shooting pain is noted down the arms and/or legs, an anterior compressive lesion may be present.
  - Hoffmann test:
    - Rapidly flex the nail of the middle finger.
    - If muscles of the hand and thumb flex, then a positive sign exists, indicative of an upper motor neuron lesion (myelopathy).
  - Static/dynamic Romberg test (2):
    - The patient stands with hands out and palms up (arms in 90° of flexion).
    - Proprioceptive deficit is present if the patient loses balance with the eyes closed or if the arms rise slowly above the parallel.

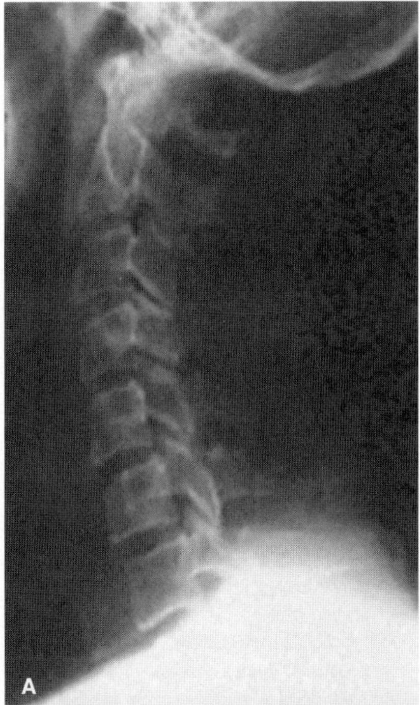


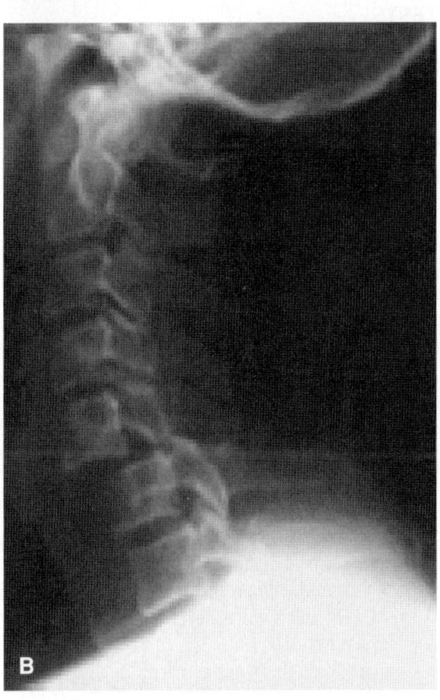


**Fig. 1.** Radiographs of an adult patient showing a normal lateral cervical spine radiograph (**A**) and bilateral C5–C6 facet dislocation (**B**).

## TESTS

### *Imaging*

- Radiography (Fig. 1):
  - AP and lateral views are used to screen for most conditions.
  - Oblique views are used to detect facet dislocation and subluxation.
  - The open-mouth view is used to detect odontoid and Jefferson burst fractures (for patients with neck pain who have struck their heads).

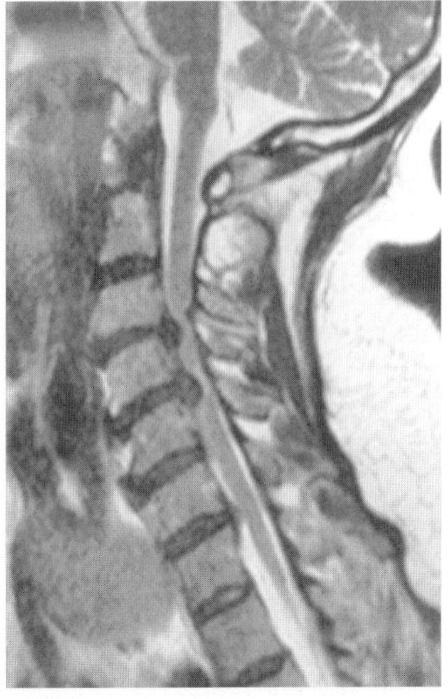

**Fig. 2.** Sagittal T2-weighted MRI scan showing severe stenosis at C3–C4 and C4–C5 secondary to large disc herniations with cord signal change at C4–C5.

  - When viewing radiographs of young children, ossification centers may be present and should not be mistaken for fractures (6).
- MRI is used to detect and define disc herniation, facet hypertrophy, or ligamentum flavum hypertrophy that may be impinging on the spinal cord or cervical nerve root foramen (Fig. 2).
- CT is used to define the anatomy of the osseous cervical spinal structures.

## REFERENCES


1. Aptaker RL. Neck pain. Part 1: Narrowing the differential. *Phys Sportsmed* 1996;24:37–46.
2. Albert TJ, Vaccaro AR. Physical examination of the cervical spine. In: *Physical Examination of the Spine*. New York: Thieme, 2005:13–63.
3. Hunt WE, Miller CA. Management of cervical radiculopathy. *Clin Neurosurg* 1986;33:485–502.
4. Tachdjian MO. The neck and upper limb. In: *Clinical Pediatric Orthopaedics: The Art of Diagnosis and Principles of Management*. Stamford, CT: Appleton and Lange, 1997:263–324.
5. Viikari-Juntura E, Porras M, Laasonen EM. Validity of clinical tests in the diagnosis of root compression in cervical disc disease. *Spine* 1989;14:253–257.
6. Fesmire FM, Luten RC. The pediatric cervical spine: developmental anatomy and clinical aspects. *J Emerg Med* 1989;7:133–142.


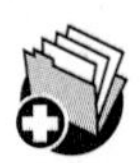

## MISCELLANEOUS

### FAQ

- Q: What is a commonly made mistake when reading a radiograph of a young child's cervical spine?
  - A: Ossification centers may still be present in young children and should not be confused with a fracture.
- Q: What does the Hoffmann sign evaluate?
  - A: The Hoffmann sign evaluates for an upper motor neuron lesion, such as cervical spinal stenosis with myelopathy.

# CERVICAL SPINE TRAUMA: DISLOCATION AND SUBLUXATION

*Dhruv B. Pateder, MD*

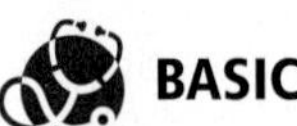

## BASICS

### DESCRIPTION

- 11,000 cases annually require surgery.
- Average hospital stay: 9.4 days (1,2); a prolonged stay partly attributable to delay in diagnosing vertebral injuries (frequently missed)
- Careful trauma-patient evaluation, increased understanding of injury patterns, and advanced imaging and treatment have decreased the morbidity and mortality associated with spinal column injuries (1,2).
- Classification:
  - The Denis 3-column theory (3,4):
    - To determine vertebral fracture stability
    - Unstable fracture: Disruption of 2 columns
  - The Ferguson-Allen classification (5):
    - Based on the mechanism of injury
    - 7 categories: Compressive flexion ("teardrop" fractures), vertical compression (burst fractures), distractive flexion (dislocations), compressive extension, distractive extension, lateral flexion, and miscellaneous cervical spine flexion

### GENERAL PREVENTION

- Seat belts and head rests on car seats
- Possibly air bags
- Strict cervical spine immobilization for all trauma patients

### EPIDEMIOLOGY

#### *Incidence*

- Up to 75% of fractures of the vertebral column occur in the cervical spine (1,2).
- 5–10% of blunt trauma patients have cervical spine injuries (1,2).
- Serious diving accidents have a 50% incidence of cervical spine injury (1,2).

### RISK FACTORS

Young males 18–25 years old

#### *Genetics*

- Many skeletal dysplasias predisposing to traumatic injuries have a genetic basis, and some atraumatic instabilities are associated with a genetic predisposition.
  - Down syndrome is associated with a chromosomal disorder (trisomy 21).
  - Rheumatoid arthritis has a genetic predisposition, which seems to be associated with certain HLA markers.
- Traumatic cervical dislocations have no genetic predisposition.

### ETIOLOGY

- Traumatic:
  - Motor vehicle collision
  - Diving in shallow water
  - Blunt trauma
- Atraumatic:
  - Rheumatoid arthritis
  - Down syndrome
  - Skeletal dysplasias

### ASSOCIATED CONDITIONS

- Neurogenic shock
- Head injury
- Cervical spine fractures
- Chest and abdominal trauma
- Extremity trauma

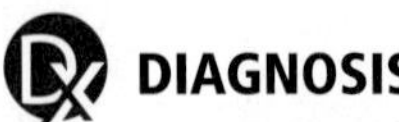

## DIAGNOSIS

### SIGNS AND SYMPTOMS

- Neck pain after trauma
- Occasionally, neck deformity, especially in rotatory subluxations or unilateral facet dislocations
- Persistent asymmetric posturing or head tilt may indicate cervical subluxation or dislocation.
- Neurologic injury may take the form of weakness, numbness, bowel or bladder incontinence, complete quadriplegia, or 1 of the incomplete spinal cord injury syndromes (Brown-Séquard, central cord, anterior cord, posterior cord).

#### *Physical Exam*

- All trauma evaluations begin with assessment of airway, breathing, and circulation (6).
- Evaluation of the cervical spine should begin only after the patient is hemodynamically stable and life-threatening injuries have been ruled out.
- Initial radiographs of the cervical spine, chest, and pelvis are useful in prioritizing therapy.
- The initial neurologic examination (with the patient in a neck collar) requires careful documentation, including time of injury, and time and details of field and hospital examinations.
  - Sensory examination: Evaluate dermatomes, light touch, pin prick, temperature, and perianal sensation.
  - Motor examination:
    - Upper extremities: Grade the deltoids, triceps, biceps, wrist flexors and extensors, finger abductors and adductors, and grip strength.
    - Lower extremities: Test the iliopsoas, quadriceps, hamstrings, hip abductors/adductors, tibialis anterior, extensor hallucis longus, and gastrocnemius–soleus complex.
    - Grade each muscle on a 0–5-point scale.
  - Do not use phrases such as "moves everything" or "feels everything" because the physical examination provides a temporal sequence for a potentially evolving neurologic injury.
  - Rectal examination: Performed by the spine surgeon to assess tone, volitional control, and sensation to light touch and pin prick.
- Examine the head and neck for tenderness and pain on motion.
  - If painful, immobilize the head and neck until adequate physical/radiologic examinations.
- Suggested motor checkpoints:
  - C4: Diaphragm
  - C5: Deltoid and elbow flexors
  - C6: Wrist extensors
  - C7: Elbow extensors
  - C8: Finger flexors (profundus)
  - T1: Intrinsics (finger abductors)
  - L2: Hip flexors
  - L3: Knee extensors
  - L4: Ankle dorsiflexors
  - L5: Great toe extensors
  - S1: Ankle plantar flexors
  - S4–5: Voluntary anal contraction
- Suggested sensory checkpoints:
  - C2: Occiput
  - C4: Tip of shoulder
  - C5: Regimental patch (lateral shoulder)
  - C6: Thumb
  - C7: Long finger
  - C8: Little finger
  - T1: Medial epicondyle
  - T4: Nipples
  - T10: Umbilicus
  - L1: Groin
  - L3: Patella
  - L4: Medial malleolus
  - L5: Great toe and first web space.
  - S1: Lateral heel
  - S2: Popliteal fossa
  - S3: Ischial tuberosity
  - S4–5: Perianal

### TESTS

#### *Lab*

- Estimated lung vital capacity of at least 20% of predicted is necessary.
- If vital capacity is <20% or 1,000 mL, a tracheostomy may be required.

#### *Imaging*

- Radiographic evaluation of the cervical spine:
  - For any potentially neurologic injury
  - The AP view allows evaluation of the interspinous distance, alignment, and symmetry of uncovertebral joints.
  - Lateral view:
    - Most important view
    - Can detect approximately 82% of injuries to the cervical vertebrae (2)
    - The C7–T1 junction must be visualized adequately because injuries at this level are not uncommon.
    - If this level cannot be visualized, a "swimmer's view" (arm abducted over the head and body slightly rotated) may be useful.
    - If C7–T1 still is not visualized, a CT scan at that level is necessary.
  - The open-mouth view is excellent for visualizing the dens and the overhanging lateral masses, but its acquisition frequently is limited by associated pain and the high degree of patient cooperation required.
  - Oblique views are excellent for visualizing the neural foramen and lamina, but their use in the trauma situation is controversial and generally is not a part of the trauma series.
  - Patient pain, cervical spine tenderness, or neurologic symptoms: Possible ligamentous injury even with negative radiographs
    - Lateral flexion–extension views may be indicated to evaluate for dynamic instability of the cervical vertebrae.

- CT:
  - Evaluates any bony abnormalities
  - Usually obtained if injury is questionable on standard cervical spine radiographs
  - Standard of care for evaluation of any loss of middle column height
  - Planar reconstructions can be very valuable in surgical planning.
- MRI:
  - Evaluates soft-tissue, pathologic, and ligamentous injuries
  - Also useful for evaluating neurologic deficits that cannot be explained radiographically
  - May be necessary for uncooperative or obtunded patients

### DIFFERENTIAL DIAGNOSIS

- Pseudosubluxation (other than normal ≤3 mm at C2 in children)
- Cervical spine fractures with instability
- Injuries at multiple levels
- Muscular torticollis

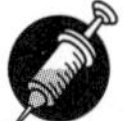

## TREATMENT

### GENERAL MEASURES

- Resuscitation and emergency measures:
  - Airway, breathing, and circulation
  - Strict immobilization during extraction and transportation (and intubation if necessary)
- Emergency department assessment:
  - Complete (with neurologic) assessment
  - Full radiographic evaluation
- Emergency treatment:
  - Traction for reduction of dislocations (MRI for facet dislocations)
  - Methylprednisolone:
    - Start within 8 hours of spinal cord injury to help preserve neuronal structures.
    - Dose: A 30-mg/kg bolus intravenously followed by 5.4 mg/kg/h for 23 hours
  - Surgery for irreducible dislocations with neurologic deficit and deterioration
- For stable injuries, immobilization may be necessary for a short period.
- The treatment of unstable injuries may vary from immobilization to surgical stabilization.

#### *Activity*

After the dislocation is stabilized, activity can be begun and advanced gradually.

### SPECIAL THERAPY

#### *Radiotherapy*

- Decreases tumor size and burden in patients with pathologic thoracolumbar fractures

#### *Physical Therapy*

- Important role in mobilizing spinal injury patients and for those with neurologic injury
- May be helpful after healing to treat residual pain and stiffness
- Wheelchairs are individualized to the patient.
- Lower extremity bracing and orthotics for upper extremity function may be beneficial.

### SURGERY

- Occipitocervical dissociation requires an occiput-to-C2 posterior fusion/instrumentation.
- Atlantoaxial instability should include bracing for children and those with ≤7 mm of translation in flexion and fusion for patients with >7 mm of persistent translation.
- Hangman's fracture–dislocation or traumatic spondylolisthesis:
  - Can be treated with closed reduction and a Minerva cast in children
  - Halo immobilization or posterior open reduction and stabilization may be necessary, depending on the type of fracture.
- Facet dislocations may require open reduction and stabilization for failed closed reduction.

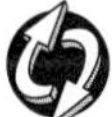

## FOLLOW-UP

Patients with neurologic injuries require long-term rehabilitation, including education, bladder and bowel program, family education, physical and occupational therapy, and psychologic counseling.

### PROGNOSIS

- Prognosis depends on injury severity.
  - Neurologically intact patients with low-energy injuries have excellent recovery.
  - Patients with neurologic injury have major issues, potentially requiring alteration in their personal and professional lives.

### COMPLICATIONS

- Surgical complications: Infection, neurologic injury, pseudarthrosis, chronic pain, and disability
- Other complications include neurologic injury, spinal deformity, chronic pain, and skin problems from pressure points on neck braces.

### PATIENT MONITORING

Neurologic monitoring (including somatosensory-evoked potentials and motor monitoring) during reduction maneuvers and surgery may increase the safety of the procedure.

### REFERENCES


1. Viano DC. Effectiveness of safety belts and airbags in preventing fatal injury. In: *Proceedings of Frontal Crash Safety Technologies, SAE Technical Paper Series*. Warrendale, PA: Society of Automotive Engineers, 1991:159–171.
2. West OC, Anbari MM, Pilgram TK, et al. Acute cervical spine trauma: diagnostic performance of single-view versus three-view radiographic screening. *Radiology* 1997;204:819–823.
3. Denis F. The three column spine and its significance in the classification of acute thoracolumbar spinal injuries. *Spine* 1983;8:817–831.
4. Denis F. Spinal instability as defined by the three-column spine concept in acute spinal trauma. *Clin Orthop Relat Res* 1984;189:65–76.
5. Ferguson RL, Allen BL, Jr. A mechanistic classification of thoracolumbar spine fractures. *Clin Orthop Relat Res* 1984;189:77–88.
6. American College of Surgeons Committee on Trauma. *Advanced Trauma Life Support Program for Doctors*, 6th ed. Chicago: American College of Surgeons, 1997.


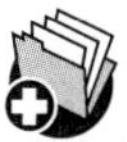

## MISCELLANEOUS

### CODES

#### *ICD9-CM*

- 839.01 C-1 dislocation
- 839.02 C-2 dislocation
- 839.03 C-3 dislocation
- 839.04 C-4 dislocation
- 839.05 C-5 dislocation
- 839.06 C-6 dislocation
- 839.07 C-7 dislocation

### PATIENT TEACHING

- Skin care and positioning to prevent flexion contractures
- Education to prevent pressure ulceration, respiratory, and urinary infections

### FAQ

- Q: What imaging modality is considered a part of the "trauma series" in evaluating a patient?
  - A: Lateral cervical spine, AP chest, and AP pelvis radiographs.
- Q: What is the last vertebrae that must be visualized for an adequate C-spine lateral radiograph?
  - A: C7–T1 junction.

# CHARCOT-MARIE-TOOTH DISEASE

*Dhruv B. Pateder, MD*

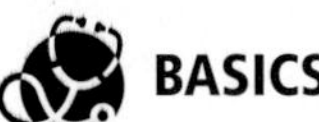

## BASICS

### DESCRIPTION

- Charcot-Marie-Tooth disease is the most common hereditary motor and sensory neuropathy.
- Involvement progresses from distal to proximal: Lower extremity wasting, weakness, and cavovarus feet develop (Fig. 1), followed in some cases by upper extremity weakness.
- 5 recognized types (1):
  - Type I (hypertrophic form):
    - The most common form (50% of patients)
    - Thickened nerves have abnormal myelin that breaks down, leading to slowed nerve conduction.
  - Type II (axonal form) is characterized by generally severe disease, with intact reflexes and a mild decrease in nerve conduction velocities secondary to axonal degeneration.
  - Type III (Dejerine-Sottas disease) shows marked segmental demyelination.
  - Type IV is autosomal recessive.
  - Charcot-Marie-Tooth-X is X-linked inheritance (~10% of cases) (2).

### RISK FACTORS

#### *Genetics*

- Charcot-Marie-Tooth disease is caused by a mutation in the gene for the peripheral myelin protein 22-kDa.

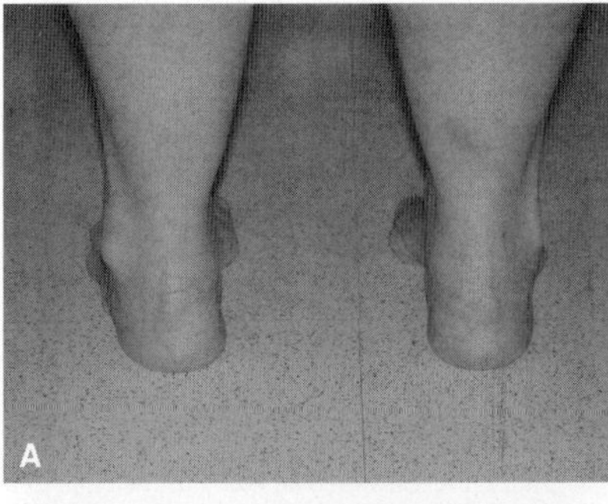


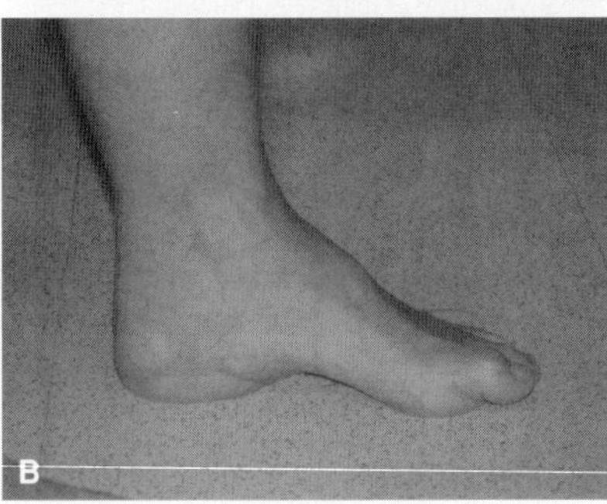


**Fig. 1.** Clinical photographs of foot deformity in Charcot-Marie-Tooth disease. Posterior view shows hindfoot varus (**A**). Medial view shows high arch and hallux clawing (**B**).

- Inheritance patterns include:
  - Autosomal dominant with variable penetrance: Types I, II, and III
  - Autosomal recessive: Type IV
  - X-linked: Type CMT-X

### PATHOPHYSIOLOGY

- Characterized by progressive weakness of the intrinsic muscles of the foot, peroneal muscles, and dorsiflexors of the foot and toes
- Intrinsic weakness leads to characteristic clawing of the toes.
- Relative weakness of the anterior tibialis and peroneus brevis leads to plantarflexion of the 1st metatarsal, which causes dynamic hindfoot inversion with gait.
- Chronic deformity leads to relative stiffness of the foot, impaired shock absorption, and arthritis.
- Long-standing hindfoot varus can lead to lateral ankle ligament attenuation and symptoms of instability.

### ASSOCIATED CONDITIONS

- Scoliosis develops in 10% of patients (3).
- Hip dysplasia develops in 6–10% of patients and presents at a later age than does the idiopathic form (4).

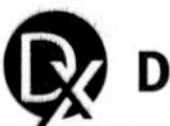

## DIAGNOSIS

### SIGNS AND SYMPTOMS

- Patients usually present at 10–20 years of age with a high arch, loss of endurance or coordination, or a "steppage" gait.
  - Their shoes wear out rapidly and unevenly because of progressive cavovarus foot alignment.
- On examination:
  - Weakness is present in the ankle evertors and dorsiflexors before the plantarflexors and invertors.
  - Sensation and proprioception are diminished.
  - There may be increased circumduction of the extremity or steppage pattern during the swing phase of gait to allow clearance of dropfoot.

#### *History*

- Identify family members with similar foot deformities.
- Note progression of deformity, weakness, and giving-way of the ankle.
- Identify site(s) of pain about the ankle and foot.

#### *Physical Exam*

- The calf usually is atrophied.
- Record and monitor foot and ankle muscle strength.
- Test sensation.
- Examine the position of the foot at rest for the presence of hindfoot varus.
  - This aspect is most strongly related to functional problems.
  - If present, assess for rigidity by placing a lift under the lateral side of the forefoot and seeing whether the hindfoot varus corrects (Coleman block test).
  - Assess passive correction of the hindfoot varus.
- Assess the lateral ankle ligaments for laxity and instability.
- Note the relative plantarflexion of the 1st metatarsals compared with that of the others.
- Record the presence or absence of toe clawing.
- Observe the patient's gait, including the presence or absence of steppage or circumduction gait.
- Examine the hips for abduction.
- Check for scoliosis with a forward bend test.
- Check the upper extremities for wasting of the ulnar-innervated hand muscles, including the abductors and interossei.

### TESTS

- Electromyography and nerve conduction velocities usually are performed for diagnosis.
  - The electromyogram shows increased duration and decreased amplitude of the motor action potentials.
  - Nerve conduction velocity testing shows decrease in motor and sensory conduction velocity.
- Biopsy:
  - Muscle biopsy shows atrophy.
  - Nerve biopsy shows loss of myelinated fibers.
  - These biopsies are not indicated routinely if the history and electrodiagnostic tests are characteristic.
- DNA testing is available through blood testing for early diagnosis or family analysis.

#### *Imaging*

- Radiography:
  - Obtain standing radiographs of the foot and ankle to assess alignment and identify arthritis.
  - Obtain spinal films in the index patient without a family history, to rule out spinal disorders.
  - Once a diagnosis is made, the physician should have a low threshold for ordering pelvic films to rule out dysplasia if limitation of abduction is present.
- Depending on the index of suspicion, MRI of the spine may be indicated because it can visualize corticospinal tract abnormalities.

#### *Pathological Findings*

- Muscle biopsy displays diffuse atrophy and replacement of muscle fibers with fibrous and adipose tissue.
- Nerve biopsy shows loss of myelinated fibers and increased fibrous tissue in the endoneurium and perineurium.
- The pathogenesis of the cavovarus foot:
  - Progressive weakness of the lumbricals, interossei, peroneals, and extensors that leaves the long toe flexors and ankle invertors unopposed.
  - Claw toes develop, and the plantar fascia and intrinsic muscles contract.

### DIFFERENTIAL DIAGNOSIS

- Tethered spinal cord
- Myelomeningocele, lipomeningocele
- Peroneal nerve palsy
- Early stages of Duchenne muscular dystrophy
- Other hereditary motor and sensory neuropathies

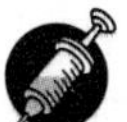

## TREATMENT

### GENERAL MEASURES

- Patients should be seen on a routine basis to monitor for worsening deformity.
- Stretching of the Achilles tendon and the plantar fascia may be helpful.
- Custom orthotic insoles with lateral heel build-up may improve hindfoot alignment, whereas forefoot accommodative padding may relieve metatarsalgia secondary to claw-toe deformities.
- Ankle bracing may assist in patients with instability symptoms.
- A custom ankle–foot orthosis may be necessary for patients with severe drop foot secondary to extensor weakness.
- Comfortable shoe wear with adequate toe boxes and cushioned heels is recommended.

### SPECIAL THERAPY

#### *Physical Therapy*

Therapy involves stretching of the Achilles tendon and plantar fascia, strengthening exercises, and proprioceptive training to assist with ankle instability.

### SURGERY

- Treatment consists of addressing individual components of deformity:
  - Claw-toe correction
    - Flexor-to-extensor transfer, MTP joint release, and PIP fusion
    - Hallux IP arthrodesis and extensor hallucis longus transfer to 1st metatarsal (Jones procedure)
  - Plantar release (plantar fascia, abductor hallucis, toe flexors) or plantar–medial release (includes posterior tibialis and long toe flexor lengthening and talonavicular capsulotomy)
  - Tendon transfer: Split or whole transfer of the posterior tibialis to assist with dorsiflexion and eversion
  - Peroneus longus tenodesis to peroneus brevis
  - Calcaneal lateral closing wedge osteotomy for rigid hindfoot varus
  - Midtarsal or metatarsal closing wedge osteotomies
  - Triple arthrodesis for rigid deformity or hindfoot arthritis
  - Ankle ligament reconstruction for instability

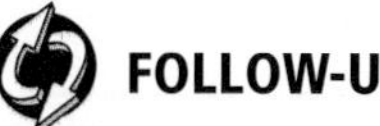

## FOLLOW-UP

### DISPOSITION

#### *Issues for Referral*

Consultation by a neurologist is warranted for electromyographic testing and peripheral blood tests for diagnosis and genetic counseling.

### PROGNOSIS

- Usually, the foot cannot be made fully normal even after surgery, and the muscle weakness progresses.
- Life expectancy is not shortened.

### COMPLICATIONS

- Missed hip dysplasia means more difficult or less successful treatment.
- May recur after surgery if soft-tissue procedures are performed in patients with a fixed bony deformity.
- Transfer of stress with degeneration of the ankle or midfoot may occur, especially after triple arthrodesis.

### PATIENT MONITORING

Patients are checked yearly for ambulatory function.

### REFERENCES


1. Kirchner JS. Charcot-Marie-Tooth disease and the cavovarus foot. In: Richardson EG, ed. *Orthopaedic Knowledge Update: Foot and Ankle 3*. Rosemont, IL: American Academy of Orthopaedic Surgeons, 2004:135–143.
2. Guyton GP, Mann RA. The pathogenesis and surgical management of foot deformity in Charcot-Marie-Tooth disease. *Foot Ankle Clin* 2000;5:317–326.
3. Hensinger RN, MacEwen GD. Spinal deformity associated with heritable neurological conditions: spinal muscular atrophy, Friedreich's ataxia, familial dysautonomia, and Charcot-Marie-Tooth disease. *J Bone Joint Surg* 1976;58A:13–24.
4. Pailthorpe CA, Benson MKD. Hip dysplasia in hereditary motor and sensory neuropathies. *J Bone Joint Surg* 1992;74B:538–540.


### ADDITIONAL READING


- Kassubek J, Bretschneider V, Sperfeld AD. Corticospinal tract MRI hyperintensity in X-linked Charcot-Marie-Tooth disease. *J Clin Neurosci* 2005;12:588–589.
- Kobsar I, Hasenpusch-Theil K, Wessig C, et al. Evidence for macrophage-mediated myelin disruption in an animal model for Charcot-Marie-Tooth neuropathy type 1A. *J Neurosci Res* 2005;81:857–864.
- McCluskey WP, Lovell WW, Cummings RJ. The cavovarus foot deformity. Etiology and management [see comments]. *Clin Orthop Relat Res* 1989;247:27–37.
- Miller MJ, Williams LL, Slack SL, et al. The hand in Charcot-Marie-Tooth disease. *J Hand Surg* 1991;16B:191–196.
- Roper BA, Tibrewal SB. Soft tissue surgery in Charcot-Marie-Tooth disease. *J Bone Joint Surg* 1989;71B:17–20.
- Wetmore RS, Drennan JC. Long-term results of triple arthrodesis in Charcot-Marie-Tooth disease. *J Bone Joint Surg* 1989;71A:417–422.


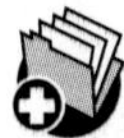

## MISCELLANEOUS

### CODES

#### *ICD9-CM*

- 356.1 Charcot-Marie-Tooth disease
- 735.5 Claw toe
- 736.75 Cavovarus foot

### PATIENT TEACHING

- Stress the importance of stretching and routine follow-up.
- DNA testing may be helpful to provide for genetic counseling.
- Discuss the risks of scoliosis and hip dysplasia.

### FAQ

- Q: What is the basic pathophysiology of Charcot-Marie-Tooth disease?
  - A: Inherited motor–sensory neuropathy with resultant preferential weakness of the intrinsic muscles of the hands and feet along with ankle extensors and evertors.
- Q: What is the typical foot deformity seen in Charcot-Marie-Tooth disease?
  - A: Cavovarus deformity and claw toes.

# CHONDROBLASTOMA

*Constantine A. Demetracopoulos, BS*
*Frank J. Frassica, MD*

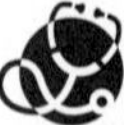

## BASICS

### DESCRIPTION
- A benign tumor of cartilaginous origin with a predilection for the epiphysis in skeletally immature patients
- Generally found in the epiphyses of long bones.
  - The humerus is most commonly affected, followed by the tibia and femur (1) (Fig. 1).
- Synonyms: Codman tumor; Epiphyseal chondromatous giant cell tumor

### EPIDEMIOLOGY
A slight male predominance (2:1) is noted (2).

#### *Incidence*
- This tumor is rare.
- In the largest series, chondroblastoma accounted for 1% of all skeletal neoplasms (3).

### RISK FACTORS
None known

#### *Genetics*
No known genetic component exists.

### ETIOLOGY
- The pathogenesis is unknown.
- Most authors agree that the neoplastic cells arise from "cartilage-forming matrix cells" or chondroblasts.
- The tumor may be related to chondromyxoid fibroma.

### ASSOCIATED CONDITIONS
Aneurysmal bone cyst

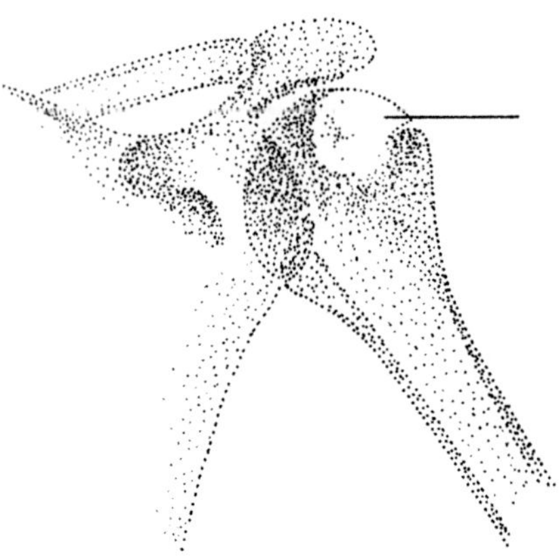

**Fig. 1.** Chondroblastoma is a lucent lesion in the immature epiphysis, most often the proximal humerus.

## DIAGNOSIS

### SIGNS AND SYMPTOMS
- Patients usually complain of mild to moderate chronic pain, often months to years in duration.
- Stiffness and effusion of the adjacent joint also are common.
- Local swelling is uncommon.

#### *Physical Exam*
- The adjacent joint may have an effusion and decreased ROM.
- A soft-tissue mass is uncommon.
- Joint tenderness is unusual.

### TESTS

#### *Lab*
- Tests are not helpful.
- All blood tests are within normal limits, including the ESR.

#### *Imaging*
- Radiography:
  - The radiographic appearance is that of a lytic lesion in the epiphysis with a thin sclerotic rim.
    - The sclerotic rim indicates the benign nature of the lesion.
    - It may expand or deform the bone.
    - Occasionally, punctate calcifications may be seen.
  - The patient's history and plain radiographs usually are sufficient for making the diagnosis.
- MRI:
  - May be used if history and radiography are not definitive
  - The boundary of the lesion on MRI scans should be distinct.

#### *Pathological Findings*
- The diagnosis requires the presence of chondroblasts on microscopic section.
  - Chondroblasts are small, round or polygonal cells with round or oval nuclei.
  - Cells are described as looking "plump" or like fried eggs.
  - A lattice of calcification extends between the cells (chicken wire) (1).
- Interspersed giant cells are a common feature and may lead to confusion with giant cell tumor.
- Areas of aneurysmal bone cyst degeneration also may be present.

### DIFFERENTIAL DIAGNOSIS
- Enchondroma
- Giant cell tumor
- Osteomyelitis
- Fibrous dysplasia

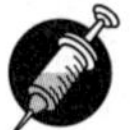

## TREATMENT

### GENERAL MEASURES
- Surgical excision is recommended to prevent progressive growth of the lesion with destruction of the epiphysis.
- Bone grafting is needed.
- Surgery is sometimes technically demanding because of the need to preserve or reconstruct the nearby joint surface.

#### *Activity*
No restrictions on activity are necessary because pathologic fracture is not a problem.

## SPECIAL THERAPY

### *Physical Therapy*

Therapy may be used to regain ROM and strength after surgery.

## SURGERY

- Because the tumor is considered benign, local measures suffice.
- Surgery generally involves curettage and bone grafting.

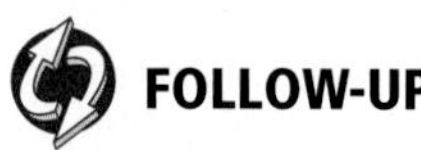

# FOLLOW-UP

## PROGNOSIS

- The recurrence rate with chondroblastoma alone is 20% at 3 years (3).
- If the tumor has an aneurysmal component, the risk of recurrence is higher (3).

## COMPLICATIONS

- Recurrence
- Joint stiffness

## PATIENT MONITORING

- Follow-up care is necessary because recurrence is common.
- Radiographs should be repeated every 6–12 months after excision for ~2 years.

## REFERENCES


1. McCarthy EF, Frassica FJ. Primary bone tumors. In: *Pathology of Bone and Joint Disorders: With Clinical and Radiographic Correlation*. Philadelphia: WB Saunders Co, 1998:195–275.
2. Spjut HJ, Dorfman HD, Fechner RE, et al. Tumors of cartilaginous origin. In: *Tumors of Bone and Cartilage*. Washington, DC: Armed Forces Institute of Pathology, 1971:33–116.
3. Huvos AG. Chondroblastoma and clear-cell chondrosarcoma. In: *Bone Tumors: Diagnosis, Treatment, and Prognosis*, 2nd ed. Philadelphia: WB Saunders Co., 1991:295–318.


## ADDITIONAL READING


- Masui F, Ushigome S, Kamitani K, et al. Chondroblastoma: a study of 11 cases. *Eur J Surg Oncol* 2002;28:869–874.
- Ramappa AJ, Lee FY, Tang P, et al. Chondroblastoma of bone. *J Bone Joint Surg* 2000;82A:1140–1145.
- Suneja R, Grimer RJ, Belthur M, et al. Chondroblastoma of bone: long-term results and functional outcome after intralesional curettage. *J Bone Joint Surg* 2005;87B:974–978.


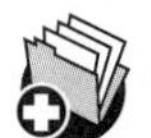

# MISCELLANEOUS

## CODES

### *ICD9-CM*

213.4 Chondroblastoma

## PATIENT TEACHING

- Patients should be counseled that the lesion is benign and rarely metastasizes (<2%).
- However, if the tumor is not removed, local morbidity may occur because of progressive enlargement of the involved epiphysis and destruction of the joint.

## FAQ

- Q: Is chemotherapy or radiation therapy needed for chondroblastoma?
  - A: Chondroblastoma is a benign bone tumor so there is no need for chemotherapy or radiation therapy.
- Q: Is there any risk of getting a viral disease or hepatitis after curettage and bone grafting for a chondroblastoma?
  - A: In general, no risk exists. The graft materials are very safe in that all the cells and nonbone proteins are removed. The exception is fresh-frozen grafts, which have the same risk of viral transmission as a blood transfusion (~1 in 500,000).

# CHONDROSARCOMA

*Derek F. Papp, MD*
*Frank J. Frassica, MD*

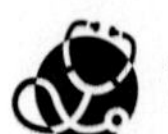

## BASICS

### DESCRIPTION

- This primary malignant tumor of bone consists of malignant chondrocytes (cartilage cells) and occurs inside a cartilage matrix.
- It most commonly affects the proximal femur, pelvic girdle, knee, and spine.
- It has a wide range of biologic behavior (1).
  - Low grade (grade 1): <5% risk of metastasis
  - Intermediate grade (grade 2): 20–30% risk of metastasis
  - Dedifferentiated (grades 3 and 4): 70% risk of metastasis
  - Mesenchymal: >50% risk of metastasis

### EPIDEMIOLOGY

#### *Incidence*

- Chondrosarcomas comprise 20% of all primary malignant bone tumors, occurring 1/2 as often as osteosarcoma (2).
- The tumor usually occurs in individuals in the 6th–8th decades of life.

### RISK FACTORS

- Multiple exostoses
- Ollier disease
- Maffucci syndrome

#### *Genetics*

- Not much is known.
- Numerous chromosomes have been implicated, including changes on chromosomes 2–11, 14, 15, and 21 (3).
- Patients with hereditary multiple exostoses and an EXT1 mutation are at higher risk than are patients with an EXT2 or EXT3 mutation.
- Myxoid chondrosarcoma is associated with a 9–22 chromosomal translocation (4).

### ETIOLOGY

- Most chondrosarcomas arise *de novo* (primary chondrosarcomas), whereas some arise in preexisting lesions (secondary chondrosarcomas).
- Secondary chondrosarcomas may arise in pre-existing lesions, such as in osteochondromas or the enchondromas in patients with Ollier disease and Maffucci syndrome.
- Dedifferentiated chondrosarcomas occur in 10% of patients (2) and are high-grade lesions.

### ASSOCIATED CONDITIONS

Multiple exostoses or enchondromatosis

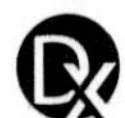

## DIAGNOSIS

### SIGNS AND SYMPTOMS

- The insidious presentation of deep pain often occurs over years to decades.
- Pain is somewhat relieved by NSAIDs or narcotic pain medication.
- A soft-tissue mass may be palpable in long-standing disease with soft-tissue extension.

#### *History*

- Physicians should have a high level of suspicion when:
  - Pain occurs at night.
  - Pain is unrelieved by rest.

#### *Physical Exam*

- Physical examination is not specific.
- Patients may have pain with deep palpation or a palpable soft-tissue mass.

### TESTS

#### *Lab*

Serum tests generally do not help establish the diagnosis.

#### *Imaging*

- Radiography:
  - Plain AP and lateral radiographs usually are diagnostic.
    - Chondrosarcoma usually is described as an intramedullary lesion with stippled and ring-like calcification.
    - Cortical bone changes usually are substantial: erosions, thickening, and bone destruction.
- Chest radiographs and CT scans usually are obtained in this age group because of the possibility of metastatic disease.
- MRI of the affected region is helpful for delineating soft-tissue extension and planning the biopsy site and the margins of resection.

#### *Pathological Findings*

- Histologically, it is difficult to differentiate between well-differentiated chondrosarcomas and chondromas (benign).
- The radiographic features are correlated with the histologic features to establish the degree of malignancy.
- Chondrosarcoma features include:
  - Permeation of the trabecular bone
  - Chondroblasts in a chondroid matrix
  - Lobular pattern of growth
  - Binucleate chondroblasts
  - Grades 1–3, based on the level of anaplasia

### DIFFERENTIAL DIAGNOSIS

- Enchondroma
- Bone infarct

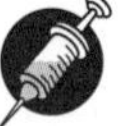

# TREATMENT

## GENERAL MEASURES

- Surgery is the mainstay of treatment.
- Chemotherapy and irradiation usually are not used.
- The goal of treatment is to minimize the chance of recurrence by resection of the entire lesion.
- For grade 1 tumors, resection and serial 6-month observation with plain radiographs are all that is necessary.
- Patients with grade 2 and 3 chondrosarcomas are followed with CT scans of the chest at 6-month intervals.
- At the 5-year disease-free interval, the frequency of clinic visits and repeated radiographs may be safely decreased.

## SPECIAL THERAPY

### *Physical Therapy*

Physical therapy is used for gait training and to regain ROM and strength.

## MEDICATION (DRUGS)

Patients who develop metastases are treated with chemotherapy, but unfortunately, no consistent benefit has been shown with this modality (3,5).

### *SURGERY*

- Wide resection involves removal of all diseased bone, with a cuff of normal tissue.
- The limb can be reconstructed using an allograft or a custom prosthesis.
- Muscle flaps are used as necessary to fill in soft-tissue defects.

# FOLLOW-UP

## PROGNOSIS

- Depends on the grade of the lesion:
  - Grade 1: Excellent (<5% incidence of metastasis)
  - Grade 2: Very good (<30% incidence of metastasis)
  - Grades 3 and 4:
    - Poor, >70% incidence of metastasis
    - In 1 study, the overall 5-year survival rate was 7.1%, and the median survival time was 7.5 months (5).
- Likewise, mesenchymal chondrosarcomas carry a poor prognosis.

## COMPLICATIONS

- Local recurrence
- Metastases in medium- and high-grade tumors
- Failure of reconstruction

## PATIENT MONITORING

Patients are followed at 1–3-month intervals until rehabilitation is complete.

## REFERENCES


1. Frassica FJ, Frassica DA, McCarthy EF, Jr. Orthopaedic pathology. In: Miller MD, ed. *Review of Orthopaedics*, 3rd ed. Philadelphia: WB Saunders, 2000:379–441.
2. Rosenberg A. Bone, joints, and soft tissue tumors. In: Cotran RS, Kumar V, Collins T, eds. *Robbins Pathologic Basis of Disease*, 6th ed. Philadelphia: WB Saunders, 1999:1215–1268.
3. Weber KL. What's new in musculoskeletal oncology. *J Bone Joint Surg* 2005;87A: 1400–1410.
4. Terek RM. Recent advances in the basic science of chondrosarcoma. *Orthop Clin North Am* 2006;37: 9–14.
5. Dickey ID, Rose PS, Fuchs B, et al. Dedifferentiated chondrosarcoma: the role of chemotherapy with updated outcomes. *J Bone Joint Surg* 2004;86A: 2412–2418.


## ADDITIONAL READING


Springfield DS, Bolander ME, Friedlaender GE, et al. Molecular and cellular biology of inflammation and neoplasia. In: Simon SR, ed. *Orthopaedic Basic Science*. Rosemont, IL: American Academy of Orthopaedic Surgeons, 1994:219–276.


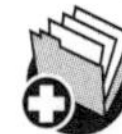

# MISCELLANEOUS

## CODES

### *ICD9-CM*

170.9 Primary bone neoplasm (malignant)

## PATIENT TEACHING

The patient should be told that this neoplasm requires correlation of histologic features with radiography for proper diagnosis and that surgery is the mainstay of treatment.

## FAQ

- Q: What is the most common symptom of chondrosarcoma?
  - A: Patients describe dull, achy pain that occurs at rest and at night.
- Q: How are chondrosarcomas treated?
  - A: Patients with chondrosarcoma are treated with wide surgical resection. Radiation therapy or chemotherapy plays no role in treatment.
- Q: What is the prognosis for patients with chondrosarcoma?
  - A: Patients with low-grade chondrosarcoma have an excellent prognosis, whereas patients with medium- and high-grade chondrosarcomas have a substantial risk of metastasis (20–30% and >50% respectively).

# CLAVICLE FRACTURES

*Henry Boateng, MD*
*James W. Wenz, Sr, MD*

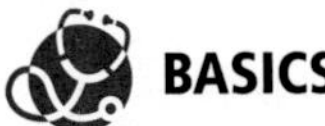

## BASICS

### DESCRIPTION
- The clavicle serves as the primary bony connection between the thorax and upper limb.
- A fracture of the clavicle also is known as a "broken collarbone."
- Classification:
  - By location in the clavicle: proximal, middle, or distal 1/3 (1)
- Fracture displacement and comminution are important factors.
- Clavicle fractures from high-energy trauma may be associated with ipsilateral scapula fractures and represent an unstable "floating shoulder."

### GENERAL PREVENTION
Avoidance of direct trauma to shoulder

### EPIDEMIOLOGY
- Distribution is trimodal:
  - Injury occurs in newborns secondary to birth trauma.
  - Fractures in adolescents and young adults is secondary to trauma.
  - Elderly patients sustain fractures secondary to osteoporosis and falls.

#### *Incidence*
- 1 of the most common fractures (2,3)
  - 5% involve the proximal 1/3 of the clavicle.
  - 70% the middle 1/3
  - 25% the distal 1/3

### RISK FACTORS
- Male gender
- Contact sports
- Large birth size (<4 kg) and older maternal age among newborns (4)
- High-energy trauma
- Falls among the elderly

### ETIOLOGY
- Primarily direct trauma to shoulder girdle
- In the adult, clavicle fractures typically result from sports or motor vehicle accidents and are caused by a direct blow to the shoulder.
- Clavicle fractures also can result from severe chest injuries with lung trauma or a dissociation of the shoulder complex from the rib cage.
- In the infant, these injuries frequently are related to difficult deliveries and can occur with brachial plexus palsy.

### ASSOCIATED CONDITIONS
- Subclavian vascular injury
- Brachial plexus injury
- Scapular fractures
- Shoulder fracture or dislocation
- Lung or rib injury
- Floating shoulder
- Ligamentous injury and disruption

## DIAGNOSIS

### SIGNS AND SYMPTOMS

#### *History*
The patient has a history of shoulder trauma, high-energy trauma, or a difficult birth.

#### *Physical Exam*
- Pain over the shoulder or clavicle
- Pain in ROM of the shoulder
- Deformity and swelling over the clavicle
- In children, refusal to move the extremity

### TESTS

#### *Imaging*
- If vascular injury is considered, obtain an arteriogram.
- Order a standard AP view of the clavicle and a view with the beam tilted 45° cephalad.
- If a shoulder disorder is suspected, then specific shoulder views, including an axillary view, are needed.
- If posterior displacement of proximal 1/3 fractures is suspected, obtain a CT scan.

#### *Pathological Findings*
- This fracture typically occurs in the middle 1/3 of the clavicle because of the bone's biomechanics and structure.
- The middle 1/3 of the clavicle experiences the largest bending moment with applied load to the shoulder and has the smallest cross-sectional area.

### DIFFERENTIAL DIAGNOSIS
- Clavicle fractures can be associated with other injuries, including pneumothorax, rib fractures, and humerus fractures.
- Posterior fracture displacement of medial fractures
- Shoulder–proximal humerus fracture or dislocation
- AC separation (tearing of the ligaments without fracture)
- AC joint arthrosis
- Rotator cuff disorders
- Pneumothorax or hemothorax
- Injury to the brachial plexus
- Injury to the great vessels
- Head injury
- Scapulothoracic dissociation
- Floating shoulder (fracture of the clavicle and scapula)

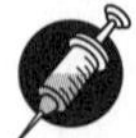

## TREATMENT

### INITIAL STABILIZATION
- Analgesics and sling immobilization
- Physical therapy for early ROM of the shoulder (Codman exercise)
- Most of these injuries can be managed nonoperatively.
- Most clavicle fractures do not require reduction maneuvers.
- Immobilization for 1 week in a sling and then gentle ROM of the shoulder are treatments of choice for most of these fractures.
- The patient should be referred to an orthopaedic surgeon if any question about treatment arises.
- Midclavicular fractures without large displacements or shortening can be treated with a sling.
- Posterior medial clavicle fractures must be evaluated for the possibility of airway compromise or concurrent injury.
  - May need immediate reduction by an orthopaedic surgeon.
- Because the medial growth physis does not close for the clavicle until the patient is ~21 years old, medial fractures in the young adult are typically Salter-Harris type II fractures and eventually remodel (5).

#### *Activity*
- The shoulder should be immobilized until comfortable, and then increasing ROM exercises should begin.
- Until tenderness resolves, limit lifting or overhead work.

#### *Nursing*
- With any shoulder injury, care should be taken that appropriate personal care of the armpit is taken.
  - Because of pain with abducting the shoulder, this area may be difficult to keep clean.

## SPECIAL THERAPY

### *Physical Therapy*

- Codman exercises should be instituted early in the course, using a pendulum-type movement of the shoulder with the trunk bent and supported.
- Passive ROM to the overhead position increases as the pain diminishes in several weeks.
- Strengthening exercises are used when pain resolves.

## MEDICATION (DRUGS)

- Analgesics should be prescribed as appropriate to the level of pain experienced.
- Narcotics may be required for pain relief.

## SURGERY

- Surgery may be needed for:
  - Displaced fractures in patients who are highly active or have jobs with overhead activity:
    - These patients may be unsatisfied with the deformity that will result from nonoperative treatment (6).
  - Comminuted or displaced midshaft fractures
  - Displaced fractures of the lateral 1/5 of the clavicle: Controversy exists as to the effectiveness of surgery (3)
  - Open fractures over the clavicle
  - Substantially displaced fractures with skin tenting
  - Nonunion of previous fractures
  - Floating shoulder
- The exact determinants for surgical intervention and the type of surgery are controversial (7).
- The most common treatment is open reduction and internal fixation with a plate and screws.
  - The plate may be placed superiorly, anteriorly, or anteroinferiorly.
  - Hardware irritation is common after surgery, requiring plate removal.
- Pin fixation is a less invasive alternative.
  - Threaded screws or titanium flexible nails may be used.
  - A serious complication of pin fixation is migration of the pin into the intrathoracic region.
  - Usually the pin must be removed after fracture healing.

## PROGNOSIS

- The prognosis is good for patients with minimally displaced fractures.
- Patients with displaced fractures develop a generally asymptomatic deformity from the fracture.
- Functional deficits are unusual but can occur with markedly displaced fractures.
- Return to full function should occur by 6–12 weeks.
- If the fracture has caused shortening or if a displaced distal clavicle fracture is present, problems with AC arthrosis or function may occur.

## COMPLICATIONS

- Skin breakdown over the fracture site
- Nonunion or malunion (may require future procedures to realign the bone and permit healing)
- Vascular injury
- Nerve injury
- Pneumothorax
- Residual pain

## PATIENT MONITORING

- Order serial radiographs at intervals of 3–4 weeks to monitor healing.
- Assess the skin carefully to ensure that it has not been compromised.
- Evaluate nerve and vascular function acutely and at follow-up intervals.

## REFERENCES


1. Robinson CM. Fractures of the clavicle in the adult. Epidemiology and classification. *J Bone Joint Surg* 1998;80B:476–484.
2. Robinson CM, Court-Brown CM, McQueen MM, et al. Estimating the risk of nonunion following nonoperative treatment of a clavicular fracture. *J Bone Joint Surg* 2004;86A:1359–1365.
3. Robinson CM, Cairns DA. Primary nonoperative treatment of displaced lateral fractures of the clavicle. *J Bone Joint Surg* 2004;86A:778–782.
4. Beall MH, Ross MG. Clavicle fracture in labor: risk factors and associated morbidities. *J Perinatol* 2001;21:513–515.
5. Salter RB, Harris WR. Injuries involving the epiphyseal plate. *J Bone Joint Surg* 1963;45A:587–622.
6. Nowak J, Holgersson M, Larsson S. Sequelae from clavicular fractures are common: a prospective study of 222 patients. *Acta Orthop* 2005;76:496–502.
7. Zlowodzki M, Zelle BA, Cole PA, et al. Treatment of acute midshaft clavicle fractures: systematic review of 2144 fractures: on behalf of the Evidence-Based Orthopaedic Trauma Working Group. *J Orthop Trauma* 2005;19:504–507.


## ADDITIONAL READING


Schmidt AH. Shoulder trauma. In: Baumgaertner MR, Tornetta P, III, eds. *Orthopaedic Knowledge Update: Trauma 3*. Rosemont, IL: American Academy of Orthopaedic Surgeons, 2005:151–161.


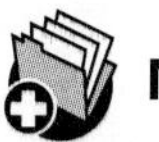

# MISCELLANEOUS

## CODES

### *ICD9-CM*

- 767.2 Clavicle fracture due to birth trauma
- 810.00 Interligamentous part clavicle fracture
- 810.01 Sternal end clavicle fracture
- 810.02 Mid shaft clavicle fracture
- 810.03 Acromial end clavicle fracture

## PATIENT TEACHING

- The physician should stress that residual bony deformity may occur after closed treatment.
- Functional limitation is unusual but may occur.

### *Activity*

Patients generally begin immediate pendulum exercises and gradually progress with ROM as tolerated.

## FAQ

- Q: How long does recovery take?
  - A: The average recovery is 4 months after injury. Some patients require >6 months to recover fully.
- Q: What factor increases the risk of late deformity or pain?
  - A: The amount of initial displacement corresponds best to ultimate outcome of closed treatment.

# CLAW TOES

*Clifford L. Jeng, MD*

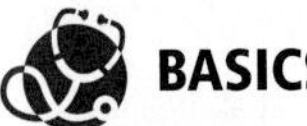

## BASICS

### DESCRIPTION

The term "claw toes" describes a hyperextension deformity of the MTP joint of the lesser toes with flexion deformity of the PIP joint (Fig. 1).

### GENERAL PREVENTION

Use of appropriate shoe wear (wide shoes with a high toe box) can prevent the development of claw toes in many cases.

### EPIDEMIOLOGY

#### *Incidence*

- Increases with advancing age
- Occurs more frequently in females than males (1).

#### *Genetics*

Patients with a hereditary motor sensory neuropathy as the cause of claw toes may have an autosomal dominant pattern of transmission.

### PATHOPHYSIOLOGY

- The most common cause is an imbalance between the intrinsic and extrinsic muscles of the foot.
  - Concurrent contracture of the long flexors and extensors of the toes without any balancing force from the intrinsic muscles
- Typically occurs secondary to underlying neurogenic or inflammatory conditions that lead to imbalance of the toe musculature and attenuation of the passive ligament restraints of the joints
- Can be idiopathic

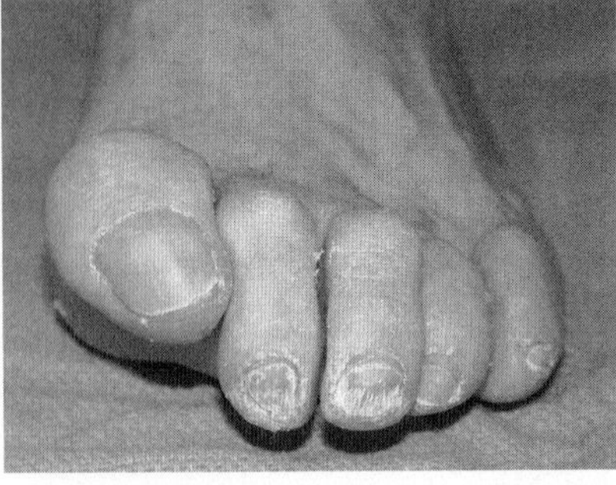

**Fig. 1.** Clinical photograph of claw toe deformity.

- Causative factors:
  - Tight shoe wear
  - Hallux valgus
  - Inflammatory arthropathy
  - Neuropathy
  - Diabetes mellitus
  - Hereditary sensorimotor neuropathies
  - Neuromuscular disease
  - Spasticity disorders
  - Compartment syndrome

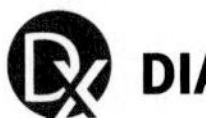

## DIAGNOSIS

### SIGNS AND SYMPTOMS

- Dorsal prominence of the PIP joint of the lesser toes
- Callosities and irritation of the overlying skin
- Pain over the dorsum of the toe or under the ball of the foot (metatarsalgia)
- Difficulty with shoe wear

#### *History*

- Patients may complain of unacceptable cosmetic appearance, difficulty with shoe wear, or a painful bursa over the dorsum of the PIP joint.
- With hyperextension of the MTP joint, the plantar fat pad subluxates distally and causes painful plantar calluses and possible ulcerations in insensate feet.

#### *Physical Exam*

- Often occurs in multiple adjacent digits, as well as bilaterally
- Often associated with cavus foot deformity
- The clinician should:
  - Manipulate the joints to determine whether the deformity is rigid or flexible
  - Perform a thorough neuromuscular exam
  - Test sensation of the foot

#### *Imaging*

Plain radiographs show subluxation of the MTP joints and flexion deformity of the PIP joint.

### DIFFERENTIAL DIAGNOSIS

- Other conditions have similar signs and symptoms but are not associated with hyperextension of the MTP joints:
  - Hammer toes
  - Mallet toes

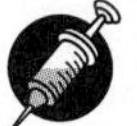

## TREATMENT

### GENERAL MEASURES

- A Budin splint may help correct flexible deformities.
- Silicone padding covering the toes may pad the symptomatic areas.
- Cushioned insoles can protect from painful metatarsalgia.
- Wide shoes with a high toe box can avoid painful rubbing of the claw toes.

### *Geriatric Considerations*
- This condition is very common in elderly females.
- If morbidities such as diabetes or peripheral vascular disease coexist, surgical management should be a last resort.

### *Pediatric Considerations*
Congenital curly toes may be present at birth and may require tendon releases at an early age.

### SURGERY
- For flexible deformities, a flexor-to-extensor tendon transfer can be performed to straighten the claw toe.
- Rigid deformities require release of the contracted MTP capsule and collateral ligaments, and extensor tendon release or lengthening.
- Claw toes with dislocation of the MTP joint are treated with oblique distal metatarsal osteotomy to achieve bony shortening and reduce the MTP joint (2,3).
- Rigid PIP joint contractures are corrected with partial phalangectomy or PIP joint fusion.

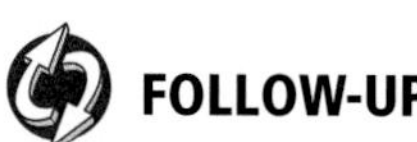

## FOLLOW-UP

### *Issues for Referral*
- Persistent pain not relieved by nonoperative care:
  - Inability to wear shoes
  - Overlying skin ulceration or impending ulceration in patients with neuropathy

### PROGNOSIS
Claw toes usually are progressive, worsening in pain and deformity over time.

### COMPLICATIONS
- Complications of surgical treatment include:
  - Stiffness
  - Wound infection
  - Persistent pain
  - Failure to correct deformity adequately
  - Recurrence of deformity

### REFERENCES

1. Coughlin MJ. Lesser toe abnormalities. *Instr Course Lect* 2003;52:421–444.
2. Hofstaetter SG, Hofstaetter JG, Petroutsas JA, et al. The Weil osteotomy: a seven-year follow-up. *J Bone Joint Surg* 2005;87B:1507–1511.
3. Trnka HJ, Muhlbauer M, Zettl R, et al. Comparison of the results of the Weil and Helal osteotomies for the treatment of metatarsalgia secondary to dislocation of the lesser MTP joints. *Foot Ankle Int* 1999;20:72–79.


### ADDITIONAL READING

- Barbari SG, Brevig K. Correction of clawtoes by the Girdlestone-Taylor flexor-extensor transfer procedure. *Foot Ankle* 1984;5:67–73.
- Barouk LS. [Weil's metatarsal osteotomy in the treatment of metatarsalgia]. *Orthopade* 1996;25:338–344.
- Mizel MS, Yodlowski ML. Disorders of the lesser MTP joints. *J Am Acad Orthop Surg* 1995;3:166–173.
- Myerson MS, Shereff MJ. The pathological anatomy of claw and hammer toes. *J Bone Joint Surg* 1989;71A:45–49.
- Taylor RG. The treatment of claw toes by multiple transfers of flexor into extensor tendons. *J Bone Joint Surg* 1951;33B:539–542.


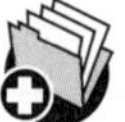

## MISCELLANEOUS

### CODES
### *ICD9-CM*
735.5 Claw toe

### PATIENT TEACHING
- Many splints and pads can be obtained at local drugstores in the foot care section.
- Medical supply stores may have a wider selection of orthoses.

### *Prevention*
Avoidance of narrow, tight-fitting shoes is the best way to prevent the development of claw toes.

### FAQ
- Q: What differentiates claw toes from hammer toes?
  - A: Claw toes involve flexion contractures of the distal and PIP joints along with hyperextension of the MTP joint. Hammer toes involve isolated PIP flexion deformity.
- Q: What is the most common underlying etiology of claw toes?
  - A: Neurologic disorders cause atrophy or weakness of the intrinsic muscles of the foot. These conditions lead to relative imbalance between the intrinsic and extrinsic muscles, leading in turn to flexion deformities of the IP joints and hyperextension of the MTP joint. Claw toes commonly are seen in conditions such as diabetes (neuropathy), spinal disorders, stroke, paralysis, and spasticity disorders, and in hereditary motor sensory neuropathies such as Charcot-Marie-Tooth disease.

# CLINODACTYLY

*John J. Hwang, MD*
*Dawn M. LaPorte, MD*

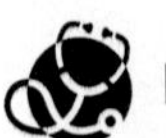

## BASICS

### DESCRIPTION
- Clinodactyly presents as a painless bent finger with angulation in a radial or ulnar direction (Fig. 1).
- It is most commonly the little finger bent in a radial direction.
- Most often, the finger has a short, delta-shaped middle phalanx.
- This condition may be associated with mental retardation, especially when clinodactyly is severe.
- Synonym: Bent finger

### GENERAL PREVENTION
No evidence suggests that the deformity may be prevented or its natural history changed by intervention.

### EPIDEMIOLOGY
- Detected at birth
- More common in males, in whom it is usually bilateral

#### *Incidence*
1–19.5% in otherwise normal children; least common in Caucasians (1)

### RISK FACTORS
- In children with Down syndrome, the incidence of clinodactyly is 35–70% (1).
- It also is seen in children with many other syndromes, especially Kline-Felter and trisomy 18.

#### *Genetics*
- The condition is autosomal dominant, with variable expressivity.
- Some cases are sporadic.

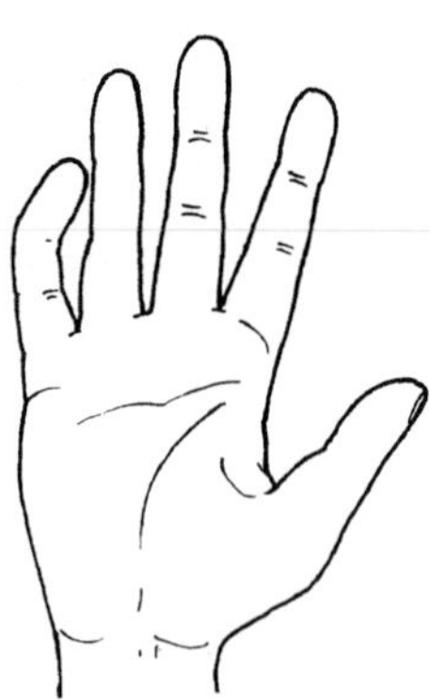

**Fig. 1.** Clinodactyly refers to bony angulation of a finger, usually the 5th.

### ETIOLOGY
Abnormal shape of the underlying phalanx develops as a result of asymmetrical longitudinal growth.

### ASSOCIATED CONDITIONS
- Symphalangism
- Brachydactyly (short fingers)
- Trisomies
- Treacher Collins syndrome
- Silver syndrome
- Holt-Oram syndrome
- Prader-Willi syndrome

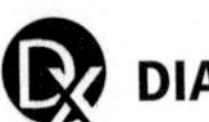

## DIAGNOSIS

### SIGNS AND SYMPTOMS
- The finger (usually the little finger) is curved in a radial or ulnar direction.
- Deviation can occur at the PIP joint, middle phalanx, or DIP joint (Fig. 1).
- It is most common in the DIP joint.
- This condition is painless.

#### *Physical Exam*
- The angle of deviation of a finger at the PIP joint, the middle phalanx, or the DIP joint should be measured.
- Active and passive motion at each joint should be recorded.
- The remainder of the skeleton also should be inspected.

### TESTS

#### *Lab*
Chromosome analysis should be undertaken if an underlying syndrome is suspected.

#### *Imaging*
- Conventional plain radiography of the affected finger is recommended, especially when considering surgical correction.
- $<10°$ of angulation is within normal limits (2).

#### *Pathological Findings*
Maldevelopment of 1 of the phalanges causes an angulation of the joint surface.

### DIFFERENTIAL DIAGNOSIS
- Delta phalanx (a wedge-shaped phalanx with a sloped joint surface)
- Malunion after fractures

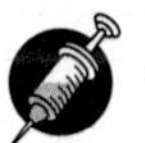

## TREATMENT

### GENERAL MEASURES
- Most cases are cosmetic problems.
- Slight deformity does not need surgical correction.
- Because nonoperative treatment, including manipulation and casting, usually is futile, and patients find such modalities difficult to tolerate, treatment choices are no intervention or surgery.
- Surgical correction can be considered for substantial deformity persisting after the age of 6 years.
- Surgical procedures are elective because the problem is mainly cosmetic.

#### *Activity*
No restrictions on activity

### SPECIAL THERAPY

#### *Physical Therapy*

Therapy may be helpful for regaining motion after surgery.

### SURGERY

- Surgical procedures include osteotomy and growth plate reconstruction with a free-fat graft.
- For a child <6 years old, a fat-graft placement should be performed after resection of the midportion of the continuous epiphysis and underlying physis (growth plate).
- After age 6, a simple closing osteotomy can be done easily and with few complications.

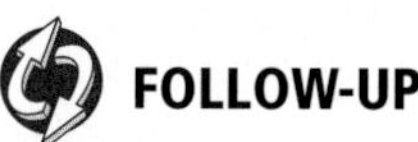

## FOLLOW-UP

### PROGNOSIS

The prognosis is good, with no evidence of degenerative joint disease.

### PATIENT MONITORING

Patients may monitor the angulation of the finger and return for surgical treatment if it becomes unacceptable.

### REFERENCES

1. Flatt AE. Crooked fingers. In: *The Care of Congenital Hand Anomalies*. St. Louis: Quality Medical Publishing, Inc., 1994:196–227.
2. Dudding BA, Gorlin RJ, Langer LO. The oto-palato-digital syndrome. A new symptom-complex consisting of deafness, dwarfism, cleft palate, characteristic facies, and a generalized bone dysplasia. *Am J Dis Child* 1967;113:214–221.

### ADDITIONAL READING

McCombe D, Kay SP. Deformities of the hand and fingers. Clinodactyly. In: Green DP, Hotchkiss RN, Pederson WC, et al., eds. *Green's Operative Hand Surgery*, 5th ed. Philadelphia: Elsevier Churchill Livingstone, 2005;1431–1434.

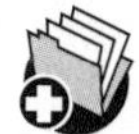

## MISCELLANEOUS

### CODES

#### *ICD9-CM*

759.59 Clinodactyly

### PATIENT TEACHING

Educating patients about the excellent prognosis and benign nature of the condition is helpful.

### FAQ

- Q: Is splinting helpful?
  - A: No. The deformity can be corrected only by surgical intervention.
- Q: Is surgery recommended for all patients?
  - A: No. Most patients do not have a functional deficit. Surgery for cosmetic improvement alone should be avoided because of the risks of scarring and stiffness.
- Q: How is clinodactyly different from camptodactyly?
  - A: Clinodactyly is angulation of the digit in a radioulnar plane distal to the MCP joint, versus camptodactyly, which is angulation in an AP plane.
- Q: What is the preferred treatment for clinodactyly?
  - A: No treatment is required for mild to moderate clinodactyly. More severe clinodactyly requires realignment of the digit through osteotomy.

# CLUBFOOT

*Paul D. Sponseller, MD*

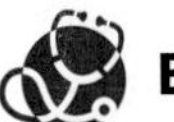

## BASICS

### DESCRIPTION

- Clubfoot, or *talipes equinovarus*, is a complex deformity seen at birth.
- It can be divided into 3 elements (1–4):
  - Equinus of the heel
  - Varus and internal rotation of the hindfoot
  - Adductus of the forefoot
- *Equinus* ("horse") is used to describe a plantarflexed position because horses walk with their heels in complete plantarflexion, and *varus* ("turned in") refers to the adducted component.
- The affected child thus bears weight along the lateral part of the foot, rather than on the sole.
- Clubfoot can be divided into 2 categories:
  - An isolated, idiopathic type
  - Associated with other congenital deformities (amniotic band syndrome, arthrogryposis, myelodysplasia, diastrophic dwarfism, Larson syndrome, Freeman-Sheldon syndrome):
    - These clubfeet have a tendency to be more severe and refractory to nonoperative therapy and more often require surgical correction.
    - The talar neck is deviated medially and in a plantar direction.
    - The foot is smaller than normal, and shortening, usually <1 cm compared with the contralateral, normal side, may occur.

### EPIDEMIOLOGY

#### Incidence

- ~1 of every 1,000 births (1)
- Male:Female ratio: ~2:1

### RISK FACTORS

- A parent with the disorder
- A sibling with the disorder
- Presence of other disorders associated with clubfoot, including:
  - Amniotic band syndrome
  - Arthrogryposis
  - Myelodysplasia
  - Mobius syndrome
  - Freeman-Sheldon syndrome
  - Larsen syndrome
  - Diastrophic dwarfism
- Drugs, such as aminopterin, taken during pregnancy

#### Genetics

- The disorder is widely believed to be polygenic with variable penetrance.
- If a child has a clubfoot, a 2–6% chance exists that the next sibling will have the disorder (1).
- If a parent has clubfoot, a 10% chance exists that each child will inherit the disorder (1).

### ETIOLOGY

The more common isolated, idiopathic form is thought to be of a genetic origin, although the genetic basis has not been identified.

### ASSOCIATED CONDITIONS

Other congenital deformities (see conditions discussed earlier)

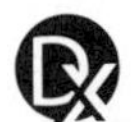

## DIAGNOSIS

### SIGNS AND SYMPTOMS

- Signs and symptoms of clubfoot are related to the findings on physical examination.
  - In general, the newborn's foot looks excessively turned inward.
  - In older children, uncorrected clubfeet may cause gait disturbances, problems with shoe fit, and painful callosities along the lateral border of the foot.
- The patient may be forced to walk on the dorsum (top) of the foot.
- Pain within the foot may develop in the older child or adult.

#### Physical Exam

- The physical examination reveals equinus of the heel, supination or varus of the hindfoot, and adductus of the midfoot and forefoot (2), which creates a foot described as "kidney shaped," with a prominent medial crease along the plantar aspect of the foot.
- The foot projects medially from the leg and resembles a club (Figs. 1 and 2).
- Check the flexibility of the foot and the correctability of its position.
- Verify the function of the ankle and toe muscles.
- Check for calf hypoplasia, which is a typical feature.

### TESTS

#### Imaging

- In routine care, radiographs may be unnecessary unless a suspicion exists for underlying bony fusion or if surgery is contemplated.
- Simulated standing AP and lateral views are most important.
  - Because of the deformity caused by clubfoot, these views may be difficult to take and may require multiple attempts.
  - The foot should be corrected to a position as close to neutral as possible and held in this position with a Plexiglas plate.
- The AP view:
  - The forefoot is noted to be in adduction.
  - In a normal foot:
    - The talus aligns roughly with the first metatarsal, and the calcaneus aligns roughly with the 5th metatarsal.
    - The angle thus formed between the axes of these 2 bones is the anterior talocalcaneal angle, or Kite angle.
    - Normal range for this angle is 20–40°.
  - In clubfoot:
    - The axes of the calcaneus and talus are nearly parallel, and thus the angle is much smaller.
- Lateral view:
  - The position of the foot is in equinus.
  - In a normal foot, the talocalcaneal angle is 35–50°.
  - In a clubfoot, that angle is considerably smaller because the 2 bones are nearly parallel in all planes.
- The assessment of these radiographic abnormalities in a clubfoot is used to determine whether a correction is acceptable after any method of correction.

#### Pathological Findings

- The essential bony change is medial deviation of the talar neck with subluxation of the talonavicular joint.
- Histologic study also has revealed smaller muscle fibers than normal on cross-section.
- Increased thickness of fascia and joint capsules is present on the medial side of the foot.

### DIFFERENTIAL DIAGNOSIS

- The differential diagnosis of clubfoot is limited because of the dramatic and characteristic appearance of this deformity.
- Some cases of metatarsus adductus varus are so severe that they are confused with clubfoot, but the equinus component of clubfoot is absent in metatarsus adductus, and the distinction should be easily made.

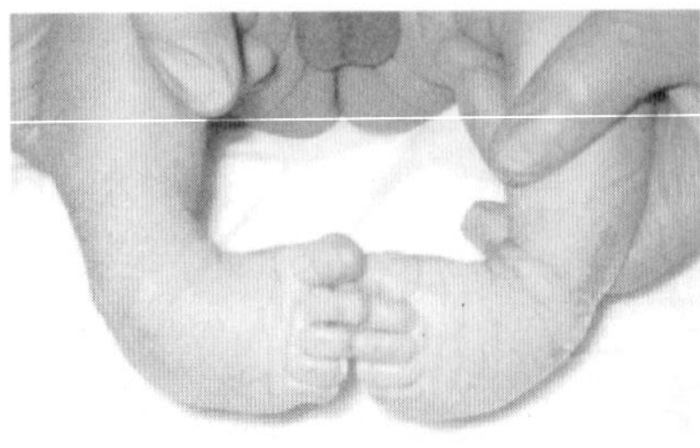

**Fig. 1.** Bilateral clubfeet in a newborn.

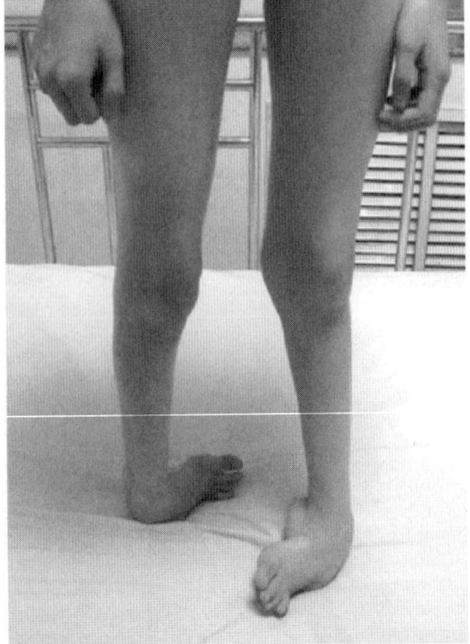

**Fig. 2.** Untreated clubfeet in a 9-year-old.

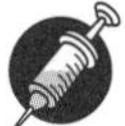

## TREATMENT

### GENERAL MEASURES

- The 1st step in management of clubfoot is taping or casting.
  - Should be started as soon as possible after birth
  - Can correct a clubfoot deformity and (for the most part) help restore normal function; it is most successful in mild cases.
  - Procedure:
    - The heel is firmly stabilized, the forefoot is brought laterally out of adductus, the foot is dorsiflexed, and the heel is externally rotated into valgus.
    - This position allows the tight tendons to stretch so that additional correction may be obtained the next time.
    - Adhesive tape or a cast from above the knee to the toes (Fig. 3) (sometimes known as the "Ponseti method") (1–3) is applied to hold the foot in this position, which essentially corrects all 3 components of clubfoot.
    - During the immediate postnatal term, the cast or taping is changed every few days; after the 1st week, the tapings are changed once to twice weekly in the office, until the position of the foot is acceptable or improvement has ceased.
  - By ~8 weeks of age, the child's foot and leg are large enough that an above-the-knee cast may be applied with the foot in the corrected position.
  - Occasionally, an Achilles tenotomy is needed.
  - After the foot is corrected (which may take 2–3 months), it should be held with reverse shoes and a Denis Browne bar between the legs full-time for 2 months and at night and nap times for 2–4 years.

### SPECIAL THERAPY

#### *Physical Therapy*

- Some clinicians believe that certain stretching exercises, particularly of the heel cord and medial ankle structures, may be of some benefit, but exercises alone usually are not sufficient.
- These exercises are most beneficial in maintaining the correction obtained by cast treatment.

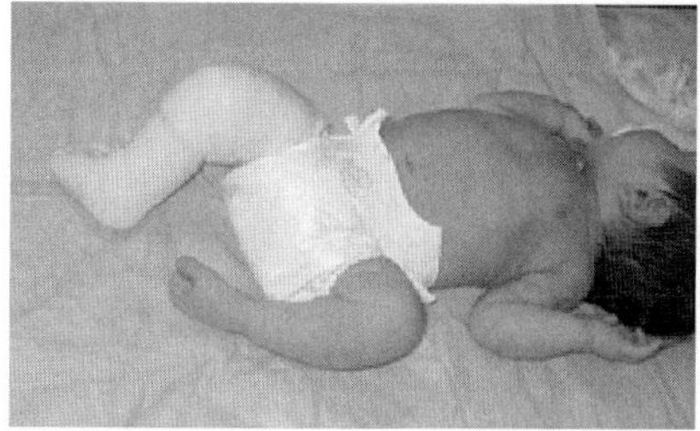

**Fig. 3.** Above-the-knee corrective cast for clubfoot.

### MEDICATION (DRUGS)

#### *First Line*

The drug botulinum toxin shows promise in combination with casting and splinting.

### SURGERY

- If cast treatment fails, surgery is needed.
  - Surgery is best performed when the child is 4–8 months old.
  - The general principle involves:
    - Releasing the tight medial structures by lengthening the flexor tendons and the PTT
    - Releasing the posterior structures by transecting the posterior joint capsule and lengthening the Achilles tendon
  - A more extensive release may be required.
  - The calcaneus also can be repositioned laterally, and a more complete correction can be achieved.
  - Pins are placed (and remain for 6 weeks) to help stabilize the correction.
- About 10–20% of children require repeat surgery in later years (4).

## FOLLOW-UP

### DISPOSITION

#### *Issues for Referral*

The patient should be referred to an orthopaedic surgeon who has expertise in treating clubfoot.

### PROGNOSIS

- Adequate treatment, whether nonoperative or surgical, likely will eliminate the positional deformity and enable to patient to ambulate adequately on the affected foot.
- Certain elements of the deformity, such as the small size of the foot, the calf hypoplasia, and the minimal shortening, cannot be corrected, but these rarely have a large effect on the patient's functional ability.

### COMPLICATIONS

- Residual deformity
- Rocker-bottom foot
- Overcorrection into valgus
- Stiffness
- Pain in later childhood or adulthood

### PATIENT MONITORING

- Children need regular follow-up care for several years to monitor for recurrence.
- Idiopathic clubfoot may recur up to age 6–7 years.
- Most recurrences occur in the 1st few years, and may be treated with repeat casting.

### REFERENCES


1. Ponseti IV. The Ponseti technique for correction of congenital clubfoot [letter]. *J Bone Joint Surg* 2002;84A:1889–1890.
2. Morcuende JA, Abbasi D, Dolan LA, et al. Results of an accelerated Ponseti protocol for clubfoot. *J Pediatr Orthop* 2005;25:623–626.
3. Morcuende JA. Congenital idiopathic clubfoot: prevention of late deformity and disability by conservative treatment with the Ponseti technique. *Pediatr Ann* 2006;35:128–136.
4. Vitale MG, Choe JC, Vitale MA, et al. Patient-based outcomes following clubfoot surgery: a 16-year follow-up study. *J Pediatr Orthop* 2005;25:533–538.


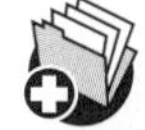

## MISCELLANEOUS

### CODES

#### *ICD9-CM*

754.51 Clubfoot

### PATIENT TEACHING

- Clubfeet tend to be slightly shorter and less supple than normal feet.
- Parents should be reassured that adequately corrected clubfeet have good long-term function.
- Parents also must monitor for signs of recurrence.

### FAQ

- Q: Will a child with a clubfoot be able to participate in sports?
  - A: With appropriate treatment, most children should be able to participate.

# COMPARTMENT SYNDROME

*Brett M. Cascio, MD*

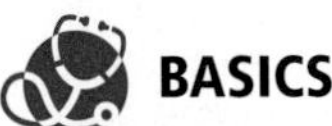

## BASICS

### DESCRIPTION
- Increase in tissue pressure within a limited space, compromising circulation and function of the contents of the space (1)
- Acute compartment syndrome is a limb-threatening emergency.
- Chronic (or exercise-induced or exertional) compartment syndrome usually is a self-limited symptomatic disorder.
- The elevated tissue pressure causes decreased perfusion, which can lead to necrosis of tissues and nerves within the enclosed space, with resulting ischemic contracture, paresis, numbness, or loss of the involved limb.
- Depending on the amount of muscle death (rhabdomyolysis), myoglobinuria, acute tubular necrosis, hyperkalemia, and kidney failure can occur.

### GENERAL PREVENTION
- A high index of suspicion is needed, especially in dealing with patients with obtunded sensorium because of trauma or pharmacologic agents, or in children in whom the history and physical examinations often are unreliable.
- Although most cases involve the legs and forearms, compartment syndromes in the thigh, hand, foot, arm, and buttock are well recognized.

### EPIDEMIOLOGY
#### *Incidence*
- 1–5% of all tibia fractures (2)
- 0.25% of distal radius fractures (2)
- 3% of forearm fracture (2)
- Up to 10% of displaced calcaneus fractures (2)

### RISK FACTORS
- Trauma, especially high-energy trauma
- Crush injury
- Prolonged unconsciousness (dependant position)
  - Anesthesia
  - Drug overdose
- Decreased mental status
- Young adult males with tibia or forearm fractures
- Displaced pediatric supracondylar humerus fractures
- Long surgical procedures
- Fractures or osteotomies
- Ischemic injuries, especially after reperfusion
- Soft-tissue trauma: Crush, contusion, snake bite
- Casts, dressings
- Tight surgical closures
- Burns
- Infiltration of intravenous fluids
- Intracompartmental hemorrhage
- Antishock trousers
- Intraosseous infusion in neonates

### PATHOPHYSIOLOGY
Local blood flow does not meet metabolic demand of tissues, leading to necrosis.

### ETIOLOGY
- Can result from any cause of increased intracompartmental pressures
- External compression from:
  - Casts
  - Positioning
- Hemorrhage from:
  - Fractures:
    - After manipulation
    - Open or closed
  - Arterial or venous injury
  - Blunt trauma
- Crush injury leading to muscle bleeding, massive cell death, and subsequent extravasation of cytoplasmic fluid
- Reperfusion injury after vascular repair
- Iatrogenic (see "Risk Factors")

### ASSOCIATED CONDITIONS
- Coagulopathy
- Altered mental state

## DIAGNOSIS

### SIGNS AND SYMPTOMS
- Classically, the 5 P's (pain, pallor, paresthesia, paralysis, and pulselessness)
- A high index of suspicion is necessary.
- Clinical signs in children and obtunded patients are not reliable.

#### *History*
- Pain out of proportion to injury:
  - Increase in need for pain medication
  - Once nerves die, pain may not be present.
  - Absence of pain in the presence of compartment syndrome is a late finding and a poor prognostic indicator.
- Numbness or tingling (paresthesias)

#### *Physical Exam*
- Note mental status.
- Assess vital signs, especially diastolic blood pressure.
- Perform motor examination.
- Perform sensory examination.
  - Hand compartment syndrome has no loss of sensation because the nerves are subcutaneous.
- Assess tenseness of compartment.
  - Compartments may be palpably tense.
  - Tenseness of the deep compartment of the leg is difficult to assess.
- Note pain with passive stretch of the muscles traversing the compartment.
- Assess for asymmetry of pulses (pulselessness is late finding).

### TESTS
- Measurement of compartment pressures
- Sterile procedure:
  - Leg: Anterior, lateral, and superficial and deep posterior compartments
  - Thigh: Anterior, posterior, medial
  - Hand: Thenar, hypothenar, interossei, adductor pollicis, carpal tunnel
  - Foot: Lateral, medial, central, intrinsic
  - Forearm: Volar, dorsal, mobile wad
  - Fingers: Clinical examination
  - Arm: Anterior and posterior, deltoid muscle
  - Buttock: Gluteus maximus
- Compartment pressure of 40 mm Hg or within 30 mm Hg of the diastolic pressure requires surgical compartment decompression.
- Recheck every few hours if needed.
- Check near fracture.
- Chronic compartment syndrome shows increased tissue pressure at rest and/or prolonged elevation of pressure after exercise.

#### *Lab*
- Basic metabolic panel/Chem 7
  - Look for hyperkalemia from muscle death.
- Serial creatine phosphokinase if the clinician suspects substantial muscle death
- Urine for myoglobin
- Hematocrit to monitor blood loss into thigh
- Routine preoperative laboratory tests

#### *Imaging*
Routine radiographs to evaluate skeletal trauma

#### *Pathological Findings*
- Bulging muscle through fasciotomy
- Tissue necrosis if diagnosis is delayed

### DIFFERENTIAL DIAGNOSIS
- Arterial occlusion (also characterized by pain and pallor):
  - Pulselessness
  - No immediate increase in compartment pressure.
- Neurapraxia (no increase in pressure or tenseness)

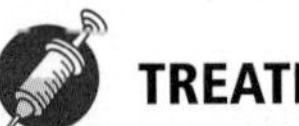

## TREATMENT

### GENERAL MEASURES
- Patients suspected of developing a compartment syndrome should have the compartment pressure monitored.
- Immediate splitting or removal of a cast or tight dressing
- For patients under surveillance for a suspected developing compartment syndrome, place limb at the level of the heart.
- Compartment syndrome is a surgical emergency requiring surgical decompression or fasciotomy to avoid additional complications.

### *Activity*
Bed rest if a compartment syndrome is suspected

### *Nursing*
Frequent neurovascular checks

## SPECIAL THERAPY

### *Physical Therapy*
Postoperative physical therapy varies, depending on soft-tissue and bony injury.

## MEDICATION (DRUGS)

### *First Line*
- Consider alkalizing urine and giving fluids to minimize renal damage if myoglobinuria is present.
- Treat hyperkalemia, if present.

### *Second Line*
- May require treatment for underlying cause of compartment syndrome:
  - Anticoagulation for DVT
  - Antibiotics for open fracture

## SURGERY
- In general, fascial tissues enveloping the affected compartment are opened in a longitudinal fashion, thereby decompressing the enclosed space and allowing tissue expansion and better perfusion.
- The wound then is left open, and delayed primary closure or skin grafting is done at a later date.
- Postoperative dressings can be moistened gauze or vacuum-assisted closure dressings.
- During the immediate postoperative period, the involved limb should be elevated to minimize swelling.
- Leg:
  - 1 lateral (for the anterior and lateral compartment) and 1 medial (for the deep and superficial posterior compartments) skin incision
- Thigh:
  - 1 lateral skin incision
  - Release the anterior compartment.
  - Release the posterior compartment if needed through the same incision.
  - Use a medial skin incision for the medial compartment as necessary.
- Hand:
  - 2 dorsal incisions, over the 2nd and 4th metacarpals
  - 2 palmar incisions, 1 over the thenar compartment, and 1 for carpal tunnel.
  - 1 incision for hypothenar compartment as needed
- Forearm:
  - Release the volar compartment with lazy-S incision.
  - This incision can be extended to release the carpal tunnel.
  - Can release dorsally, but usually not necessary
- Foot:
  - Release with medial incision.
  - Add 2 dorsal incisions as necessary, over the 2nd and 4th metatarsals.
- Arm:
  - Medial incision, especially if exploration of vessels is necessary
- Fingers:
  - Release ulnarly for the 2nd and 3rd digits, radially for the 4th and 5th digits.
- Gluteus:
  - Release with 1 incision over the gluteus maximus.

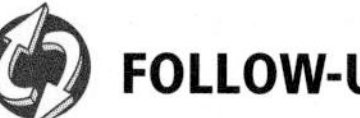

# FOLLOW-UP

## DISPOSITION

### *Issues for Referral*
- Prosthetic referral for limb loss
- Referral for orthotic splints such as ankle-foot orthosis for foot drop
- Occupational therapy for treatment of hand weakness, specialized splints
- Physical therapy for regaining strength and mobility
- Plastic surgery for wound issues

## PROGNOSIS
- In general, complications can be minimized with rapid diagnosis and fasciotomy.
- Fasciotomies are not benign procedures.
  - They can leave large, painful scars, especially if they cannot be closed primarily.
  - Chronic venous stasis can develop (3).
- Paresis does not usually improve.
- Numbness usually does not improve.

## COMPLICATIONS
- Motor deficit:
  - Weakness or paresis
  - Foot drop
  - Volkmann contracture
- Sensory deficits:
  - Complications, such as ulcers, infections, and burns, secondary to an insensate limb
- Kidney failure from rhabdomyolysis
- Infection from fasciotomy with necrotic muscle
- Chronic venous stasis
- Loss of limb
- Reflex sympathetic dystrophy

## PATIENT MONITORING
- Intraoperatively, compartment pressure can be measured after fasciotomy to confirm that the compartment has been decompressed appropriately.
- After closure, monitoring for redevelopment of compartment syndrome is important.

## REFERENCES

1. Matsen FA, III. A practical approach to compartmental syndromes. Part I. Definition, theory, and pathogenesis. *Instr Course Lect* 1983;32:88–92.
2. McQueen MM, Gaston P, Court-Brown CM. Acute compartment syndrome. Who is at risk? *J Bone Joint Surg* 2000;82B:200–203.
3. Fitzgerald AM, Gaston P, Wilson Y, et al. Long-term sequelae of fasciotomy wounds. *Br J Plast Surg* 2000;53:690–693.


## ADDITIONAL READING

- Archdeacon, MT. Knee and leg: bone trauma. In: Vaccaro AR, ed. *Orthopaedic Knowledge Update 8*. Rosemont, IL: American Academy of Orthopaedic Surgeons, 2005:433–441.
- Kostler W, Strohm PC, Sudkamp NP. Acute compartment syndrome of the limb. *Injury* 2004;35:1221–1227.
- Olson SA, Rhorer AS. Orthopaedic trauma for the general orthopaedist: avoiding problems and pitfalls in treatment. *Clin Orthop Relat Res* 2005;433: 30–37.




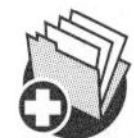

# MISCELLANEOUS

## CODES

### *ICD9-CM*
958.8 Compartment syndrome

## PATIENT TEACHING
- The patient must be informed about the need for subsequent delayed primary closure or skin grafting.
- Inform the patient of the risk for weakness, numbness, and loss of limb.
- For high-risk orthopaedic procedures, such as tibial nailing and high tibial osteotomy, patients must be advised of the risk of compartment syndrome and the possible need for fasciotomy.

### *Activity*
Activity depends on the underlying injury.

### *Prevention*
- Repositioning patients during long procedures in the operating room
- Care with applying casts and dressings
- Monitoring fluid extravasation with arthroscopy or pulsatile lavage
- High index of suspicion

## FAQ
- Q: How can you have tissue ischemia with palpable pulses?
  - A: The elevated tissue pressure causes an increase in venous pressure. The capillary bed blood flow loses its flow gradient, and flow through the capillary bed can decrease to the point where it does not meet metabolic demand. Arterial pressure usually is greater than the elevated tissue pressure; flow is maintained through the compartment and can be felt as a pulse.
- Q: Can compartment syndrome develop with an open fracture?
  - A: Yes. Open fractures alone do not decompress a compartment and are often high-energy, crushing-type injuries.
- Q: What is the most common symptom of compartment syndrome?
  - A: Pain out of proportion to the injury.

# COMPARTMENT SYNDROME OF THE FOOT

*Clifford L. Jeng, MD*

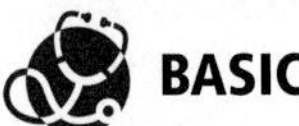

## BASICS

### DESCRIPTION

Compartment syndrome of the foot occurs when bleeding and interstitial edema in the muscle compartments of the foot cause a substantial decrease in capillary perfusion, resulting in myoneural ischemia and eventual necrosis.

### GENERAL PREVENTION

Prevention of the long-term sequelae of compartment syndrome requires a high level of suspicion for the diagnosis.

### EPIDEMIOLOGY

#### *Incidence*

Occurs in up to 17% of patients with calcaneus fracture (1)

### PATHOPHYSIOLOGY

- Blood flow ceases when local tissue pressure exceeds diastolic blood pressure.
- Tissue ischemia develops.
- Myoneural necrosis results, with long-term sequelae of pain, paresthesias, stiffness, claw toes, and foot deformity.

### ETIOLOGY

- Frequently occurs with calcaneus fracture, midfoot/forefoot fractures, or crush injury of the foot (1,2)
- May occur with open foot injuries

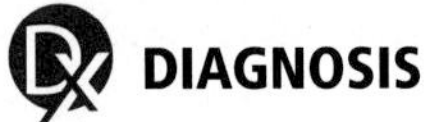

## DIAGNOSIS

### SIGNS AND SYMPTOMS

- Severe pain
- Massive swelling
- Pain with passive stretching of the toes
- Diminished sensation or pulses less reliable

#### *Imaging*

Plain radiographs of the foot and ankle are necessary for diagnosing fractures or dislocations that may be causing the massive swelling.

#### *Diagnostic Procedures/Surgery*

- Invasive pressure measurement of the foot compartments is helpful for diagnosing compartment syndrome.
- Needle insertion sites for compartment pressure monitoring:
  - Medial (abductor) compartment: Directly inferior to the 1st metatarsal
  - Deep compartment: Advance the needle from the medial compartment ~1 cm deeper under the arch of the foot
  - Interosseous compartment: Dorsal foot between the 3rd and 4th metatarsals
  - Lateral compartment: Plantar to the 5th metatarsal
- Compartment syndrome commonly is defined as compartment pressure >30 mm Hg (2,3).

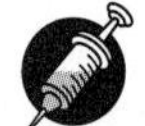

## TREATMENT

### INITIAL STABILIZATION

No circumferential bandages should be applied to the area while monitoring for possible compartment syndrome because doing so may worsen the condition.

### GENERAL MEASURES

- A pneumatic foot pump often is useful in decreasing foot swelling early after trauma (4).
- Oral or intravenous diuretics may help reduce edema.
- If compartment syndrome is suspected, invasive pressure measurements of the compartments should be performed.
- Early fasciotomy is the most reliable way to avoid the complications of compartment syndrome.
  - Future fixation of these fractures must be considered when selecting the fasciotomy approach.

#### *Activity*

If massive swelling is present, a patient should be kept at bed rest with the foot at heart level.

#### *Nursing*

- Vigilant monitoring of the patient with a traumatic foot injury is necessary; worsening or unremitting pain should prompt request for evaluation by physician.
- Frequent testing of the foot for pain with passive stretching of the toes
- If any change in the condition of the foot occurs, the physician should be called to check invasive pressure measurements.

### SPECIAL THERAPY

#### *Physical Therapy*

Stretching exercises and desensitization may be useful in a patient who has long-term sequelae of foot compartment syndrome.

### SURGERY

- Perform fasciotomy (compartment release):
  - Surgical emergency once diagnosis is made
  - Standard technique (5,6):
    - 2 dorsal incisions over the 2nd and 4th metatarsals to release adjacent interosseous spaces and lateral abductor compartment
    - Medial arch incision to release abductor hallucis and deep muscle compartments
  - Alternative technique (6):
    - Single medial incision to release abductor hallucis and deep compartments
    - Muscles reflected plantarly
    - Interosseous compartments released through medial approach

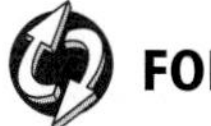

## FOLLOW-UP

- Foot fasciotomy incisions usually can be closed 5–7 days after the original surgery, once severe edema has subsided.
- Split-thickness skin graft may be required to cover the wounds if the skin edges cannot be approximated.

### *Issues for Referral*

Patients with severe foot trauma or massive swelling of the foot should prompt urgent orthopaedic consultation.

### PROGNOSIS

- The prognosis after a missed or untreated compartment syndrome of the foot is poor.
  - Such patients typically have chronic pain and stiffness that can be disabling.
  - Cavus or cavovarus foot deformities can occur secondary to myonecrosis and fibrosis of intrinsic foot muscles.
  - Claw toes that require surgical release may develop.
  - Complex regional pain syndrome can develop after compartment syndrome or crush injury.

### COMPLICATIONS

- Pain
- Paresthesias
- Stiffness
- Claw toes
- Foot deformities

### REFERENCES

1. Myerson MS. Management of compartment syndromes of the foot. *Clin Orthop Relat Res* 1991;271:239–248.
2. Manoli A, II. Compartment syndromes of the foot: current concepts. *Foot Ankle* 1990;10:340–344.
3. Myerson M. Diagnosis and treatment of compartment syndrome of the foot. *Orthopaedics* 1990;13:711–717.
4. Gardner AMN, Fox RH, Lawrence C, et al. Reduction of post-traumatic swelling and compartment pressure by impulse compression of the foot. *J Bone Joint Surg* 1990;72B:810–815.
5. Manoli A, II, Weber TG. Fasciotomy of the foot: an anatomical study with special reference to release of the calcaneal compartment. *Foot Ankle* 1990;10:267–275.
6. Myerson MS. Experimental decompression of the fascial compartments of the foot—the basis for fasciotomy in acute compartment syndromes. *Foot Ankle* 1988;8:308–314.

### ADDITIONAL READING

Myerson M, Manoli A. Compartment syndromes of the foot after calcaneal fractures. *Clin Orthop Relat Res* 1993;290:142–150.

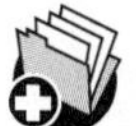

## MISCELLANEOUS

### CODES

#### *ICD9-CM*

958.8 Compartment syndrome

### FAQ

- Q: What is the pathophysiology of compartment syndrome?
  - A: Trauma or severe intramuscular edema causes impairment of intracompartmental microcirculation, leading to cell ischemia, necrosis, and intracellular fluid leakage, which propagates additional increase in compartment pressure. Muscle and nerve tissue is susceptible to ischemia, leading to myonecrosis and nerve injury.
- Q: Which group of patients is especially at risk for a compartment syndrome of the foot?
  - A: Patients with crush injuries or calcaneal fractures are at greatest risk.

# COMPUTED TOMOGRAPHY

*William J. Didie, MD*
*Laura M. Fayad, MD*

## BASICS

### DESCRIPTION

- CT is a noninvasive diagnostic technique that uses a rotational radiographic source to generate cross-sectional images.
- CT is particularly advantageous for musculoskeletal imaging when used with multiplanar, volume-rendered reconstruction techniques.

### ETIOLOGY

- Chronology of development (1):
  - 1972: Introduction
  - 1974–1976: 1st clinical scanners installed
  - 1980: Became widely available
  - 1985–1986: Introduction of modern applications, such as dynamic imaging, multiplanar reformatting, and 3D CT with volume rendering and shaded surface display
  - 1989: Beginning of routine spiral scanning

## DIAGNOSIS

- Advantages:
  - Rapid image acquisition, particularly useful in pediatric, trauma, and very ill patients, with reduced need for sedation
  - Clear evaluation of anatomically complex areas not always well evaluated by plain radiographs, such as the axial skeleton and small joints (ankle and wrist)
  - Multiplanar reformatted and 3D capabilities: For 16-slice multidetector CT and beyond, acquisition in only 1 plane is required because the data set may be reconstructed into different planes and perspectives.
  - May virtually eliminate streak artifact secondary to metal hardware through volume rendering of a multidetector CT axial database (Fig. 1).
    - MRI evaluation in such patients often is extremely limited.
  - Can safely image patients with contraindications to MRI, such as aneurysm clips, pacemaker, or orbital metallic fragments
  - Cost-effective modality for a wide range of clinical problems
  - Widely available
- Disadvantages:
  - Inferior to MRI for bone marrow and soft-tissue details
  - Requires ionizing radiation exposure
  - More expensive than plain radiography
  - If contrast is necessary, a risk of allergic reaction or contrast nephropathy exists.

### TESTS

- Skeletal pathology:
  - Typically imaged with thin-section collimation (0.75 mm for a 16-slice multidetector CT).
  - Postprocessing of data into multiplanar reformatted images and 3D reconstructions is performed on a workstation.
- Soft tissues:
  - Thin-section imaging is not as crucial as for the evaluation of the skeleton.
  - Reconstructed slice thickness typically is set at 2–3 mm.
  - Studies performed to evaluate a soft-tissue mass, potential abscess, or vascular injury typically require the administration of intravenous contrast material, requiring injection rates of 3 mL/sec.
    - Intravenous contrast should be used with caution in patients with renal insufficiency.
    - Patients with potential allergies to intravenous contrast should be identified, premedicated, or not injected.

### DIFFERENTIAL DIAGNOSIS

- Postoperative indications:
  - Identification of complications of hardware implantation, such as osteomyelitis or fracture
  - Identification of potential tumor recurrence in the presence of hardware
  - Detection of retained foreign body

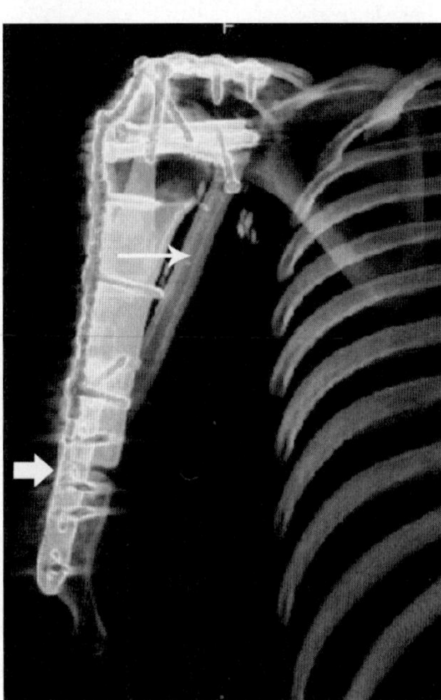

**Fig. 1.** Coronal oblique volume-rendered 3D CT showing reconstruction of the humerus with an allograft (*thick arrow* marks allograft–host junction). Healing is augmented by a vascularized fibular graft (*thin arrow*). Note the minimized streak artifact around the metal hardware on this 3D CT.

- Oncology indications:
  - Detection of calcification within a lesion: Distinction of myositis ossificans and neoplasm by detecting pattern of mineralization
  - Characterization of cortical and periosteal changes for distinguishing benign and malignant processes
  - Assessment of bone destruction and fracture risk
  - Definitive treatment of osteoid osteomas with CT-directed radiofrequency ablation of the nidus
  - Detection of compartmental and neurovascular involvement, although typically more commonly assessed by MRI
- Trauma indications:
  - Definition or exclusion of a fracture that is equivocal on plain radiograph: 3D CT and multiplanar reconstructions are particularly useful for detecting fractures oriented in the axial plane.
  - Determination of extent of fracture, including physeal and intra-articular involvement
  - Identification of intra-articular fracture fragments
  - Identification of fracture nonunion
  - Detailed cervical spine evaluation in moderate- and high-risk trauma patients
- Evaluation of anatomically complex areas, such as pelvis, scapula, wrist, ankle, and spine (Fig. 2)

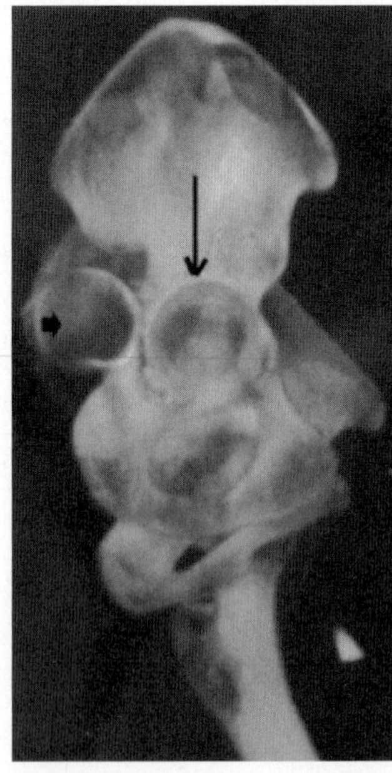

**Fig. 2.** Sagittal oblique volume-rendered 3D CT image of the pelvis shows posterior dislocation of the right hip. The femoral head (*short arrow*) and empty acetabular fossa (*long arrow*) are marked.

- Infection indications:
  - Determination of compartments of tissue involvement (bone, muscle, fascia, subcutaneous tissue) necessary for patient triage as medical or surgical candidates
  - Assessment of response to antibiotic therapy
- Pediatric indications (2):
  - Skeletal dysplasias:
    - Useful for applications, such as dysplasias, that require imaging of a large field of view to define the anatomy and evaluate the skeleton postoperatively
    - Such cases often are difficult to image completely by radiography or MRI.
  - DDH:
    - Diagnosis usually is made by physical examination, plain radiographs, and ultrasound.
    - CT may be used in difficult cases or, with low-dose scanning, as an imaging alternative.
    - CT more commonly is used to define success of reduction after cast placement.
  - SCFE:
    - Detection of contralateral involvement with coronal and sagittal display
    - Exclusion of other causes of hip pain, such as osteoid osteoma or septic joint
  - Legg-Calvé-Perthes disease:
    - Presurgical: Planning for identification of severity of disease
    - Postoperative: Assessment for determination of success of intervention or evaluation of new symptoms
  - Pectus deformities:
    - Surgical approach and anatomic definition, especially if initial repair was unsuccessful
  - Tarsal coalition:
    - CT reconstruction in multiple planes to define the different osseous and nonosseous coalitions

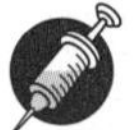

## TREATMENT

### ALERT

#### *Pediatric Considerations*

- Children are more sensitive to radiation than are adults and are more likely to develop radiation-induced neoplasm over a lifetime (3–5).
- CT exposure parameters should be adjusted, and only necessary examinations performed (3–5).
- Multiphase imaging (both with and without contrast) should be avoided.
- Multidetector technology with volume visualization and postprocessing minimizes radiation exposure.

#### *Pregnancy Considerations*

- Scan volume should be limited to necessary anatomy.
- Multiphase imaging should be avoided.
- Establish protocols that appropriately use radiation and are tested regularly by departmental medical physicists.
- The magnitude of leukemogenic fetal risk is uncertain.
- No long-term effects of intravenous contrast on fetus are known, but the usual dose should be reduced by 59% to 0.5 mL/kg (6).
- Consider nonionizing alternative modalities, such as MRI or ultrasound, if possible.
- Lead shield the abdomen and pelvis, if possible.
- Nursing mothers should wait 24 hours after intravenous contrast administration to resume breast-feeding.

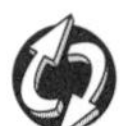

## FOLLOW-UP

### COMPLICATIONS

- Contrast allergy:
  - Risk factors include history of asthma and previous reactions.
  - Option to premedicate at-risk patients with steroids and diphenhydramine
- Contrast nephropathy:
  - Risk factors include pre-existing renal disease, multiple myeloma, diabetes, and dehydration
  - Aggressive hydration and use of low-osmolar agents

### REFERENCES


1. Siemens Medical. CT: Its History and Technology. (PDF file available at http://www.medical.siemens.com/siemens/en_US/gg_ct_FBAs/files/brochures/CT_History_and_Technology.pdf). Accessed 10/12/05.
2. Fayad LM, Johnson P, Fishman EK. Multidetector CT of musculoskeletal disease in the pediatric patient: principles, techniques, and clinical applications. *Radiographics* 2005;25:603–618.
3. Boice JD, Jr, Miller RW. Childhood and adult cancer after intrauterine exposure to ionizing radiation. *Teratology* 1999;59:227–233.
4. Brenner DJ, Elliston CD, Hall EJ, et al. Estimated risks of radiation-induced fatal cancer from pediatric CT. *AJR Am J Roentgenol* 2001;176:289–296.
5. Boone JM, Geraghty EM, Seibert JA, et al. Dose reduction in pediatric CT: a rational approach. *Radiology* 2003;228:352–360.
6. Wagner LK, Huda W. When a pregnant woman with suspected appendicitis is referred for a CT scan, what should a radiologist do to minimize potential radiation risks? *Pediatr Radiol* 2004;34:589–590.


### ADDITIONAL READING


- Fishman EK, Kuszyk B. 3D imaging: musculoskeletal applications. *Crit Rev Diagn Imaging* 2001;42:59–100.
- Karcaaltincaba M, Akata D, Aydingoz U, et al. Three-dimensional MDCT angiography of the extremities: clinical applications with emphasis on musculoskeletal uses. *AJR Am J Roentgenol* 2004;183:113–117.


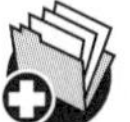

## MISCELLANEOUS

### PATIENT TEACHING

- The patient should expect to be in the CT scanner, motionless, for up to several minutes during the acquisition of images, but with modern-day scanners, a typical CT examination may require <30 seconds.
- Intravenous contrast may be administered, depending on the indication, and informed consent should be obtained.

### FAQ

- Q: How much time does a CT scan require?
  - A: Depending on the type of scanner available, as short as 10 seconds (64-slice multidetector CT) and usually <1 minute.
- Q: Can I order a CT scan on a pregnant patient?
  - A: Yes, if clinically necessary. However, the protocol is adjusted to reduce radiation exposure.
- Q: Can I order a CT scan for a patient with a pacemaker, aneurysm clips, or other metal hardware?
  - A: Yes. Metal is not a contraindication for CT.
- Q: How does metal hardware affect CT imaging?
  - A: Metal creates streak artifact. This artifact can be reduced or eliminated with volume-rendered 3D CT.
- Q: How do I order a 3D CT?
  - A: 3D CT is most effective with advanced CT technology (16-slice multidetector CT and beyond). A discussion of imaging equipment and techniques with the radiologist is the 1st step.

# CONGENITAL PSEUDARTHROSIS

*Paul D. Sponseller, MD*

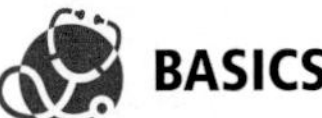

## BASICS

### DESCRIPTION

- Congenital pseudarthrosis is a rare defect of the distal tibia (at the junction of the middle 1/3 and distal 1/3) in which the bone is cystic and bowed and eventually fractures.
  - The bone is dysplastic from birth.
  - The deformity often increases with age.
  - The abnormality may not be noticed unless anterior bowing becomes prominent or fracture occurs.
  - It has no spontaneous healing potential, and it may require surgery to attempt union.
  - Multiple surgical procedures sometimes are required.
  - It is almost always unilateral.
  - After maturity, the bone behaves more normally.
- About 1/2 of cases are associated with NF; in those cases, other skeletal findings may be present.
- Congenital pseudarthrosis also may occur in other bones, such as the forearm and clavicle.
  - These occurrences are even rarer than those in the tibia.
  - Other sites are not affected concurrently in the patient with tibia pseudarthrosis.
  - Congenital pseudarthrosis of the clavicle affects only the right side unless the patient has dextrocardia.
- Classification (1–3):
  - Congenital pseudarthrosis is associated in some cases with NF.
  - Isolated congenital pseudarthrosis has been subclassified (1–3) into 3 types:
    - Dysplastic
    - Cystic
    - Sclerotic
- Synonyms: Congenital kyphoscoliotic tibia; Dysplastic tibia

### EPIDEMIOLOGY

Males and females are affected equally with all types of congenital pseudarthroses.

#### *Incidence*

~1 per 100,000–1 per 200,000 in the population are affected (3,4).

### RISK FACTORS

- NF
- Bowing of the tibia

#### *Genetics*

- NF is an autosomal dominant disorder.
- Its gene is located on the long arm of chromosome 17, and normally codes for a tumor suppressor, neurofibromin.
- Otherwise, congenital pseudarthrosis in the absence of NF is not an inherited disorder.

### ETIOLOGY

- The cause is unknown.
- Fracture usually occurs with minor or unrecognized trauma.
- The distal segment of the tibia is in the most poorly vascularized region of the bone
- NF tissue is not found in pseudarthrosis.

### ASSOCIATED CONDITIONS

NF

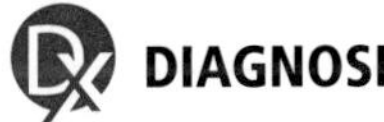

## DIAGNOSIS

### SIGNS AND SYMPTOMS

- Signs:
  - Increasing anterior and lateral bow of distal tibia (Fig. 1)
  - Mild limp
  - Possible signs of NF may be present, such as:
    - >5 café-au-lait spots
    - Subcutaneous NF
    - Scoliosis
  - In pseudarthrosis of the clavicle, bump in the right midclavicle with clicking
  - Mild leg-length difference possible
- Symptom:
  - Minimal to no pain

#### *Physical Exam*

- Inspect for signs of NF.
- Assess for limb-length discrepancy and stability.
- Assess the foot for size, stability, and plantigrade status.

### TESTS

#### *Lab*

No characteristic laboratory findings are noted, and no special tests are indicated routinely.

#### *Imaging*

- Radiography:
  - Plain AP and lateral films display the lesion in the distal tibia and fibula.
- MRI is not routinely indicated.
- Even before fracture, 1 or both of the following signs may be evident:
  - Cyst formation and sclerosis in the lesion
  - Local tapering (Fig. 2)
- Once the fracture appears, it may be characterized as atrophic or hypertrophic.
- A search for NF should be conducted, but the full-blown signs of NF may not appear until later in the 1st decade of life.
- If vascularized bone grafting is indicated, a preoperative angiogram is useful for showing vascular anatomy.

#### *Pathological Findings*

- The pseudarthrosis resembles that of any other cause.
- A thick cuff of hamartomatous tissue encircles the tibia.
- This cuff contains inactive fibroblasts, with no findings of NF such as Schwann cells, axons, or perineural cells.

### DIFFERENTIAL DIAGNOSIS

- Ossifying fibroma: A multiple cystic lesion affecting the anterior cortex of the tibia in older children
- Fibrous dysplasia: May produce bowing, but rarely fracture
- Posteromedial bow of the tibia: Benign, self-correcting bow in the same region of the tibia but in the opposite direction
- Focal fibrocartilaginous dysplasia: Rare, usually self-correcting bow of the proximal tibial metaphysis that rarely fractures
- Nonunion after fracture or osteotomy of the distal tibia

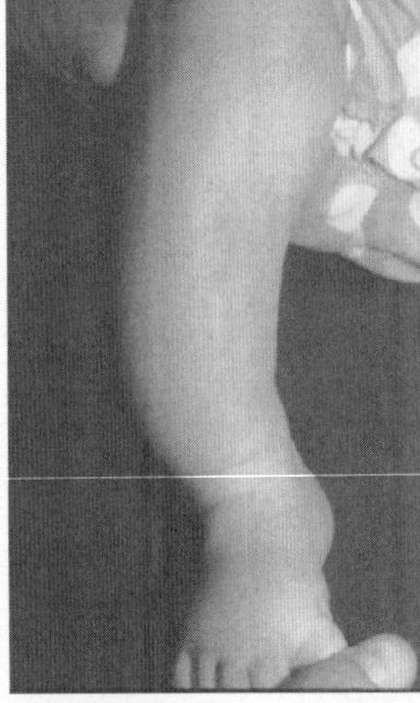

**Fig. 1.** Clinical appearance of anterolateral bow of the tibia secondary to congenital pseudarthrosis. Note the distal location of the bow.

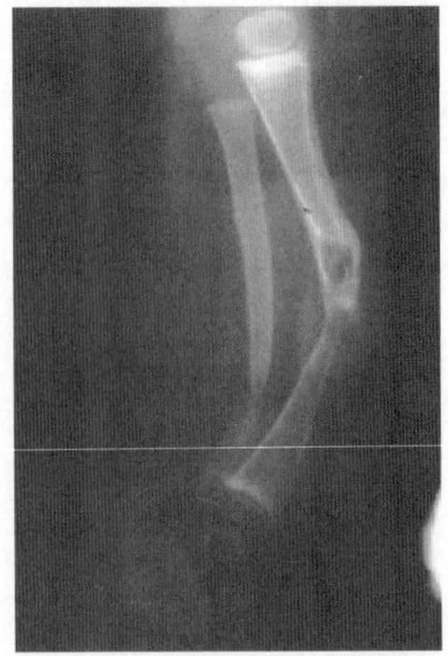

**Fig. 2.** Lateral radiograph of the tibia showing the tapering and cyst formation typical of congenital pseudarthrosis.

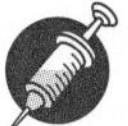

## TREATMENT

### GENERAL MEASURES

- The leg should be splinted and monitored to rule out increasing deformity.
- If the lesion has not fractured, a brace should be provided for protection.
- If the lesion has fractured, surgery always is required.

### SPECIAL THERAPY

#### *Physical Therapy*

Physical therapy is not necessary.

### MEDICATION (DRUGS)

- Medications do not affect the success of treatment.
- A recent article has suggested that rhBMP2 does not seem to improve the results of surgical treatment (5).

### SURGERY

- Intramedullary nail with bone graft: The nail is left in place until maturity (6,7).
- Ilizarov treatment: Distraction and compression of the fracture site stimulates a healing response (4).
- Free vascularized fibula graft: A segment of living, normal fibula with its blood supply is transferred to increase chances of success (8).
- As a last resort, if many different treatments do not succeed, Syme amputation through the ankle may be elected by the family to allow the child to proceed with physical activities (4).

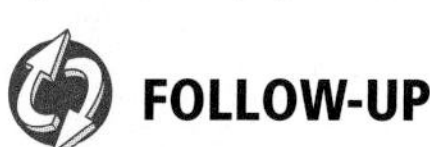

## FOLLOW-UP

### PROGNOSIS

- Good: 80–90% may heal (4–8).
- Refracture may occur even after union.
- Refracture rate and nonunion rate decline after puberty (3).

### COMPLICATIONS

- Nonunion of defect after surgical procedure
- Angular deformity because of the small size and bowing of the distal fragment (9)
- Recurrence of fracture, even months to years after apparent healing
- Foot and ankle stiffness
- Limb-length inequality

### PATIENT MONITORING

The patient should be seen every 3–6 months to rule out progressive bowing and leg-length inequality and to check brace fit.

### REFERENCES


1. Boyd HB, Sage FP. Congenital pseudarthrosis of the tibia. *J Bone Joint Surg* 1958;40A:1245–1270.
2. Boyd HB. Pathology and natural history of congenital pseudarthrosis of the tibia. *Clin Orthop Relat Res* 1982;166:5–13.
3. Morrissy RT, Riseborough EJ, Hall JE. Congenital pseudarthrosis of the tibia. *J Bone Joint Surg* 1981;63B:367–375.
4. Schoenecker PL, Rich MM. The lower extremity. In: Morrissy RT, Weinstein SL, eds. *Lovell and Winter's Pediatric Orthopaedics,* 6th ed. Philadelphia: Lippincott Williams & Wilkins, 2006:1157–1211.
5. Lee FYI, Sinicropi SM, Lee FS, et al. Treatment of congenital pseudarthrosis of the tibia with recombinant human bone morphogenetic protein-7 (rhBMP-7). A report of five cases. *J Bone Joint Surg* 2006;88A:627–633.
6. Dobbs MB, Rich MM, Gordon JE, et al. Use of an intramedullary rod for treatment of congenital pseudarthrosis of the tibia. A long-term follow-up study. *J Bone Joint Surg* 2004;86A:1186–1197.
7. Dobbs MB, Rich MM, Gordon JE, et al. Use of an intramedullary rod for the treatment of congenital pseudarthrosis of the tibia. Surgical technique. *J Bone Joint Surg* 2005;87A:33–40.
8. Weiland AJ, Weiss APC, Moore JR, et al. Vascularized fibular grafts in the treatment of congenital pseudarthrosis of the tibia. *J Bone Joint Surg* 1990;72A:654–662.
9. Kristiansen LP, Steen H, Terjesen T. Residual challenges after healing of congenital pseudarthrosis in the tibia. *Clin Orthop Relat Res* 2003;414:228–237.


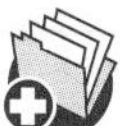

## MISCELLANEOUS

### CODES

#### *ICD9-CM*

733.82 Congenital pseudarthrosis

### PATIENT TEACHING

- The family should be educated about the natural history of the lesion—the propensity for fracture, the need for bracing, the tendency to nonunion, treatment options, improvement in biology (increased chance of healing and less likelihood of refracture) after puberty.
- With this knowledge, they will be more understanding of the multiple procedures sometimes needed for healing.
- Rough play should be avoided as much as possible.
- Prevention of fracture or refracture by use of a brace is common practice.

### FAQ

- Q: What is the cause of congenital pseudarthrosis of the tibia?
  - A: The cause is unknown.
- Q: Which of the surgical treatments listed is better?
  - A: No superiority of one over the other is proven. Treatment choice depends on the experience and preference of the surgeon.

# CUBITAL TUNNEL SYNDROME

*Dawn M. LaPorte, MD*

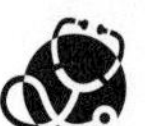

## BASICS

### DESCRIPTION

- Cubital tunnel syndrome consists of pain and paresthesias over the medial border of the forearm and hand, as well as weakness in an ulnar nerve distribution from compression of the ulnar nerve as it passes through the cubital tunnel at the elbow.
- It affects the elbow, forearm, and hand in the ulnar nerve distribution and is most commonly seen in adults.
- Synonym: Ulnar tunnel syndrome

### EPIDEMIOLOGY

#### *Incidence*

- The 2nd most common entrapment neuropathy (after CTS) in the upper extremity
- Males and females are affected equally.

### RISK FACTORS

Diabetes

### ETIOLOGY

- The ulnar nerve is compressed as it passes through the cubital tunnel at the medial side of the elbow, which may compress the blood vessels that feed the nerve and create symptoms.
- Possible causes of the compression include:
  - Enlarged medial head of the triceps muscle
  - Trauma
  - Recurrent dislocation of the nerve from the tunnel
  - Arthritis (bony spurs)
  - Ganglia
  - Abnormal muscles (anconeus epitrochlearis)

### ASSOCIATED CONDITIONS

TOS

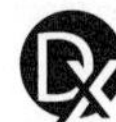

## DIAGNOSIS

The diagnosis is made clinically, with aid from nerve conduction studies.

### SIGNS AND SYMPTOMS

- Vague, aching pain
- Paresthesias
- Numbness over the medial forearm, hand, and (occasionally) upper arm

#### *Physical Exam*

- Note decreased sensation in the ulnar nerve distribution.
- Check for intrinsic weakness by placing a sheet of paper between the patient's thumb and 1st finger and attempting to pull the paper away as the patient resists.
- Look for intrinsic muscle wasting, especially of the 1st dorsal interosseous muscle.
- Percussion test (Tinel sign): Tapping over the ulnar nerve at the elbow causes a reproduction of symptoms (Fig. 1).
- Elbow flexion test: Keeping the elbow fully flexed (and the wrist in neutral or extension to avoid carpal tunnel symptoms) for 1 minute causes a reproduction of the symptoms.
- Order nerve conduction studies (nerve conduction is slowed across the elbow).

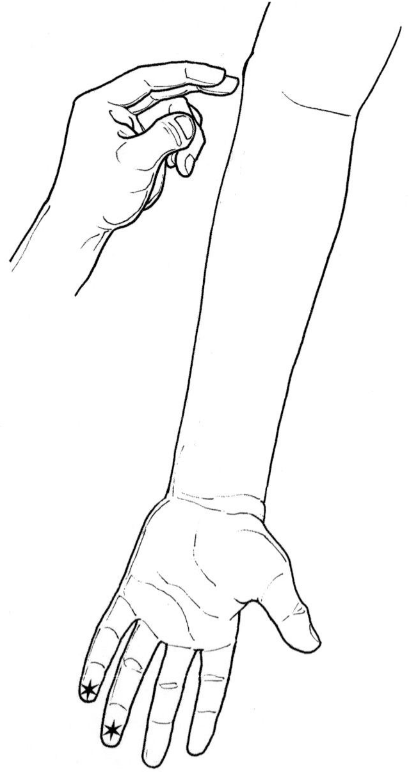

**Fig. 1.** Tinel sign. Tapping over the ulnar nerve at the cubital tunnel produces paresthesias in the small and ring fingers.

### TESTS

#### *Imaging*

AP radiography of the elbow may be indicated.

#### *Pathological Findings*

- At decompression, specific sites of nerve compression usually can be found.
- Inspect the arcade of Struthers, intermuscular septum, cubital tunnel, and Osborne fascia (between 2 heads of flexor carpi ulnaris).

### DIFFERENTIAL DIAGNOSIS

- Thoracic outlet syndrome
- C8–T1 cervical root compression
- Compression of the ulnar nerve at the wrist (Guyon canal)
- CTS
- Guillain-Barré syndrome
- Amyotrophic lateral sclerosis

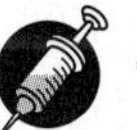

## TREATMENT

### GENERAL MEASURES

- Nonoperative treatment involves splinting the elbow in extension to relieve acute symptoms.
- Patients wear the splint when sleeping.
- Nighttime elbow extension splints with the forearm held in neutral or supination
- Avoid prolonged elbow flexion.

### SURGERY
- Consider surgery if symptoms continue after 3 months of nonoperative therapy.
- Many procedures have been described (1–6):
  - Procedures usually consist of some form of decompression of the nerve in the canal.
  - Operations often involve transposition of the nerve out of the canal in an anterior direction.

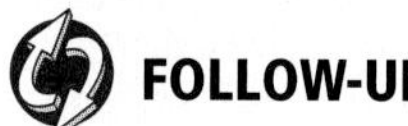

## FOLLOW-UP

### PROGNOSIS
- Nonoperative therapy: 50% excellent results (7)
- Surgical therapy: Good to excellent results in nearly all patients

### COMPLICATIONS
- Reflex sympathetic dystrophy and nerve irritation may occur after surgery.
  - If left untreated, severe ulnar neuropathy can lead to clawing of the small finger and ring finger, atrophy of intrinsic muscles, and positive Froment and/or Wartenberg signs.

### PATIENT MONITORING
Motor and sensory examinations are performed at follow-up visits.

### REFERENCES

1. Dellon AL, Coert JH. Results of the musculofascial lengthening technique for submuscular transposition of the ulnar nerve at the elbow. Surgical technique. *J Bone Joint Surg* 2004;86A: 169–179.
2. Dinh PT, Gupta R. Subtotal medial epicondylectomy as a surgical option for treatment of cubital tunnel syndrome. *Tech Hand Up Extrem Surg* 2005;9:52–59.
3. Eaton RG, Crowe JF, Parkes JC, III. Anterior transposition of the ulnar nerve using a non-compressing fasciodermal sling. *J Bone Joint Surg* 1980;62A:820–825.
4. Gervasio O, Gambardella G, Zaccone C, et al. Simple decompression versus anterior submuscular transposition of the ulnar nerve in severe cubital tunnel syndrome: a prospective randomized study. *Neurosurgery* 2005;56:108–117.
5. Learmonth JR. A technique for transplanting the ulnar nerve. *Surg Gynecol Obstet* 1942;75:792–793.
6. Nabhan A, Ahlhelm F, Kelm J, et al. Simple decompression or subcutaneous anterior transposition of the ulnar nerve for cubital tunnel syndrome. *J Hand Surg* 2005;30B:521–524.
7. Padua L, Aprile I, Caliandro P, et al. Natural history of ulnar entrapment at elbow. *Clin Neurophysiol* 2002;113:1980–1984.


### ADDITIONAL READING

- Mackinnon SE, Novak CB. Compression neuropathies. In: Green DP, Hotchkiss RN, Pederson WC, et al., eds. *Green's Operative Hand Surgery*, 5th ed. Philadelphia: Elsevier Churchill Livingstone, 2005;999–1045.
- Jobe MT, Martinez SF. Peripheral nerve injuries. In: Canale ST, ed. *Campbell's Operative Orthopaedics*, 10th ed. St. Louis: Mosby, 2005:3221–3283.


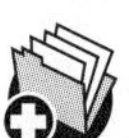

## MISCELLANEOUS

### CODES
#### *ICD9-CM*
354.2 Cubital tunnel syndrome

### PATIENT TEACHING
Patients are counseled to avoid activities that exacerbate their symptoms.

#### *Prevention*
- Avoid:
  - Repetitive work activities if they cause symptoms
  - Prolonged elbow flexion

### FAQ
- Q: Is there a nonoperative treatment for cubital tunnel syndrome?
  - A: Mild or mild/moderate cubital tunnel syndrome can be treated with a nighttime elbow extension splint to minimize elbow flexion during sleep. Patients also are advised to avoid prolonged activity with the elbow flexed. Nerve glides (active exercises that help to prevent scarring around the nerve) may be of some benefit.
- Q: Once a patient has intrinsic wasting, what can be done to restore intrinsic strength?
  - A: Once intrinsic atrophy occurs, nothing can be done specifically to restore the intrinsic motor loss. Ulnar nerve decompression and transposition can halt additional progression of motor loss and, if the patient has a functional deficit, tendon transfers could be considered.
- Q: What are the symptoms of cubital tunnel?
  - A: Patients typically present with complaints of numbness and tingling in their small and ring fingers. Symptoms frequently are worse during extended periods of elbow flexion, for example, talking on the phone or blow-drying hair.

# DE QUERVAIN (THUMB EXTENSOR) TENOSYNOVITIS

*Dawn M. LaPorte, MD*
*Peter R. Jay, MD*

## BASICS

### DESCRIPTION

- Thumb extensor or de Quervain tendinitis is stenosing tenosynovitis of the 1st dorsal compartment of the wrist, which contains the abductor pollicis longus and the extensor pollicis brevis.
- Patients present with pain and discomfort on the radial aspect of the wrist.
- It often occurs in middle-aged females, although males and females of all ages can be affected.

### EPIDEMIOLOGY

#### *Incidence*

This condition is common—up to 6 times more common in females than in males (1,2).

### RISK FACTORS

Frequently seen in new mothers, in part secondary to repetitive lifting and setting down of the baby.

### ETIOLOGY

- Repetitive motions of thumb or wrist
- Associated with:
  - Racquet sports
  - Fly fishing
  - Golf (often affecting the nondominant hand in golfers)
  - Infant care
- Can be associated with rheumatoid arthritis

### ASSOCIATED CONDITIONS

Rheumatoid arthritis

## DIAGNOSIS

### SIGNS AND SYMPTOMS

- Pain and tenderness on the radial aspect of the wrist, often isolated to directly over the 1st dorsal compartment
- Pain and discomfort exacerbated by extension or abduction of the thumb with simultaneous ulnar deviation of the wrist
- Repetitive activities particularly painful

#### *Physical Exam*

- Note pain, tenderness, swelling, bogginess, and crepitus over the 1st dorsal compartment of the wrist—the radial aspect of the radial styloid.
- A positive Finkelstein test (Fig. 1) helps confirm the diagnosis: Exacerbation of the symptoms (pain) with the thumb clenched in the palm and ulnar deviation of the wrist (2,3).

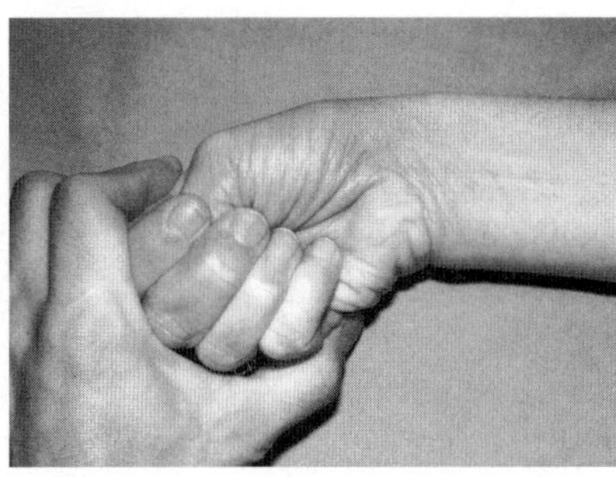

**Fig. 1.** Finkelstein test. Test is considered positive if it produces sharp pain when the thumb is clasped in the palm and the wrist is forced into ulnar deviation.

- Examine the 1st CMC joint, use the grind test, and assess ROM to rule out degenerative joint disease; degenerative joint disease and de Quervain syndrome can coexist:
  - Intersection syndrome is rarer than de Quervain and often is associated with more severe symptoms.
  - On physical examination, the pain localizes 4 cm proximal to the wrist, rather than over the radial styloid, as in de Quervain syndrome.

### TESTS

#### *Lab*

No serum laboratory tests are needed.

#### *Imaging*

AP and lateral views of the wrist and 1st CMC views are helpful in ruling out other disorders and in differentiating between degenerative joint disease of the 1st CMC and de Quervain syndrome.

#### *Pathological Findings*

- The dorsum of the wrist is divided anatomically into 6 separate extensor tendon compartments.
  - The 1st compartment contains the abductor pollicis longus and extensor pollicis brevis, which can become inflamed and irritated as they enter and pass through the rigid fibro-osseous tunnel of the 1st compartment.
  - Intersection syndrome is thought to be an inflammatory condition that exists at the point where the 1st and 2nd dorsal compartment (the ECRL and ECRB) cross; this site of "intersection" is ~4 cm proximal to the wrist.

### DIFFERENTIAL DIAGNOSIS

- Degenerative joint disease of the 1st (thumb) CMC joint
- Intersection syndrome (much rarer)
- Radiocarpal arthritis

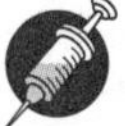

# TREATMENT

## GENERAL MEASURES

As with most types of tendinitis, rest and avoidance of aggravating conditions are the mainstays of treatment.

## SPECIAL THERAPY

### *Physical Therapy*

- Splinting often is helpful to put the tendon at rest.
- Iontophoresis (ultrasound through a corticosteroid cream) can help decrease the inflammation.
- Stretching the wrist also may be helpful.

## MEDICATION (DRUGS)

### *First Line*

- The 1st line of therapy is nonoperative care, which includes:
  - Immobilization of thumb and wrist, usually in a thumb spica splint.
  - NSAIDs
  - Steroid injection into the 1st dorsal compartment; success rates for steroid injection range from 50–80% (4,5).
- Recalcitrant or recurrent symptoms often require surgical release of the 1st dorsal compartment.
- Decrease activity until symptoms resolve.

### *Second Line*

Patients who have persistent pain despite nonoperative measures are candidates for surgical release of the 1st dorsal compartment.

## SURGERY

- Positive response to injection should precede decision for surgery.
- Make a radial incision over the 1st dorsal compartment with release of the fibro-osseous tunnel and all its septa, as well as the release of the fascial sheaths of each tendon and the compartment.
- Incise the sheath on dorsal margin to prevent tendon subluxation.
- Multiple anatomic variations are present.

# FOLLOW-UP

## PROGNOSIS

The prognosis is good.

## COMPLICATIONS

- The most serious complication of surgical intervention is transection of the dorsal sensory radial nerve, which lies in proximity to the 1st dorsal compartment.
- This complication can leave the patient with a small area of numbness/absence of sensation or, more seriously, with a painful neuroma, which often requires surgical resection.

## PATIENT MONITORING

Patients are followed at 3-month intervals until their symptoms resolve.

## REFERENCES


1. Harvey FJ, Harvey PM, Horsley MW. De Quervain's disease: surgical or nonsurgical treatment. *J Hand Surg* 1990;15A:83–87.
2. Piver JD, Raney RB. De Quervain's tendovaginitis. *Am J Surg* 1952;83:691–694.
3. Finkelstein H. Stenosing tendovaginitis at the radial styloid process. *J Bone Joint Surg* 1930;12A:509–540.
4. Phalen GS. Stenosing tenosynovitis: trigger fingers, trigger thumb, and de Quervain's disease. Acute calcification in wrist and hand. In: Jupiter JB, ed. *Flynn's Hand Surgery,* 4th ed. Baltimore: Williams & Wilkins, 1991:439–447.
5. Weiss APC, Akelman E, Tabatabai M. Treatment of de Quervain's disease. *J Hand Surg* 1994;19A:595–598.


## ADDITIONAL READING


Wolfe SW. Tenosynovitis. In: Green DP, Hotchkiss RN, Pederson WC, et al., eds. *Green's Operative Hand Surgery*, 5th ed. Philadelphia: Elsevier Churchill Livingstone, 2005:2137–2159.


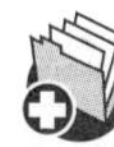

# MISCELLANEOUS

## CODES

### *ICD9-CM*

727.04 de Quervain tendinitis

## PATIENT TEACHING

- Patients are counseled to avoid repetitive activities that worsen the pain.
- Attention to workplace ergonomics also is important.

## FAQ

- Q: What is the 1st line of treatment for de Quervain syndrome?
  - A: Thumb spica splint immobilization, anti-inflammatory medication, and therapy with modalities.
- Q: Are any risks associated with corticosteroid injection?
  - A: Some localized hypopigmentation may occur after injection.
- Q: What other diagnoses can cause radial-side wrist pain?
  - A: The differential diagnosis for de Quervain syndrome includes thumb CMC arthritis and radiocarpal arthritis. Thumb CMC arthritis is distinguished by pain over the thumb CMC joint, a positive grind test, and a negative Finkelstein test. Radiocarpal arthritis may be distinguished by pain over the radiocarpal joint and pain with radial deviation of the wrist, as compared with pain with ulnar deviation with de Quervain syndrome.

# DEEP VENOUS THROMBOSIS

*Misty A. Moore, MSN, FNP*
*Michelle Cameron, MD*

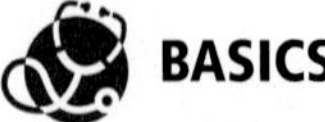

## BASICS

### DESCRIPTION
- DVT is a blood clot in the deep venous plexus of the legs.
- Venous thrombus may embolize and result in fatal PE.
- Classification:
  - DVTs are classified by location using ultrasound.
    - Thrombi below the popliteal fossa usually do not embolize.
    - 50% of thrombi at or above the popliteal fossa will embolize (1).

### GENERAL PREVENTION
- Pharmacologic prophylaxis
- Pneumatic compression
- Early mobilization

### EPIDEMIOLOGY
#### *Incidence*
- The DVT rate in orthopaedic patients without prophylaxis is:
  - 15–25% after total hip arthroplasty (2)
  - As high as 50% after total knee arthroplasty (3)
  - 20–60% after pelvic, acetabular, or hip fracture (4)
  - 0.3–26% after spinal surgery
  - 0.25% after foot and ankle surgery
- Affects males and females equally

### RISK FACTORS
- Age >60 years
- Prolonged immobility or paralysis
- History of DVT or PE
- Family history of DVT or PE
- Cancer
- Obesity
- Varicose veins
- Congestive heart failure
- Myocardial infarction
- Stroke
- Major lower extremity trauma, including fractures of the pelvis and hip
- Hypercoagulable states
- Sepsis
- Hormone therapy
- Inherited thrombophilia
- Smoking
- Pregnancy and giving birth

#### *Genetics*
- The risk of DVT is increased by inherited thrombophilia, including the presence of:
  - Protein C and S deficiency
  - Heparin cofactor II deficiency
  - G20210A prothrombin gene polymorphism
  - Dysfibrinogenemia
  - Factor V Leiden deficiency

### ETIOLOGY
The Virchow triad (endothelial injury, blood injury, and clotting abnormalities) can result in venous thromboembolism.

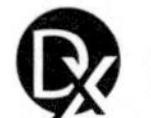

## DIAGNOSIS

### SIGNS AND SYMPTOMS
- DVT and PE manifest few specific symptoms; the clinical diagnosis is neither sensitive nor reliable (5).
  - DVT:
    - Pain and swelling in the leg and thigh
    - Possible phlebitis
    - Fever
  - PE:
    - Dyspnea
    - Pleuritic chest pain
    - Hemoptysis
    - Tachypnea
    - Acute right ventricular strain
    - Rubs or cackles in the lung fields
    - Tachycardia

#### *History*
A history of risk factors should be obtained to risk-stratify the patient.

#### *Physical Exam*
- Calf pain
- Swelling of the calf (may be measured and compared with the other side)
- Tachypnea and hypoxia
- Tachycardia

### TESTS
- Electrocardiography:
  - Classic findings after massive PE are S waves in lead I, and a Q wave with T-wave inversion in lead III.
  - In less severe PE, sinus tachycardia and new arrhythmias may be present.

#### *Lab*
- DVT: None
- PE:
  - Arterial blood gas
  - D-dimer

#### *Imaging*
- DVT:
  - Doppler ultrasonography:
    - Sensitive for detection of DVT
    - Sensitivity decreases in the upper thigh and pelvic veins.
    - Operator-dependent
  - Venography:
    - 100% sensitive and specific
    - Provides visualization of the entire deep venous system
    - Expensive and invasive
  - Magnetic resonance venography:
    - May be difficult to interpret and is operator-dependent
    - Visualizes pelvic thrombi
- PE:
  - Chest radiography:
    - Results generally are normal, but a pleural effusion or wedge-shaped pulmonary infarction may be noted.
  - Ventilation-perfusion scan:
    - A normal ventilation-perfusion scan excludes PE.
    - An abnormal scan showing perfusion defects does not confirm PE.
  - Pulmonary angiography:
    - 100% sensitive and specific, but expensive and invasive.
  - Spiral chest CT:
    - Sensitive and specific for PE detection
    - Replaced pulmonary angiography

#### *Pathological Findings*
- A clot develops in the lower extremity veins and enlarges proximally.
- The clot can embolize and fill the pulmonary arteries.

### DIFFERENTIAL DIAGNOSIS
- Lower leg thrombosis:
  - Phlebitis
  - Cellulitis
  - Deep or superficial wound infection
  - Ruptured Baker cyst
- PE:
  - Acute myocardial infarction
  - Congestive heart failure
  - Pneumonia
  - Fat emboli syndrome

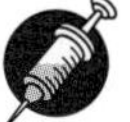

# TREATMENT

All patients undergoing major orthopaedic surgery (e.g., hip/knee arthroplasty) or who have had pelvic fractures or major lower extremity trauma should be placed on routine prophylaxis.

## GENERAL MEASURES

- Prophylaxis:
  - Anticoagulants are effective in reducing DVT incidence (1).
  - Pneumatic compression devices applied intraoperatively and postoperatively are effective (3).
  - Vena cava filter may be used for high-risk patients in whom anticoagulation is contraindicated (6).
- DVT above the popliteal fossa:
  - Patients should be anticoagulated immediately.
  - Bleeding risks should be considered, especially if the patient is within several days of surgery, because wound hematoma or uncontrolled bleeding may occur.
  - Patients should be placed on bed rest to decrease the chance of embolization.
- DVT below the popliteal fossa:
  - Blood clots may resolve over time without treatment.
  - Prophylactic doses of anticoagulant should be continued, and clots should be followed with Doppler ultrasonography to rule out propagation (7).

### *Activity*

To decrease the risk of embolization, patients with above-the-knee clots should be placed on bed rest until anticoagulation is achieved.

## MEDICATION (DRUGS)

### *First Line*

- Prophylaxis:
  - Patients at risk of DVT should be treated with prophylaxis.
  - Guidelines for prophylaxis were published in *Chest* and are widely followed (1).
  - Patients should be risk-stratified according to their risk factors and the type of surgery.
- For patients at high risk of DVT, the following treatments are thought to have the highest evidence for use:
  - Low molecular weight heparin:
    - Enoxaparin, 30 mg subcutaneously every 12 hours
    - Dalteparin, 5,000 IU subcutaneously every 24 hours
  - Warfarin:
    - Dose given nightly after surgery
    - Goal: Prothrombin time INR of 2.0–3.0
  - Pentasaccharides:
    - Approved for use after hip fracture
    - Fondaparinux sodium, 2.5 mg subcutaneously every 24 hours
- Duration of prophylaxis:
  - Should be continued for at least 2 weeks after surgery for high-risk patients
  - Should be continued for at least 4 weeks for patients at very high risk of DVT
- Treatment of DVT or PE:
  - Enoxaparin, 1 mg/kg subcutaneously every 24 hours
  - Warfarin:
    - Goal: Prothrombin time INR of 2.0–3.0
    - Length of treatment varies, but current recommendation is for at least 3 months (8).
  - Heparin, intravenous drip, dose-adjusted to an activated partial thromboplastin time of 2.0–3.0 times control values

### *Second Line*

- Evidence is not as substantial for DVT prophylaxis with aspirin or with mechanical devices, such as sequential compression devices (9).
- Sequential compression devices and graded compression stockings may be useful in the early period after surgery before anticoagulants are given.
- Compliance with these devices is difficult to enforce.
- The use of these methods alone for DVT prophylaxis is not recommended by the *Chest* guidelines (1).

# FOLLOW-UP

## COMPLICATIONS

- Increased risk of DVT in the future
- Chronic venous stasis
- PE
- Death

## PATIENT MONITORING

Monitoring varies, depending on the anticoagulant chosen.

## REFERENCES


1. Geerts WH, Pineo GF, Heit JA, et al. Prevention of venous thromboembolism: the Seventh ACCP Conference on Antithrombotic and Thrombolytic Therapy. *Chest* 2004;126:338S–400S.
2. Freedman KB, Brookenthal KR, Fitzgerald RH, Jr, et al. A meta-analysis of thromboembolic prophylaxis following elective total hip arthroplasty. *J Bone Joint Surg* 2000;82A:929–938.
3. Lieberman JR, Hsu WK. Prevention of venous thromboembolic disease after total hip and knee arthroplasty. *J Bone Joint Surg* 2005;87A:2097–2112.
4. Geerts WH, Jay R, Code KI, et al. A comparison of low-dose heparin with low-molecular-weight heparin as prophylaxis against venous thromboembolism after major trauma. *N Engl J Med* 1996;335:701–707.
5. Goodacre S, Sutton AJ, Sampson FC. Meta-analysis: the value of clinical assessment in the diagnosis of deep venous thrombosis. *Ann Intern Med* 2005;143:129–139, W-33–W-35.
6. Girard P, Stern JB, Parent F. Medical literature and vena cava filters: so far so weak. *Chest* 2002;122:963–967.
7. Wang CJ, Wang JW, Weng LH, et al. Outcome of calf deep-vein thrombosis after total knee arthroplasty. *J Bone Joint Surg* 2003;85B:841–844.
8. Nijkeuter M, Hovens MMC, Davidson BL, et al. Resolution of thromboemboli in patients with acute pulmonary embolism: a systematic review. *Chest* 2006;129:192–197.
9. Lotke PA, Palevsky H, Keenan AM, et al. Aspirin and warfarin for thromboembolic disease after total joint arthroplasty. *Clin Orthop Relat Res* 6;324:251–258.


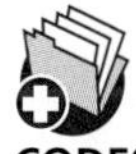

# MISCELLANEOUS

## CODES

### *ICD9-CM*

- 415.1 Pulmonary embolus
- 453.9 Venous embolism and thrombosis, of unspecified site

## PATIENT TEACHING

- Patients at risk are told the warning signs of DVT and PE, including:
  - Calf pain and calf and foot swelling that persist despite elevation
  - Chest pain, cough, and shortness of breath
- Patients should be educated about early mobilization.
- Medication teaching:
  - Low-molecular-weight heparin: Subcutaneous injection, side effects, bleeding precautions
  - Coumadin: Diet instructions, limiting vitamin K, bleeding precautions, importance of lab monitoring (INR)

### *Prevention*

Patients should be risk-stratified and treated with prophylaxis according to the *Chest* guidelines (1).

## FAQ

- Q: Is immobility a risk for DVT?
  - A: Yes. Immobility, such as long travel in a car or plane or periods of bed rest or casting, place a patient at risk for DVT.

# DESMOID TUMOR (EXTRA-ABDOMINAL)

*Frank J. Frassica, MD*
*Deborah A. Frassica, MD*

## BASICS

### DESCRIPTION

- A common benign soft-tissue tumor that occurs in young patients
- Although this tumor never metastasizes, a high rate of local recurrence occurs in the following locations (1):
  - Neck: 8%
  - Shoulder: 22%
  - Upper arm: 6%
  - Chest wall/back: 17%
  - Buttock/hip: 6%
  - Thigh: 12%
  - Knee: 7%
  - Lower leg: 5%
- Synonyms: Desmoid tumor; Extra-abdominal fibromatosis; Well-differentiated fibrosarcoma; fibromatosis

### GENERAL PREVENTION

No preventive measures

#### *Incidence*

3–4 per 1,000,000 in the United States (1)

### RISK FACTORS

Trauma (possible, but not definitely proven)

#### *Genetics*

No genetic factors are known.

### PATHOPHYSIOLOGY

Unknown (may be associated with trauma)

### ASSOCIATED CONDITIONS

May be associated with trauma

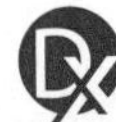

## DIAGNOSIS

### SIGNS AND SYMPTOMS

Usually a nonpainful or moderately painful soft-tissue mass

#### *History*

Patients may report a history of a slowly growing soft-tissue mass

#### *Physical Exam*

Palpate for a hard and usually fixed soft-tissue mass.

### TESTS

Imaging is the major testing modality.

#### *Lab*

No pertinent laboratory tests

#### *Imaging*

- Plain radiographs and MRI scans should be obtained.
- Radiography:
  - Inspect plain films for cortical erosion or periosteal reaction.
- MRI:
  - Shows anatomic features of the tumor:
    - T1-weighted images: Low signal, excellent anatomic detail
    - T2-weighted images: Moderate to high signal with low signal areas

#### *Diagnostic Procedures/Surgery*

Diagnosis can be established only by needle or open biopsy.

#### *Pathological Findings*

- Mature fibroblasts with large amounts of collagen:
  - No cellular atypia
  - Few if any mitoses
  - No herringbone pattern
  - Highly infiltrative to muscle and other soft tissues

### DIFFERENTIAL DIAGNOSIS

- Must differentiate from soft-tissue sarcomas and benign reactive conditions
  - May be confused with fibrosarcoma
  - May be confused with posttraumatic conditions, nodular fasciitis

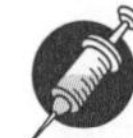

## TREATMENT

#### *Nursing*

Reassure the patient and family that the process is completely benign.

#### *Radiotherapy*

- Commonly used for recurrent or unresectable tumors
  - 5200 cGy over 5 weeks with 5–10-cm margins

### SPECIAL THERAPY

#### *Physical Therapy*

Often used to gain ROM and strength after surgical excision

### MEDICATION (DRUGS)

- Because of the high recurrence rate, many different medication regimens have been tried, with variable results, but none of these measures have been definitely shown to be effective.
- 3 therapies generally are used for patients with recurrent tumors:
  - Low-dose chemotherapy (vincristine/methotrexate)
  - Tamoxifen
  - NSAIDs

### SURGERY

- Wide surgical resection with negative margins is the preferred modality.
  - Often difficult to achieve secondary to the invasive nature of the tumor

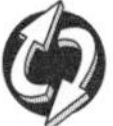

# FOLLOW-UP

- Patients are followed every 6–12 months:
  - MRI with contrast is the best modality.

### *Issues for Referral*
Patients should be referred to an orthopaedic oncologist.

## PROGNOSIS
- The prognosis is excellent with regard to survival, but the local recurrence rate is very high.
  - Rarely will a patient die from this tumor.
  - Local recurrence rate is >50% (1).

## COMPLICATIONS
- The major complication is local recurrence.
- Delayed wound healing occurs after wide resection.

## PATIENT MONITORING
Patients are followed every 6 months with MRI scans.

## REFERENCES
1. Weiss SW, Goldblum JR. Fibromatoses. In: Weiss SW, Goldblum JR, eds. *Enzinger and Weiss's Soft Tissue Tumors*, 4th ed. St. Louis: Mosby, 2001:309–346.

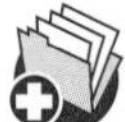

# MISCELLANEOUS

## CODES
### *ICD9-CM*
215._Neoplasm, benign, connective tissue

## PATIENT TEACHING
- Patients are taught the major features of this tumor.
  - The tumor never metastasizes.
  - Local recurrence rate is high.
  - Important to regain ROM and strength after surgery

### *Activity*
Patients may return to full activity after wound healing.

### *Prevention*
No preventive measures

## FAQ
- Q: Do desmoid tumors ever spread to other parts of the body?
  - A: Desmoid tumors never metastasize. However, they may threaten a patient's life through invasive local growth.
- Q: What is the best way to treat recurrent tumors?
  - A: Recurrence is a very difficult problem. Patients often are treated with a combination of repeat surgery and irradation.
- Q: Can the desmoid tumor be diagnosed without a biopsy?
  - A: The diagnosis of this tumor cannot be made without a needle or open biopsy.

# DEVELOPMENTAL DYSPLASIA OF THE HIP

*Paul D. Sponseller, MD*

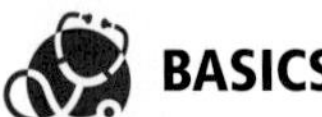

## BASICS

### DESCRIPTION

- DDH covers a spectrum of varying degrees of superolateral displacement of the femur and deformation of the acetabulum, developing mostly *in utero* or, rarely, in infancy.
- It usually is discovered on routine screening in early childhood.
- It occasionally is discovered in teens with a limp or pain, in which case it probably represents a mildly subluxed hip that could not be detected on physical examination.
- Classification by spectrum of severity (1):
  - A subluxable hip is reduced but can be subluxated with pressure and goes back to the reduced position.
  - A dislocatable hip can be fully dislocated and reduced.
- A dislocated hip rests in a dislocated position and reduces only with manual effort.
- Synonyms: DDH; Congenital dislocation of the hip (old term); Hip dysplasia; Unstable hip

### GENERAL PREVENTION

- No effective preventive means exist.
- Early detection is most important (2–5).
- Patients with hip dysplasia should have their children examined carefully at birth (5).

### EPIDEMIOLOGY

Females are affected 4 times as often as males because of increased ligamentous laxity (1).

#### *Incidence*

- For all degrees of instability, 1 per 200 births (1,5)
- For full dislocation, 1 per 1,000 births (1,5)

### RISK FACTORS

- Breech position
- 1st-born status
- Female gender
- Oligohydramnios
- Family history
- Ehlers-Danlos or Marfan syndromes

#### *Genetics*

Increased risk occurs in persons with a positive family history, but no established Mendelian pattern.

### ETIOLOGY

- Dysplasia occurs because of unfavorable forces on the hip *in utero* (1).
- Adduction of the limb, such as with oligohydramnios, directs the femoral head to the edge of the acetabulum.
- Breech position increases hamstring tension and thus the force across the hip.
- Ligamentous laxity, greater in females and in some families, also increases the risk.
- The earlier *in utero* these factors develop, the more severe the dysplasia.
- Postpartum factors, such as a contralateral abduction contracture or swaddling of the limbs, prevent some hips from stabilizing on their own.

### ASSOCIATED CONDITIONS

- Muscular torticollis
- Foot deformities
- Genetic syndromes (especially connective-tissue disorders and skeletal dysplasia)

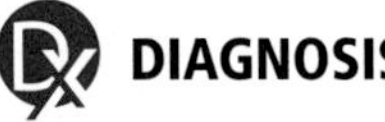

## DIAGNOSIS

### SIGNS AND SYMPTOMS

- No symptoms appear during the 1st few years of life (4).
- Only careful physical examination for a gentle clunk of the hip out of (Barlow sign) or into (Ortolani sign) the acetabulum shows the problem.
- The affected hip may rest in slight adduction and may have a deeper proximal thigh crease, but these signs are not constant.
- The abduction of the affected limb usually is <50° because of the changed center of rotation.
  - The parent may note this adduction limitation while changing the infant's diapers (Fig. 1).
  - A click may be felt in the hip, but it is a nonspecific sign because a click often is felt in normal hips and comes from the meniscus of the knee, fascia lata, or a synovial fold.
  - The clunk of instability usually is lost after ~6 months, when the dislocation becomes more fixed.
- The child with a dysplastic hip may begin to walk on time or just a few months late.
  - After walking age, the thigh crease may become more pronounced, and the circumference may be decreased.
  - A Trendelenburg limp may be noted (the pelvis drops when the patient stands on the dysplastic side).
  - If both sides are affected, increased lumbar lordosis may be present (4).
  - Pain develops only after cartilage degeneration starts at 18 years of age at the earliest, and often much later.
  - Associated conditions should raise the suspicion of hip dysplasia.

#### *Physical Exam*

- Hip abduction is assessed.
  - Document Ortolani and Barlow tests on all newborns and repeat during well-baby checks.
    - Baby warm, quiet, and relaxed on parent's lap
    - 1 hip at a time
    - Gentle downward pressure on knee or thigh with adduction
    - Feel whether hip goes partially or fully out (Barlow test).
    - Abduct to feel it slide back in (Ortolani test).
    - Check for hip abduction (<60° is suspicious).
- With the patient's pelvis flat, note any difference in the height of the 2 knees with the thighs together (Galeazzi or Allis sign).
- Check gait in the older child.

### TESTS

#### *Imaging*

- If abnormal examination or risk factors exist, an ultrasound study is indicated in the first 6 months, before cartilage ossifies; this procedure requires an ultrasonographer experienced in hips (3,6).
- Arthrography shows the depth of reduction with a 90% good outcome if <5 mm of space exists between the femoral head and acetabulum.
- Plain radiographs are most useful after 5 months.
  - Both the shape of the acetabulum and its relation to the femur should be assessed.
  - The Shenton line should form a smooth arc from the neck of the femur to the superior ramus of the pubis.
  - The femoral epiphysis should be medial to the outer edge of the acetabulum.
- MRI and CT have only limited roles in usual cases of DDH (Fig. 2).

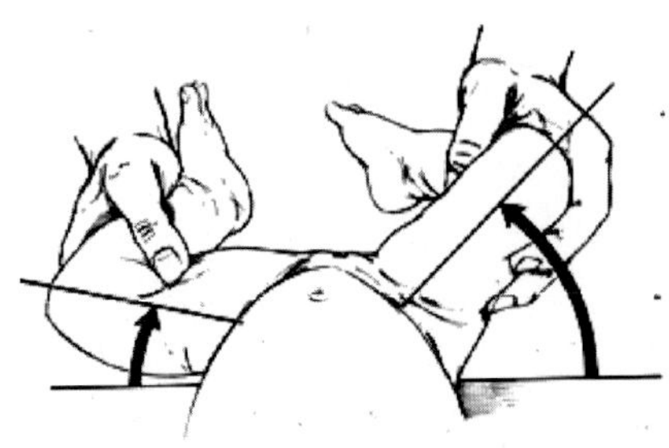

**Fig. 1.** Asymmetrical abduction of the hip is the most sensitive sign of DDH across all age groups.

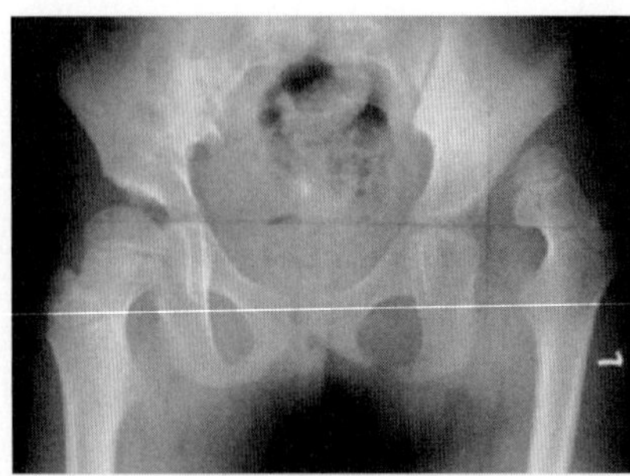

**Fig. 2.** DDH was not diagnosed until age 5 in this patient. Note the extensive proximal migration and dysplasia of both femur and acetabulum.

### *Pathological Findings*

- The acetabulum is flattened posterosuperiorly.
- The femoral head is flattened anteriorly, and femoral anteversion is increased.
- Cartilage erosion and arthritis develop after the 2nd decade.

## DIFFERENTIAL DIAGNOSIS

- Benign soft-tissue click from hip or knee fascia
- Neuromuscular hip dysplasia from muscle imbalance in cerebral palsy or spina bifida
- Congenital short femur and coxa vara, but with located hip

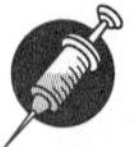

# TREATMENT

## GENERAL MEASURES

- The hip should be reduced within the 1st 6 weeks if the dislocation is recognized.
- The earlier the diagnosis is made, the easier and safer the treatment will be.
- Even up until age 6–8 years, reduction is worthwhile but requires surgery.
- Treatment varies according to age.
  - Newborn:
    - Click and subluxation are followed with serial examinations.
    - Many patients improve within 1 week.
  - Newborn–6 months:
    - Full dislocation or persistent instability is treated with an abduction brace, such as the Pavlik harness, which flexes the hip beyond 90° (Fig. 3).
    - Bracing should be done by an orthopaedist familiar with pediatrics.
    - The hip should reduce within 3 weeks, which should be confirmed with ultrasound or radiography.
    - A full-time brace is used until the hip is clinically stable; then, a part-time brace is used until the hip is radiographically normal.
    - After 6 months: Closed versus open reduction

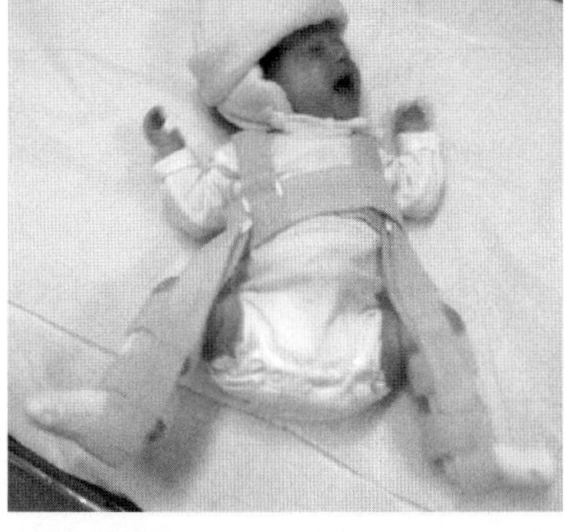

**Fig. 3.** Treatment of DDH with a Pavlik harness.

## SPECIAL THERAPY

### *Physical Therapy*

Minimal need exists for physical therapy because, with time, children regain strength and motion on their own.

## SURGERY

- A medial or lateral approach to the hip joint is used to release the structures inside the joint that are blocking reduction.
- Osteotomy of the pelvis or femur is done to realign the joint surface.
- The approach depends on patient age.
  - 6–24 months:
    - Many surgeons proceed with a period of skin traction first to stretch the soft tissues.
    - Closed or open reduction with the patient under anesthesia
    - After reduction, spica cast for 3–6 months
  - >24 months:
    - Open reduction, usually including a femoral osteotomy or iliac osteotomy
    - The results of surgical reduction decline with the increasing age of the child (7).

# FOLLOW-UP

## PROGNOSIS

- Untreated complete dislocation results in a permanent waddling (Trendelenburg) gait and pain by age 30–50 years at the latest (1,7).
- Patients with subluxed, but not dislocated, hips may have pain earlier.
- Hips that are successfully treated early may have normal function.

## COMPLICATIONS

- Redislocation (5%) (1–3)
- Residual dysplasia (25%) (1–3)
- AVN (10%) (1–3):
  - If the blood supply to the upper femur is disturbed by the process of reduction
  - It may be impossible to reverse this process fully.

## PATIENT MONITORING

- After treatment of a dysplastic hip, follow-up care is needed until the patient reaches maturity.
- Even after successful hip reduction, a 10–25% chance exists of incomplete remodeling of the femur and acetabulum that may require osteotomy (1–3,7)

## REFERENCES

1. Weinstein SL, Mubarak SJ, Wenger DR. Developmental hip dysplasia and dislocation: Part I. *Instr Course Lect* 2004;53:523–530.
2. Cady RB. DDH: definition, recognition, and prevention of late sequelae. *Pediatr Ann* 2006;35:92–101.
3. Harcke HT. Imaging methods used for children with hip dysplasia. *Clin Orthop Relat Res* 2005;434:71–77.
4. Ilfeld FW, Westin GW, Makin M. Missed or developmental dislocation of the hip. *Clin Orthop Relat Res* 1986;203:276–281.
5. US Preventive Services Task Force. Screening for developmental dysplasia of the hip: recommendation statement. *Pediatrics* 2006;117:898–902.
6. Harcke HT, Kumar SJ. The role of ultrasound in the diagnosis and management of congenital dislocation and dysplasia of the hip. *J Bone Joint Surg* 1991;73A:622–628.
7. Kim YH, Kim JS. Total hip arthroplasty in adult patients who had developmental dysplasia of the hip. *J Arthroplasty* 2005;20:1029–1036.

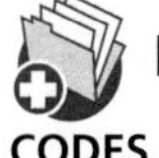

# MISCELLANEOUS

## CODES

### *ICD9-CM*

- 754.31 Congenital dislocation of the hip (unilateral)
- 754.32 Congenital dislocation of the hip (bilateral)
- 754.33 Congenital subluxation of the hip (unilateral)
- 754.34 Congenital subluxation of the hip (bilateral)

## PATIENT TEACHING

- The monitoring of skin around casts and braces is important.
- Infants in Pavlik harness should wear the device continuously until the hip is stable.
- Older children are treated in a spica (body) cast, so walking is not possible.
- Special car seats and wheelchairs are available.

## FAQ

- Q: Are all cases of developmental dysplasia detectable by physical examination?
  - A: No. Physical screening tests are useful for detecting many cases in infancy, but physical tests are neither completely sensitive nor specific. On the other hand, the rarity of hip dysplasia means that routine ultrasound or radiography are not indicated for all children.
- Q: Is double-diapering effective in treating DDH?
  - A: Most experts believe that double diapering is not enough because the diapers do not control the position of the hips accurately enough. It may be a useful temporizing maneuver while awaiting the results of a repeat ultrasound or obtaining a brace.

# DISCITIS

*Paul D. Sponseller, MD*
*Andrew P. Mansita, MD*

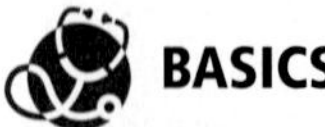

## BASICS

### DESCRIPTION

- Discitis is an infection of the disc space and vertebral endplate that is caused by hematogenous or postoperative inoculation.
- It affects intervertebral discs of the spine.
  - The lower lumbar discs are most commonly involved.
  - However, the infection may occur in any disc.
- Classification:
  - Spontaneous (hematogenous)
  - Iatrogenic (after discectomy or discogram)

### EPIDEMIOLOGY

- Hematogenous infection is uncommon.
- The mean age of occurrence of hematogenous (spontaneous) discitis is 7 years (1), but it may affect individuals of any age.

#### *Incidence*

The incidence of infection after discectomy is <1% (2).

### RISK FACTORS

- Compromised host (patients with diabetes, alcohol abuse, transplants)
- Intravenous drug abuse
- Procedures involving the disc (discography, discectomy, spinal anesthesia)

### ETIOLOGY

- Bacterial infection:
  - The causative organism most commonly is *Staphylococcus*, except in the compromised host or intravenous drug abuser, in whom Gram-negative aerobic bacteria and *Candida* are more common (for these patients, biopsy is indicated) (3).
- Vascularity issues in children <8 years old:
  - The blood supply to the disc comes from the adjacent vertebral body.
  - Vessels cross the cartilaginous endplate in children until they are approximately 8 years old, and the resultant vascularity renders younger children susceptible to infection in the area.

### ASSOCIATED CONDITIONS

Vertebral osteomyelitis

## DIAGNOSIS

### SIGNS AND SYMPTOMS

- Symptoms:
  - Back pain, usually insidious in onset but increasing with time
  - Abdominal pain
  - Loss of appetite
  - Malaise
- Signs:
  - Back stiffness
  - Refusal to walk
  - Pain on spinal percussion
  - Loss of lordosis
  - Fever: Usually low-grade, but may be absent

#### *Physical Exam*

- Note the presence or absence of normal lumbar lordosis.
- Look for pain or refusal to bend forward.
- Look for pain on paraspinal percussion.
- Look for pain on abdominal palpation in lumbar discitis.
- Neurologic examination remains normal, except in late presentations of fulminant discitis.

### TESTS

#### *Lab*

- White blood cell count, ESR, and C-reactive protein usually are mildly elevated but may be normal.
- Obtain a blood culture even though it is positive <30% of the time (4)
- No specific laboratory tests exists for this disorder.

#### *Imaging*

- Plain films are positive only after several weeks; they show irregularity and narrowing of the disc space, with mild osseous involvement.
- MRI:
  - For suspected cases of discitis, shows the pathologic features before abnormalities are visible radiographically.
  - Gives more detailed anatomic information than a bone scan, but a bone scan is an acceptable alternative

#### *Pathological Findings*

- Chronic inflammation
- Destruction of disc structure and endplates

### DIFFERENTIAL DIAGNOSIS

- Tuberculosis (usually shows more destruction of adjacent bone)
- Vertebral osteomyelitis (more destruction of bone than disc, but these 2 entities may merge)

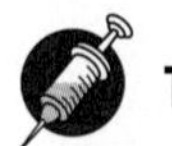

## TREATMENT

### GENERAL MEASURES

- Rest
- Immobilization
- Antibiotics
- For childhood spontaneous discitis, no biopsy or débridement is needed because treatment of staphylococcal infection is virtually always successful.
  - This treatment should be given intravenously if the patient is severely ill, orally if the patient is only mildly symptomatic.
  - Bed rest and bracing may be used if pain is pronounced.
  - For discitis in the compromised host, biopsy and drainage should be performed.

### SPECIAL THERAPY

#### *Physical Therapy*

Therapy is useful for adults with severe back stiffness after treatment has begun.

### MEDICATION (DRUGS)

- For routine spontaneous discitis, oxacillin, dicloxacillin, and cephalosporin are indicated.
- For complicated cases or in compromised hosts, broad-spectrum antibiotics effective against Gram-negative and anaerobic organisms should be added.
- NSAIDs or mild narcotics may help patients with severe pain initially until the infection is controlled.

### SURGERY
- Biopsy may be required in the immunocompromised patient, or one for whom medical therapy has failed.
  – Anterolateral or posterolateral approach with fluoroscopic guidance
- Drainage may be required for patients who fail to respond to medical management alone.
  – Usually obtained via an anterior approach to allow adequate visualization, débridement, and safety
- Surgical reconstruction of the spine segment may be indicated for adults with substantial disc space destruction or endplate compromise.

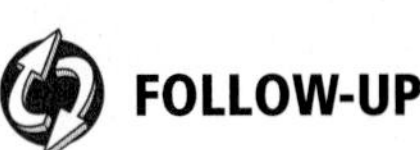

## FOLLOW-UP

### PROGNOSIS
- Prognosis is good once the infection has cleared.
- After childhood discitis, the vertebrae adjacent to the infected disc usually develop a spontaneous painless fusion.
- In adults, spontaneous fusion does not always occur, and back pain may persist.

### COMPLICATIONS
Persistence of infection (lack of symptom improvement in 1–2 weeks) requires accurate identification of the organism and adequate débridement.

### PATIENT MONITORING
- Physical examination is the most useful means for monitoring infection healing.
- The examiner should check for tenderness to percussion and range of forward flexion.
- Radiographs and ESR lag far behind the clinical course.

### REFERENCES

1. Cushing AH. Diskitis in children. *Clin Infect Dis* 1993;17:1–6.
2. Schnoring M, Brock M. [Prophylactic antibiotics in lumbar disc surgery: analysis of 1,030 procedures]. *Zentralbl Neurochir* 2003;64:24–29.
3. Berbari EF, Steckelberg JM, Osmon DR. Osteomyelitis. In: Mandell GL, Bennett JE, Dolin R, eds. *Mandell, Douglas, and Bennett's Principles and Practice of Infectious Diseases,* 6th ed. New York: Churchill Livingstone, 2005:1322–1332.
4. Fernandez M, Carrol CL, Baker CJ. Discitis and vertebral osteomyelitis in children: an 18-year review. *Pediatrics* 2000;105:1299–1304.


### ADDITIONAL READING

- Eastlack RK, Kauffman CP. Pyogenic infections. In: Bono CM, Garfin SR, Tornetta P, et al., eds. *Spine.* Philadelphia: Lippincott Williams & Wilkins, 2004:73–80.
- Gutierrez KM. Diskitis. In: Long SS, ed. *Principles and Practice of Pediatric Infectious Diseases*, 2nd ed. New York: Churchill Livingstone, 2003:481–484.
- Lifeso RM, Weaver P, Harder EH. Tuberculous spondylitis in adults. *J Bone Joint Surg* 1985;67A:1405–1413.
- Stans A. Osteomyelitis and septic arthritis. In: Morrissy RT, Weinstein SL, eds. *Lovell and Winter's Pediatric Orthopaedics*, 6th ed. Philadelphia: Lippincott Williams & Wilkins, 2006:439–491.
- Wenger DR, Bobechko WP, Gilday DL. The spectrum of intervertebral disc-space infection in children. *J Bone Joint Surg* 1978;60A:100–108.


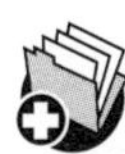

## MISCELLANEOUS

### CODES
#### *ICD9-CM*
722.90 Discitis

### PATIENT TEACHING
#### *Activity*
- The patient may resume activity according to symptom level.
- Activities such as jumping, lifting, and bending forward should be discouraged until symptoms subside.

### FAQ
- Q: Does lack of a positive blood culture rule out discitis in a symptomatic child?
  – A: No. Blood cultures are positive in only a minority of reported cases of discitis.
- Q: What is the preferred imaging study for the evaluation of a patient with suspected or known discitis?
  – A: MRI is preferred because it shows changes within the disc and endplate before conventional radiographic images do, and because the information it provides is more specific than that provided by a 3-phase bone scan.

# DISCOID MENISCUS

*Jason W. Hammond, MD*

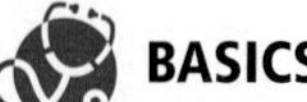

## BASICS

### DESCRIPTION

- Discoid meniscus is a thickened, pancake-shaped lateral meniscus of developmental origin (Fig. 1).
- It often causes clicking or locking of the knee in childhood or early adulthood.
- It may be unilateral or bilateral.
- Classification:
  - General (1):
    - Complete: Meniscus covers entire lateral tibial plateau
    - Incomplete: Meniscus larger than normal but does not cover the entire lateral plateau
  - Wrisberg (1):
    - Ligament type
    - Unstable
    - Lacks posterior attachment of meniscus to tibia
- Synonym: Wrisberg meniscus

### EPIDEMIOLOGY

#### *Incidence*

- The approximate incidence is <1% in the United States and up to 26% in Japan (2).
- Most cases present in late childhood or early adolescence.

#### *Prevalence*

The United States prevalence is ~4–5% (1).

### ETIOLOGY

This condition is an anatomic or developmental abnormality.

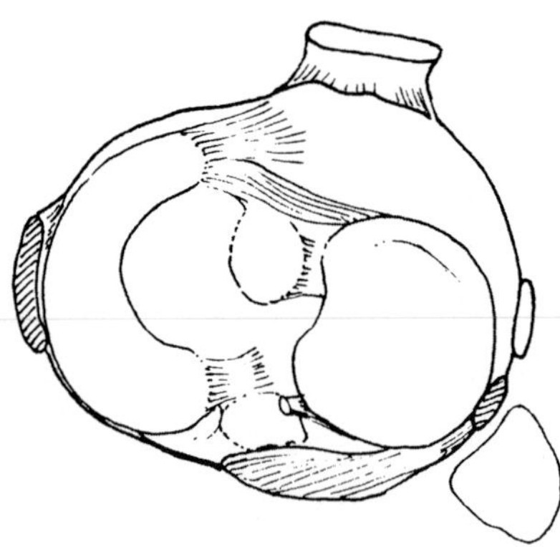

**Fig. 1.** A diseased lateral meniscus lacks the normal semilunar shape and covers the entire lateral side of the tibia.

## DIAGNOSIS

### SIGNS AND SYMPTOMS

- Many patients are asymptomatic.
- Presentation is highly variable, depending on the type of meniscus and the presence or absence of a tear.
- The classic snapping-knee syndrome is characterized by a "clunk" at the terminal limits of flexion and extension.
- May be associated with pain, clicking, swelling, locking, popping, and blocks to motion
- The onset often is insidious, without a history of trauma.
- If symptoms are acute or associated with trauma, an acute tear may be the cause.

#### *Physical Exam*

- Usually, little to no effusion is present in the knee.
- Mild tenderness may be present at the lateral joint line, but not as severe as that with an acute meniscus tear.
- Often, a pop or click is noted with the McMurray test (rotating the knee while it is in a fully flexed position).
- The examiner may note a block to full extension or the patient's apprehension when the knee is straightened.

### TESTS

- The McMurray test: Extension and rotation of a maximally flexed knee:
  - A positive test is pain or popping at the lateral joint line.

#### *Imaging*

- Plain radiography:
  - Wide lateral joint space (3)
  - Lateral joint lipping
  - Cupping of the lateral tibial plateau
  - Flattening of the lateral femoral condyle
- MRI:
  - 3 or more contiguous 5-mm sagittal sections showing continuity between the anterior and posterior horns
  - Block "bow tie" appearance on the coronal view with increased width of the mid-AP diameter

#### *Pathological Findings*

- Disc-shaped meniscus
- Stable variant: Normal tibial ligaments
- Unstable variant: Absence of the posterolateral tibial attachments

### DIFFERENTIAL DIAGNOSIS

- Acute meniscus tear
- OCD or osteochondral fracture
- Physeal fracture
- Fracture of the tibial eminence
- ACL tear

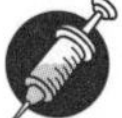

## TREATMENT

### GENERAL MEASURES

- Asymptomatic patients should be observed.
- Symptomatic patients often require surgical treatment, which varies depending on whether a tear is present and whether the meniscus is stable or unstable.
- Nonoperative methods are rarely helpful in the patient with symptomatic discoid meniscus, although a trial of immobilization may be attempted in patients with acute-onset cases.
- Patients may resume normal activity when symptoms resolve.

### SURGERY

- Stable meniscus: Partial meniscectomy or saucerization (trimming) to form a more normal-appearing meniscus (4)
- Unstable meniscus:
  - Saucerization and reattachment to the posterolateral capsule in an attempt to preserve the meniscus
  - Complete meniscectomy is indicated if the patient has degenerative changes or a large meniscal tear.

## FOLLOW-UP

### PROGNOSIS

Patients with a stable discoid meniscus have good results with saucerization.

### COMPLICATIONS

- Degenerative joint disease is possible with complete meniscectomy.
- Recurrent meniscal tears

### PATIENT MONITORING

Patients should be followed until symptoms resolve.

### REFERENCES


1. Jordan MR. Lateral meniscal variants: evaluation and treatment. *J Am Acad Orthop Surg* 1996;4:191–200.
2. Miller RH, III. Knee injuries. In: Canale ST, ed. *Campbell's Operative Orthopaedics,* 9th ed. St. Louis: Mosby-Year Book Inc., 1998:1113–1299.
3. Asik M, Sen C, Taser OF, et al. Discoid lateral meniscus: diagnosis and results of arthroscopic treatment. *Knee Surg Sports Traumatol Arthrosc* 2003;11:99–104.
4. Youm T, Chen AL. Discoid lateral meniscus: evaluation and treatment. *Am J Orthop* 2004;33:234–238.


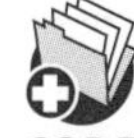

## MISCELLANEOUS

### CODES

#### *ICD9-CM*

717.5 Discoid meniscus

### PATIENT TEACHING

- Observation, if the discoid meniscus is asymptomatic
- Increased risk of degenerative changes after total meniscectomy

### FAQ

- Q: Do patients with discoid lateral meniscus require surgery?
  - A: If the discoid lateral meniscus is truly asymptomatic or is noted incidentally on MRI or at the time of arthroscopy, surgical repair is not necessary. If the discoid meniscus is symptomatic (lateral knee pain, locking, swelling), it should be saucerized to resemble a normal lateral meniscus. Degenerative tears should be débrided, but unstable peripheral tears should be repaired after saucerization.

# DISLOCATION IN THE ADULT

*Simon C. Mears, MD, PhD*

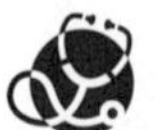

## BASICS

### DESCRIPTION

- Dislocation occurs when a force across a joint disrupts the restraining capsule, ligaments, and muscles.
- Dislocated joints may reduce spontaneously or remain unreduced.
- Dislocations can be associated with periarticular fractures, ruptured ligaments, capsular damage, and cartilage damage (1).
- The dislocation may result in stretch or injury to the arteries or nerves that cross the joint.
- Dislocation may occur after prosthetic joint replacement, particularly of the hip.

### GENERAL PREVENTION

Use of protective devices and equipment during sporting activity

### EPIDEMIOLOGY

#### *Incidence*

- In 1 study, the rate of shoulder dislocation was 17 in 100,000 per year (2).
- In another study, the rate of dislocation after hip replacement was 3.9% (3).

### RISK FACTORS

- Sports
- Car accidents
- Falls
- Trauma
- Joint replacement
- Skateboarding and in-line skating

### PATHOPHYSIOLOGY

- The vector of force on a limb results in particular patterns of injury to the joint (4).
  - When a hip is flexed, a force on the axis of the femur results in a posterior hip dislocation.
  - Force on a hip in an extended position results in an anterior dislocation.

### ETIOLOGY

### ASSOCIATED CONDITIONS

- Periarticular fractures
- Nerve and vessel injury
- Osteonecrosis
- Cartilage damage

## DIAGNOSIS

### SIGNS AND SYMPTOMS

- Pain and deformity of the joint
- Inability to bear weight on the affected limb
- Neurologic compromise

#### *History*

Traumatic injury, as from a fall or car accident

#### *Physical Exam*

- A complete neurologic examination is important, and the strength and sensation distally should be noted.
- Pulses should be palpated and, if not found, Doppler ultrasound should be performed.
- The remainder of the extremity should be evaluated for swelling or deformity.

### TESTS

#### *Imaging*

- Radiography:
  - Plain radiographs of the joint should be taken in 2 planes to show the direction of dislocation.
  - Radiographs are repeated after reduction.
- CT is used to evaluate intra-articular fracture patterns.
- MRI is used to evaluate ligament and soft-tissue damage around the joint.

### DIFFERENTIAL DIAGNOSIS

- Fracture
- Joint effusion
- Joint infection

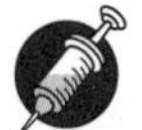

## TREATMENT

### INITIAL STABILIZATION

- All joint dislocations should be reduced as soon as possible.
- Radiographs should be taken 1st to confirm the dislocation and to show fractures.

### GENERAL MEASURES

- Depending on the nature of the injury, reduction may require no anesthesia, intra-articular joint injection, conscious sedation, or full anesthesia.
  - The hip joint often requires sedation or a full anesthetic with muscle relaxant because the muscle forces around the joint can be great.
- After reduction, joint stability should be confirmed by taking the joint through its ROM.
- Unstable joints should be braced or placed in traction after reduction and usually require surgical stabilization.
- Plain radiographs should be taken in 2 views to confirm reduction.
- CT is used in dislocations of the hip and shoulder to assess for fractures or intra-articular fragments (5).

#### *Activity*

- Dislocations that are stable after reduction and do not have fractures usually should be mobilized quickly.
- Immobilization for a week may help with soft-tissue pain and swelling.

### SPECIAL THERAPY

#### *Physical Therapy*

Patients with stable dislocations should begin an assisted program in ROM and joint strengthening.

### SURGERY

- Indications for surgery include:
  - Unstable joint dislocations
  - Periarticular fractures:
    - Joint injuries do best when ROM exercises can be started early.
    - Fractures must be stabilized to allow for early ROM.
    - Fractures also must be reduced anatomically to decrease the risk of posttraumatic arthritis.
  - In some cases, ruptured or torn periarticular soft tissue may be treated with surgery.
    - Acute shoulder dislocations in young adults have a high risk of recurrent instability.
  - Irreducible joint dislocations:
    - Soft tissues such as tendons, nerves, or arteries may be caught in the joint.
    - Open reduction is required.
  - Intra-articular osteochondral fragments

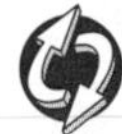

## FOLLOW-UP

- Confirmation should be made after reduction, taking care to assure joint congruity.
- Patients should be reassessed in 1–2 weeks.
  - If the joint is stable, early ROM should be started.
- Dislocation may put the patients at risk for instability, osteonecrosis, or posttraumatic arthritis.

## PROGNOSIS

- Prognosis depends on the particular joint dislocated and the injuries to surrounding tissues.
- Injuries to nerves and arteries around the joint have a poor prognosis.
- Periarticular fractures are at risk for posttraumatic arthritis and the need for later joint replacement (6).
- Missed joint dislocations have a poor prognosis.
- Shoulder dislocations have a high rate of redislocation in young adults (7).
- In active patients, early surgery may be helpful in preventing chronic instability (7).

## COMPLICATIONS

- Stiffness
- Osteonecrosis:
  - Most common after hip dislocations.
  - Thought to be secondary to damage to the blood supply of the femoral head (8).
  - The length of time to reduction is directly related to the risk of osteonecrosis.
    - Hips should be reduced within 6 hours (6).
- Posttraumatic arthritis:
  - Depends on the reduction of the fracture and the amount of chondral damage to the joint at the time of injury
    - In 1 study of the outcomes after posterior fracture-dislocations of the hip, poor outcome was seen in 18% of patients (6).
  - Common after hindfoot subtalar dislocation (9)
- Joint instability:
  - The presence of fracture and damage to surrounding supportive structures of the joint increases the risk of late instability (10).
  - Joints with less innate stability, such as the shoulder, have a higher risk of late instability than do joints with more stable bony structures, such as the elbow.
- Nerve damage:
  - Early reduction reduces the amount of time that nerves are stretched.
  - After hip dislocation, patients with longer times to reduction have worse nerve injuries (11).

## PATIENT MONITORING

- Patients should be monitored with radiographs to check that the joint is reduced concentrically.
- Additional follow-up is based on the individual injury.
  - Patients with hip dislocations should be followed radiographically for the 1st year to assess for posttraumatic arthritis and osteonecrosis.

## REFERENCES


1. te Slaa RL, Wijffels MPJM, Brand R, et al. The prognosis following acute primary glenohumeral dislocation. *J Bone Joint Surg* 2004;86B:58–64.
2. Kroner K, Lind T, Jensen J. The epidemiology of shoulder dislocations. *Arch Orthop Trauma Surg* 1989;108:288–290.
3. Phillips CB, Barrett JA, Losina E, et al. Incidence rates of dislocation, pulmonary embolism, and deep infection during the first six months after elective total hip replacement. *J Bone Joint Surg* 2003;85A:20–26.
4. Monma H, Sugita T. Is the mechanism of traumatic posterior dislocation of the hip a brake pedal injury rather than a dashboard injury? *Injury* 2001;32:221–222.
5. Brooks RA, Ribbans WJ. Diagnosis and imaging studies of traumatic hip dislocations in the adult. *Clin Orthop Relat Res* 2000;377:15–23.
6. Moed BR, Willson Carr SE, Watson JT. Results of operative treatment of fractures of the posterior wall of the acetabulum. *J Bone Joint Surg* 2002;84A:752–758.
7. Bottoni CR, Wilckens JH, DeBerardino TM, et al. A prospective, randomized evaluation of arthroscopic stabilization versus nonoperative treatment of acute, traumatic, first-time shoulder dislocations. *Am J Sports Med* 2002;30:576–580.
8. Yue JJ, Wilber JH, Lipuma JP, et al. Posterior hip dislocations: a cadaveric angiographic study. *J Orthop Trauma* 1996;10:447–454.
9. Bibbo C, Anderson RB, Davis WH. Injury characteristics and the clinical outcome of subtalar dislocations: a clinical and radiographic analysis of 25 cases. *Foot Ankle Int* 2003;24:158–163.
10. Robinson CM, Kelly M, Wakefield AE. Redislocation of the shoulder during the first six weeks after a primary anterior dislocation: risk factors and results of treatment. *J Bone Joint Surg* 2002;84A:1552–1559.
11. Hillyard RF, Fox J. Sciatic nerve injuries associated with traumatic posterior hip dislocations. *Am J Emerg Med* 2003;21:545–548.
12. Everett WW. Skatepark injuries and the influence of skatepark design: a one year consecutive case series. *J Emerg Med* 2002;23:269–274.


## ADDITIONAL READING


Dirschl DR, Marsh JL, Buckwalter JA, et al. Articular fractures. *J Am Acad Orthop Surg* 2004;12:416–423.


D

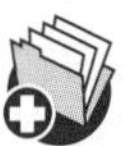

# MISCELLANEOUS

## CODES

### *ICD9-CM*

- 718.3 Recurrent dislocation
- 831.00 Shoulder dislocation
- 832.00 Elbow dislocation
- 833.00 Wrist dislocation
- 835.00 Hip dislocation
- 836.50 Knee dislocation
- 837.1 Ankle dislocation

## PATIENT TEACHING

### *Activity*

Early ROM is started for stable joint dislocations.

### *Prevention*

- Design of skate parks may reduce the risk of injuries (12).
- Use of protective equipment may reduce the risk of injuries after falls during sporting events.

## FAQ

- Q: When should a joint be reduced?
  - A: Joint dislocations should be reduced as quickly as possible to reduce the risk of osteonecrosis, joint damage, and stretch to nerves and blood vessels.

# DUPUYTREN CONTRACTURE

*Darryl B. Thomas, MD*
*Dawn M. LaPorte, MD*

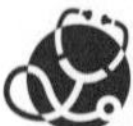

## BASICS

### DESCRIPTION

- Dupuytren contracture is a proliferative disorder of subcutaneous palmar fibrous tissue (fascia) that occurs in the form of nodules and cords and results in contractures of the finger joints (Fig. 1).
- It occurs typically in men in the 5th to 7th decades.
- Younger patients are more likely to have rapid progression of disease with poorer long-term results and frequent recurrences.
- Aggressive, early onset is seen in a subgroup of patients with Dupuytren diathesis.
- Synonym: Dupuytren disease

### EPIDEMIOLOGY

#### *Incidence*

- Greatest in Northern Europe and in immigrants of Celtic origin
- Incidence in the United States is 2–3% that of the general population.
- Hand dominance not a factor
- More frequent and severe in patients with diabetes
- Increased incidence in patients with epilepsy and chronic obstructive pulmonary disease
- Possible link to alcoholism and tobacco is controversial (1,2).
- More common in males than in females (2:1–10:1)
- In females, usually later onset and less severe disease

### RISK FACTORS

- Caucasian
- Northern European descent
- Increased age
- Family history

#### *Genetics*

- The disorder is autosomal dominant with variable penetrance.
- Only 10% of patients with Dupuytren contractures have a positive family history.

### ETIOLOGY

- Unknown
- Strong evidence for hereditary factors, possibly through transmission of defective genes responsible for collagen formation

### ASSOCIATED CONDITIONS

- Alcoholism (controversial)
- Epilepsy
- Diabetes
- Chronic obstructive pulmonary disease

## DIAGNOSIS

### SIGNS AND SYMPTOMS

- Usually begins with 1 or more nodules in the palmar fascia of the ring and little finger rays
- Often associated with skin dimpling over or around the nodules
- Often bilateral (45%) (3)
- Rarely symmetric
- As the disease progresses, the digital fascia becomes involved, usually producing contractures, first of the MCP joints, and then of the PIP joints (Fig. 2).
- Web space contractures can occur.
- Knuckle pads over the dorsum of the PIP joints are present in ~20% of patients.
  - These usually are unnoticeable, but if large and prominent, they may be painful when hit.
- In the subgroup of patients with Dupuytren diathesis, the disease involves the hands, feet, and penis.
  - Often associated with knuckle pads, plantar fibromatosis (Ledderhose disease), and penile fibromatosis (Peyronie disease)

#### *Physical Exam*

- The Hueston table-top test (4) is positive when the palm is placed on a flat surface and the digits, because of joint contractures, cannot be simultaneously placed fully on the same surface.
- A positive test often is an indication for the consideration of surgical management.

### TESTS

#### *Pathological Findings*

- Histologically, the important cells are the myofibroblasts, which seem to undergo pathologic proliferation.
- An increase in the ratio of type III to type I collagen is found in Dupuytren disease (5).

### DIFFERENTIAL DIAGNOSIS

- Arthritis
- Joint capsule contractures

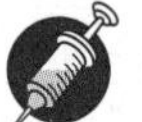

## TREATMENT

### GENERAL MEASURES

In the absence of contracture, or when a contracture is progressing slowly and is not disabling, the patient should be observed every 3–6 months.

### SPECIAL THERAPY

#### *Physical Therapy*

- The goals are to maintain the extension gained by the surgical procedure and to restore preoperative flexion and function of the hand.
- A comfortable, well-fitted splint is an important adjunct to therapy.
- Physical therapists play a major role in recovery, and their programs should stress performance of independent exercises.

### MEDICATION (DRUGS)

- Nonoperative management:
  - Vitamin E and splinting have been ineffective (5).
  - Cortisone injection of nodules that have not yet formed cords has been shown to suppress their development (6).
  - Injection also may be helpful in treating knuckle pads (6).

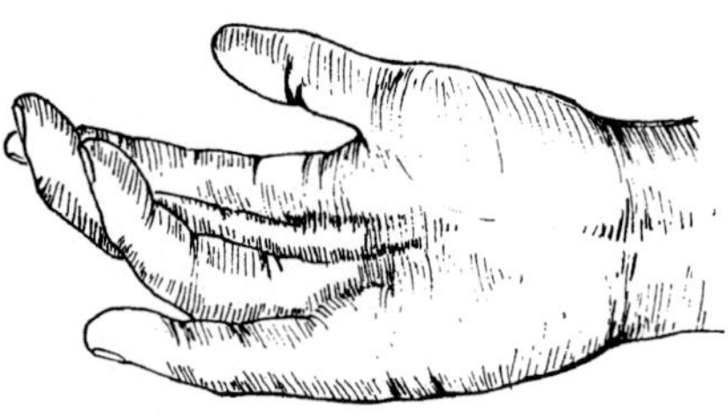

**Fig. 1.** Dupuytren contracture most commonly involves the ring and small fingers and produces cordlike tightening over the flexion tendon.

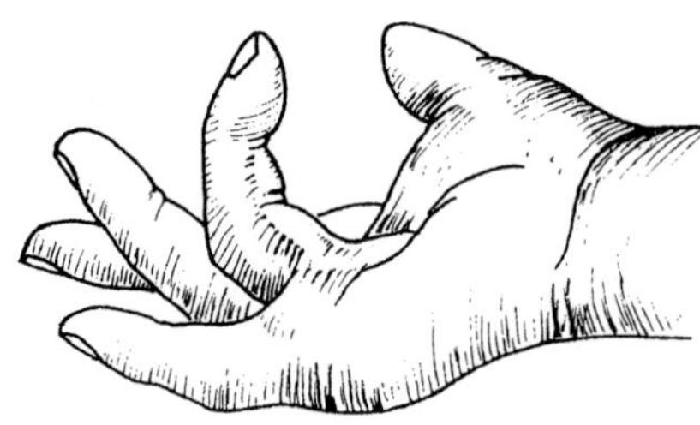

**Fig. 2.** In advanced Dupuytren contracture, the finger is drawn up and impairs the use of the hand.

### SURGERY

- Not indicated for static, painless nodules and rarely for knuckle pads
- Early surgical intervention is indicated for any degree of proximal IP joint involvement or in the presence of progression of contracture or loss of function.
- 5 surgical procedures are used in treating Dupuytren contractures:
  - Subcutaneous fasciotomy
  - Partial (selective) fasciectomy
  - Complete fasciectomy
  - Fasciectomy with skin grafting
  - Amputation
- To choose the best procedure for a given patient, the clinician must consider:
  - The degree of contracture
  - Patient's age, occupation, and general health
  - Nutritional status of the palmar skin
  - Presence or absence of arthritis
- The frequency and duration of splinting after surgery vary with the severity of the disease.
  - A minimum of 3 months usually is required; many patients are instructed to wear a splint at night for up to an additional 3 months.
  - Return to normal activity usually is anticipated within 2–3 months after surgical intervention.

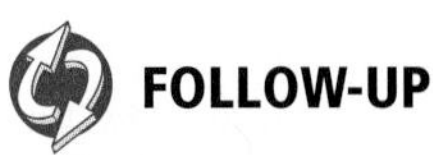

## FOLLOW-UP

### PROGNOSIS

- The normal postoperative expectation is a full range of flexion and extension in 80% of patients seen primarily.
- The disease is likely to progress more rapidly and to recur more frequently in young male patients with a strong family history.
- Patients with epilepsy, diabetes, and alcoholism tend to develop more severe disease.
- Although long-term recurrence rates vary from 26–80%, often only the young patient with a strong diathesis will need multiple repeat procedures.

### COMPLICATIONS

- Joint stiffness usually can be prevented with early physical therapy and patient education.
- 1–3% risk of nerve injury during surgery
- 50% risk of recurrence after 5–10 years
- Unfortunately, long-term complications often depend on the diathesis of the patient.

### PATIENT MONITORING

- Patients must be followed closely (each week during the 1st postoperative month) to help assess wound healing and to prevent stiffness.
- Once healed, follow-up may be on an as-needed basis.

### REFERENCES


1. Burge P, Hoy G, Regan P, et al. Smoking, alcohol and the risk of Dupuytren's contracture. *J Bone Joint Surg* 1997;79B:206–210.
2. Hurst LC, Badalamente MA. Associated diseases. In: McFarlane RR, McGrouther DA, Flint MH, eds. *Dupuytren's Disease: Biology and Treatment.* Edinburgh: Churchill Livingstone, 1990:253–260.
3. Calandruccio JH. Dupuytren contracture. In: Canale ST, ed. *Campbell's Operative Orthopaedics,* 9th ed. St. Louis: Mosby-Year Book Inc., 1998:3675–3684.
4. Hueston JT. Dupuytren's contracture. In: Jupiter JB, ed. *Flynn's Hand Surgery,* 4th ed. Baltimore: Williams & Wilkins, 1991: 864–889.
5. Hurst LC. Dupuytren's disease. In: Manske PR, ed. *Hand Surgery Update.* Rosemont, IL: American Society for Surgery of the Hand, 1994:271–279.
6. Ketchum LD, Donahue TK. The injection of nodules of Dupuytren's disease with triamcinolone acetonide. *J Hand Surg* 2000;25A:1157–1162.


### ADDITIONAL READING


McGrouther DA. Dupuytren's contracture. In: Green DP, Hotchkiss RN, Pederson WC, et al., eds. *Green's Operative Hand Surgery*, 5th ed. Philadelphia: Elsevier Churchill Livingstone, 2005:159–185.


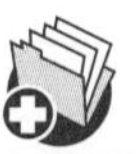

## MISCELLANEOUS

### CODES

#### *ICD9-CM*

728.6 Dupuytren contracture

### PATIENT TEACHING

- Patients should be aware that although MCP deformities usually can be corrected surgically, PIP deformities often may not.
- The patient also must realize that surgery cannot cure Dupuytren disease.

#### *Prevention*

No effective means of prevention is known.

### FAQ

- Q: When is surgery indicated for a Dupuytren contracture?
  - A: Surgery is not indicated unless the patient has a functional disability and progression of the contracture. Typically, surgery is not considered until a >30° contracture is present at the MCP joint and/or some contracture at the PIP joint.
- Q: Why is recurrence frequent?
  - A: The goal of surgery is release of contracture. Dupuytren contracture is a genetic condition, and surgery does not alter the genes, so recurrence is to be expected.

# EHLERS-DANLOS SYNDROME

*Paul D. Sponseller, MD*

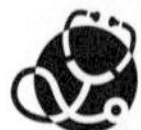

## BASICS

### DESCRIPTION

- Ehlers-Danlos syndrome is a family of disorders involving abnormal collagen that produces connective tissue laxity, with many resultant abnormalities in the skeleton, vasculature, eyes, and other systems.
  - At least 11 subtypes of Ehlers-Danlos syndrome have been identified, with varying patterns of inheritance and genetic causes (1,2).
  - The age at diagnosis varies from infancy to adulthood.
- Classification (1–3):
  - Type I: Gravis (classic):
    - Aneurysms
    - Rupture of hollow viscus
    - Skin hyperextensibility
    - Bruising
    - Pigmented areas
    - Hernias
  - Type II: Mitis:
    - Similar manifestations but milder
  - Type III: Benign hypermobility syndrome:
    - Laxity
    - Joint dislocations
    - Mitral valve prolapse
    - Positive family history
  - Type IV: Ecchymotic:
    - Thin skin
    - Normal joints
    - Aneurysms
    - Viscus rupture
  - Type V: X-linked:
    - Intramuscular hemorrhagia
    - Floppy baby characteristics
  - Type VI: Ocular-scoliotic
  - Type VII: Arthrochalasis multiplex congenital:
    - Extreme joint laxity
    - Short stature
    - Hip dislocations
  - Type VIII: Periodontosis (progressive periodontal disease)
  - Type IX: Occipital horns and skeletal dysplasia
  - Type X: Platelet dysfunction
  - Type XI: Familial joint laxity (patellar and hip dislocation)

### GENERAL PREVENTION

- Prevention of cardiovascular and bleeding emergencies should be the goal of treatment.
- Reduction in frequency of joint dislocations also may be possible.

### EPIDEMIOLOGY

#### *Incidence*

- Overall, males and females are affected equally (2,3).
- Incidence is impossible to calculate accurately because of the numerous forms of this disorder and their varying degrees of severity.

### RISK FACTORS

A positive family history of the syndrome or of its major manifestations is a risk factor.

#### *Genetics*

- Types I, IV, VIII, and XI are autosomal dominant.
- Types V and IX are X-linked.
- The remainder are autosomal recessive in transmission.
- Many patients present as having a new mutation without a family history.

### ETIOLOGY

- Type IV, the ecchymotic variety, is secondary to a disorder of type III collagen.
- Type VI (ocular-scoliotic) is the best characterized.
  - It is caused by a defect in lysine hydroxylase that affects collagen.
  - This change results in decreased collagen cross-linking.
- Type VII (arthrochalasis multiplex congenital) is secondary to a defect in type I collagen.
- Type X (with platelet dysfunction) also results from a defect in type I collagen.

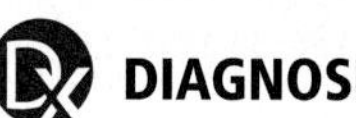

## DIAGNOSIS

The diagnosis is made by a medical geneticist on a clinical basis, with verification in some types by use of molecular testing.

### SIGNS AND SYMPTOMS

- Signs:
  - Lax skin (Fig. 1)
  - Joint hypermobility (Fig. 2)
  - Joint instability (1)
  - Scoliosis (4,5)
  - Ability of some affected persons to perform skeletal contortions impossible for nonaffected persons
- Symptoms:
  - Multiple joint pains
  - Vague musculoskeletal pains

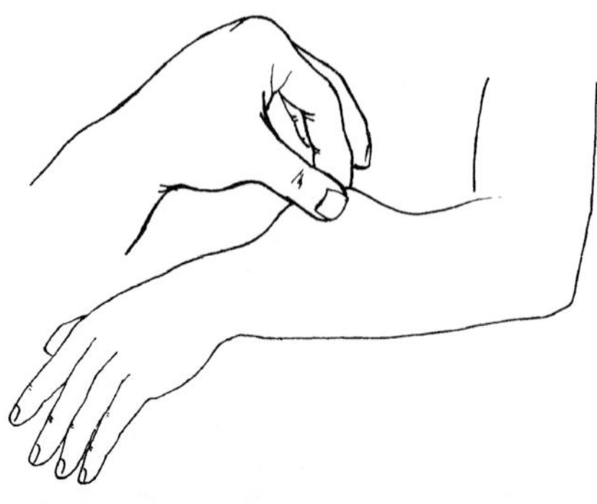

**Fig. 1.** Ehlers-Danlos syndrome is one of several conditions characterized by cutaneous laxity.

#### *Physical Exam*

- Record height.
- Observe the proportions of the skeleton.
- Systematically measure joint ROM.
- Note the ability to hyperextend the fingers and the knees.
- Check the shoulders, elbows, and knees for stability.
- Feel the quality of the skin.
- Note any bruising.
- Pursue an ocular examination if any symptoms of deficit are present.
- Observe the spine for kyphosis.
- Conduct a forward-bend test for scoliosis.

### TESTS

- Molecular testing is available to confirm many, but not all, types of Ehlers-Danlos syndrome.
- An experienced genetics laboratory should be consulted.

#### *Imaging*

- Imaging of the heart and aorta should be obtained periodically for patients with type I and type IV disorders.
- Plain radiographs should be obtained when physical examination suggests scoliosis, kyphosis, or spondylolisthesis.

#### *Pathological Findings*

- Light microscopic examination of fibroblasts of the skin shows irregular collagen fibers.
- Gross examination of the aorta may show dissecting aneurysms in type I, myxomatous changes in the cardiac valves, and redundant chordae tendineae.

### DIFFERENTIAL DIAGNOSIS

- Marfan syndrome also is characterized by laxity of major joints, but it is rarely symptomatic, and it has well-defined diagnostic criteria.
- Larsen syndrome also presents with multiple joint dislocations, but contractures also are present, and cervical kyphosis is common.
- Cutis laxa and pseudoxanthoma elasticum also should be ruled out in patients with predominant skin findings.

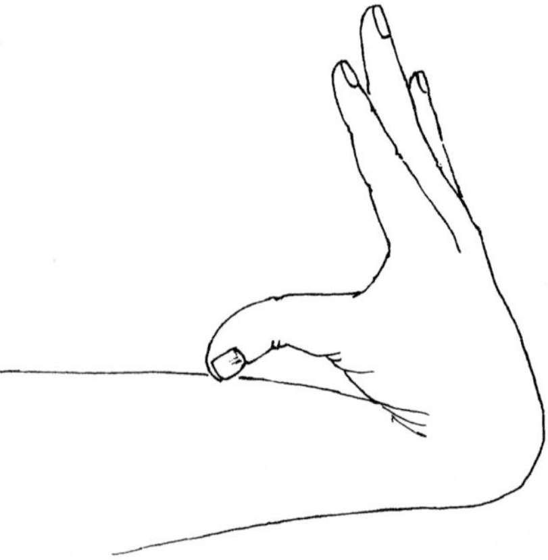

**Fig. 2.** Hypermobile joints are characteristic of Ehlers-Danlos syndrome.

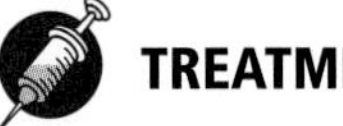

## TREATMENT

### GENERAL MEASURES

- Specialist referral for the systems listed earlier is indicated when problems are manifested by the patient.
- One should use caution when recommending surgery for joint instability because the failure rate is higher than normal.
- Surgical treatment should not be undertaken in Ehlers-Danlos syndrome unless symptoms are severe.
- Fusion of joints may be necessary to provide stability.

### SPECIAL THERAPY

#### *Physical Therapy*

- Muscle conditioning may ameliorate some of the symptoms of joint instability, even if these symptoms are not eliminated.
- Physical therapy also should be helpful in educating patients about how to decrease the frequency of joint dislocations.

### SURGERY

- Fusion for scoliosis is indicated if curves are $>45^\circ$ (approximately) and the patient's medical condition is otherwise satisfactory (4,5).
- Physical activity usually is encouraged, but should be tailored to the patient and focused on low-impact sports.

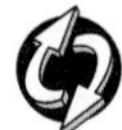

## FOLLOW-UP

### DISPOSITION

#### *Issues for Referral*

The best specialist for the routine follow-up of patients with Ehlers-Danlos syndrome is usually a medical geneticist.

### PROGNOSIS

The listed complications lead to a moderate decline in the mean life expectancy.

### COMPLICATIONS

- Sudden death from cardiovascular complications
- Osteoarthritis of joints
- Visual deficits

### REFERENCES


1. Badelon O, Bensahel H, Csukonyi Z, et al. Congenital dislocation of the hip in Ehlers-Danlos syndrome. *Clin Orthop Relat Res* 1990;255:138–143.
2. McKusick VA. Ehlers-Danlos syndrome. In: *Heritable Disorders of Connective Tissue,* 4th ed. St. Louis: CV Mosby Co., 1972:292–371.
3. Beighton P, De Paepe A, Steinmann B, et al. Ehlers-Danlos syndromes: revised nosology, Villefranche, 1997. *Am J Med Genet* 1998;77:31–37.
4. Akpinar S, Gogus A, Talu U, et al. Surgical management of the spinal deformity in Ehlers-Danlos syndrome type VI. *Eur Spine J* 2003;12:135–140.
5. Vogel LC, Lubicky JP. Neurologic and vascular complications of scoliosis surgery in patients with Ehlers-Danlos syndrome. A case report. *Spine* 1996; 21:2508–2514.


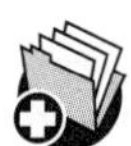

## MISCELLANEOUS

### CODES

#### *ICD9-CM*

756.83 Ehlers-Danlos syndrome

### PATIENT TEACHING

- Genetic counseling should be offered.
- Understanding the nature of any cardiovascular abnormality should be taught, in case of medical emergency.
- Contact or high-impact sports should be discouraged.

#### *Activity*

Activity is encouraged but should be limited to noncontact sports that do not cause pain.

### FAQ

- Q: Are braces helpful in Ehlers-Danlos syndrome?
  - A: They may be in some cases, but in others they produce more inefficient movement. A trial can help determine applicability.
- Q: Is any medication available that can improve the tissue laxity?
  - A: No, not at this time.
- Q: How does one deal with the pain felt by some patients with Ehlers-Danlos syndrome?
  - A: If standard measures fail, referral to a pain specialist may be helpful.

# ELBOW ANATOMY AND EXAMINATION

*Timothy S. Johnson, MD*
*Constantine A. Demetracopoulos, BS*

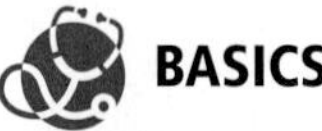

## BASICS

### DESCRIPTION

- Bones (Figs. 1 and 2)
  - Ulnohumeral joint:
    - The trochlea of the humerus articulates with the trochlear notch of the proximal ulna.
    - The olecranon process of the ulna lies posterior to the joint.
    - Allows for elbow flexion and extension
  - Radiohumeral joint:
    - The capitulum of the humerus articulates with the radial head.
    - Allows for forearm supination and pronation
- Ligaments:
  - UCL: Stabilizes the elbow medially
  - RCL: Stabilizes the elbow laterally

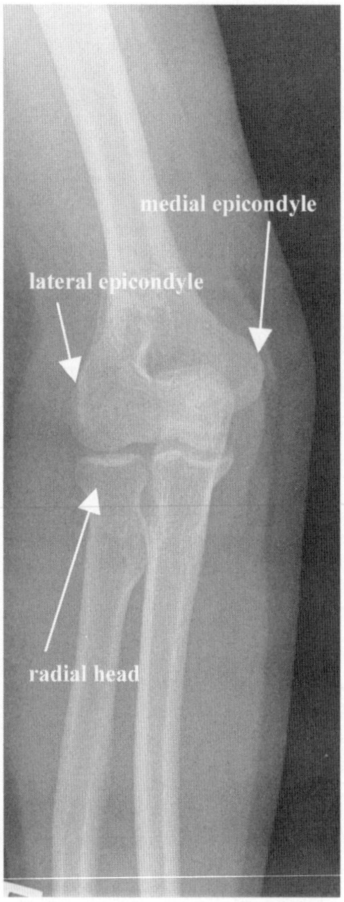

Fig. 1. AP radiograph of a normal elbow.

- Muscles:
  - Biceps: Flexor and supinator
  - Brachialis: Flexor
  - Triceps brachii: Extensor
  - Pronator teres: Flexor and pronator
- Nerves:
  - Median nerve:
    - Crosses the elbow anteriorly, superficial to the brachialis muscle, and medial to the brachial artery
    - Innervates the flexors of the forearm
  - Ulnar nerve:
    - Crosses the elbow superficially and posterior to the medial epicondyle in cubital tunnel
    - Innervates the intrinsic muscles of the hand
  - Radial nerve:
    - Crosses the elbow anteriorly to the lateral epicondyle
    - Innervates wrist, hand, and elbow extensors

### SIGNS AND SYMPTOMS

#### *Physical Exam*

- Initial assessment:
  - Assess completely the contralateral elbow for comparison.
  - Assess the neck, shoulder, and wrist.
  - Perform a complete neurovascular examination of the extremities.
- Inspection:
  - Expose both upper extremities from the shoulder girdle to the hand, inspecting for asymmetry anteriorly and posteriorly.
  - The elbow-carrying angle should be 5–10° of valgus for males and 10–15° of valgus for females.

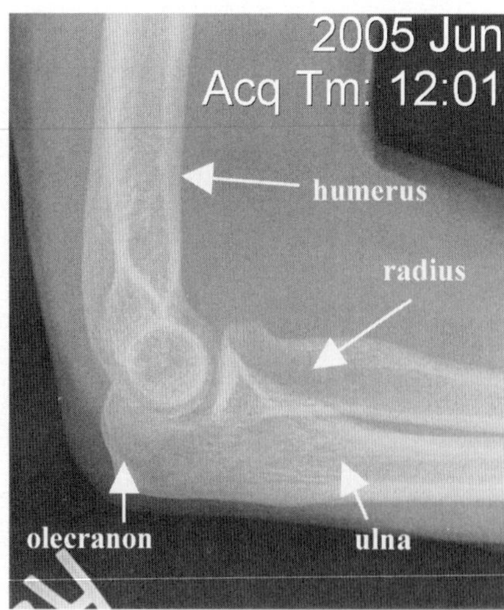


Fig. 2. Lateral radiograph of a normal elbow.

- Palpation:
  - Localize pain to an anatomic structure with digital palpation.
- ROM and strength testing:
  - Compare active and passive ROM.
    - Flexion: 140–150°
    - Extension: 0–10° of hyperextension
    - Supination: 90°
    - Pronation: 80–90°
  - Activities of daily living require 30–130° of flexion, 50° of supination, 50° of pronation.
  - Test isometric strength, testing bilaterally
- Elbow effusion:
  - Palpate elbow laterally in the center of the anatomic triangle formed by the lateral epicondyle, radial head, and tip of the olecranon.
  - Effusion may indicate intra-articular abnormality and can be accompanied by loss of elbow extension.

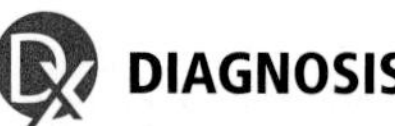

## DIAGNOSIS

- Lateral epicondylitis (tennis elbow) (1):
  - Repetitive overuse of the wrist and finger extensors
  - Tenderness to palpation of lateral epicondyle
  - Resisted wrist extension test:
    - Test resisted dorsiflexion of the wrist with forearm in pronation.
    - Test is positive if it reproduces pain near the lateral epicondyle.
- Medial epicondylitis (golfer's elbow):
  - Resisted flexion/supination test:
    - Place the patient's elbow in slight flexion and the forearm in full supination.
    - Test resisted wrist flexion and/or pronation against resistance.
    - The test is positive if pain is reproduced at the medial epicondyle.
- Olecranon bursitis:
  - Bursa lies subcutaneous and posterior to the olecranon process.
  - Bursitis may be secondary to trauma, hemorrhage, sepsis, or a rheumatologic condition.
  - Effusion can present with or without erythema and may be tender to palpation over the tip of the olecranon.

- Instability (2):
  - UCL insufficiency (valgus stress test):
    - Secure the wrist between the examiner's forearm and trunk.
    - Flex the elbow to 30° and apply a valgus stress.
    - Palpate the UCL along its course from the medial epicondyle toward the proximal ulna during this maneuver.
    - Increased medial joint-space opening with loss of a firm endpoint suggests UCL insufficiency.
  - RCL insufficiency (posterolateral rotatory instability test) (3):
    - With the patient supine and the shoulder flexed overhead, externally rotate the humerus to stabilize it.
    - Grasp the forearm in full supination.
    - Starting with forearm supination and elbow extension, slowly flex the elbow while applying a slight valgus.
    - A positive test results in a palpable clunk, a posterior prominence of the radial head, and an obvious dimple in the skin proximal to the radial head as the elbow subluxates.

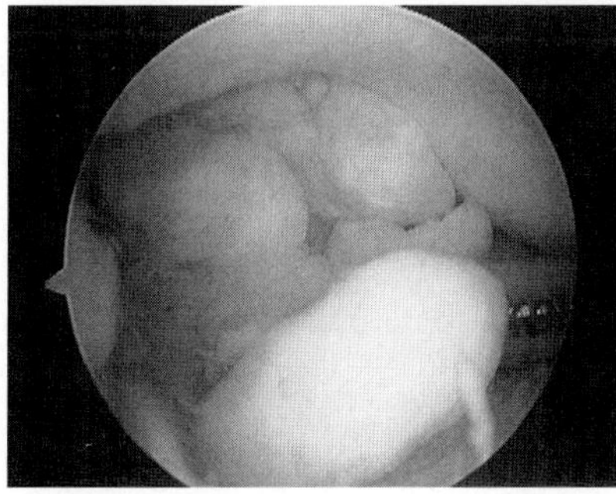

**Fig. 3.** Arthroscopic view of loose bodies in the posterior elbow.

- Valgus extension overload (2):
  - Overuse injury associated with a throwing athlete
  - Often associated with UCL insufficiency, intra-articular loose bodies, and radiocapitellar articular cartilage injury (Fig. 3)
  - Caused by posterior medial impingement of ulnohumeral articulation and compression of radiocapitellar joint during throwing motion
  - Passive hyperextension of the elbow reproduces pain posteromedially.
- Elbow arthritis:
  - Commonly presents with flexion contracture (incomplete passive and active extension) and pain at terminal extension
  - Can present with limitation in elbow flexion
  - Elbow effusion can be variable.
- Cubital tunnel syndrome:
  - Created by compression of ulnar nerve at the elbow
  - Usually presents with pain
  - May be associated with numbness and paresthesias in distribution of the ulnar nerve
  - Symptoms worsen with prolonged elbow flexion
  - Positive Tinel sign: Tapping of the ulnar nerve at the posterior aspect of lateral epicondyle reproduces radicular pain and or paresthesia down the ulnar aspect of forearm/hand.
- Distal biceps rupture:
  - Nonpalpable biceps tendon
  - Pain to palpation in the antecubital space
  - Popeye sign:
    - The biceps resembles a "Popeye" muscle when resisted elbow flexion is tested.
    - Note: The Popeye sign also occurs with proximal biceps tendon rupture.

## REFERENCES


1. Jobe FW, Ciccotti MG. Lateral and medial epicondylitis of the elbow. *J Am Acad Orthop Surg* 1994;2:1–8.
2. Chen FS, Rokito AS, Jobe FW. Medial elbow problems in the overhead-throwing athlete. *J Am Acad Orthop Surg* 2001;9:99–113.
3. Mehta JA, Bain GI. Posterolateral rotatory instability of the elbow. *J Am Acad Orthop Surg* 2004;12:405–415.


## ADDITIONAL READING


- Hoppenfeld S. Physical examination of the elbow. In: *Physical Examination of the Spine & Extremities.* Norwalk, CT: Appleton & Lange, 1976:35–57.
- Hoppenfeld S, deBoer P. The elbow. In: *Surgical Exposures in Orthopaedics: The Anatomical Approach*, 3rd ed. Philadelphia: Lippincott Williams & Wilkins, 2003:105–139.
- Morrey BF. Anatomy of the elbow joint. In: Morrey BF, ed. *The Elbow and its Disorders*, 2nd ed. Philadelphia: WB Saunders Co, 1993:16–52.


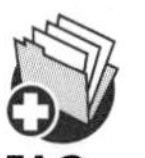

## MISCELLANEOUS

### FAQ

- Q: What are 3 common causes of atraumatic elbow pain?
  - A: Lateral epicondylitis, olecranon bursitis, and ulnar neuritis.

# ELBOW ARTHRITIS

*Jinsong Wang, MD*
*Mark Clough, MD*

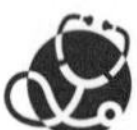

## BASICS

### DESCRIPTION

- The elbow can be affected by inflammatory and noninflammatory arthropathies.
- Regardless of the underlying pathologic process, elbow arthritis generally presents with pain on ROM and loading of the affected joint.

### EPIDEMIOLOGY

#### *Incidence*

- Uncommon
- Primary osteoarthritis accounts for 1–2% of all elbow arthritis; the remainder are inflammatory or posttraumatic (1).
- Can occur in any age group
- Males and females are affected equally.
- Most authorities recommend reserving total elbow arthroplasty for patients >60 years old.

### RISK FACTORS

- Rheumatoid arthritis
- History of septic arthritis
- Previous injury

### ETIOLOGY

- Inflammatory arthropathies
- Trauma

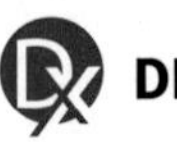

## DIAGNOSIS

### SIGNS AND SYMPTOMS

- Degenerative joint disease of the elbow presents as pain at the extremes of motion that is generally greater in extension than in flexion.
  - A history of trauma often is present.
    - Carrying an object, such as a briefcase or groceries, is possible only for short periods.
  - In later stages, pain can be present with reduced ROM, and a flexion contracture may develop.
  - AP and lateral radiographs show osteophyte formation and bony sclerosis of the elbow.
- Inflammatory arthropathy can present with a similar pain profile.
  - Patients also have signs of inflammation, such as effusion and warmth.
  - Early in the disease, radiographs may be normal because only intense synovitis and effusion are present.

#### *Physical Exam*

- Pain and limited ROM are the earliest findings.
- Effusions are palpated most easily on the lateral side of the elbow.
- Contractures may be seen.
- Ulnar neuropathy can be seen in late presentations.
- Ankylosis of the elbow develops with advanced disease.

### TESTS

#### *Lab*

- Rheumatologic workup is indicated if an inflammatory arthropathy is suspected.
- Joint aspiration with cell count and differential is warranted if a septic joint is a concern.
- Joint fluid may be sent for crystal analysis if crystalline arthropathy is suspected.

#### *Imaging*

Routine AP and lateral radiographs of the elbow

#### *Pathological Findings*

- With rheumatoid arthritis, the synovium proliferates and progressive destruction of the joint occurs.
- The radial head often is destroyed, and valgus deformity occurs.

### DIFFERENTIAL DIAGNOSIS

- Septic joint
- Elbow instability
- Tendinitis
- Nerve entrapment syndromes

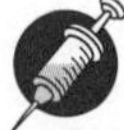

## TREATMENT

### GENERAL MEASURES

- Operative treatment should be reserved for those patients for whom nonoperative measures have failed and who continue to have debilitating pain.
- Activity should be modified to suit the level of symptoms.

### SPECIAL THERAPY

#### *Radiotherapy*

- Radioactive synovectomy:
  - Via sterile intra-articular injection of a radioisotope

#### *Physical Therapy*

- Strengthening and ROM exercises are helpful for patients who respond to nonoperative management.
- A similar postoperative physical therapy regimen is critical to obtaining the highest level of functioning possible after arthroplasty or elbow replacement.

### MEDICATION (DRUGS)

- Initial management should be nonoperative, with NSAIDs, rest, and bracing or supportive devices.
- In addition to NSAIDs, antimalarial agents, gold salts, immunosuppressive drugs, and corticosteroids are used.
- Caution should be used with bracing and immobilization of the elbow because elbow stiffness and even ankylosis may occur quickly.
- Patients who are unresponsive to systemic anti-inflammatory drugs may benefit from intra-articular steroid injections.
  - Care must be exercised with this treatment option because improper aseptic technique can result in joint infection.
  - Frequent injections can weaken tendinous and ligamentous structures.

### SURGERY

- A variety of surgical options are possible, depending on presentation:
  - Arthroscopy represents an early surgical option for elbow arthritis; in addition to an arthroscopic synovectomy for pain relief, osteophytes can be excised to improve ROM (2).
  - Osteotomy (Outerbridge-Kashiwagi arthroplasty, an excision of olecranon and coronoid osteophytes) for decompression in an area of impingement in osteoarthritis (3)
  - Interpositional arthroplasty in patients <60 years old with posttraumatic arthritis (4)
  - Total elbow arthroplasty for (5):
    - Patients for whom nonoperative interventions have failed
    - Patients undergoing less invasive surgical treatments or who have osteoarthrosis involving more than the ulnohumeral joint
  - Resection arthroplasty for salvage (i.e., cases of failed total elbow arthroplasty)
  - Arthrodesis may be considered for intractable sepsis or when revision arthroplasty is not possible.
- Ulnar nerve decompression is indicated in all of the above if evidence of nerve irritation is present.

## FOLLOW-UP

### COMPLICATIONS

- Nonoperative treatment:
  - Ankylosis
  - Ulnar nerve palsy
- Total elbow arthroplasty:
  - Infection
  - Ulnar nerve irritation
  - Aseptic loosening

### PATIENT MONITORING

Patients with rheumatoid arthritis are followed at 6–12-month intervals with AP and lateral radiographs.

### REFERENCES


1. Wada T, Isogai S, Ishii S, et al. Debridement arthroplasty for primary osteoarthritis of the elbow. *J Bone Joint Surg* 2004;86A:233–241.
2. Ramsey ML. Elbow arthroscopy: basic setup and treatment of arthritis. *Instr Course Lect* 2002;51:69–72.
3. O'Driscoll SW. Elbow arthritis: treatment options. *J Am Acad Orthop Surg* 1993;1:106–116.
4. Morrey BF. Nonreplacement reconstruction of the elbow joint. *Instr Course Lect* 2002;51:63–67.
5. Kozak TK, Adams RA, Morrey BF. Total elbow arthroplasty in primary osteoarthritis of the elbow. *J Arthroplasty* 1998;13:837–842.


### ADDITIONAL READING


- King GJ. New frontiers in elbow reconstruction: total elbow arthroplasty. *Instr Course Lect* 2002;51:43–51.
- Yamaguchi K, Adams RA, Morrey BF. Infection after total elbow arthroplasty. *J Bone Joint Surg Am* 1998;80:481–491.


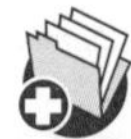

## MISCELLANEOUS

### CODES

#### *ICD9-CM*

716.92 Elbow arthritis

### PATIENT TEACHING

#### *Activity*

Patients are shown how to avoid aggravating activities and are encouraged to maintain a functional ROM.

### FAQ

- Q: Does arthroscopy have any role in the treatment of elbow arthritis?
  - A: Arthroscopy provides a minimally invasive way of performing a synovectomy to reduce pain and swelling and to improve the ROM. It also allows for early physical therapy.

# ELBOW DISLOCATION

*Simon C. Mears, MD, PhD*
*Jinsong Wang, MD*

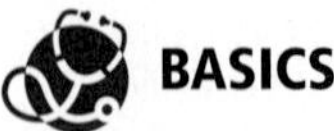

## BASICS

### DESCRIPTION

- Dislocation of the elbow mostly results from trauma.
- Posterior dislocation is most common.
- It most frequently involves people <20 years of age.
- Rarely, elbow dislocation can occur in elderly patients after a fall.
- Most elbow dislocations occur at the ulnohumeral joint.
- Classification: Usually refers to the position of the ulna relative to the humerus after injury:
  - Dislocations can be classified as posterior, anterior, medial, lateral, and divergent.
  - Fracture dislocations of the elbow are associated with radial head and coronoid fractures: the "terrible triad of the elbow" (1).
  - Classification of coronoid fractures (2):
    - I: Avulsion of the tip
    - II: ≤50% of the coronoid
    - III: >50% of the coronoid
    - Large coronoid fractures are thought to be associated with anterior and posterior fracture dislocations, whereas small transverse fractures are associated with the terrible triad (3).

### EPIDEMIOLOGY

#### *Incidence*

- The highest incidence is in persons <20 years old (4).
- It represents 3–6% of all children's fractures and dislocations (5).

### RISK FACTORS

- Snowboarders have a higher risk of elbow dislocation than do skiers (6).
- Sports activities (7)

### PATHOPHYSIOLOGY

- Posterior dislocations are most common and thought to be secondary to a fall on an outstretched hand.
- The collateral ligaments usually are ruptured, with injury to the brachialis muscle and coronoid.

### ASSOCIATED CONDITIONS

- Fracture of the radius
- Fracture of the ulna
- Fracture of the humerus
- Ulnar and median nerve injury
- Brachial artery injury

## DIAGNOSIS

### SIGNS AND SYMPTOMS

- Elbow dislocation occurs mostly after trauma.
- The patient presents with pain, swelling, elbow deformity, and inability to move the elbow.

#### *Physical Exam*

- Assess the patient's neurovascular status.
  - Examine the functions of the radial, median, and ulnar nerves before reduction.
    - The median nerve can be injured at the time of reduction by becoming entrapped in the joint.
    - It is crucial to check nerve function before and after reduction.
  - Evaluate the patient for brachial artery injury before reduction.
    - The brachial artery may be trapped in the joint along with the median nerve.
    - Vascular injury is an indication for immediate surgery.
- The upper extremity should be inspected for other injuries, such as Monteggia fracture-dislocation.
- Palpate the forearm for increased swelling or signs of compartment syndrome.

### TESTS

#### *Imaging*

- Radiography:
  - AP and lateral views of the elbow are sufficient for diagnosis.
  - They should be obtained with the elbow out of the splint, to rule out subtle intra-articular fractures and dislocations.
- CT is used for fracture dislocation of the elbow to determine the precise fracture pattern.
- MRI scan is useful for diagnosing ligamentous injury.

### DIFFERENTIAL DIAGNOSIS

The main differential diagnosis is associated fracture.

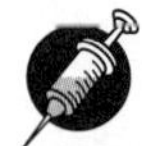

## TREATMENT

### GENERAL MEASURES

- The injured arm should be immobilized and elevated, with ice packs applied to the elbow.
- The patient should be sent to the emergency department immediately.
- The patient's neurovascular status must be evaluated before and after reduction.
- The examiner rules out associated fractures.
- Most dislocations can be treated with closed reduction, with the patient under sedation.
- Open reduction is indicated in irreducible dislocation, i.e., one caused by soft-tissue entrapment and free fragment in the joint, or changes in neurovascular status.
- Longitudinal traction, with gradual flexion and downward pressure on the forearm, usually reduces posterior or posterolateral dislocations.
- After reduction, elbow ROM and stability should be checked with gentle ROM and valgus and varus stress.
  - Neurovascular function also should be examined.
- Immobilization of the elbow in 90° of flexion with a posterior splint is recommended.
- Duration of immobilization varies, depending on elbow stability, but generally is 1 week.
- >3 weeks of immobilization should be avoided to prevent stiffness.
- If any neurovascular injury is detected, a vascular or orthopaedic surgeon should be notified.

#### *Activity*

- Gradual passive and active ROM and strengthening physical therapy should be started as soon as the immobilization device is removed.
- No lifting is allowed for 2 weeks.

### SPECIAL THERAPY

#### *Physical Therapy*

Therapy involves ROM and muscle strengthening.

### SURGERY

- Surgery is indicated for:
  - Irreducible dislocation
  - Open dislocation
  - Neurovascular entrapment
  - Certain types of associated fractures
  - Complex fracture dislocations
- Open reduction and internal fixation are recommended for:
  - Displaced radial head fractures
  - Olecranon fractures
  - Supracondylar humerus fractures
- Repair of complex fracture dislocations should be based on restoring stability to the elbow.
  - Should be accomplished by repair of the coronoid (if possible), restoration of the radial head or radial head replacement, or repair of the collateral ligaments (1,8)
- Total elbow arthroplasty has been used for severe fracture dislocation or missed injuries (9).

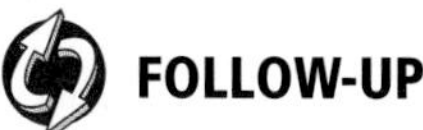

## FOLLOW-UP

### PROGNOSIS

- Most patients do well after closed reduction.
- The most common residual condition after dislocation is decreased ROM (loss of 10–15° of extension).
- Medial instability leads to late arthritis and persistent pain (10).
- Surgery has not been shown to be beneficial for dislocations without fracture (11).
- Complex fracture dislocations have a worse prognosis but benefit from an aggressive surgical approach (8).

### COMPLICATIONS

- Decreased ROM
- Neurovascular injury
- Persistent pain
- Arthritis
- Instability
- Heterotopic ossification

### PATIENT MONITORING

- The follow-up frequency varies with the individual surgeon.
- In general, immobilization should continue for ~1 week, depending on the stability of elbow.
- Immobilization should be no longer than 3 weeks.
- Clinical monitoring of compartment status and of neurovascular function is recommended for the first 12–24 hours.

### REFERENCES


1. Ring D, Jupiter JB, Zilberfarb J. Posterior dislocation of the elbow with fractures of the radial head and coronoid. *J Bone Joint Surg* 2002;84A:547–551.
2. Regan W, Morrey BF. Classification and treatment of coronoid process fractures. *Orthopedics* 1992; 15:845–848.
3. Doornberg JN, Ring D. Coronoid fracture patterns. *J Hand Surg* 2006;31A:45–52.
4. Josefsson PO, Nilsson BE. Incidence of elbow dislocation. *Acta Orthop Scand* 1986;57: 537–538.
5. Rasool MN. Dislocations of the elbow in children. *J Bone Joint Surg* 2004;86B:1050–1058.
6. Matsumoto K, Miyamoto K, Sumi H, et al. Upper extremity injuries in snowboarding and skiing: a comparative study. *Clin J Sport Med* 2002;12: 354–359.
7. Rettig AC. Traumatic elbow injuries in the athlete. *Orthop Clin North Am* 2002;33:509–522.
8. Pugh DMW, Wild LM, Schemitsch EH, et al. Standard surgical protocol to treat elbow dislocations with radial head and coronoid fractures. *J Bone Joint Surg* 2004;86A: 1122–1130.
9. Mighell MA, Dunham RC, Rommel EA, et al. Primary semi-constrained arthroplasty for chronic fracture-dislocations of the elbow. *J Bone Joint Surg* 2005;87B:191–195.
10. Eygendaal D, Verdegaal SHM, Obermann WR, et al. Posterolateral dislocation of the elbow joint. Relationship to medial instability. *J Bone Joint Surg* 2000;82A:555–560.
11. Josefsson PO, Gentz CF, Johnell O, et al. Surgical versus non-surgical treatment of ligamentous injuries following dislocation of the elbow joint. A prospective randomized study. *J Bone Joint Surg* 1987;69A:605–608.


### ADDITIONAL READING


- Morrey BF. The posttraumatic stiff elbow. *Clin Orthop Relat Res* 2005;431:26–35.
- Tashjian RZ, Katarincic JA. Complex elbow instability. *J Am Acad Orthop Surg* 2006;14: 278–286.


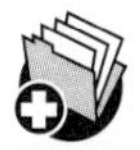

## MISCELLANEOUS

### CODES

#### *ICD9-CM*

832.0 Elbow dislocation

### PATIENT TEACHING

- Monitor for signs of compartment syndrome.
- Emphasize ROM exercises at home.

#### *Prevention*

- Snowboarding is a risky sport for complex elbow fracture dislocations.
  - –No methods are available to lessen this risk.

### FAQ

- Q: What is the long-term outcome of elbow dislocation?
  - A: Outcomes of dislocations without fracture are generally good. Some patients will develop arthritis symptoms and medial instability of the elbow. Outcomes of complex fracture dislocations are not as good.

# ENCHONDROMA

*Frank J. Frassica, MD*

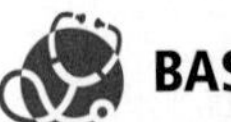

## BASICS

### DESCRIPTION
- A common benign lesion of mature hyaline cartilage in the medullary canal of the metaphysis or metadiaphysis of bone
- Commonly involves the short tubular bones (usually proximal phalanx) of adult hands and feet:
  - Also may involve the distal femur, proximal humerus, and tibia
  - Rare in the spine and pelvis
  - Does not form in bones that develop by membranous ossification
- Nongrowing lesion
- Small peripheral cartilage tumors tend to be benign, whereas large axial tumors have the greatest risk of malignancy.

### EPIDEMIOLOGY
#### *Incidence*
- One of the most common benign bone tumors
- Most common bone tumor of the hand
- Most common destructive bone lesion in hand

#### *Prevalence*
- Found in all age groups but more commonly recognized in adults
- The Male:Female ratio is equal.

### ETIOLOGY
- May result from epiphyseal growth cartilage that does not remodel and persists in the metaphysis, or may be the persistence of the original cartilage anlage
- Cartilage stops growing in adulthood.

### ASSOCIATED CONDITIONS
- Enchondroma protuberans: Eccentric enchondroma may cause bulging of the cortex.
- Enchondromatosis (Ollier disease): Multiple enchondromas:
  - Widespread involvement of the skeletal system by chondromas that occur principally in the medullary cavity but also on the surface of the bone
  - Typically occurs in a unilateral distribution
  - May involve any bone
  - Occurrence in multiple siblings has been documented, but no genetic basis has been found.
- Maffucci syndrome: Multiple enchondromas with soft-tissue hemangiomas

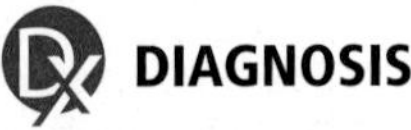

## DIAGNOSIS

### SIGNS AND SYMPTOMS
- General features:
  - Most lesions are asymptomatic.
    - Enchondromas of the long bones do not cause pain.
    - Patients with intramedullary cartilage lesions and pain should be evaluated carefully for another source of pain, possibly a chondrosarcoma.
  - Pain sometimes is present in patients with enchondromas in the hand from pathologic fractures.
  - If lesions occur in the hand, some enlargement of the digit may be noted if the cortex is expanded.
  - The lesion usually is diagnosed incidentally on a routine radiograph or bone scan and frequently is "hot" on a bone scan.
  - Rarely, a chondrosarcoma may develop in a pre-existing enchondroma (typically in the long bones).
- Enchondromatosis:
  - Usually recognized clinically by 10 years of age because of the development of palpable masses, unilateral shortening of an extremity, or angular deformity
  - Most cases are bilateral, but involvement usually predominates on 1 side.
    - Within an extremity, the lesions may be asymmetric (i.e., affecting the radial side more than the ulnar side, or vice versa).
  - Affected bones are shortened or deformed by epiphyseal involvement.
  - The disease regresses after puberty.
- Maffucci syndrome:
  - Vascular phleboliths are apparent in the associated soft-tissue hemangiomas.

#### *Physical Exam*
Palpate the bone for tenderness and a soft-tissue mass.

### TESTS
#### *Imaging*
- Children: Plain radiographs in 2 planes and a bone scan should be obtained to evaluate for other lesions.
- Radiography:
  - Serial radiographs taken every 3–6 months or review of old radiographs can help determine whether the lesion is inactive.
  - Well-defined, solitary, lytic lesions occur in the central portions of the metaphysis or metadiaphysis, with occasional endosteal scalloping and variable intralesional calcifications.
  - The calcification pattern is described as rings and stipple, popcornlike, and punctate.
  - In small tubular bones (e.g., the hand), the entire shaft usually is involved.
  - The cortex usually is intact, but it may be expanded mildly (by lack of remodeling in the metaphysis, not by expansion of the bone by tumor).
    - It often is radiolucent in children (may look like a unicameral bone cyst).
  - As patients age, the normally radiolucent cartilage begins to ossify and calcify, and ring-and-stipple calcifications are observed.
  - Occasionally, the mineralization is so dense that the lesion may suggest a bone infarct.
  - No periosteal reaction occurs.
  - Enchondromatosis:
    - Radiolucent areas of cartilage are seen in the metaphysis, with irregular calcification in a longitudinal or streaking pattern extending from the physis.
    - The cortices are expanded from within, inhibiting normal metaphyseal remodeling.
    - Affected bones cannot tubulate, so ends have a clubbed appearance.
    - The chondroma may be intracortical, subcortical, or in the epiphysis.
    - The tendency is to spare the epiphysis and diaphysis, but in severe cases, the entire bone may be involved.
- MRI:
  - Well-circumscribed lobular lesion is bright on T2-weighted images.
  - Low signal intensity on T1-weighted images
- Bone scanning:
  - Enchondromas take up radionuclide tracer and may be "hot" on a bone scan.
  - Positive bone scans should be interpreted cautiously because they do not, by themselves, indicate malignant change.
  - Although they do not grow, enchondromas are constantly remodeling.
  - Increased uptake and activity are not indications of malignant degeneration unless the lesion had less uptake on a previous scan.
  - Initial scans are used for baselines if any symptoms change.

#### *Pathological Findings*
- Microscopic features:
  - Nests of cartilage cells without atypia are separated by normal marrow.
  - Foci of calcification usually are present.
  - A thin layer of lamellar cartilage may be observed.
  - Negative Ki-67 stain is noted.
  - Evidence of invasive infiltration of bone marrow suggests chondrosarcoma.
  - Low magnification: Hypocellular lesions with a blue-gray aura and inconspicuous nuclei.
  - High magnification: Lesions have uniform nuclei (small, regular, darkly stained), and binucleated cells are rare.
- Hand lesions:
  - May be hypercellular
  - May have slight myxoid change
  - Nuclei may show atypical features.
  - Double nucleated cells are common.

### DIFFERENTIAL DIAGNOSIS
- Radiographic features:
  - Bone infarct
  - Chondrosarcoma

- Benign versus malignant lesions:
  - Distinguishing a benign latent enchondroma and an active enchondroma or low-grade chondrosarcoma is a common and difficult clinical problem.
  - Because the histologic characteristics of an enchondroma overlap those of a low-grade chondrosarcoma, biopsy often is not helpful.
  - The correct diagnosis depends on observing and correlating clinical and radiographic features of the lesion.
    - Is the lesion growing?
    - Is the lesion painful?
- Enchondroma:
  - Painless condition
  - Lack of growth
  - Bone scan variability
  - Uniform matrix calcification
  - Lack of endosteal erosion
  - Uniform small bland cells
  - Low cellularity
- Low-grade chondrosarcoma:
  - Painful condition
  - Slow-growing lesion
  - Bone scan variability
  - Presence of lucent regions
  - Endosteal erosion
  - Mild cellular atypia
  - Moderate to high cellularity
  - Ki-67-positive status

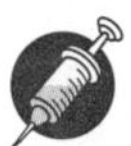

## TREATMENT

### GENERAL MEASURES

- Enchondromas do not cause pain, so other causes need to be sought (e.g., those in Table 1).
- Serial radiographs are obtained to ensure that the cartilage lesion is not growing.
  - Enchondromas show no changes except for increased mineralization.
  - Chondrosarcomas show:
    - Cortical erosions
    - Cortical thickening
    - Cortical destruction
- Activity modification is not necessary regardless of the size of the enchondroma.
- Patients with enchondromas of the hand often require curettage because of weakening of the bone.
- If the bone has fractured, the fracture is allowed to heal before curettage and grafting.

**Table 1. Possible Causes of Pain**

| Enchondroma Site | Associated Conditions |
|---|---|
| Proximal humerus | Rotator cuff tendinitis, rotator cuff tear, glenohumeral arthritis |
| Proximal femur | Trochanteric bursitis, hip arthritis |
| Distal femur | Patellofemoral syndrome, knee arthritis |

### SURGERY

- General principles:
  - Surgery usually is not necessary for enchondromas of long bones.
  - Enchondromas of the hand, which often present with pathologic fracture, should be treated with curettage.
- Hand lesions:
  - Make a small window in the lateral aspect of the phalanx for curettage and bone grafting.
    - Replace the cortical window.
  - Amputation may be necessary if finger function is compromised by the lesion.
- Enchondromatosis:
  - Surgery may be necessary for angular deformities.
  - Osteotomies may be performed through the enchondroma.
  - Leg-length discrepancy may require epiphysiodesis or limb-lengthening procedures.
  - Hand lesions may require curettage and bone grafting because of their large size and interference with function.

## FOLLOW-UP

- Patients with long-bone enchondromas are followed with serial radiographs every 3–6 months for 1–2 years.
- Patients are counseled to return for evaluation if the extremity becomes painful.

### DISPOSITION

#### *Issues for Referral*

- Patients with enchondromas often have other sources of musculoskeletal pain (e.g., those in Table 1).
- Patients with enchondroma and musculoskeletal pain should be referred to an orthopaedic oncologist.

### COMPLICATIONS

- General complications: Malignant degeneration (look for pain and growth of lesion)
- Enchondromatosis:
  - Of these patients, ~30% develop low-grade chondrosarcoma (1).
  - Usually occurs in patients in the 3rd and 4th decades of life
  - Look for changes on plain radiographs or MRI/CT scans.
- Maffucci syndrome:
  - Almost 100% develop low-grade chondrosarcoma (1).
  - Malignant brain tumors and liver and pancreatic carcinomas also may develop.

### REFERENCE

1. Dorfman HD, Czerniak B. Benign cartilage lesions. In: *Bone Tumors*, St. Louis: Mosby, 1998:253–352.

### ADDITIONAL READING

- Biermann JS. Musculoskeletal neoplasms. In: Richards BS, ed. *Orthopaedic Knowledge Update: Pediatrics*. Rosemont, IL: American Academy of Orthopaedic Surgeons, 1996:55–64.
- Cole WG. Genetic aspects of orthopaedic conditions. In: Morrissy RT, Weinstein SL, eds. *Lovell and Winter's Pediatric Orthopaedics*, 6th ed. Philadelphia: Lippincott Williams & Wilkins, 2006:145–165.
- Gitelis S, Soorapanth C. Benign chondroid tumors. In: Menendez LR, ed. *Orthopaedic Knowledge Update: Musculoskeletal Tumors*. Rosemont, IL: American Academy of Orthopaedic Surgeons, 2002:103–112.
- Mackenzie WG, Gabos PG. Localized disorders of bone and soft tissue. In: Morrissy RT, Weinstein SL, eds. *Lovell and Winter's Pediatric Orthopaedics*, 6th ed. Philadelphia: Lippincott Williams & Wilkins, 2006:315–356.
- McCarthy EF, Frassica FJ. Primary bone tumors. In: *Pathology of Bone and Joint Disorders: With Clinical and Radiographic Correlation*. Philadelphia: WB Saunders, 1998:195–275.

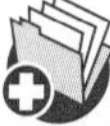

## MISCELLANEOUS

### CODES

#### *ICD9-CM*

756.4 Enchondroma, enchondromatosis, Maffucci syndrome

### FAQ

- Q: Do enchondromas cause pain?
  - A: In general, enchondromas do not cause pain. Often associated conditions are present, such as tendinitis, bursitis, or arthritis.
- Q: Are plain radiographs enough to establish the diagnosis of enchondroma?
  - A: In general, plain radiographs are sufficient. If concern exists, a CT or MRI scan can be performed to ensure that no large cortical erosions, cortical destruction, or soft-tissue masses are present.
- Q: Is there a substantial risk of a long-bone enchondroma converting into a chondrosarcoma?
  - A: The risk of an enchondroma transforming into a low- or high-grade chondrosarcoma is extremely low. Patients can and should be assured that the risk of malignancy is minimal.

# EOSINOPHILIC GRANULOMA

*Frank J. Frassica, MD*

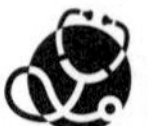

## BASICS

### DESCRIPTION

- EOG is the bony, and most common, manifestation of a group of nonneoplastic disorders known as "LCH."
- 3 basic scenarios occur:
  - Solitary site bone disease
  - Multiple bone lesions without visceral disease
  - Multiple bone lesions and visceral disease
- EOG commonly affects the skull, ribs, pelvis, spine, diaphysis of long bones, and mandible, but any bone may be involved.
- It more commonly affects a single bone rather than multiple bones.
- LCH:
  - Spectrum of disease involvement rather than separate specific entries
  - In the past, divided into 3 separate conditions:
    - EOG: Single intramedullary site of bone disease
    - Hand-Schüller Christian disease: Multiple sites of bone disease and visceral disease (skin, lymph nodes, liver, spleen, etc.); the classic triad (Christian triad) (uncommon by itself) involves lytic skull disease, exophthalmos, and diabetes insipidus.
  - Letter-Siwe disease: Fulminant condition in young children (<2 years old) with widespread involvement that often results in death (lymphadenopathy, hepatosplenomegaly, and extensive pulmonary disease)
- Synonyms: Histiocytosis X; Langerhans cell histiocytosis; Reticuloendotheliosis

### EPIDEMIOLOGY

#### Incidence

Rare

#### Prevalence

- Usually seen in patients <30 years old, with a peak incidence at age 5–10 years (1)
- Male:Female ratio of 2:1 (1)

### ETIOLOGY

- The cause of the accumulation of abnormal metabolic products in the reticuloendothelial cells is unknown.
- An inflammatory response occurs around these cells and produces the lytic destruction of bone.

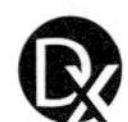

## DIAGNOSIS

- 3 diagnostic criteria for LCH of the spine (2)
- Percutaneous needle biopsy is a very effective method of establishing the diagnosis (3).

### SIGNS AND SYMPTOMS

- Local pain
- Swelling, tenderness
- Warmth at the site of involvement
- Occasional fever

#### Physical Exam

- The skull and skeleton should be palpated for areas of tenderness.
- Note the position of the eyes within the orbit.
- The spine should be percussed for tenderness.
- The patient's gait should be observed for the presence of a limp.

### TESTS

#### Lab

- Elevated ESR
- Peripheral eosinophilia

#### Imaging

- Radiography:
  - Plain radiographs show sharply circumscribed, "punched-out" lytic lesions.
  - As the lesion heals, a thick rim of reactive bone forms around the periphery.
  - The cortex may be destroyed with endosteal scalloping, periosteal reaction, and expansion of the bone.
  - If the cortex is destroyed unevenly (EOG attacks cortex from within the canal, but 1 side of the cortex may be more involved than the other), a "hole within a hole" appearance ensues.
  - In the vertebra, the body may collapse to a slender sclerotic wafer of bone called *vertebra plana*.
  - In the mandible and maxilla, the lytic lesion appears as a "floating tooth."
- Bone scanning usually is not recommended because the lesions may not be "hot" on bone scan.

#### Pathological Findings

- Sheets of "foamy" (lipid-filled) histiocytes:
  - Coffee-bean-shaped nucleus
  - Crisp nuclear membrane
  - Abundant pale eosinophilic cytoplasm
  - Staining with S-100 and Cd1a stains (1)
- Inflammatory cells found around these histiocytes:
  - Predominantly eosinophils, but also a few lymphocytes, neutrophils, and giant cells

### DIFFERENTIAL DIAGNOSIS
- Ewing sarcoma
- Lymphoma
- Osteomyelitis
- EOG appropriately is called the "great imitator," because it may mimic infection or neoplasm.

## TREATMENT

### GENERAL MEASURES
- Most lesions are self-limiting and resolve spontaneously.
- Options include:
  - Observation
  - Curettage and bone grafting
  - Injection with steroids
- If a pathologic fracture is impending, or the articular surface is in danger, curettage and bone grafting are necessary.
- Biopsy often is necessary except for characteristic spine lesions.

### MEDICATION (DRUGS)
- Methylprednisolone acetate injected into the lesion is effective in >90% of patients, with excellent bone healing (3).
- For patients with systemic disease with constitutional symptoms, chemotherapy with methylprednisolone, methotrexate, doxorubicin (Adriamycin), and other agents is indicated.
- Vertebra plana usually heals itself, and vertebral body height is restored with time.

### SURGERY
- Surgery is unnecessary in most cases.
- However, curettage and bone grafting with or without internal fixation are indicated if nonoperative measures fail and pathologic fracture seems imminent.

## FOLLOW-UP

### COMPLICATIONS
- Pathologic fractures may occur.
  - Usually heal well with closed or operative treatment

### PATIENT MONITORING
Observation with plain radiographs is indicated if the diagnosis is clear-cut and the patient has no impending fracture, until lesions resolve (usually 6 months).

### REFERENCES

1. Dorfman HD, Czerniak B. Immunohematopoietic tumors. In: *Bone Tumors*. St. Louis: Mosby, 1998: 664–728.
2. Garg S, Mehta S, Dormans JP. Langerhans cell histiocytosis of the spine in children. Long-term follow-up. *J Bone Joint Surg* 2004;86A: 1740–1750.
3. Yasko AW, Fanning CV, Ayala AG, et al. Percutaneous techniques for the diagnosis and treatment of localized Langerhans-cell histiocytosis (eosinophilic granuloma of bone). *J Bone Joint Surg* 1998;80A:219–228.


### ADDITIONAL READING

McCarthy EF, Frassica FJ. Skeletal manifestations of systemic disease. In: *Pathology of Bone and Joint Disorders: With Clinical and Radiographic Correlation*. Philadelphia: WB Saunders, 1998:119–133.


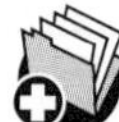

## MISCELLANEOUS

### CODES
#### *ICD9-CM*
277.8 EOG

### PATIENT TEACHING
- Reassure the patient and family about the self-limiting nature of most lesions.
- Make sure that the child and parents understand the need for close follow-up care.
- Make sure disease progression is not occurring.
- Ensure that this is not the initial presentation of widespread disease.

#### *Activity*
No restrictions are placed on activity unless the patient has an impending pathologic fracture.

### FAQ
- Q: Is EOG or LCH a malignant condition?
  - A: No. It is a self-limited inflammatory process.
- Q: What is the prognosis when a single bone is involved?
  - A: The prognosis is excellent.
- Q: Do patients with complete vertebral collapse need surgery?
  - A: Patients with complete vertebral collapse can be treated symptomatically, and only ∼10% of patients with LCH of the spine need reconstructive surgery at long-term follow-up.

# EWING SARCOMA

*Frank J. Frassica, MD*

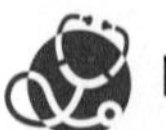

## BASICS

### DESCRIPTION

- Ewing sarcoma is a malignant bone tumor of the long bones, pelvis, and spine usually seen in childhood (1).
- Bone pain is the most common finding.
- Fever and an elevated white blood cell count and ESR sometimes are found.
- Nerve root irritation may be noted in patients with spinal lesions.
- It most commonly involves the diaphysis or metaphysis of long bones.
- Classification:
  - Classified according to the system of the Musculoskeletal Tumor Society (known as the "Enneking" system) (2,3)
  - Most are stage II-B (high-grade, extracompartmental tumors), but up to 20–25% of children present with lung or bone metastases (4).
- Synonym: Round cell sarcoma

### EPIDEMIOLOGY

#### *Incidence*

- The second most common malignant bone tumor of childhood, after osteosarcoma
- Affects males more often than females
- Is most common in persons <25 years old but rarely occurs in children <3 years old
- Rare in non-Caucasion individuals

### RISK FACTORS

#### *Genetics*

Reciprocal translation t(11;22)(q24;q12) [fusion transcription factor EWS/FL1-1 product] (4)

### ETIOLOGY

The causes of this tumor are not known.

## DIAGNOSIS

### SIGNS AND SYMPTOMS

- A localized mass with pain and tenderness for several weeks or months is common.
- The patient often presents with systemic symptoms of fever, malaise, and weight loss.
- Occasionally, the tumor is associated with a pathologic fracture.

#### *Physical Exam*

- In the early course of the disease, the physical examination is normal.
- As the soft-tissue component of the tumor grows, a soft-tissue mass may be palpated.

### TESTS

#### *Lab*

- Complete blood count
- Electrolyte determinations
- ESR
- Bone marrow aspiration and biopsy:
  - Biopsy of the soft-tissue portion of the lesion (if present) avoids the need to penetrate the bone.

#### *Imaging*

- Plain radiographs are indicated.
  - Often show a large lytic lesion that usually affects the diaphysis or metaphysis of long bones (frequently the fibula)
  - May show a variable amount of reactive new bone formation
  - May show a periosteal reaction, with a characteristic "onion skin" appearance
  - May show tumor invading the soft tissue
  - May appear normal in the early stage of the disease
- Patients with lesions suspected of being Ewing sarcoma should undergo staging studies, including:
  - MRI of the primary lesion
  - Chest radiography
  - Chest CT
  - Bone scanning
  - Bone marrow aspiration

#### *Pathological Findings*

- Numerous small, round cells are blue on hematoxylin and eosin staining.
- The uniform, densely packed cell population has scant cytoplasm.
- The outlines of cells and nuclei are indistinct and may appear "out of focus."
- Special immunochemical stains are used to confirm the diagnosis (e.g., HBA-71) (4).

### DIFFERENTIAL DIAGNOSIS

- Most commonly confused with osteomyelitis
- Histologically similar to:
  - Metastatic neuroblastoma (especially in patients <5 years old)
  - Lymphoma (especially in patients <5 years old)
  - Rhabdomyosarcoma
- One must also consider EOG and metastatic disease (especially in patients >30 years old).
- If the patient is <5 years old, lymphoma and metastatic neuroblastoma must be excluded.

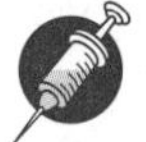

## TREATMENT

### GENERAL MEASURES

- Multiagent chemotherapy and external beam irradiation
- Wide surgical resection in certain cases, especially when the bone is "expendable," such as the fibula, iliac wing, and clavicle

### SPECIAL THERAPY

#### *Radiotherapy*

External beam irradiation can be used definitively for local control or as an adjunct to surgery.

#### *Physical Therapy*

Physical therapy is used to maintain ROM and muscle strength.

### MEDICATION (DRUGS)

Drugs of choice are various chemotherapeutic agents, according to the most current protocols.

### SURGERY

- Surgery has become an important modality for achieving local control.
- If surgery is indicated, a wide surgical margin is necessary.
- Limb salvage is performed in almost all cases.

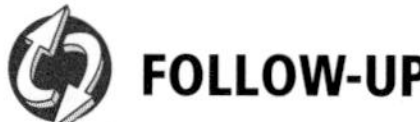

## FOLLOW-UP

### PROGNOSIS
- 5-year survival of 60–70% with current treatment (4)
- Less favorable outcome with tumors in the pelvis or spine

### COMPLICATIONS
- Postirradiation sarcomas may occur 2–5 years after external beam irradiation (4).
- After treatment with chemotherapy and external beam irradiation:
  - Fracture: The proximal femur is the most at-risk bone.
  - Osteonecrosis of the hip in patients with pelvic or proximal femur lesions

### PATIENT MONITORING
- Metastasis:
  - May develop in 30–40% of patients (4)
  - Pulmonary:
    - CT scans are obtained every 3–4 months for 2–3 years, then every 6 months up to 5 years, annually thereafter
  - Bone:
    - Technetium bone scans are used to detect bone metastaseas and are obtained every 3–6 months for 2–3 years, then annually
- Local recurrence:
  - May develop in 10–30% of patients treated with irradiation and chemotherapy and in 5–10% of patients treated with chemotherapy and surgery (4)
  - MRI/CT is used when a prosthesis is not present.
  - Radiographs and serial physical examinations are used for patients with prosthetic devices.

### REFERENCES

1. Dorfman HD, Czerniak B. Ewing's sarcoma and related entities. In: *Bone Tumors*. St. Louis: Mosby, 1998:607–663.
2. Enneking WF. Malignant skeletal neoplasms. In: *Clinical Musculoskeletal Pathology*, 3rd ed. Gainsville: University of Florida Press, 1990:358–421.
3. McCarthy EF, Frassica FJ. Primary bone tumors. In: *Pathology of Bone and Joint Disorders: With Clinical and Radiographic Correlation*. Philadelphia: WB Saunders, 1998:195–275.
4. Hornicek FJ. Ewing's sarcoma. In: Menendez LR, ed. *Orthopaedic Knowledge Update: Musculoskeletal Tumors*. Rosemont, IL: American Academy of Orthopaedic Surgeons, 2002:195–202.


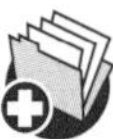

## MISCELLANEOUS

### CODES
***ICD9-CM***

170.9 Ewing sarcoma

### PATIENT TEACHING
- Patients and family members are taught the importance of systemic chemotherapy to prevent metastasis.
- Protected weightbearing is important during induction chemotherapy.
- Compliance with posttreatment surveillance is necessary to monitor for metastasis and local recurrence.

### FAQ
- Q: Is surgery better for local control than radiation therapy?
  - A: Surgery to remove the tumor has the advantage of a better local control rate, and it obviates the risk of a postirradiation sarcoma. Compared with chemotherapy, surgical resection may not be associated with a survival benefit.
- Q: Can patients still be cured if they present with metastatic disease?
  - A: Although the prognosis is much worse for such patients, 10–25% can still be cured.

# EXTENSOR TENDON LACERATION

*John J. Carbone, MD*
*Dawn M. LaPorte, MD*

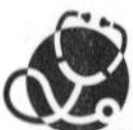

## BASICS

### DESCRIPTION

- Extensor tendon lacerations are common because of the superficial location of the extensor tendons on the back of the hand (1).
- Tendon disruption often is indicated by a change in the posture of the hand or fingers.
- The most distal injury, at the DIP joint, shows a mallet-type of deformity.
- An injury over the PIP joint may result in a boutonniere deformity.
- Extensor injuries usually are repaired surgically, either in the emergency department or in the operating room within 2 weeks of injury.
- These injuries, most common in young adults, affect active finger extension and wrist extension.
- Males are affected more commonly than are females.
- Classification: Partial or complete laceration, as noted during wound exploration

### EPIDEMIOLOGY

#### *Incidence*

This laceration is less common than flexor tendon injuries.

### ETIOLOGY

- Laceration on dorsum of hand or wrist, coupled with the superficial location of the extensor mechanism
- Possible association with bite injuries

### ASSOCIATED CONDITIONS

Open fractures and joints

## DIAGNOSIS

### SIGNS AND SYMPTOMS

- Laceration on the dorsum of the hand:
  - Tendon ends frequently visible in wound with minimal exploration
  - Change in posture of finger or hand
  - Inability to extend actively the joints distal to the injury
- Mallet deformity:
  - Inability to extend the distal joint of the finger (The finger droops downward.)
- Boutonniere deformity:
  - The PIP joint goes into flexion, whereas the DIP joint extends or hyperextends.
- Decrease in extension strength or ROM of the index or the small finger, both of which have small secondary independent extensor muscle and tendon units

#### *Physical Exam*

- Examine all fingers for active extension and the wrist for strength and ROM.
- Carefully explore the wound for evidence of tendon lacerations (partial or complete).

### TESTS

#### *Lab*

If operative treatment is necessary, standard preoperative tests are performed, depending on the health of the patient.

#### *Imaging*

AP and lateral radiographs are obtained to rule out foreign body or fracture.

### DIFFERENTIAL DIAGNOSIS

Fracture or avulsion injury of extensor mechanism (Fig. 1)

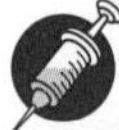

## TREATMENT

### GENERAL MEASURES

- Tetanus booster or toxoid as needed
- Intravenous antibiotics, typically a 3rd-generation cephalosporin, if the wound is contaminated
- Skin closure until definitive surgery is performed
- Hand splinted in wrist or finger extension (Fig. 1)
- Wound irrigation and débridement as needed
- Orthopaedic surgery or hand surgery consult

### SPECIAL THERAPY

#### *Physical Therapy*

- Physical therapy regimens are based on injury type and location and on the type of repair.
- The goal is to achieve a repair that allows early passive and active ROM.

### SURGERY

- The tendon ends are isolated, approximated, and repaired with 4-0 Prolene or 4-0 Ticron (Sherwood-Davis & Geck, St. Louis, MO).
  - Mattress sutures are used.
  - If the injury is at the level of the wrist, then the repair usually is performed in the operating room.
  - The repair is less surgically demanding than a repair of a flexor tendon lacerated at the same level because no tendon pulley is present around extensor tendons.
  - This anatomy also allows delayed surgical repair for up to 2 weeks without any adverse effects on outcome.
  - Postoperative splinting is necessary while the tendon heals.

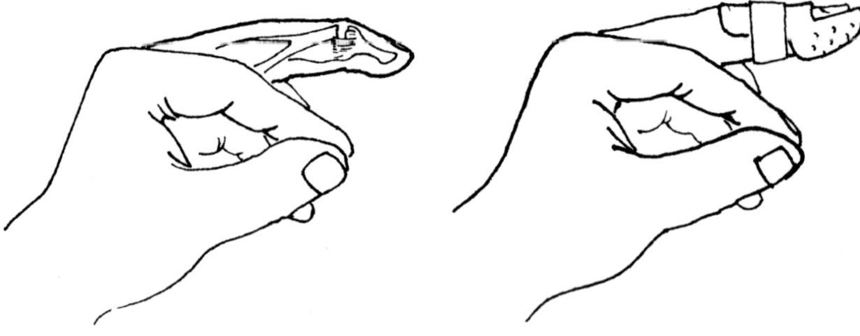

**Fig. 1.** An extensor tendon laceration or avulsion over the DIP joint will heal with a finger splint.

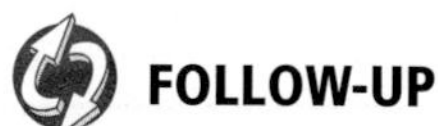

## FOLLOW-UP

### PROGNOSIS
Good with complete surgical repair

### COMPLICATIONS
- Infection
- Open joint injuries
- Failure of tendon repair/tendon rupture
- Scarring
- Adhesions
- Loss of function

### REFERENCE
1. Newport ML. Extensor tendon Injuries in the hand. *J Am Acad Orthop Surg* 1997;5:59–66.

### ADDITIONAL READING
- American Society for Surgery of the Hand. *The Hand: Primary Care of Common Problems*, 2nd ed. New York: Churchill Livingstone, 1990.
- Ariyan S. *The Hand Book*. New York: McGraw-Hill, 1989.
- Baratz ME, Schmidt CC, Hughes TB. Extensor tendon injuries. In: Green DP, Hotchkiss RN, Pederson WC, et al., eds. *Green's Operative Hand Surgery*, 5th ed. Philadelphia: Elsevier Churchill Livingstone, 2005:187–217.

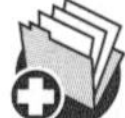

## MISCELLANEOUS

### CODES
#### *ICD9-CM*
884.2 Tendon laceration with open wound, upper extremity

### PATIENT TEACHING
- Patient compliance with splinting, wound care, and physical therapy is critical to good functional outcome.
- It is important to stress the fact that, with a complete laceration, the tendon will not heal or repair itself for normal function.

### FAQ
- Q: What should be done for a patient with an extensor tendon laceration if the surgeon is not available?
  - A: The wound should be washed out and, if clean, the skin should be reapproximated and the joint splinted in full extension. The patient should be seen promptly in follow-up with a surgeon for operative exploration and repair within 7–10 days.
- Q: What is the most common complication after extensor tendon repair?
  - A: The most common complication is formation of adhesions between the repair site and adjacent tissue, which can restrict joint motion. Therapy helps to minimize adhesion formation and to improve tendon gliding, but occasionally surgical tenolysis is necessary.

E

# FEMORAL ANTEVERSION

*Eric D. Shirley, MD*
*Jinsong Wang, MD*

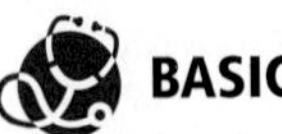

## BASICS

### DESCRIPTION

- Femoral torsion is the angular difference between the femoral neck axis and the transcondylar axis of the knee (1).
- Increased femoral anteversion can result in in-toeing.
- Synonym: Pigeon toes

### EPIDEMIOLOGY

- In-toeing from increased femoral anteversion usually increases until age 5 years and then resolves by age 8 years (1).
- Increased femoral anteversion is symmetric and tends to occur in females (1).

#### *Incidence*

Increased femoral anteversion is the most common cause of in-toeing in early childhood (1).

### RISK FACTORS

Positive family history

### ETIOLOGY

- Many infants are born with a substantial amount of femoral anteversion, an external rotation contracture of the hip, and internal tibial torsion (1).
- The external hip contracture initially masks increased femoral anteversion (1).
- Femoral anteversion at birth is ~40°.
- Femoral anteversion decreases until adult values (10–15°) are reached by age 8 years (1).
- Differences in inheritance and connective tissue account for the variation in anteversion among patients.

### ASSOCIATED CONDITIONS

Internal tibial torsion

## DIAGNOSIS

### SIGNS AND SYMPTOMS

- In-toeing and abnormal appearance of the child's legs during walking or running (1)
- Parents will note that the child sits in the "W" or reverse-tailor position that is characteristic of patients with increased anteversion.

#### *History*

- Tripping, shoe wear difficulty, and falling are common reasons that parents seek medical attention (1).
- Knee pain is associated with increased femoral anteversion and external tibial torsion (miserable malalignment syndrome) (2).
- A birth history should be obtained to ascertain risk factors for cerebral palsy (1).
- A family history should obtain information about rotational disorders, rickets, and skeletal dysplasias (1).

#### *Physical Exam*

- Diagnosis typically can be made by physical examination.
- Physical examination begins with inspection of the gait and progresses to an assessment from the hips to the toes.
- Affected children run with an egg-beater-type motion (1).
- In-toeing and medial-facing patellar alignment are seen during walking.
- The rotational profile and its 5 components should be recorded (3).
- The sum total of the entire extremity alignment is quantified by the foot progression angle (i.e., the angle of the foot relative to an imaginary straight line in the patient's path) (3).
- Hip rotation, measured in the prone position, reflects the degree of femoral anteversion (3).
- Normal hip rotation by age (3):
  - Infants:
    - Internal: Average, 40° (range, 10–60°)
    - External: Average, 70° (range, 45–90°) (3).
  - By age 10 years:
    - Internal: Average, 50° (range, 25–65°)
    - External: Average, 45° (range, 25–65°)
- Hip internal rotation of 70°, 80°, or 90° is evidence of a mild, moderate, or severe increase in femoral anteversion, respectively (4).
- Increased femoral anteversion is associated with decreased hip external rotation (4).
- The thigh–foot axis, in the prone position, is the angle subtended by the longitudinal axis of the thigh and the foot; this angle reflects the amount of tibial torsion present (3).
- The transmalleolar axis, the angle formed at the intersection of a line between the malleoli and a line between the femoral condyles, also reflects the amount of tibial torsion (3).
- The final component of the rotational profile, the heel-bisector line, identifies forefoot abduction and adduction; this line goes through the mid-axis of the hindfoot and forefoot (3).
- A rotational profile 2 standard deviations outside the mean for that child's age is considered abnormal (4).

### TESTS

#### *Imaging*

- Radiography:
  - Are indicated in children with highly abnormal rotational profiles, short stature, marked asymmetry, or pain.
  - A pelvic radiograph is indicated if the patient has an abnormal hip examination.
- CT may be used to quantitate the degree of femoral anteversion and for preoperative planning.

#### *Pathological Findings*

- A progressive or asymmetric deformity suggests a possible underlying pathology and should be investigated.
- A gait with equinus and in-toeing may suggest cerebral palsy.
- A Trendelenburg gait or abnormal hip examination may suggest DDH.

### DIFFERENTIAL DIAGNOSIS

- Tibial torsion
- Associated conditions that may lead to femoral anteversion and should be excluded:
  - DDH
  - Cerebral palsy

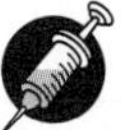

# TREATMENT

## GENERAL MEASURES

- Pathologic processes (cerebral palsy or hip dysplasia) should be addressed.
- Because increased femoral anteversion tends to resolve by age 8 years, no treatment is indicated for most cases.
- Care consists of reassurance and education about the natural history.
- Bracing and shoe modifications are unnecessary.
- Some cases of increased femoral anteversion may persist, and remodeling after age 8 years is minimal, but most patients with persistent increased anteversion are asymptomatic.
- Surgical intervention may be indicated in a child >8 years old with a marked functional deformity (tripping and falling during sports or activities of daily living) and femoral anteversion of >50° (5); careful patient selection is critical.
- Surgery also may be indicated in children with increased femoral anteversion associated with external tibial torsion, patella alta, increased Q-angle, and anterior knee pain (miserable malalignment syndrome) (6); again, careful patient selection is critical.

## SPECIAL THERAPY

### *Physical Therapy*

Physical exercises do not affect the natural history of anteversion.

## SURGERY

- Femoral (proximal, diaphyseal, or distal) derotation osteotomy rarely is required.
- Fixation of a diaphyseal derotation osteotomy can be achieved with a rigid, bent nail inserted through the lateral aspect of the greater trochanter (5).
  - Patients may bear weight as tolerated after the procedure.
- Derotational osteotomies of the femur and tibia may be performed for miserable malalignment syndrome (6).

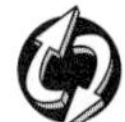

# FOLLOW-UP

## PROGNOSIS

- Prognosis is good, and most cases resolve by age 8 years (1).
- No relationship exists between increased femoral anteversion and hip arthritis (7).
- No relationship exists between increased femoral anteversion and knee osteoarthritis, but decreased anteversion does place the knee at risk for osteoarthritis (7).

## COMPLICATIONS

- The potential postoperative complications of derotation osteotomy are:
  - Nonunion, malunion
  - Implant prominence
  - Overcorrection or undercorrection
  - Failure to relieve pain or other symptoms

## PATIENT MONITORING

For patients with severe cases, annual or biannual observation and examination are recommended to document expected rotational change with growth.

## REFERENCES


1. Lincoln TL, Suen PW. Common rotational variations in children. *J Am Acad Orthop Surg* 2003;11:312–320.
2. Delgado ED, Schoenecker PL, Rich MM, et al. Treatment of severe torsional malalignment syndrome. *J Pediatr Orthop* 1996;16:484–488.
3. Staheli LT. Rotational problems in children. *J Bone Joint Surg* 1993;75A:939–949.
4. Staheli LT, Corbett M, Wyss C, et al. Lower-extremity rotational problems in children. Normal values to guide management. *J Bone Joint Surg* 1985;67A:39–47.
5. Gordon JE, Pappademos PC, Schoenecker PL, et al. Diaphyseal derotational osteotomy with intramedullary fixation for correction of excessive femoral anteversion in children. *J Pediatr Orthop* 2005;25:548–553.
6. Bruce WD, Stevens PM. Surgical correction of miserable malalignment syndrome. *J Pediatr Orthop* 2004;24:392–396.
7. Eckhoff DG, Kramer RC, Alongi CA, et al. Femoral anteversion and arthritis of the knee. *J Pediatr Orthop* 1994;14:608–610.


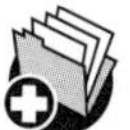

# MISCELLANEOUS

## CODES

### *ICD9-CM*

755.63 Femoral anteversion

## PATIENT TEACHING

Explanation of the expected resolution and benign natural history of increased femoral anteversion

### *Activity*

No limitation of activity

## FAQ

- Q: What is the natural history of increased femoral anteversion?
  - A: In-toeing from increased femoral anteversion usually increases until age 5 years, then resolves by age 8 years.
- Q: How is increased femoral anteversion diagnosed?
  - A: By physical examination. The rotational profile shows medially directed patellae and increased hip internal rotation.
- Q: What is the treatment for increased femoral anteversion?
  - A: Primarily observation. There is no role for bracing or physical therapy. In rare cases, correctional derotational osteotomy may be indicated for increased femoral anteversion that persists after age 8 years and causes functional impairment.

# FEMORAL NECK FRACTURE

*Daniel L. Miller, BS*
*Tung B. Le, MD*

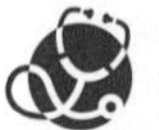

## BASICS

### DESCRIPTION

- Femoral neck fracture is the most common cause of a "broken hip."
- The femoral neck is the intracapsular portion of the proximal femur between the femoral head and the lesser and greater trochanters.
- Femoral neck fractures are most common in elderly patients, although younger patients involved in high-energy trauma also are affected.
- In the elderly, immobilization from these injuries can lead to secondary cardiopulmonary complications, severe morbidity, and mortality.
- Classification (4):
  - Stable (nondisplaced fracture): May be impacted or incomplete
  - Unstable: Complete and displaced fracture

### EPIDEMIOLOGY

#### *Incidence*

- The occurrence of femoral neck fractures per 100,000 person years is 27.7 in males and ~63.3 in females (1,2).
- Rates of fracture have leveled off, perhaps secondary to the use of antiresorptive agents (3).

#### *Prevalence*

- In the young population, more males than females sustain this injury.
- In elderly patients, females are affected 2–3 times more often than are males (3).

### RISK FACTORS

- Osteoporosis, which is the major risk factor for femoral neck fractures in the elderly
- Factors that increase the risk of falling, such as an unsteady gait
- Female gender (postmenopausal)
- Physical inactivity
- Caucasian race

### ETIOLOGY

- In patients <50 years old, femoral neck fractures often are the result of high-energy trauma with a direct force along the femoral shafts.
- In the older population, these fractures are caused by low-energy trauma, such as a fall from a standing height.

### ASSOCIATED CONDITIONS

- Osteoporosis
- Conditions that increase the risk of a fall:
  - Poor vision and macular degeneration
  - Urinary incontinence or frequency
  - Poor balance
  - Polypharmacy
  - Syncope
  - Use of benzodiazepams

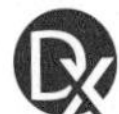

## DIAGNOSIS

### SIGNS AND SYMPTOMS

- Patients have severe pain in the groin area and, with unstable fractures, the leg is shortened.
- The patient may be unable to ambulate.
- Patients hold their hips slightly flexed and externally rotated.
- Pain is worsened with attempted ROM or axial loading.
- Patients with stable fractures will not have shortening or rotational deformity.

#### *History*

A history of pain in the hip before the fracture is worrisome for metastatic disease.

#### *Physical Exam*

- Perform an examination for pain on ROM, especially internal rotation.
- With unstable fractures, the leg often is rotated externally and shortened.
- Examine the pelvis with direct palpation and radiography to exclude a concomitant pelvic fracture.
- Active straight-leg raise will provoke pain.

### TESTS

#### *Lab*

Preoperative laboratory tests, blood type and screen, chest radiographs, and an electrocardiogram are needed at time of admission.

#### *Imaging*

- Radiography:
  - AP pelvic radiographs
  - AP and cross-table lateral radiographs of the affected hip and femur
- MRI to diagnose occult femoral neck fractures in patients with negative radiographs
- Dedicated hip CT is useful for patients with ipsilateral femoral shaft fractures.

#### *Pathological Findings*

Elderly patients may have comminution of the femoral neck, especially in the subcapital region.

### DIFFERENTIAL DIAGNOSIS

- When a fracture is not obvious on the plain films of a patient with hip pain secondary to trauma, an occult (nondisplaced) fracture should be suspected.
- Other causes of hip pain include:
  - Pelvic fracture
  - Intertrochanteric fracture
  - Infection
  - Greater trochanter bursitis
  - Metastatic disease

## TREATMENT

### GENERAL MEASURES

- Stable fractures should be stabilized internally with cannulated lag screws.
- Treatment of unstable femoral neck fractures is controversial (5):
  - In general, displaced fractures in young (<50 years old), active patients should be reduced by closed or open means and stabilized internally with screws.
  - Because of the high rate of osteonecrosis of the femoral head, fractures in young patients (<50 years old) are considered orthopaedic emergencies.
  - In the multiply injured patient, attention to other organ systems and concurrent care with other members of the trauma team are essential.
  - In older (physiologic age >70 years) patients, more sedentary patients, or in those with Paget disease or neurologic diseases such as Parkinson disease or hemiplegia, partial or total arthroplasty is the treatment of choice.
- In older patients with isolated femoral neck injuries, rapid medical consultation to optimize surgical outcomes is important.
- Delayed treatment of femoral neck fractures in elderly patients can lead to major cardiopulmonary complications.

#### *Activity*

- Patients are at bed rest.
- Use of traction does not give pain relief and can cause skin complications.

#### *Nursing*

- Avoid decubitus ulcers of the buttock and heels.
  - Turn the patient frequently.
  - Use heel protectors and specialized beds.
- Avoid delirium in the elderly by:
  - Constant reorientation of the patient
  - Appropriate use of calendars and clocks
  - Avoidance of medicines that can provoke delirium (e.g., long-acting benzodiazepams)

### SPECIAL THERAPY

#### *Physical Therapy*

- Begin physical therapy the day after surgery.
- Elderly patients are allowed to bear weight as tolerated after fracture repair.
- In younger patients, weightbearing is restricted until the fracture heals (6).

### MEDICATION (DRUGS)

- Analgesics
- In the elderly, one should observe for a change in mental status and constipation with the use of narcotic analgesics.
- Young patients need adequate narcotic doses to facilitate rehabilitation.

## SURGERY

- The patient is placed supine on a fracture table, and the fracture is visualized through a small incision or percutaneously under fluoroscopy; alternatively, a lateral approach on a radiolucent table may be used.
  - In young patients or those with stable fractures:
    - 3 screws are placed with the aid of the image intensifier.
    - Screws should be spread out in a triangular pattern.
    - Screws must be inserted deeply into the subchondral bone of the femoral head.
  - Unstable fracture patterns, in which the fracture line is closer to the trochanters (basicervical fractures):
    - A hip screw and side plate are required.
    - Precise reduction of the fracture is crucial to a good outcome (7).
  - 6–9% of patients with femoral shaft fractures have an ipsilateral femoral neck fracture; fixation of the femoral neck takes precedence over that of the shaft (8).
- Prosthetic replacement can be done through a lateral or posterior approach with uncemented or cemented devices, depending on bone geometry and surgeon comfort.
  - In minimally active patients, hemiarthroplasty (replacing only the femoral head and neck) is performed.
  - In active patients or those with pre-existing osteoarthritis, consider total hip replacement (replacement of both the acetabulum and the femoral head and neck) (9).

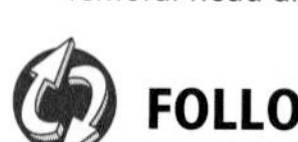

# FOLLOW-UP

## PROGNOSIS

- The mortality rate in the elderly population ranges from 4–31% at 30 days after hip fracture (10).
- This rate is highest during the first 6 months and in patients with multiple medical problems or prolonged immobilization.

## COMPLICATIONS

- Osteonecrosis of the femoral head
- Nonunion or malunion of bone
- Prosthetic dislocation or loosening
- Persistent pain
- Infection
- Cardiopulmonary complications
- Postoperative delirium
- DVT

## PATIENT MONITORING

- Intensive cardiovascular monitoring in multiply injured patients or in patients with multiple medical problems should be instituted during the perioperative period.
- In patients with internally stabilized fractures, radiographs are obtained once a month until union is achieved.
- In patients who have undergone arthroplasty, radiographs are obtained at 3 and 12 months.

## REFERENCES


1. Cummings SR, Rubin SM, Black D. The future of hip fractures in the United States. Numbers, costs, and potential effects of postmenopausal estrogen. *Clin Orthop Relat Res* 1990;252:163–166.
2. Hedlund R, Lindgren U, Ahlbom A. Age- and sex-specific incidence of femoral neck and trochanteric fractures. An analysis based on 20,538 fractures in Stockholm County, Sweden, 1972–1981. *Clin Orthop Relat Res* 1987;222:132–139.
3. Chang KP, Center JR, Nguyen TV, et al. Incidence of hip and other osteoporotic fractures in elderly men and women: Dubbo Osteoporosis Epidemiology Study. *J Bone Miner Res* 2004;19:532–536.
4. Rodriguez-Merchan EC. In situ fixation of nondisplaced intracapsular fractures of the proximal femur. *Clin Orthop Relat Res* 2002;399:42–51.
5. Bhandari M, Devereaux PJ, Swiontkowski MF, et al. Internal fixation compared with arthroplasty for displaced fractures of the femoral neck. A meta-analysis. *J Bone Joint Surg* 2003;85A:1673–1681.
6. Koval KJ, Sala DA, Kummer FJ, et al. Postoperative weight-bearing after a fracture of the femoral neck or an intertrochanteric fracture. *J Bone Joint Surg* 1998;80A:352–356.
7. Haidukewych GJ, Rothwell WS, Jacofsky DJ, et al. Operative treatment of femoral neck fractures in patients between the ages of fifteen and fifty years. *J Bone Joint Surg* 2004;86A: 1711–1716.
8. Watson JT, Moed BR. Ipsilateral femoral neck and shaft fractures: complications and their treatment. *Clin Orthop Relat Res* 2002;399:78–86.
9. Blomfeldt R, Tornkvist H, Ponzer S, et al. Comparison of internal fixation with total hip replacement for displaced femoral neck fractures. Randomized, controlled trial performed at four years. *J Bone Joint Surg* 2005;87A:1680–1688.
10. Roberts SE, Goldacre MJ. Time trends and demography of mortality after fractured neck of femur in an English population, 1968–98: database study. *Br Med J* 2003;327:771–775.


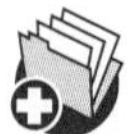

# MISCELLANEOUS

## CODES

### *ICD9-CM*

820.8 Femoral neck fracture

## PATIENT TEACHING

- Patients should be informed about the high incidence of osteonecrosis (also known as "AVN") of the femoral head associated with this type of injury.
- The risk of osteonecrosis depends on the type of injury and on the timing of diagnosis and treatment.
- A multiply injured patient has a higher risk of osteonecrosis than does a patient with an isolated injury.

### *Prevention*

- In the elderly:
  - Calcium, vitamin D, bisphosphonates, and physical therapy should be used to reduce osteoporosis and minimize the risk of femoral neck fracture.
  - Fall prevention should be emphasized.
  - Ambulatory aids, such as walkers or canes to increase stability, are helpful.
  - Home modification strategies, such as handrails or single level homes, should be considered.
  - Externally worn hip protectors may decrease the incidence or fracture.

## FAQ

- Q: How likely is an elderly person to get back to the previous level of ambulation?
  - A: ~1/2; the other 1/2 require more aids to ambulate.
- Q: What is the outcome of unstable fractures in the elderly treated with internal fixation?
  - A: Patients treated with internal fixation may heal their fractures and save their native hip. However, risk exists that either the fracture will not heal or AVN will develop. More patients with internal fixation require a 2nd surgery than do those with replacement.

F

# FEMORAL SHAFT FRACTURE IN THE ADULT

*Matthew D. Waites, AFRCS (Ed)*

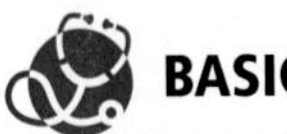

## BASICS

### DESCRIPTION

- Femoral shaft fractures occur in the diaphysis of the bone.
- High-energy trauma such as vehicular accidents, falls, or gunshots are the common causes of these fractures in normal bone.
- Low-energy trauma may cause femoral shaft fractures in pathologic or osteoporotic bone.
- Classification:
  - Winquist and Hansen (1) assessed fractures according to the proportion of cortical contact between proximal and distal fragments:
    - Type I: >75% bony contact
    - Type II: At least 50% cortical contact
    - Type III: <50% contact
    - Type IV: No bone contact
  - The AO/Orthopaedic Trauma Association (2) classifies these fractures as:
    - Type 32A (simple), 32B (wedge), or 32C (complex)
    - Each type is subdivided as 1, 2, or 3 according to the inherent instability of the fracture configuration.

### GENERAL PREVENTION

- Accident prevention and safety measures for both pedestrians and vehicle occupants
- Reduction and prevention of gun crime
- Preemptive stabilization of impending pathologic fractures

### EPIDEMIOLOGY

#### *Incidence*

- Bimodal incidence, <25 years old and >65 years old (3)
- Estimated to be 1 per 10,000 persons per year (3).

### RISK FACTORS

- Young adult males
- Urban living
- Alcohol or drug abuse

### ETIOLOGY

- Mechanism of injury:
  - Motor vehicle accident
  - Pedestrian hit by car
  - Fall from height
  - Gunshot
  - Low-energy falls or twisting injuries in pathologic bone

### ASSOCIATED CONDITIONS

- Trauma patients with a femoral shaft fracture must be assessed for injuries in all other systems.
- Orthopaedic injuries:
  - Ipsilateral femoral neck fracture is relatively infrequent, but up to 30% are missed (3).
  - Ligamentous derangement of the knee
  - Lower leg and foot trauma
  - Pelvic and spinal fractures

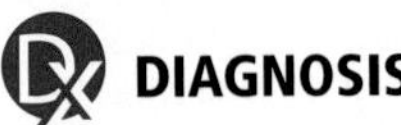

## DIAGNOSIS

### SIGNS AND SYMPTOMS

- Signs of hemorrhagic shock:
  - Average blood loss from an isolated femoral shaft fracture is estimated to be >1,200 mL (4).
- 5–10% are open fractures.
- The injured limb appears swollen and shortened.

#### *History*

It is vital to understand the mechanism of injury to recognize possible associated injuries.

#### *Physical Exam*

- Perform the ATLS (5) primary survey to eliminate associated life-threatening injuries.
- Carefully check and document the neurovascular status of the lower limb.
- Examine for associated fractures, especially of the hip and knee.
- Examine the knee for ligamentous injuries after stabilization of the fracture.

### TESTS

#### *Lab*

- All preoperative trauma laboratory tests
- Blood must be made available by type and cross-matching.
- Hematocrit checks for blood loss anemia

#### *Imaging*

- AP and lateral, full-length radiographs of the affected femur
- Internal rotation view or CT scan of ipsilateral femoral neck to rule out neck fracture
- Cervical spine, chest, and pelvis radiographs
- Full-length contralateral femur films are useful for length determination with comminuted or long oblique femoral fractures.

#### *Pathological Findings*

- Injured tissues: Bone, muscle, and fascia
- Rarely, injury to femoral artery or sciatic nerve

### DIFFERENTIAL DIAGNOSIS

- Suspicion of a pathologic cause should be raised if a femur fracture occurs in the presence of any of the following criteria:
  - Spontaneous fracture (zero or very-low-energy trauma)
  - History of pain before fracture
  - Destructive or permeative lesion on radiograph

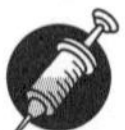

## TREATMENT

### INITIAL STABILIZATION

- Treat life-threatening airway and breathing injuries.
- Control hemorrhage: Resuscitate with intravenous fluids and cross-matched blood.
- Splint the limb with a Thomas-type splint to help reduce blood loss from the fracture and relieve pain.
- Intravenous antibiotics and saline dressings for open fractures
- Narcotic pain medicines

### GENERAL MEASURES

- "Damage-control" orthopaedics has emerged in the polytrauma patient (6):
  - Intramedullary nailing compounds the systemic inflammatory response by increasing inflammatory mediators and toxic metabolites in patients with high Injury Severity Scores (7).
  - Life-threatening hemorrhage should be controlled, and the skeleton should be stabilized with external fixation.
  - A few days later, when the initial systemic inflammatory response has subsided, the external fixator can be exchanged for definitive skeletal stabilization.
- Most femoral shaft fractures are treated operatively with intramedullary nailing.

#### *Activity*

- Before skeletal stabilization, patients should be restricted to bed rest.
- Skeletal traction should be used if a delay in operative fixation is anticipated.

#### *Nursing*

- Care should be taken to avoid pressure sores on the heel and buttocks before surgery.
- Traction pins must be monitored carefully to avoid pressure necrosis or osteomyelitis.

### SPECIAL THERAPY

#### *Physical Therapy*

- Early physical therapy to regain motion and strength of the hip, knee, and ankle

### MEDICATION (DRUGS)

#### *First Line*

Oral narcotic analgesics

### SURGERY

- External fixation:
  - Initial stabilization in polytrauma patients (damage-control orthopaedics)
  - Severe open fractures
  - Vascular injury
- Plating:
  - Rarely indicated for femoral shaft fractures
  - Periprosthetic fractures where implant is well fixed
- Intramedullary nailing:
  - Reamed anterograde nailing is the standard treatment for most femoral shaft fractures.
  - Retrograde reamed nail may be indicated for patients with:
    - Distal femoral shaft fractures
    - Ipsilateral acetabular fractures
    - Ipsilateral femoral neck fractures
    - Obese patients in whom access to the piriformis fossa for antegrade nailing may prove too difficult.
    - Bilateral femur fractures

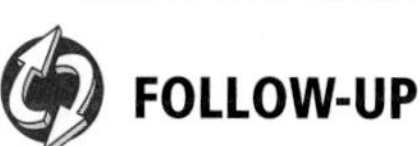

## FOLLOW-UP

### DISPOSITION

- Patients may bear weight early in the postoperative period (8).
- Physical therapy should focus on gait training, hip and knee ROM, and strengthening of the leg.

### PROGNOSIS

95% of femoral shaft fractures unite without complications.

### COMPLICATIONS

- Fat embolization, adults respiratory distress syndrome, and pulmonary complications can result from reamed femoral nailing, particularly in the polytrauma patient with chest and head trauma.
- Nonunion is uncommon and usually is treated successfully by exchange nailing.
  - Rotational malunions and limb-length inequalities can occur, particularly in comminuted shaft fractures.
  - Rotational malalignments of $>15°$ and length discrepancies of $>2$ cm should be corrected (3,9).
- Vascular injuries are uncommon in femoral shaft fractures, except in those caused by penetrating trauma.
- Nerve injuries resulting at the same time as shaft fracture are uncommon, although there are reported cases of pudendal nerve palsies resulting from the peroneal post while the patient is on the traction table (10).
- Heterotopic ossification can occur around the hip after anterograde nailing, particularly in a patient with a head injury.
- Compartment syndrome in the thigh may occur pre- or postoperatively.

### PATIENT MONITORING

- Neurovascular check postoperatively to assess for compartment syndrome
- Radiographs are taken every 6–8 weeks until bony union.

### REFERENCES


1. Winquist RA, Hansen ST, Jr, Clawson DK. Closed intramedullary nailing of femoral fractures. A report of five hundred and twenty cases. *J Bone Joint Surg* 1984;66A:529–539.
2. Orthopaedic Trauma Association Committee for Coding and Classification. Fracture and dislocation compendium. *J Orthop Trauma* 1996;10:v–154.
3. Bennett FS, Zinar DM, Kilgus DJ. Ipsilateral hip and femoral shaft fractures. *Clin Orthop Relat Res* 1993;296:168–177.
4. Lieurance R, Benjamin JB, Rappaport WD. Blood loss and transfusion in patients with isolated femur fractures. *J Orthop Trauma* 1992;6:175–179.
5. American College of Surgeons Committee on Trauma. *Advanced Trauma Life Support Program for Doctors,* 6th ed. Chicago: American College of Surgeons, 1997.
6. Pape HC, Hildebrand F, Pertschy S, et al. Changes in the management of femoral shaft fractures in polytrauma patients: from early total care to damage control orthopaedic surgery. *J Trauma* 2002;53:452–461.
7. Harwood PJ, Giannoudis PV, van Griensven M, et al. Alterations in the systemic inflammatory response after early total care and damage control procedures for femoral shaft fracture in severely injured patients. *J Trauma* 2005;58:446–452 [disc 452–454].
8. Brumback RJ, Toal TR, Jr, Murphy-Zane MS, et al. Immediate weight-bearing after treatment of a comminuted fracture of the femoral shaft with a statically locked intramedullary nail. *J Bone Joint Surg* 1999;81A:1538–1544.
9. Jaarsma RL, Pakvis DFM, Verdonschot N, et al. Rotational malalignment after intramedullary nailing of femoral fractures. *J Orthop Trauma* 2004;18:403–409.
10. Brumback RJ, Ellison TS, Molligan H, et al. Pudendal nerve palsy complicating intramedullary nailing of the femur. *J Bone Joint Surg* 1992;74A:1450–1455.


### ADDITIONAL READING


- Bradford HM. Fractures of the femoral shaft and subtrochanteric region. In: Brinker MR, ed. *Review of Orthopaedic Trauma.* Philadelphia: WB Saunders, 2001:67–86.
- Ricci WM. Femur: trauma. In: Vaccaro AR, ed. *Orthopaedic Knowledge Update 8.* Rosemont, IL: American Academy of Orthopaedic Surgeons; 2005;425–431.


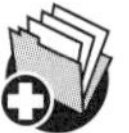

## MISCELLANEOUS

### CODES

#### *ICD9-CM*

- 821.0 Closed femoral shaft fracture
- 821.1 Open femoral shaft fracture

### PATIENT TEACHING

#### *Activity*

Most patients can bear weight as tolerated and resume activities gradually.

#### *Prevention*

- High-energy injuries should be prevented.
- Seat belt and airbag use help prevent injury in car crashes.

### FAQ

- Q: How long do femoral shaft fractures take to heal?
  - A: Closed fractures heal faster than open ones, usually within 3 months. Open fractures may take 3–6 months to heal.

# FEMORAL SHAFT FRACTURE IN THE CHILD

*Paul D. Sponseller, MD*

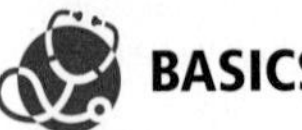

## BASICS

### DESCRIPTION

- Femoral shaft fractures are defined as those $>5$ cm below the lesser trochanter, but above the distal metaphyseal (wider) portion of the lower femur.
- The location usually is specified as:
  - Proximal
  - Midshaft
  - Distal
- Although the femur usually requires a large amount of energy to fracture, fractures can occur with low amounts of energy in infants and toddlers, and in those with a weak area in the bone (1).

### GENERAL PREVENTION

- Appropriate supervision
- Avoidance of contact sports if a substantial weakness of the bone or a known lesion in the femur is present

### EPIDEMIOLOGY

- Fractures of the femur are more common:
  - In areas of high population density or low socioeconomic level
  - In children 0–3 and 12–16 years old

### PATHOPHYSIOLOGY

- Femur fractures may occur in different patterns, which are suggestive of, but do not prove, a particular mechanism (1).
  - "Buckle" fracture suggests direct impact.
  - Spiral fracture suggests twisting.
  - Transverse fracture suggests a hit from the side.
  - Comminuted (shattered) and/or open fracture suggests very high energy or weak bone.
- Femur fractures in children usually are followed by a 1.0–1.5 cm "overgrowth" during the 18 months after healing, which accommodates some shortening during fracture treatment.

### ETIOLOGY

- The most common mechanisms by age are:
  - 0–2 years old:
    - Nonaccidental injury (child abuse) in those $<12$ months old
    - Fall from a height
  - 2–5 years old:
    - Fall from a height
    - Fall while playing
    - Pedestrian–motor vehicle accident
  - 5–16 years old:
    - Bicycle
    - Pedestrian–motor vehicle accident
    - Motor vehicle occupant
    - Sports

### ASSOCIATED CONDITIONS

- Some underlying bone disorders:
  - OI
  - Bone cyst
  - Fibrous cortical defect or NOF
  - Cerebral palsy
  - Fibrous dysplasia
- Other injuries that occur with femur fractures:
  - Head injury
  - Spine fracture
  - Upper extremity fracture

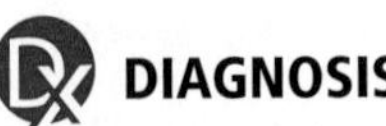

## DIAGNOSIS

### SIGNS AND SYMPTOMS

#### *History*

- Patients should be asked about antecedent pain if a question of a pathologic lesion arises.
- In cases of possible nonaccidental injury, caregivers or witnesses should be questioned about specifics of the event, including:
  - Child's position before the injury
  - Mechanism of injury
  - What happened after the injury

#### *Physical Exam*

- The thigh is swollen with a femur fracture.
- If the fracture is displaced, it usually is shortened and externally rotated.
- Any internal or external rotation motion of the lower extremity causes pain.
- The knee may be swollen, even in the absence of a ligament injury.
- Pulses and muscle function below the knee should be checked.
- If nonaccidental injury is suspected, check for other bruises or tenderness, including fundus of the eye.

### TESTS

#### *Imaging*

- Plain radiographs usually are sufficient.
- MRI or CT scan may be needed if a nondisplaced or stress fracture is suspected.
- If nonaccidental injury is suspected, a skeletal survey or bone scan may be necessary to rule out other injuries.

#### *Diagnostic Procedures/Surgery*

If a malignant lesion is suspected, a biopsy is indicated before surgical treatment, but this scenario is rare.

#### *Pathological Findings*

- Thin cortices and bowing suggest OI.
- Broad loss of cortical definition suggests fibrous dysplasia.
  - Focal lesions suggest unicameral cyst (centrally) or fibrous cortical defect (eccentrically)

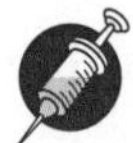

## TREATMENT

### INITIAL STABILIZATION

If the fracture is displaced and unstable, a Hare traction apparatus or a long splint should be used for comfort.

### GENERAL MEASURES

#### *Physical Therapy*

- Physical therapy is helpful in children $>8$–10 years old.
- Younger children usually do well on their own.
- Weightbearing depends on treatment and stage of healing, and should be prescribed by the orthopaedist.

### MEDICATION (DRUGS)

- Usually strong (narcotic) analgesics are needed in the early stages after fracture.
- Pain usually is minimal after 2–3 weeks.
- NSAIDS may slow healing.

### SURGERY

- Many different options for treatment of a femoral shaft fracture (1–9):
  - Choice depends on patient age and fracture characteristics.
  - All options produce good results.
- Immediate spica cast (3):
  - Best for children $\leq 6$ years old, $<32$ kg
  - Leg(s) is immobilized in a cast that extends distally from just below the ribs.
  - Applied in the emergency department or operating room with the patient sedated or anesthetized
  - $\leq 2.5$ cm of shortening and 10–15° of angulation can be accepted because of remodeling and overgrowth.
  - Healing usually is complete by 6–8 weeks.
- Traction (2–3 weeks) followed by spica cast (3):
  - Controls length and angulation well
  - Requires substantial hospital stay
  - No age limit
  - Not commonly used today because of desire for early mobilization
- Flexible intramedullary nails (Fig. 1) (5,7):
  - Used mostly for children ~5–11 years old
  - Not for fractures near the proximal or distal ends or those with comminution
  - Sometimes no cast needed
  - Nail removal necessary at 3–6 months
- External fixation (9):
  - Mostly for severe open fractures
  - Ages ~5–16 years
  - Slightly slower healing than that with nails (10–16 weeks) and, therefore, a higher risk of refracture

- Plate fixation (2,8):
  - May be open or minimally invasive
  - Slight risk of plate failure
  - Usually used in comminuted or emergent situations
- Rigid intramedullary nails (4,6):
  - Usually for children >10–11 years old
  - Avoid piriformis entry, which could cause AVN.
  - Allows early weightbearing
  - Subsequent nail removal recommended for young teens

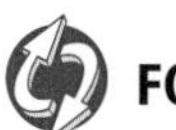

## FOLLOW-UP

- Patients usually are seen every 4–8 weeks until healing.
  - Radiographs usually are needed.
  - No sports are allowed until the fracture is well healed.
  - Implant removal usually is required.
  - Follow-up may continue for 2 years to assess overgrowth.

### *Issues for Referral*

Physical therapy referral is needed if the patient is not progressing well or has special complications.

### PROGNOSIS

- Most children have full return to function.
- Concomitant internal knee ligament injury in a child <12 years old may produce long-term impairment.
  - Examine at time of stabilization and healing.
  - MRI if indicated

### COMPLICATIONS

- Nonunion:
  - Occurs in <1% of closed pediatric femur fractures (5–9)
  - Occurs in 10–20% of open fractures (5–9)
- Malunion:
  - Up to 15–20° are acceptable proximally.
  - 10° are acceptable distally.
  - Remodeling usually is good if the patient is <10 years old.
- Shortening:
  - 2.5–3 cm of shortening are acceptable if the patient is <10 years old.
  - Overgrowth compensates for up to 1.5 cm.
  - Contralateral epiphysiodesis is an option.
- Neurovascular injury:
  - Most common with open fractures
  - Risk of femoral artery injury or compartment syndrome
- Infection:
  - 1% risk with operative treatment (5–9)
  - Risk is higher with open than with closed fractures.
- AVN:
  - Risk with adult-type nails inserted through the piriformis fossa
  - Do not use in children <15 years old.
- Ligament injury:
  - May coexist with fracture
  - Check for this injury when the fracture is stable.

### PATIENT MONITORING

Neurovascular checks for the first 1–2 days

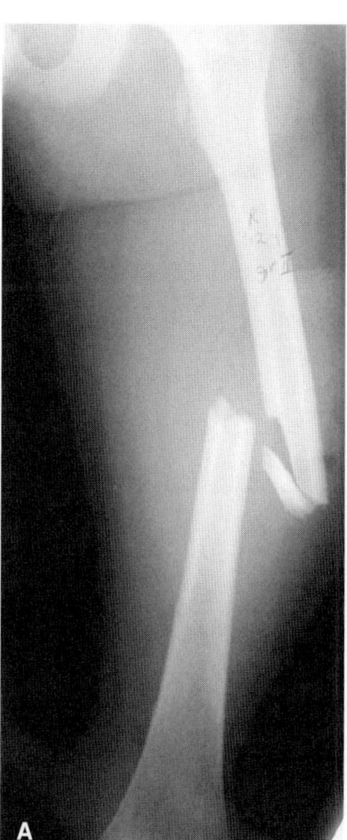


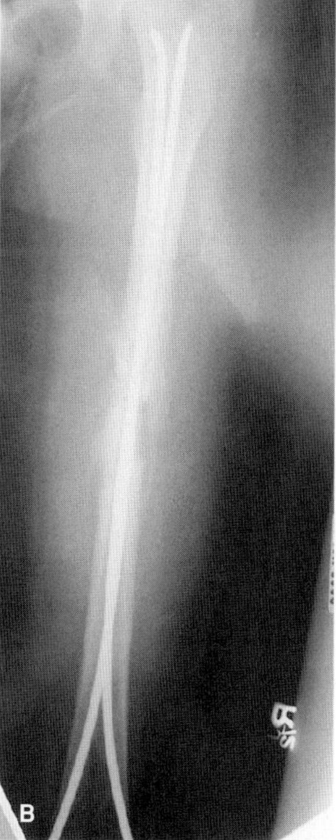


**Fig. 1.** Femur fracture in a 10-year-old (A) treated with flexible intramedullary nails (B).

### REFERENCES


1. Pierce MC, Bertocci GE, Janosky JE, et al. Femur fractures resulting from stair falls among children: An injury plausibility model. *Pediatrics* 2005;115:1712–1722.
2. Caird MS, Mueller KA, Puryear A, et al. Compression plating of pediatric femoral shaft fractures. *J Pediatr Orthop* 2003;23:448–452.
3. Epps HR, Molenaar E, O'Connor DP. Immediate single-leg spica cast for pediatric femoral diaphysis fractures. *J Pediatr Orthop* 2006;26:491–496.
4. Gordon JE, Swenning TA, Burd TA, et al. Proximal femoral radiographic changes after lateral transtrochanteric intramedullary nail placement in children. *J Bone Joint Surg* 2003;85A:1295–1301.
5. Ho CA, Skaggs DL, Tang CW, et al. Use of flexible intramedullary nails in pediatric femur fractures. *J Pediatr Orthop* 2006;26:497–504.
6. Kanellopoulos AD, Yiannakopoulos CK, Soucacos PN. Closed, locked intramedullary nailing of pediatric femoral shaft fractures through the tip of the greater trochanter. *J Trauma* 2006;60:217–223.
7. Sink EL, Gralla J, Repine M. Complications of pediatric femur fractures treated with titanium elastic nails: A comparison of fracture types. *J Pediatr Orthop* 2005;25:577–580.
8. Sink EL, Hedequist D, Morgan SJ, et al. Results and technique of unstable pediatric femoral fractures treated with submuscular bridge plating. *J Pediatr Orthop* 2006;26:177–181.
9. Skaggs DL, Leet AI, Money MD, et al. Secondary fractures associated with external fixation in pediatric femur fractures. *J Pediatr Orthop* 1999;19:582–586.




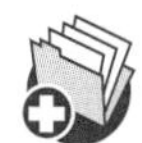

## MISCELLANEOUS

### CODES

#### *ICD9-CM*

821.01 Femur shaft fracture

### PATIENT TEACHING

- Early in the treatment, it is helpful to explain the concepts of remodeling and overgrowth to the parents, so that they can understand when they see an acceptable alignment on their child's radiographs.
- Illustrative radiographs are helpful.
- Parents of children treated in a spica cast require special teaching about hygiene and transportation.

### ACTIVITY

Children may return to school as the environment allows.

### PREVENTION

The management of motor vehicle traffic, as well as appropriate intervention in instances of nonaccidental injury, may prevent future injuries.

### FAQ

- Q: Are there specific fracture patterns that prove nonaccidental injury?
  - A: Not really. Only multiple unreported fractures in different stages of healing, or metaphyseal "corner" fractures, are diagnostic.
- Q: Will a child who fractures a femur be able to return to sports?
  - A: Yes, barring complications, no sequelae should present.

# FIBROUS CORTICAL DEFECT/NONOSSIFYING FIBROMA

*Frank J. Frassica, MD*

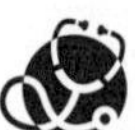

## BASICS

### DESCRIPTION

- NOF is a common developmental abnormality in children and adolescents with open physes; it is not seen in adults (1).
  - Despite the name, this condition mineralizes and disappears with skeletal maturity.
  - When the lesion is very small, it is called a "fibrous cortical defect."
  - Occurs eccentrically in the metaphyses of long bones, most commonly in the distal femur, proximal tibia, or distal tibia
- The lesion is seen in children and adolescents, but not in adults.
- Staging (as with other benign lesions) (2):
  - Stage 1: Latent (~96%)
  - Stage 2: Active (~2–3%)
  - Stage 3: Aggressive (<1%)
- Natural history:
  - Active stage 2 during childhood
  - Becoming latent stage 1 at skeletal maturation
- Synonyms: Benign metaphyseal cortical defect; Metaphyseal fibrous defect; Benign fibrous histiocytoma; Fibrous xanthoma

### EPIDEMIOLOGY

A common skeletal lesion

#### *Incidence*

Estimated to occur in 35% of healthy children with open physes (3)

### ETIOLOGY

The cause is hypothesized to be a focal area of increased periosteal resorption during growth.

### ASSOCIATED CONDITIONS

- NF:
  - NOF-appearing lesions may be found (~5%) (3).
- Jaffe-Campanacci syndrome (3):
  - Rare, congenital disorder
  - Multiple NOFs (widespread and symmetric)
  - Café-au-lait pigmentation
  - Nonskeletal abnormalities
  - Mental retardation

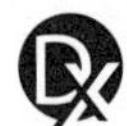

## DIAGNOSIS

### SIGNS AND SYMPTOMS

- Most lesions are asymptomatic and are found incidentally on radiographs.
- Occasionally, the condition is painful if a pathologic fracture occurs through the lesion or if such a fracture is impending.

#### *Physical Exam*

- Usually, the lesion is nontender.
- No swelling or tenderness should be present with weightbearing, unless a fracture is impending.
- NOF-like lesions may occur in NF.
- Jaffe-Campanacci syndrome

### TESTS

#### *Imaging*

- On plain radiographs, a lytic (radiolucent) lesion is seen eccentrically in the metaphyses of long bones (usually the distal femur, proximal tibia, or distal tibia).
  - Based in the cortex
  - Overlying cortex if thinned
  - Surrounded by a scalloped, reactive rim of sclerotic (radiopaque) bone
  - Often appears multiloculated, producing a "bubbling" appearance
  - Ranges in size from a few millimeters to a few centimeters
  - Usually solitary
  - If a bone scan is obtained, the lesion will appear "hot" early on from the reactive rim of bone.
    - As the lesion heals, the bone scan will become normal.

#### *Pathological Findings*

- The lesion is filled with fibrous connective tissue arranged in a whirled, "starry night" pattern.
- Also seen are multinucleated giant cells, foam-filled histiocytes, and hemosiderin pigmentation.
- Cystic spaces are not typical.

### DIFFERENTIAL DIAGNOSIS

- Chondromyxoid fibroma
- Giant cell tumor
- Fibrous dysplasia

## TREATMENT

### GENERAL MEASURES

- In general, full, unrestricted activity is allowed.
- If weightbearing pain develops, AP and lateral radiographs should be obtained to look for stress fractures.
- MRI is effective in detecting stress fractures.

### MEDICATION (DRUGS)

- The treatment for large lesions is radiographic monitoring according to the physician's judgment because the lesion is self-healing at skeletal maturity.
- Patients with large lesions should be seen every 6 months.
  - This monitoring may continue until growth is complete.
- If >50% of the cortex is involved, and the patient is symptomatic (pain), a pathologic fracture is possible.
  - In this case, treatment is surgery with curettage and bone grafting.
  - If the lesion is small and asymptomatic (<25% of the width of the cortex), no monitoring is needed.
- No restrictions are placed on activity unless a pathologic fracture is impending (>50% of the cortex is involved in a symptomatic child), in which case the child should be nonweightbearing or have protected weightbearing on the affected extremity.

### SURGERY

- For impending pathologic fracture, curettage (scraping the lesion) followed by bone grafting (placing bone graft into the lesion) should be performed.
- Internal fixation usually is not necessary.

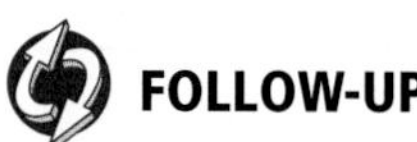

## FOLLOW-UP

### PROGNOSIS
All these lesions are self-healing at skeletal maturity.

### COMPLICATIONS
- Pathologic fracture is seen rarely.
- Pathologic fractures usually occur only in lesions involving >50% of the cortex in symptomatic patients or in patients who have had severe trauma.

### PATIENT MONITORING
- Serial radiography:
  - AP and lateral views of the affected part

### REFERENCES

1. Enneking WF. Benign skeletal lesions. In: *Clinical Musculoskeletal Pathology*, 3rd ed. Gainsville, FL: University of Florida Press, 1990:302–357.
2. McCarthy EF, Frassica FJ. Primary bone tumors. In: *Pathology of Bone and Joint Disorders: With Clinical and Radiographic Correlation*. Philadelphia: WB Saunders, 1998:195–275.
3. Dorfman HD, Czerniak B. Fibrous and fibrohistiocytic lesions. In: *Bone Tumors*. St. Louis: Mosby, Inc, 1998:492–558.


### ADDITIONAL READING

Frassica FJ, Frassica DA, McCarthy EF, Jr. Orthopaedic pathology. In: Miller MD, ed. *Review of Orthopaedics*, 3rd ed. Philadelphia: WB Saunders, 2000:379–441.


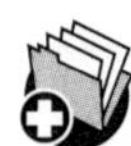

## MISCELLANEOUS

### CODES
#### *ICD9-CM*
213.9 Fibrous cortical defect

### PATIENT TEACHING
- Tell children that they must report pain or limp to their parents.
- Reassure the child and parents regarding the benign nature of the lesion, the natural course of self-healing, and the prevalence of the lesion in healthy children (35%).
- If the lesion is small, no follow-up is needed.
- If it is large, follow-up should be obtained every 6–12 months.

### FAQ
- Q: If a child has a large NOF and is completely asymptomatic, is protected weightbearing or surgery necessary?
  - A: In general, if the child is completely asymptomatic, protected weightbearing is not necessary. A small risk of fracture is likely with trauma. Surgery is not necessary.
- Q: What are the disadvantages of surgery?
  - A: A major disadvantage is the scar and the need for protected weightbearing for 3–6 months after surgery.

# FIBROUS DYSPLASIA

*Frank J. Frassica, MD*

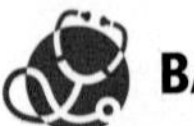

## BASICS

### DESCRIPTION

- Fibrous dysplasia is a benign bone process in which there is a failure to produce mature lamellar bone.
- The condition:
  - Causes focal defects in bone quality
  - Is characterized by multiple, gradual bone deformities; a risk of endocrinopathy (in the polyostotic variety); and a tendency toward pain in the lesions
- Café-au-lait spots are common signs in multifocal disease.
- Physical findings require some time to develop.
- Precocious puberty may occur as early as the 1st year of life.
- Classification:
  - Monostotic: Involves only 1 bone
  - Polyostotic: Involves multiple bones, usually more on 1 side of the body
- Synonym: Osteitis fibrosa cystica

### EPIDEMIOLOGY

#### *Incidence*

- Rare
- Occurs equally in males and females

### RISK FACTORS

McCune-Albright syndrome (the triad of polyostotic fibrous dysplasia, café-au-lait spots, and precocious puberty) is an age-related risk factor.

#### *Genetics*

(See "Etiology")

### ETIOLOGY

- A defect in the gene occurs for a subunit of a certain G-protein, a type of protein that couples cell-surface receptors to extracellular signals and activates intracellular synthesis of cyclic adenosine monophosphate.
- The extent and severity of the disease are related to the period in embryonic life when the mutation occurred.

### ASSOCIATED CONDITIONS

- Endocrinopathy
- Osteosarcoma
- Fibrosarcoma

## DIAGNOSIS

The diagnosis is made from the characteristic plain radiograph.

### SIGNS AND SYMPTOMS

- Signs:
  - Progressive distortion of bone, as in the proximal femur, pelvis, and cranium
  - Possible neurologic compromise, caused by cranial or spinal deformity
  - Café-au-lait spots in the polyostotic form (spots have irregular margins likened to the coast of Maine)
  - Pain and a waddling gait
  - Scoliosis
- Symptoms: Constant aches from bones affected by dysplasia under loading

#### *Physical Exam*

- Measure the patient's height.
- Check for scoliosis, because sometimes it may develop in this condition.
- Measure limb-length and angular deformities.
- Check all 4 extremities for bowing.
- Document the ROM, especially about the hip.
- Palpate tender areas of bone.
- Observe the patient's gait.

### TESTS

#### *Lab*

- Specific tests for any of the described endocrinopathies should be performed if clinically indicated.
  - May include measurement of growth hormone, thyroid function, and adrenal function

#### *Imaging*

- Radiography:
  - The internal appearance of bone with fibrous dysplasia on radiographs is so homogeneous that it is called "ground glass."
    - This finding is not surprising, given the histologic findings of multiple small disorganized trabeculae.
  - Fibrous dysplasia usually is seen occupying a large segment of the diaphysis, and sometimes the entire diaphysis, of a bone.
  - The classic teaching is that fibrous dysplasia is a "long lesion in a long bone" (1).
  - A characteristic deformity is the "shepherd's crook" appearance of the proximal femur:
    - A diffuse, severe bowing of the entire proximal end, secondary to bone weakening
- Technetium bone scans may be used to locate other lesions of fibrous dysplasia, if needed.
  - The lesions are usually "hot" on bone scans, although not universally so.
- CT is useful for imaging cranial or spinal disorders.

#### *Pathological Findings*

- Bone lesions show multiple small, disorganized bony trabeculae, not organized to provide normal mechanical support.
  - Likened to "alphabet soup" in their disorganized appearance
- The marrow is filled with fibrous tissue.
- Osteoblastic rimming of the trabeculae is absent; the bone forms from fibro-osseous metaplasia.

### DIFFERENTIAL DIAGNOSIS

- Unicameral bone cyst
- Fibrous cortical defect
- Ollier disease

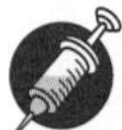

# TREATMENT

## GENERAL MEASURES

- Correct progressive skeletal deformity when painful.
- Treat endocrinopathy appropriately.
- Perform craniofacial reconstruction in patients with severe deformity.
- Manage pain with analgesics, or consult a pain management specialist.
  - Early trials of diphosphonate agents are promising.

## SPECIAL THERAPY

### *Physical Therapy*

- Therapy is useful for postoperative rehabilitation.
- The involvement of multiple limbs often poses special challenges to the therapist.

## MEDICATION (DRUGS)

- Pain should be managed with analgesics, or a pain management specialist should be consulted.
  - Early trials of diphosphonates are promising.
- No evidence suggests that increasing a patient's activity level will strengthen the dysplastic bone.
  - Generally, pain should be the patient's guide to what is allowed.
  - High-impact or endurance activities pose an increased risk of fracture.

## SURGERY

- Orthopaedic principles:
  - A marked bowing deformity should be straightened to minimize additional bending forces.
  - In the proximal femur, this procedure involves a valgus osteotomy or a medial displacement osteotomy.
  - Diseased bone should be supported with a stronger material, such as cortical bone or a metal implant.
  - An intramedullary device usually is better than a plate because it can protect the length of the bone and is more centrally located and therefore more effective (less subject to fatigue fracture).
  - Lesions of fibrous dysplasia often recur after simple bone grafting.
- Lesions often bleed copiously during surgery.
- Autogenous cancellous grafts are not used because this graft material is remodeled quickly into fibrous dysplasia.

# FOLLOW-UP

## PROGNOSIS

- Progression of dysplasia and new lesions may occur in adulthood.
- About 1/3 of patients have chronic pain.
- Life expectancy is shortened in patients with the polyostotic form because of pneumonia, thrombosis, and malignant transformation.

## COMPLICATIONS

- Fracture
- Chronic pain
- Depression
- Malignant transformation, most commonly to osteosarcoma (~1% [2])

## PATIENT MONITORING

- Patients should be seen periodically by the same physician or set of specialists to detect progressive deformity.
- In particular, this regimen should include yearly visits to the orthopaedic surgeon to track femoral bowing and scoliosis.
- Patients also should be told about the risk and warning signs of malignant transformation to sarcoma:
  - Increase in pain, size, or warmth of the lesion

## REFERENCES


1. McCarthy EF, Frassica FJ. Primary bone tumors. In: *Pathology of Bone and Joint Disorders: With Clinical and Radiographic Correlation*. Philadelphia: WB Saunders, 1998:195–275.
2. Dorfman HD, Czerniak B. Fibroosseous lesions. In: *Bone Tumors*. St. Louis: Mosby, 1998:441–491.


## ADDITIONAL READING


Stephenson RB, London MD, Hankin FM, et al. Fibrous dysplasia. An analysis of options for treatment. *J Bone Joint Surg*. 1987;69A:400–409.


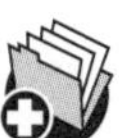

# MISCELLANEOUS

## CODES

### *ICD9-CM*

- 733.29 Monostotic fibrous dysplasia
- 756.54 Polyostotic fibrous dysplasia

## PATIENT TEACHING

- Patients should be supported because of the chronic nature of the disease.
- Sports restrictions, specific to the patient's individual lesions, should be discussed.
- Career counseling should be given.

### *Prevention*

Avoid irradiation of the lesions because of the risk of malignant transformation.

## FAQ

- Q: Is the solitary form of fibrous dysplasia painful?
  - A: In general, no pain is present, but some patients do have unexplained pain.
- Q: Is it necessary to perform curettage and bone grafting in patients with no symptoms?
  - A: Patients who have no symptoms should be treated with observation.
- Q: Will the bone heal in fibrous dysplasia after a fracture?
  - A: Yes, it will heal in ~6–12 weeks. If a marked deformity is present, the risk of repeat fracture is high.

# FIBULA FRACTURE

*Simon C. Mears, MD, PhD*
*Nicholas Ahn, MD*

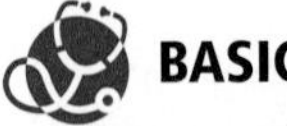

## BASICS

### DESCRIPTION

- Fractures of the fibula can be described by anatomic position as proximal, midshaft, or distal.
- Fractures may involve the knee, tibiofibular syndesmosis, tibia, or ankle joint.
- Rarely, a fracture of the fibula may be isolated but, in general, the force required to fracture the fibula also breaks other structures in the leg.
- Distal fibula fractures that involve the ankle joint are by far the most common fibula fractures (see "Ankle Fracture" chapter).
- Fractures of the fibular shaft occurring without ankle injury nearly always are associated with tibial shaft fractures.
- Fractures of the proximal head and neck of the fibula are associated with substantial damage to the knee (1).
  - These fractures may be isolated, caused by a direct blow to the area, or caused by an avulsion injury at the insertion of the biceps femoris tendon or LCL.
- Fractures of the fibula often involve a syndesmotic injury (called "Maisonneuve fractures").
  - Damage along the medial aspect of the ankle joint by external rotation forces may be associated with rupture of the deltoid and tibiofibular ligaments, which may, in turn, cause a tear in the interosseous membrane between the shafts of the tibia and fibula.
  - As this tear progresses up the interosseous membrane, all the forces are placed more proximally along the fibula at the area where the tear ends, causing a proximal fibula fracture (2).

### EPIDEMIOLOGY

#### *Incidence*

Fibula fractures, including ankle fractures, are among the most commonly encountered fractures in orthopaedics (3).

### ETIOLOGY

- Trauma (direct blow or gunshot wound)
- Falls
- Missteps
- Sports injuries

### ASSOCIATED CONDITIONS

- Fractures of the tibial shaft
- Compartment syndrome of the leg
- Tibial plateau fractures
- MCL injury of the knee
- LCL injury of the knee
- Biceps femoris tendon injury
- Common peroneal nerve palsy
- Interosseous membrane rupture
- Deltoid ligament of the ankle injury
- Medial malleolar ankle fracture

### CLASSIFICATION

- Proximal fracture
- Midshaft fracture
- Distal (ankle) fracture

## DIAGNOSIS

### SIGNS AND SYMPTOMS

- Patients with fibular shaft or head fractures generally present with tenderness and swelling in the area of injury.
  - Numbness or paresthesias may arise if damage to the peroneal nerve has occurred.
- With an associated knee injury, patients have pain and swelling of the knee joint.
- Maisonneuve fractures present with swelling and pain, not only proximally in the area of the fibula fracture, but also about the medial aspect of the ankle joint.

#### *Physical Exam*

- Physical examination shows point tenderness and swelling in the area of fracture.
- Always assess stability and medial tenderness of the ankle because a possible deltoid tear with a proximal fibula fracture may be present (Maisonneuve fracture).
- Always assess the stability and tenderness of the knee, particularly in proximal fibula fractures, including examination of all ligaments.

### TESTS

#### *Lab*

No serum laboratory tests are indicated.

#### *Imaging*

- Radiography:
  - Obtain AP and lateral views of the shafts of the tibia and fibula.
  - Obtain AP and lateral views of the knee to look for associated injury to the knee.
  - Obtain 3 views of the ankle (AP, lateral, and mortise) to look for ankle fracture or syndesmotic disruption.

#### *Pathological Findings*

- The fibula fracture may have several different patterns:
  - Spiral
  - Transverse
  - Comminuted
- Fractures secondary to tumors are rare.

### DIFFERENTIAL DIAGNOSIS

- Muscle tears (gastrocnemius, soleus)
- Tendon rupture
- Syndesmotic injury
- Knee or ankle injury

## TREATMENT

### GENERAL MEASURES

- Isolated fibular shaft fractures that do not involve the ankle or knee are relatively unimportant because the fibula supports only 17% of body weight and is not essential to stability (4).
- The shaft of the fibula tends to heal well on its own because it is encompassed completely by vascularized muscle.
- A splint or cast may be applied to increase comfort but is not essential.
  - The RICE protocol, with elastic wrap compression and pain medication, may be sufficient.
- Pain and swelling usually are diminished in 1–2 weeks, at which time the patient is allowed to return to regular activity as tolerated.
- Full healing usually is accomplished by 6–8 weeks.
- Fractures that involve syndesmotic injury or ankle or knee fracture often require surgical treatment.

#### *Activity*

Weightbearing on the involved leg may be allowed as tolerated by the patient.

### SPECIAL THERAPY

#### *Physical Therapy*

- Patients with isolated fibular shaft fractures are instructed to bear partial weight.
- Patients with fractures of the distal fibula and ankle instability are nonweightbearing until the fracture heals.

### MEDICATION (DRUGS)

#### *First Line*

Patients require pain medicine as appropriate.

### SURGERY

- If a fibula fracture is associated with a tibial shaft fracture or a tibial plateau fracture, then the tibial fracture is repaired, and the fibula usually heals without fixation.
- For distal tibial fractures, fixation of the fibula:
  - May aid in realignment or length restoration of the tibial fracture
  - Increases the stability of the tibial fracture repair (5,6)
  - Is performed with a 3.5-mm compression plate
- Maisonneuve fractures with syndesmotic injury imply injury to the medial side of the ankle joint.
  - These fractures should be treated operatively with open plating of the fibula fracture and syndesmotic screw placement.
  - If a medial malleolar fracture is present, it should be repaired with open fixation.

- Repair of the deltoid ligament tear is not believed to be necessary (7).
- The need for syndesmotic screw fixation should be determined by the use of an intraoperative external rotation stress test under fluoroscopy (8).
- Type of screw fixation for repairing the syndesmosis:
  - Choice is debated.
  - Differences have not been found between syndesmotic screws that engage 3 or 4 cortices (9).
  - Debate also exists as to whether these screws should be removed or should remain in place indefinitely or until they break and require removal.
- The position of the ankle when fixation is applied is not important, but the syndesmosis must be reduced anatomically (10).
- The use of bioabsorbable screws may obviate the need for screw removal (11).

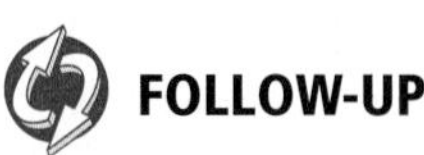

## FOLLOW-UP

### DISPOSITION

#### *Issues for Referral*

Patients with tibia fractures, syndesmosis injuries, or ankle fractures should be referred to an orthopaedic surgeon.

### PROGNOSIS

Generally, fibula fractures do well, and most patients have normal function at long-term follow-up (12,13).

### COMPLICATIONS

- Nonunion
- Chronic pain
- Malunion
- Hardware pain or breakage
- Compartment syndrome

### PATIENT MONITORING

Patients are followed at 1-month intervals with plain radiographs until the fractures are healed.

### REFERENCES


1. Bozkurt M, Turanli S, Doral MN, et al. The impact of proximal fibula fractures in the prognosis of tibial plateau fractures: a novel classification. *Knee Surg Sports Traumatol Arthrosc* 2005;13:323–328.
2. Nielson JH, Sallis JG, Potter HG, et al. Correlation of interosseous membrane tears to the level of the fibular fracture. *J Orthop Trauma* 2004;18:68–74.
3. van Staa TP, Dennison EM, Leufkens HGM, et al. Epidemiology of fractures in England and Wales. *Bone* 2001;29:517–522.
4. Wang Q, Whittle M, Cunningham J, et al. Fibula and its ligaments in load transmission and ankle joint stability. *Clin Orthop Relat Res* 1996;330:261–270.
5. Egol KA, Weisz R, Hiebert R, et al. Does fibular plating improve alignment after intramedullary nailing of distal metaphyseal tibia fractures? *J Orthop Trauma* 2006;20:94–103.
6. Kumar A, Charlebois SJ, Cain EL, et al. Effect of fibular plate fixation on rotational stability of simulated distal tibial fractures treated with intramedullary nailing. *J Bone Joint Surg* 2003;85A:604–608.
7. Stromsoe K, Hoqevold HE, Skjeldal S, et al. The repair of a ruptured deltoid ligament is not necessary in ankle fractures. *J Bone Joint Surg* 1995;77B:920–921.
8. Jenkinson RJ, Sanders DW, Macleod MD, et al. Intraoperative diagnosis of syndesmosis injuries in external rotation ankle fractures. *J Orthop Trauma* 2005;19:604–609.
9. Hoiness P, Stromsoe K. Tricortical versus quadricortical syndesmosis fixation in ankle fractures: a prospective, randomized study comparing two methods of syndesmosis fixation. *J Orthop Trauma* 2004;18:331–337.
10. Tornetta P, III, Spoo JE, Reynolds FA, et al. Overtightening of the ankle syndesmosis: is it really possible? *J Bone Joint Surg* 2001;83A:489–492.
11. Thordarson DB, Samuelson M, Shepherd LE, et al. Bioabsorbable versus stainless steel screw fixation of the syndesmosis in pronation-lateral rotation ankle fractures: a prospective randomized trial. *Foot Ankle Int* 2001;22:335–338.
12. Sproule JA, Khalid M, O'Sullivan M, et al. Outcome after surgery for Maisonneuve fracture of the fibula. *Injury* 2004;35:791–798.
13. Weening B, Bhandari M. Predictors of functional outcome following transsyndesmotic screw fixation of ankle fractures. *J Orthop Trauma* 2005;19:102–108.
14. Boden BP, Lohnes JH, Nunley JA, et al. Tibia and fibula fractures in soccer players. *Knee Surg Sports Traumatol Arthrosc* 1999;7:262–266.


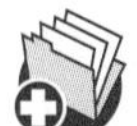

## MISCELLANEOUS

### CODES

#### *ICD9-CM*

823.8 Fibula fracture

### PATIENT TEACHING

Patients are counseled that, although fibula fractures heal well, tenderness and swelling may persist for several months after injury.

#### *Prevention*

In 1 recent study, shin guards did not seem to prevent tibia and fibula fractures in soccer players (14).

### FAQ

- Q: Do syndesmotic screws require removal?
  - A: The removal of screws after healing is controversial. Some surgeons recommend routine removal to avoid breakage; others believe that screws should be removed only if they become painful.

# FLATFOOT

*Kris J. Alden, MD, PhD*

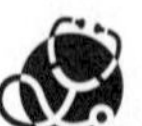

## BASICS

### DESCRIPTION

- Flatfoot, or pes planus, is a deformity of the foot in which the normal medial longitudinal arch of the foot has been lost (1–4).
- It may present as an asymptomatic incidental finding or as a painful condition secondary to an associated anatomic abnormality or pathologic condition of the foot.
- Classification:
  - Rigid versus flexible:
    - A flexible flatfoot lacks an arch only when patient is weightbearing, not when nonweightbearing or toe-standing.
    - A rigid flatfoot lacks an arch at all times.
  - Pediatric versus adult:
    - Onset may indicate underlying potential cause.

### EPIDEMIOLOGY

#### *Incidence*

- Congenital flexible flatfoot after infancy:
  - Is a trait that often runs in families, although the pattern of inheritance is not known
  - Is present in ~15% of adults (5)
- Tarsal coalition, the most common type of congenital rigid flatfoot, is inherited in an autosomal dominant pattern (6).
  - The exact overall incidence is unknown, but it is <1% (7).
- PTT deficiency is the most common cause of acquired flatfoot in adults, although its precise incidence is not known.
- The exact incidence of other patterns of acquired flatfeet is not known.

### RISK FACTORS

- For persistent congenital flexible flatfoot: Other family members with the same condition
- For congenital rigid flatfoot secondary to tarsal coalition: Female gender and other family members with the same condition
- For acquired flexible flatfoot secondary to PTT synovitis or rupture: Hypertension, diabetes, and a history of trauma
- Other conditions that can lead to flatfoot:
  - Tight Achilles tendon
  - Neurologic diseases (e.g., poliomyelitis, spina bifida, myelodysplasia, NF, stroke)
  - Osteoarthritis, posttraumatic arthritis, or inflammatory arthritis
  - Charcot arthropathy secondary to diabetes or other peripheral neuropathy

### ETIOLOGY

- Congenital flexible flatfoot and tarsal coalition are the result of genetic inheritance.
- PTT dysfunction is secondary to tendon degeneration and attenuation.
- Flatfoot deformity from Charcot neuroarthropathy is secondary to bone fragmentation, resorption, and fracture.
- Other causes to consider: Congenital vertical talus, peroneal spastic flatfoot, and trauma (8–12)

## DIAGNOSIS

### SIGNS AND SYMPTOMS

- Flatfoot with low or no arch
- Pain over medial arch
- Deformity may progress with time.
- May be exacerbated by walking, sports, high level of activity, or traumatic event
- Abnormal shoe wear pattern

#### *History*

- The onset of deformity, family history, associated diseases, activity level, and history of previous trauma should be noted for all patients.
- The patient or parents may complain of tenderness and swelling along the medial part of the foot, a diminished endurance in the foot, a decreased ability to participate in sports, and, eventually, a progressive difficulty in ambulating.
- Increased wear on medial aspect of the shoe
- Pediatric flatfoot deformity often is present from an early age.
- Adult acquired flatfoot caused by arthritis or rupture of the PTT presents as a gradual, progressive aching and swelling along the medial aspect of the foot and ankle.

#### *Physical Exam*

- Of primary importance is the determination of whether the condition is rigid or flexible.
  - Rigid flatfoot:
    - Loss of the normal longitudinal arch of the foot at all times
    - Restricted motion of the hindfoot
  - Flexible flatfoot:
    - Loss of arch only on standing on the affected foot, with reconstitution of the arch when the foot is dependent or when the patient toe-stands
    - Normal motion of the hindfoot
- Increasing severity is associated with forefoot abduction and the "too many toes" sign when the patient is viewed from behind.
- Inversion against resistance may be absent or diminished in patients with PTT dysfunction.
  - The patient may have pain or difficulty when attempting a single-limb heel rise on the affected side.
- The foot should be inspected for deformity or swelling and then palpated for tenderness.
- Gait pattern should be assessed.
  - An antalgic gait may indicate a painful condition such as arthritis or tendinitis.
  - The patient may have impaired propulsion with PTT abnormality.
  - An awkward, foot-slapping gait may suggest a neurologic or neuromuscular disease (e.g., spina bifida or poliomyelitis).
- The Achilles tendon should be examined to test whether the heel cord is tight.

### TESTS

#### *Imaging*

- Radiography:
  - 3 standing radiographic views of the patient's ankle (AP, lateral, and mortise) and 3 views of the patient's foot (AP, lateral, and oblique) should be obtained.
  - The calcaneal pitch is diminished and may approach 0° with more severe flatfoot deformity.
  - The talus-1st metatarsal angle increases with loss of arch.
    - This angle should normally be 0° with the talus and metatarsal collinear.
    - Angle measurements: ≤15°, minor pes planus deformity; 15–30°, moderate deformity; >30°, severe deformity
  - When tarsal coalition is suspected:
    - Assess oblique radiograph for a calcaneonavicular coalition.
    - Obtain a CT scan to rule out a talocalcaneal coalition.
  - Assess the degree of hindfoot or midfoot arthritis.
  - Rule out bony fragmentation indicative of Charcot arthropathy.
- An MRI scan may be useful for visualizing PTT abnormality.

#### *Pathological Findings*

- Secondary to underlying cause:
  - Charcot arthropathy: Fragmentation, resorption of bone
  - PTT dysfunction: Degeneration, tearing, hypertrophy
  - Tarsal coalition: Fibrous, fibrocartilaginous, or osseous coalition

### DIFFERENTIAL DIAGNOSIS

- Pediatric flatfoot:
  - Benign flexible flatfoot
  - Tarsal coalition
  - Congenital vertical/oblique talus
  - Accessory navicular
- Adult acquired flatfoot:
  - PTT dysfunction or tear
  - Midfoot arthritis
  - Charcot arthropathy
  - Neuromuscular disorders

## TREATMENT

### GENERAL MEASURES
- No treatment needed if asymptomatic
- Pediatric:
  - Benign flexible flatfoot:
    - Shoes with good arch support
    - Consider orthotic device (e.g., prefabricated or custom-made medial arch support).
  - Tarsal coalition:
    - Initially, immobilization with a below-the-knee cast or boot brace
    - Rest and temporary activity restriction
  - Flatfoot secondary to a tight Achilles tendon may be relieved by physical therapy and heel-cord stretching.
- Adult:
  - PTT dysfunction or tear:
    - NSAIDs and rest
    - Short-term immobilization with a below-the-knee cast or boot brace
    - Long-term maintenance with custom orthotic arch support or ankle-foot orthosis (brace)
    - Injection of corticosteroids is not recommended because it may weaken or rupture the tendon.
    - Weight loss
  - Midfoot arthritis:
    - Orthotic arch support
    - NSAIDs
    - Foot wear modifications (e.g., rocker-bottom and steel shank)
    - Intra-articular corticosteroid injections
  - Charcot arthropathy:
    - Acutely: Total contact cast and restricted weightbearing
    - Long-term: Orthotics and/or bracing
  - Surgical treatment is indicated for failure of nonoperative treatment.

### SPECIAL THERAPY
#### *Physical Therapy*
- Physical therapy can be used to increase ankle and foot ROM and to stretch a tight Achilles tendon.
- Orthotists can fabricate appropriate orthotic devices.

### MEDICATION (DRUGS)
- NSAIDs:
  - Can be used if swelling and pain are substantial
  - Are most useful for acute injuries or for patients with posterior tibial tendinitis.

### SURGERY
- Indicated for failure of nonoperative treatment, progression of deformity, or instability (13)
  - Surgical treatment may entail fusion, osteotomies, and possible soft-tissue procedures.
  - Age, activity level, degree of deformity, and comorbid conditions play a role in determining the extent of surgical treatment.
- Pediatric flexible flatfoot:
  - Surgical treatments usually consist of osteotomies that realign the foot to correct valgus and improve mechanical alignment of the foot and ankle.
- Rigid flatfoot from tarsal coalition:
  - Resection of tarsal coalition with interposition of fat or muscle
  - For patients with talocalcaneal coalition involving >50% of the joint surface or those with degenerative joint arthritis, subtalar arthrodesis is indicated.
- Flatfoot secondary to a tight Achilles tendon:
  - Tendon lengthening involves a Z-lengthening procedure or partial sectioning of the tendon.
- Acquired flatfoot secondary to PTT synovitis:
  - In early stages of the disease, synovectomy may be sufficient.
  - Flexible deformities are corrected with tendon transfers, calcaneal and midfoot osteotomies, and/or limited hindfoot arthrodesis.
- Fusion is necessary for arthritis or rigid flatfoot deformity.

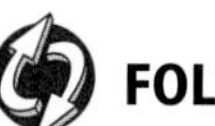

## FOLLOW-UP

### PROGNOSIS
Most patients do not develop progressive deformities and do not need corrective surgery.

### COMPLICATIONS
- Most patients have little risk of complications with nonoperative treatment.
- 1 major exception is patients with PTT dysfunction (acquired flatfoot) because they may develop a rigid flatfoot.

### PATIENT MONITORING
Patients should be followed at 3-month intervals to monitor their discomfort and function and to check whether their deformity is stable or progressive.

### REFERENCES

1. Chang FM. The flexible flatfoot. *Instr Course Lect* 1988;37:109–110.
2. Chu IT, Myerson MS, Nyska M, et al. Experimental flatfoot model: the contribution of dynamic loading. *Foot Ankle Int* 2001;22: 220–225.
3. Jones LJ, Todd WF. Abnormal biomechanics of flatfoot deformities and related theories of biomechanical development. *Clin Podiatr Med Surg* 1989;6:511–520.
4. Kitaoka HB, Ahn TK, Luo ZP, et al. Stability of the arch of the foot. *Foot Ankle Int* 1997;18: 644–648.
5. Gould N, Schneider W, Ashikaga T. Epidemiological survey of foot problems in the continental United States: 1978–1979. *Foot Ankle* 1980;1:8–10.
6. Leonard MA. The inheritance of tarsal coalition and its relationship to spastic flat foot. *J Bone Joint Surg* 1974;56B:520–526.
7. Palladino SJ, Schiller L, Johnson JD. Cubonavicular coalition. *J Am Podiatr Med Assoc* 1991;81:262–266.
8. Harris EJ. The oblique talus deformity. What is it, and what is its clinical significance in the scheme of pronatory deformities? *Clin Podiatr Med Surg* 2000;17:419–442.
9. Hefti F. [Foot pain]. *Orthopade* 1999;28: 173–179.
10. Kumar SJ, Cowell HR, Ramsey PL. Vertical and oblique talus. *Instr Course Lect* 1982;31: 235–251.
11. Sullivan JA. Pediatric flatfoot: evaluation and management. *J Am Acad Orthop Surg* 1999;7: 44–53.
12. Tonnis D. [Skewfoot ]. *Orthopade* 1986;15: 174–183.
13. Henceroth WD, II, Deyerle WM. The acquired unilateral flatfoot in the adult: some causative factors. *Foot Ankle* 1982;2:304–308.


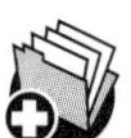

## MISCELLANEOUS

### CODES
#### *ICD9-CM*
- 734.0 Acquired flat foot
- 754.61 Congenital flat foot

### PATIENT TEACHING
- Patient education is crucial because cosmesis in the absence of symptoms is not an appropriate indication for surgery.
- Stretching exercises can help patients with tight Achilles tendons, and foot orthoses may be useful for patients who want to be active.

### FAQ
- Q: What are 3 causes of flatfoot deformity in pediatric patients?
  - A: Benign flexible flatfoot, tarsal coalition, and congenital vertical talus.
- Q: What are 3 causes of flatfoot deformity in adults?
  - A: PTT dysfunction (most common cause of adult acquired flatfoot), neuroarthropathy, and degenerative or inflammatory arthritis.

# FLEXOR TENDON LACERATION

*John J. Carbone, MD*
*Dawn M. LaPorte, MD*

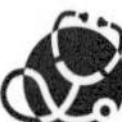

## BASICS

### DESCRIPTION

- Flexor tendon laceration may require emergency surgical repair, depending on:
  - Location of the laceration
  - Hand dominance
  - Age and occupation of the patient
- Lacerations located between the distal transverse palmar crease and the PIP joint flexor crease represent an area of increased risk from scarring or adhesions and poor functional outcome resulting from the complex and precise anatomy in this area ("no-man's land") (1,2).
- The superficial and deep flexors are at risk at different locations in the hand because each has a superficial course on the palmar surface.
- Each tendon adds to the strength and independent function of the fingers in flexion.
- Classification is by the name of the tendon lacerated (superficial versus deep) and the location of the laceration.
- The level of the laceration is described most easily by the zone of the injury (3).
  - Zone 1: Fingertip to PIP flexor crease
  - Zone 2: PIP flexor crease to distal palmar transverse crease
  - Zone 3: Distal palmar transverse crease to distal wrist flexor crease

### EPIDEMIOLOGY

#### *Incidence*

This injury is one of the most common types of tendon lacerations.

### RISK FACTORS

Working with sharp objects

### ETIOLOGY

The cause of the injury is sharp laceration to the tendon (e.g., via knife, glass).

### ASSOCIATED CONDITIONS

- Digital nerve laceration
- Digital artery laceration

## DIAGNOSIS

### SIGNS AND SYMPTOMS

- Laceration to the palmar aspect of the hand
- Change in the resting posture of the finger relative to the other fingers (e.g., slight extension of the injured finger)
- Loss of independent flexion of the distal digital joint when tested
- Loss of ability to flex the finger
- Decreased strength of finger flexion
- Evidence of tendon injury during wound exploration
- Evidence of tendon sheath or pulley laceration during wound exploration

#### *Physical Exam*

- Test independent DIP and PIP flexor flexion (Figs. 1 and 2).
- Test for lacerations of adjacent nerves.
- Test the strength of each finger.
- Explore the wound for a tendon or pulley injury.

### TESTS

#### *Imaging*

Obtain radiographs to rule out foreign body, fracture, dislocation, or avulsion injury.

### DIFFERENTIAL DIAGNOSIS

- Fracture-dislocation
- Avulsion injury of tendon
- Rupture of tendon

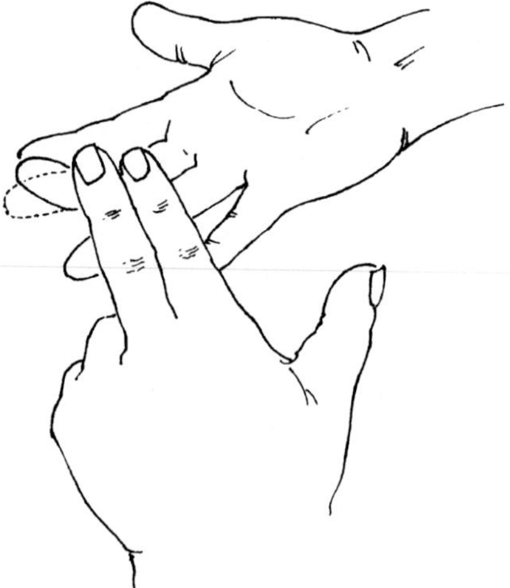

**Fig. 1.** Testing for an intact profundus tendon is performed by holding the proximal joints straight and asking the patient to flex only the distal joint.

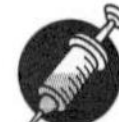

## TREATMENT

### GENERAL MEASURES

- Tetanus shot
- Wound washout using normal saline
- Antibiotics (usually 3rd-generation cephalosporin IV)
- Elevation and splinting of the hand until surgical evaluation is performed
- Orthopaedic consultation and preoperative laboratory tests
- Digital nerve and artery laceration:
  - Careful and complete neurovascular examination, including 2-point discrimination and Doppler study of the neurovascular bundle on each side of the tendon in question

### SPECIAL THERAPY

#### *Physical Therapy*

- Postoperative ROM depends on the lesion location and the type and quality of repair.
- Usually, the goal is passive ROM as soon as the skin repair tolerates motion.
  - Children and adults who cannot follow restrictions should be immobilized postoperatively.

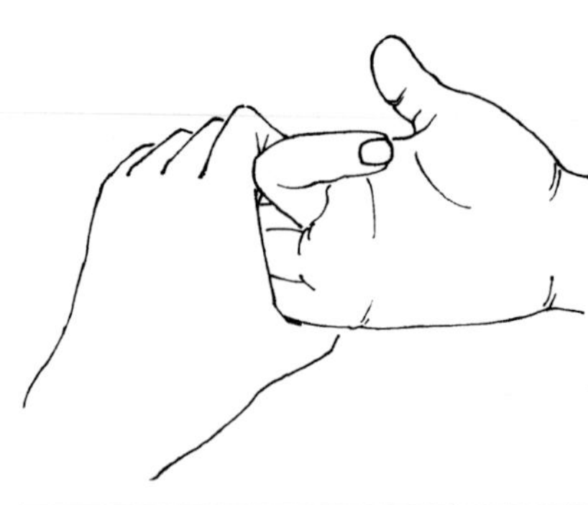

**Fig. 2.** Testing for an intact sublimis flexor tendon is done by asking patient to flex an individual finger while holding the other fingers in full extension. The finger then will flex only at the proximal joint.

### MEDICATION (DRUGS)

Antibiotic choice may be related to the contamination at the time of injury.

### SURGERY

- Flexor tendon repair and results depend on the location, level, and type of injury.
- Primary acute repair has provided the most functional results (4).
- Repair should be performed within 1–2 weeks after injury.
- In the presence of a flexor tendon sheath injury, early repair may be done to minimize scarring and adhesions and to give the best functional result.

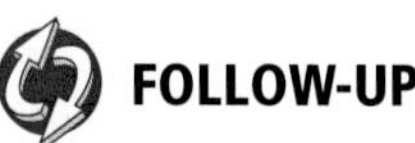

## FOLLOW-UP

### PROGNOSIS

- Prognosis depends heavily on the type and location of the injury.
- Injuries located between the distal transverse palmar crease and the most distal digit flexor crease often result in finger stiffness.
- In other areas, results are better.

### COMPLICATIONS

- Infection
- Decreased ROM secondary to scarring or adhesions
- Loss of strength
- Need for delayed repair or reconstruction
- Tendon rupture

### REFERENCES


1. Amadio PC, Hunter JM. Prognostic factors in flexor tendon surgery in zone 2. In: Hunter JM, Schneider LH, Mackin EJ, eds. *Tendon Surgery in the Hand*. St. Louis: CV Mosby, 1987:138–147.
2. Tang JB. Flexor tendon repair in zone 2C. *J Hand Surg* 1994;19B:72–75.
3. Boyer MI. Flexor tendon injury. Acute injuries. In: Green DP, Hotchkiss RN, Pederson WC, et al., eds. *Green's Operative Hand Surgery,* 5th ed. Philadelphia: Elsevier Churchill Livingstone, 2005: 219–240.
4. Strickland JW. Development of flexor tendon surgery: twenty-five years of progress. *J Hand Surg* 2000;25A:214–235.


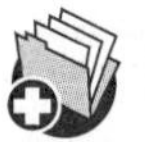

## MISCELLANEOUS

### CODES

#### *ICD9-CM*

840.9 Upper limb tendon laceration

### PATIENT TEACHING

- The patient should understand the severity of the injury even though the laceration may appear small.
- Functional outcome strongly depends on the compliance and cooperation of the patient.
- Postoperative hand therapy is critical to a good result.

#### *Prevention*

United States Occupational Safety and Health Administration guidelines should be used when working with sharp objects.

### FAQ

- Q: Do partial flexor tendon lacerations need to be repaired?
  - A: If the laceration involves $>60\%$ of the tendon, repair is recommended. If it involves $\leq 60\%$ of the tendon, repair is not necessary and débridement is indicated only for entrapment of the tendon under the pulley system (e.g., triggering).
- Q: What are the timing requirements for flexor tendon repair?
  - A: Repair should be performed in the operating room within 3 weeks, optimally in $<2$ weeks, of the laceration. Primary repair usually is not recommended in presentations delayed $>5$–6 weeks.

# FOOT AND ANKLE ANATOMY AND EXAMINATION

*Marc D. Chodos, MD*

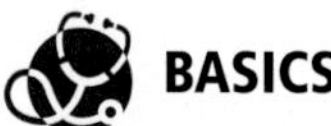

## BASICS

### DESCRIPTION

- The major function of the foot and ankle is to allow even stress distribution between the foot and lower extremity during walking and running.
- For adequate function, the foot must be plantigrade (i.e., rest evenly flat on the ground) and painless.
- The muscles that control foot and ankle function include extrinsic (originating outside the foot) and intrinsic (originating within the foot) groups.
- Extrinsic muscles: 4 groups of muscles and tendons (dorsiflexors, evertors, plantarflexors, and invertors):
  - Dorsiflexors:
    - Extensor tendons: Tibialis anterior, extensor digitorum longus, and extensor hallucis longus
    - Easily palpable crossing the ankle; can be lacerated by sharp objects
  - Evertors:
    - Peroneus longus and brevis
    - Situated on the lateral aspect of the leg
    - Tendons run posterior to the lateral malleolus.
    - Injury to tendon sheath can cause tendon subluxation over malleolus.
  - Plantarflexors and invertors:
    - Travel posteromedial to the ankle
    - The PTT, the main invertor, is prone to tenosynovitis and rupture in the adult, a condition leading to acquired flatfoot.
    - The extrinsic toe flexors include the flexor digitorum longus and flexor hallucis longus.
- Intrinsic foot muscles include 1 dorsal layer and three plantar layers, all of which help to control toe motion.
- An imbalance between extrinsic and intrinsic muscle strength can contribute to toe deformities such as mallet toes, claw toes, and hammer toes.
- Foot and ankle bones are easily palpable.
  - The ankle joint:
    - Consists of the articulation between the distal tibia, fibula, and talus
    - Predominantly allows plantar- (40°) and dorsiflexion (20°)
    - Is supported by several ligaments:
      - Anterior and posterior tibiofibular ligaments stabilize the syndesmosis; if injured, "high ankle sprain" results.
      - The superficial and deep deltoid ligaments connect the medial malleolus to the hindfoot.
      - The ATFL, CFL, and PTFL support the lateral ankle; the ATFL commonly is injured in inversion ankle sprains.
  - The hindfoot:
    - Consists of the talus and calcaneus, which articulate at the subtalar joint
    - Allows inversion and eversion (40° arc of motion), which is important when walking on uneven surfaces.
    - The talus is covered almost completely with cartilage; its blood supply frequently is disrupted during subtalar dislocation or talar fracture, leading to AVN.
    - The calcaneus acts as a shock absorber; axial loading from a fall is a common mechanism of calcaneal fracture.
  - The midfoot:
    - Consists of 2 rows of bones:
      - Proximally, the navicular and the cuboid articulate with the hindfoot through the Chopart joint.
      - Distally, the 3 cuneiform bones and cuboid articulate with the metatarsals via the tarsometatarsal (Lisfranc) joint.
    - Ligaments attach all but the 1st and 2nd metatarsal bases to the adjacent metatarsals.
    - The strong Lisfranc ligament connects the 2nd metatarsal to the medial cuneiform.
  - The forefoot consists of the 5 metatarsals and 14 phalanges (2 phalanges in the hallux and 3 in each of the lesser toes).
- The gait cycle consists of the stance and swing phases.
  - Stance phase: Heel strike, foot flat, toe-off:
    - Heel strike:
      - Tibialis anterior and long toe extensors are active.
      - The foot is pronated, which unlocks the Chopart joint, makes the midfoot flexible, and helps with energy absorption and load acceptance.
    - Foot flat:
      - Tibialis posterior and peroneals are active.
      - The leg rotates externally, which supinates and locks the midfoot and stabilizes the foot for weightbearing.
    - Toe-off:
      - Gastrocnemius–soleus complex is active.
      - Dorsiflexion of the toes tightens the plantar fascia (windlass mechanism), increasing the midfoot arch and locking the midfoot, which allows the foot to act as a lever during push-off.
  - Swing phase: Tibialis anterior and long toe extensors are active.

## DIAGNOSIS

### SIGNS AND SYMPTOMS

#### *History*

- Address the patient's symptoms:
  - Mechanism of injury for acute trauma
  - Pain: Severity, location, quality, radiation, and alleviating/aggravating factors
  - Mechanical symptoms (locking/catching) and instability
  - Neurologic symptoms: Numbness, dysesthesia, paresthesias
- Pertinent medical and surgical history:
  - Diabetes, neurologic disorders, vascular disease, inflammatory arthritides
  - Previous foot or leg surgery
- Shoe wear
- Occupation
- Sport or recreational activities

#### *Physical Exam*

- Physical examination findings of the involved extremity should be compared with those of the contralateral extremity.
- Patient in standing position:
  - Evaluate the patient's gait pattern and stance to assess ankle/foot alignment.
    - Viewed from behind, alignment of the hindfoot can be determined as varus, neutral, or valgus.
    - More lateral toes seen on the affected side than on the uninvolved foot is called the "too-many-toes" sign, and implies the presence of flatfoot with arch collapse and midfoot abduction.
    - Assess gait pattern for steppage (dropfoot), circumduction, scissoring, or antalgia.
  - Double- and single-limb heel rises allow for evaluation of dynamic foot function, including tibialis posterior strength, arch reconstitution, and balance.
- Patient in seated position:
  - Vascular assessment:
    - Palpate the dorsalis pedis on the dorsum of the foot lateral to extensor hallucis longus, and the posterior tibial pulse behind the medial malleolus.
    - Examine for venous stasis, pitting edema.
  - Sensory and neurologic examination:
    - Dorsal foot (superficial peroneal nerve)
    - 1st dorsal web space (deep peroneal nerve)
    - Medial border of foot (saphenous nerve)
    - Lateral border of foot (sural nerve)
    - Plantar foot (tibial nerve)
    - Patient's ability to feel the 5.07 Semmes-Weinstein monofilament on the plantar foot correlates with having protective sensation (1).
    - Check reflexes and evaluate for Babinski sign and clonus.
  - Motor examination: Test strength and palpate tendons.
    - Ankle dorsiflexion (tibialis anterior)
    - Ankle plantarflexion (gastrocnemius–soleus complex)
    - Eversion (peroneals)
    - Inversion in plantarflexion (tibialis posterior)
    - Flexion and extension of the distal phalanx of the great toe (flexor and extensor hallucis longus); evaluate active and passive motion.
    - Ankle plantar and dorsiflexion, with any hindfoot deformity passively corrected

- Hindfoot inversion and eversion to assess subtalar motion
- Chopart joint abduction/adduction while stabilizing the hindfoot
- Assess Lisfranc joint with palpation and plantar- and dorsiflexion of the tarsometatarsal joints.
- Assess motion at the MTP and toe joints.

– Palpation:
  - Medial and lateral malleoli (fracture)
  - Ankle joint for tenderness, effusion (osteochondral lesion, synovitis)
  - PTT along its course posterior to the medial malleolus to insertion on navicular (tendinitis)
  - Navicular tuberosity ~2 cm distal and plantar to medial malleolus (accessory navicular, stress fracture, talonavicular pathology)
  - Achilles tendon and retrocalcaneal bursa along the posterior ankle and hindfoot for defects, nodules, thickening, swelling, and tenderness (tendinitis, tear)
  - Peroneal tendons posterior to the lateral malleolus to the brevis insertion on the base of the 5th metatarsal, and where the longus passes through the plantar groove of the cuboid (tendinitis, 5th metatarsal base fracture); also assess for tendon subluxation with foot circumduction.
  - Sinus tarsi ~1 cm distal to lateral malleolus (subtalar joint pathology)
  - Tenderness along the tip of medial or lateral malleolus (ligament sprain)
  - Tenderness between the tibia and fibula proximal to the ankle joint (syndesmosis injury)
  - Palpate the plantar fascia, originating at the base of the heel (plantar fasciitis, especially if tenderness is accentuated with toe dorsiflexion).
  - Base of the 2nd metatarsal (Lisfranc injury)
  - Plantar MTP joint of the great toe (sesamoiditis, sesamoid fracture)
  - Plantar lesser toe MTP joints (metatarsalgia)
  - Metatarsal interspaces (neuroma)

- Specific tests and examinations:
  – Anterior drawer test (ankle instability):
    - Try to sublux the talus anteriorly from tibia.
    - Foot dorsiflexed stresses the ATFL.
  – Thompson test:
    - With the patient in the prone position, squeeze the posterior calf.
    - Loss of foot plantarflexion implies disruption of the Achilles tendon (2).
  – Coleman block test:
    - Helps determine if varus hindfoot deformity is flexible or rigid
    - The patient stands on a block with the 1st ray unsupported; if the hindfoot deformity corrects, then it is flexible (3).
  – Lesser toe deformities:
    - Assess the location of the calluses.
    - Assess if the deformity is correctable or not (flexible versus rigid).
    - Assess MTP joint stability with modified drawer test, trying to sublux and reduce proximal phalanx on metatarsal head.
  – Hallux valgus:
    - Assess the location of the calluses.
    - Assess tenderness over the medial eminence.
    - Assess MTP motion with the deformity corrected.
    - Assess for hypermobility of the 1st tarsometatarsal joint by stabilizing the lateral foot and attempting to translate the 1st metatarsal plantar and dorsal.
    - Assess for lesser toe deformities that could contribute to symptoms.

## TESTS

### Lab

- If concern for infection exists, consider obtaining ESR, C-reactive protein, and white blood cell count.
- Joint aspirations should be sent for cell count, differential, Gram stain, evaluation for crystals, and culture.

### Imaging

- Plain radiographs:
  – If the patient has acute trauma, and fracture or dislocation is being considered, obtain nonweightbearing films.
  – If the patient is able to stand, then weightbearing radiographs should be obtained.
    - Standing radiographs show bony relationships in the physiologic state and are much more likely to reveal foot disorders than are nonweightbearing views.
  – Stress view radiographs help to evaluate indirectly the integrity of ligamentous structures.
- CT is helpful for identifying and delineating fracture patterns and bony pathology, especially of the midfoot and hindfoot.
- MRI helps to show soft-tissue disorders, including tendon and ligament pathology, soft-tissue lesions, subtle fractures, and infection.
- Technetium-99m bone scans:
  – Useful for localizing problems when the complaint is vague or multifocal
  – Can help locate stress fractures, tumors, and other pathology
- Indium-labeled white blood cell scans:
  – Useful for identifying infection
  – Combined with a marrow scan, can help differentiate infection and Charcot arthropathy

## REFERENCES

1. Olmos PR, Cataland S, O'Dorisio TM, et al. The Semmes-Weinstein monofilament as a potential predictor of foot ulceration in patients with noninsulin-dependent diabetes. *Am J Med Scin* 1995;309:76–82.
2. Thompson TC. A test for rupture of the tendo Achilles. *Acta Orthop Scand* 1962;32:461–465.
3. Coleman SS, Chesnut WJ. A simple test for hindfoot flexibility in the cavovarus foot. *Clin Orthop Relat Res* 1977;123:60–62.

## ADDITIONAL READING

- Mann RA. Principles of examination of the foot and ankle. In: Mann RA, Coughlin MJ, eds. *Surgery of the Foot and Ankle*, 6th ed. St. Louis: Mosby-Year Book Inc., 1993:45–60.
- Michelson J. Foot and ankle biomechanics. In: Mizel MS, Miller RA, Scioli MW, eds. *Orthopaedic Knowledge Update: Foot and Ankle 2*. Rosemont, IL: American Academy of Orthopaedic Surgeons, 1998:1–9.
- Resch S. Functional anatomy and topography of the foot and ankle. In: Myerson MS, ed. *Foot and Ankle Disorders*. Philadelphia: WB Saunders, 2000:25–49.
- Shuler FD. Anatomy. In: Miller MD, ed. *Review of Orthopaedics*, 4th ed. Philadelphia: WB Saunders, 2004:660–668.

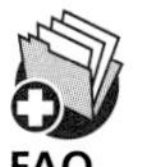

## MISCELLANEOUS

### FAQ

- Q: What anatomic structure causes a Tillaux fracture?
  – A: In adolescents, fusion of the distal tibial physis begins centrally and progresses medially. The lateral portion of the physis is the last area to fuse. The *ATFL* attaches to this part of the tibia. A twisting injury to the ankle at this stage of development can cause this ligament to avulse the unfused segment of tibial physis, with extension of the fracture into the ankle joint.
- Q: What is the main blood supply to the talar body?
  – A: The artery of the tarsal canal, a branch of the tibial artery, is the main blood supply to the talar body. Branches of the dorsalis pedis and peroneal artery also provide limited blood supply to the talus. Injury to this vascular network can cause AVN of the talar body.

# FOREARM FRACTURE

*Simon C. Mears, MD, PhD*
*Darryl B. Thomas, MD*

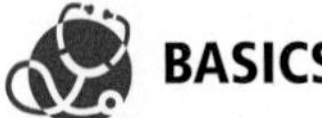

## BASICS

### DESCRIPTION

- Forearm fractures involve the bones of the forearm (the radius and ulna), and sometimes the fractures are associated with elbow and wrist injuries.
- In addition to the bone injury, soft-tissue injuries may include compartment syndrome, neurapraxia, and vascular damage.
- Adults are more susceptible than children to more severe injuries.
- Adults also require a more exact reduction because they have less potential for bony remodeling, and the fractures have no innate stability.
- Children <12 years old do not require anatomic reduction of forearm fractures.
- Classification:
  - Multiple classification schemes
  - Important factors include:
    - Fracture location
    - Fracture configuration
    - Presence of any radioulnar or radiohumeral articular involvement
    - Isolated ulna shaft fractures are called "nightstick"' fractures because they often are caused by blunt trauma.
- Synonyms: Monteggia fracture (forearm fracture with radial head dislocation); Galeazzi fracture (forearm fractures with distal radioulnar joint dislocation); Both-bone forearm fracture

### EPIDEMIOLOGY

No particular gender predilection

#### *Incidence*

Drivers involved in motor vehicle accidents are more likely to have forearm fractures than passengers, especially with front airbag deployment (1).

#### *Prevalence*

- In children, forearm fractures are a common result of skateboarding, roller skating, and scooter riding (2).
- Forearm fractures occur most frequently in boys aged 11–14 years and in girls aged 8–11 years (3).

### RISK FACTORS

- High-energy trauma
- Osteoporosis
- Gunshot wounds

### ETIOLOGY

- High-energy trauma (e.g., motor vehicle accidents, fall from a height, crushing injury)
- Low-energy trauma (e.g., falls)

### ASSOCIATED CONDITIONS

- Fractures of the ulna may be associated with dislocation of the radial head, an injury called the "Monteggia fracture."
- Fractures of the radius may be associated with dislocation of the distal radioulnar joint, an injury termed the "Galeazzi fracture."

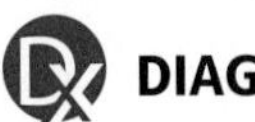

## DIAGNOSIS

### SIGNS AND SYMPTOMS

- Pain
- Swelling
- Loss of elbow or wrist motion
- Deformity
- Important: Assessment of forearm for skin and soft-tissue (neurovascular) compromise

#### *Physical Exam*

- Careful examination of the entire involved extremity is mandatory, including:
  - Detailed neurologic and vascular evaluations
  - Assessment of the soft tissues
- Compartments, anterior (flexor) and posterior (extensor), are checked for evidence of compartment syndrome.
- Compartment pressure is measured if the forearm feels "tight" or if the patient displays pain out of proportion to the injury.

### TESTS

#### *Imaging*

- AP, lateral, and oblique views of the wrist and the entire forearm, as well as AP and lateral views of the ipsilateral elbow, are mandatory.
  - Fracture of one bone often is accompanied by dislocation of another.
  - Radiographic signs of injury to the distal radioulnar joint include:
    - Fracture at the base of the ulnar styloid
    - Widening of the joint space on the AP view
    - Dislocation of the radius relative to the ulna on the lateral view
    - Radial shortening >5 mm
  - If the radial head is located properly, a line drawn through the radial head and shaft on any radiographic projection should align with the capitellum of the elbow.
  - If dislocation of the radial head is suspected clinically, a lateral radiograph of the elbow with the arm in supination may be helpful.

#### *Pathological Findings*

- Most forearm fractures are either transverse or short oblique in configuration.
- Comminution is variable (none to moderate).

### DIFFERENTIAL DIAGNOSIS

Look for associated wrist or elbow dislocations and interosseous membrane rupture.

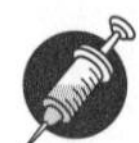

## TREATMENT

### GENERAL MEASURES

- Pain medication should be administered only after a careful physical examination, including documentation of neurovascular status.
- The forearm should be elevated, with application of ice to the fracture site to help to reduce swelling.
- In general, closed treatment of diaphyseal fractures is best used for stable (<50% of the shaft diameter displaced), isolated fractures of the distal 2/3 of the ulna with $\leq 10°$ of angular deformity.
- Fractures of the proximal 1/3 of the ulna and fractures of the distal 2/3 of the ulna with $>10°$ angulation are best treated operatively.
- Pediatric both-bone fractures do not remodel well and should be treated with surgery if reduction cannot be maintained (4).
- In addition, most radial shaft fractures, except those that are nondisplaced, and virtually all both-bone forearm fractures in adults (prone to shortening and angulation) require surgical management.
- Closed forearm fractures of 1 or both bones that are displaced minimally should be splinted in a neutral position to prevent additional displacement and possible neurovascular injury.
- In general, forearm fractures with associated ligamentous injuries, either distally (wrist) or proximally (elbow), are unstable injuries.
  - They are not always evident initially, and a high index of suspicion is required.
  - These more severe injuries require early surgical intervention for reduction and stabilization of both the forearm fractures and the associated ligamentous injuries.

### SPECIAL THERAPY

#### *Physical Therapy*

Early ROM of the elbow and fingers is important to help to reduce soft-tissue scarring and to prevent contractures.

### MEDICATION (DRUGS)

Acetaminophen plus a mild narcotic are used most often in the immediate postinjury period for pain control.

### SURGERY

- Surgical options include percutaneous Kirschner wire fixation, external fixation, intramedullary nailing, and plate and screw fixation.
- Acute bone grafting is unnecessary (5).
- For open fractures, irrigation and débridement with the administration of intravenous antibiotics should be performed on an emergent basis.
  - If the open wound is not massively contaminated, the fractures are stabilized after débridement.
  - With massive contamination, fixation is performed in a delayed fashion.
- Radial and ulnar fractures usually are stabilized rigidly with 3.5-mm dynamic compression plates.
- Locking plates seem to have no advantages compared with nonlocking plates (6).
- Pediatric fractures may be treated with plating or with intramedullary nailing.
  - Results with intramedullary nail fixation seem to be superior (7,8).

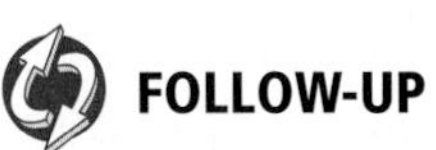

## FOLLOW-UP

### PROGNOSIS

- In general, most nondisplaced or minimally displaced fractures in children who undergo closed treatment heal well, with good return of forearm function (9).
- Minimally displaced isolated ulna fracture have excellent results when treated with functional bracing (10).
- The prognosis in adults with displaced fractures of the radius and ulna and closed treatment is poor.
- For fractures treated with open reduction and rigid internal fixation, the prognosis for achieving union is ~95% (5).
- Because rigid fixation allows early ROM, patients who have no associated severe soft-tissue injuries should experience only mild loss of forearm rotation.

### COMPLICATIONS

- Nonoperative treatment:
  - Decreased ROM (supination and pronation)
  - Synostosis (fusion of the radius and ulna)
  - Malunion (defined as any fracture healing with >20° of angulation or 1 cm of shortening) leads to loss of forearm motion (11).
  - Nonunion
- Operative treatment complications include (in addition to those for nonoperative treatment):
  - Late infections
  - Iatrogenic nerve injuries
  - Vascular injuries
  - Loss of fixation
- Compartment syndrome:
  - Compartment syndrome is a risk after any treatment.
  - It is manifested by exquisite pain on passive stretch of the digits.
  - Constrictive dressings should be released down to the skin at the 1st symptom or sign of compartment syndrome.
    - If pain is not improved, compartment pressure should be measured.
    - Confirmation of the diagnosis requires emergent fasciotomy of the forearm.

### PATIENT MONITORING

- Follow-up care should be arranged within 1 week after injury for repeat physical examination and repeat radiographs before and after the application of a cast, to verify fracture position when cast treatment is chosen.
- Additional follow-up every 2–3 weeks then is necessary to assess healing of the fracture site and to guide early ROM of the fingers and elbow.
- Healing of closed forearm fractures usually takes 4–6 weeks for a child and 6–12 weeks for an adult.

### REFERENCES


1. Conroy C, Schwartz A, Hoyt DB, et al. Upper extremity fracture patterns following motor vehicle crashes differ for drivers and passengers. *Injury* 2006;Epub (doi:10.1016/j.injury.2006.03.017):1–8.
2. Zalavras C, Nikolopoulou G, Essin D, et al. Pediatric fractures during skateboarding, roller skating, and scooter riding. *Am J Sports Med* 2005;33:568–573.
3. Khosla S, Melton LJ III, Dekutoski MB, et al. Incidence of childhood distal forearm fractures over 30 years: a population-based study. *JAMA* 2003;290:1479–1485.
4. Johari AN, Sinha M. Remodeling of forearm fractures in children. *J Pediatr Orthop B* 1999; 8:84–87.
5. Wright RR, Schmeling GJ, Schwab JP. The necessity of acute bone grafting in diaphyseal forearm fractures: a retrospective review. *J Orthop Trauma* 1997;11:288–294.
6. Leung F, Chow SP. A prospective, randomized trial comparing the limited contact dynamic compression plate with the point contact fixator for forearm fractures. *J Bone Joint Surg* 2003;85A:2343–2348.
7. Fernandez FF, Egenolf M, Carsten C, et al. Unstable diaphyseal fractures of both bones of the forearm in children: plate fixation versus intramedullary nailing. *Injury* 2005;36:1210–1216.
8. Jubel A, Andermahr J, Isenberg J, et al. Outcomes and complications of elastic stable intramedullary nailing for forearm fractures in children. *J Pediatr Orthop B* 2005;14:375–380.
9. Zionts LE, Zalavras CG, Gerhardt MB. Closed treatment of displaced diaphyseal both-bone forearm fractures in older children and adolescents. *J Pediatr Orthop* 2005;25:507–512.
10. Sarmiento A, Latta LL, Zych G, et al. Isolated ulnar shaft fractures treated with functional braces. *J Orthop Trauma* 1998;12:420–423.
11. Dumont CE, Thalmann R, Macy JC. The effect of rotational malunion of the radius and the ulna on supination and pronation. *J Bone Joint Surg* 2002;84B:1070–1074.


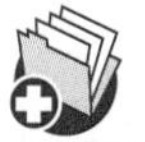

## MISCELLANEOUS

### CODES

#### *ICD9-CM*

813.8 Forearm fractures

### PATIENT TEACHING

Patients should be told about the potential for loss of pronation and supination of the forearm, depending on the severity of the initial injury and the final angulation at the fracture site.

### FAQ

- Q: How long does a forearm fracture take to heal?
  - A: Forearm fractures in adults treated with plating take ~3–4 months to heal.
- Q: Should plates be removed after healing?
  - A: Unless residual pain occurs, plates should be left intact. The reported risk of refracture after plate removal is 3–25%.

# FRACTURE TREATMENT

*Derek F. Papp, MD*
*Simon C. Mears, MD, PhD*

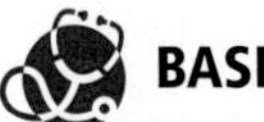

## BASICS

### DESCRIPTION

- Fractured or broken bones are a common result of trauma.
- Treatment of fractures may be with or without surgery and depends on the location and severity of the fracture.
- Nondisplaced:
  - 1 or both cortices may be involved, but the fracture has not moved.
  - Nondisplaced fractures may be difficult to detect.
- Displaced:
  - Displacement
  - Angulation:
    - A clear way to describe this deformity is to state the direction of the apex of the fracture, such as "fracture apex anterior"
    - Another method is to state the type of deformity, such as "varus angulation"
  - Shortening
  - Rotation
  - Translation

### ALERT

- Open versus closed:
  - One of the most important determinations to make when evaluating a patient with a fracture
  - Any wound anywhere on a limb with a fracture must be suspect!
    - If one believes that a wound could communicate with the fracture site, the fracture must be considered to be open.
  - To decrease bacterial colonization, open wounds should be covered with an antiseptic-soaked sterile dressing until the patient is in the operating room.
- Open fractures: Gustilo Anderson classification (1):
  - I: Low energy, laceration <1 cm
  - II: Moderate energy, laceration >1 cm and <10 cm
  - III: High energy, laceration >10 cm:
    - IIIA: Adequate soft-tissue coverage (muscle flap not necessary)
    - IIIB: Massive soft-tissue destruction, bony exposure (muscle flap necessary)
    - IIIC: Fractures associated with a vascular injury
- Fracture sites:
  - Diaphysis: May describe by relative anatomic level (i.e., proximal 1/3, middle 1/3, and distal 1/3)
  - Metaphysis: Intra-articular (i.e., within a joint, with low tolerance for any incongruence or step-off)
- Fracture patterns:
  - Transverse: Perpendicular to the bone
  - Oblique: Oblique across the bone
  - Spiral: Spirals around the bone
  - Comminuted: Fragments at fracture site
  - Segmental: The same bone is fractured in 2 places, resulting in a "floating segment of bone"
  - Impacted
  - Avulsion: A tendon or ligament has pulled a section of bone free after trauma.
  - Compression

#### *Pediatric Considerations (2)*

- Greenstick fracture: The cortex and periosteum on the concave side are intact, whereas the cortex and often the periosteum on the convex side are fractured.
- Buckle (torus fracture): This metaphyseal compression injury is relatively stable and is splinted for comfort.
- Growth-plate injuries are defined according to the Salter-Harris classification (3):
  - I: Transverse fracture through the physis
  - II: Fracture through the physis with a metaphyseal fragment
  - III: Fracture through the physis and the epiphysis (intra-articular)
  - IV: Fracture through the epiphysis, physis, and metaphysis (intra-articular)
  - V: Crush injury of the physis
  - VI: Injury to the perichondral ring (not part of the original classification)

### GENERAL PREVENTION

- Avoidance of trauma
- Osteoporosis prevention

### PATHOPHYSIOLOGY

- Force applied to a bone may result in fracture.
- Bones that are weaker from osteoporosis require less force to fracture.

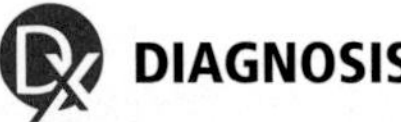

## DIAGNOSIS

### SIGNS AND SYMPTOMS

#### *History*

- Most often traumatic, whether secondary to a motor vehicle crash, fall, or direct blow to the affected area
- Fractures in the elderly may occur with minimal trauma.

### ALERT

- When the mechanism reported seems mild in comparison to the injury (e.g., humerus fracture while throwing a ball or femur fracture while stepping off a curb), one must consider a pathologic fracture (through a tumor or metabolic process) in the differential diagnosis.
- Suspect child abuse when fractures and bruises of different ages are seen, or when the story is not consistent with the injury.
  - In decreasing order of incidence, fractures of the humerus, tibia, and femur are most commonly seen in child abuse (4).

#### *Physical Exam*

Look for gross deformity, swelling, and pain to palpation and, with movement of the affected area, bruising, warmth, and possibly fracture blisters.

### TESTS

#### *Imaging*

- Plain radiographs in 2 planes are mandatory and should include the joint above and below the injury.
- CT is better than radiography at identifying fractures of the spine and showing the joint involvement in intra-articular fractures.
- MRI or bone scans may be used to detect nondisplaced fractures.

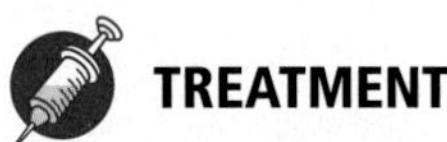

## TREATMENT

### GENERAL MEASURES

- Begin ice, elevation, and immobilization as soon as the patient is in the emergency department (5).
- Reduce displaced fractures under sedation or anesthesia.
  - Immobilization protects soft tissue and allows the bone to heal.
  - The goal of immobilization is to maintain the alignment of the reduction of the fracture until it heals.

- For early treatment with closed therapy, splinting is preferred to casting because of a lower risk of compartment syndrome and soft-tissue injury.
- Regardless of whether the final treatment is nonoperative or operative, definitive fracture management depends on basic principles:
  - Adequate fracture reduction (restored as close to the anatomic position as possible)
  - Fracture stabilization
- Cast:
  - Used for many nondisplaced or simple fractures
  - Univalved or bivalved models reduce the risk of compartment syndrome.
  - Must be molded with 3-point fixation to maintain fracture reduction
- Functional bracing has been successful in the treatment of humerus and tibial fractures (6).

### *Activity*
Depends on method of treatment, but operative management often leads to earlier return to motion and weightbearing.

### *Nursing*
Awareness of complications such as compartment syndrome and cast problems is important.

## MEDICATION (DRUGS)
### *First Line*
- Patients with open fractures should be treated with intravenous antibiotics to prevent deep infection (7).
  - Gram-positive coverage (often cefazolin, 1 g in adults and 25 mg/kg in children) and tetanus prophylaxis
  - For Gustilo type II fractures, an aminoglycoside also should be given for Gram-negative coverage
  - For patients with fractures that occurred in a farm environment, with vascular compromise or with extensive soft-tissue crush, 4–5 million units of aqueous penicillin G every 4–6 hours should be given (1st-generation cephalosporin plus an aminoglycoside plus penicillin).
- Patients may require pain medicines, depending on the severity of the fracture.

## SURGERY
- The decision to proceed to operative management depends on several issues, including:
  - The severity of the fracture
  - The need to return to activity more quickly
  - The need to avoid stiffness that comes with casting
- Intra-articular fracture with displacement requires reduction and fixation to avoid posttraumatic arthritis and to allow for joint motion (8).
  - Diaphyseal fractures may require fixation to allow for early mobilization or to correct deformity.
- Types of surgical fixation:
  - Plates and screws:
    - Used for intra-articular fractures after reduction
  - Intramedullary nails:
    - Used for long-bone diaphyseal fractures
    - Allows for early weightbearing
  - External fixation:
    - This approach is used in situations of tenuous blood supply, marked soft-tissue injury, and gross contamination, and for comminuted distal radius fractures.
    - Polytrauma patients with multiple fractures may be treated with damage-control orthopaedics: Temporary external fixators are applied and, later, when the patient is stabilized, staged definitive fixation is performed (9).

# FOLLOW-UP

## DISPOSITION
### *Issues for Referral*
When a question of child abuse arises, a social worker and pediatrician should be involved.

## PROGNOSIS
Intra-articular injuries and injuries with substantial soft-tissue damage have poorer prognoses than do injuries to the diaphysis.

## COMPLICATIONS
- Delayed union: Healing has not occurred in 3–4 months
- Nonunion: Healing has not occurred in 6 months
- Malunion: Healing with malalignment
- Osteonecrosis (AVN):
  - This condition occurs secondary to the disruption of the blood supply to the bone.
  - Most commonly seen with fractures of the femoral neck and head, femoral condyles, proximal scaphoid, proximal humerus, and talar neck.
- Osteomyelitis
- Compartment syndrome
- Pulmonary disorders:
  - Adult respiratory distress syndrome
  - Fat emboli syndrome
  - DVT/PE
- Reflex sympathetic dystrophy
- Posttraumatic arthritis

### *Geriatric Considerations*
It is important to consider carefully operative versus nonoperative management in the elderly, given their higher rates of comorbidities such as diabetes, coronary artery disease, and vascular disease.

## PATIENT MONITORING
A patient with a fracture should be followed carefully with serial radiographs to ensure fracture stability and healing.

## REFERENCES

1. Gustilo RB, Anderson JT. Prevention of infection in the treatment of one thousand and twenty-five open fractures of long bones: retrospective and prospective analysis. *J Bone Joint Surg* 1976;58A:453–458.
2. Rodriguez-Merchan EC. Pediatric skeletal trauma: a review and historical perspective. *Clin Orthop Relat Res* 2005;432:8–13.
3. Salter RB, Harris WR. Injuries involving the epiphyseal plate. *J Bone Joint Surg* 1963;45A: 587–622.
4. Kocher MS, Kasser JR. Orthopaedic aspects of child abuse. *J Am Acad Orthop Surg* 2000;8:10–20.
5. Lee C, Porter KM. Prehospital management of lower limb fractures. *Emerg Med J* 2005;22: 660–663.
6. Sarmiento A, Latta L. The evolution of functional bracing of fractures. *J Bone Joint Surg* 2006;88B: 141–148.
7. Zalavras CG, Patzakis MJ. Open fractures: evaluation and management. *J Am Acad Orthop Surg* 2003;11:212–219.
8. Dirschl DR, Marsh JL, Buckwalter JA, et al. Articular fractures. *J Am Acad Orthop Surg* 2004;12:416–423.
9. Pape HC, Giannoudis P, Krettek C. The timing of fracture treatment in polytrauma patients: relevance of damage control orthopedic surgery. *Am J Surg* 2002;183:622–629.


## ADDITIONAL READING

Cole PA, Bhandari M. What's new in orthopaedic trauma. *J Bone Joint Surg* 2004;86A:2782–2795.


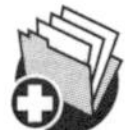

# MISCELLANEOUS

## CODES
### *ICD9-CM*
829.0 Fracture

## FAQ
- Q: Which fractures require surgery?
  - A: No definitive rule exists. However, in general, open fractures require surgery for débridement of foreign material; intra-articular fractures require surgery to correct displacement, avoid arthritis, and allow for early joint motion; displaced fractures may require surgery to correct deformity; and patients with multiple injuries may require surgery for early mobilization.

# FREIBERG DISEASE (FREIBERG INFRACTION)

*John T. Campbell, MD*

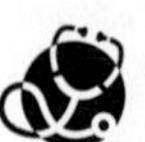

## BASICS

### DESCRIPTION

- "Freiberg infraction" is an eponym for osteonecrosis of the 2nd metatarsal head (1).
- The most common presentation is in a young or middle-aged adult with a history of well-localized pain to the 2nd MTP joint that is aggravated with activities and relieved with rest.
  - It primarily affects the 2nd metatarsal head (2).
  - Rarely, the 3rd or other metatarsal heads may be involved.
  - It may be unilateral or bilateral.
- Stages of involvement:
  - Early stages may show mottling of the metatarsal head or central collapse on radiographs.
  - Moderate disease shows flattening or collapse of the metatarsal head along with osteophytes or loose ossicles.
  - Late stages include loss of joint space and arthritis.

### EPIDEMIOLOGY

Occurs more often in females than in males

#### *Incidence*

The true incidence is unknown because many cases are asymptomatic and discovered incidentally on radiographs (2).

#### *Prevalence*

Most common in 13–18-year-olds, with symptoms occasionally persisting into adulthood (1,2)

### RISK FACTORS

- Running
- Dancing
- Long 2nd metatarsal

### ETIOLOGY

- This disorder is characterized by AVN of the involved metatarsal head (Fig. 1).
- Impaired microcirculation to bone (3,4)
- Acute trauma
- Repetitive microtrauma or overuse
- The fact that the 2nd metatarsal is the longest metatarsal and is relatively immobile subjects it to increased stress (3).

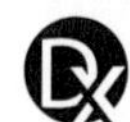

## DIAGNOSIS

### SIGNS AND SYMPTOMS

- Pain about the 2nd MTP joint is aggravated with activity and alleviated by rest.
- Running or sports often is associated with increased pain.
- Tenderness and soft-tissue thickening about the MTP joint may occur.
- Stiffness of affected MTP joint may develop.

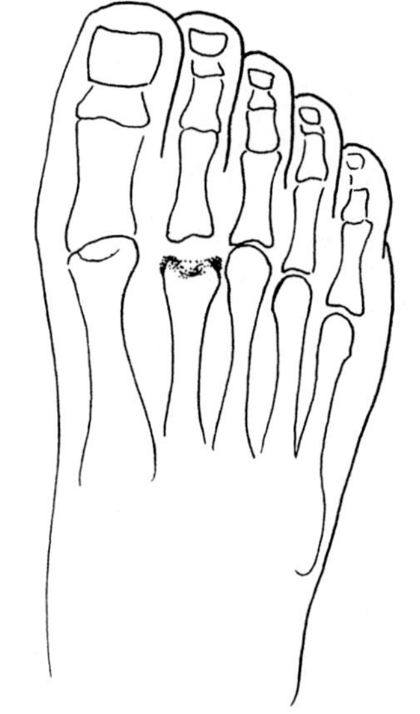

**Fig. 1.** Freiberg disease involves AVN of the 2nd metatarsal head.

#### *Physical Exam*

- Decreased joint ROM
- Tenderness to palpation
- Swelling after activity
- Pain on toe-raising

### TESTS

#### *Imaging*

- Radiography: Standing foot radiographs:
  - AP, oblique, and lateral views
  - Early findings include osteopenia and mild subchondral lucency.
  - Later stages show enlargement and flattening of the metatarsal head, sclerosis, cystic changes, and osteophytes.
  - End-stage disease shows arthritic narrowing and destruction of the joint.
- Occasionally, in early or occult cases, radiographs may be unremarkable and technetium bone scan or MRI may help confirm the diagnosis.
  - Bone scan shows focal intense uptake at the involved metatarsal head (3).
  - MRI shows bony edema with osteonecrosis of head.

#### *Pathological Findings*

- Typical findings include:
  - Synovitis, loose bodies, osteophytes
  - Metatarsal head osteonecrosis, with fibrosis of the marrow space, spicules of dead bone, resorption, and collapse (2)
  - Arthritic changes with loss of cartilage

### DIFFERENTIAL DIAGNOSIS

- Idiopathic synovitis
- Inflammatory arthritides
- Acute fracture
- Sprain of MTP joint
- Metatarsal stress fracture
- Morton neuroma

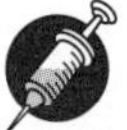

# TREATMENT

## GENERAL MEASURES

- Patients should avoid or limit activities that cause pain, especially running, jumping, and dancing.
- Early disease may be treated with a hard-soled shoe, fracture boot brace, or a walking cast.
- Symptoms may be relieved by using a metatarsal pad just proximal to the involved metatarsal head (1).
- Taping or strapping the toe can help to immobilize the joint.
- Judicious use of intra-articular corticosteroid injections may relieve synovitis.
- Late stages of the disease may require surgery.

## MEDICATION (DRUGS)

NSAIDs may alleviate swelling and pain.

## SURGERY

- Surgery is indicated if nonoperative measures are unsuccessful.
- Treatment options include (2):
  - Synovectomy
  - Joint debridement, including removal of fibrosis, loose bodies, and osteophytes (3)
  - Bone grafting of the metatarsal head if no flattening or joint surface collapse is present (3)
  - Dorsiflexion osteotomy of the involved metatarsal to rotate healthier plantar cartilage to articulate with the phalanx (4)
  - Metatarsal head resection arthroplasty (3)
  - Prosthetic joint replacement is not recommended because of transfer metatarsalgia, bony resorption, and implant failure.

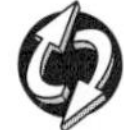

# FOLLOW-UP

## PROGNOSIS

In most patients, symptoms abate after the acute period and are replaced by an occasional ache.

## COMPLICATIONS

- Collapse of joint surface
- Arthritis of the second MTP joint
- Mechanical unloading of the joint with transfer metatarsalgia

## REFERENCES


1. Freiberg AH. The so-called infraction of the second metatarsal bone. *J Bone Joint Surg* 1926;8A: 257–261.
2. Katcherian DA. Treatment of Freiberg's disease. *Orthop Clin North Am* 1994;25:69–81.
3. Helal B, Gibb P. Freiberg's disease: a suggested pattern of management. *Foot Ankle* 1987;8: 94–102.
4. Kinnard P, Lirette R. Dorsiflexion osteotomy in Freiberg's disease. *Foot Ankle* 1989;9:226–231.


## ADDITIONAL READING


Daniels TR. Osteochondroses of the foot. In: Myerson MS, ed. *Foot and Ankle Disorders*. Philadelphia: WB Saunders, 2000:785–799.


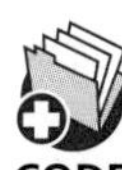

# MISCELLANEOUS

## CODES

### *ICD9-CM*

732.5 Freiberg disease (osteochondrosis, metatarsal head)

## PATIENT TEACHING

### *Activity*

- Explain the concept of AVN, including the slow process of revascularization, and warn that joint collapse may occur if weight is borne prematurely.
- Describe activities likely to exacerbate the disorder, such as running and jumping.
- Suggest substitute activities such as swimming.

## FAQ

- Q: What are the possible causes of Freiberg infraction (osteonecrosis of metatarsal head)?
  - A: Overuse, trauma, vascular impairment, inflammatory disease, increased 2nd metatarsal length, and immobility of 2nd metatarsal leading to increased stress.
- How is Freiberg infraction treated?
  - Rest, unloading or protection of the MTP joint, NSAIDs, and corticosteroid injections are standard nonoperative measures. Surgery is considered after failure of these methods.

# FRIEDREICH ATAXIA

*Paul D. Sponseller, MD*

## BASICS

### DESCRIPTION
- Friedreich ataxia is an uncommon, heritable disorder causing progressive spinocerebellar degeneration (1,2).
- Scoliosis, ataxia, and foot deformities are the most common findings (Fig. 1).
- Systems affected: Central nervous system; Heart; Skeleton
- Classification:
  - No subclassifications are used in Friedreich ataxia.
  - It is classified under the category *spinocerebellar degeneration*, and it is the most common example of this class.
  - Another disorder in this class is *spinocerebellar ataxia*.
- Synonym: Spinocerebellar degeneration

### EPIDEMIOLOGY

#### *Incidence*
Prevalence is ~1 per 50,000 persons (1).

#### *Prevalence*
- It may become apparent anytime from 5–25 years of age.
- Males and females are affected equally.

### RISK FACTORS
The condition is more common in people of French Canadian descent (1).

#### *Genetics*
Transmission is autosomal recessive.

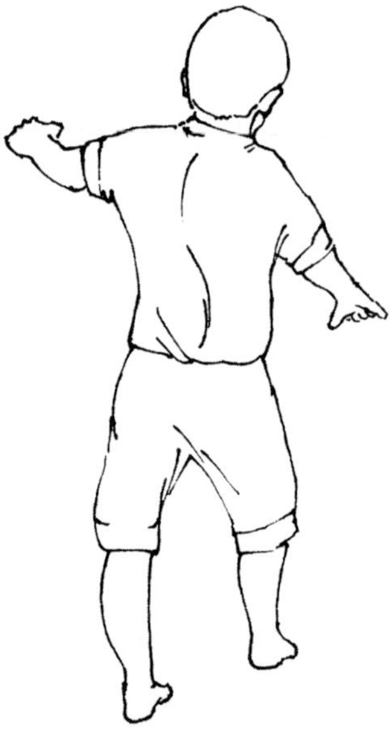

Fig. 1. Scoliosis, cavovarus feet, and ataxia as seen in Friedreich ataxia.

### ETIOLOGY
- The cause is a defect in a gene for a protein, frataxin, found on chromosome 9 (1).
- The pathogenesis of the findings is not well known.
- Variations in characteristics of the disease (e.g., age at onset and rate of progression) may be caused by different mutations at one of the loci.

### ASSOCIATED CONDITIONS
- Diabetes mellitus
- Cardiomyopathy
- Scoliosis
- Foot deformity

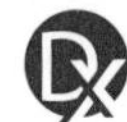

## DIAGNOSIS

The diagnosis is made on a clinical basis, usually confirmed by a neurologist.

### SIGNS AND SYMPTOMS
- Common signs:
  - Ataxia
  - Wide-based gait
  - Weakness and loss of position sense in the lower extremities
  - Frequently, loss of upper extremity reflexes
- Less common signs:
  - Pes cavus
  - Optic atrophy
  - Nystagmus is possible.
- Symptoms:
  - Partial deafness, depression, loss of coordination, painful muscle spasms, and weakness
  - Symptoms of diabetes mellitus also may be related because of the increased coexistence of these disorders.

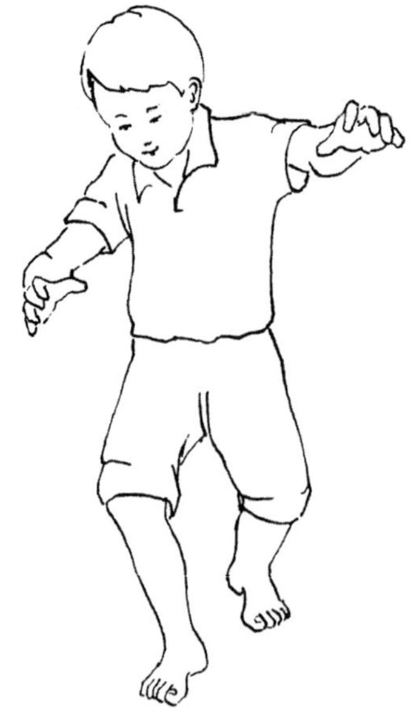

Fig. 2. Ataxia and cavovarus feet in Friedreich ataxia.

#### *Physical Exam*
- Examine heel-to-toe walking and finger-to-nose positioning (Fig. 2).
- Look for the presence of increased kyphosis on routine standing.
- Perform the forward-bend test for scoliosis.
- Test upper and lower extremity reflexes.
- Note the flexibility of the feet and the correctability of any deformity.
- Test muscle strength (proximal muscles are affected earlier are than distal muscles).
- The gluteus maximus is the 1st muscle to be affected clinically.

### TESTS

#### *Lab*
- Creatine phosphokinase levels are normal.
- Fasting serum glucose for diabetes mellitus should be obtained.
- Other tests:
  - Electrocardiography should be performed before surgery, with echocardiography as indicated, because of the increased incidence of hypertrophic cardiomyopathy.
  - Electromyography shows polyphasic potentials and mild slowing of nerve conduction velocity.

#### *Imaging*
- Standing posteroanterior and lateral radiographs of the spine should be ordered when scoliosis and kyphosis are found.
  - Periodic monitoring then is indicated, even after maturity.
- Foot radiographs may be indicated.

### DIFFERENTIAL DIAGNOSIS
- Cerebellar tumors
- Chiari malformation
- Muscular dystrophy
- Spinal dysraphism (as a cause of scoliosis and foot deformity)

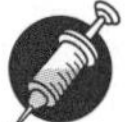

## TREATMENT

### GENERAL MEASURES

- Foot and spine deformities should be followed by an orthopaedic surgeon, even if surgery is not contemplated.
- Brace treatment of scoliosis is appropriate for curves of 25–45° and may slow the rate of progression.
- Stretching and night bracing may be helpful in preventing worsening of the foot deformities.
- Walking should be maintained as long as possible.

### SPECIAL THERAPY

#### *Physical Therapy*

- Therapy is essential, to keep up strength and skills after surgery.
- Stretching of plantar fascia and ankle muscles help to prevent deformity.

### MEDICATION (DRUGS)

- No medical treatment currently is available.
- If painful muscle spasms occur, baclofen or diazepam may be helpful.

### SURGERY

- Scoliosis:
  - A cardiopulmonary evaluation is indicated preoperatively.
  - To prevent progressive decompensation of the spine, posterior fusion and instrumentation with 2 contoured rods is indicated for curves of >50°.
  - If the curve is large, rigid, and unbalanced, an anterior release also may be indicated to increase the correctability (2–4).
  - Spinal cord monitoring may be more challenging and should include sensory and motor modalities.
  - Postoperative immobilization usually is unnecessary.
- Cavovarus feet: Correction may include:
  - Plantar fasciotomy
  - Achilles tendon lengthening and transfer or lengthening of the PTT
  - Possible osteotomy

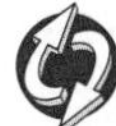

## FOLLOW-UP

### DISPOSITION

#### *Issues for Referral*

A neurologist is the best specialist for coordinating the overall care of these patients.

### PROGNOSIS

- If scoliosis develops before the patient is 15 years old, it most likely will become severe and require surgery.
- Most affected individuals stop walking by 20–30 years of age and are wheelchair dependent.
- Death usually occurs by the 4th or 5th decade; causes most often include pneumonia, aspiration, and cardiomyopathy.

### COMPLICATIONS

- Cardiomyopathy
- Calluses or skin breakdown on the foot
- Pneumonia

### PATIENT MONITORING

- This disease is progressive.
- Walking distance and status of all physical findings should be monitored every 3–6 months.
- Scoliosis, if present, should be checked every 6 months.

### REFERENCES


1. Cady RB, Bobechko WP. Incidence, natural history, and treatment of scoliosis in Friedreich's ataxia. *J Pediatr Orthop* 1984;4:673–676.
2. Delatycki MB, Paris DBBP, Gardner RJM, et al. Clinical and genetic study of Friedreich ataxia in an Australian population. *Am J Med Genet* 1999;87: 168–174.
3. Labelle H, Tohme S, Duhaime M, et al. Natural history of scoliosis in Friedreich's ataxia. *J Bone Joint Surg* 1986;68A:564–572.
4. Shapiro F, Bresnan MJ. Orthopaedic management of childhood neuromuscular disease. Part II: Peripheral neuropathies, Friedreich's ataxia, and arthrogryposis multiplex congenita. *J Bone Joint Surg* 1982;64A:949–953.


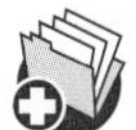

## MISCELLANEOUS

### CODES

#### *ICD9-CM*

334.0 Friedreich ataxia

### PATIENT TEACHING

- Patients should be counseled about the natural history of the disease, which consists of slow degeneration, so they can plan appropriately.
- Patient support groups often are helpful.
- Genetic counseling should be offered.

### FAQ

- Q: Will physical therapy help to restore coordination?
  - A: No. Coordination depends most on the progression of the disease.

# GENU VALGUM (KNOCK-KNEE)

*Paul D. Sponseller, MD*

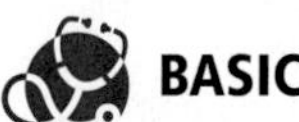

## BASICS

### DESCRIPTION
- Genu valgum, or knock-knee, is a normal phase of development in children 2–4 years old.
- Girls normally have slightly more valgus of the knee than do boys.
- The valgus straightens to achieve the adult position by 6–7 years of age (1,2).
- Rickets, trauma, and genetic disorders also may cause genu valgum.
- Some patients have an idiopathic valgus, not resulting from any of the foregoing disorders, that falls outside the normal limits and persists beyond 10 years of age.
- Areas affected include the distal femoral and proximal tibial growth plates.

### EPIDEMIOLOGY
#### *Incidence*
- The condition is rare.
- Pathologic valgus occurs in <1 per 1,000 (2).

#### *Prevalence*
- It occurs in young children, usually 3–11 years old (1).
- Physiologic genu valgum is more common in females than in males.

### RISK FACTORS
- Family history of genu valgum
- Proximal tibia metaphysic fracture in children (Cozen fracture); asymmetric overgrowth occurs and deformity is possible (parents should be warned about this possibility).

#### *Genetics*
- Many forms of rickets are transmitted genetically.
- Idiopathic valgus may be transmitted in families.

### ETIOLOGY
- Physiologic genu valgum (Fig. 1)
- Metabolic disorder (e.g., rickets)
- Steroid dependence
- Proximal tibia fracture (3,4)
- Skeletal dysplasias
- Chromosome disorders (e.g., Klinefelter syndrome)

### ASSOCIATED CONDITIONS
- Proximal tibia fracture
- Pseudoachondroplasia
- Renal osteodystrophy
- Metaphyseal dysplasia
- Rickets
- Down syndrome

## DIAGNOSIS

### SIGNS AND SYMPTOMS
- Parental concern about the appearance of the child's legs is the most common reason for presentation.
- It is usually asymptomatic.
- The knees usually are not painful in childhood but the physical appearance is sometimes bothersome; occasionally, valgus knees are associated with patellar discomfort.
- In adulthood, valgus knees are more likely to produce arthritic symptoms outside of the joint.

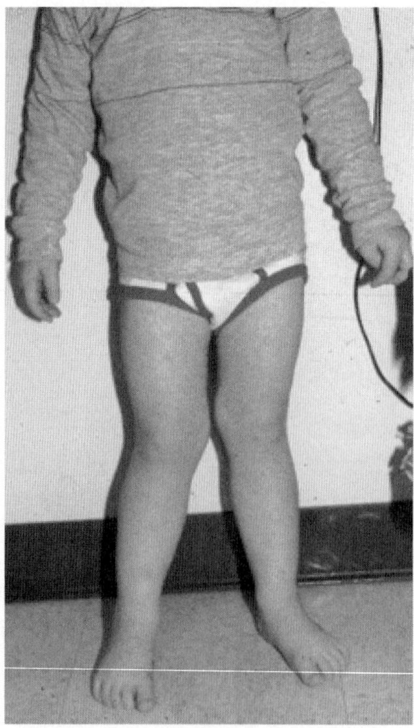

**Fig. 1.** This 3-year-old had typical physiologic genu valgum. It resolved with growth within 1 year.

#### *Physical Exam*
- Measure the ROM of the knee.
- Determine and plot height and weight percentiles for the patient's age.
- Measure the angle between the tibia and the femur with a goniometer.
- Measure the distance between the ankles when the knees are touching (intermalleolar distance).
- Assess the alignment and ROM in the adjacent hip and ankle.
- Check the rotation of the limb and the gait.
- Check the collateral ligaments of the knee for laxity.

### TESTS
#### *Lab*
- Serum levels of calcium, phosphate, alkaline phosphatase, urea nitrogen, and creatinine should be measured if rickets or a metabolic problem is suspected.
- The most common type of rickets in developed countries is familial hypophosphatemic rickets.
- If rickets is to be evaluated, check vitamin D levels (25-hydroxy and 1,25-dihydroxy) as well as the other parameters.

#### *Imaging*
- Imaging of genu valgum, which is thought to be physiologic, is unnecessary for children <6 years old unless the patient has an asymmetric deformity or a pathologic condition is suspected.
- An AP view of the lower extremity from the hip to ankle obtained while the patient is standing should be the 1st imaging study.
  - The knee should be pointing straight ahead.
  - The film cassette should be long enough to accommodate the entire extremity.
  - The femorotibial angle should be measured, and the site of the deformity should be identified as femoral, tibial, or both.

### DIFFERENTIAL DIAGNOSIS
- The main differential diagnosis is to determine whether the condition is physiologic or pathologic.
- Physiologic genu valgum occurs without underlying rickets, dysplasia, or other known cause.
- The most common skeletal dysplasias causing valgus are metaphyseal dysplasia and pseudoachondroplasia, as well as multiple osteochondromas.

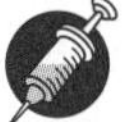

# TREATMENT

## GENERAL MEASURES

- Physiologic valgus:
  - No treatment is indicated for physiologic genu valgum in patients <7 years old.
  - If the deformity persists after 7 years of age, hemiepiphysiodesis (at age 11–12 years) may be considered to achieve normal alignment.
    - Epiphysiodesis consists of slowing or stopping the growth plate on the medial side to allow the lateral side to catch up.
    - This relatively simple procedure does not substantially weaken the bone and allows early weightbearing.
- Pathologic valgus:
  - For metabolic disorders, including renal osteodystrophy, the underlying condition should be treated.
  - Bracing has not been effective in preventing or reversing the deformity.
  - Single- or multiple-level osteotomy may be necessary to correct the deformity; medical control of the disease is needed first.
  - Usually, therapy is directed by a renal or endocrine specialist.
- Fracture:
  - Follow-up of proximal tibia fracture should extend for several years after the injury (3).
  - Early tibial osteotomy should be avoided because of the high incidence of recurrence of valgus deformity (3).
  - If an unacceptable degree of valgus remains after 1–2 years follow-up, hemiepiphysiodesis or osteotomy may be indicated (5,6).
- Dysplasia:
  - Children with pseudoachondroplasia and metaphyseal dysplasias are likely to develop genu valgum.
  - Osteotomy may be necessary to correct the deformity.

### *Activity*

No activity restrictions are necessary.

## SPECIAL THERAPY

### *Physical Therapy*

Not indicated, because therapy and exercises cannot affect the growth of the limb

## SURGERY

- 2 types of surgery commonly are used to correct valgus deformity when it persists: Hemiepiphysiodesis and varus osteotomy.
  - Epiphysiodesis aims to achieve satisfactory mechanical alignment at the end of growth.
  - Proximal tibia osteotomy should be considered if epiphysiodeses is not feasible.
    - Osteotomy involves a more difficult recovery period than epiphysiodesis because, in the former procedure, the bone is divided completely.
- The overall success rate of surgery is >90%.

# FOLLOW-UP

## PROGNOSIS

Physiologic genu valgum resolves by age 7–10 years as long as it is mild (<15°) and no metabolic problems are present.

## COMPLICATIONS

- Untreated genu valgum: If severe, the patient may develop patellofemoral pain and late degenerative arthritis from stresses on the lateral joint surface.
- Surgical complications:
  - Infection
  - Compartment syndrome
  - Recurrence of deformity or overcorrection and neurovascular injury

## PATIENT MONITORING

Children with idiopathic genu valgum may be followed every 12–24 months to determine whether the deformity is improving before a treatment decision is made.

## REFERENCES


1. Arazi M, Ogun TC, Memik R. Normal development of the tibiofemoral angle in children: a clinical study of 590 normal subjects from 3 to 17 years of age. *J Pediatr Orthop* 2001;21:264–267.
2. White GR, Mencio GA. Genu valgum in children: diagnostic and therapeutic alternatives. *J Am Acad Orthop Surg* 1995;3:275–283.
3. Balthazar DA, Pappas AM. Acquired valgus deformity of the tibia in children. *J Pediatr Orthop* 1984;4:538–541.
4. Brougham DI, Nicol RO. Valgus deformity after proximal tibial fractures in children. *J Bone Joint Surg* 1987;69B:482.
5. Bowen JR, Torres RR, Forlin E. Partial epiphysiodesis to address genu varum or genu valgum. *J Pediatr Orthop* 1992;12:359–364.
6. Ferrick MR, Birch JG, Albright M. Correction of non-Blount's angular knee deformity by permanent hemiepiphyseodesis. *J Pediatr Orthop* 2004;24:397–402.


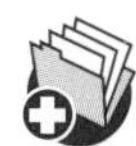

# MISCELLANEOUS

## CODES

### *ICD9-CM*

736.41 Genu valgum

## PATIENT TEACHING

Inform parents that most cases of physiologic genu valgum begin to resolve spontaneously by 7 years of age.

## FAQ

- Q: Is bracing indicated in genu valgum?
  - A: Bracing for valgus has never been shown to be effective. It is very cumbersome because the knee cannot bend in a corrective brace.
- Q: Is valgus a cosmetic problem or a functional one?
  - A: In the more severe degrees, it can impair running and increase the risk of arthritis.

# GENU VARUM (BOWED LEGS)

*Paul D. Sponseller, MD*

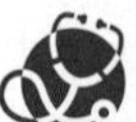

## BASICS

### DESCRIPTION
- The knee goes through normal phases of changing alignment in childhood: Genu varum (bowed legs) is physiologic in infants and young children up to 2 years of age, and its appearance is maximal at 12–18 months of age (1–3).
- Bowing is most obvious when children start walking.
- It may be combined with internal tibial torsion, which makes it appear more pronounced.
- Bowing may seem greater with weightbearing.
- This condition usually resolves by 2 years of age and changes to physiologic genu valgum (knock-knee) (2).
- Tibia vara (Blount disease) (see "Blount Disease" chapter), rickets, fibrocartilaginous dysplasia of the proximal tibia, and other genetic disorders can cause pathologic genu varum (Fig. 1).

### EPIDEMIOLOGY
- Physiologic (normal) bowing is ~1,000 times more common than pathologic bowing (e.g., Blount disease) (1,3).
- It occurs equally in boys and girls.

### RISK FACTORS
Family history

#### *Genetics*
- Some causes of bowed legs are familial:
  - Blount disease
  - Renal rickets
  - Skeletal dysplasia

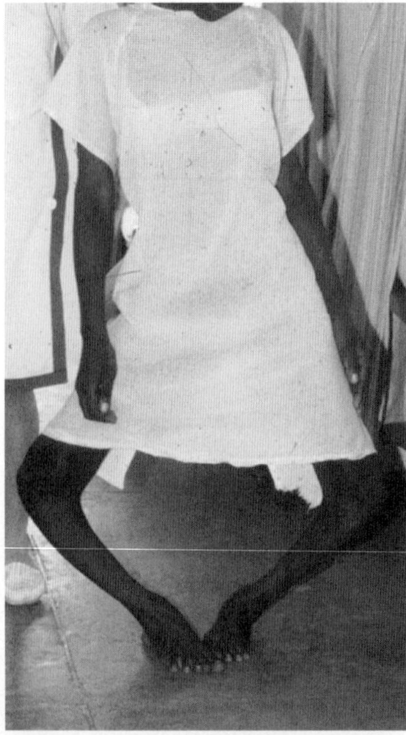

**Fig. 1.** Patient with severe untreated infantile varus now in adolescence.

### ETIOLOGY
- Bowing is an imbalance between the load and growth plate development.
- It may be caused by:
  - Overweight
  - Rickets (4)
  - Skeletal dysplasia
- Physiologic causes: Normal growth patterns of the femoral and tibial growth plates include a period of normal varus in early infancy.
- Pathologic causes:
  - Tibia vara (Blount disease)
  - Rickets (nutritional or renal)
  - Achondroplasia
  - Epiphyseal and metaphyseal dysplasias
  - Focal fibrocartilaginous dysplasia
- In most of these conditions, the varus results from inability of the growth plate to respond normally to load (3).

### ASSOCIATED CONDITIONS
- Early walker
- Heavy weight

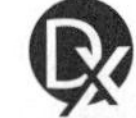

## DIAGNOSIS

### SIGNS AND SYMPTOMS
- Parental concern about the appearance of the legs is the most common reason for the presentation of children.
- The patient should be pain free; if pain exists, another cause should be sought.
- Genu varum may develop spontaneously in the overweight adolescent who previously had straight legs (adolescent Blount disease), and it usually requires treatment (Fig. 2).

#### *History*
If a patient has physiologic bowing, the parents should start to notice improvement after the 2nd birthday (3).

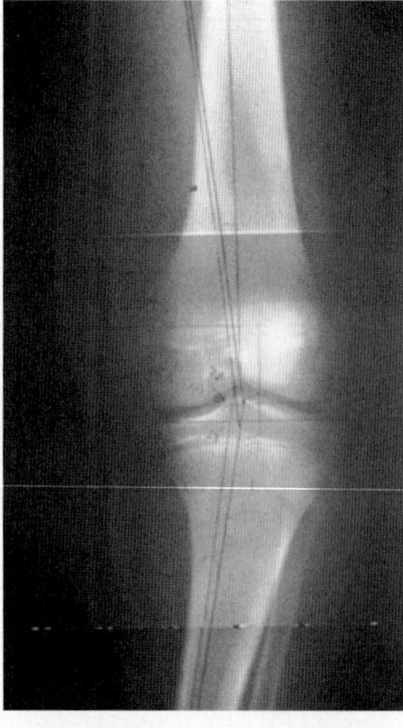

**Fig. 2.** 13-year-old boy with adolescent genu varum. Note the widened medial physis.

#### *Physical Exam*
- Obtain a medical, family, and developmental history.
- Determine the patient's height and weight percentiles.
- Estimate the angulation of the knee.
- Check the rotation of the tibia and femur.
- To monitor the patient's progress, document the distance between the medial surfaces of the knees (intercondylar distance) (5,6).

### TESTS

#### *Lab*
- In routine cases, tests are not indicated if varus appears mild and physiologic.
- If metabolic causes are suspected, serum calcium, phosphate, alkaline phosphatase, 1,25-vitamin D, and creatinine levels may be measured (3,4).

#### *Imaging*
- Radiographic evaluation of bowed legs in children <18 months old should be reserved for asymmetric bowing or for patients suspected of having a pathologic condition other than benign physiologic varus.
- A single AP radiograph of the lower extremity from hip to ankle on a standing film is the most appropriate 1st imaging study; care should be taken that the knee is pointing straight ahead.
- Widening of physis suggests rickets; delayed ossification of the distal femoral and proximal tibial epiphyses may be a result of excessive pressure on 1 side of the knee.
- The femorotibial angle and the metaphyseal–diaphyseal angle of the tibia should be measured (5).
- If the metaphyseal–diaphyseal angle is <11°, physiologic bowing is assured.
- If the metaphyseal-diaphyseal angle is >16°, the child has Blount disease.
- If the metaphyseal bowing in the femur is equal to or greater than that in the tibia, the bowing is more likely to be physiologic (1) (Fig. 3).

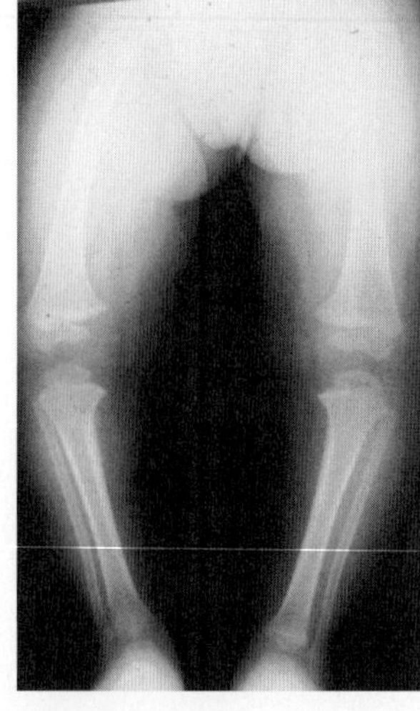

**Fig. 3.** This 2-year-old patient had bowed legs. The metaphyseal–diaphyseal angle is 10° on each side. The bowing is more pronounced on the femoral than the tibial metaphysis. It resolved without treatment.

## DIFFERENTIAL DIAGNOSIS

- Achondroplasia
- Rickets
- Infantile or adolescent Blount disease
- Metaphyseal or epiphyseal dysplasia

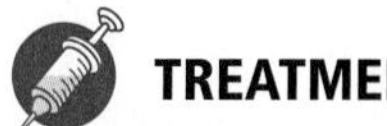

# TREATMENT

## GENERAL MEASURES

- Physiologic conditions:
  - Physiologic bowing always resolves without treatment; bracing is not needed
  - At ≥18 months of age, follow-up examination and imaging are needed to differentiate physiologic bowing from tibia vara (may be difficult) (6).
- Pathologic conditions:
  - Rickets or other metabolic bone disease:
    - The underlying disease is treated, with osteotomy reserved for those patients with persisting varus after treatment.
  - Achondroplasia and epiphyseal or metaphyseal dysplasia:
    - The patient may need surgical treatment, depending on the degree of deformity.
  - Tibia vara (Blount disease):
    - Brace treatment is appropriate for children <3 years old; a knee-ankle-foot brace may be used for walking.
    - If the patient is >4 years of age, osteotomy is recommended.

## SPECIAL THERAPY

### *Physical Therapy*

- Not necessary for physiologic bowing
- Not an effective treatment for pathologic varus

## SURGERY

- Many different types of osteotomy are available for correcting varus deformity, including dome, oblique, closing wedge, or opening wedge osteotomy.
- The tibia or the femur may require surgery, depending on the site of the deformity.
- Physeal bar resection or hemiepiphysiodesis may be indicated for some cases.

# FOLLOW-UP

## PROGNOSIS

- Physiologic genu varum has an excellent prognosis for spontaneous improvement.
- The prognosis of pathologic genu varum varies.
- Knee pain and worsening of the bow are likely in adulthood if the deformity is >10–15° (5).

## COMPLICATIONS

- Untreated genu varum may cause pain on the medial part of the knee and eventual arthritis during adulthood.
- Adolescent genu varum may be painful.
- Complications occasionally seen from surgery may include:
  - Infection
  - Compartment syndrome
  - Recurrence of deformity
  - Growth disturbance

## PATIENT MONITORING

- The frequency of follow-up varies, depending on the individual surgeon or pediatrician.
- Physiologic bowing does not need frequent follow-up unless the condition is not improving; resolution is a slow process and may take a year.
- Pathologic bowing needs more prolonged follow-up.

## REFERENCES


1. Bowen RE, Dorey FJ, Moseley CF. Relative tibial and femoral varus as a predictor of progression of varus deformities of the lower limbs in young children. *J Pediatr Orthop* 2002;22:105–111.
2. Salenius P, Vankka E. The development of the tibiofemoral angle in children. *J Bone Joint Surg* 1975;57A:259–261.
3. Schoenecker PL, Rich MM. The lower extremity. In: Morrissy RT, Weinstein SL, eds. *Lovell and Winter's Pediatric Orthopaedics,* 6th ed. Philadelphia: Lippincott Williams & Wilkins, 2006:1157–1211.
4. Biser-Rohrbaugh A, Hadley-Miller N. Vitamin D deficiency in breast-fed toddlers. *J Pediatr Orthop* 2001;21:508–511.
5. Gordon JE, King DJ, Luhmann SJ, et al. Femoral deformity in tibia vara. *J Bone Joint Surg* 2006;88A:380–386.
6. Langenskiold A. Tibia vara. A critical review. *Clin Orthop Relat Res* 1989;246:195–207.


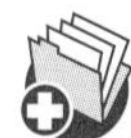

# MISCELLANEOUS

## CODES

### *ICD9-CM*

736.42 Genu varum

## PATIENT TEACHING

- Parents should be told that physiologic genu varum will resolve spontaneously and slowly; if it is not starting to improve at least by 2–3 years of age, additional evaluation is needed.
- No restriction on activity is recommended.
- Exercises do not help genu varum resolve.

## FAQ

- Q: Do infant "jumper" devices contribute to bowed legs?
  - A: No evidence suggests that they do. The children are supported in these devices, so the load on the legs is controlled.
- Q: When should a child with bowing be referred to a specialist?
  - A: If the bowing gets worse after 18 months or persists after the 2nd birthday.

# GIANT CELL TUMOR

*Uma Srikumaran, MD*
*Frank J. Frassica, MD*

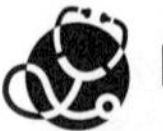

## BASICS

### DESCRIPTION (1–3)

- A benign but often locally aggressive neoplasm, characterized by large numbers of uniformly distributed, osteoclastlike giant cells and a background population of plump, epithelioid-to-spindle mononuclear cells (Fig. 1)
- The vast majority of these tumors are located near the articular end of a tubular bone; ~50% occur in the knee.
- Other frequently involved sites:
  - Distal radius
  - Proximal femur
  - Proximal humerus
  - Distal tibia
  - Sacrum
- Flat-bone involvement tends to occur in the sacrum and pelvis.
- Giant cell tumors complicating Paget disease often involve the flat bones, particularly those of the craniofacial region.
- Multifocal giant cell tumors are rare.
- Classification: Musculoskeletal Tumor Society surgical staging system (also known as the "Enneking" system [1,4]), a grading system that may have prognostic importance:
  - Stage I (<5% of patients):
    - Virtually asymptomatic and often discovered incidentally
    - Occasionally may cause pathologic fracture
    - Has a sclerotic rim on a plain radiograph or CT scan
    - Is relatively inactive on a bone scan
    - Is histologically benign
  - Stage II (70–85% of patients):
    - Symptomatic
    - May be associated with pathologic fracture
    - Has an expanded cortex but no breakthrough on a plain radiograph
    - Is active on a bone scan
    - Is histologically benign
  - Stage III (10–15% of patients):
    - Symptomatic, rapidly growing mass
    - Has cortical perforation with an accompanying soft-tissue mass on a plain radiograph or CT scan
    - Its activity on a bone scan extends beyond the lesion seen on a plain radiograph.
    - Shows intense hypervascularity on angiography
    - Is histologically benign, although one may see tumor infiltration of the peritumoral capsule with violation of the cortex and extension into the surrounding soft tissues

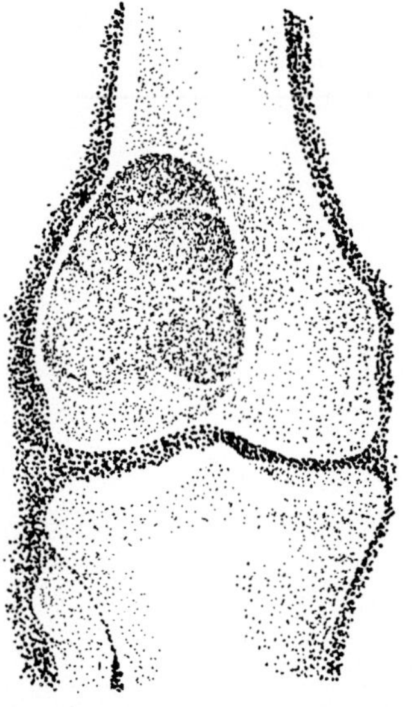

**Fig. 1.** A giant cell tumor arises in the epiphysis but may expand into the metaphysis. The distal femoral epiphysis is one of the most common sites.

### EPIDEMIOLOGY

#### *Incidence*

The peak incidence is in the 3rd decade of life, with a gradual decline into late adulthood (3).

#### *Prevalence (3)*

- Accounts for 5% of biopsied primary bone tumors and ~20% of benign bone tumors
- It is the 6th most common primary osseous neoplasm.
- It almost always affects the mature skeleton with closed epiphyseal plates.
- ~10–15% of patients are <20 years old, but almost all are skeletally mature.
- The onset of giant cell tumor after 55 years of age is rare.
- <2% of these tumors occur adjacent to open epiphyses; the diagnosis of giant cell tumor in a skeletally immature patient therefore must be questioned.
- Females are affected 1.3–1.5 times as often as males.

### RISK FACTORS

Paget disease (rare association)

### ETIOLOGY

Rare cases may result as a complication of pre-existing Paget disease of bone.

### ASSOCIATED CONDITIONS

- Rarely, giant cell tumors may complicate Paget disease of bone.
- More frequently, secondary aneurysmal bone cyst formation may be associated with giant cell tumors.

## DIAGNOSIS

### SIGNS AND SYMPTOMS (2,3)

- Complaints usually are nonspecific, and patients often have joint symptoms.
- 90% of patients complain of pain, often with accompanying mass or swelling.
- 5–10% of patients present with pathologic fracture.
- Serum chemistry studies typically are normal.

#### *Physical Exam*

- A physical examination is not specific for this condition.
- In general, tenderness over the epiphyseal end of a bone adjacent to a joint is noted.
- An effusion or restriction of joint motion may be present if the tumor has nearly violated the cortex.

### TESTS

#### *Lab*

Serum calcium and phosphate levels should be checked to exclude hyperparathyroidism.

#### *Pathological Findings (1)*

- The tumor has a background of proliferating, homogeneous mononuclear cells, which are round to ovoid, have relatively large nuclei with inconspicuous nucleoli, and display multinucleated giant cells dispersed evenly throughout the tissue.
- Mitotic figures may be common.
- It may have an aneurysmal bone cyst component, and it may invade blood vessels.
- Involutional changes with lipid-filled histiocytes may be observed.

#### *Imaging (1,2)*

- Radiography:
  - Plain radiographs show an eccentric, expanding zone of radiolucency, frequently at the end of a long bone.
  - Usually, no reactive sclerosis is present.
  - The tumor often begins in the metaphysis and extends to the articular surface.
  - Almost invariably, it involves the epiphysis, usually with metaphyseal extension.
  - If the spine is affected, it usually is the anterior vertebral body.
  - The tumor is multicentric in only 1% of cases.
  - Chest radiography is performed because 2% of patients may have pulmonary metastases.
- A bone scan often is positive, but the lesion may be inactive on a bone scan.

### DIFFERENTIAL DIAGNOSIS

- Giant cell reparative granuloma, or "brown tumor" of hyperparathyroidism (The giant cell reparative granuloma tumor contains a more uniform distribution of larger giant cells with many more nuclei.)
- NOF
- Benign fibrous histiocytoma
- Aneurysmal bone cyst
- Telangiectatic osteosarcoma

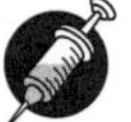

## TREATMENT (5,6)

### GENERAL MEASURES

Patients with large lesions are placed on crutches until definitive surgery.

### SPECIAL THERAPY

#### *Radiotherapy*

Radiotherapy should be used only rarely for giant cell tumors because its use increases the risk of malignant transformation of the tumor.

#### *Physical Therapy*

Patients undergo physical therapy to regain their ROM and strength.

### SURGERY

- Current technique involves a combination of marginal resection and curettage using power burrs on the margins of the cavity, followed by painting with full-strength phenol.
- Polymethylmethacrylate cement augmentation may be used to fill the cavity and to provide a rigid construct.
- Cancellous bone grafting is used to restore the subchondral surface.
- Internal fixation may be necessary to provide a rigid construct.
- When the tumor is in an expendable bone, such as the fibula, or is a recurrent lesion with joint destruction, wide resection may be necessary.
- Reconstruction around the knee may involve resection arthrodesis, osteoarticular allograft, or prosthetic implantation.
- Amputation may be indicated for neglected tumors with substantial soft-tissue extension and, in rare instances, for recurrent tumors.

## FOLLOW-UP (2,6)

### PROGNOSIS

- Recurrence may occur in 40–60% of giant cell tumors treated by simple curettage alone.
- Most recurrences occur within 2 years, and nearly all occur within 5 years.
- The recurrence rate with modern treatment (exteriorization, power burr curettage, and adjuvant therapy) is ~10–15%.

### COMPLICATIONS

- A secondary malignant giant cell tumor results when a sarcoma develops at the site of a previously treated giant cell tumor.
- In the past:
  - 10–15% of patients with giant cell tumors treated with irradiation developed postirradiation sarcomas.
  - In comparison, ~5% of recurrent giant cell tumors not subjected to irradiation developed sarcomatous transformation.

### PATIENT MONITORING

- Because recurrence is common, patients should be followed closely postoperatively (every 3 months for 2 years).
- A chest radiograph is taken once a year.

### REFERENCES


1. McCarthy EF, Frassica FJ. Primary bone tumors. In: *Pathology of Bone and Joint Disorders: With Clinical and Radiographic Correlation*. Philadelphia: WB Saunders, 1998:195–275.
2. Turcotte RE. Giant cell tumor of bone. *Orthop Clin North Am* 2006;37:35–51.
3. Unni KK. Giant cell tumor (osteoclastoma). In: *Dahlin's Bone Tumors: General Aspects and Data on 11,087 Cases*, 5th ed. Philadelphia: Lippincott-Raven Publishers, 1996:263–283.
4. Enneking WF. Malignant skeletal neoplasms. In: *Clinical Musculoskeletal Pathology*, 3rd ed. Gainsville: University of Florida Press, 1990:358–421.
5. Mendenhall WM, Zlotecki RA, Scarborough MT, et al. Giant cell tumor of bone. *Am J Clin Oncol* 2006;29:96–99.
6. Ward WG, Sr, Li G, III. Customized treatment algorithm for giant cell tumor of bone: Report of a series. *Clin Orthop Relat Res* 2002;397:259–270.


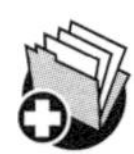

## MISCELLANEOUS

### CODES

#### *ICD9-CM*

170.9 Giant cell tumor

### PATIENT TEACHING

- The patient should understand the frequency of recurrence and the need for continued follow-up.
- The patient also should understand that the tumor is considered benign, but that in rare instances it may metastasize to the lungs (2% risk).

### FAQ

- Q: Is a giant cell tumor a cancer?
  - A: Although giant cell tumors of bone may behave in an aggressive local fashion, the tumor is benign.
- Q: Can a giant cell tumor spread to other sites?
  - A: Occasionally (~2% of the time), a giant cell tumor can spread to the lungs. This spread is a benign metastasis because only ~20% of patients will die because of the spread.
- Q: Can a giant cell tumor come back after surgery?
  - A: Giant cell tumors are prone to recurrence. With the best treatment, the rate of recurrence is ~10–15%.

# GROWING PAINS

*Paul D. Sponseller, MD*

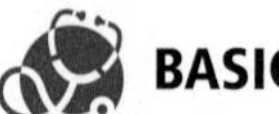

## BASICS

### DESCRIPTION

- This poorly understood syndrome is characterized by a long history of lower extremity pains that usually occur at night and worsen after active days.
- Pain:
  - Resolves completely each time it occurs
  - Occurs predominantly in the lower extremities
  - Occurs in 1 or both legs with random frequency
- No objective physical findings are seen.
- Synonyms: Leg aches; Night pains

### EPIDEMIOLOGY

#### *Incidence*

- Very common
- An estimated 15–36% of children complain of these pains at some time (1).

#### *Prevalence*

- Occurs in children 3–10 years old (1)
- Slightly more common in girls than in boys

### RISK FACTORS

High activity levels in normal young children

### ETIOLOGY

- The condition is believed to be secondary to stretch or fatigue of muscle.
- Support for this theory:
  - The fact that bones grow primarily when they are unloaded
  - The beneficial response that many children have to a stretching program (2,3)

## DIAGNOSIS

### SIGNS AND SYMPTOMS

- Signs:
  - Nonspecific for this condition
  - No localized tenderness
  - No limp
  - Full ROM
- Symptoms:
  - Pains occur after periods of activity, most often at night.
  - Pains come and go spontaneously.
  - Pains most often are bilateral, vague, and poorly localized.
  - Symptoms are often of long, though intermittent, duration, a feature that helps to rule out more serious causes.

#### *Physical Exam*

- Usually, with a careful history and physical examination, one can rule out more serious causes and define a typical picture.
- The child should be observed while walking into the office, especially before the child knows that the examiner is watching; there should not be any stiffness or limp.
- The lower extremities should be palpated systematically for tenderness; growing pains do not manifest tenderness.
- The ROM of the hips, knees, and ankles should be checked.
  - The hips, in particular, should show no stiffness or guarding on gentle rolling (the "roll test").
  - ROM should be full and symmetric.

### TESTS

#### *Lab*

- If the history is not typical:
  - Complete blood count and ESR may be done.
  - An appropriate workup tailored to the possibilities listed in the differential diagnosis should then be undertaken.

#### *Imaging*

- Bone scans and plain radiographs may help to define the site of pain if the history is not typical.
- However, these tests are not needed in most cases.

### DIFFERENTIAL DIAGNOSIS

- Perthes disease
- Chronic or subacute osteomyelitis
- Leukemia
- Sickle cell anemia
- Juvenile rheumatoid arthritis
- Lyme disease
- OSD (older child)
- Restless leg syndrome (4)

## TREATMENT

### GENERAL MEASURES

- If the diagnosis of growing pains fits the history, reassuring the parent and child is the 1st step.
- A program of stretching for the hamstrings, quadriceps, and calf muscles at night before bed has been shown to decrease the number of complaints, perhaps by mechanical means or by virtue of increased parent–child interaction.
- Activity levels may need to be modified to bring symptoms into a tolerable range.

## SPECIAL THERAPY

### *Physical Therapy*

The stretching program described under "General Measures" may be guided by parents and does not require a trained therapist.

## MEDICATION (DRUGS)

Analgesics may be used periodically, but not continuously.

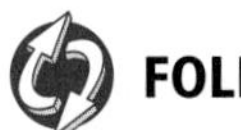

# FOLLOW-UP

## PROGNOSIS

Spontaneous resolution is the rule as the patient matures.

## PATIENT MONITORING

- Several successive office visits may be needed to show the character of the pain or to determine the direction of the workup.
- The stretching program is maintained, and the activity level is adjusted as needed.

## REFERENCES


1. Evans AM, Scutter SD. Prevalence of "growing pains" in young children. *J Pediatr* 2004;145:255–258.
2. Baxter MP, Dulberg C. "Growing pains" in childhood—a proposal for treatment. *J Pediatr Orthop* 1988;8:402–406.
3. Noonan KJ, Farnum CE, Leiferman EM, et al. Growing pains: are they due to increased growth during recumbency as documented in a lamb model? *J Pediatr Orthop* 2004;24:726–731.
4. Rajaram SS, Walters AS, England SJ, et al. Some children with growing pains may actually have restless legs syndrome. *Sleep* 2004;27:767–773.


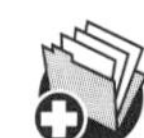

# MISCELLANEOUS

## CODES

### *ICD9-CM*

729.5 Growing pains

## PATIENT TEACHING

- Describe the nature of the process.
- Instruct in stretching exercises.
- Offer to see the patient any time the symptoms change.

## FAQ

- Q: Is growing pains a real condition?
  - A: Although the pathogenetic mechanism is lacking, most specialists agree that a constellation of symptoms, with a history of spontaneous resolution, is seen frequently by pediatricians and orthopaedic surgeons everywhere.
- Q: Is physical therapy necessary?
  - A: It is better to maximize parent–child interaction by stretching.

# HAMMER TOES

*Clifford L. Jeng, MD*

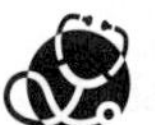

## BASICS

### DESCRIPTION

- The term "hammer toe" describes a flexion deformity of the PIP joint of the lesser toes (Fig. 1).
- It may be a flexible or rigid deformity.

### GENERAL PREVENTION

Because the most common cause of hammer toes is poor shoe wear with a tight, narrow toe box, the best prevention is to wear shoes with a wide, high toe box that does not constrain the forefoot area.

#### *Incidence*

More common in females than in males

### ETIOLOGY

- Most commonly from poorly fitting shoes
- Neuromuscular disease
- Diabetes mellitus
- Inflammatory arthropathy
- Compartment syndrome

### ASSOCIATED CONDITIONS

- Hallux valgus
- MTP dorsiflexion deformity (claw toe)

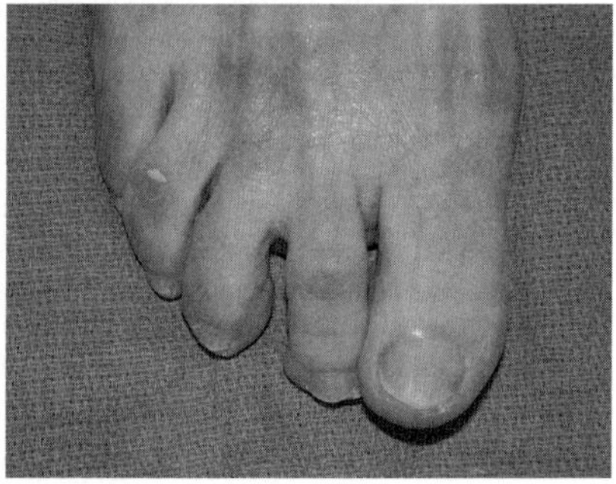

**Fig. 1.** Clinical photograph of hammer toe deformity.

## DIAGNOSIS

### SIGNS AND SYMPTOMS

- Dorsal prominence over the lesser-toe PIP joints
- Toe may be erythematous from shoe irritation.
- Overlying callus may be present from pressure of the shoe on the toe.

#### *History*

- Patients complain of pain over the dorsal prominence of the hammer toe with shoe wear.
- Patients also may have pain under the metatarsal heads (metatarsalgia).

#### *Physical Exam*

- Determine if the flexion deformity of the toe is flexible or rigid.
- Determine if an associated dorsal subluxation of the MTP joint is present.
- Look for an associated hallux valgus deformity (bunion).

#### *Imaging*

Plain radiographs of the foot show the flexion deformity of the PIP joint of the lesser toes consistent with the examination.

### DIFFERENTIAL DIAGNOSIS

- Claw toes have a concomitant dorsiflexion deformity of the MTP joint.
- Mallet toes have a flexion deformity at the DIP joint.

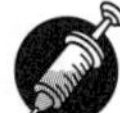

## TREATMENT

### GENERAL MEASURES

- If the deformity is flexible, a Budin splint may help straighten the dorsal prominence of the toe and diminish symptoms.
- If the deformity is rigid, then padding, including "doughnut" pads, and silicone gel toe sleeves help decrease pressure over the dorsal prominence.

#### *Geriatric Considerations*

- Hammer toes are a common diagnosis in elderly females.
- In patients with coexisting morbidities, such as diabetes or peripheral vascular disease, nonoperative management should be exhausted before considering surgery.

### SURGERY

- For flexible hammer toes, a flexor-to-extensor tendon transfer may be used to correct the deformity (1).
- Resection arthroplasty of the distal end of the proximal phalanx with pinning can straighten a rigid hammer toe (2,3).
- PIP fusion (4):
  - Is an alternative option for treating painful hammer toes
  - Can be used for primary surgery or for revision surgery on recurrent deformities

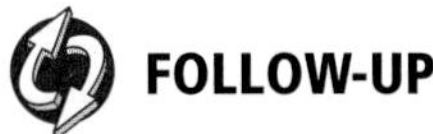

## FOLLOW-UP

### *Issues for Referral*

- Patients for whom nonoperative interventions, such as padding or splinting, fail may require surgical consultation.
- Diabetic patients need early consultation to prevent the development of neuropathic ulceration.

### PROGNOSIS

Hammer toes usually worsen over time, with increasing deformity and pain.

### COMPLICATIONS

- Complications of surgical treatment include:
  - Stiffness
  - Wound infection
  - Persistent pain
  - Failure to correct deformity adequately
  - Recurrence

### REFERENCES


1. Barbari SG, Brevig K. Correction of clawtoes by the Girdlestone-Taylor flexor-extensor transfer procedure. *Foot Ankle* 1984;5:67–73.
2. Coughlin MJ, Dorris J, Polk E. Operative repair of the fixed hammertoe deformity. *Foot Ankle Int* 2000;21:94–104.
3. O'Kane C, Kilmartin T. Review of proximal interphalangeal joint excisional arthroplasty for the correction of second hammer toe deformity in 100 cases. *Foot Ankle Int* 2005;26:320–325.
4. Lehman DE, Smith RW. Treatment of symptomatic hammertoe with a proximal interphalangeal joint arthrodesis. *Foot Ankle Int* 1995;16:535–541.


### ADDITIONAL READING


- Cahill BR, Connor DE. A long-term follow-up on proximal phalangectomy for hammer toes. *Clin Orthop Relat Res* 1972;86:191–192.
- Coughlin MJ, Mann RA. Lesser toe deformities. In: Coughlin MJ, Mann RA, eds. *Surgery of the Foot and Ankle*, 7th ed. St. Louis: Mosby, 1999:320–391.
- Coughlin MJ. Lesser toe abnormalities. *Instr Course Lect* 2003;52:421–444.
- Myerson MS, Shereff MJ. The pathological anatomy of claw and hammer toes. *J Bone Joint Surg* 1989;71A:45–49.
- Taylor RG. The treatment of claw toes by multiple transfers of flexor into extensor tendons. *J Bone Joint Surg* 1951;33B:539–542.


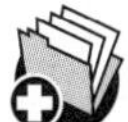

## MISCELLANEOUS

### CODES

#### *ICD9-CM*

735.4 Hammer toe

### FAQ

- Q: What are simple nonsurgical measures to relieve symptoms of painful hammer toes?
  - A: Shoes with low heels and a wide toe box are recommended to relieve pressure. Taping or strapping devices may improve alignment, whereas foam or gel pads can relieve focal pressure or calluses caused by the shoe.
- Q: What is the key physical finding of hammer toes?
  - A: Determining the flexibility or rigidity of hammer toes is crucial to determining nonoperative treatment options and surgical strategies.

# HAMSTRING STRAIN

*Brett M. Cascio, MD*
*Melanie Kinchen, MD*

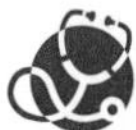

## BASICS

### DESCRIPTION
- The hamstrings are long muscles in the posterior thigh that extend from the ischial tuberosity behind the hip, down to the knee.
- A hamstring strain is a stretch-induced muscle injury.
- Tears result from the hamstring muscle suddenly changing from a stabilizing flexor to an extensor.
- It usually is caused by quick starts with sudden hamstring contraction.
- Strain classification (1):
  - Mild: Muscle spasm only, with no evidence of tear, with minimal discomfort and with only minimal loss of strength
  - Moderate: Muscle fiber tear that results in a loss of strength and pain
  - Severe: A tear across the entire muscle or tendon

### GENERAL PREVENTION
- Stretching the hamstrings while muscles are fatigued
- Anaerobic interval training
- Sport-specific training drills (2)

### EPIDEMIOLOGY
- Common in athletes, especially those who sprint or jump
- 12% of the injuries in professional football players (3,4)
- 34% of injuries have a later recurrence.

### RISK FACTORS
- Age
- Low muscular strength
- Previous hamstring injury
- Tight hamstrings

### PATHOPHYSIOLOGY
- The hamstring muscles are the biceps femoris, the semitendinosus, and the semimembranosus muscles.
  - All 3 arise from the ischial tuberosity and extend in the posterior aspect of the thigh and cross the knee.
  - The biceps femoris also has a short head that inserts into the femur.
  - The hamstring muscles contract eccentrically to absorb kinetic energy during gait.
  - Muscle strain most commonly occurs at the proximal musculotendinous junction of the biceps femoris (5).
- Children and adolescents may avulse the bone at the hamstring origin, resulting in an ischial fracture.
- Adults may avulse the tendon.

### ETIOLOGY
- Predisposing factors:
  - Poor flexibility
  - Inadequate warm-up
  - Fatigue
  - Dehydration
  - Deficiency in the reciprocal actions of opposing muscle groups
  - Strength imbalance between the quadriceps and hamstring muscles
- Movements that commonly result in strain:
  - Flexing the leading hip during a hurdle
  - Sprinting out of the start-up blocks
  - Charging by a football lineman
  - Take-off by a jumper
  - Water-skiing falls

### ASSOCIATED CONDITIONS
- Back strain
- Groin strain

## DIAGNOSIS

### SIGNS AND SYMPTOMS
#### *History*
- The patient has a sudden onset of pain and tenderness in the posterior thigh.
- 10% of patients have an insidious onset of pain.
- With more severe strains, a pop may be felt, with an immediate loss of function.

#### *Physical Exam*
- Look for tenderness and swelling in the posterior thigh over one of the hamstring muscles.
- Bruising or hematoma may be visible in the posterior thigh.
- Look for pain on resisted knee flexion or hip extension.

### TESTS
#### *Pathological Findings*
This symptom complex may represent a partial or a complete tear of one of the hamstring muscles (biceps, semitendinosus, or semimembranosus).

#### *Imaging*
- Imaging usually is not indicated if the diagnosis is straightforward.
- Radiography:
  - Radiographs of the pelvis may show an ischial avulsion in a young athlete.
  - Radiographs of the knee may show a fibular avulsion if the symptoms are in this area.
  - Plain radiographs of the femur may be helpful if a fracture is suspected.
- MRI:
  - Can differentiate a stress fracture from a hamstring strain.
  - Can show the location and extent of the muscle tear.
    - Bone scintigraphy can differentiate a stress fracture from a hamstring strain.

### DIFFERENTIAL DIAGNOSIS
- Acute fracture
- Stress fracture
- Muscle contusion

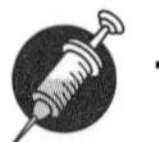

## TREATMENT

### GENERAL MEASURES
- Acute (1st week after injury):
  - RICE protocol
  - Early gentle motion
- Subacute (up to 3 weeks):
  - After inflammation resolves, concentric strength exercises should begin with cross-training.
- Remodeling phase (2–6 weeks):
  - More aggressive stretching (6)
  - Eccentric strengthening
  - Progressive agility and trunk stabilization exercises (7)
- Functional stage (up to 6 months):
  - Gentle return to running and sports activities when the patient is pain free
- Competitive phase:
  - Focus on prevention, strengthening, and stretching (1)

#### *Activity*
Rest, return to activity gradually as tolerated

### SPECIAL THERAPY
#### *Physical Therapy*
- Ice massage and ultrasound are advised after swelling is controlled.
- Exercise in water may help ROM.
- The patient may begin active ROM followed by knee curls and extensions once soreness is resolved.

### MEDICATION (DRUGS)
#### *First Line*
- NSAIDs: Ibuprofen, Naprosyn, COX-2 inhibitors:
  - Not shown to improve outcome, but help symptoms

#### *Second Line*
Acetaminophen for analgesia

### SURGERY
- Surgery is not indicated for musculotendinous junction injuries.
- Ischial avulsion fractures:
  - >2 cm displacement: May be considered for internal fixation (8)
  - >2 cm displacement can lead to a symptomatic nonunion.
- Tendinous avulsions may be considered for operative repair.

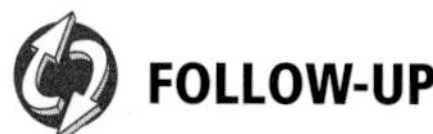

# FOLLOW-UP

## DISPOSITION

### *Issues for Referral*

Evidence of complete tendinous avulsion or rupture should lead to referral to an orthopaedic sports-medicine specialist.

## PROGNOSIS

- Mild strains heal in a few days to a week.
- Moderate strains heal in 1–3 weeks.
- Severe strains involving avulsion fractures at the ischial tuberosity or fibular head may take a month or more to heal.

## COMPLICATIONS

- Patients with a hamstring strain are at high risk for recurrent strain.
- Patients with ischial avulsion fractures with substantial displacement are at risk for chronic symptomatic nonunion.

## PATIENT MONITORING

Patients with hamstring strain must continue an active program of stretching and strengthening to prevent additional injury.

## REFERENCES


1. Petersen J, Holmich P. Evidence based prevention of hamstring injuries in sport. *Br J Sports Med* 2005;39:319–323.
2. Verrall GM, Slavotinek JP, Barnes PG. The effect of sports specific training on reducing the incidence of hamstring injuries in professional Australian Rules football players. *Br J Sports Med* 2005;39:363–368.
3. Orchard J, Seward H. Epidemiology of injuries in the Australian Football League, seasons 1997–2000. *Br J Sports Med* 2002;36:39–44.
4. Woods C, Hawkins RD, Maltby S, et al. The Football Association Medical Research Programme: an audit of injuries in professional football—analysis of hamstring injuries. *Br J Sports Med* 2004;38:36–41.
5. Koulouris G, Connell D. Evaluation of the hamstring muscle complex following acute injury. *Skeletal Radiol* 2003;32:582–589.
6. Malliaropoulos N, Papalexandris S, Papalada A, et al. The role of stretching in rehabilitation of hamstring injuries: 80 athletes follow-up. *Med Sci Sports Exerc* 2004;36:756–759.
7. Sherry MA, Best TM. A comparison of 2 rehabilitation programs in the treatment of acute hamstring strains. *J Orthop Sports Phys Ther* 2004;34:116–125.
8. Wootton JR, Cross MJ, Holt KWG. Avulsion of the ischial apophysis. The case for open reduction and internal fixation. *J Bone Joint Surg* 1990;72B: 625–627.


## ADDITIONAL READING


- Almekinders LC. Muscle pathophysiology. In Arendt EA, ed. *Orthopaedic Knowledge Update. Sports Medicine 2.* Rosemont, IL: American Academy of Orthopaedic Surgeons, 1999:37–42.
- Bull RC. *Handbook of Sports Injuries.* New York: McGraw-Hill, 1999.
- Goitz HT, Johnsen SDS, Armstrong LJ. The torso, pelvis, hip, and thigh. In: Perrin DH, ed. *The Injured Athlete,* 3rd ed. Philadelphia: Lippincott–Raven, 1999:329–351.


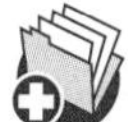

# MISCELLANEOUS

## CODES

### *ICD9-CM*

843.8, 843.9 Sprain or strain of hip and thigh

## PATIENT TEACHING

- Explain the importance of hamstring stretch before activity.
- Explain the importance of maintaining strength in these muscles as well as the quadriceps.

### *Activity*

Patients are prone to reinjury.

### *Prevention*

- Stretching, strengthening
- Hydration
- Proper training
- Team-wide prevention with stretching and strengthening, especially in high-risk sports

## FAQ

- Q: Ice or heat?
  - A: Neither is shown to decrease time to return to sport. Ice is recommended after activity and in the early days after injury. Heat is recommended before activity to help loosen muscles.
- Q: Who is most prone to hamstring strains?
  - A: Patients with a history of previous strains who are involved in sports are most susceptible. These patients must actively follow a program of stretching and strengthening to prevent reinjury.

H

# HAND ANATOMY AND EXAMINATION

*John J. Hwang, MD*
*Dawn M. LaPorte, MD*

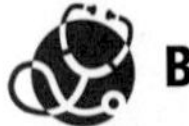

## BASICS

### DESCRIPTION

- The hand is a unique organ that allows humans to work and to create.
- The hand can be conveniently divided into the palmar (volar) and dorsal parts.
- The volar portion of the hand contains the major digital nerves, the flexor tendons, and the muscles that allow finger movement.
- The bony architecture is complex: The distal surface of the radius (the major portion of the wrist); 8 carpal bones; 5 metacarpals; 3 phalanges for each of the fingers; and a proximal and distal phalanx for the thumb.

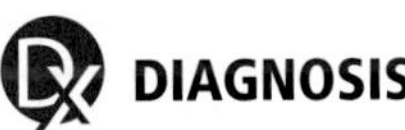

## DIAGNOSIS

### SIGNS AND SYMPTOMS

#### *Physical Exam*

- General considerations:
  - Examination of the hand is extremely complex.
  - It is essential to understand the anatomy and biomechanics of the hand.
  - An examiner should have his or her own system of examining the key components of hand anatomy and function.
- Vascular assessment:
  - Palpate the radial and ulnar arteries (Doppler examination as needed).
  - Examine the digital arteries using a Doppler technique.
  - Check the capillary refill in each finger (should be <2 sec).
  - Some hand surgeons examine individual digits by measuring the temperature of fingers and by placing a pulse oximeter to measure oxygen saturation.
  - Perform the Allen test (1) to check the competence of the palmar arch:
    - Press firmly on radial and ulnar arteries and have the patient open and close the fingers actively several times.
    - Take pressure off 1 artery and observe for vascular refill in the digits within 15 seconds. (A slow or absent refill suggests vascular obstruction or an incomplete arch.)
- Neurologic assessment:
  - Check the median nerve.
    - Examine the sensation on the volar tip of the thumb.
    - Perform a 2-point examination (normal: <5 mm).
    - Ask the patient to appose the thumb to the little finger to test the motor function of the median nerve.
  - Check ulnar nerve.
    - Examine the sensation on the volar tip of the little finger.
    - Ask the patient to cross the fingers (the motor branches of the ulnar nerve innervate the intrinsic muscles of the hand) to test the motor function of the ulnar nerve.
  - Check radial nerve.
    - The radial nerve has no motor branch in the hand.
    - The sensation of the radial nerve is tested on the dorsal aspect of the hand in the first web space.
- Assessment of bones, tendons, and ligaments:
  - Each bone is palpated to rule out a fracture.
  - Swelling can be variable.
  - Check each joint for active and passive ROM (2):
    - IP thumb joint: Normal ROM, 0–80°
    - MCP thumb joint: Normal ROM, 0–50°
    - DIP and MCP finger joints: Normal ROM, 0–90°
    - PIP finger joints: Normal ROM, 0–100°
    - Wrist: Normal values, 80° of flexion and 70° of extension

### TESTS

- Tinel sign:
  - Percussion over the median nerve at the wrist produces numbness, tingling, and pain in the thumb and index and middle fingers.
  - Test for CTS.
- Phalen test:
  - Flexion of the wrist completely for 1 min produces numbness, tingling, and pain in the hand.
  - Test for CTS.
- Aspiration of the wrist joint (2 approaches):
  - Dorsal approach: Insert a needle between the 3rd compartment (extensor pollicis longus) and the 4th compartment (extensor digitorum communis and extensor indicis proprius).
  - Palpate the Lister tubercle (bony prominence in distal radius) and introduce the needle just distal to it; flexing the wrist facilitates entry.
- Finkelstein test:
  - Passive hyperflexion of thumb MCP and IP joints (thumb in fist) with ulnar deviation of wrist causes pain over abductor pollicis longus and extensor pollicis brevis.
  - Test for de Quervain tenosynovitis.
- Grind test:
  - Hold the proximal phalanx and the MCP joint and forcefully push against the trapeziometacarpal joint.
  - Pain during this maneuver is consistent with arthritis in the trapeziometacarpal joint.

#### *Imaging*

AP, lateral, and oblique radiographs should be obtained as the 1st step in imaging.

### REFERENCES

1. Trumble TE. Anatomy and examination of the hand. In: Trumble TE, ed. *Principles of Hand Surgery and Therapy.* Philadelphia: WB Saunders, 2000:1–18.
2. Hoppenfeld S. Physical examination of the wrist and hand. In: *Physical Examination of the Spine & Extremities.* Norwalk, CT: Appleton & Lange, 1976: 59–104.

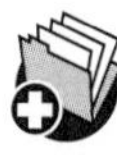

## MISCELLANEOUS

### FAQ

- Q: What structures run through the carpal canal? What is released in carpal tunnel surgery?
  - A: The long finger flexors and the median nerve are contained in the carpal canal. The transverse carpal ligament, which forms the roof of the carpal tunnel, is released during carpal tunnel surgery.
- Q: What ligament injury predisposes to a dorsal intercalated segment instability deformity and/or a wrist with a scapholunate dissociation advanced collapse pattern of arthritis?
  - A: The scapholunate ligament, when injured, causes a diastasis of the scaphoid and lunate, a resultant dorsal intercalated segment instability deformity, and likely a wrist with scapholunate dissociation advanced collapse.

H

# HEEL PAIN (PLANTAR FASCIITIS)

*Dhruv B. Pateder, MD*

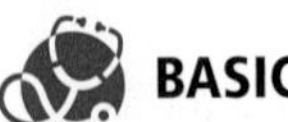

## BASICS

### DESCRIPTION

- Plantar fasciitis is the most common cause of plantar heel pain.
- Other causes include:
  - Compression of the 1st branch of the LPN
  - Fat pad atrophy of the heel
  - Pain and enthesopathy associated with seronegative spondyloarthropathies
  - Tarsal tunnel syndrome
  - Calcaneal stress fracture

#### *Geriatric Considerations*

Plantar heel pain in geriatric patients often is secondary to atrophy of the heel pad or degenerative changes of the plantar fascia origin.

#### *Pediatric Considerations*

- Heel pain in pediatric patients usually is secondary to apophysitis of the calcaneus (Sever disease), a self-limited condition related to tension of the insertion area of the Achilles tendon.
- It usually responds to rest, NSAIDs, restriction from running or sports, and short-term immobilization with a cast.
- It virtually always resolves once skeletal maturity is achieved, resulting in fusion of the calcaneal apophysis.

#### *Pregnancy Considerations*

- Heel pain often is secondary to plantar fasciitis or enthesopathy from hormonal changes or mechanical stress secondary to weight gain during pregnancy.
- It also can occur from nerve compression of the tarsal tunnel or 1st branch of the LPN because of increased fluid retention.
- It often improves once pregnancy ends.

### GENERAL PREVENTION

The condition is not always preventable, but it may be limited by avoiding excessive weight gain, prolonged standing, and sudden increases in running or jumping stresses.

### EPIDEMIOLOGY

#### *Incidence*

- Extremely common in adults
- Most common in the 3rd to 5th decades

### RISK FACTORS

- Decreased ankle dorsiflexion/tight heel cord
- Obesity/body mass index >30
- Prolonged standing
- Running
- Jumping sports
- Lupus or inflammatory spondyloarthropathy
- Diabetes
- Thyroid dysfunction

### ETIOLOGY

- The term "fasciitis" represents a misnomer; fasciitis is a degenerative condition without histologic evidence of chronic inflammation (Fig. 1).
- May have repetitive contracture and adhesions of the plantar fascia, with painful microscopic tearing with daily activity

### ASSOCIATED CONDITIONS

- Flatfoot
- Achilles contracture or tight heel cord
- Inflammatory arthropathies
- Obesity
- Cavus foot that results in contracture of plantar fascia and plantar soft tissues

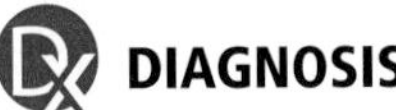

## DIAGNOSIS

### SIGNS AND SYMPTOMS

#### *History*

- Plantar fasciitis commonly is diagnosed with the history and physical examination.
- Patients commonly complain of heel pain that is worse in the morning with the "1st step" or after prolonged sitting.
- Symptoms may ease as the person walks and "loosens up."
- Symptoms may worsen as the day progresses.
- Pain is described as sore, aching, burning, or stabbing.

#### *Physical Exam*

- Assess alignment for planus or cavus foot deformity.
- Assess ankle dorsiflexion with the knee flexed and extended to rule out contracture of Achilles tendon or gastrocnemius.
- Palpate to localize tenderness to the plantar-medial heel at the origin of the plantar fascia.
- Tenderness may worsen with the toes passively dorsiflexed by the examiner, a maneuver that stretches the plantar fascia.
- Palpate and percuss (Tinel sign) over the tarsal tunnel and 1st branch of the LPN deep to the abductor hallucis muscle to identify nerve compression.
- Pain central and directly plantar under the calcaneal tuberosity, along with thinning of the heel pad, may indicate fat pad atrophy.
- Medial-lateral compression may be suggestive of calcaneal stress fracture.

### TESTS

#### *Lab*

- Chronic cases may necessitate lab tests, including rheumatoid factor, antinuclear antibody screen, thyroid function, blood glucose and hemoglobin A1C levels.
- HLA-B27 determination may be obtained if spondyloarthropathy is suspected.

#### *Imaging*

- Radiography:
  - Standing radiographs of the foot should be obtained for patients with persistent pain.
  - The presence of a heel spur at the calcaneal tuberosity is not diagnostic; the spur is located within the flexor hallucis brevis muscle rather than the plantar fascia.
  - In addition, the literature reports a high incidence of spur in asymptomatic patients.
- Bone scans may show increased uptake at the origin of the plantar fascia; more diffuse uptake may indicate calcaneal stress fracture.
- MRI:
  - May show thickening and degenerative changes of the plantar fascia origin, along with bony edema adjacent to it.
  - In calcaneal stress fracture, MRI shows more extensive bony edema.

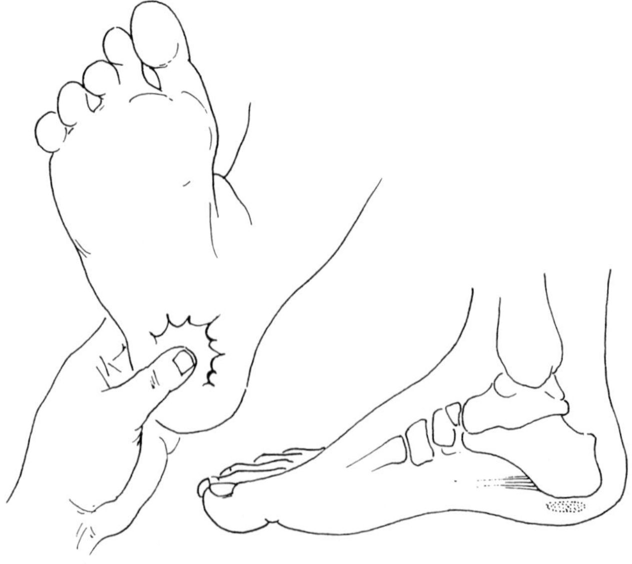

**Fig. 1.** In a patient with plantar fasciitis, the area of tenderness is in the insertion of the plantar fascia into the calcaneus.

### *Pathological Findings*

- Chronic degeneration is noted at the plantar fascia origin.
- Usually no evidence of inflammation is present.

## DIFFERENTIAL DIAGNOSIS

- Calcaneal apophysitis (Sever disease) in children
- Calcaneal stress fracture
- Central heel pad atrophy
- Tarsal tunnel syndrome or entrapment of the 1st branch of LPN
- Inflammatory enthesopathy
- Spinal radiculopathy

# TREATMENT

## GENERAL MEASURES

- Nonoperative treatment is the cornerstone for this problem, and surgery rarely is indicated.
- Stretching exercises of the heel cord should be performed multiple times daily and before and after sports.
- NSAIDs
- Off-the-shelf gel heel pad or wedge may improve cushioning of the heel.
- A dorsiflexion night splint has been shown to alleviate symptoms in chronic cases (1).
- An orthotic arch support may be indicated if the patient has pes planus.
- Deep tissue massage and ice application may help symptoms.
- Immobilization in a walking cast or fracture boot may rest the plantar fascia.
- Injections into the plantar fascia origin can be administered if the pain does not respond to other measures.
  - The patient should be immobilized for 1–2 weeks in a boot or cast to prevent rupture after injection.
- After successful treatment, the patient may be allowed to resume activities gradually, taking care not to resume running or jumping sports too quickly or too strenuously.
- Extracorporeal shock-wave treatment shows promise in the treatment of recalcitrant plantar fasciitis
  - Success rates of ~80%, with low complications (2)
  - May prove to be an alternative or last resort before surgical treatment (2)
- A calcaneal stress fracture or apophysitis (Sever disease) usually responds to rest, restriction from sports, NSAIDs, and short-term immobilization for severe symptoms.
- Heel pad atrophy is treated with a comfortable shoe with absorptive heel cushioning or off-the-shelf gel cushion.

## SPECIAL THERAPY

### *Physical Therapy*

Physical therapy may be helpful in teaching patients to stretch and in supervising their return to physical activity.

## MEDICATION (DRUGS)

NSAIDs are useful for patients with severe pain.

## SURGERY

- Indicated only after nonoperative methods have failed for at least 6–9 months
- Consists of partial release of plantar fascia origin
  - Some authors recommend removal of a bone spur, although most believe doing so is not necessary in most cases.
- For resistant tarsal tunnel syndrome or entrapment of the 1st branch of the LPN, decompression of the nerve is indicated at the time of partial plantar fascia release (3).
- Contraindicated in patients with Sever disease.

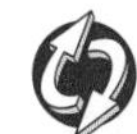

# FOLLOW-UP

## PROGNOSIS

>90% of cases respond to nonoperative treatments, with generally good prognosis for return to activities (4).

## COMPLICATIONS

Rupture of the plantar fascia after a steroid injection or excessive (total) surgical release can result in arch collapse and painful mechanical overload of the lateral midfoot (5).

## REFERENCES


1. Wapner KL, Sharkey PF. The use of night splints for treatment of recalcitrant plantar fasciitis. *Foot Ankle* 1991;12:135–137.
2. Ogden JA, Alvarez RG, Marlow M. Shockwave therapy for chronic proximal plantar fasciitis: a meta-analysis. *Foot Ankle Int* 2002;23:301–308.
3. Baxter DE, Pfeffer GB. Treatment of chronic heel pain by surgical release of the first branch of the lateral plantar nerve. *Clin Orthop Relat Res* 1992;279:229–236.
4. Gill LH. Plantar fasciitis: diagnosis and conservative management. *J Am Acad Orthop Surg* 1997;5:109–117.
5. Acevedo JI, Beskin JL. Complications of plantar fascia rupture associated with corticosteroid injection. *Foot Ankle Int* 1998;19:91–97.


## ADDITIONAL READING


- Pfeffer GB. Plantar heel pain. In: Myerson MS, ed. *Foot and Ankle Disorders*. Philadelphia: WB Saunders, 2000:834–850.
- Riddle DL, Pulisic M, Pidcoe P, et al. Risk factors for plantar fasciitis: a matched case-control study. *J Bone Joint Surg* 2003;85A:872–877.


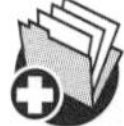

# MISCELLANEOUS

## CODES

### *ICD9-CM*

355.5 Tarsal tunnel syndrome
355.8 First branch lateral plantar nerve entrapment
726.73 Heel pain
728.71 Plantar fasciitis
732.5 Sever's disease/apophysitis
733.95 Calcaneal stress fracture

## PATIENT TEACHING

- Instruct the patient about the anatomy of the plantar fascia and its role in stabilizing the foot.
- Review the pathophysiology and degenerative nature of this condition, with its tendency for recurrent episodes.
- Remind the patient about the importance of stretching and of moderation during a return to sports.
- Reassure patients that, in most cases, this condition is self-limited.

## FAQ

- Q: What is the most common cause of heel pain in children?
  - A: Sever disease, or apophysitis of the calcaneus at the insertion of the Achilles tendon. This self-limited condition resolves once the apophysis fuses to the remainder of the calcaneus at skeletal maturity.
- Q: What is the pathophysiology of plantar fasciitis?
  - A: This condition is degenerative rather than inflammatory. Microscopic tears and adhesions of the plantar fascia result in pain with weight bearing activity.
- Q: When is surgery indicated for plantar fasciitis?
  - A: Only after a trial of nonsurgical methods for 6–9 months has failed.

# HEEL SORES

*Gregory Gebauer, MD, MS*

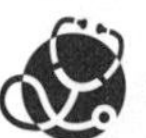

## BASICS

### DESCRIPTION
- Heel sores occur when the skin over the heel breaks down because of pressure.
- Generally caused by prolonged lying in bed, as in patients in intensive care units or nonambulatory bedridden individuals
- Also can occur in a patient in a lower extremity cast
- Classification (1) by depth is used most commonly.
  - Stage I: Nonblanchable erythema of the skin, intact epidermis
  - Stage II: Partial-thickness skin loss involving the epidermis and possibly the dermis; may involve cracking or blistering of the skin
  - Stage III: Full-thickness skin loss extending to but not through the fascia
  - Stage IV: Extensive full-thickness ulceration extending to bone, tendon, or other deep structures
- Synonyms: Bedsores; Heel or foot ulcers

#### *Geriatric Considerations*
Geriatric patients are at high risk for heel sores because of their thinner skin and their higher probability of being immobilized in bed.

### GENERAL PREVENTION
- Instruct patients and nursing staff to prevent progression of early partial-thickness lesions.
- Avoid prolonged periods of recumbency in the same position.
  - Bed-bound patients should be repositioned frequently and have their heels elevated off the bed.
- Do not allow patients in casts to rest on their heels for lengthy periods.

### EPIDEMIOLOGY
- One of the most common complications in the postoperative or rehabilitative setting
- More common in elderly or debilitated patients

#### *Incidence*
In hospitalized patients, the incidence of heel ulcers is reported to be up to 18% (2,3).

### RISK FACTORS
- Diabetes mellitus
- Lower extremity neuropathy
- Lower extremity vascular disease
- Poor nutrition
- Nonambulatory
- Bed-bound status

### ETIOLOGY (2,4,5)
- Direct pressure from the weight of the foot and shear forces from movement create trauma to the heel's capillary bed and small vessels, which can lead to local ischemia and tissue necrosis.
- These sores generally occur in patients who have limited mobility, neuropathic skin, vascular disease, or diabetes.
- They also can occur in postoperative patients with limited mobility who are bed-bound and are subjected to prolonged pressure over the heels.
- They may occur in patients with casts because of excess pressure or decreased padding.

### ASSOCIATED CONDITIONS
- Paralysis
- Diabetes mellitus
- Loss of sensation/neuropathy
- Contracture

## DIAGNOSIS

#### *History*
- Initially presents as pain and softening over the heel region
- May occur without the warning symptom of pain in the patient with decreased or impaired sensation
- Particular attention should be paid to at-risk individuals, including immobilized patients or those with predisposing risk factors.

#### *Physical Exam*
- The skin over the heel should be inspected for changes, including signs of early alteration (erythema) or more progressive injury (cracks, ulcers, and skin breakdown).
- The heel may be tender to palpation, even if no obvious skin changes are present.
  - A dark purple or red lesion that does not blanch with pressure is a sign that breakdown will occur eventually.
- More advanced lesions will have increasing levels of damage, including exposure of tendon and bone in stage IV lesions.
- The wound should be inspected for surrounding cellulitis and purulent drainage.
- Pain with ROM of the foot or ankle joints may suggest joint involvement and septic arthritis.
- A thorough motor and sensory examination should be performed.

### TESTS

#### *Lab*
- If the wound appears infected, check the complete blood count, differential, ESR, and C-reactive protein.
- If poor nutrition is suspected, albumin and prealbumin levels should be checked.

#### *Imaging*
- Radiography:
  - Routine AP and lateral foot and ankle films are helpful in distinguishing bone destruction and osteomyelitis.
  - Superficial soft-tissue breakdown may show no radiographic change.
- Suspected osteomyelitis should be evaluated with MRI and/or tagged white-blood cell nuclear medicine imaging.

#### *Diagnostic Procedures/Surgery*
- Areas of necrotic tissue should be débrided to enhance healing and to determine the full extent of the ulceration.
- Progression of these ulcerations to osteomyelitis and systemic infection may necessitate more aggressive débridement or amputation.

#### *Pathological Findings*
- Heel sores are caused primarily by ischemia from prolonged pressure over the heel.
- As the ischemia and pressure persist, the skin and soft tissues overlying the heel become necrotic, break down, and ulcerate.
- In chronically debilitated and diabetic patients, these lesions easily become infected and can eventually result in osteomyelitis or septic arthritis.

### DIFFERENTIAL DIAGNOSIS
- Osteomyelitis
- Soft-tissue abscess
- Cellulitis
- Fracture
- Septic arthritis

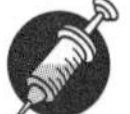

# TREATMENT

## GENERAL MEASURES (4)

- Prevention is key: At-risk patients must be instructed in meticulous foot care and shoe selection.
  - Bed-bound patients need good heel padding and frequent turning.
- Patients with diabetes or neuropathy should wear appropriate shoes and perform daily inspection of the feet.
- Treatment should be initiated at the earliest signs of skin breakdown.
- Superficial heel sores generally respond to pressure relief and padding over the affected area.
- Deeper ulcerations generally require surgical débridement and may require removal of infected bone or partial amputation.
- Broad-spectrum antibiotics are indicated for infected ulcers.
  - Such infections often are polymicrobial, including aerobic, anaerobic, and Gram-negative species.
- Patients in casts complaining of heel pain should have the cast removed to assess the skin adequately.

### *Nursing*

- The nursing staff is critical to the prevention of heel ulceration.
  - Prevention is assisted by changing patient position and removing pressure from the heels.
  - The presence of heel ulcers should be identified and conveyed to physician staff for treatment.

## SPECIAL THERAPY

### *Physical Therapy*

- Whirlpool therapy to débride necrotic tissue may be helpful.
- Physical therapists can be integral in monitoring for pressure relief.

## MEDICATION (DRUGS)

Antibiotics with broad-spectrum coverage are required to manage the polymicrobial infections associated with these types of foot ulceration.

## SURGERY

- Generally, soft-tissue débridement of the affected tissues is indicated.
- This débridement usually can be done in an outpatient or clinic setting.
- Extensive necrotic tissue or the presence of osteomyelitis may require formal surgical débridement in the operating room.

# FOLLOW-UP

## DISPOSITION

### *Issues for Referral*

- Because poor nutrition may contribute to the formation of ulcers and may inhibit healing, a nutrition consultation should be considered.
- Consulting a wound care specialist also may be helpful.

## PROGNOSIS

- Stage I and Stage II ulcers have a good prognosis.
- Stage III and Stage IV ulcers have a poorer prognosis.
- Prognosis also depends on the severity of underlying disease, patient age (younger is better), presence of deep infection, activity level (e.g., bedridden), and nutritional deficit.

## COMPLICATIONS

- Osteomyelitis
- Septic arthritis

## PATIENT MONITORING

Heel ulcers should be monitored closely because patients are at high risk for disease progression if the ulcer is not treated aggressively.

## REFERENCES

1. Maklebust J. Pressure ulcer assessment. *Clin Geriatr Med* 1997;13:455–481.
2. Wong VK, Stotts NA. Physiology and prevention of heel ulcers: the state of science. *J Wound Ostomy Continence Nurs* 2003;30:191–198.
3. Cuddigan J, Berlowitz DR, Ayello EA. Pressure ulcers in America: prevalence, incidence, and implications for the future: An executive summary of the National Pressure Ulcer Advisory Panel monograph. *Adv Skin Wound Care* 2001;14: 208–215.
4. Brem H, Lyder C. Protocol for the successful treatment of pressure ulcers. *Am J Surg* 2004;188:9S–17S.
5. Hampton S. The complexities of heel ulcers. *Nurs Stand* 2003;17:68–79.

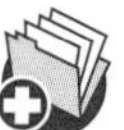

# MISCELLANEOUS

## CODES

### *ICD9-CM*

707.13 Decubitus ulcer of heel

## PATIENT TEACHING

Patients at risk for heel sores should be educated in foot care and shoe selection.

### *Prevention (2,4,5)*

- Prevention is key: Careful attention should be paid to the heels of at-risk patients, including those bed-bound, diabetic, neuropathic, and with casts.
- Bed-bound patients should be rotated frequently.
- Patients with early changes or heel pain should be treated aggressively with removal of pressure from the heels.
- Patients' heels should be well padded when casts are applied.

## FAQ

- Q: What can be done to prevent heel ulcers?
  - A: Heel position should be changed frequently and patients should be monitored for early signs of ulceration.
- Q: Which patients are at risk for heel ulcers?
  - A: Patients who are bed-bound or who have a history of vascular disease, diabetes, or neuropathy are at high risk. People who have casts also are at increased risk.
- Q: What should be done for patients who have ulcers?
  - A: The pressure should be removed from the heel. Any necrotic tissue should be débrided. Patients with signs of infection should be treated aggressively with antibiotics. Deep ulcerations and infections may require surgical management.

# HEMANGIOMA

*Frank J. Frassica, MD*

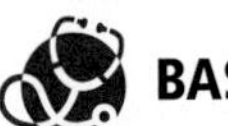

## BASICS

### DESCRIPTION
- This benign tumor of vascular origin usually affects the skeletal system, but it also may occur in the soft tissues (1,2).
- Found in all age groups, this tumor most commonly is diagnosed in the middle decades of life.

### EPIDEMIOLOGY
#### *Incidence*
This tumor is uncommon.

#### *Prevalence*
No substantial gender difference has been noted.

### RISK FACTORS
None are known.

#### *Genetics*
No known correlation exists.

### ETIOLOGY
- The cause is unknown.
- Hemangioma is considered a benign lesion without metastatic potential.
- Many pathologists consider it a hamartoma, rather than a true neoplasm.

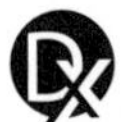

## DIAGNOSIS

### SIGNS AND SYMPTOMS
- It may present with local pain and swelling of insidious onset and indolent progression.
- Soft-tissue hemangioma often presents without pain but with intermittent swelling.
- Occasionally, pathologic fracture may be the initial presentation.
- Hemangioma in the vertebra may lead to vertebral collapse, with local pain and neurologic findings.

#### *Physical Exam*
- When palpated, soft-tissue hemangiomas have a fluctuant or springy feel.
  - They are composed of a large number of blood vessels, which compress when palpated and then refill with blood.
- Hemangiomas often increase in size when the limb is placed in the dependant position.

### TESTS
#### *Lab*
No diagnostic serum tests

#### *Imaging*
- Soft tissue:
  - Lesions in the soft tissue may erode the adjacent bone and may show characteristic "phleboliths" on radiographs.
    - These lesions are easily confused with a variety of other lesions.
  - Soft-tissue hemangiomas are best imaged with gadolinium contrast-enhanced MRI.
    - Round, vascular channels that have a serpiginous shape and that enhance
    - Contain large amounts of fat
- Bone:
  - Lesions frequently are multiple, expansile, and trabeculated and show little periosteal reaction.
  - The typical radiographic appearance is osteopenia, with parallel vertical streaks described as a "corduroy cloth" appearance.
  - The radiographic appearance is variable, from "soap bubble" to purely lytic appearance.
  - Multiple lesions and the lack of periosteal reaction may provide clues to the diagnosis.

#### *Pathological Findings*
- Tumors are grossly bloody and traversed by bony trabeculae.
- Microscopically, conglomerates of thin-walled capillaries filled with red cells typically are seen.
- Lymphatics also may be prominent.

### DIFFERENTIAL DIAGNOSIS
- Myeloma
- Infection
- Bone cyst
- Malignant primary bone neoplasm
- Metastatic disease

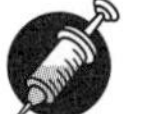

## TREATMENT

### GENERAL MEASURES

- Soft-tissue hemangiomas can recur after surgical excision.
- Surgery should be avoided when possible.
- Compressive dressings can aid in nonoperative treatment.
- Sclerosing therapy (using alcohol) is the preferred method of treatment.
- Hemangiomas of bone seldom need surgical treatment.

### SPECIAL THERAPY

#### *Physical Therapy*

Not indicated.

### SURGERY

Surgery should be avoided unless biopsy is needed.

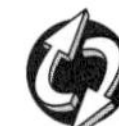

## FOLLOW-UP

### PROGNOSIS

- Good overall
- Recurrence not uncommon

### COMPLICATIONS

Pathologic fracture

### PATIENT MONITORING

- Patients with bone lesions seldom need treatment unless pathologic fracture occurs.
- Soft-tissue lesions are monitored with serial physical examinations and MRI scans every 3–6 months.

### REFERENCES


1. McCarthy EF, Frassica FJ. Primary bone tumors. In: *Pathology of Bone and Joint Disorders: With Clinical and Radiographic Correlation*. Philadelphia: WB Saunders, 1998:195–275.
2. Weiss SW, Goldblum JR. Benign tumors and tumor-like lesions of blood vessels. In: Weiss SW, Goldblum JR, eds. *Enzinger and Weiss's Soft Tissue Tumors*, 4th ed. St. Louis: Mosby, 2001:837–890.


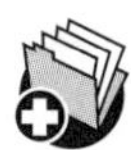

## MISCELLANEOUS

### CODES

#### *ICD9-CM*

228.0 Hemangioma

### PATIENT TEACHING

Patients with soft-tissue lesions are instructed to avoid provocative activities such as prolonged standing.

### FAQ

- Q: Is surgery necessary for soft-tissue hemangiomas?
  - A: Surgery usually is not necessary or effective. Local recurrence is common after surgical treatment.
- Q: Is a biopsy necessary to establish the diagnosis of intramuscular hemangioma?
  - A: Most intramuscular hemangiomas have characteristic features on MRI scan so that biopsy is not necessary to establish the diagnosis.

H

# HEMOPHILIA

*Paul D. Sponseller, MD*

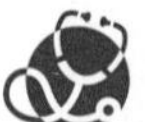

## BASICS

### DESCRIPTION
- This disorder of clotting factor results in easy bleeding.
- Secondary effects may occur in any system (most importantly brain, joint, muscle, and nerve) secondary to bleeding (1).
- Depending on its severity, it usually is diagnosed in early childhood.
- Classification (1–3):
  - Severe: <1% clotting factor activity
  - Moderate: 1–5% clotting factor activity
  - Mild: >5% clotting factor activity
- Synonyms: Hemophilia A (Classic Hemophilia [factor VIII deficiency]); Hemophilia B (Christmas Disease [factor IX deficiency])

### GENERAL PREVENTION
Prevent the development of "target joints" by a home maintenance program and by observing activity restrictions (1).

### EPIDEMIOLOGY
#### *Incidence*
- The combined incidence of hemophilia is ~1 per 10,000 population (1).
- Males are affected much more commonly than are females.

#### *Prevalence*
- 75% of this group have hemophilia A (4).
- 12% of this group have hemophilia B (4).
- The rest have rare deficiencies in other coagulation factors.

### RISK FACTORS
Positive family history

#### *Genetics*
Hemophilia A and B are both inherited as sex-linked recessive disorders, leading to the typical picture of multiple affected males on the maternal side of a family.

### ETIOLOGY
- Hemophilia A: Defect in gene for factor VIII
- Hemophilia B: Defect in gene for factor IX

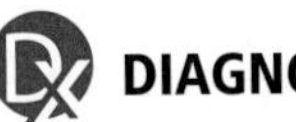

## DIAGNOSIS

### SIGNS AND SYMPTOMS
- In patients with severe hemophilia, failure to clot after circumcision, immunizations, or lip lacerations sustained in falls often brings the diagnosis to light.
- In persons affected more mildly, major cuts or surgery may be required to show the defect.
- Later problems include repeated episodes of bleeding in a joint or muscle, possibly with only mild trauma.
- The joints most affected include the knee, ankle, and elbow.
- Once a joint has sustained a bleeding episode, it is much more likely to be affected again; this is called a "target joint."
- The internal bleeding episodes are noted 1st because of pain, before swelling occurs.
- Muscle bleeding is noted because of swelling and nerve compression, most commonly affecting the psoas muscle and the femoral nerve.
- Repeated bleeding episodes eventually cause degenerative change, with stiffness and pain in a target joint over several years (2).

#### *Physical Exam*
- Check all major joints for effusion and ROM.
- Remember that knees, ankles, shoulders, and elbows are the joints most commonly involved.
- Note that the presence of an effusion in an ankle is heralded initially by obliteration of the "hollow" around the malleoli.
- In examining the knees, document the symmetry of flexion and the presence or absence of the normal hyperextension of 5–10°.
- Look for apparent enlargement of the joints, secondary to epiphyseal hypertrophy of hyperemia or atrophy of the surrounding muscles.
- Observe the patient's gait.
- Ask the patient to keep a log of joint bleeding to allow detection of a target joint.
- Look for any neurologic sequelae of bleeding, such as hemiparesis from a previous intracranial hemorrhage or neuropathy from a femoral or sciatic hemorrhage.

### TESTS
#### *Lab*
- Factor levels should be quantitated in terms of percentage of normal.
  - It takes a surprisingly small percentage of normal factor VIII (as little as 5–10%) to preserve normal clotting function.
- If factor levels do not rise with replacement as expected, an inhibitor should be suspected (1,3).
  - This inhibitor is an antibody to factor VIII and is a relative contraindication to any elective surgery.
- For all patients with hemophilia, the clinician should be aware of the status of the following:
  - Hepatitis
  - Inhibitor
  - HIV

#### *Pathological Findings*
- On gross examination of a hemophilic joint, the synovium is brown and appears velvety.
- The joint surface loses its luster and, with advanced disease, becomes eroded in rivet-like tracts.
- On light microscopy, the synovial lining of the joint is hypertrophic and hypervascular; the hypervascularity renders it more likely to bleed with additional trauma.
- Eventually, the synovium becomes fibrotic, thus accounting for the loss of motion.

#### *Imaging*
- Plain radiographs show the following sequence of changes in a hemophilic target joint (2):
  - 1: Soft-tissue swelling and osteopenia
  - 2: Epiphyseal enlargement, followed by joint space narrowing and irregularity
  - 3: Degenerative arthritis

### DIFFERENTIAL DIAGNOSIS
- von Willebrand disease
- PVNS
- Transient inhibitor of coagulation
- Thrombocytopenia

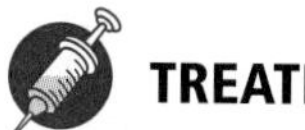

# TREATMENT

## GENERAL MEASURES

- For acute bleeding episodes:
  - Factor replacement
  - Rest and brief immobilization followed by ROM exercises
- Synovectomy for chronic hemarthropathy (1,5)
- Arthroplasty (or occasionally, arthrodesis) for painful end-stage joint disease (6,7)
- Factor replacement and observation for psoas bleeding causing femoral neurapraxia
- For compartment syndrome, decompression as in any other situation
- Home maintenance programs, which have shown benefit in terms of decreasing joint bleeding and damage:
  - Should be considered if the patient and family are capable of handling it
  - When a hemorrhage does occur, factor should be infused immediately.
  - If a large joint effusion develops, aspiration and irrigation should be considered, once adequate factor replacement has been achieved.
  - Rest and compression also should be recommended.

## MEDICAL TREATMENT

- Factor replacement
- Rest and brief immobilization
- Factor replacement and observation for a psoas hemorrhage causing femoral neurapraxia
- Decompression for compartment syndrome
- Discouragement of the use of salicylates and other NSAIDs, except acetaminophen

## SPECIAL THERAPY

### *Radiotherapy*

Synovectomy of target joints may be accomplished by injection of a radionuclide, which may decrease the frequency of bleeding episodes (5).

### *Physical Therapy*

- May assist in monitoring ROM in target joints
- Also indicated after a major bleeding episode or surgery

## MEDICATION (DRUGS)

### *First Line*

- Avoid use of NSAIDs for pain because their antiplatelet action may facilitate bleeding.
  - Disalcid and Tylenol are acceptable.
- When aspirating a hemarthrosis, instilling bupivacaine with epinephrine as well as corticosteroid may help to arrest the risk of rebleed and the joint inflammatory response.

## SURGERY

- Synovectomy (removal of hypertrophic synovial lining to decrease bleeding in target joints):
  - May be done through the arthroscope in some joints
  - May even be done nonsurgically, using injected radioisotopes in high-risk or juvenile patients
- Knee replacement arthroplasty involves replacement of joint surface with metal and plastic articulation to relieve pain.
- Ankle fusion can be done for end-stage degeneration in this joint.

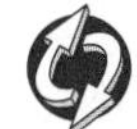

# FOLLOW-UP

## PROGNOSIS

Life expectancy may be diminished by catastrophic bleeding and infectious diseases.

## COMPLICATIONS

- Neurologic: Bleeding into the central nervous system or major peripheral nerves
- Joints: Stiffness, contracture, and arthritis
- Compartment syndrome
- Blood-borne infections

## PATIENT MONITORING

- Ideally, patients should be followed in a multidisciplinary fashion by specialists in hematology, orthopaedics or physical therapy, and dentistry.
- Social work may be helpful in obtaining needed services and medical coverage.

## REFERENCES


1. Luck JV, Jr, Silva M, Rodriguez-Merchan EC, et al. Hemophilic arthropathy. *J Am Acad Orthop Surg* 2004;12:234–245.
2. Arnold WD, Hilgartner MW. Hemophilic arthropathy. Current concepts of pathogenesis and management. *J Bone Joint Surg* 1977;59A: 287–305.
3. Hvid I, Rodriguez-Merchan EC. Orthopaedic surgery in haemophilic patients with inhibitors: an overview. *Haemophilia* 2002;8:288–291.
4. Cornwall R, Dormans JP. Diseases of the hematopoietic system. In: Morrissy RT, Weinstein SL, eds. *Lovell and Winter's Pediatric Orthopaedics*, 6th ed. Philadelphia: Lippincott Williams & Wilkins, 2006:357–404.
5. Siegel HJ, Luck JV, Jr, Siegel ME. Advances in radionuclide therapeutics in orthopaedics. *J Am Acad Orthop Surg* 2004;12:55–64.
6. Goddard NJ, Rodriguez-Merchan EC, Wiedel JD. Total knee replacement in haemophilia. *Haemophilia* 2002;8:382–386.
7. Kamineni S, Adams RA, O'Driscoll SW, et al. Hemophilic arthropathy of the elbow treated by total elbow replacement. A case series. *J Bone Joint Surg* 2004;86A:584–589.


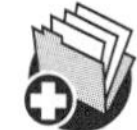

# MISCELLANEOUS

## CODES

### *ICD9-CM*

958.2 Hemophilia

## PATIENT TEACHING

- Stress sports restrictions, especially sports involving contact or twisting.
- Advise that the school be notified of the patient's sports restrictions.
- Encourage substitute pastimes.
- Offer genetic counseling early at diagnosis.

### *Prevention*

Consider a home maintenance program.

## FAQ

- Q: What is the role of synovectomy in arresting the progression to arthritis?
  - A: Synovectomy may decrease the frequency of bleeding episodes and slow the progression toward arthritis, but it does not totally arrest the process.

# HETEROTOPIC OSSIFICATION

*Constantine A. Demetracopoulos, BS*
*Frank J. Frassica, MD*

## BASICS

### DESCRIPTION
- Pathologic bone formation as a consequence of direct trauma or central nervous system injuries
- Bone formed in heterotopic locations such as muscle, subcutaneous tissues, or nerves
- Most commonly occurs at the hip, elbow, and shoulder joints (1).

### EPIDEMIOLOGY
Less common in children than in adults, and more common in males than in females (1)

#### *Incidence*
Occurs in 10–20% of patients with central nervous system or traumatic injuries, with an average onset of 2 months after injury (1).

### RISK FACTORS (2)
- Central nervous system injury
- Osteoarthrosis
- Osteophyte formation
- Surgical approach
- Previous surgical procedures
- Trochanteric osteotomy
- AS

#### *Genetics*
No genetic link can successfully predict patient susceptibility to heterotopic ossification.

### ETIOLOGY
- Traumatic brain injury
- Spinal cord injury
- Trauma

### ASSOCIATED CONDITIONS
- Fibrodysplasia ossificans progressiva
- Primary osteoma cutis

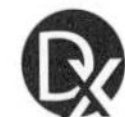

## DIAGNOSIS

### SIGNS AND SYMPTOMS
- Unexplained increase in pain, spasticity, or muscle guarding
- Decreased ROM
- Stiffness
- Radiographic evidence of ectopic bone

#### *Physical Exam*
- Limited ROM is the most common and earliest sign (1).
- Erythema, swelling, and signs of inflammation also may be noted.

### TESTS

#### *Lab*
- Serum alkaline phosphatase levels are elevated.
  - Value begins to rise 2–3 weeks after injury (1).
  - Although nonspecific and not absolute, elevated serum alkaline phosphatase may be the earliest test for detection.

#### *Imaging*
- On plain radiographs, new bone formation may be 1st visible at 3– 6 weeks; but radiographs generally are not confirmatory until 3 months.
- Bone scans allow for earlier detection and show intense uptake.
- CT may be used for preoperative planning and to show the zonal pattern: Mineralized in the periphery and lucent in the center.

#### *Pathological Findings*
- Initially, an intense inflammatory response occurs with myofibroblasts and osteoblasts.
- Such a high degree of cellular activity occurs that the inflammatory response can be mistaken for a neoplasm.

### DIFFERENTIAL DIAGNOSIS
- Septic joint
- Thrombophlebitis
- Neoplasm in the soft tissues

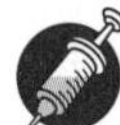

## TREATMENT

### GENERAL MEASURES
- Joint motion is maintained to allow normal functioning.
- Most patients are treated successfully with nonoperative measures, including physical therapy, analgesics, and NSAIDs.
- Few patients require surgical excision.

### SPECIAL THERAPY

#### *Radiotherapy*
- Radiation therapy is ineffective once heterotopic ossification has been documented.
  - When used for prophylaxis, it must be delivered within 72 hours (2).

#### *Physical Therapy*
Use ROM exercises and treatment modalities that are designed to increase joint mobility.

### MEDICATION (DRUGS)

#### *First Line*
- Anti-inflammatories are used to prevent or to lessen the amount of heterotopic ossification formation after the initial insult and to prevent recurrence after surgical excision.
  - Indomethacin, naproxen, or other NSAIDs for 6 weeks (3)

### SURGERY

- Surgery is indicated to restore joint motion or to correct contractures in disabled patients.
- Heterotopic ossification should not be resected earlier than 6 months after injury.
- Excision after 2 years increases the likelihood of permanent contractures.
- After resection of heterotopic ossification, patients are treated with low doses of irradiation (must be delivered within 72 hours) (2).
- Some patients elect to take NSAIDs (e.g., indomethacin) for 6 weeks after resection.
  - For effective prophylaxis, the medications must be taken.
  - Gastric intolerance prevents 10–20% of patients from taking these medications (3).

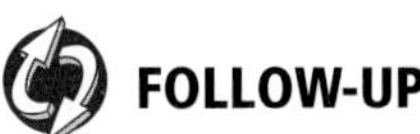

## FOLLOW-UP

### PROGNOSIS

- Prognosis varies, depending on the location of heterotopic ossification and its cause.
- Most patients with nonneurogenic heterotopic ossification maintain reasonable function and do not require surgical intervention.

### COMPLICATIONS

- Loss of mobility
- Ankylosis

### PATIENT MONITORING

Serial radiographs are obtained at 1–3-month intervals for 6 months.

### REFERENCES

1. Garland DE. A clinical perspective on common forms of acquired heterotopic ossification. *Clin Orthop Relat Res* 1991;263:13–29.
2. Ayers DC, Pellegrini VD Jr, Evarts CM. Prevention of heterotopic ossification in high-risk patients by radiation therapy. *Clin Orthop Relat Res* 1991;263: 87–93.
3. Kjaersgaard-Andersen P, Schmidt SA. Total hip arthroplasty. The role of antiinflammatory medications in the prevention of heterotopic ossification. *Clin Orthop Relat Res* 1991;263: 78–86.

### ADDITIONAL READING

- McCarthy EF, Sundaram M. Heterotopic ossification: a review. *Skeletal Radiol* 2005;34:609–619.
- Pape HC, Marsh S, Morley JR, et al. Current concepts in the development of heterotopic ossification. *J Bone Joint Surg* 2004;86B:783–787.

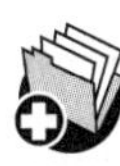

## MISCELLANEOUS

### CODES

#### *ICD9-CM*

728.89 Heterotopic ossification

### PATIENT TEACHING

- Joint motion should be encouraged.
- Immobilization is not recommended and can worsen the prognosis.

#### *Activity*

Patients are encouraged to use involved joints.

#### *Prevention*

Heterotopic ossification can be prevented in at-risk patients (e.g., trauma patients) with external beam irradiation or NSAIDs.

### FAQ

- Q: Which patients are at greatest risk for heterotopic ossification?
  - A: Patients who have substantial heterotopic ossification from a previous arthroplasty and patients who have AS (20–50% risk).
- Q: Why are patients with a neurologic injury, such as head or spinal trauma, at such high risk?
  - A: Patients with a severe closed head injury or a spinal cord injury have a high risk of heterotopic ossification of the hip, shoulder, and elbow. Unfortunately, the cause of the heterotopic bone formation is unknown.

# HIP ARTHRITIS

*Kris J. Alden, MD, PhD*
*Simon C. Mears, MD, PhD*

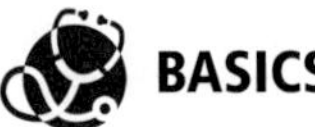

## BASICS

### DESCRIPTION

- Hip arthritis is caused by loss of the articular cartilage of the acetabulum and proximal femur.
- As the cartilage is lost, the subchondral bone of the proximal femur and the acetabulum rub, causing pain with ambulation, loss of motion, and disability.

### GENERAL PREVENTION

- Low-impact exercise (swimming, biking, walking)
- Activity modification
- Weight loss

### EPIDEMIOLOGY

- Hip arthritis is caused by loss of the articular cartilage of the acetabulum and proximal femur.
- Some hips are more susceptible to arthritis than others, which is thought to be secondary to subtle differences in hip alignment, such as hip dysplasia or femoroacetabular impingement.

#### *Prevalence*

It is estimated that 12% of the population in the United States suffers from arthritis (1,2).

### RISK FACTORS

- Trauma
- Osteonecrosis
- Infections
- Hemophilia
- Hip dysplasia
- Femoroacetabular impingement
- Perthes disease
- SCFE
- Inflammatory arthritis:
  - Rheumatoid arthritis
  - Systemic lupus erythematosus
  - Psoriatic arthritis

### ETIOLOGY

- The cause of primary osteoarthritis is unknown, but it is thought to be secondary to a combination of factors:
  - Differences in cartilage properties
  - Mechanical differences of alignment of the joint, such as hip dysplasia or femoroacetabular impingement (3,4)

### CLASSIFICATION

- Hip arthritis is classified broadly as:
  - Primary osteoarthritis
  - Inflammatory arthritis
  - Secondary osteoarthritis

### ASSOCIATED CONDITIONS

- Spine degenerative disc disease
- Knee arthritis

## DIAGNOSIS

### SIGNS AND SYMPTOMS

- Patients present with a diffuse ache over the hip.
- Classically, pain occurs in the anterior groin, often with radiation of pain to the buttock and knee, especially on the medial side.
- Occasionally, knee pain is the predominant symptom.
- Patients often describe limping and fatigue with walking.
- As patients lose ROM, they have difficulty tying their shoes and getting in and out of cars.

#### *History*

- Typically, the pain is gradual in onset, of long duration, and relieved by rest.
- Night pain or constant pain implies cancer or infection.
- Pain with activity is typical of hip arthritis.
- Primary osteoarthritis is a disorder of patients >50 years old.
- Hip arthritis in a young person is usually secondary to trauma, osteonecrosis, or developmental causes.

#### *Physical Exam*

- Assess the patient's ROM.
  - Loss of internal fixation is one of the earliest signs of hip arthritis.
  - Hip flexion also is limited.
- Check for flexion contracture, gait abnormalities, leg-length discrepancy, and muscle weakness.
- A resisted straight-leg raise (Stinchfield test) loads the joint and reproduces the pain.
- Palpate the greater trochanter to assess for trochanteric bursitis.
- Perform a careful neurologic examination and straight-leg-raise test to assess for radicular signs.
- Assess for leg-length discrepancy and pelvic tilt.
- Evaluate the spine for scoliosis or tenderness.

### TESTS

#### *Lab*

Rheumatologic screening tests should be ordered if one suspects inflammatory arthritis.

#### *Imaging*

- Plain radiographs (the 1st step):
  - An AP view of the pelvis and AP and lateral views of the involved hip to rule out fracture and assess joint space narrowing, osteophyte formation, sclerosis, and subchondral cysts
  - AP and lateral views of the lumbosacral spine if any suggestion of radiculopathy is present
- Special imaging:
  - Technetium bone scans to screen the entire body for occult bone disease in the presence of severe pain and no apparent areas of disease
  - MRI of the hip and pelvis:
    - An excellent modality for excluding bone and soft-tissue disease of the pelvis and hip
    - Ensure that the pathologic area is in the field of the scan.

#### *Diagnostic Procedures/Surgery*

Intra-articular injection of local anesthetic agents may be used as a test for diagnosing hip arthritis when the diagnosis is unclear.

### DIFFERENTIAL DIAGNOSIS

- The differential diagnosis is extensive:
  - Neoplasms:
    - Young patients (4–20 years old): Osteosarcoma, Ewing sarcoma
    - Patients >50 years old: Metastatic bone disease, multiple myeloma
  - Stress fractures of the femoral neck:
    - Runners and osteoporotic patients
  - Greater trochanteric bursitis:
    - Lateral hip pain
  - Radiculopathy:
    - Pain distal to the knee

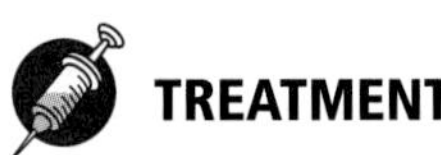

## TREATMENT

### GENERAL MEASURES

- Weight reduction and activity modification are the major general measures.
- Initial arthritis care begins with:
  - Activity modification and avoidance of provocative activities, such as running and heavy lifting
  - NSAIDs
  - Cortisone injection
  - Tylenol for patients with contraindications to NSAIDs
  - Cane support in the opposite hand
  - Weight reduction if appropriate

### SPECIAL THERAPY

#### *Physical Therapy*

- Patients are instructed on the use of a cane and on appropriate exercises to prevent contractures.
- Strengthening of the hip and leg muscles may help pain symptoms and strengthen the limb for later surgery (5).

### Complementary and Alternative Therapies

- Randomized trials have not been performed for many therapies.
- Alternative medicines with some evidence of effectiveness include:
  - Devil's claw (*Harpagophytum procumbens*) (6)
  - Avocado-soybean unsaponifiables (7)
  - Capsaicin cream (8)
  - Phytodolor (8)
- Little evidence exists for magnet or laser therapy.
- The role of acupuncture is unclear and therefore should not be performed in patients susceptible to infections.

## MEDICATION (DRUGS)

- Acetaminophen
- NSAIDs (3,9)
- Occasional intra-articular steroid injections
- Glucosamine

## SURGERY

- Surgery is indicated for patients for whom activity modification, NSAIDs, and other medical treatments have failed.
- Core decompression may be used for patients with osteonecrosis of the femoral head.
- Hip fusion may be indicated in young, active patients.
- In some young patients with acetabular or proximal femoral dysplasia, acetabular or proximal femoral osteotomy can be used to reduce the joint forces and improve cartilage physiology.
- Young patients with symptomatic femoroacetabular impingement may benefit from a femoral reshaping procedure.
- Total hip replacement is the main surgical procedure.

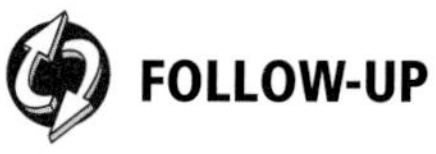

# FOLLOW-UP

## PROGNOSIS

- In patients with early arthritis, acetaminophen or NSAIDs may relieve all pain and substantially improve function.
- The prognosis after total hip replacement is excellent: Virtually all such patients attain pain relief, good motion, and functional improvement.

## COMPLICATIONS

- Complications of nonoperative care:
  - Hip stiffness
  - Leg-length discrepancy
  - Limp
  - Muscle weakness
  - Inability to ambulate
  - Pain
- Complications of total hip replacement:
  - Hip stiffness
  - Infection
  - Dislocation (more common in revision hip arthroplasty surgery)
  - Femoral or acetabular fracture
  - Nerve palsy (sciatic nerve most commonly)
  - DVT, PE
  - Heterotopic ossification
  - Loosening of components
  - Wear of the acetabular liner
  - Osteolysis or bone loss around the components

## PATIENT MONITORING

Patients with hip arthritis should be reassessed if symptoms change or pain worsens.

## REFERENCES


1. Berenbaum F, Hochberg MC, Cannon GW. Osteoarthritis. In: Klippel JH, ed. Primer on the Rheumatic Diseases, 12th ed. Atlanta, GA: Arthritis Foundation, 2001:285–297.
2. Lawrence RC, Helmick CG, Arnett FC, et al. Estimates of the prevalence of arthritis and selected musculoskeletal disorders in the United States. *Arthritis Rheum* 1998;41:778–799.
3. Beck M, Kalhor M, Leunig M, et al. Hip morphology influences the pattern of damage to the acetabular cartilage: femoroacetabular impingement as a cause of early osteoarthritis of the hip. *J Bone Joint Surg* 2005;87B:1012–1018.
4. Jacobsen S, Sonne-Holm S. Hip dysplasia: a significant risk factor for the development of hip osteoarthritis. A cross-sectional survey. *Rheumatology (Oxford)* 2005;44:211–218.
5. Roddy E, Zhang W, Doherty M, et al. Evidence-based recommendations for the role of exercise in the management of osteoarthritis of the hip or knee—the MOVE consensus. *Rheumatology (Oxford)* 2005;44:67–73.
6. Gagnier JJ, Chrubasik S, Manheimer E. Harpagophytum procumbens for osteoarthritis and low back pain: a systematic review. *BMC Complement Altern Med* 2004;4:1–10.
7. Ernst E. Avocado-soybean unsaponifiables (ASU) for osteoarthritis—a systematic review. *Clin Rheumatol* 2003;22:285–288.
8. Soeken KL. Selected CAM therapies for arthritis-related pain: the evidence from systematic reviews. *Clin J Pain* 2004;20:13–18.
9. Zhang W, Doherty M, Arden N, et al. EULAR evidence based recommendations for the management of hip osteoarthritis: report of a task force of the EULAR Standing Committee for International Clinical Studies Including Therapeutics (ESCISIT). *Ann Rheum Dis* 2005;64:669–681.


## ADDITIONAL READING


Felson DT. An update on the pathogenesis and epidemiology of osteoarthritis. *Radiol Clin North Am* 2004;42:1–9.


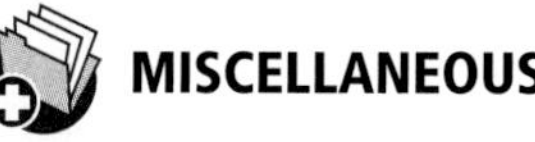

# MISCELLANEOUS

## CODES

### ICD9-CM

715.95 Arthropathy not otherwise specified, pelvis

## PATIENT TEACHING

- Patients are instructed on the importance of compliance with weight reduction, the use of NSAIDs, and the avoidance of painful activities.
- The role of hip replacement is discussed.

### Activity

- Patients can perform activities as tolerated but should avoid those that cause pain and may hasten the arthritic changes, such as running, racquetball, and heavy lifting.
- Water therapy is an effective exercise for patients with hip arthritis.

### Prevention

Prevention is achieved in some young patients with recognized hip dysplasia or femoroacetabular impingement by surgery to realign the joint or to reshape the femoral head.

## FAQ

- Q: When is a patient ready for hip replacement?
  - A: This decision is individualized and made by the patient in discussion with the surgeon. Every patient has different levels of pain and disability that does not correlate with the radiographic progression of disease. Patients must understand the risks of surgery and believe that the chance of improving their disability and pain is worth those risks.
- Q: Does progressive wear make a hip replacement harder to perform?
  - A: In general, wear does not happen quickly, and the hip replacement can be performed with little difficulty. Progressive hip stiffness, limp, and muscular weakness do make the postsurgical recovery of function more difficult.

# HIP AVASCULAR NECROSIS

*Ricardo A. Gonzales, MD*
*Michelle Cameron, MD*

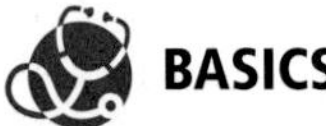

## BASICS

### DESCRIPTION

- AVN is osteonecrosis, or death of the bone.
  - All major joints can be affected.
  - In the pediatric population, this condition is called "Legg-Calvé-Perthes disease" and, in general, has a better prognosis than osteonecrosis in the adult.
- AVN of the hip is osteonecrosis of the femoral head.
- Synonyms: Osteonecrosis; Aseptic necrosis; Chandler disease
- Classification:
  - Ficat and Arlet (1) described 4 stages:
    - Stage I: No changes on radiograph, changes noted on MRI
    - Stage II: Sclerotic or cystic changes on radiographs in the femoral head, no collapse
    - Stage III: Subchondral fracture, crescent sign on radiographs
    - Stage IV: Degenerative changes in the hip joint with involvement of the femoral head
  - Steinberg et al. (2) modification of the Ficat and Arlet classification (all stages except stage 0 + advanced degenerative changes):
    - Stage 0: Normal radiograph, normal bone scan
    - Stage I: Normal radiograph, abnormal bone scan
    - Stage II: Sclerosis or cyst formation in the femoral head (A = mild, <20%; B = moderate, 20–40%; C = severe, >40%)
    - Stage III: Subchondral collapse (crescent sign) without flattening (A = mild, <15%; B = moderate, 15–30%; C = severe, >30%)
    - Stage IV: Flattening of the head without joint narrowing or acetabular involvement (A = mild, <15% of surface and <2 mm of depression; B = moderate, 15–30% of surface or 2–4 mm of depression)
    - Stage V: Flattening of head with joint narrowing or acetabular involvement (A = mild; B = moderate; C = severe [acetabular involvement])
  - One of the most predictive findings on radiography or MRI is the actual size of the lesion (3).

### GENERAL PREVENTION

- Limited systemic corticosteroid use
- Avoidance of alcohol abuse
- Early fixation of femoral neck fractures or reduction of hip dislocations

### EPIDEMIOLOGY

- Most common in young adults 20–40 years old and in children 6–10 years old.
- The average age of patients with osteonecrosis who require hip arthroplasty is 38 years (4).
- The distribution between males and females is equal (4).
- Patients with atraumatic osteonecrosis of one hip have a >50% chance of developing osteonecrosis of the contralateral side (5).

#### *Prevalence*

~2.5% of total hip replacements are performed for the diagnosis of AVN (6).

### RISK FACTORS

- Femoral neck fractures
- Steroid use
- Alcohol abuse
- Hemoglobinopathies (e.g., sickle cell anemia)
- Clotting abnormalities
- Dysbarism ("bends")
- Ionizing radiation
- Pancreatitis
- Gout

#### *Genetics*

A genetic pattern may be related to a clotting disorder with protein S deficiency.

### ETIOLOGY

- Osteonecrosis is most commonly alcohol-related or induced by incremental and cumulative doses of corticosteroids (90%) (4).
  - Alcohol: The threshold of alcohol ingestion reported to be associated with osteonecrosis is the equivalent of 400 mL or more per week of 100% ethyl alcohol (~3 beers per day) (4).
  - Corticosteroids:
    - A total dose of 2,800 mg of oral prednisone over 4 months significantly increases the risk of bone infarction (7).
    - Some researchers believe that patients who have idiosyncratic reactions to steroids, with systemic changes such as acute weight gain or moon faces, have an increased risk of developing osteonecrosis.
- Other causes include:
  - Traumatic injuries such as hip fractures
  - Subclinical clotting disorders
  - Exposure to atmospheric pressure variations

### ASSOCIATED CONDITIONS

- Hip fracture
- Hemoglobinopathy
- Alcohol abuse
- Perthes disease

## DIAGNOSIS

### SIGNS AND SYMPTOMS

- Onset of pain in the hip without antecedent trauma
- Pain is usually in the groin.

#### *History*

- The patient often initially complains of vague pain in the groin for 4–6 months before evaluation.
- Pain increases with internal rotation of the hip.
- A high index of suspicion should exist in a young patient with hip pain and other risk factors.

#### *Physical Exam*

- Look for groin pain with ROM of the hip (internal rotation), which is not typically tender with direct palpation.
- The patient has a limp but a normal neurologic examination.
- The combination of history and physical examination should lead to a suspicion of osteonecrosis of the hip.

### TESTS

#### *Lab*

- Complete blood count
- ESR
- Coagulation profile (research tool at present)

#### *Imaging*

- Plain radiographs, including AP and lateral projections of the hip
- MRI of the hip is the single best test for diagnosing osteonecrosis of the hip (specificity, 98%) (8).

#### *Pathological Findings*

- Although osteonecrosis has many possible causes, a common final pathway leads to the typical pathologic findings, including death of the osteoblast and osteocytes with empty lacunae in the trabecula of the necrotic area.
- An area of sclerotic margin also commonly is present in the area of necrosis.

### DIFFERENTIAL DIAGNOSIS

- Fracture
- Infection
- Transient osteoporosis of the hip
- Neurogenic pain
- Sports hernia
- Acetabular labral tear
- Psoas bursitis
- Synovitis or adhesions of the capsule

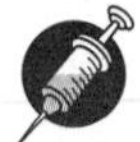

## TREATMENT

### GENERAL MEASURES

- The diagnosis of osteonecrosis of the hip should be made as early as possible.
- Other joints, including the contralateral hip, knees, shoulders, and ankles, should be evaluated.
- Patients with this diagnosis should be evaluated by an orthopaedic surgeon who is experienced in treating osteonecrosis of the hip.
- Nonoperative treatment typically is not successful for symptomatic lesions.
  - The failure rate is ~80%, depending on the size and classification of the lesion (4).
- Small lesions have a higher rate of spontaneous resolution than do large lesions (9).

## SPECICAL THERAPY

### *Physical Therapy*

Physical therapy can be useful for maintaining ROM but usually is of little benefit.

## MEDICATION (DRUGS)

### *First Line*

- Anticoagulants, antihypertensives, and lipid-lowering agents are all being investigated for the treatment of early-stage disease.
- Currently, use of these pharmacologic agents should be considered experimental.
- Evidence exists that diphosphonate may be helpful in preventing collapse (10).

## SURGERY

- Surgery for the treatment of osteonecrosis of the hip can be divided into procedures that preserve the femoral head and arthroplasty options.
- Head-preserving techniques:
  - Core decompression:
    - Indicated for small- to medium-sized precollapse lesions
    - Weightbearing should be protected for 5 weeks after surgery to avoid fracture.
    - Variable satisfactory outcomes have been reported (range, 40–90%) (5).
  - Osteotomy: Rotates the affected area of the head away from the weightbearing portion (11).
  - Vascularized fibular grafts: 1 study indicated an 83% success at 17-year follow-up in specialized centers (12).
  - Nonvascularized bone-graft:
    - Dead bone is removed and replaced with bone graft through a trapdoor in the femoral neck.
    - Reported success rate of 80–83% at 2.5–5 years follow-up (13)
- Arthroplasty options:
  - Resurfacing arthroplasty:
    - Indicated for patients with severe femoral head collapse and minimal acetabular changes
    - Variable results have been reported (14).
  - Total hip arthroplasty:
    - Indicated for patients with femoral head collapse and acetabular involvement
    - A lower success rate is reported for patients with osteonecrosis than patients with osteoarthritis (4).

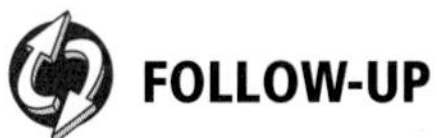

# FOLLOW-UP

## PROGNOSIS

- <50% of asymptomatic hips progress to end-stage disease requiring hip arthroplasty (5).
- Nonoperative treatment of symptomatic lesions result in 79% failure rate (5).
- Patients with diagnoses or risk factors thought to contribute to the development of osteonecrosis have worse outcomes with head-preserving procedures (5).

## COMPLICATIONS

- Progressive collapse of the hip can lead to debilitating arthritis and the need for total hip arthroplasties.
- Risk of fracture exists with weightbearing after core decompression.
  - Risk is increased if the core tract is made through diaphyseal bone.
- Risk of donor site morbidity exists with vascularized fibular grafting (15).
- Hip arthroplasty in patients with osteonecrosis has a higher failure rate, owing to loosening, than in patients with osteoarthritis (20% versus 5%, respectively, at 10 years) (16).
  - With modern implants, bearing surfaces may become the limiting factor of replacements in younger patients (16).

## PATIENT MONITORING

- Serial radiographs are used to note any progression of joint involvement every 3–4 months.
- Clinical symptoms are equally important, especially if nonoperative management is selected with the end point of total hip arthroplasty.

## REFERENCES


1. Ficat RP, Arlet J. Functional investigation of bone under normal conditions. In: *Ischemia and Necrosis of Bone*. Baltimore: Williams & Wilkins, 1980:29–52.
2. Steinberg ME, Hayken GD, Steinberg DR. A quantitative system for staging avascular necrosis. *J Bone Joint Surg* 1995;77B:34–41.
3. Hungerford DS, Lennox DW. Diagnosis and treatment of ischemic necrosis of the femoral head. In: Evarts CM, ed. *Surgery in the Musculoskeletal System,* 2nd ed. New York: Churchill Livingstone, 1990:2757–2794.
4. Mont MA, Jones LC, Hungerford DS. Nontraumatic osteonecrosis of the femoral head: ten years later. *J Bone Joint Surg* 2006;88A: 1117–1132.
5. Lieberman JR, Berry DJ, Mont MA, et al. Osteonecrosis of the hip: management in the 21st century. *Instr Course Lect* 2003;52: 337–355.
6. Pedersen AB, Johnsen SP, Overgaard S, et al. Total hip arthroplasty in Denmark: incidence of primary operations and revisions during 1996–2002 and estimated future demands. *Acta Orthop* 2005;76:182–189.
7. Shpall EJ, Efremidis AP, Kasambalides E, et al. Case report 352: osteonecrosis of the femoral shaft (probably steroid-induced). *Skeletal Radiol* 1986;15:170–174.
8. Thickman D, Axel L, Kressel HY, et al. Magnetic resonance imaging of avascular necrosis of the femoral head. *Skeletal Radiol* 1986;15: 133–140.
9. Cheng EY, Thongtrangan I, Laorr A, et al. Spontaneous resolution of osteonecrosis of the femoral head. *J Bone Joint Surg* 2004;86A: 2594–2599.
10. Lai KA, Shen WJ, Yang CY, et al. The use of alendronate to prevent early collapse of the femoral head in patients with nontraumatic osteonecrosis. A randomized clinical study. *J Bone Joint Surg* 2005;87A:2155–2159.
11. Shannon BD, Trousdale RT. Femoral osteotomies for avascular necrosis of the femoral head. *Clin Orthop Relat Res* 2004;418:34–40.
12. Urbaniak JR, Harvey EJ. Revascularization of the femoral head in osteonecrosis. *J Am Acad Orthop Surg* 1998;6:44–54.
13. Mont MA, Einhorn TA, Sponseller PD, et al. The trapdoor procedure using autogenous cortical and cancellous bone grafts for osteonecrosis of the femoral head. *J Bone Joint Surg* 1998;80B: 56–62.
14. Adili A, Trousdale RT. Femoral head resurfacing for the treatment of osteonecrosis in the young patient. *Clin Orthop Relat Res* 2003;417: 93–101.
15. Vail TP, Urbaniak JR. Donor-site morbidity with use of vascularized autogenous fibular grafts. *J Bone Joint Surg* 1996;78A:204–211.
16. Hartley WT, McAuley JP, Culpepper WJ, et al. Osteonecrosis of the femoral head treated with cementless total hip arthroplasty. *J Bone Joint Surg* 2000;82A:1408–1413.


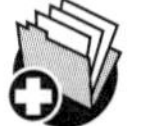

# MISCELLANEOUS

## CODES

### *ICD9-CM*

733.42 Osteonecrosis (aseptic necrosis), femoral head

## PATIENT TEACHING

Patients are counseled on the natural history of the disease and are asked to call the physician's attention to bone or joint pain.

## FAQ

- Q: Will osteonecrosis of the hip get better?
  - A: Spontaneous resolution occurs more often in patients with small lesions. Larger lesions and those that have collapsed are unlikely to improve spontaneously.
- Q: Which patients should have total hip replacement?
  - Collapse of the femoral head and arthritic changes in the joint are indications for arthroplasty.

# HIP DISLOCATION, TRAUMATIC

*Gregory Gebauer, MD, MS*

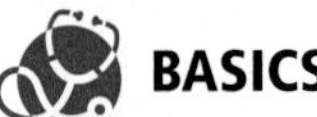

## BASICS

### DESCRIPTION

- Dislocations and fracture-dislocations of the hip are orthopaedic emergencies.
  - Serious, high-energy injuries in which the femoral head becomes completely dislodged from the acetabulum
- A thorough examination must be performed to assess for other possible injuries.
  - Up to 50% of patients suffer other fractures at the time of injury (1).
  - Associated acetabular or femoral head or neck fractures are common.
- Classification is based on the direction of dislocation (anterior versus posterior) and associated fractures in the femoral head or femoral neck (Fig. 1).

### GENERAL PREVENTION

Seat belts should be used in conjunction with air bags.

### EPIDEMIOLOGY

- Most common in young adults (1)
- More males than females are affected (1).

#### *Incidence*

- Anterior dislocation: 10–15% (1)
- Posterior dislocation: 85–90% (1)

### RISK FACTORS

- Motor vehicle accidents
- Falls from substantial heights

### ETIOLOGY

- 70–90% of traumatic hip dislocations are caused by motor vehicle accidents (2).
  - As the car decelerates, the flexed knee strikes the dashboard, forcing the femoral head out posteriorly (2).
- Other mechanisms include automobile versus pedestrian accidents, falls from heights, industrial injuries, and sporting accidents.

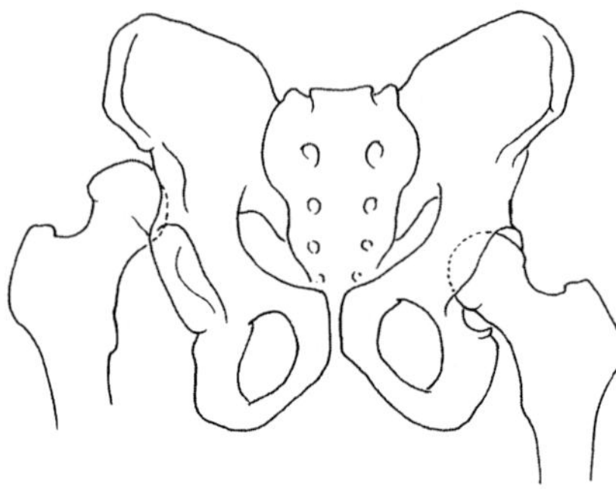

**Fig. 1.** In an acute hip dislocation, the femoral head usually is displaced posteriorly and superiorly. The acetabulum should be inspected for fractures.

### ASSOCIATED CONDITIONS

- Because hip dislocations usually are secondary to high-energy trauma, other severe injuries are common, including:
  - Neurologic injuries: Sciatic nerve palsy and herniated discs
    - Sciatic nerve injury occurs in 10–20% of posterior dislocations (3).
    - Sciatic nerve injury appears to be related to the length of time that the hip is dislocated (3).
  - Musculoskeletal injuries:
    - Femoral head, neck, and acetabular fractures
    - Common: Ipsilateral knee and foot injuries
  - Intra-abdominal or chest injuries

## DIAGNOSIS

### SIGNS AND SYMPTOMS

- Severe pain over the hip or numbness along the posterior thigh
- Altered resting lower extremity position:
  - In posterior dislocation, the hip is fixed in a position of flexion, internal rotation, and adduction.
  - In anterior dislocation, the hip is in marked external rotation with mild flexion and abduction.
- Shortening of the extremity
- Many patients suffering traumatic hip dislocations are obtunded or unconscious on arrival at the emergency department and, therefore, cannot assist the physician in the initial evaluation.

#### *Physical Exam*

- Examination must include a full trauma survey, because concomitant injuries are common.
- Motor and sensory nerve function as well as the presence or absence of pulses should be documented before and after reduction of the dislocation.
- In particular, sciatic nerve function should be assessed.

### TESTS

#### *Lab*

A standard series of lab tests for a trauma workup should be obtained.

#### *Imaging*

- All patients with traumatic hip dislocations should have routine trauma radiographs, including cervical spine, chest, and AP pelvic films.
  - Plain films of painful extremities or other pelvic views (internal or external oblique-Judet views) should be obtained if associated fractures are suspected.
  - A cross-table lateral view of the hip will determine if the dislocation is anterior or posterior.
  - Judet views may help identify any acetabular fracture.
  - In a posterior dislocation, the femoral head appears smaller radiographically than on the contralateral, uninjured side.
  - In an anterior dislocation, the femoral head appears slightly larger than in the uninjured hip.
  - Careful evaluation of the femoral neck must rule out the presence of a femoral neck fracture before any manipulative reduction is undertaken.
    - The acetabulum should be inspected carefully to ascertain the presence or absence of intra-articular osteochondral fragments and asymmetry of the joint space.
- CT scans:
  - Should be obtained routinely after successful closed reductions or before surgery, if open reduction is planned.
  - Valuable in showing the presence of small intra-articular fragments and in assessing the congruence of the femoral head and acetabulum (4)
- The role of MRI in posttraumatic evaluation of the hip has not yet been established, and this technique is not currently used.

### DIFFERENTIAL DIAGNOSIS

- Femoral neck and head fracture
- Acetabular and pelvic fractures

## TREATMENT

### INITIAL STABILIZATION

- Assess the patient for concomitant injuries, which are common.
- Determine whether closed reduction can be done.
- Sedation is required for reduction.
- Document the affected limb's neurovascular status before and after reduction.

### GENERAL MEASURES

- Emergent orthopaedic consultation should be obtained because urgent reduction of the dislocated hip is necessary to prevent long-term complications.
- It is important to assess patients fully for concomitant injuries secondary to high-energy trauma.
- The management of a patient with a hip dislocation is divided into 2 phases:
  - Initial phase: Identify and reduce the dislocation:
    - Perform reduction quickly to reduce the risk of femoral head osteonecrosis.
    - If possible, closed reduction in the emergency department or operating room with the patient under general anesthesia and with complete muscle paralysis
    - If general anesthesia is not immediately feasible, attempt reduction with the patient under intravenous sedation.

- Regardless of the direction of the dislocation, attempt reduction with inline traction with the patient lying supine (5).
- During the reduction, assess stability.
- Obtain confirmatory radiographs after reduction.
- After successful closed reduction and completion of the stability examination, place the patient in traction to await CT evaluation.
  - If the hip has been shown to be stable, simple traction using a Buck traction boot or skin traction is sufficient.
  - If the hip is unstable, it is preferable to use skeletal traction with a tibial pin.

– Secondary phase: Plan and perform definitive care:
- Once the femoral head has been reduced, urgency is diminished, and an appropriate diagnostic workup, including CT analysis, can be completed.
- Surgical intervention, if indicated, can be undertaken after the patient has become hemodynamically stable and safe for operative management.
- Indications for surgical treatment include inability to obtain adequate closed reduction, nonconcentric reduction, ipsilateral femur fracture, or presence of an associated acetabular fracture requiring surgical treatment (6).

#### *Activity*

- Weightbearing status depends on the stability of the hip and the presence of any associated fractures.
- Early active ROM is ideal.
- Patients with postreduction stable hips should be mobilized and allowed to bear weight (7).

### SPECIAL THERAPY

#### *Physical Therapy*

Often required for gait training with protected weightbearing and ROM

### MEDICATION (DRUGS)

#### *First Line*

Narcotic analgesics

### SURGERY

- If closed reduction cannot be achieved, then open reduction is indicated.
- The standard posterior approach, or a lateral decubitus position, is used with or without a fracture (traction) table, depending on the surgeon's preference.

## FOLLOW-UP

### PROGNOSIS

- Posterior dislocations:
  - 70–80% of simple posterior hip dislocations (without associated fractures) have good or excellent outcomes (1).
  - When posterior dislocations are associated with femoral head fractures or acetabular fractures, the outcome is not as favorable.
- Anterior dislocations:
  - Patients with anterior dislocations have been noted to have a high incidence of femoral head injuries, and long-term outcome is not as good as with posterior dislocations.
- Long-term prognosis worsens if the time to reduction is >12 hours.

### COMPLICATIONS

- Posttraumatic arthritis is the most frequent long-term complication.
  - The incidence of arthritis is higher in patients with associated acetabular or femoral head fractures.
  - Secondary arthritis may develop as a result of AVN.
- Osteonecrosis (AVN) occurs in 1–17% of these patients (8).
  - A risk exists for osteonecrosis of the hip, even with prompt hip reduction, secondary to injury to the femoral head's blood supply.
  - The risk increases when the hip remains dislocated for a period of time.
  - Threshold time is reported to be ~6–24 hours (5).
- Sciatic nerve injury occurs in 8–19% of patients and is caused by stretching of the nerve from a posteriorly dislocated femoral head or from a displaced fracture fragment.
  - The peroneal component of the nerve is affected most commonly.
  - Electromyography and nerve conduction studies are indicated at 3–4 weeks for baseline information, documentation of precise level, and prognostic guidance.
  - Prognosis is unpredictable, with 40–50% reporting full recovery (3).
- Recurrent dislocation is rare (<2%) (1).
- Heterotopic ossification is a rare complication of hip dislocation.

### PATIENT MONITORING

- In the 1st year, serial hip radiographs every 3–4 months
- MRI will diagnose osteonecrosis.

### REFERENCES


1. Sahin V, Karakas ES, Aksu S, et al. Traumatic dislocation and fracture-dislocation of the hip: a long-term follow-up study. *J Trauma* 2003;54: 520–529.
2. Monma H, Sugita T. Is the mechanism of traumatic posterior dislocation of the hip a brake pedal injury rather than a dashboard injury? *Injury* 2001;32: 221–222.
3. Hillyard RF, Fox J. Sciatic nerve injuries associated with traumatic posterior hip dislocations. *Am J Emerg Med* 2003;21:545–548.
4. Brooks RA, Ribbans WJ. Diagnosis and imaging studies of traumatic hip dislocations in the adult. *Clin Orthop Relat Res* 2000;377:15–23.
5. Yang EC, Cornwall R. Initial treatment of traumatic hip dislocations in the adult. *Clin Orthop Relat Res* 2000;377:24–31.
6. Alonso JE, Volgas DA, Giordano V, et al. A review of the treatment of hip dislocations associated with acetabular fractures. *Clin Orthop Relat Res* 2000;377:32–43.
7. Schlickewei W, Elsasser B, Mullaji AB, et al. Hip dislocation without fracture: traction or mobilization after reduction? *Injury* 1993;24: 27–31.
8. Rodriguez-Merchan EC. Osteonecrosis of the femoral head after traumatic hip dislocation in the adult. *Clin Orthop Relat Res* 2000;377:68–77.


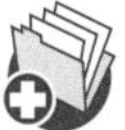

## MISCELLANEOUS

### CODES

#### *ICD9-CM*

835.00 Hip dislocation

### PATIENT TEACHING

#### *Activity*

Patients should be counseled on safe driving practices, including the use of seat belts and airbags.

#### *Prevention*

The use of seat belts and airbags may help prevent hip dislocations.

### FAQ

- Q: Will I be at risk for dislocation in the future?
  - A: No. The risk of recurrent dislocation is low (<2%).
- Q: What problems may I have in the future?
  - A: The most common long-term problems after hip dislocation are osteonecrosis and traumatic arthritis, both of which may lead to chronic hip pain. These problems may ultimately lead to total hip replacement.
- Q: My sciatic nerve was injured during the dislocation; can I expect to get function back?
  - A: 40–50% of patients report full recovery, but recovery can take months to a year.

# HIP EXAMINATION IN THE CHILD

*Ryan K. Takenaga, BS*
*Paul D. Sponseller, MD*

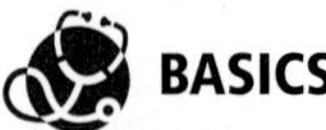

## BASICS

### DESCRIPTION

- Because many pediatric hip disorders develop only in certain age groups, it is important that the clinician, when performing a hip examination, keep in mind the child's age and have an understanding of the following age-specific pediatric hip disorders (1):
  - DDH:
    - Spectrum of conditions resulting in an unstable fit between the femoral head and acetabulum
    - Most cases are detectable at birth by performing the Ortolani and Barlow maneuvers.
    - If not seen at birth, it is usually found when the pediatrician notes asymmetrical abduction or parents notice limp or abnormal gait.
    - Risk factors include: Breech delivery, oligohydramnios, female gender (Male:Female ratio, 1:4) (1), 1st born, positive family history or ethnic background (e.g., Native American).
  - Septic arthritis:
    - Pyogenic infection of the hip
    - Most cases occur before the age of 5 years.
    - Patient is acutely ill and nonweightbearing.
  - Legg-Calvé-Perthes syndrome
    - Idiopathic AVN of the femoral head in children
    - Occurs most commonly at age 4–8 years (range, 2–12 years) (1,2)
    - 90% unilateral (1)
    - Male:Female ratio, 4–5:1 (1).
    - Typical presentation is the insidious onset of a limp that is worsened by activity.
  - Transient synovitis:
    - Self-limited, idiopathic inflammation of the hip joint
    - Most common cause of hip pain in children
    - Occurs most commonly in children 5–6 years old (range, 3–8 years) (1)
    - 95% unilateral (1)
    - Male:Female ratio, 2:1 (1,2)
    - Presents as an acute onset painful limp
  - SCFE:
    - Displacement of the upper femoral epiphysis from the metaphysis through the physeal plate
    - Age at onset: 9–14 years in girls and 10–16 years in boys (1,2)
    - Male:Female ratio, 1.4–2:1 (1,2)
    - More prevalent in the obese
    - Typical presentation is the insidious onset of pain and limp exacerbated by activity.

## DIAGNOSIS

### SIGNS AND SYMPTOMS

#### *History*

- Onset of pain:
  - Acute: Fracture, septic arthritis, transient synovitis, osteomyelitis
  - Chronic: Legg-Calvé-Perthes syndrome, SCFE, idiopathic chondrolysis of the hip
  - Associated with activity: Legg-Calvé-Perthes syndrome, SCFE
  - Location: Hip pain can be referred to the medial thigh and knee.
- Limp:
  - Acute: Transient synovitis, septic arthritis
  - Chronic: DDH, Legg-Calvé-Perthes syndrome, SCFE, developmental coxa vara, idiopathic chondrolysis of the hip, limb-length discrepancy
- Nonweightbearing:
  - Fracture
  - Septic arthritis
  - Transient synovitis
  - Osteomyelitis
- Constitutional symptoms:
  - Septic arthritis
  - Osteomyelitis
- Snapping sound: Iliopsoas snapping hip

#### *Physical Exam: Preambulatory Infants*

- General notes:
  - An upset or crying infant may tighten these muscles, decreasing the value of the examination.
  - To help relax the baby, the family should be allowed to feed or soothe the infant.
- Inspection and palpation:
  - Excess thigh folds on 1 side may indicate a limb-length discrepancy.
- Tests and measurements:
  - Ortolani and Barlow maneuvers detect hip instability in newborns $\leq$3 months old.
    - After ~3 months, capsule laxity decreases and muscle tightness increases so that the hip cannot be relocated by the Ortolani maneuver.
  - Ortolani maneuver: A "sign of entry" as the femoral head reduces into the acetabulum:
    - With the baby supine and the knees fully flexed, flex the hips to a right angle and place the long finger of each hand laterally along the axis of the femur over the greater trochanter.
    - Place the thumb of each hand on the inner side of the thigh opposite the lesser trochanter.
    - Lift the thighs into midabduction and exert forward pressure behind the greater trochanter, using the middle finger on 1 side, while the other hand holds the opposite femur and pelvis steady.
    - If the femoral head "clunks" or slides forward into the acetabulum, the hip has been relocated into the acetabulum.
  - Barlow maneuver: A "sign of exit" as the femoral head subluxates or dislocates from the acetabulum:
    - With fingers in the same position as for the Ortolani maneuver, exert backward and outward pressure with the thumb on the inner side of the thigh as the hip is adducted.
    - If the femoral head "clunks" or slips out over the posterior lip of the acetabulum the hip is "unstable."
- Galeazzi (Allis) sign: Indicates limb-length discrepancy, which can be secondary to a unilateral hip problem:
  - With the baby supine on a firm table, flex the knees and hips and put the feet flat on the table.
  - The knee on the side of the shorter limb will be lower than the knee of the normal limb.
- ROM (2–4):
  - Abduction and adduction:
    - With the baby supine on a firm table, flex the knees and hips to 90°.
    - Abduct the legs (average, 78°)
  - Flexion and internal and external rotation:
    - Extension should be 0–20°
    - Average flexion: 140°
    - Average internal/external rotation: 58–80°

#### *Physical Exam: Ambulatory Children*

- The child's capacity to walk and to understand and follow instructions allows for a broader hip examination than in the preambulatory infant, which provides information on strength, balance, stability, and pain.
- Standing examination:
  - Measure pelvic tilt.
    - Place hands on the patient's iliac crests.
    - Any difference in level represents a pelvic tilt and may indicate a limb-length discrepancy
  - Trendelenburg test:
    - Ask the patient to stand on 1 leg.
    - Any contralateral pelvic tilting is a positive Trendelenburg test, which indicates weak abductors or an irritable hip.
- Gait examination:
  - Observe from in front of and behind the patient.
  - For younger children, ask parents to walk the child down the hall and back.
  - Note any asymmetries (e.g., stride lengths, duration of stance or swing phases).

- Pathologic gaits:
  - Antalgic (painful) gait: Short strides and a shortened stance phase on the painful side
  - Trendelenburg gait: Swaying or bending of the trunk over the affected hip because the patient shifts the center of gravity to compensate for weak hip abductors or to decrease the joint reactive forces that irritate the affected hip
  - Gluteus maximus gait: Lurching backward during the stance phase of the involved side, which shifts the center of gravity posteriorly to compensate for weak hip extensors.
  - Limb-length discrepancy gait: Abnormal up-and-down motion because the patient with a true limb-length discrepancy of $>2$ cm bends the longer leg excessively or stands on the toes of the shorter leg.
- Positioning and leg lengths:
  - With the patient supine, inspect the leg position for symmetric rotation, flexion, and adduction.
  - With the patient supine, measure from the inferior edge of the anterior superior iliac spine to the inferior edge of the ipsilateral medial malleolus.
- Isolating hip pathology (1):
  - Roll test:
    - With the patient supine, gently roll the leg internally and externally.
    - Guarding or stiffness on 1 side indicates hip abnormality.
- ROM (4):
  - Flexion (average: 120–130°) (4):
    - With the patient lying supine and the knee fully flexed, place 1 hand on the contralateral pelvis.
    - Flex the hip until movement in the contralateral pelvis is noted.
    - The angle between the femur and examining table is the hip flexion.
  - Internal and external rotation:
    - With the patient in the prone position, flex the knees to 90°.
    - Rotate the legs outward for internal rotation and inward for external rotation.
    - The angle between each leg and the line perpendicular to the tabletop is the degree of rotation.
    - Normal internal rotation: Average, 45–50° (range, 20–70°)
    - Normal external rotation: Average, 40° (range, 25–60°)
  - Abduction (average, 40–50°):
    - With the patient lying supine and hip in extension, place 1 finger on the contralateral anterior superior iliac spine.
    - Abduct the hip until the finger feels the pelvis start to tilt.
- Flexion contracture:
  - Thomas test (normal, 0°):
    - With the patient lying supine, maximally flex both hips.
    - Allow the femur on the ipsilateral side to fall into as much extension as possible, while holding the other hip up.
    - The angle between the femur and examining table is the residual flexion and represents the flexion contracture.
  - Staheli test (normal: 0°):
    - Particularly suitable for the spastic patient
    - The patient is positioned prone, providing a way to flatten the lumbar spine and level the pelvis.
    - Have the patient lie in the prone position with the hip flexed over the end of the table.
    - 1 hip remains flexed at 90°.
    - Gradually extend the other hip while palpating the ipsilateral pelvis.
    - As soon as pelvic motion is detected, measure the amount of residual hip flexion, which represents the flexion contracture.
    - Normal values in the infant: Birth, 21°; 3 months, 11°; $\geq$6 months: 3°
- Muscle strength:
  - Hip flexors (iliopsoas supplied by L1–L3):
    - Have patient sit with knees flexed to 90°.
    - Push against the anterior aspect of the thigh while the patient flexes 1 hip.
  - Hip extensors (gluteus maximus supplied by S1):
    - With the patient in the prone position, push against the posterior thigh while the patient elevates the femur off the table.
  - Hip abductors (gluteus medius and minimus supplied by L5):
    - Have the patient lie on 1 side.
    - Push against the lateral knee of the top leg while the patient elevates it.
  - Hip adductors (adductors longus, brevis, and magnus, gracilis and pectineus supplied by L2–L4):
    - With the patient lying supine, push against the medial aspect of 1 thigh while the patient pushes that leg toward the midline.

## TESTS

### *Imaging*

- AP radiographs of the pelvis and/or AP and frog-lateral radiographs of the hip usually are sufficient for diagnosing many common pediatric hip disorders.
- If plain films are normal, an MRI, CT, or bone scan may be helpful.
- Common pediatric hip disorders and the imaging modalities that contribute to their diagnoses:
  - Hip fracture or dislocation:
    - AP pelvis/hip radiographs may show upward and lateral displacement of the femoral shaft.
    - In newborns, ultrasound may be helpful in showing a dislocation.
  - DDH:
    - The physical examination usually is sufficient for diagnosing and initiating treatment.
    - Radiographs of the hip in neonates are difficult to interpret because the femoral head is cartilaginous.
    - Ultrasound can show an unstable or dislocated hip joint, and is particularly useful before the femoral head has ossified.
  - Septic arthritis:
    - Plain films usually are normal, but ultrasound may show widening of joint space secondary to swelling.
    - Fluoroscopy may aid in the aspiration of joint fluid for culture.
  - Legg-Calvé-Perthes syndrome:
    - AP and frog-lateral radiographs of the pelvis aid in diagnosis and help guide treatment.
    - Plain radiographs may be normal early in the disease, but increased density of the femoral head is an early sign of Legg-Calvé-Perthes syndrome.
    - MRI helps show osteonecrosis.
    - Bone scan may help distinguish between Legg-Calvé-Perthes syndrome and transient synovitis early in the disease.
    - If bilateral involvement is present, screen hand and knee radiographs to rule out epiphyseal dysplasia or thyroid disease.
  - Transient synovitis:
    - If symptoms have been present for several days, then AP and frog-lateral radiographs are appropriate to rule out a latent osteomyelitis or other chronic processes.
    - Radiographs are normal, but ultrasound may reveal swelling of the capsule and adjacent soft tissue and slight widening of the joint space.
  - SCFE:
    - AP and frog-lateral radiographs of each hip confirm the diagnosis.
    - Early in the disorder, an abnormal widening of the physis is seen.
    - As the slip progresses, the metaphysis appears more lateral relative to the acetabular teardrop.

## REFERENCES


1. Pizzutillo PD (section ed.). Section 9: Pediatric orthopaedics. In: Griffin LY, ed. *Essentials of Musculoskeletal Care*, 3rd ed. Rosemont, IL: American Academy of Orthopaedic Surgeons, 2005:791–957.
2. Aronsson DD. The pediatric orthopaedic examination. In: Morrissy RT, Weinstein SL, eds. *Lovell and Winter's Pediatric Orthopaedics*, 6th ed. Philadelphia: Lippincott Williams & Wilkins, 2006:113–143.
3. Mercier LR. The hip. In: *Practical Orthopaedics*, 4th ed. St. Louis: Mosby, 1995:183–206.
4. Schwarze DJ, Denton JR. Normal values of neonatal lower limbs: an evaluation of 1,000 neonates. *J Pediatr Orthop* 1993;13:758–760.


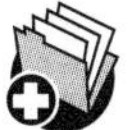

## MISCELLANEOUS

### FAQ

- Q: Can DDH always be detected by physical examination?
  - A: No. It is usually, but not always, possible to detect it on routine physical examination. Situations that make detection more difficult include a child who is irritable or who has ligamentous laxity, bilateral abnormalities, or a very mild degree of dysplasia.
- Q: Should all newborns have screening ultrasound for DDH?
  - A: Ultrasound leads to some false-positive results and consequent overtreatment. Therefore, it should be used only in the presence of a clinical suspicion of dysplasia, such as an abnormal physical examination, positive family history, or breech birth.

# HIP FRACTURE IN THE CHILD

*Paul D. Sponseller, MD*

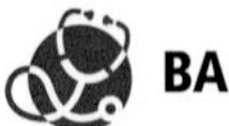

## BASICS

### DESCRIPTION

- Fracture of the femoral neck, in the intertrochanteric or subtrochanteric region
- Classification: Delbet system as popularized by Colonna (1):
  - Type I
    - Transphyseal separation (femoral head separates from neck through the growth plate)
    - Can be nondisplaced (widened physis), displaced, or dislocated
    - Least common type
    - Occurs in young children
    - Many patients have dislocation of the femoral head from the acetabulum.
  - Type II:
    - Transcervical
  - Type III:
    - Cervicotrochanteric
  - Type IV:
    - Intertrochanteric
- Initial displacement seems to affect the risk of osteonecrosis most.
- Anatomy:
  - Blood supply:
    - At birth, the blood supply to the femoral head travels through the metaphyseal vessels traversing the neck, deriving from the medial and lateral femoral circumflex arteries.
    - The growth plate of the proximal femur prevents these vessels from penetrating the femoral head.
    - By 4 years of age, the contribution by the metaphyseal blood supply is negligible, and the medial femoral circumflex artery provides the major blood supply to the head.
    - Capsulotomy of the hip does not damage the femoral head's blood supply unless the procedure violates the intertrochanteric notch or damages the posterosuperior or posteroinferior vessels along the femoral neck.
    - The ligamentum teres contributes only a small percentage of the blood supply to the femoral head.
  - Bone:
    - ~1/2 of pediatric hip fractures are nondisplaced.
    - If the fracture is displaced, it is likely to be unstable.

### EPIDEMIOLOGY

#### *Incidence*

This injury accounts for <1% of all pediatric fractures, far less than the percentage in adults (2) because the bone is so strong.

### ETIOLOGY

- 75% of pediatric hip fractures are caused by severe trauma and high-velocity injuries (e.g., motor vehicle accidents, falls).
- The remainder result from some underlying pathologic process (e.g., fracture through a unicameral bone cyst, aneurysmal bone cyst, or fibrous dysplasia) or child abuse.

### ASSOCIATED CONDITIONS

- Infants:
  - Suspect child abuse.
  - If the injury is a result of an automobile accident, look for associated injuries.
- Children:
  - Great force is required.
  - Look for associated injuries.
- Adolescents:
  - Acute fracture occurs through the growth plate (SCFE), or it is a pathologic slip (look for hypothyroidism, renal osteodystrophy).

## DIAGNOSIS

### SIGNS AND SYMPTOMS

- Sudden pain in the hip
- Inability to stand or walk
- Swelling in the inguinal crease, gluteal, proximal thigh
- Limb held in external rotation, flexion, and adduction to relieve capsular distention
- Resistance to any movement: Active hip motion is impossible if the fracture is displaced, and passive motion (especially flexion, abduction, and internal rotation) is restricted and painful.
- Pain and sometimes crepitus with hip motion
- Pseudoparalysis of the affected limb in infants
- Extremity possibly shortened 1–2 cm

#### *Physical Exam*

- Most children with femoral neck fractures are in extreme pain.
- For the minority who do not have a complete fracture, pain is elicited most by internal rotation, abduction, and flexion.

### TESTS

#### *Imaging*

- AP and lateral radiographic views of the hip may show upward and lateral displacement of the femoral shaft.
- CT can be helpful for determining the direction of the femoral head dislocation.
- In newborns, ultrasound may be helpful in showing a femoral neck fracture.

### DIFFERENTIAL DIAGNOSIS

- SCFE
- Developmental coxa vara (this condition has a vertical cleft in the femoral neck)

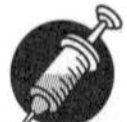

## TREATMENT

### GENERAL MEASURES

- Treatment is aimed at achieving anatomic reduction, either open or closed.
- Use smooth pins or cannulated 4.0–4.5-mm screws in children ~2–6 years old and cannulated 6.5–7.0-mm screws in children ≥7 years old.
- Usually, a spica cast is used postoperatively because the smaller diameter of the femoral neck in these younger patients limits the size and number of screws that can be placed.
- If the injury is type I and one must cross the physis, use smooth pins followed by a spica cast.
- For types II–IV, screws should not cross the physis unless the fracture cannot be stabilized without doing so; the physis of the proximal femur grows only 3 mm per year, so fear of limb-length discrepancy should not compromise fixation.
- If the hip is dislocated, make one attempt at closed reduction, then try open reduction.
- If open reduction is attempted, the surgical approach should be in the direction of the dislocation: Posterior for posterior dislocation, anterior for anterior dislocation.

### SURGERY

- Type I:
  - Without dislocation:
    - Gentle closed or open reduction and fixation with a screw or a pin
  - With dislocation:
    - Nearly 100% develop osteonecrosis, and 80% are at risk for developing degenerative joint disease.
    - Attempt gentle closed reduction using longitudinal traction, abduction, and internal rotation; if that is unsuccessful, try immediate open reduction and pin fixation.
- Type II:
  - Most common type
  - Most fractures are displaced.
  - Osteonecrosis in ~50% (displaced fractures at higher risk than nondisplaced)
  - Closed or open reduction and pin or screw fixation for both displaced and nondisplaced fractures
- Type III:
  - 2nd most common type
  - Osteonecrosis in 25%
  - Displaced:
    - Gentle closed reduction or open reduction and internal fixation
  - Nondisplaced:
    - Abduction spica cast possibly adequate in children <8 years old, although late displacement or coxa vara is possible; close observation is necessary.

- Type IV:
  - Open reduction and internal fixation with pediatric hip compression screw fixation.
- Surgical pearls:
  - Use a fluoroscopy table or a fracture table and an image intensifier.
  - A straight lateral approach is used.
    - If intracapsular open reduction is needed, types II and III can be via a proximal extension of the tensor fascia lata–gluteus interval.
    - Type I and high type II: Use the anterior iliofemoral approach
  - The reduction maneuver includes traction and internal rotation.
  - Unacceptable reduction is indicated by a varus position or excessive displacement on AP and lateral views.
  - No displacement of the width of the femoral neck should be accepted because additional varus angulation is likely.
  - Instrumentation:
    - Types I, II, and III: Use 2–3 cannulated screws of appropriate size for age (3).
    - Type IV: Use a hip compression screw device with a side plate.
  - Nonoperative option: Reduce with 3–6 weeks of skeletal traction and then immobilization in hip abduction cast for a total treatment course of 12 weeks.
  - Patient age:
    - For patients 7–12 years old, use pediatric hip screw fixation, followed by hip spica cast for 8–12 weeks after surgery, depending on the stability of fixation.
    - For patients ≥13 years old, treat as an adult: The hip screw and side plate may cross the physis, and no postoperative immobilization is required.
  - Timing of surgery:
    - Within 24 hours
    - Type I fracture with dislocation requires immediate treatment
    - No conclusive data on the effect of timing on osteonecrosis
  - Implant removal:
    - No absolute time limit exists for removal of hardware.
    - However, it usually is removed within 12–18 months of injury, if the fracture has healed, to prevent bony overgrowth or refracture at the base of the implant.

### *Pediatric Considerations*

- Neonatal epiphysiolysis:
  - If recognized initially, use skin traction to restore alignment.
  - If recognized after callus formation is visible radiographically, use simple immobilization.
  - Open surgical reduction is not advised because these injuries in newborns tend to remodel if the physis does not close prematurely.
  - Close observation is necessary; a low incidence of osteonecrosis is noted.

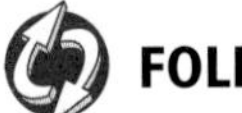

## FOLLOW-UP

### PROGNOSIS

The outcome is determined by the degree of damage to the blood supply.

### COMPLICATIONS

- Complications occur in as many as 60% of patients (3,4).
- Most complications of pediatric hip fractures are influenced by the changing blood supply of the proximal femoral epiphysis.
- AVN (osteonecrosis):
  - Most common, most devastating complication
  - May affect epiphysis, both epiphysis and metaphysis, or metaphysis alone
  - Develops in 42% of hip fractures in children within 9–12 months after injury (4):
    - Type I, nearly 100%
    - Type II, 52%
    - Type III, 27%
    - Type IV, 14%
  - Initial displacement of the fracture, fracture types I and II, and age (>10 years) are associated with increased risk.
  - Treatment:
    - Motion and containment are maintained.
    - Osteotomies to rotate the less-deformed or less-involved portion into the weightbearing region may improve congruity and symptoms.
  - Ratliff (5) classification of osteonecrosis in children, with current commentary (3,4):
    - Type I: Total involvement and collapse of the femoral head; worst prognosis; most common injury; injury to all lateral epiphyseal vessels
    - Type II: Involvement of a portion of the epiphysis accompanied by minimal collapse of the femoral head; localized injury to the anterolateral femoral head
    - Type III: Increased sclerosis of the femoral neck from the fracture line to the physis, but sparing of the femoral head; injury to the metaphyseal vessels
- Nonunion:
  - Occurs in 5–8% of fractures (similar to the risk in adults) (3,4).
  - Closed treatment of types II and III is associated with an increased incidence of coxa vara and nonunion (3,4).
  - Internal fixation after acceptable reduction decreases the incidence of nonunion because it does not allow varus angulation or late displacement.
- Coxa vara:
  - Secondary to growth-arrest of the proximal femoral physis or to malunion
  - If the neck shaft angle is <110°, it will not correct with remodeling.
  - Subtrochanteric valgus osteotomy, bone grafting, and internal fixation can give excellent long-term results if no osteonecrosis is present.
- Premature closure of the physis:
  - A slight leg-length inequality results.
  - It occurs even without internal fixation crossing the physis.
  - Closure often is related to osteonecrosis.
  - The proximal femoral physis contributes growth of only 3 mm per year (~15% of total length of extremity) but, if osteonecrosis and premature closure occur, a substantial limb-length discrepancy can develop.
  - Follow with yearly scanograms and hand and wrist radiographs for bone age, with plotting on Moseley charts; consider epiphysiodesis of contralateral limb if substantial limb-length inequality develops.
  - In rare cases, symptomatic trochanteric overgrowth in children >8 years old can require trochanteric transfer.

### REFERENCES


1. Colonna PC. Fracture of the neck of the femur in children. *Am J Surg* 1929;7:793–797.
2. Pring ME, Rang M, Wenger DR. Pelvis and hip. In: Rang M, Pring ME,Wenger DR, eds. *Rang's Children's Fractures,* 3rd ed. Philadelphia: Lippincott Williams & Wilkins, 2005:165–179.
3. Cheng JCY, Tang N. Decompression and stable internal fixation of femoral neck fractures in children can affect the outcome. *J Pediatr Orthop* 1999;19:338–343.
4. Morsy HA. Complications of fracture of the neck of the femur in children. A long-term follow-up study. *Injury* 2001;32:45–51.
5. Ratliff AHC. Fractures of the neck of the femur in children. *J Bone Joint Surg* 1962;44B:528–542.


### ADDITIONAL READING


Gray DW. Trauma to the hip and femur in children. In: Sponseller PD, ed. *Orthopaedic Knowledge Update: Pediatrics 2.* Rosemont, IL: American Academy of Orthopaedic Surgeons, 2002:81–91.


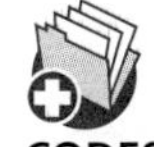

## MISCELLANEOUS

### CODES

#### *ICD9-CM*

820.08 Pediatric hip fracture

### FAQ

- Q: What is the most serious complication of femoral neck fracture in children?
  - A: AVN, which is an increased risk with greater displacement and with more proximal fracture.

# HIP PAIN IN THE CHILD

*Paul D. Sponseller, MD*

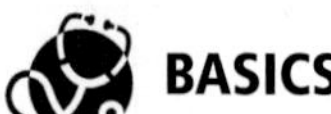

## BASICS

### DESCRIPTION

- "Hip pain" is a term used to describe discomfort in the groin, which receives sensory innervation provided by the obturator and femoral nerves.
- This pain can be produced by a lesion anywhere in the region of the hip joint, such as:
  - Capsule and synovial lining
  - Bone of the pelvis or proximal femur
  - Muscles, nerves, and vascular structures in the region of hip, buttock, groin, or pelvis
- Regardless of cause, hip pain usually is localized to the region of the anterior groin, the greater trochanter, or the anterolateral thigh down to the knee.
- Because many of the causes of hip pain need urgent treatment or carry a poor prognosis if left untreated, hip pain must be evaluated thoroughly.

### EPIDEMIOLOGY

- Transient synovitis is reported to be the most common cause of hip pain in children (1).
- Male predominance:
  - Septic arthritis, slight; transient synovitis, 2:1 (1); SCFE, 2.5:1 (2); osteomyelitis, 4:1 (3); Legg-Calvé-Perthes disease, 6:1 (3).

#### *Incidence*

- Transient synovitis of the hip: 3% risk for a child to have at least 1 episode (3).
- Legg-Calvé-Perthes disease:
  - Peak incidence at 6 years of age (3)
  - ~1 per 1,500 (3)
- SCFE (2):
  - Almost always occurs during preadolescence or adolescence
  - 1 per 10,000

### RISK FACTORS

- Juvenile rheumatoid arthritis
- Closed trauma
- Impaired host immune defense
- Obesity, trauma, and age (all shown to be related to the development of SCFE)

#### *Genetics*

A genetic association is not clearly shown, except in conditions such as SCFE, in which ~4% of patients have a family history (2).

### ETIOLOGY

- The 2 most common causes are transient synovitis and septic arthritis.
  - Transient synovitis:
    - Average age of onset of symptoms is 6 years, with most cases occurring in children 3–8 years old.
    - Associated with current or recent illness, trauma, or allergic reaction
  - Septic arthritis:
    - ~2/3 of all cases occur in children <3 years old.
    - Mechanism of onset: Direct extension of osteomyelitis from the proximal metaphysis of the femur into the hip joint or hematogenous dissemination of organisms through the blood supply of the synovial membrane
    - During a child's first 12–18 months, little resistance exists to the extension of infection across the physis in the proximal femur because of vascular channels in the growth plate, so osteomyelitis and septic arthritis are more common in this group than in others.
    - In newborns, most commonly caused by *Staphylococcus*, *Streptococcus*, or *Haemophilus influenzae* type B
    - In those >6 months old, predominantly caused by *Staphylococcus aureus*
    - In adolescents, possibly caused by *Neisseria gonorrhoeae*
  - Legg-Calvé-Perthes disease: Cause unknown, although trauma, hypercoagulability, and thrombosis have been postulated
  - SCFE:
    - Physeal weakness during adolescent growth spurt and trauma probably are related.
    - ~80% of patients are obese; hormonal factors most likely are involved (2).
- Other types of hip pain:
  - Infectious
  - Traumatic
  - Neoplastic
  - Idiopathic

### ASSOCIATED CONDITIONS

Current or recent illness, trauma, and allergic reactions are associated with transient synovitis.

## DIAGNOSIS

### SIGNS AND SYMPTOMS

- Pain referred to the groin, trochanter, anterolateral thigh, or knee
- Involuntary guarding or spasm of muscles around the hip joint
- Limitation of active and passive hip motion (i.e., loss of internal rotation and abduction in Legg-Calvé-Perthes disease or hip dysplasia; external rotation of the hip with attempted flexion pathognomonic for SCFE)
- Refusal to walk or bear weight on the affected extremity
- Limp, possibly antalgic or painless
- Atrophy of the thigh or buttock muscles
- Fever in septic arthritis, osteomyelitis

#### *Physical Exam*

- Inspect and palpate the tissues around the hip, buttock, lower back, and thigh to detect warmth, erythema, swelling, bruising, or specific areas of point tenderness (e.g., bursae).
- Note the lower extremity's general position.
- Measure and document passive and active ROM of the hip and knee joints, especially internal and external rotation.
- Document a complete neurovascular extremity examination, noting any weakness or numbness.
- If possible, examine the gait, including toe- and heel-walking.
- If septic arthritis is a distinct possibility, perform a hip aspiration, usually under fluoroscopic or sonographic guidance; if no fluid is obtained, an arthrogram should be performed to confirm needle placement.

### TESTS

#### *Lab*

- In transient synovitis, Legg-Calvé-Perthes disease, SCFE, and hip dysplasia, results of routine tests usually are nonspecific and within normal limits but, to rule out infection, it is important to order these tests.
- In septic arthritis:
  - The cell count of the aspirated joint fluid is the most sensitive test, with >50,000 cells/mm$^3$.
  - The serum leukocyte count is elevated, and a left shift may occur.
- Blood cultures:
  - Positive in 40% of children with osteomyelitis or septic arthritis (3)
  - Should always be obtained during the initial stages of the workup

#### *Imaging*

- Plain radiographs in septic arthritis may show obliteration of fat planes and soft-tissue swelling.
- With early osteomyelitis, one may see mottling of bone density; later, sclerosis (new bone formation) and lytic lesions (additional bony destruction) are more prevalent, with destruction of the femoral head being the end result.
- In transient synovitis, plain films of the hip (AP and lateral views) are nonspecific, but they may help rule out other diagnoses.
- In Legg-Calvé-Perthes disease, plain film findings include:
  - Early: Failure of epiphyseal growth and loss of bone density
  - Later: Crescent-shaped subchondral fracture in the femoral head, shortening of the femoral neck, and flattening or (ultimately) enlargement of the femoral head
- Widening of the growth plate, mild osteopenia of the proximal femur, or displacement of the epiphysis is seen in SCFE.

#### *Pathological Findings*

- In septic arthritis, synovial hypertrophy initially; later, cartilage destruction
- In SCFE, posterior and inferior displacement of the femoral head on the metaphysis
- In Perthes disease, flattened and extruded femoral head

## DIFFERENTIAL DIAGNOSIS

- Transient synovitis (although the most common cause of hip pain) should be a diagnosis of exclusion only.
- Infections of the hip joint, proximal femur, pelvis, intervertebral discs, SI joint
- Legg-Calvé-Perthes disease (AVN of the femoral head)
- SCFE
- Juvenile rheumatoid arthritis, early osteoarthritis
- Tumors of the pelvis, spine, or proximal femur
- Bursitis of psoas or trochanter
- Sickle cell crisis
- Nonarticular processes
- SI joint septic arthritis
- Pyomyositis around the hip
- Psoas septic bursitis
- Leukemia or lymphoma

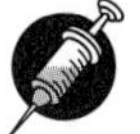

# TREATMENT

## GENERAL MEASURES

- Transient synovitis:
  - Rapidly resolve underlying inflammation with rest and anti-inflammatory agents.
  - Prescribe bed rest and no weightbearing on the involved joint until pain resolves and full motion returns.
  - Spontaneous resolution is the natural course: This condition usually is self-limiting.
- Septic arthritis:
  - Perform immediate surgical drainage and administer antibiotic therapy.
  - Antibiotics:
    - Give broad-spectrum antibiotic coverage until culture results are available.
    - Oral antibiotics, if appropriate, usually are given for 3 weeks, until the clinical examination and/or ESR has returned to normal.
    - Splint hips in abduction if capsular distention has occurred.
    - After infection is controlled and drainage has ceased, begin ROM exercises.
- Legg-Calvé-Perthes disease:
  - Prevent subluxation.
  - Preserve the sphericity of the femoral head.
  - Order bed rest, if needed, and traction to reduce spasms and synovitis.
  - Surgical reconstruction sometimes is necessary to maintain the femoral head within the acetabulum.
- SCFE:
  - Prevent additional slipping while minimizing the risk of AVN or chondrolysis.
  - Provide the necessary immobilization for acute slips with prompt *in situ* pin fixation with threaded screws.

## SPECIAL THERAPY

### *Physical Therapy*

Not usually required

## MEDICATION (DRUGS)

### *First Line*

- Appropriate antibiotics are essential for the treatment of septic arthritis and osteomyelitis.
- NSAIDs are appropriate for transient synovitis.

## SURGERY

- An anterior or posterior approach to the hip may be used, with irrigation, débridement, and insertion of drain.
- For osteomyelitis:
  - A small window is cut in the bone for curettage of material for culture and open drainage.
  - Chronic osteomyelitis, although rare, often requires surgical débridement.
- Legg-Calvé-Perthes disease may require surgical reconstruction of the femur or acetabulum for severe cases.
- *In situ* percutaneous pinning is required for SCFE to prevent additional slips and the associated complications.

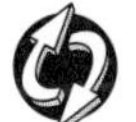

# FOLLOW-UP

## PROGNOSIS

- Septic arthritis and osteomyelitis:
  - Early detection, may have good prognosis
  - Chronic osteomyelitis often results in residual deformity.
- Legg-Calvé-Perthes disease:
  - The smaller the amount of avascular bone and the younger the child at the onset of disease, the better the prognosis, although some residual deformity always is seen on radiographs.
  - Other good prognostic signs include lack of lateralization or extrusion and adequate ROM.
- SCFE:
  - Long-term prognosis depends on the amount of displacement.
  - Patients with more severe slips have a greater likelihood of developing degenerative arthritis later in life.

## COMPLICATIONS

- Untreated septic arthritis and osteomyelitis can be devastating for a growing child and can result in limb shortening, joint-surface irregularities, stiffness, and early degenerative changes. (Cartilage destruction begins as early as 8 hours after the onset of infection.)
- SFCE:
  - Either the slip itself or reduction attempts may result in AVN or chondrolysis, a condition in which the cartilage of the femoral head degenerates and produces joint narrowing, stiffness, contracture, pain, and limping.
  - Patients with SCFE have a higher-than-normal risk of developing degenerative arthritis.

## PATIENT MONITORING

- ESR or C-reactive protein value:
  - Shown to be a reliable marker to guide the length of antibiotic therapy after surgical management for septic arthritis and osteomyelitis
  - Should return to within normal limits before antibiotics are discontinued.
- Observation only is appropriate for all patients with transient synovitis and for patients with Legg-Calvé-Perthes disease with minimal involvement of the femoral head (<50%).

## REFERENCES


1. Dobbs MB, Morcuender JA. Other conditions of the hip. In: Morrissy RT, Weinstein SL, eds. *Lovell and Winter's Pediatric Orthopaedics,* 6th ed. Philadelphia: Lippincott Williams & Wilkins, 2006: 1126–1155.
2. Kay M. Slipped capital femoral epiphysis. In: Morrissy RT, Weinstein SL, eds. *Lovell and Winter's Pediatric Orthopaedics,* 6th ed. Philadelphia: Lippincott Williams & Wilkins, 2006:1085–1124.
3. Weinstein SL. Legg-Calve-Perthes syndrome. In: Morrissy RT, Weinstein SL, eds. *Lovell and Winter's Pediatric Orthopaedics,* 6th ed. Philadelphia: Lippincott Williams & Wilkins, 2006:1039–1083.


## ADDITIONAL READING


Johnson K, Haigh SF, Ehtisham S, et al. Childhood idiopathic chondrolysis of the hip: MRI features. *Pediatr Radiol* 2003;33:194–199.


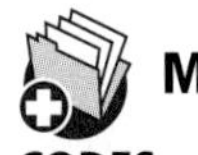

# MISCELLANEOUS

## CODES

### *ICD9-CM*

- 711.0 Septic arthritis
- 719.45 Hip pain, not otherwise specified
- 732.1 Perthes disease
- 732.2 SCFE

## PATIENT TEACHING

- The parents of a patient who is presumed to have synovitis of the hip should be able to observe the child and ensure that improvement continues.
- They should maintain regular follow-up and should contact the physician if the child's status worsens.

## FAQ

- Q: What is transient synovitis of the hip?
  - A: It is an idiopathic inflammation of the hip that resolves spontaneously.
- Q: What is chondrolysis?
  - A: It is loss of joint cartilage; it may occur from infection, inflammation, abrasion, or unknown causes.

# HIP REPLACEMENT

*Kris J. Alden, MD, PhD*
*Simon C. Mears, MD, PhD*

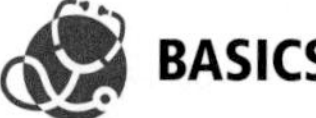

## BASICS

### DESCRIPTION

- Many forms of arthritis lead to destruction of the articular cartilage of the hip joint, resulting in pain and loss of function.
- End-stage arthritis can be treated with surgical replacement of the joint.
- Elderly patients may have a greater risk of cardiac complications and more associated medical problems than younger patients.
- Patients <50 years old:
  - Are likely to need revision surgery because their life expectancy may exceed the longevity of the prosthesis
  - Other treatment options, such as medical management, hip fusion, and femoral osteotomy, should be strongly considered in the younger, high-demand patient.
- Hip replacements may be anchored to the bone with bone cement or with uncemented techniques that allow the bone to grow into the implant.

### GENERAL PREVENTION

Weight loss and limitation of activity may postpone the need for hip replacement.

### EPIDEMIOLOGY

Most hip replacements are performed in patients >65 years old, but the procedure is being performed more commonly in younger patients than in the past (1).

#### *Incidence*

- >200,000 total hip replacements are performed in the United States each year (2).
- The number of hip replacements continues to increase (3).

### RISK FACTORS

- Primary osteoarthritis may be more common in high-demand athletes and obese patients.
- Osteonecrosis has been linked to prolonged steroid use, alcoholism, radiation, and trauma.
- Osteoporosis often leads to femoral neck fractures in elderly patients.

#### *Genetics*

- Possible familial predisposition to primary osteoarthritis
- No Mendelian pattern of inheritance

### PATHOPHYSIOLOGY

#### *Pathological Findings*

The common denominators in all forms of arthritis are breakdown of the articular cartilage, loss of the proteoglycan, and gradual cartilage dissolution.

### ETIOLOGY

- Primary osteoarthritis is the most common cause of disabling hip arthritis.
- Traumatic arthritis, osteonecrosis, rheumatoid arthritis, sickle cell anemia, recurrent hemarthrosis, Paget disease, and AS all may lead to degenerative destruction of the hip joint.
- Developmental conditions such as SCFE, DDH, and Legg-Calvé-Perthes disease all may lead to degenerative joint disease later in life.
- Some acute hip fractures also may be treated with partial or total hip replacement.

### ASSOCIATED CONDITIONS

Degenerative joint disease of the contralateral hip, either knee, the lumbar spine, and the upper extremities often is seen in patients requiring hip replacement.

## DIAGNOSIS

- Primary osteoarthritis of the hip may result in pain in the groin, the lateral thigh, or radiating to the knee.
- Pain is more common with activity but may eventually become present at rest and at night.
- In advanced stages, pain may limit the patient to needing rest after walking <1 block.
- Limitation of ROM, especially of flexion, extension, and internal rotation, may be present.
- With ambulation, abductor lurch may be evident.

### SIGNS AND SYMPTOMS

- Incapacitating arthritis of the hip commensurate with physical and radiographic findings
- Failure to walk more than a few blocks without stopping
- Pain unrelieved by standard arthritis medication
- Pain after activity
- Difficulty with activities of daily living, including dressing, grooming, and climbing stairs

#### *Physical Exam*

- Perform a neurovascular examination of the affected extremity.
- Record the ROM of the hip.
- Pay special attention to contractures, leg-length discrepancy, and gluteal muscle strength.
- Assess the patient's gait.
- Pain at extremes of motion
- Positive Trendelenburg test
- Groin or anterior thigh pain with active straight-leg raises

### TESTS

#### *Lab*

- For total hip replacement, order the following before surgery:
  - Complete blood count
  - Blood chemistry studies
  - Coagulation times
- Electrocardiogram, chest radiographs, and urinalysis should be obtained when appropriate.
- Many patients are able to donate autologous units of blood 4–6 weeks before surgery.

#### *Imaging*

- Radiography:
  - AP pelvis and frog-leg lateral hip radiographs usually are adequate for assessing the hip joint.
  - Long, standing films of the lower extremities and pelvis may be helpful.

### DIFFERENTIAL DIAGNOSIS

- Hip pain may be caused by spinal stenosis or a herniated lumbar disc.
- Low back pain of any cause may radiate to the lateral thigh and hip.
- Trochanteric bursitis may result in lateral hip pain.
- Stress fracture
- Occult neoplasms, such as metastatic bone disease, multiple myeloma, and primary mesenchymal tumors, also can cause hip pain.

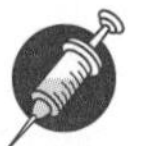

## TREATMENT

### SPECIAL THERAPY

#### *Physical Therapy*

- Postoperative patients are instructed in strengthening exercises, especially hip flexion, extension, and abduction.
- Transfer and gait training with a standup walker are emphasized.

### MEDICATION (DRUGS)

#### *First Line*

- Analgesics in the acute postoperative period
- Postoperative patients require prolonged treatment for prophylaxis of DVT with warfarin (Coumadin) or low-molecular-weight heparin (4).

### SURGERY

- Total hip replacement consists of a metal femoral component and a head that replaces the proximal femur.
  - The acetabulum most commonly is replaced with a metal shell that has a high-density polyethylene plastic insert.
  - The components may be fixed to the bone with or without cement.
    - Uncemented components have a rough surface to allow for bony ingrowth.

- Surgical approaches (5):
  - Anterior (Smith-Peterson)
    - Superficial interval: Sartorius and tensor fascia lata
    - Deep interval: Rectus femoris and gluteus medius
    - Lateral femoral cutaneous nerve is in danger because it penetrates the sartorial fascia.
  - Anterolateral (Watson-Jones approach):
    - Interval between the gluteus medius muscle and the tensor fascia lata
  - Lateral (Hardinge):
    - The anterior 1/3 of the gluteus medius and minimus are reflected off the greater trochanter.
    - The superior gluteal nerve and artery can be injured with anterior reflection of the gluteus medius.
    - Slower abductor rehabilitation
  - Posterior (Langenbeck/Moore):
    - Splitting of the gluteus maximus with release of short external rotators
    - The sciatic nerve should be identified and protected.
    - Higher dislocation rate than with other approaches, especially without capsular repair (6)
- Bearing surfaces: The acetabular liner and the femoral head ball can be made of different materials to prevent wear.
  - Metal on polyethylene:
    - Standard option
    - Newer highly cross-linked polyethylenes are thought to decrease wear rates.
    - Polyethylene wear debris leads to osteolysis and component loosening.
  - Metal on metal:
    - Very low wear rates
    - Metal ion debris can accumulate in the bloodstream and organs.
    - Very large head size may decrease dislocation rates and increase ROM.
  - Ceramic on ceramic:
    - Very low wear rates
    - Very low rate of ceramic fracture
    - No liner options
- Minimally invasive surgery:
  - Some approaches may limit muscle damage.
  - Multimodal approaches to anesthesia and therapy have hastened recovery (7).
  - Some evidence suggests that smaller incisions are not responsible for faster recovery (8).

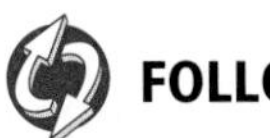

## FOLLOW-UP

### PROGNOSIS

- Hip arthroplasty has excellent long-term results, with many patients ambulating without external support and resuming previously impossible activities (9).
- A long-term study has shown that 85% of cemented prostheses survive for 20 years (10).
- Uncemented components also have an excellent long-term performance.

### COMPLICATIONS

- Postoperative medical complications:
  - Myocardial infarction
  - Pneumonia
  - Urinary retention
  - Ileus
  - Death
- Leg-length discrepancy
- DVT and PE
- Infection
- Revision surgery
- Polyethylene wear
- Osteolysis
- Dislocation
- Periprosthetic fracture
- Heterotopic ossification
- Loosening
- Nerve palsy (11)

### PATIENT MONITORING

- The importance of long-term radiographic monitoring must be stressed.
  - Radiographs should be taken at 1–2-year intervals to look for polyethylene wear and osteolysis.
- After hip replacement, patients should receive antibiotic prophylaxis before dental work.

### REFERENCES


1. Crowninshield RD, Rosenberg AG, Sporer SM. Changing demographics of patients with total joint replacement. *Clin Orthop Relat Res* 2006;443:266–272.
2. American Academy of Orthopaedic Surgeons Department of Research and Scientific Affairs. Information About Hip Replacements: 1999 to 2003. http://www.aaos.org/wordhtml/research/stats/hip_all.htm#source. Accessed on May 15, 2006.
3. Kurtz S, Mowat F, Ong K, et al. Prevalence of primary and revision total hip and knee arthroplasty in the United States from 1990 through 2002. *J Bone Joint Surg* 2005;87A: 1487–1497.
4. Lieberman JR, Hsu WK. Prevention of venous thromboembolic disease after total hip and knee arthroplasty. *J Bone Joint Surg* 2005;87A: 2097–2112.
5. McGann WA. Surgical approaches. In: Callaghan JJ, Rosenberg AG, Rubash HE, eds. *The Adult Hip*. Philadelphia: Lippincott-Raven, 1998: 663–718.
6. Morrey BF. Results of reoperation for hip dislocation: the big picture. *Clin Orthop Relat Res* 2004;429:94–101.
7. Inaba Y, Dorr LD, Wan Z, et al. Operative and patient care techniques for posterior mini-incision total hip arthroplasty. *Clin Orthop Relat Res* 2005;441:104–114.
8. Ogonda L, Wilson R, Archbold P, et al. A minimal-incision technique in total hip arthroplasty does not improve early postoperative outcomes. A prospective, randomized, controlled trial. *J Bone Joint Surg* 2005;87A:701–710.
9. Ethgen O, Bruyere O, Richy F, et al. Health-related quality of life in total hip and total knee arthroplasty. A qualitative and systematic review of the literature. *J Bone Joint Surg* 2004;86A:963–974.
10. Berry DJ, Harmsen WS, Cabanela ME, et al. Twenty-five-year survivorship of two thousand consecutive primary Charnley total hip replacements: factors affecting survivorship of acetabular and femoral components. *J Bone Joint Surg* 2002;84A:171–177.
11. Farrell CM, Springer BD, Haidukewych GJ, et al. Motor nerve palsy following primary total hip arthroplasty. *J Bone Joint Surg* 2005;87A: 2619–2625.


### ADDITIONAL READING


Clohisy JC, Calvert G, Tull F, et al. Reasons for revision hip surgery: a retrospective review. *Clin Orthop Relat Res* 2004;429:188–192.


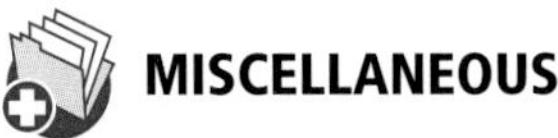

## MISCELLANEOUS

### CODES

#### *ICD9-CM*

715.95 Hip osteoarthritis

### PATIENT TEACHING

- Patients must understand that hip arthroplasty is a major surgical procedure that requires months of substantial activity limitation and may require a full year to achieve full benefit.
- They must be prepared to adhere to the hip precautions taught in physical therapy and to contribute to the rehabilitation process.

#### *Activity*

- Weightbearing after surgery depends on surgeon technique and preference, but as-tolerated is common.
- Patients may be given motion restrictions to prevent dislocation; most commonly, avoidance of hip flexion >90° and crossing the legs.

### FAQ

- Q: When should I have a hip replacement?
  - A: Hip replacement has an excellent chance of reducing pain and improving function. However, it is major surgery with serious potential complications, including death. A patient should have severe pain and disability before considering surgery.

# HIP TRANSIENT SYNOVITIS

*Paul D. Sponseller, MD*

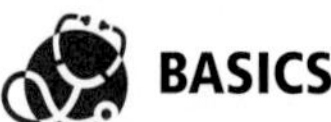

## BASICS

### DESCRIPTION

- Transient synovitis is characterized by the acute onset of monarticular hip pain, limp, and restricted hip motion.
- It must be distinguished from septic arthritis.
- Gradual but complete resolution over several days to weeks is the norm.
- Synonyms: Toxic synovitis; Irritable hip

### EPIDEMIOLOGY

- Transient synovitis is the most common cause of hip pain in children.
- It is a diagnosis of exclusion.
- Transient synovitis of the hip can occur from 9 months of age to adolescence; most cases occur in children 3–8 years old (1–3).
- The risk of a child having at least 1 episode of transient synovitis of the hip is 1–3% (3).
  - This risk is 3 times greater in patients with a stocky or obese physique (3).
- Right and left involvement is essentially equal; concurrent bilateral involvement has not been reported.
- Male:Female ratio is 2:1.

#### *Incidence*

- Transient synovitis accounts for 0.5% of annual pediatric orthopaedic admissions (1).
- The incidence is much lower among African Americans (2).

### RISK FACTORS

- Male gender
- Upper respiratory infection or other active infection

#### *Genetics*

This condition is not genetic.

### ETIOLOGY

- The true cause is unknown; it appears to be an immune-mediated inflammation, not an infection.
- It has been proposed that transient synovitis of the hip may be associated with active infection elsewhere, trauma, or allergic hypersensitivity (1,3).
- Nonspecific upper respiratory infection, pharyngitis, and otitis media have been associated with the occurrence of transient synovitis in as many as 70% of cases (1,2).
- An association is noted with minor trauma in up to 30%, and with allergic predisposition in up to 25% (3).

### ASSOCIATED CONDITIONS

Legg-Calvé-Perthes disease (~1.5%) (3)

## DIAGNOSIS

### SIGNS AND SYMPTOMS

- An acute onset of unilateral hip pain occurs in an otherwise healthy child.
- Pain usually is confined to the ipsilateral groin and hip area, but it may present as anterior thigh and knee pain.
- Limp and antalgic gait are common, with some patients refusing to bear weight on the involved extremity.
- The hip is held in a flexed and externally rotated position and has restricted ROM.
- The patient may have a low-grade fever.
- Laboratory values are nonspecific and are often within normal limits (4,5).

#### *Physical Exam*

- The patient usually indicates unilateral hip pain confined to the ipsilateral groin, anterior thigh, or knee.
- ROM often is decreased and painful.
- The patient does not have as much pain as a patient with a septic hip.
  - If the hip ROM is tested slowly, it is usually at least 50% of normal.
- While walking, patients often display a limp or an antalgic gait; some children refuse to walk (4,5).
- Ipsilateral muscle atrophy is seen rarely, but when present, it implies a longstanding duration of symptoms, and a diagnosis other than transient synovitis should be considered.

### TESTS

#### *Lab*

- Results are usually nonspecific and within normal limits, but they may help to rule out other diagnoses (1).
  - The peripheral white blood cell count is normal to slightly elevated.
  - The ESR averages 20 mm/hour but may be slightly higher.
  - Urinalysis, blood culture, rheumatoid factor, and Lyme titers and tuberculin skin test results are usually within normal limits.
  - Analysis of joint fluid for complement levels or other tests has been nonspecific.

#### *Imaging*

- Radiography:
  - Plain films of the hip should include AP and lateral views.
- In transient synovitis, these films are normal but may help rule out other diagnoses, such as Legg-Calverthes disease and SCFE (3,6–8).
- Ultrasound may be useful to determine if an effusion exists, and to guide aspiration, if infection cannot be ruled out clinically.
- MRI is needed only in cases of persistent pain, when infection has been excluded.
- A bone scan often is not helpful because this condition is not a bony process.

#### *Pathological Findings*

- Biopsy specimens have shown synovial hypertrophy secondary to nonspecific, nonpyogenic inflammatory reaction.
- Hip joint aspirates have shown a culture-negative synovial effusion, usually 1–5 mL.

### DIFFERENTIAL DIAGNOSIS

- Transient synovitis of the hip is a diagnosis of exclusion (1,4,5).
- Conditions to rule out include:
  - Pyogenic arthritis (4,5)
  - Osteomyelitis in the adjacent femoral neck or pelvis (4)
  - Tuberculous arthritis
  - Psoas abscess
  - Other muscle infection about the hip
  - Juvenile rheumatoid arthritis
  - Acute rheumatic fever
  - Legg-Calvé-Perthes disease (3,8)
  - Tumor
  - SCFE
  - Dislocation
  - SI joint infection

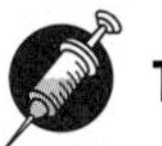

## TREATMENT

### GENERAL MEASURES

- Transient synovitis usually has a limited duration of symptoms, averaging <7 days (2).
  - Most studies report complete resolution of all signs and symptoms with no immediate residual clinical or radiographic abnormalities.
  - Long-term studies have shown mild radiographic changes in the involved hip.
- Traction and routine joint aspiration are not always needed.
  - If traction is used, it is to promote rest and comfort.
  - The hip should be in ~30° of flexion to avoid increasing intra-articular pressure.
- The important point in management of this condition is to establish the diagnosis: Pyogenic arthritis must be excluded, on clinical grounds or with laboratory tests.
- Treatment is directed at rapidly resolving the underlying inflammatory synovitis with its symptoms.

### Activity

- Bed rest until initial acute pain resolves
- Weightbearing after pain resolves and full ROM returns, followed by a period of refraining from strenuous activities

## SPECIAL THERAPY

### Physical Therapy

- Usually not necessary
- Parents can moderate child's activity adequately.

## MEDICATION (DRUGS)

### First Line

- Anti-inflammatory drugs:
  - Some experts believe these medications should be withheld to avoid masking an infection, but others believe they may have diagnostic value in speeding the natural resolution of inflammatory symptoms.

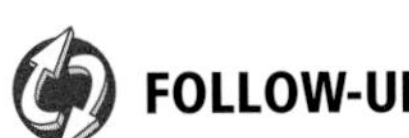

# FOLLOW-UP

## PROGNOSIS

The prognosis is good because transient synovitis is self-limiting, without any clinically significant sequelae.

## COMPLICATIONS

- 1 study has reported that Legg-Calvé-Perthes disease or AVN of the femoral head may develop several months after an episode of transient synovitis of the hip (3).
  - This finding probably represents a delay in establishing the correct diagnosis.

## PATIENT MONITORING

- A physician should be available for re-evaluation at all times until the possibility of infection is excluded.
- The child should be re-examined in ~1–2 weeks to determine return of motion before resuming full weightbearing and normal activity.
- Parents should bring the child back if symptoms recur or increase.

## REFERENCES


1. Dobbs MB, Morcuender JA. Other conditions of the hip. In: Morrissy RT, Weinstein SL, eds. *Lovell and Winter's Pediatric Orthopaedics,* 6th ed. Philadelphia: Lippincott Williams & Wilkins, 2006: 1126–1155.
2. Haueisen DC, Weiner DS, Weiner SD. The characterization of "transient synovitis of the hip" in children. *J Pediatr Orthop* 1986;6:11–17.
3. Landin LA, Danielsson LG, Wattsgard C. Transient synovitis of the hip. Its incidence, epidemiology and relation to Perthes' disease. *J Bone Joint Surg* 1987;69B:238–242.
4. Kocher MS, Mandiga R, Murphy JM, et al. A clinical practice guideline for treatment of septic arthritis in children. Efficacy in improving process of care and effect on outcome of septic arthritis of the hip. *J Bone Joint Surg* 2003;85A:994–999.
5. Kocher MS, Mandiga R, Zurakowski D, et al. Validation of a clinical prediction rule for the differentiation between septic arthritis and transient synovitis of the hip in children. *J Bone Joint Surg* 2004;86A:1629–1635.
6. Johnson K, Haigh SF, Ehtisham S, et al. Childhood idiopathic chondrolysis of the hip: MRI features. *Pediatr Radiol* 2003;33:194–199.
7. Kay RM. Slipped capital femoral epiphysis. In: Morrissy RT, Weinstein SL, eds. *Lovell and Winter's Pediatric Orthopaedics*, 6th ed. Philadelphia: Lippincott Williams & Wilkins, 2006:1085–1124.
8. Weinstein SL. Legg-Calvé-Perthes syndrome. In: Morrissy RT, Weinstein SL, eds. *Lovell and Winter's Pediatric Orthopaedics*, 6th ed. Philadelphia: Lippincott Williams & Wilkins, 2006:1039–1083.


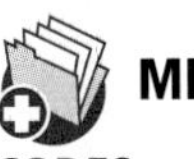

# MISCELLANEOUS

## CODES

### ICD9-CM

727.0 Synovitis

## PATIENT TEACHING

- Transient hip synovitis is a self-limiting process without major consequences.
- Some authorities have suggested an increased incidence of later Legg-Calvé-Perthes disease in such patients, but this finding has not been proven conclusively.

## FAQ

- Q: Do all patients with transient synovitis require aspiration of the hip?
  - A: No. Although the essence of management is to rule out infection, in many cases this goal can be accomplished clinically by noting that transient synovitis involves a more mild degree of guarding, more mild elevation of infection and inflammatory markers. Most often, patients with transient synovitis will be able to bear some weight on the involved side.
- Q: If aspiration is needed to rule out infection, where and how should it be done?
  - A: Aspiration requires sedation. It should be done with imaging (ultrasound or fluoroscopy) to be certain that the aspirate is from the hip joint. A radiologist or orthopaedic surgeon may perform this procedure. Anterior, medial, or lateral approaches are used. Fluid should be sent for cell count with differential and culture.

# HUMERAL SHAFT FRACTURE

*Simon C. Mears, MD, PhD*
*Chris Hutchins, MD*

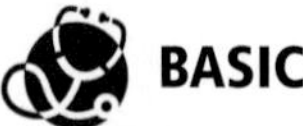

## BASICS

### DESCRIPTION

- Fractures of the diaphysis (shaft) of the humerus
- Occur at all ages
- Classification:
  - AO classification method (1)
  - Anatomic location:
    - Proximal 1/3 of the shaft
    - Medial 1/3 of the shaft
    - Distal 1/3 of the shaft
- Fracture characteristics:
  - Fracture pattern (transverse versus oblique versus comminuted)
  - Fractures may be open or closed.
  - Pathologic (secondary to underlying bone disease)
  - Spiral fractures of the distal 1/3 have been termed "Holstein-Lewis" fractures and are associated with radial nerve injury.

### EPIDEMIOLOGY

#### *Incidence*

- Fracture rate is 0–2 per 10,000 per year with no gender differences (2).
- Midshaft fractures comprise ~40% of all humerus fractures (3).
- In children, humerus fractures cause 17% of admissions for fracture (4).
- Fracture incidence peaks in the 3rd decade, but a 2nd peak occurs in females in their 7th decade (5).

### RISK FACTORS

- Osteoporosis in the elderly
- High-energy trauma, such as motor vehicle accidents or falls from heights, in younger patients
- Sports with rotational forces, such as wrestling or baseball

### ETIOLOGY

- Usually results from direct force to the upper extremity
- May occur:
  - From violent muscle contractions and twisting arm injuries
  - After relatively minor trauma in patients with underlying bone disease
  - In young adults when throwing balls while playing softball or baseball

### ASSOCIATED CONDITIONS

- Look for other associated upper extremity fractures or injuries.
- Carefully examine the neurovascular status.

## DIAGNOSIS

### SIGNS AND SYMPTOMS

- Pain
- Deformity
- Bruising
- Crepitus
- Swelling

#### *Physical Exam*

- Assess for skin integrity (ensure that no open fracture exists).
- Examine the shoulder and elbow joints and the forearm, hand, and clavicle for associated trauma.
- Check the function of the median, ulnar, and, particularly, the radial nerves.
- Assess for the presence of the radial pulse.

### TESTS

#### *Lab*

No serum or laboratory test is diagnostic.

#### *Imaging*

AP and lateral views of the humerus, including the joints below and above the injury, are obtained.

### DIFFERENTIAL DIAGNOSIS

- Pathologic fractures through abnormal bone
- Muscular contusions
- Muscle tear or strain

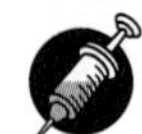

## TREATMENT

- Most closed fractures of the humeral shaft may be managed nonoperatively.
- Reduction should be attempted if there is >20–30° of angulation, >3 cm of shortening, or >15° of rotational deformity.
  - Lesser degrees of shortening or angulation are tolerated satisfactorily.
- Splinting:
  - Fractures are splinted with a "U" splint, which is from the axilla, under the elbow, postioned to the top of the shoulder (Fig. 1).
  - The U splint is supplemented by a posterior splint, which originates at the proximal humerus and extends behind the elbow to the forearm.
  - The splinted extremity is supported by a sling.
- Fracture brace:
  - After 1–2 weeks, swelling will have subsided, and the extremity is placed in a fracture brace.
  - Immobilization by fracture bracing is continued for at least 2 months or until clinical and radiographic evidence of fracture healing is observed.
- With this treatment regimen, union rates of ~90% can be attained (6,7).
- Occasionally, humeral shaft fractures require operative fixation; indications include:
  - Open fractures
  - Articular injury
  - Neurovascular injury
  - Ipsilateral forearm fractures
  - Impending pathologic fractures
  - Segmental fractures
  - Multiple extremity fractures
  - Fractures in which reduction is unable to be achieved or maintained
  - Fractures with nerve palsy after reduction maneuvers

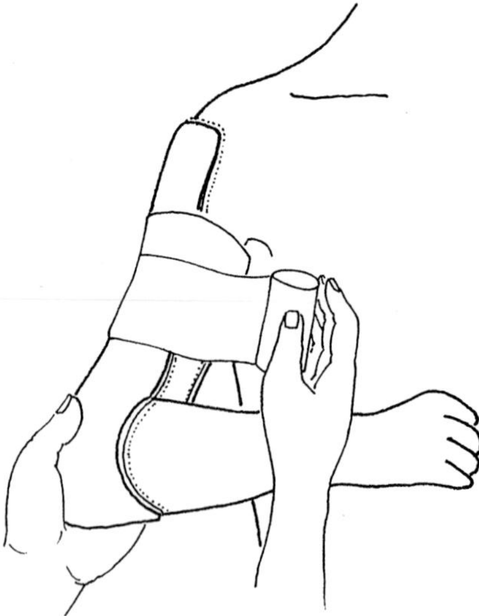

**Fig. 1.** Applying a sugar tong splint for humeral shaft fractures.

## GENERAL MEASURES

### Activity

Support the arm in a sling.

### Nursing

- In the acute period, apply ice to the region for 20 min every 3–4 hours to help decrease swelling.
- Sensation of movement of the fracture ends is common.
- The axillary area must be cleaned after splinting.

## SPECIAL THERAPY

### Physical Therapy

- None is required in the initial period.
- When pain has subsided (~1–2 weeks), gentle ROM of the shoulder and elbow should be started.

## MEDICATION (DRUGS)

### First Line

Narcotic analgesics may be required for pain control.

## SURGERY

- Surgery involves fixation of the bone fragments with a plate and screws or intramedullary fixation with a metal nail.
  - Plating with a 4.5-mm dynamic compression plate or a locking plate
  - Intramedullary fixation with an anterograde or a retrograde starting point
    - Anterograde starting points are associated with a higher rate of late shoulder pain than are retrograde starting points (8).
- If severe soft-tissue injury exists, external fixation may be necessary.

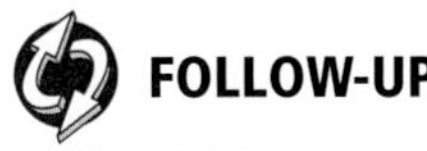

# FOLLOW-UP

## PROGNOSIS

~90% of humeral shaft fractures treated without surgery heal (6,7).

## COMPLICATIONS

- Injury to the radial nerve:
  - Occurs in ~11% of humerus fractures
  - Can occur at the time of initial injury, during closed reduction, or during operative repair (9)
  - If radial nerve palsy is identified after fracture reduction, operative exploration with plate fixation usually is recommended.
  - ~70% of these injuries are neurapraxias (contusions to the nerve fibers) that improve over time (9).
- Nonunion rates are thought to be higher when fractures are treated with intramedullary nailing (10).
- Malunion is thought be well tolerated.
- Shoulder pain has been reported when fractures are treated with nails and with plates (11).
- Elbow or shoulder stiffness

## PATIENT MONITORING

- Serial radiographs are obtained at 4–6-week intervals to ensure progressive healing and angulation of <30°.
- ROM of the shoulder and elbow must be checked so that adjustments can be made in the physical therapy program.

## REFERENCES


1. Muller ME. Appendix A to chapter 1: The comprehensive classification of long bones. In: Muller ME, Allgower M, Schneider R, et al., eds. *Manual of Internal Fixation. Techniques Recommended by the AO-ASIF Group*, 3rd ed. New York: Springer-Verlag,1991:118–150.
2. Singer BR, McLauchlan GJ, Robinson CM, et al. Epidemiology of fractures in 15,000 adults: the influence of age and gender. *J Bone Joint Surg* 1998;80B:243–248.
3. Igbigbi PS, Manda K. Epidemiology of humeral fractures in Malawi. *Int Orthop* 2004;28: 338–341.
4. Galano GJ, Vitale MA, Kessler MW, et al. The most frequent traumatic orthopaedic injuries from a national pediatric inpatient population. *J Pediatr Orthop* 2005;25:39–44.
5. Tytherleigh-Strong G, Walls N, McQueen MM. The epidemiology of humeral shaft fractures. *J Bone Joint Surg* 1998;80B:249–253.
6. Koch PP, Gross DFL, Gerber C. The results of functional (Sarmiento) bracing of humeral shaft fractures. *J Shoulder Elbow Surg* 2002;11: 143–150.
7. Sarmiento A, Zagorski JB, Zych GA, et al. Functional bracing for the treatment of fractures of the humeral diaphysis. *J Bone Joint Surg* 2000;82A:478–486.
8. Scheerlinck T, Handelberg F. Functional outcome after intramedullary nailing of humeral shaft fractures: comparison between retrograde Marchetti-Vicenzi and unreamed AO antegrade nailing. *J Trauma* 2002;52:60–71.
9. Shao YC, Harwood P, Grotz MRW, et al. Radial nerve palsy associated with fractures of the shaft of the humerus: a systematic review. *J Bone Joint Surg* 2005;87B:1647–1652.
10. McCormack RG, Brien D, Buckley RE, et al. Fixation of fractures of the shaft of the humerus by dynamic compression plate or intramedullary nail. A prospective, randomised trial. *J Bone Joint Surg* 2000;82B:336–339.
11. Flinkkila T, Hyvonen P, Siira P, et al. Recovery of shoulder joint function after humeral shaft fracture: a comparative study between antegrade intramedullary nailing and plate fixation. *Arch Orthop Trauma Surg* 2004;124:537–541.


## ADDITIONAL READING


- Caviglia H, Garrido CP, Palazzi FF, et al. Pediatric fractures of the humerus. *Clin Orthop Relat Res* 2005;432:49–56.
- DeFranco MJ, Lawton JN. Radial nerve injuries associated with humeral fractures. *J Hand Surg* 2006;31A:655–663.
- Sarmiento A, Waddell JP, Latta LL. Diaphyseal humeral fractures: treatment options. *Instr Course Lect* 2002;51:257–269.


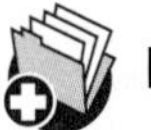

# MISCELLANEOUS

## CODES

### ICD9-CM

812.21 Humeral shaft fracture

## PATIENT TEACHING

- Once in a fracture brace, the patient may commence gentle active ROM of the shoulder and the elbow.
- Activities of daily living are encouraged.
- During the initial healing period, many patients find that sleeping in a chair is more comfortable than sleeping in a bed.

### Activity

Patients treated with open plating may bear weight on the affected arm.

## FAQ

- Q: How long does it take to heal a humerus fracture?
  - A: Most fractures are treated without surgery and take ~3–4 months to heal. After healing, continued work is needed to improve arm motion and strength.

# INTERCONDYLAR ELBOW FRACTURE

*Peter R. Jay, MD*
*Simon C. Mears, MD, PhD*

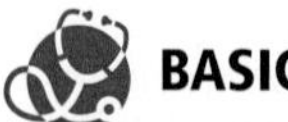

## BASICS

### DESCRIPTION

- Intra-articular fracture of the distal humerus, which may occur with a supracondylar fracture
- Biomechanically and anatomically, the distal humerus forms a triangle composed of a medial column and a lateral column that support the articular surface of the trochlea.
- The trochlea articulates with the ulna.
- The capitellum is the part of the humerus that articulates with the radius and is part of the lateral column.
- Classification:
  - No single classification system is uniformly accepted or used.
  - Many of the newer classification systems simply substitute the word "column" for "condylar" because this is believed to be more appropriate, given current understanding of the anatomy.
  - Single-column fractures:
    - Divided into medial or lateral fractures
    - High fractures involve most of the trochlea and are unstable.
  - Milch classification (1): Based on whether the fracture includes the lateral aspect of the trochlea
    - Type I: Analogous to a low, single-column fracture
    - Type II: Analogous to a high, single-column fracture
  - Bicolumn fractures: A more complex descriptive classification by Jupiter and Mehne (2) is based on the fracture pattern as it traverses the columns and the articular surface.
    - T pattern
    - Y pattern
    - H pattern
    - Lambda pattern
  - Synonyms: Unicondylar fracture; Bicondylar fracture; Intra-articular distal humerus fracture

### EPIDEMIOLOGY

- This fracture occurs in all age groups.
- In adults, the distal humerus fracture rate is ~5.7 cases per 100,000 in the population with an equal gender distribution (3).
- Single-column fractures (unicolumnar, unicondylar) are more common in children than in adults.
- Lateral column fractures are more common than medial column fractures.

#### *Incidence*

- A single-column fracture is rare (3–4% of fractures of the distal humerus) (2).
- The reported incidence of bicolumn fractures varies markedly, ranging from 5–62% of all distal humerus fractures (2).

#### *Prevalence*

A bimodal age distribution is noted: Young patients (often male) involved in high-velocity trauma, or elderly osteoporotic patients (often female) with a lesser mechanism (3).

### RISK FACTORS

- Persons at risk for high-energy trauma
- Elderly persons: Risks for falls and osteoporosis

### ETIOLOGY

- Falls: From a height; on an outstretched arm
- Automobile versus pedestrian accidents
- Motor vehicle accidents
- Direct blows to the elbow

### ASSOCIATED CONDITIONS

- Neurapraxia
- Vascular injury
- Polytrauma

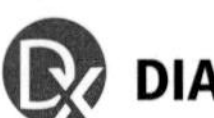

## DIAGNOSIS

### SIGNS AND SYMPTOMS

- Severe pain, swelling, and a decreased ability or inability to move the extremity at the elbow
- Ischemia, dysesthesia, or paresthesia also possible (not common, but important to assess)

#### *Physical Exam*

- These injuries often are associated with substantial energy, and the patient requires a thorough examination.
- Extremity:
  - Evaluate soft tissues to establish open versus closed fracture status.
  - Marked swelling often is present.
  - Assess the limb for vascular status and signs of ischemia (pallor, capillary refill, peripheral pulses).
- Neurologic status:
  - Evaluate and clearly document the neurologic status of the extremity in the ulnar, median (and anterior interossei), and radial (and posterior interossei) nerve distributions, including specific muscle testing and 2-point discrimination.
  - Often the patient cannot or will not move, or allow passive movement of, the elbow.
  - If the patient does move it, or allow it to be moved, marked crepitus often is present.

### TESTS

#### *Imaging*

- Radiography:
  - Plain radiographs include AP and lateral views of the elbow and humerus and forearm views if indicated by examination.
  - Subtle signs, such as posterior or anterior fat pad signs, may be indicative of fracture.
  - Special views, such as the radiocapitellar view, can differentiate other fractures (e.g., radial head or capitellar fractures).
- CT is useful for operative planning for partial articular fractures or fractures with severe comminution.

### DIFFERENTIAL DIAGNOSIS

- Humerus shaft fracture
- Supracondylar fracture
- Transcondylar fracture
- Elbow dislocation
- Elbow sprain
- Capitellum fracture
- Trochlea fracture
- Olecranon fracture
- Proximal single or both bones of the forearm fracture or dislocation
- Radial head fracture or dislocation
- Monteggia fracture or dislocation

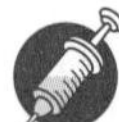

## TREATMENT

### GENERAL MEASURES

- The key to success in all these fractures is stability and early motion.
  - The current trend is to treat most of these injuries surgically.
- The RICE protocol should be initiated even during evaluation.
- If operative care is indicated, surgery preferably is performed early (within 2–3 days).
- If the limb has a diminished or absent pulse, reduction with immobilization or traction should be performed.
  - If this procedure does not improve the status of the limb, angiography or surgical exploration should be performed.
- The sequence of angiography versus immediate surgery depends on warm ischemia time, other injuries, availability of angiography, and the surgeon's preference and experience.
- Single-column fractures:
  - Nondisplaced fractures:
    - Rare and may be treated nonsurgically, but clinical and radiographic vigilance on the part of the physician is required
    - The duration of immobilization should be <2 weeks.
    - Treatment should include gentle passive ROM and placement in a hinged brace with gradually increasing motion.
  - Displaced fractures should be treated surgically.
- Bicolumn fractures:
  - Treat surgically.
  - In rare cases (severe fracture comminution in an elderly patient or other patient unable to tolerate surgery), treat with immobilization.

#### *Activity*

- Early motion is essential.
- A period of 10–14 days of immobilization is considered by many to be the maximal acceptable duration.
- Loaded motion (heavy lifting, repetitive loading) must be avoided until fracture healing has occurred.

### SPECIAL THERAPY

#### *Physical Therapy*

- Early and carefully monitored ROM exercises are necessary to regain a functional arc of motion (100° of flexion).
- A hinged brace is useful for guiding motion.

### MEDICATION (DRUGS)

In the acute setting, the patient requires analgesia and postoperative antibiotics.

### SURGERY

- Surgical therapy for the different types of intercondylar fractures is similar.
  - Most commonly, a posterior approach is used.
  - An olecranon osteotomy is useful for exposure.

- 3.5-mm reconstruction plates and screws are used for rigid fixation.
  - 2 plates at right angles to each other give maximal strength to the repair.
    - The most common configuration is a plate placed posteriorly on the lateral column and medially on the medial column.
  - Newer plates are precontoured for the bones of the distal humerus.
- It often is necessary to reconstruct the articular surface with screws before or concomitantly with plating 1 or both columns, to use bone graft, and to transpose the ulnar nerve.
- Some single-column fractures are far less complex and require simpler constructs, sometimes a single screw or multiple Kirschner wires.
- Elderly patients with severe comminution and osteoporotic bone can be treated with primary total elbow arthroplasty (4).

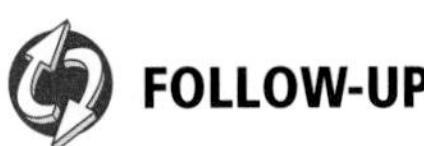

## FOLLOW-UP

### PROGNOSIS

- Despite the technical challenges, studies with the newer techniques have reported remarkably good results (~75% good to excellent results even with the most complex fractures) (5).
- For ROM, a good to excellent result is in the range of 15–30° to 120–130° (6).

### COMPLICATIONS (7)

- Loss of ROM (all patients: usually 10–20° of extension, 10–20° of flexion)
- Nonunion
- Malunion
- Posttraumatic arthritis
- Loss of fixation
- Symptomatic hardware
- Osteonecrosis
- Neurovascular injury
- Ulnar neuropathy
- Infection
- Heterotopic ossification

### PATIENT MONITORING

The patient must be monitored acutely and postoperatively for neurovascular status and compartment syndrome.

### REFERENCES


1. Milch H. Fractures and fracture dislocations of the humeral condyles. *J Trauma* 1964;4:592–607.
2. Jupiter JB, Mehne DK. Trauma to the adult elbow and fractures of the distal humerus. In: Browner BD, Jupiter JB, Levine AM, et al, eds. *Skeletal Trauma. Fractures, Dislocations, Ligamentous Injuries*. Philadelphia: WB Saunders Co., 1992: 1125–1176.
3. Robinson CM, Hill RMF, Jacobs N, et al. Adult distal humeral metaphyseal fractures: epidemiology and results of treatment. *J Orthop Trauma* 2003;17:38–47.
4. Kamineni S, Morrey BF. Distal humeral fractures treated with noncustom total elbow replacement. *J Bone Joint Surg* 2004;86A:940–947.
5. Ring D, Jupiter JB, Gulotta L. Articular fractures of the distal part of the humerus. *J Bone Joint Surg* 2003;85A:232–238.
6. McKee MD, Wilson TL, Winston L, et al. Functional outcome following surgical treatment of intra-articular distal humeral fractures through a posterior approach. *J Bone Joint Surg* 2000;82A: 1701–1707.
7. Sodergard J, Sandelin J, Bostman O. Postoperative complications of distal humeral fractures. 27/96 adults followed up for 6 (2–10) years. *Acta Orthop Scand* 1992;63:85–89.


### ADDITIONAL READING


- Jupiter JB. Complex fractures of the distal part of the humerus and associated complications. *Instr Course Lect* 1995;44:187–198.
- Pajarinen J, Bjorkenheim JM. Operative treatment of type C intercondylar fractures of the distal humerus: results after a mean follow-up of 2 years in a series of 18 patients. *J Shoulder Elbow Surg* 2002;11:48–52.


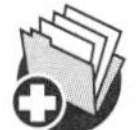

## MISCELLANEOUS

### CODES

#### *ICD9-CM*

- 812.41 Closed supracondylar fracture
- 812.42 Lateral condyle fracture
- 812.43 Medial condyle fracture
- 812.51 Open supracondylar fracture

### PATIENT TEACHING

The patient must be informed that he or she will lose ROM at the elbow, and that the functional outcome greatly depends on patient compliance with ROM protocols and strict compliance with lifting and activity restrictions.

### FAQ

- Q: How are intercondylar fractures treated?
  - A: Most fractures are treated surgically to reduce the joint surface. Rigid fixation allows for early motion, without which elbow stiffness is inevitable.



I

# INTERTROCHANTERIC HIP FRACTURE

*Daniel L. Miller, BS*
*Scott Berkenblit, MD, PhD*

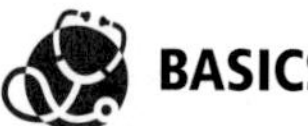

## BASICS

### DESCRIPTION

- Fractures of the proximal femur located between the greater and lesser trochanters and external to the capsule of the hip joint
  - The greater and lesser trochanters may be avulsed as separate fragments.
- Many classification systems have been developed that are unreliable in identifying fracture types (1), but in general, they are classified as stable or unstable.
  - Stable fractures:
    - Nondisplaced or those in which the femur is broken into 2 or 3 fragments
    - A large lateral buttress must exist, and the lesser trochanter must be intact.
  - Unstable fractures:
    - The femur is broken into $\geq$4 fragments
    - The lateral buttress is not intact, or the fracture is reverse oblique.
  - Synonyms: Trochanteric hip fracture; Pertrochanteric hip fracture

### GENERAL PREVENTION

- Use of calcium and vitamin D or bisphosphonates and physical therapy to preserve bone mass
- Prevention of falls in the elderly:
  - Use of ambulatory aids, such as canes or walkers
  - Home modification strategies, such as hand railings
- External hip protectors

### EPIDEMIOLOGY

Intertrochanteric hip fractures are 2–8 times as common in females than in males, presumably because of postmenopausal loss of bone mass (2).

#### *Incidence*

- Intertrochanteric fractures occur in 34 per 100,000 person years in males and in 63 per 100,000 person years in females (2).
- Intertrochanteric fractures account for 40–50% of hip fractures (2).
- The increased incidence with advanced age is likely secondary to osteoporosis and the increased risk of falling.

### RISK FACTORS

- Osteoporosis is a substantial risk factor.
- Any factor that increases the risk of falling (e.g., unsteady gait) increases the risk.
- Pathologic fractures may occur in the presence of tumor or metastatic bone lesions.

### ETIOLOGY

- Nearly all intertrochanteric fractures are the result of falls.
- Motor vehicle accidents comprise the 2nd most common cause of this injury.
- Mechanism of injury:
  - Typically direct axial loading of the femur or direct force over the greater trochanter
  - Indirect forces from muscle insertion on the trochanters also may contribute to the injury and deformity.

### ASSOCIATED CONDITIONS

- Osteoporosis
- Frailty
- Other fractures and soft-tissue injuries of the affected limb, as well as associated neural and vascular injuries, can occur in patients with these fractures.

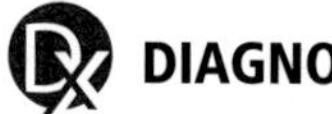

## DIAGNOSIS

### SIGNS AND SYMPTOMS

- Stable fractures:
  - Patients may be ambulatory and experience minimal pain.
  - Patients have pain with weightbearing and motion of the hip.
- Unstable fractures:
  - The patient is in severe pain and is unable to ambulate.
  - The affected leg is shortened and externally rotated to as much as 90° (more marked than seen with femoral neck fractures) because of the action of the iliopsoas at its insertion distal to the fracture site.
- Swelling may occur over the hip, and ecchymosis over the greater trochanter.

#### *History*

Most commonly, the patient has a history of a low-energy fall.

#### *Physical Exam*

- In addition to assessing the deformity of the proximal femur, the clinician should examine the ipsilateral knee for evidence of ligamentous injury.
- Neurovascular status of the limb should be assessed carefully.

### TESTS

#### *Imaging*

- Radiography:
  - Obtain AP radiographs of the affected hip and the pelvis, with the affected hip internally rotated.
  - Obtain a cross-table lateral hip radiograph.
- If a fracture is not visible on the plain radiographs, obtain an MRI scan.

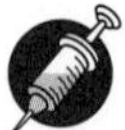

## TREATMENT

### GENERAL MEASURES

#### *Activity*

- Patients with fractures should be kept nonweightbearing and at rest until fracture fixation.
- Traction has not been found to be helpful preoperatively.

#### *Nursing*

- Care must be taken to avoid pressure points and decubitus ulcers of the sacrum and heels.
- In the elderly, nursing precautions to avoid delirium, including reorientation and avoidance of sedatives

### SPECIAL THERAPY

#### *Physical Therapy*

- Strengthening and ambulation are the main goals.
- After surgical fixation, patients should be mobilized quickly and allowed to bear weight as tolerated.

### MEDICATION (DRUGS)

#### *First Line*

Pain should be controlled with opioid analgesics and acetaminophen.

#### *Second Line*

- Most patients are treated surgically.
- Rarely, nonoperative treatment is selected.
  - Patients who are nonambulatory and at high surgical risk are candidates for nonoperative treatment.
  - Patients must be padded carefully and gently mobilized to avoid pressure sores.

### SURGERY

- After open or closed reduction of the fracture, the reduction is maintained by internal fixation.
- A sliding hip screw with side plate device or an intramedullary hip screw may be used, depending on fracture geometry.
- The most important factor in fracture fixation is placement of the screw into the femoral head.
  - The lag screw is positioned under fluoroscopy so that the tip-to-apex distance is $\leq$24 mm.
    - The tip-to-apex distance is the sum of the distances from the tip of the lag screw to the apex of the femoral head, as measured on AP and lateral radiographs, adjusted for magnification.
    - If the tip-to-apex distance is >24 mm, the rate of failure of fixation increases (3).
- A sliding hip screw allows the lag screw to slide through the plate so that the fracture can partially collapse.
  - Sliding of the screw compresses the fracture fragments and promotes healing.
  - For a sliding screw and side plate to be effective, a lateral buttress of bone in the greater trochanteric region must be present to provide a stop point for the screw when sliding (4).
  - If the buttress does not exist, the fracture is classified as unstable and is best treated with an intramedullary hip screw, which serves as the lateral buttress to stop sliding.

- Intramedullary fixation devices are indicated when the fracture is unstable, especially those with a reverse oblique pattern or those with subtrochanteric extension.
- Hip replacement may be considered in patients with extreme comminution or for pre-existing arthritis.
- Replacement is challenging and requires special techniques (5).

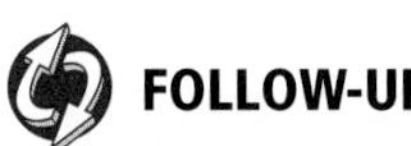

## FOLLOW-UP

### DISPOSITION

- Early mobilization is the key goal of rehabilitation after operative treatment.
  - The patient should commence weightbearing as tolerated, using a walker, crutches, or a cane as necessary, on postoperative day 1 (6).
  - Elderly patients often require a postoperative rehabilitation stay to increase strength and ability to ambulate.

### PROGNOSIS

- Although most patients can expect satisfactory results, only ~50% return completely to their previous level of function (7).
- Morbidity and mortality are substantial, mainly because of the patients' advanced age (8).

### COMPLICATIONS

- The mortality rate in the 1st year is high (secondary to coexisting morbidities), ranging from 10–30% (8).
- Mental status change is common during the acute phase of hospitalization.
  - Precautions should be taken to avoid and treat postoperative delirium.
- DVT is common, and prophylaxis should be given: Warfarin, low-molecular-weight heparin, or factor Xa inhibitors combined with mechanical prophylaxis.
- Mechanical complications include failure of fixation (usually resulting in impaction or varus angulation), penetration of the fixation device into the hip joint, and stress fractures of the femoral neck, resulting from poor positioning of the fixation device within the femoral head.
- Nonunion and osteonecrosis are uncommon complications (<2%) because these fractures occur through well-vascularized cancellous bone (7).
- Mechanical complications and nonunion usually are treated with a complex total hip replacement.
- Postoperative wound infection rates of 1–17% have been reported (7).

### PATIENT MONITORING

- Patient radiographs should be monitored for at least 1 year after fixation.
- Fracture healing may be difficult to visualize, and CT scan may be necessary to reveal nonunion.

### REFERENCES


1. Jin WJ, Dai LY, Cui YM, et al. Reliability of classification systems for intertrochanteric fractures of the proximal femur in experienced orthopaedic surgeons. *Injury* 2005;36:858–861.
2. Lofman O, Berglund K, Larsson L, et al. Changes in hip fracture epidemiology: redistribution between ages, genders and fracture types. *Osteoporos Int* 2002;13:18–25.
3. Baumgaertner MR, Curtin SL, Lindskog DM, et al. The value of the tip-apex distance in predicting failure of fixation of peritrochanteric fractures of the hip. *J Bone Joint Surg* 1995;77A:1058–1064.
4. Gotfried Y. The lateral trochanteric wall. A key element in the reconstruction of unstable pertrochanteric hip fractures. *Clin Orthop Relat Res* 2004;425:82–86.
5. Kim SY, Kim YG, Hwang JK. Cementless calcar-replacement hemiarthroplasty compared with intramedullary fixation of unstable intertrochanteric fractures. A prospective, randomized study. *J Bone Joint Surg* 2005;87A: 2186–2192.
6. Koval KJ, Sala DA, Kummer FJ, et al. Postoperative weight-bearing after a fracture of the femoral neck or an intertrochanteric fracture. *J Bone Joint Surg* 1998;80A:352–356.
7. Lindskog DM, Baumgaertner MR. Unstable intertrochanteric hip fractures in the elderly. *J Am Acad Orthop Surg* 2004;12:179–190.
8. Dobbs RE, Parvizi J, Lewallen DG. Perioperative morbidity and 30-day mortality after intertrochanteric hip fractures treated by internal fixation or arthroplasty. *J Arthroplasty* 2005;20: 963–966.


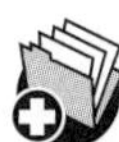

## MISCELLANEOUS

### CODES

#### *ICD9-CM*

820.21 Intertrochanteric hip fracture

### PATIENT TEACHING

#### *Activity*

Exercise is helpful in increasing bone density.

#### *Prevention*

- Patients at risk for osteoporosis should be screened with bone densitometry and treated with calcium and diphosphonate.
- Fall prevention techniques and a home visit to assess fall risk are important.

### FAQ

- Q: How are intertrochanteric hip fractures treated?
  - A: Most fractures are treated with surgery to reduce the fracture, using a hip screw and side plate or an intramedullary hip screw.
- Q: How well do patients recover after surgery?
  - A: ~50% of patients return to their previous level of function. The other 1/2 require more ambulatory aids.
- Q: Why do some fracture heal with a shortened leg?
  - A: The sliding hip screw is designed to slide in line with the femoral neck. Controlled collapse of the fracture gives more bony contact and allows for healing. Collapse of the hip does shorten the leg and may result in the need for a heel wedge. Shortening of the hip may result in weakness to the hip abductors and a Trendelenburg-type of limping gait.

I

# JONES FRACTURE

*Bill Hobbs, MD*
*Simon C. Mears, MD, PhD*

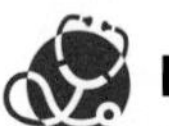

## BASICS

### DESCRIPTION

- Fracture of the base of the 5th metatarsal of the foot
  - Injuries may be acute or stress fractures.
- Classification is by location of the fracture (1).
  - Tuberosity avulsion fracture: No involvement of the 4th to 5th intermetatarsal joint
  - True Jones fracture: Proximal metaphyseal fracture with involvement of the 4th to 5th intermetatarsal joint up to the metaphyseal–diaphyseal junction
  - Diaphyseal fracture (pseudo-Jones fracture): At the proximal diaphysis, distal to the tuberosity of the peroneus tertius insertion

### GENERAL PREVENTION

Early radiographs for athletes complaining of lateral foot pain so that treatment measures can be initiated to decrease prolonged symptoms.

### EPIDEMIOLOGY

- Common in athletes
- Metatarsal fractures occur at all ages (mean age, 42 years) (2).
- Occurs more often in females than males
- 63% of all metatarsal fractures involve the 5th metatarsal (2).

#### *Incidence*

1.8% of professional football players sustain a Jones fracture (3).

### RISK FACTORS

- Athletics
- Falls
- Osteoporosis is a risk factor for foot fractures (4).

### ETIOLOGY

- Avulsion fracture: Inversion or internal rotation injury of the foot
- Jones or diaphyseal fractures: Indirect trauma (inversion or internal rotation injuries) or direct trauma, such as dropping a heavy object on the foot

## DIAGNOSIS

### SIGNS AND SYMPTOMS

Pain and swelling along the lateral border of the foot occur with point tenderness at the base of the 5th metatarsal.

#### *Physical Exam*

- Pain over the lateral forefoot with palpation and weightbearing
- Swelling and redness also common

### TESTS

#### *Imaging*

Plain, AP, lateral, and oblique radiographs of the foot are obtained to determine the level and displacement of the fracture.

#### *Pathological Findings*

The watershed blood supply to the metaphyseal–diaphyseal junction makes fractures in this area more susceptible to nonunion and requires more aggressive treatment of the Jones fracture than do other metatarsal fractures.

### DIFFERENTIAL DIAGNOSIS

- Lisfranc injury (dislocation of tarsometatarsal joints)
- Stress fracture of the 5th metatarsal diaphysis (Fig. 1)

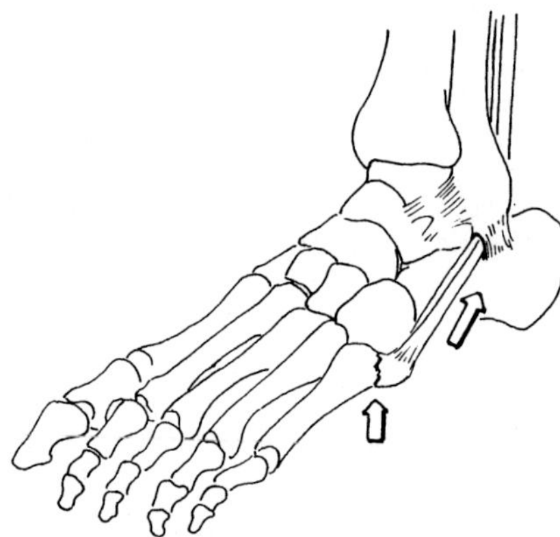

**Fig. 1.** Avulsion fracture of the 5th metatarsal bone (as shown here) must be differentiated from Jones fracture, which occurs more distally.

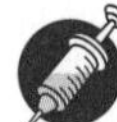

## TREATMENT

### GENERAL MEASURES

- Treatment varies by fracture type.
  - Tuberosity avulsion:
    - Symptomatic management involves weightbearing as tolerated with a hard-soled shoe, cast, or splint, even with considerable displacement (>1 cm).
    - Clinical union often occurs by 3 weeks.
    - Nonunion is rarely symptomatic; if problematic, resect the fragment and reattach the peroneus brevis tendon.
  - Diaphyseal fracture:
    - The patient is nonweightbearing in a below-the-knee cast until radiographic union occurs (usually 8 weeks), followed by 6 weeks of limited activity.
  - Jones fracture:
    - Most are treated with a nonweightbearing below-the-knee cast for 4–6 weeks.
    - Competitive athletes may undergo percutaneous screw fixation with weightbearing after 2 weeks and may return to sports after pain and tenderness have resolved (8 weeks).

#### *Activity*

Activity is as-tolerated with the previously mentioned external supports, except for diaphyseal fractures, for which patients should remain nonweightbearing for 6–8 weeks.

### SPECIAL THERAPY

#### *Physical Therapy*

Rarely indicated

### SURGERY

- Diaphyseal fractures:
  - May be treated with percutaneous placement of a malleolar screw for earlier return to activity
- Jones fracture:
  - Screw fixation for Jones fractures in competitive athletes
  - A cannulated screw can be placed percutaneously.
- Avulsion fracture
  - Symptomatic nonunion may be treated with excision of the fragment and reattachment of the peroneus brevis tendon.

## FOLLOW-UP

### PROGNOSIS

- The prognosis is excellent for avulsion fractures (5).
- Jones fractures treated nonoperatively have approximately a 40% chance of not healing (6).
- Treatment of Jones fractures with intramedullary fixation is thought to result in a higher rate of healing and earlier return to function for athletes (7).

### COMPLICATIONS

- Nonunion of fracture
- Recurrent fractures are more common in highly competitive athletes.
- Returning to sport before full healing is thought to increase the rate of nonunion even with surgical treatment (8).

### PATIENT MONITORING

- Patients are followed at 1-month intervals until the fracture heals and they return to full weightbearing.
- Delayed union occurs when the healing at the fracture site has not occurred by 6–8 weeks.
- The fracture is judged to be a nonunion if no evidence of additional healing is noted and pain is present at the fracture site.

### REFERENCES

1. Torg JS, Balduini FC, Zelko RR, et al. Fractures of the base of the fifth metatarsal distal to the tuberosity. Classification and guidelines for non-surgical and surgical management. *J Bone Joint Surg* 1984;66A:209–214.
2. Petrisor BA, Ekrol I, Court-Brown C. The epidemiology of metatarsal fractures. *Foot Ankle Int* 2006;27:172–174.
3. Low K, Noblin JD, Browne JE, et al. Jones fractures in the elite football player. *J Surg Orthop Adv* 2004;13:156–160.
4. Hasselman CT, Vogt MT, Stone KL, et al. Foot and ankle fractures in elderly white women. Incidence and risk factors. *J Bone Joint Surg* 2003;85A: 820–824.
5. Konkel KF, Menger AG, Retzlaff SA. Nonoperative treatment of fifth metatarsal fractures in an orthopaedic suburban private multispeciality practice. *Foot Ankle Int* 2005;26:704–707.
6. Mologne TS, Lundeen JM, Clapper MF, et al. Early screw fixation versus casting in the treatment of acute Jones fractures. *Am J Sports Med* 2005; 33:970–975.
7. Rosenberg GA, Sferra JJ. Treatment strategies for acute fractures and nonunions of the proximal fifth metatarsal. *J Am Acad Orthop Surg* 2000;8: 332–338.
8. Larson CM, Almekinders LC, Taft TN, et al. Intramedullary screw fixation of Jones fractures. Analysis of failure. *Am J Sports Med* 2002;30: 55–60.

### ADDITIONAL READING

Fetzer GB, Wright RW. Metatarsal shaft fractures and fractures of the proximal fifth metatarsal. *Clin Sports Med* 2006;25:139–150.

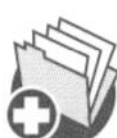

## MISCELLANEOUS

### CODES

#### *ICD9-CM*

825.25 Metatarsal fracture

### PATIENT TEACHING

- Stress the importance of following weight limitations to prevent nonunion and delay in return to normal activities.
- Stress to athletes that training should not begin after a Jones fractures until healing can be seen radiographically.

#### *Activity*

Patients with stress injuries should resume activity slowly.

#### *Prevention*

Athletes should monitor training activity to avoid repetitive stress injury.

### FAQ

- Q: Is a cast or splint needed for a fracture of the base of the 5th metatarsal?
  - A: The need for immobilization depends on the fracture type. Avulsion fractures require only symptomatic treatment. A splint may be used if the patient has a lot of pain. Jones fractures should be treated with immobilization; consideration should be given to intramedullary fixation.

J

# JUMPER'S KNEE (PATELLAR TENDINOPATHY)

*Gregory Gebauer, MD, MS*
*John H. Wilckens, MD*

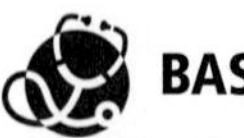

## BASICS

### DESCRIPTION
- Patellar tendinopathy, also known as "Jumper's knee," is an overuse injury of the patellar tendon.
- Children develop a similar condition known as OSD.

### GENERAL PREVENTION
Avoidance of repetitive jumping exercises without proper quad strengthening

### EPIDEMIOLOGY
Equally common among males and females

#### *Incidence*
Overall incidence in the community is unknown, but it is very common and usually self-limiting.

#### *Prevalence*
- Most prevalent in young athletes, particularly dancers and basketball and volleyball players
- Also commonly seen during basic training of military recruits

### RISK FACTORS
- Participation in repetitive jumping sports.
- Repetitive leg extension exercises
- Training errors
- Limb malalignment

### ETIOLOGY
- Recurrent microtrauma from overuse
- Can develop areas of mucoid degeneration and fibrinous necrosis of the tendon

### ASSOCIATED CONDITIONS
Achilles tendinitis

## DIAGNOSIS

### SIGNS AND SYMPTOMS

#### *History*
- Patients often complain of dull, aching pain (insidious in onset) over the patellar tendon.
- Pain is exacerbated by active and resisted knee extension.

#### *Physical Exam*
- Tenderness is localized most commonly over the tendinous insertion at the inferior pole of the patella.
- May have tenderness over the tendon insertion on the proximal tibia and the tendon itself
- Quadriceps, hamstring, Achilles, and hip flexor tightness

### TESTS

#### *Imaging*
- AP and lateral views of the knee should be obtained to rule out other pathologic processes.
- Ultrasound and MRI are helpful in recalcitrant cases, identifying areas of mucoid degeneration.

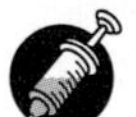

## TREATMENT

### GENERAL MEASURES

#### *Activity*
- Relative rest:
  - Patients should refrain from activities that exacerbate the pain, particularly jumping and knee extension exercises.
  - However, patients should not be immobilized.
- Gradual resumption of low-impact exercise, including swimming and cycling, and resumption of normal activity as symptoms permit

#### *Nursing*
Icing the affected area may help relieve some of the discomfort.

### SPECIAL THERAPY

#### *Physical Therapy*
- As the symptoms improve, physical therapy, including stretching and quadriceps and hamstring strengthening, should be initiated, with particular attention to eccentric strengthening.
- Special attention should be paid to limb alignment and core strength.

#### *Complementary and Alternative Therapies*
Patients also may respond to modalities such as ultrasound, phonophoresis, and iontophoresis.

### MEDICATION (DRUGS)

#### *First Line*
NSAIDs may help relieve some of the discomfort.

#### *Second Line*
Corticosteroid injection should not be considered because of the unacceptable risk of patellar tendon rupture.

### SURGERY
Refractory symptoms after 6 months of documented physical therapy may respond to open or arthroscopic débridement of the patellar tendon.

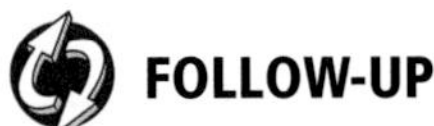

## FOLLOW-UP

### DISPOSITION

- Patients should be seen again at 6 weeks after diagnosis to assess the effects of therapy.
- Patients may resume regular activity after symptoms resolve.

### PROGNOSIS

- Prognosis is good for patients compliant with activity restriction and physical therapy.
- For patients with persistent disease (>6 months) and for those who require surgery, 50–80% report resolution of symptoms (1).

### REFERENCE


1. Coleman BD, Khan KM, Kiss ZS, et al. Open and arthroscopic patellar tenotomy for chronic patellar tendinopathy. A retrospective outcome study. *Am J Sports Med* 2000;28:183–190.


### ADDITIONAL READING


- Duri ZA, Aichroth PM, Wilkins R, et al. Patellar tendonitis and anterior knee pain. *Am J Knee Surg* 1999;12:99–108.
- Panni AS, Tartarone M, Maffulli N. Patellar tendinopathy in athletes. Outcome of nonoperative and operative management. *Am J Sports Med* 2000;28:392–397.
- Shalaby M, Almekinders LC. Patellar tendinitis: the significance of MRI findings. *Am J Sports Med* 1999;27:345–349.
- Witvrouw E, Bellemans J, Lysens R, et al. Intrinsic risk factors for the development of patellar tendinitis in an athletic population. A two-year prospective study. *Am J Sports Med* 2001;29:190–195.


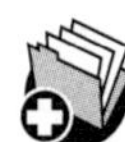

## MISCELLANEOUS

### CODES

#### *ICD9-CM*

726.64 Patellar tendonitis

### PATIENT TEACHING

#### *Activity*

- Patients should be educated about:
  - Avoiding exacerbating (at-risk) activities, such as knee squats, knee extension exercises, and jumping, to promote healing and prevent recurrence
  - Stretching, and quadriceps-, hamstring- and core-strengthening exercises (and proper technique) as symptoms begin to resolve

#### *Prevention*

Core and quadriceps strengthening, hamstring flexibility, and limb-alignment improvement

### FAQ

- Q: When can I return to play/normal activity?
  - A: Athletes can return to normal activity/play when they are symptom-free.
- Q: What can I do to prevent this in the future?
  - A: Quadriceps- and core-strengthening exercises and avoidance of exacerbating activities are the best ways to avoid recurrence.

J

# KIENBÖCK DISEASE

*Marc W. Hungerford, MD*
*Dawn M. LaPorte, MD*

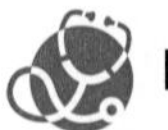

## BASICS

### DESCRIPTION

- Kienböck disease is AVN of the lunate of the wrist with collapse of the bone and arthritis in the advanced stage (Fig. 1).
- The classification system by Stahl (1), which was later modified by Lichtman et al. (2), is based on the radiographic appearance of the lunate:
  - Stage 1: Radiographically normal lunate or with small fracture lines
  - Stage 2: Sclerosis of the lunate
  - Stage 3a: Collapse of the lunate
  - Stage 3b: Lunate collapse with proximal migration of the capitate and fixed rotation of the scaphoid
  - Stage 4: Generalized wrist arthrosis
- Modification (3,4):
  - Stage 0: MRI evidence of AVN of the lunate and no plain radiographic findings
- Synonym: Lunatomalacia

### EPIDEMIOLOGY

- Most common in young adults (20–40 years old)
- Gender predominance uncertain
- Disease onset usually in young to middle adulthood

#### *Incidence*

~1 per 1,000

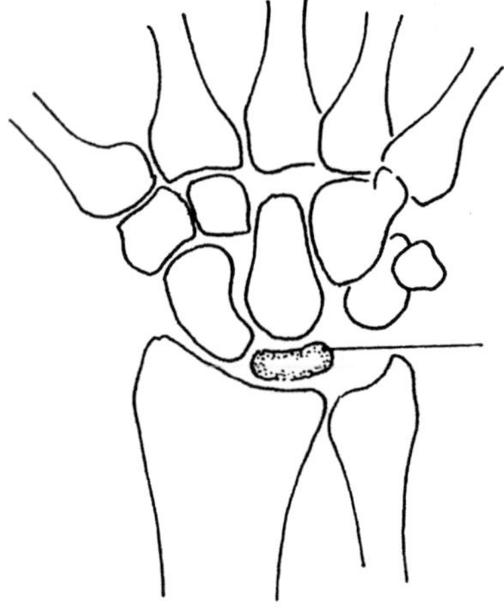

**Fig. 1.** Kienböck disease is AVN of the lunate, usually followed by flattering of this bone (*stippled*).

### RISK FACTORS

- Ulnar-negative wrist:
  - The carpal bones of the wrist, which are supported by the distal radius and ulna, should be the same length.
  - The term "ulnar-negative wrist" refers to a short ulna, which causes more pressure to be borne by the radial side of the wrist.
  - The ulnar-negative variant wrist is thought to overload the lunate and predispose to Kienböck disease.
  - Similarly, the lunate is perfused through a single nutrient artery, so it is thought to be at higher risk (5).
- Disorders leading to ischemia of the lunate, such as sickle cell anemia
- Traumatic ligamentous disruption of the intercarpal ligaments

#### *Genetics*

No known correlation exists.

### ETIOLOGY

- Although this disease was originally described by Kienböck in 1910 (6), the precise cause has yet to be determined.
- Theories proposing a primary ischemic or traumatic origin are supported in the literature.
- Current consensus supports repetitive microtrauma in the lunate at risk.

## DIAGNOSIS

### SIGNS AND SYMPTOMS

- Most patients complain of pain and stiffness with tenderness over the dorsal lunate (middle of the wrist) on physical examination.
- Alternatively, patients may have little pain but markedly decreased grip strength.
- If untreated, the pain may increase progressively and develop into arthritis of the wrist.

#### *History*

Many patients give a history of a recent hyperextension injury of the wrist.

#### *Physical Exam*

Tenderness with palpation over the anatomic snuffbox and/or dorsal lunate is noted.

### TESTS

#### *Imaging*

- Radiography:
  - Plain AP radiographs of the wrist often establish the diagnosis.
    - The lunate may show a lucent line.
    - In more advanced cases, sclerosis or collapse may be seen.
  - An ulnar variance view with the shoulder in 90° of abduction, the elbow in 90° of flexion, and the wrist in neutral rotation should be obtained.
- In patients with a strong clinical suspicion and normal radiographs, MRI may show characteristic changes of AVN.
- Bone scanning sometimes is used to establish the diagnosis, and it shows a cold spot (less technetium uptake) over the lunate.

#### *Pathological Findings*

- A transverse internal fracture of the lunate has been described in 75% of cases, but it rarely is recognized clinically.
- Changes characteristic of AVN are seen in biopsy specimens.

### DIFFERENTIAL DIAGNOSIS

- Scapholunate ligament tear
- Scaphoid fracture
- Perilunate dislocation
- Wrist arthritis
- Ulnar impaction syndrome

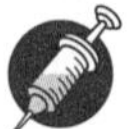

## TREATMENT

### GENERAL MEASURES

- The optimal treatment for patients with Kienböck disease is debated, but the following generally are accepted:
  - The wrist should be splinted and the patient referred to a hand specialist for additional treatment.
  - Untreated, the condition may follow a course of relentless radiologic progression, but the clinical course is variable.
  - Most practitioners favor some surgical intervention in the young, active patient with early-stage disease.
  - Radial shortening or ulnar lengthening may be considered if the ulna is short.
  - Proximal row carpectomy, limited fusion, arthroplasty, or another reconstructive procedure may be considered for advanced cases.

## SPECIAL THERAPY

### *Physical Therapy*

- Physical therapy usually is not necessary except in the postoperative period.
- Splinting of the wrist helps relieve discomfort.

## SURGERY

- Stage 1 and 2 disease:
  - Surgery is aimed at lunate load reduction or improvement of lunate perfusion.
  - Load reduction may be achieved by joint-leveling procedures (in the case of the ulnar-negative wrist) or limited intercarpal fusion.
  - Perfusion may be improved through vascularized bone grafts.
- Stage 3 disease:
  - A proximal row carpectomy may provide symptomatic relief while maintaining ROM.
- Stage 4:
  - Wrist fusion is the treatment of choice.

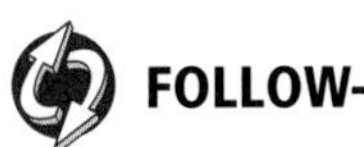

# FOLLOW-UP

## PROGNOSIS

Degenerative arthritis usually results if left untreated.

## COMPLICATIONS

- Increasing pain, clicking
- Wrist arthritis

## PATIENT MONITORING

Even if no surgery is performed initially, the patient should be followed periodically with serial radiographs to determine whether collapse and arthritis are progressive.

## REFERENCES


1. Stahl F. On lunatomalacia (Kienbock's disease): a clinical and roentgenological study, especially on its pathogenesis and the late results of immobilization treatment. *Acta Chir Scand Suppl* 1947;95:1–133.
2. Lichtman DM, Mack GR, MacDonald RI, et al. Kienbock's disease: the role of silicone replacement arthroplasty. *J Bone Joint Surg* 1977; 59A:899–908.
3. Amadio PC, Hanssen AD, Berquist TH. The genesis of Kienbock's disease: evaluation of a case by magnetic resonance imaging. *J Hand Surg* 1987;12A:1044–1049.
4. Cristiani G, Cerofolini E, Squarzina PB, et al. Evaluation of ischaemic necrosis of carpal bones by magnetic resonance imaging. *J Hand Surg* 1990; 15B:249–255.
5. Gelberman RH, Bauman TD, Menon J, et al. The vascularity of the lunate bone and Kienbock's disease. *J Hand Surg* 1980;5A:272–278.
6. Kienbock R. Uber traumatische Malazie des Mondbeins und ihre Folgezustande: Entartungsformen und Kompressionsfrakturen. *Fortschr Geb Rontgenstr* 1910;16:77–103.


## ADDITIONAL READING


- Almquist EE. Kienböck's disease. *Hand Clin* 1987;3:141–148.
- Amadio PC, Moran SL. Fractures of the carpal bones. In: Green DP, Hotchkiss RN, Pederson WC, et al, eds. *Green's Operative Hand Surgery*, 5th ed. Philadelphia: Elsevier Churchill Livingstone, 2005;711–768.
- Weiland AJ. Avascular necrosis of the carpus. In: *Hand Surgery Update*. Rosemont, IL: American Academy of Orthopaedic Surgeons, 1994:85–92.


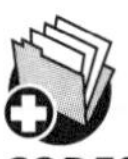

# MISCELLANEOUS

## CODES

### *ICD9-CM*

732.3 Kienböck's disease

## PATIENT TEACHING

The patient should be counseled about the natural history of the disease and the need for rest or activity restriction.

## FAQ

- Q: What are signs and symptoms of Kienböck disease?
  - A: Patients typically present with complaints of wrist pain localized to the region of the lunate; this pain is present at rest as well as with activity. Decreased wrist ROM also is seen frequently in Kienböck disease. Swelling and tenderness dorsally in the area of the lunate also may be seen.
- Q: How is the diagnosis of Kienböck disease made?
  - A: The diagnosis usually is made with radiographs. In the early stages, radiographs can be negative, and MRI or bone scan can support the diagnosis if Kienböck disease is strongly suspected.

# KNEE ANATOMY AND EXAMINATION

*Timothy S. Johnson, MD*
*Constantine A. Demetracopoulos, BS*

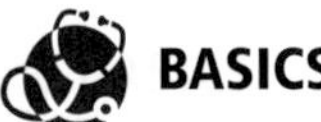

## BASICS

### DESCRIPTION

- Anatomy of the knee consists of compartments, bones, menisci, ligaments, muscles, and nerves.
- 3 compartments:
  - Medial, lateral, and patellofemoral
- Bones: Patella:
  - Serves as fulcrum to aid knee extension
- Medial and lateral menisci:
  - Fibrocartilaginous structures in medial and lateral femorotibial compartments
  - Aid in joint lubrication and nutrition and in load distribution across articular cartilage
- Ligaments/tendons:
  - Patellar ligament/tendon: Distal part of quadriceps tendon originating from the apex of the patella and inserting on the tibial tuberosity
  - ACL:
    - Originates from the posteromedial aspect of the lateral femoral condyle and attaches to the tibia's anterior intercondylar spine
    - Prevents anterior displacement of the tibia on the femur
  - PCL:
    - Originates from the anterolateral aspect of the medial femoral condyle and inserts on the posterior intercondylar spine of the tibia
    - Prevents posterior displacement of the tibia on the femur during knee flexion
  - MCL:
    - Originates on the medial femoral epicondyle and inserts on the medial tibial plateau and medial meniscus
    - Stabilizes the knee against valgus loads
  - LCL and posterolateral corner complex:
    - Originates on the lateral femoral epicondyle and inserts on the fibular head
    - Stabilizes the knee against varus loads
    - Resists tibial external rotation
- Muscles:
  - Quadriceps (extensors): Rectus femoris, vastus lateralis, vastus intermedius, vastus medialis
  - Hamstrings (flexors): Biceps femoris, semimembranosus, semitendinosus, gracilis
- Nerves:
  - Femoral: Innervates quadriceps
  - Sciatic: Bypasses knee posteriorly with popliteal vessels
  - Common peroneal: Major branch of the sciatic that travels laterally around the fibular neck

## DIAGNOSIS

### SIGNS AND SYMPTOMS

#### *History and Physical Exam*

- Initial assessment:
  - Assess the contralateral knee for comparison.
  - Assess for referred pain from the spine or hip.
  - Perform a complete neurovascular examination of the extremities.
  - ROM:
    - Normal = 0–155°
    - Flexion contracture: Incomplete passive and active extension
    - Extension lag: Full passive extension with incomplete active extension
- Inspection:
  - Observe knees for erythema, effusion, and skin abrasion.
  - Observe for muscular atrophy.
  - Assess standing varus/valgus alignment.
    - Physiologic alignment is approximately 5° of valgus for males and 7° of valgus for females.
  - Assess gait.
    - Antalgic gait: Shortened stride and decreased stance phase on the affected leg
- Palpation:
  - With the knee at 90° of flexion, palpate along the course of the patellar and quadriceps tendons, medial and lateral joint lines, the MCL, the LCL, and the iliotibial band.
  - Localize painful structures.
- Knee effusion:
  - Marked effusion can be secondary to hemarthrosis (fracture, ligamentous or meniscal tear) or inflammation (arthritis, gout, infection).
  - Assess the knee joint for warmth, which may indicate active inflammation.
  - Blot test:
    - Press the patella against the femoral groove.
    - If a large effusion is present, the fluid will be forced out of the groove and cause the patella to rebound as it flows back in.
- Prepatellar bursitis:
  - A fluctuant, painful subcutaneous swelling anterior to the patella with anterior knee pain
- Popliteal cyst (Baker cyst):
  - Painful swelling of the popliteal fossa.
  - Usually indicates intra-articular pathology
- ITBS:
  - Lateral knee pain, localized specifically over the lateral epicondyle commonly seen as an overuse injury in runners and cyclists
  - Ober test:
    - With the patient lying on the unaffected side, and with the unaffected hip and knee flexed to 90°, stabilize the pelvis.
    - With the affected leg abducted and extended, lower it into adduction.
    - If the iliotibial band is tight, the leg will remain in the abducted position and/or the patient may complain of lateral knee pain.
- Patellar fracture, patellar tendon/quadriceps tendon rupture:
  - Palpable defect of affected structure
  - Extension lag
- Patellofemoral syndrome
  - Anterior knee pain with standing from a seated position, squatting, or stair-climbing
  - Q angle:
    - Angle of the anterior superior iliac spine, patella, and tibial tubercle
    - An angle >15° may suggest patellar instability.
  - Medial and lateral glide test:
    - With the affected knee extended, determine the number of quadrants the patella will translate over the trochlear groove.
    - <1 quadrant medially suggests lateral patellofemoral compression syndrome.
  - Apprehension test:
    - With the affected knee in full extension, translate the patella laterally.
    - Apprehension during this maneuver suggests patella instability.
  - Grind test:
    - Press the patella distally against the trochlear groove.
    - Then have the patient contract the quadriceps while palpating for crepitus indicative of patellofemoral arthrosis (Fig. 1).

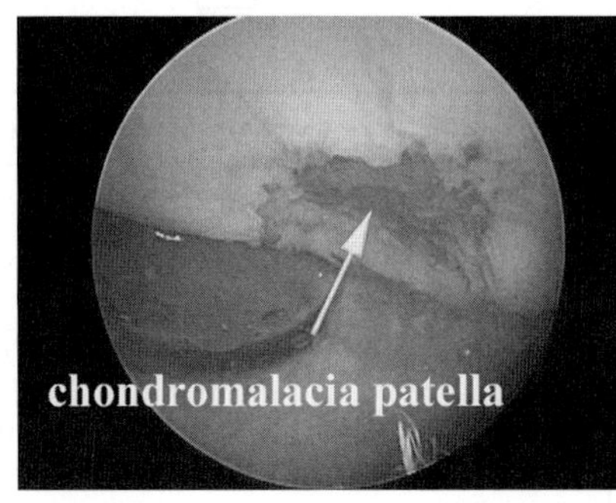


**Fig. 1.** Arthroscopic photo of an articular cartilage injury on the patella.

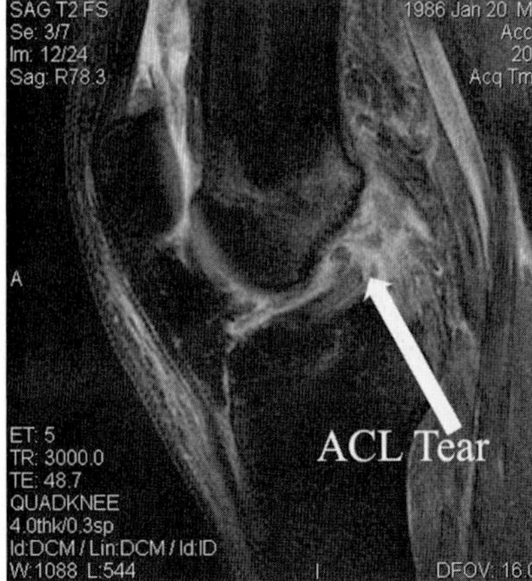


**Fig. 2.** MRI of an ACL rupture of the femur.

- Ligamentous instability:
  - Mechanism of injury may indicate cause of instability.
    - ACL: Noncontact, twisting/pivoting motion with foot firmly planted and audible "pop"
    - PCL: Dashboard injuries
    - MCL/LCL: Extreme valgus/varus force about the knee
  - Ligament tears frequently are accompanied by an acute hemarthrosis.
  - Knee feels like it "gives out" or "buckles."
  - Varus and valgus stress test (MCL/LCL) (1):
    - With the knee flexed to 30°, place 1 hand on the patient's distal thigh and with the other, grasp the patient's ankle.
    - Apply varus/valgus stress in coronal plane with the knee in 30° of flexion.
    - If instability is detected, the collateral ligament has been injured.
    - Grades: 1, <5 mm; 2, 5–10 mm; 3, >10 mm
  - Lachman test (ACL) (Fig. 2):
    - Most sensitive test for ACL integrity
    - With the patient's knee relaxed and flexed at 30°, place 1 hand on the distal thigh and the other on the proximal tibia.
    - Then translate the tibia anteriorly.
    - Test is abnormal if there is >5 mm of translation and/or >3 mm difference between the values for the affected and uninjured knees.
  - Anterior and posterior drawer test (ACL/PCL) (2):
    - Place the knee in 90° of flexion and neutral rotation, and stabilize the foot.
    - Place both hands around the proximal tibia and attempt to translate the tibia anteriorly and posteriorly on the femur.
    - Subluxation anteriorly suggests ACL instability. Similarly, subluxation posteriorly suggests PCL instability.
    - Grades: 1, <5 mm; 2, 5–10 mm; 3, >10 mm
  - External rotation test (posterolateral corner):
    - Test with the patient prone.
    - Simultaneously compare the affected and normal knees.
    - Starting at 0° of knee flexion, externally rotate the tibia and observe the thigh–foot angle.
    - Look for excessive external rotation (>10°) on the affected side.
    - Repeat at 30° and 90°.
    - Increased external rotation only at ≤30° of knee flexion indicates an isolated PLC injury.
    - Increased external rotation at ≤30° and at 90° of knee flexion indicates posterolateral corner and PCL insufficiency.
- Meniscal pathology (3) (Fig. 3):
  - Patient complains of episodic painful "mechanical symptoms" that may present with the knee locked in flexion.
  - Patient presents with focal tenderness to palpation on the affected joint line (best examined with the knee flexed at 90°).
  - McMurray test:
    - With the patient supine and the knee in full flexion, internally rotate the tibia and apply a valgus force to load the lateral meniscus.
    - Then passively extend the knee to 0° of flexion while palpating the lateral joint line.
    - The test is positive if an audible or palpable click is produced during extension.
    - Reposition the knee in full flexion and repeat the test with the tibia in external rotation by applying varus force and palpating the medial joint line to test the medial meniscus.
    - Pain may be associated with this maneuver.
  - Apley compression and dislocation test:
    - With the patient prone and the knee flexed at 90°, grasp the heel and axially load the tibia while simultaneously externally and internally rotating the foot.
    - Pain localized to the medial joint line with compression and rotation suggests medial meniscus abnormality.
    - Pain localized to the lateral joint line with compression and rotation suggests lateral meniscus abnormality.
- Knee arthritis (Fig. 4):
  - Patients complain of morning stiffness and soreness.
  - Intra-articular swelling can be variable.
  - Osteophytes and crepitus may be palpable.
  - Flexion contractures with reduced ROM and marked functional limitations are common.
  - Late stages of degenerative arthritis are associated with pseudolaxity on valgus/varus testing.
  - Radiographs show joint space narrowing and osteophytes (Fig. 3).

## REFERENCES


1. Grood ES, Noyes FR, Butler DL, et al. Ligamentous and capsular restraints preventing straight medial and lateral laxity in intact human cadaver knees. *J Bone Joint Surg* 1981;63A:1257–1269.
2. Cosgarea AJ, Jay PR. Posterior cruciate ligament injuries: evaluation and management. *J Am Acad Orthop Surg* 2001;9:297–307.
3. Greis PE, Bardana DD, Holmstrom MC, et al. Meniscal injury: I. Basic science and evaluation. *J Am Acad Orthop Surg* 2002;10:168–176.


## ADDITIONAL READING


- Hoppenfeld S. Physical examination of the knee. In: *Physical Examination of the Spine and Extremities*. Norwalk, CT: Appleton-Century-Crofts, 1976:171–196.
- Hoppenfeld S, deBoer P. The knee. In: *Surgical Exposures in Orthopaedics: The Anatomical Approach*, 3rd ed. Philadelphia: Lippincott, Williams & Wilkins, 2003:493–568.


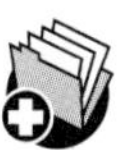

## MISCELLANEOUS

### FAQ

- Q: In addition to pain, of what do people with knee ligament injuries complain most commonly?
  - A: Instability or buckling of the knee.
- Q: In addition to pain, what is the classic chief complaint of a person with an unstable meniscus tear?
  - A: Locking of the knee in a flexed position.

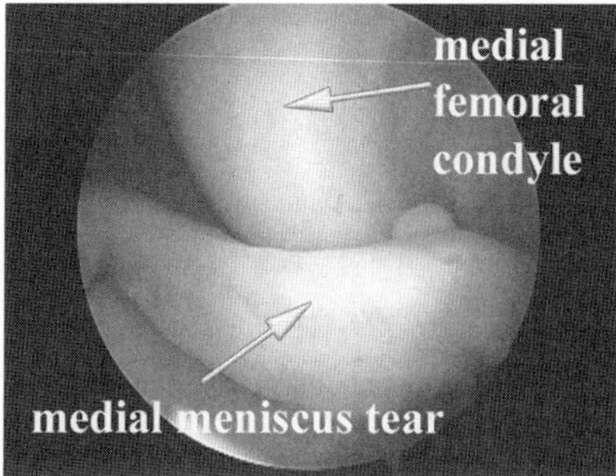


**Fig. 3.** Arthroscopic photograph of an unstable bucket-handle medial meniscus tear.

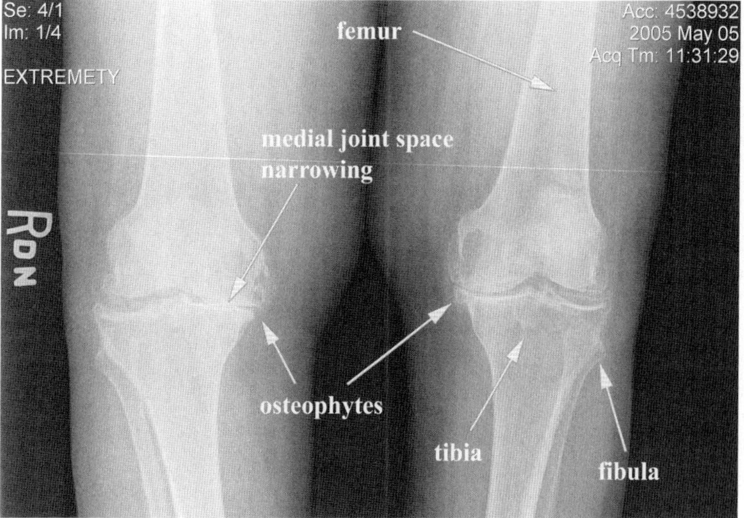


**Fig. 4.** Radiograph of advanced knee osteoarthritis.

# KNEE DISLOCATION

*Gregory Gebauer, MD, MS*
*John H. Wilckens, MD*

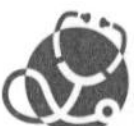

## BASICS

### DESCRIPTION

- Dislocation of the knee is an orthopaedic emergency.
- The most common causes are motor vehicle accidents, followed by sports and falls from heights.
- Classification:
  - Anterior
  - Posterior
  - Medial
  - Lateral
  - Rotary: Subclassified as anteromedial, anterolateral, posteromedial, posterolateral

### GENERAL PREVENTION

Seat belts and airbags are the best methods of prevention.

### EPIDEMIOLOGY

#### *Incidence*

Rare

### ASSOCIATED CONDITIONS

- Neurovascular injury, particularly to the popliteal artery or peroneal nerve
- Fractures of the tibia or femur
- Rupture of the collateral and/or cruciate ligaments

## DIAGNOSIS

### SIGNS AND SYMPTOMS

#### *History*

- Classically, patients with knee dislocations present with obvious deformity, swelling, pain, and inability to move the knee.
- Many knee dislocations are reduced before examination by a physician; thus, deformity may not be present.
- It is critical to assess the neurovascular status of all patients with possible knee dislocations because:
  - Injury to the popliteal artery occurs in 32–45% of cases (1,2).
  - Nerve injury (most commonly the peroneal nerve) occurs in 16–40% of all knee dislocations (3,4).
- Urgent vascular evaluation is required for absent pulses; ecchymosis in the popliteal fossa; a cold, cyanotic extremity; or loss of sensorimotor function.

#### *Physical Exam*

- Inspect the extremity for obvious deformity, swelling, and ecchymosis.
- Perform a thorough neurovascular examination.
  - Palpate pulses or assess them by Doppler, note warmth of skin, and examine sensory and motor function.
- The presence of pulses does not rule out vascular injury because an intimal flap tear of the vessel may be present.
- Any sign of vascular injury necessitates an emergent vascular surgery consultation.
- Examination for laxity of the knee should be performed systematically for injury to any of the 4 knee ligaments (ACL, PCL, MCL, or LCL).
- Laxity of 2 or more knee ligaments leads to a presumptive diagnosis of knee dislocation.
- Patients should be examined carefully at regular intervals to exclude the possibility of compartment syndrome.
  - The most reliable signs for compartment syndrome are intractable, unrelenting pain out of proportion to the injury and pain with passive stretch of the ankle and toes.

### TESTS

#### *Imaging*

- Radiography:
  - AP and lateral views of the knee should be obtained, but doing so should not delay reduction of an obvious dislocation.
- MRI:
  - May be useful in assessing soft-tissue and ligamentous injury, but it should not be performed acutely.
  - Also allows visualization of the vascular system

#### *Diagnostic Procedures/Surgery*

Any patient with a vascular injury should undergo angiography or MRI.

### DIFFERENTIAL DIAGNOSIS

- Dislocation of the patella
- Neurovascular injury unrelated to dislocation
- Fracture of the tibia or femur

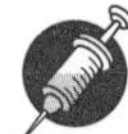

## TREATMENT

### GENERAL MEASURES

- Many knee dislocations are the result of motor vehicle crashes; therefore, all such patients should be assessed by a trauma protocol.
  - Initial assessment should include evaluation of airway, breathing, circulation, and vital signs.
- Immediate reduction is recommended.
  - Anterior dislocations are reduced with longitudinal traction and the lifting of the femur anteriorly.
  - Posterior dislocations are reduced with longitudinal traction and the lifting upward of the proximal tibia while extending the knee.
  - Medial and lateral dislocations are reduced with longitudinal traction and the appropriate medial or lateral pressure on the tibia and femur.
- The neurovascular status should be assessed before and after reduction.
- Orthopaedic and vascular surgeons should be notified.
- The knee should be immobilized in a splint or spanning external fixator, with careful attention to the neurovascular status and the development of compartment syndrome.
- Nonoperative treatment:
  - Indicated for patients who are sedentary or elderly or who have substantial comorbidities preventing surgical repair.
  - A splint should be followed by 6–8 weeks of protected immobilization.

#### *Activity*

- Nonoperatively treated patients:
  - 6–8 weeks of protected immobilization
  - May begin quadriceps setting exercises in the splint, followed by active leg-lifting exercises after the immobilizer is removed
- Operatively treated patients:
  - Activity is determined by which structures were injured, repaired, and reconstructed.
  - After 6 weeks, patients may begin active ROM exercises.
- Average return to previous activity for both treatments:
  - Sports, 9–12 months
  - Sedentary jobs, 2 months
  - Heavy labor, 6–9 months

## SPECIAL THERAPY

### *Physical Therapy*

- ROM and strengthening exercises should be started after immobilization.
- Quadriceps setting exercises can begin in the splint/fixator.

## MEDICATION (DRUGS)

### *First Line*

Narcotics

## SURGERY

- Emergent surgery is required for patients with vascular injury; saphenous vein grafting often is required.
- Fasciotomies may be required for patients with prolonged ischemic time or with compartment syndrome.
- Open dislocation requires immediate surgical intervention.
- Definitive surgical repair usually is performed 10–14 days after the injury, to allow swelling to diminish and to facilitate arthroscopic procedures.
- Methods of repair and reconstruction depend on the extent and nature of the injuries.

# FOLLOW-UP

## DISPOSITION

Patients should be followed at 4–6-week intervals until they achieve maximum recovery.

### *Issues for Referral*

- An orthopaedic surgeon should be consulted emergently.
- Any vascular injuries require immediate consultation with a vascular surgeon.

## PROGNOSIS

- Prognosis depends on the associated limb injuries and the interventions for those injuries.
- Viability of the limb in the presence of vascular compromise is directly related to the time between injury and revascularization.
- The most common residual effects are arthrofibrosis (knee stiffness) and postoperative arthritis.

## COMPLICATIONS

- Loss of limb:
  - Usually secondary to prolonged ischemia
  - The amputation rate is 86% when ischemia lasts >8 hours (1).
- Arthrofibrosis (stiff knee):
  - In nonoperative treatment, residual stiffness provides stability for injured ligaments.
  - Operative treatment may increase the incidence of arthrofibrosis unless reconstruction is strong enough to allow early ROM.
- Neurologic deficit:
  - Nerve injury, most often the peroneal nerve, is a common sequela of knee dislocation.
  - Recovery may take months to years, and prognosis varies.
- Knee instability:
  - Secondary to injury to the ligamentous structures
  - Redislocation is rare.
- Posttraumatic arthritis:
  - Secondary to cartilage injury during the trauma
  - Can lead to long-term disability

## REFERENCES


1. Green NE, Allen BL. Vascular injuries associated with dislocation of the knee. *J Bone Joint Surg* 1977;59A:236–239.
2. Jones RE, Smith EC, Bone GE. Vascular and orthopaedic complications of knee dislocation. *Surg Gynecol Obstet* 1979;149:554–558.
3. Almekinders LC, Logan TC. Results following treatment of traumatic dislocations of the knee joint. *Clin Orthop Relat Res* 1992;284:203–207.
4. Welling RE, Kakkasseril J, Cranley JJ. Complete dislocations of the knee with popliteal vascular injury. *J Trauma* 1981;21:450–453.


## ADDITIONAL READING


- Giannoulias CS, Freedman KB. Knee dislocations: management of the multiligament-injured knee. *Am J Orthop* 2004;33:553–559.
- Rihn JA, Groff YJ, Harner CD, et al. The acutely dislocated knee: evaluation and management. *J Am Acad Orthop Surg* 2004;12:334–346.
- Schenck RC Jr, ed. *Multiple Ligamentous Injuries of the Knee in the Athlete*. Rosemont, IL: American Academy of Orthopaedic Surgeons, 2002.
- Stannard JP, Sheils TM, Lopez-Ben RR, et al. Vascular injuries in knee dislocations: the role of physical examination in determining the need for arteriography. *J Bone Joint Surg* 2004;86A: 910–915.
- Wong CH, Tan JL, Chang HC, et al. Knee dislocations—a retrospective study comparing operative versus closed immobilization treatment outcomes. *Knee Surg Sports Traumatol Arthrosc* 2004;12:540–544.


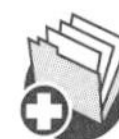

# MISCELLANEOUS

## CODES

### *ICD9-CM*

- 836.5 Closed knee dislocation
- 836.6 Open knee dislocation

## PATIENT TEACHING

### *Activity*

Emphasize ROM and, later, strengthening exercises.

## FAQ

- Q: Do all patients with a knee dislocation require an arterial study to document the status of the popliteal artery?
  - A: No. Although as many as 50% of knee dislocations from high-energy motor vehicle accidents have a popliteal artery injury, <10% of athletic knee dislocations have an arterial injury. Patients with diminished distal pulses before surgical evaluation require urgent vascular consultation.

# KNEE EXAMINATION IN THE CHILD

*Ryan K. Takenaga, BS*
*Paul D. Sponseller, MD*

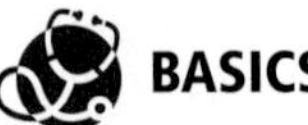

## BASICS

### DESCRIPTION

- It is important, during a knee examination, to keep in mind the child's age and to understand the age-specific pediatric knee disorders.
- Congenital hyperextension or dislocation of the knee:
  - Varies from simple hyperextension to anterior dislocation of the tibia on the femur
  - Hyperextended knee presents at birth.
  - A hyperextensible knee resolves spontaneously, whereas a dislocated knee requires surgery.
- Blount disease (infantile tibia vara and adolescent tibial vara) (1–4):
  - Abnormality of the proximal tibial growth plate causes excessive varus alignment of the knees (bowed legs) in children.
  - Varus/valgus natural history:
    - Birth: Normal bowing of 10–15°
    - 12–18 months: Varus decreases to 0°.
    - 3–5 years: Maximum valgus reached (10–15°).
    - Early adolescence: Valgus decreases to normal adult values (5–10°).
  - Infantile tibia vara, a common cause of pathologic bowed legs in children, usually presents at age 2–4 years and is painless.
  - Adolescent tibial vara, which is becoming more common, usually presents after age 9–10 years.
- Discoid meniscus (5,6):
  - Congenital abnormality in which the lateral meniscus does not acquire a discoid shape during embryologic development, which makes it more susceptible to tearing.
- Septic arthritis of the knee:
  - Pyogenic infection of the knee
  - 2/3 of all cases occur before 3 years of age.
  - Patient is acutely ill and nonweightbearing.
- Popliteal cyst (1–4):
  - Cyst arising from the posterior knee joint
  - Typically presents as an asymptomatic mass on the posteromedial aspect of the knee at the popliteal crease
- Tibial spine fracture (1–4): Avulsion of the tibial attachment of the ACL, usually from a bicycle fall, sporting injuries, or other indirect trauma to the knee
- Genu valgum:
  - Valgus of the knee that increases after age 7 years is not physiologic.
  - Knee pain is a common feature.
- JIA (1–4)
- OSD:
  - Traction apophysitis of the tibial tubercle
  - Occurs during time of rapid growth (ages 9–14 years)
  - Typical presentation is pain over the tibial tubercle exacerbated by running, jumping, and kneeling
- Osteochondritis dissecans: Condition of unknown cause in which a segment of subchondral bone undergoes AVN
- ITBS:
  - Most common cause of lateral knee pain in athletes
  - An overuse condition secondary to friction of the iliotibial band over the lateral femoral condyle
  - Presents as pain over the lateral femoral condyle that is worsened by activity
- ACL injury (1–4):
  - 2 general mechanisms:
    - Direct trauma to the anterior aspect of the knee (more in young children)
    - Indirect injury by twisting motion
- Lyme disease: Early in the disease, presents as fever and migratory arthralgia, with little or no joint swelling
- Lyme arthritis:
  - Occurs months to years after the initial infection
  - Typically a low-grade inflammatory synovitis with a large and relatively painless joint effusion
- SCFE:
  - Overweight child, aged 6–14 years
  - Pain referred to the knee (often missed)
  - Obtain hip radiographs in such children.

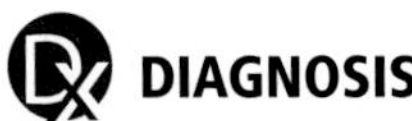

## DIAGNOSIS

### SIGNS AND SYMPTOMS

#### *History*

- Pain:
  - Acute: Ligament and meniscal tears, fractures, septic arthritis
  - Chronic: Genu valgum, JIA, OSD, Sinding-Larsen-Johansson syndrome, osteochondritis dissecans, ITBS, Lyme disease, tendinitis, neoplasm
  - Specific location:
    - Anterior (patellofemoral pain syndrome): Patellar maltracking, pathologic plica, symptomatic bipartite patella.
    - Lateral: ITBS
    - Tibial tubercle: OSD
    - Inferior pole of the patella: Sinding-Larsen-Johansson syndrome
  - At night: Neoplasm (osteosarcoma, Ewing sarcoma)
- Swelling:
  - Acute: Ligament and meniscal tears, fractures, septic arthritis
  - Chronic: JIA, Lyme disease, synovitis, neoplasm
- Mechanical factors:
  - Catching or locking: Meniscal tears, articular cartilage damage, loose bodies (e.g., as in osteochondritis dissecans)
  - Giving way or coming apart:
    - Complete ligamentous injuries

#### *Physical Exam*

- General considerations:
  - The entire lower extremity should be exposed.
  - When palpating, start with the normal knee to facilitate comparison and patient relaxation.
  - Start with examination steps not likely to hurt.
- Inspection:
  - Anterior:
    - Inspect for valgus or varus deformity.
    - In adolescence, normal standing alignment is slight valgus (5–10°)
    - Look for evidence of effusion.
  - Lateral:
    - Look for incomplete extension resulting from flexion contracture or excessive hyperextension (recurvatum deformity).
    - Look for symmetry of the tibial tuberosities.
  - Palpation: Assess for warmth and check for tenderness along the medial and lateral joint lines, medial and collateral ligaments, patella and its supporting ligaments, femoral and tibial condyles, and tibial tubercles.
- Hip examination: Because knee pain often is referred from the hip, any child presenting with knee pain should have an evaluation of hip ROM (see "Hip Examination of the Child" chapter).
- Testing for effusion:
  - In marked effusions, the landmarks are obscured and the patella is ballotable, as seen with hemarthrosis, arthritis, and synovitis.
  - Mildly obscured landmarks suggest a mild joint effusion or fluid collection in the bursae (see "Knee Anatomy and Examination" chapter for details of the Blot and Milk tests for knee effusions).
- Patellar assessment:
  - Inhibition test:
    - To determine if anterior knee pain is secondary to pressure in the patellofemoral joint
    - With the patient supine and knee extended, have the patient do a straight-leg raise.
    - Hold the patella to prevent it from ascending along the femoral sulcus.
    - Any pain is a positive test, which may indicate a patellofemoral disorder.
  - J sign:
    - Observe the patella as the patient actively extends the knee.
    - As the knee extends, the patella remains in the femoral sulcus as it ascends along the axis of the femur.
    - As the knee reaches full extension, the patella deviates laterally like an upside-down "J," a positive J sign.
- Menisci assessment:
  - McMurray test:
    - Flex the knee and hip maximally, and apply a valgus (varus) force to the knee.
    - Externally (internally) rotate the foot and passively extend the knee.
    - A palpable, painful snap or pop during extension suggests a tear of the medial (lateral) meniscus.
- ROM:
  - Flexion (normal, 130–140°):
    - Have the patient sit or lie prone and fully flex each knee.
    - The angle between the leg and the thigh is the degrees of flexion.
  - Extension (normal, 5°):
    - With the patient lying supine with extended knees, stabilize the thigh and lift the foot.
    - The angle between leg and table is degrees of extension.

- Ober test:
  - Assesses the flexibility of the iliotibial band.
  - With the patient lying on the unaffected side, stabilize the pelvis with 1 hand and abduct and extend the hip with the knee flexed.
  - Support the patient's ankle and allow the thigh to drop.
    - If the thigh does not become parallel to the table, the test is positive.
  - A positive test is associated with ITBS.
- Stability tests:
  - AP stability is provided by the ACL and PCL.
  - Mediolateral stability is provided by the MCL and LCL.
  - See the "Knee Anatomy and Examination" chapter for details of the Lachman test, anterior and posterior drawer tests, and varus and valgus stress tests.
- Neurovascular examination: Especially important for acute injuries
  - Sensation: Test sensation to light touch and pinprick in the peroneal, superficial peroneal, and tibial nerve distributions.
  - Motor: Apply resistance while the patient:
    - Dorsiflexes and plantarflexes the foot
    - Inverts and everts the foot
    - Dorsiflexes and plantarflexes the great toe
  - Pulses: Check popliteal, dorsalis pedis, and posterior tibial pulses.

## TESTS

### *Imaging*

- General considerations:
  - Standard radiographs of the knee joint: AP, lateral, tunnel, and patellar views
  - Skyline (Merchant, patellar) view:
    - Shows the location of the patella in the femoral groove and the thickness of the cartilage, which may be beneficial in identifying causes of anterior knee pain
    - Is an axial view of the patellofemoral joint with the knee flexed to 35–45°.
  - 25° AP (tunnel) view aids in the detection of osteochondritis dissecans.
  - A standing view of entire femur and tibia is needed to assess ligament alignment accurately.
  - MRI is best for evaluating soft-tissue masses and injury to menisci or ligaments.
- Congenital knee dislocation: Radiographs help differentiate mild from the more severe hyperextension deformity characterized by a fixed anterior dislocation of the tibia on the distal femur.
- Blount disease and genu valgum: AP, standing, long cassette radiograph of both lower extremities, which includes the hips, knees, and ankles, is best for assessing the mechanical axis and any deviation in joint alignment.
- Discoid meniscus:
  - MRI is the most useful imaging modality.
  - Plain radiographs may reveal a widened lateral joint space with squaring of the lateral femoral condyle.
- Septic arthritis of the knee:
  - Plain films usually are not useful because they may show only widening of joint space secondary to swelling.
- Popliteal cyst:
  - Plain films show no bony abnormality and are needed only in the presence of pain.
  - Transillumination with a penlight confirms benign cystic nature.
  - Ultrasound is another option for documenting the cystic nature of the lesion and ruling out solid soft-tissue lesions.
  - MRI is indicated if ultrasound or transillumination does not show a typical homogenous fluid-filled cyst.
- Tibial spine fracture:
  - AP and lateral radiographs are essential for evaluating the degrees of displacement of the anterior tibial spine.
  - Fracture is best seen on a lateral radiograph.
- JIA:
  - Often no specific radiologic findings early in the course of JIA
  - As it progresses, periarticular osteopenia, localized soft-tissue swelling and, occasionally, joint space widening from effusion or synovial hypertrophy often are present.
- OSD/Sinding-Larsen-Johansson syndrome:
  - Radiographs confirm the clinical diagnosis.
  - If bilateral involvement, radiographs usually are not needed.
  - If unilateral involvement, obtain radiographs to rule out neoplasms.
- Osteochondritis dissecans:
  - Radiography:
    - Diagnostic
    - Reveals a fragment of avascular bone demarcated from the adjacent femur by a radiolucent line
    - AP, lateral, and a tunnel view, which is best for seeing the lesion in the classic location on the lateral aspect and posterior 2/3 of the medial femoral condyle
  - MRI is a useful adjunct for determining the extent of articular cartilage involvement and the stability of the lesion.
- ITBS: Radiographs are unnecessary because diagnosis is based on the patient's symptoms.
- ACL injury:
  - Diagnosis is based primarily on the physical examination.
  - Plain radiographs should be obtained for all patients suspected of knee ligament injury.
  - MRI is indicated only for the patient in whom ROM does not improve and who has a persistent effusion after conventional therapy, or in whom the physical examination is difficult to interpret.
- Patella alta:
  - Position of the patella is best seen on a lateral radiograph with the knee flexed to 30°.
  - Patellar height:
    - Can be assessed via the Insall ratio (length of patella ligament = diagonal length of patella).
    - Variations of >20% are deemed abnormal.
- Lyme disease:
  - Plain films rule out other causes.
  - Diagnosis usually is based on clinical findings and positive blood serology.

## REFERENCES


1. Aronsson DD. The pediatric orthopaedic examination. In: Morrissy RT, Weinstein SL, eds. *Lovell and Winter's Pediatric Orthopaedics*, 6th ed. Philadelphia: Lippincott Williams & Wilkins, 2006: 113–143.
2. Schoenecker PL, Rich MM. The lower extremity. In: Morrissy RT, Weinstein SL, eds. *Lovell and Winter's Pediatric Orthopaedics*, 6th ed. Philadelphia: Lippincott Williams & Wilkins, 2006:1157–1211.
3. Willis RB. Sports medicine in the growing child. In: Morrissy RT, Weinstein SL, eds. *Lovell and Winter's Pediatric Orthopaedics*, 6th ed. Philadelphia: Lippincott Williams & Wilkins, 2006:1383–1428.
4. Wright DA. Juvenile idiopathic arthritis. In: Morrissy RT, Weinstein SL, eds. *Lovell and Winter's Pediatric Orthopaedics*, 6th ed. Philadelphia: Lippincott Williams & Wilkins, 2006:405–437.
5. Tearse DS. Examination of the knee. In: Clark CR, Bonfiglio M, eds. *Orthopaedics: Essentials of Diagnosis and Treatment*. New York: Churchill Livingstone, 1994:75–80.
6. Pizzutillo PD (section ed). Section 9: Pediatric orthopaedics. In: Griffin LY, ed. *Essentials of Musculoskeletal Care*, 3rd ed. Rosemont, IL: American Academy of Orthopaedic Surgeons, 2005:791–957.


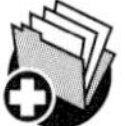

## MISCELLANEOUS

### FAQ

- Q: Is an MRI needed if I suspect a popliteal cyst?
  - A: Not if the history is typical, and the swelling transilluminates.
- Q: Where is the tenderness located in OSD?
  - A: Over the tibial tubercle only.

K

# KNEE INJECTION

*Timothy S. Johnson, MD*

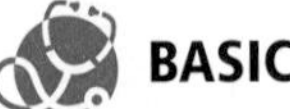

## BASICS

### DESCRIPTION

- Knee aspiration commonly is used for diagnostic purposes for effusions of unclear cause.
- Injections are used most commonly to treat arthritis.
- Indications
  - Effusion
  - Hemarthrosis
  - Infection/septic joint
  - Synovitis/arthritis
- Equipment
  - 18-gauge needle
  - 20–60-mL syringes
  - Sterile gloves
  - Sterile antiseptic solution

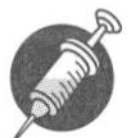

## TREATMENT

- Aspiration technique (Fig. 1):
  - The superolateral approach is the most reliable for aspiration (1).
  - Position the patient supine on the examination table with the knee fully extended or with a pillow under the knee.
  - Perform a wide sterile preparation of the knee.
  - Identify the aspiration site ~1 finger breadth proximal to the superior pole of the patella and 1 finger breadth lateral to the lateral border of the patella.
  - Advance a needle through the skin, subcutaneous tissue, and lateral retinaculum into the suprapatellar pouch between the anterior femur and the quadriceps tendon from lateral to medial.
  - Aspirate the entire fluid collection.
    - When the syringe is full, clamp the hub of the needle with a sterile clamp.
    - Hold the hub and unscrew the syringe from the needle without removing the needle from the joint.
    - Apply a new syringe to the needle hub and continue aspirating.
    - Repeat these steps as many times as necessary to aspirate the effusion completely.
  - Remove the needle and apply a bandage.
  - Store the fluid for laboratory analysis (see "Arthrocentesis" chapter)
- Pearls
  - A wide sterile skin preparation allows for manipulation of the knee and patella during aspiration.
  - Milking the effusion up into the suprapatellar pouch allows for a more complete aspiration of fluid.
  - Synovium can easily clog the needle tip during aspiration; use a large-bore needle (18-gauge or higher) to minimize this problem.
  - Injecting the skin with lidocaine at the injection/aspiration site is an option for patients concerned about pain.
    - It may allow the patient to tolerate the procedure better.
    - However, it does require an additional needle stick.
    - Alternatively, ethyl chloride sprayed on the skin immediately before the aspiration has a similar effect.
  - Never aspirate or inject through cellulitic skin.
- Therapeutic injection:
  - Injection of corticosteroid:
    - Commonly performed after aspiration of synovial fluid that is not infected
    - The superolateral approach is the most reliable (1).
  - If an aspiration was performed:
    - Do not remove the needle from the joint.
    - Simply exchange the aspiration syringe with the syringe filled with the injectable and inject the medication without changing the needle's location within the joint.
  - If an aspiration was not performed:
    - Identify the landmarks and insertion location as described for the superolateral approach into the suprapatellar pouch.
    - Advance the needle into the pouch.
    - Aspirate a small amount of synovial fluid to confirm intra-articular placement.
    - Once confirmed, inject the medication into the joint.
  - Remove the needle and apply a bandage.

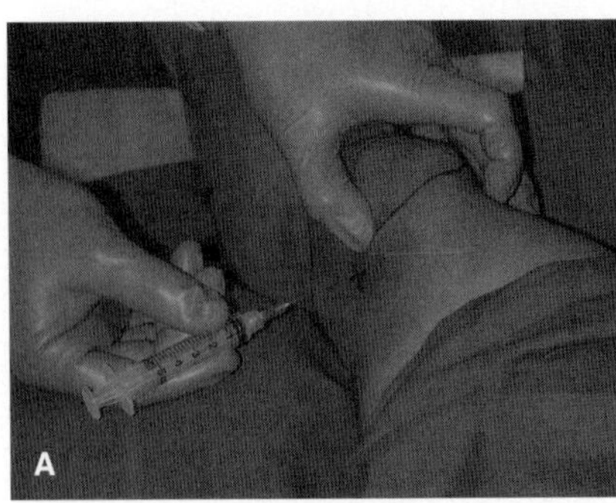


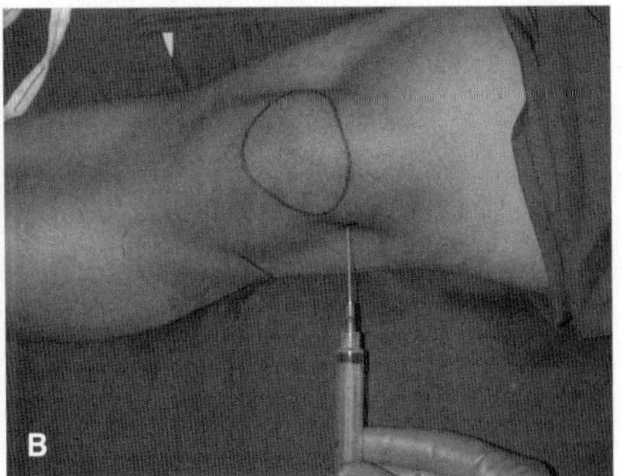


**Fig. 1.** Knee injection. **A**: Lateral view. **B**: Superior view.

## MEDICATION (DRUGS)

- Lidocaine:
  - Can be helpful in controlling pain caused by the injection.
  - Also can facilitate diagnostic procedures.
    - Painful knees are examined more easily after injection because of lidocaine's numbing effect.
    - This effect is particularly helpful in determining the cause of a traumatic knee effusion.
    - Bupivicaine also may be used for a longer numbing effect.
    - On the day of injection, limit activity on the affected knee to activities of daily living.
- Corticosteroid:
  - Can be useful for controlling pain and inflammation from noninfectious arthritis
  - Contraindicated if a septic knee has not been ruled out
  - A typical dose for the knee is 1 mL of kenalog (40 mg/mL), usually injected with 4 mL of 1% lidocaine.
  - Steroid medication usually takes 2–3 days to have an effect.
    - Manage the patient's expectations by discussing this delayed pain relief at the time of the injection.
- Hyaluronates (2) are indicated for treatment of mild osteoarthritis.

## REFERENCES

1. Wind WM, Jr, Smolinski RJ. Reliability of common knee injection sites with low-volume injections. *J Arthroplasty* 2004;19:858–861.
2. Miller EH. Viscosupplementation: therapeutic mechanisms and clinical potential in osteoarthritis of the knee. *J Am Acad Orthop Surg* 2001;9: 146–147.

## ADDITIONAL READING

Cole BJ, Schumacher HR, Jr. Injectable corticosteroids in modern practice. *J Am Acad Orthop Surg* 2005; 13:37–46.

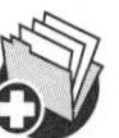

## MISCELLANEOUS

### FAQ

- Q: Which approach is least reliable in successfully injecting therapeutic agents into the knee joint?
  - A: The lateral joint line approach.
- Q: Viscosupplementation therapy of the knee is indicated for which type of arthritis?
  - A: Osteoarthritis.

# KNEE PAIN

*John H. Wilckens, MD*
*Bill Hobbs, MD*

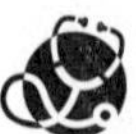

## BASICS

### DESCRIPTION

- Knee pain has many causes, including pathologic processes in the knee and disorders in distant locations with referral to the knee area.
- Diffuse or located in a specific region
- A characteristic history and physical examination frequently narrow the diagnosis (1).
- Classification:
  - Traumatic
  - Acquired

### RISK FACTORS

- Athletic activity (2)
- Obesity
- Sedentary lifestyle

### ETIOLOGY

- Traumatic injury
- Overuse injury
- Disease process(es) in or around the knee

### ASSOCIATED CONDITIONS

- Rheumatoid arthritis
- Active lifestyle

## DIAGNOSIS

### SIGNS AND SYMPTOMS

- General:
  - Swelling
  - Locking
  - Popping
  - Difficulty with stairs and rising from a chair
  - Chronic pain with increased activity
- Patellofemoral conditions:
  - Patellofemoral syndrome:
    - Typically occurs in young adults
    - Involves articular cartilage softening
    - Pain is most frequent in the anterior knee and is worse with stairs.
    - Knee ROM often has a grating sensation, and pain is elicited by pressing firmly on the patella.
  - Patellar subluxation–dislocation:
    - Traumatic
    - Can be related to a combination of structural variations (compared with normal anatomy) in the knee and leg: Femoral anteversion and valgus (a configuration that increases the Q angle) and a laterally moving patella with an extended knee ("J sign")
  - Articular cartilage injury:
    - Frequently related to a traumatic event
    - Pain is worse with activity.
- Meniscal injuries (3):
  - Can be degenerative (with an incidental initial event) or traumatic (with a clear injury)
  - Swelling develops slowly and is activity related.
  - Locking or giving-way of the knee, along with medial or lateral joint line pain, is common.
- Arthritis:
  - Symptoms frequently are gradual in onset and progressive.
  - Pain is worse with increased activity and improves with rest.
  - Pain at night after an active day is common.
- Ligament tears:
  - ACL:
    - Prevents anterior translation of the tibia on the femur
    - Injured predominantly from noncontact decelerations such as stopping suddenly, pivoting, or landing after jumping
  - PCL:
    - Primary stabilizer to posterior translation of the tibia on the femur
    - Direct trauma to anterior knee ("dashboard injury")
    - Knee pain and swelling occur after the injury, with improvement in generalized pain symptoms at several weeks.
    - Develop medial compartment and patellofemoral symptoms over time
  - MCL:
    - The primary restraint to valgus stress on the knee
    - Pain is felt along the medial aspect of the knee, typically extending proximally and distally along the region of the MCL.
    - Isolated MCL injuries occur from a direct blow to the lateral knee.
    - Can be associated with ACL and meniscal tears.
  - LCL:
    - Extends from the lateral femoral condyle to the fibular head
    - Isolated injury to the LCL is rare.
    - LCL Injury frequently is associated with a cruciate ligament injury.
    - Assessment of the peroneal nerve is important.
- Quadriceps or patellar tendon rupture (4):
  - Causes a loss of extension of the leg
  - Symptoms include the inability to extend the knee actively, pain, and knee effusion.
  - Often a palpable defect and a patella that appears more distal (quadriceps) or more proximal (patellar) than normal
  - Most frequent cause is direct trauma to the knee or forced flexion of the knee that is resisted by maximal quadriceps contraction.
- Bursitis and tendinitis:
  - Inflammatory changes occur in the bursa or tendon insertions around the knee, typically with tenderness to direct palpation over the anatomic location.
- Osteochondritis dissecans:
  - Observed in children and young adults who are active and participate in sports
  - Result of localized bone necrosis with loss of overlying cartilage support
  - Symptoms include knee pain, effusion, tenderness over the lesion, and (occasionally) locking or catching of the knee if the fragment has become a loose body in the joint.
  - Pain often is insidious and related to activity.
- OSD:
  - An overuse syndrome from repetitive stress on the tubercle, resulting in an apophysitis of the patellar tendon insertion
- Baker cyst (popliteal cyst):
  - Caused by a distended capsule in the posterior fossa of the knee, often directly connected to the joint space
  - Most often associated with intra-articular disease
  - Presents as a mass in the popliteal fossa of the knee
  - The intra-articular disorder may not be symptomatic; therefore, the patient may complain only of posterior knee fullness.
- Fracture:
  - Fracture about the knee should be ruled out in any patient with a traumatic injury.
  - Can occur in the distal femur, proximal tibia, and patella
  - Usually, plain AP and lateral radiographic views are sufficient.
- Bone tumor:
  - Rare, but should be a differential diagnosis in patients with night pain
  - Most patients have musculoskeletal pain.
    - Typically described as dull, deep, aching
    - Often becomes constant
    - Many patients experience pain at night.
    - May not be related to activity
  - Patients also may complain of swelling, loss of function at the involved site, weight loss, or acute symptoms of a pathologic fracture.

#### *Physical Exam*

- Palpate the joint for:
  - Effusion and localized swelling
  - Joint line tenderness (Medial and lateral tenderness suggests meniscal tear or arthritis.)
- Compare ROM of the affected knee with that of the contralateral knee.
- Observe patellar tracking as the knee is ranged from flexion to extension.
- Check joint stability (MCL, LCL, ACL, PCL).

### TESTS

#### *Lab*

- Order serum laboratory tests based on a suspicion for specific clinical entities, as follows:
  - Septic arthritis: Complete blood count with differential ESR, C-reactive protein
  - Rheumatoid arthritis or other inflammatory arthritis: Rheumatoid screen, including rheumatoid factor and antinuclear antibody
  - Gout: Serum uric acid level

#### *Imaging*

- The 1st step is plain radiographs (including weightbearing posteroanterior, lateral, and tangential [Merchant] views) of the patella.
- MRI is used to detect meniscal tears, ligament injury, synovial proliferative disorders, tumors, and AVN.

#### *Diagnostic Procedures/Surgery*

- Arthrocentesis often can aid in establishing a definitive diagnosis.
  - With septic arthritis, findings include positive culture and elevated white blood cell count (>50,000).
  - With gout, findings include uric acid crystals.
  - Fat droplets suggest intra-articular fracture.

#### *Pathological Findings*

Depend on causative factors

### DIFFERENTIAL DIAGNOSIS

- A complete differential diagnosis is beyond the scope of this chapter (5), but most common:
  - Patellofemoral conditions
  - Articular cartilage injury
  - Meniscal disorders
  - Arthritis
  - Ligament tears
  - Tendinitis and tendon ruptures
  - Osteochondritis dissecans
  - OSD
  - Baker cyst
  - Gout
  - Fracture
  - Tumor
- The diagnosis can be made by symptoms and history in conjunction with the physical examination and imaging studies (Table 1).

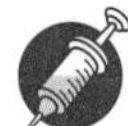

## TREATMENT

### GENERAL MEASURES

- Patellofemoral syndrome: Anti-inflammatory medication and exercise
- Patellar subluxation-dislocation: Often improved by extensive physical therapy and patellar bracing
- Arthritis: Initially, analgesics, activity modification, injections, unloader bracing
- Bursitis and tendinitis: Analgesics, topical treatments, activity modification
- OSD: Rest and activity modification
- Ligamentous and meniscal injuries: Protected ROM and weightbearing, ice, analgesics, and orthopaedic referral

### SPECIAL THERAPY

#### *Physical Therapy*

- Excellent for treating patients with knee pain (6)
- Therapists:
  - Concentrate on ROM; quadriceps, hamstring, and core strengthening; and stretching.
  - May include modalities such as cryotherapy, electrical stimulation, and ultrasound

### MEDICATION (DRUGS)

- NSAIDs
- Acetaminophen
- Mild narcotic analgesics
- Intra-articular hyalurans

### SURGERY

- 3 main categories of knee surgery (7):
  - Arthritis: Arthroscopic meniscal and cartilage débridement, tibial and femoral osteotomy, total and hemi knee replacement
  - Sports medicine: Arthroscopic evaluation and treatment of meniscal and ligament injuries, patellar mechanism realignment
  - Trauma: Internal fracture fixation, tendon rupture repair

## FOLLOW-UP

### PROGNOSIS

Excellent with well-defined diagnoses and appropriate surgical and nonsurgical treatment

### COMPLICATIONS

- Loss of motion
- Loss of function, particularly weightbearing
- Chronic pain

### PATIENT MONITORING

Patients are followed at 4–6-week intervals until they regain strength and ROM.

### REFERENCES


1. Jensen JE, Conn RR, Hazelrigg G, et al. Systematic evaluation of acute knee injuries. *Clin Sports Med* 1985;4:295–312.
2. Collins HR. Screening of athletic knee injuries. *Clin Sports Med* 1985;4:217–230.
3. Henning CE, Lynch MA. Current concepts of meniscal function and pathology. *Clin Sports Med* 1985;4:259–265.
4. Carson WG, Jr. Diagnosis of extensor mechanism disorders. *Clin Sports Med* 1985;4:231–246.
5. Wilckens JH, Mears SC, Byank RP. Knee, lower leg, and ankle pain. In: Barker LR, Burton JR, Zieve PD, eds. *Principles of Ambulatory Medicine*, 7th ed. Philadelphia: Lippincott Williams & Wilkins, 2006, in press.
6. Montgomery JB, Steadman JR. Rehabilitation of the injured knee. *Clin Sports Med* 1985;4: 333–343.
7. Feagin JA, Jr. Operative treatment of acute and chronic knee problems. *Clin Sports Med* 1985;4: 325–331.


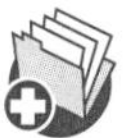

## MISCELLANEOUS

### CODES

#### *ICD9-CM*

- 719.46 Pain in joint
- 719.6 Knee pain

### PATIENT TEACHING

#### *Activity*

Depends on causative pain factors

### FAQ

- Q: What is a sensitive physical finding for intra-articular knee pathology?
  - A: In addition to localized tenderness, a knee effusion suggests intra-articular abnormality.
- Q: How do meniscal tears occur?
  - A: Meniscal tears can occur with an acute ligament injury, such as an ACL injury, or in chronically ligament-deficient knees because the menisci serve as secondary knee joint stabilizers. Degenerative tears can occur in the meniscus from malalignment, overuse, and repetitive trauma.

**Table 1**

| Symptom/History | Location of Pain | Diagnosis |
|---|---|---|
| Locking | Medial or lateral knee | Meniscus tear |
| Pop and sudden turn | Entire knee with swelling | ACL injury |
| Stairs and getting out of chair | Anterior knee | Patellofemoral cause |
| Striking knee hard against dashboard | Entire knee with swelling | PCL injury |
| Side contact to knee | Medial or lateral knee | Collateral ligament |
| Chronic pain with increased activity | Medial or lateral knee | Arthritis |

# KNEE REPLACEMENT

*Tariq A. Nayfeh, MD, PhD*
*Peter R. Jay, MD*

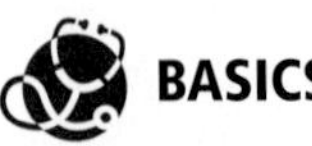

## BASICS

### DESCRIPTION
- Total knee arthroplasty—resurfacing of the articular surfaces of the knee with metal and interposed plastic liner—is a highly effective treatment for patients with disabling knee arthritis.
- The components are shaped to conform to the previous joint geometry.
- Classification is by involved compartment.
  - Medial compartment (tibial femoral)
  - Lateral compartment (tibial femoral)
  - Patellofemoral

### EPIDEMIOLOGY
#### *Incidence*
- 61% of total knee replacements occur in females (1).
- In 2003, 418,000 surgeries were performed in the United States (2).
  - The number of knee replacements performed per year continues to rise.
  - Patients had an average age of 67 years at the time of replacement.

### RISK FACTORS
- Trauma
- Meniscectomy
- Obesity

### ETIOLOGY
- Osteoarthritis: Often idiopathic
- Posttraumatic: Athletic injuries, falls, motor vehicle accidents
- Inflammatory arthritis: Rheumatoid arthritis, pseudogout, or gout

### ASSOCIATED CONDITIONS
- Many patients have associated hip arthritis.
- Foot and ankle arthritis with and without severe deformity is common in patients with rheumatoid arthritis.

## DIAGNOSIS

### SIGNS AND SYMPTOMS
- Signs:
  - Effusions
  - Medial joint line tenderness
  - Varus (osteoarthritis) or valgus (rheumatoid arthritis)
  - Deformity
  - Limp
- Symptoms:
  - Pain
  - Start-up pain
  - Swelling
  - Catching
  - Giving way

#### *History*
Pain not responsive to medications

#### *Physical Exam*
- The knee is examined for signs of osteoarthritis, including:
  - Effusions
  - Joint line tenderness (suggests meniscal disorder)
  - Areas of tenderness
  - ROM
  - Gait disruption

### TESTS
#### *Lab*
- When infectious causes are considered, the C-reactive protein and ESR are useful tests.
- Serum uric acid levels are determined if the clinician suspects gouty arthritis.

#### *Imaging*
- Plain radiographs are the 1st step in imaging.
  - Standing AP view of both knees: Can detect subtle loss of the articular cartilage thickness.
  - Lateral view: Can assess for arthritic changes in the patellofemoral joint.
- MRI can be used to detect meniscal tears, synovial proliferative disorders such as PVNS, and cartilage loss.

#### *Diagnostic Procedures/Surgery*
Arthrocentesis is an easy and effective method for screening for septic arthritis and gout or pseudogout.

#### *Pathological Findings*
- The common denominator in all forms of arthritis is breakdown of the articular cartilage with loss of the proteoglycan and gradual loss of thickness.
- As the cartilage thins, the joint deformity increases, and patients often experience the painful sensation of bone rubbing on bone.

### DIFFERENTIAL DIAGNOSIS
- Arthritis
- Infections: Septic arthritis or osteomyelitis
- Patellofemoral syndrome or patellofemoral instability
- Meniscal tears
- Tumors

## TREATMENT

### GENERAL MEASURES
- Patients with knee arthritis first should be treated with nonoperative means, including NSAIDs, pain medicines, ambulatory aids, braces, and intra-articular injections.
- Patients <50 years old should be considered for realignment surgery or arthroscopy.
- After failure of nonoperative treatments and an extensive discussion of surgical risks and expectations, the patient may elect to proceed with surgery.
- Patients are prepared for knee replacement with a careful medical examination.
  - They may consider autologous blood donation.
  - NSAIDs and, if medically safe, blood thinners are halted 6–7 days before the procedure.

### SPECIAL THERAPY
#### *Physical Therapy*
- The focus of this integral component of care after knee replacement is on the following:
  - ROM (attaining 0–110° within 4–8 weeks)
  - Quadriceps strengthening
  - Full weightbearing

### MEDICATION (DRUGS)
- After knee reconstruction, adequate narcotic analgesics are necessary to allow patients to participate fully in physical therapy.
- Most patients do not require long-term analgesics, although intermittent courses of NSAIDs may be used for minor aches and pains about the knee.

## SURGERY

- Knee replacement can be partial or total.
  - Partial or unicompartmental replacement:
    - Can be performed through a smaller incision
    - Is indicated if only 1 compartment of the knee has arthritis and the cruciate ligaments are functioning
    - Can be performed for the medial or lateral compartments of the knee
    - Patellofemoral compartment replacement is being developed.
  - Total knee replacement:
    - Is performed through a midline incision over the knee
    - Bony cuts are made with the use of specialized jigs to obtain correct alignment.
    - The components are cemented onto the bone or are press fit (the bone then will grow into the pores).
    - The articular surface of the patella also may be resurfaced.
    - The actual joint articulation is between metal and high-density polyethylene.
- Two replacement designs are available.
  - In 1 design, the PCL is retained.
  - In the other, the PCL is excised.
    - A peg is built into the polyethylene liner of these knee replacement designs (3).
- Computer-assisted surgery is under development (4).
  - Allows for alignment to be checked precisely intraoperatively
  - May allow for improvements in component placement
- After surgery, all patients should be treated with low-molecular-weight heparin or Coumadin to prevent DVT (5).
  - In the hospital, mechanical prophylaxis and early mobilization also should be used.

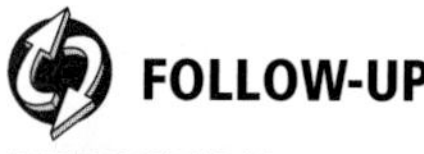

# FOLLOW-UP

## DISPOSITION

### *Issues for Referral*

Severe pain, swelling, redness, or instability after surgery

## PROGNOSIS

- The long-term results of total knee replacement are excellent.
  - ~91% of knee replacements are functioning well at 10 years (6).
  - At 20 years, 78% are functioning well (6).
- Newer prosthetic designs have shown a 96% survival rate at 8-year follow-up (7).
- No differences have been found in the results of cruciate-retaining and cruciate-sacrificing total knee designs (8).
- 1 study has shown a 95% survival rate for unicompartmental replacement at 10 years, but that arthritic changes slowly continued in the knee (9).

## COMPLICATIONS

- Infection
- Aseptic loosening
- Polyethylene wear and osteolysis
- Patellofemoral problems:
  - Subluxation
  - Dislocation
- Periprosthetic fracture:
  - Femoral
  - Tibial
  - Patellar
- Tendon ruptures:
  - Quadriceps
  - Patellar
- DVT and pulmonary embolus
- Medical complications:
  - Heart attack
  - Pneumonia
  - Urinary infection
  - Death
- Stiffness
- Numbness around the incision
- Pain
- Pes bursitis

## PATIENT MONITORING

- After surgery, patients are followed at 1-month intervals until they attain a functional ROM, after which they are followed once a year.
- Plain radiographs are used to monitor the metal and cement interfaces with the bone and to check for polyethylene wear.

## REFERENCES


1. SooHoo NF, Lieberman JR, Ko CY, et al. Factors predicting complication rates following total knee replacement. *J Bone Joint Surg* 2006;88A: 480–485.
2. American Academy of Orthopaedic Surgeons Department of Research and Scientific Affairs. Information About Knee Replacements: 1999 to 2003. http://www.aaos.org/wordhtml/research/stats/knee_all.htm#patients. Accessed on June 3, 2006.
3. Morgan H, Battista V, Leopold SS. Constraint in primary total knee arthroplasty. *J Am Acad Orthop Surg* 2005;13:515–524.
4. Haaker RG, Stockheim M, Kamp M, et al. Computer-assisted navigation increases precision of component placement in total knee arthroplasty. *Clin Orthop Relat Res* 2005;433:152–159.
5. Lieberman Jr, Hsu WK. Prevention of venous thromboembolic disease after total hip and knee arthroplasty. *J Bone Joint Surg* 2005;87A: 2097–2112.
6. Rand JA, Trousdale RT, Ilstrup DM, et al. Factors affecting the durability of primary total knee prostheses. *J Bone Joint Surg* 2003;85A:259–265.
7. Bozic KJ, Kinder J, Meneghini RM, et al. Implant survivorship and complication rates after total knee arthroplasty with a third-generation cemented system: 5 to 8 years followup. *Clin Orthop Relat Res* 2005;435:277.
8. Jacobs WCH, Clement DJ, Wymenga AB. Retention versus sacrifice of the posterior cruciate ligament in total knee replacement for treatment of osteoarthritis and rheumatoid arthritis. *Cochrane Database Syst Rev* 2005;4(CD004803):1–30.
9. Berger RA, Meneghini RM, Jacobs JJ, et al. Results of unicompartmental knee arthroplasty at a minimum of ten years of follow-up. *J Bone Joint Surg* 2005;87A:999–1006.


## ADDITIONAL READING


Insall JN, Scott WN, eds. *Surgery of the Knee*, 3rd ed. New York: Churchill Livingstone, 2001.


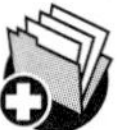

# MISCELLANEOUS

## CODES

### *ICD9-CM*

- 714.0 Rheumatoid arthritis
- 7715.96 Osteoarthritis of the knee

## PATIENT TEACHING

Early on, patients must perform their ROM exercises rigorously to attain functional ROM and to prevent contractures.

### *Activity*

- To ensure the longevity of the replacement, patients must modify their activities.
- Activities can be grouped as follows:
  - Good activities:
    - Walking
    - Bicycling
    - Golf
    - Swimming
  - Bad activities:
    - Running
    - Racquetball
    - Heavy lifting
    - Singles tennis

## FAQ

- Q: How long will a knee replacement last?
  - A: At the 10-year follow-up, ~91% of total knee replacements are functioning well. At 20 years, this number is reduced to 78%.
- Q: When should I get a knee replacement?
  - A: Knee replacement is indicated for patients with severe arthritis of the knee and degenerative changes. Patients must have made extensive attempts at nonoperative treatment and be ready to take the risks of major surgery. Patients also must be ready to change their lifestyle and stop activities (e.g., running) that may lead to failure of the knee replacement.

# KNEE SUPRACONDYLAR FRACTURE

*Carl Wierks, MD*
*David Solacoff, MD*

## BASICS

### DESCRIPTION

- These fractures involve the supracondylar (metaphyseal) area of the distal femur.
- Classification AO/ASIF (1):
  - Type A: Extra-articular:
    - A1: Simple fracture
    - A2: Metaphyseal wedge
    - A3: Comminuted metaphyseal fracture
  - Type B: Unicondylar:
    - B1: Lateral condyle
    - B2: Medial condyle
    - B3: Fracture in the frontal plane
  - Type C: No part of the joint is attached to the shaft.
    - C1: Simple articular fracture with simple metaphyseal fracture
    - C2: Simple articular fracture with comminuted metaphyseal fracture
    - C3: Fractures with articular comminution
- Synonym: Distal femur fracture

### EPIDEMIOLOGY

#### *Incidence*

- Up to 30% of all femur fractures (2)
- Less common than femoral shaft fractures
- Most pediatric supracondylar femur fractures occur in adolescents.
- 2 peaks (3):
  - Young (<35 years old): High-energy fractures
  - Older (>50 years old): Low-energy fractures
- In the young, high-energy group, males are affected more commonly than females.
- In the older, low-energy group, females are affected more often than males.
- Osteopenia is prevalent in the older, low-energy group.

### RISK FACTORS

Risk factors in the older group are osteopenia and previous age-related fractures.

### ETIOLOGY

- Young group: High-energy trauma (e.g., motor vehicle collision, falls from heights)
- Older group: Low-energy trauma (e.g., falls on flexed knee)
- Rarely, a complication of total knee arthroplasty
- In pediatric patients, injuries usually are traumatic, with the fracture exiting at the metaphysis on the compression side, resulting in a Salter-Harris type II fracture (4).

### ASSOCIATED CONDITIONS

- Acetabular fractures
- Hip dislocations
- Femoral neck and shaft fractures
- Knee ligamentous injuries
- Tibial plateau and shaft fractures
- Femoral artery disruptions

## DIAGNOSIS

### SIGNS AND SYMPTOMS

- Pain
- Tenderness to palpation
- Edema
- Deformity
- Inability to walk
- Ecchymosis

#### *Physical Exam*

- Complete musculoskeletal and neurovascular examination is essential.
- Full examination of the knee is difficult until after fracture fixation.

#### *Pathological Findings*

- Muscle spasm often leads to shortening of the femur and limb.
- The femoral shaft often overrides anteriorly as the gastrocnemius pulls the distal fragment posteriorly into an apex-anterior deformity.
- The adductors often cause a varus deformity.

### TESTS

#### *Imaging*

- Radiography:
  - Knee:
    - AP and lateral radiographs of the knee and supracondylar region
    - 45° oblique radiographs if intercondylar involvement is present
  - Pelvis:
    - AP radiograph (to rule out other fractures) in trauma settings
  - Hip and femur:
    - AP and lateral radiographs of the hip and the whole femur (to rule out other fractures) in trauma settings
- Angiogram if distal vascular status is questionable
- CT may be beneficial for operative planning for complex fractures.
- Pediatric patients:
  - Standard trauma radiographs should be obtained.
  - Stress views may be taken when occult injury to the epiphysis is suspected.
  - The physeal line should be 3–5 mm thick until adolescence.

### DIFFERENTIAL DIAGNOSIS

- Bruise
- Knee ligamentous injury
- Fracture of the patella or proximal tibia

## TREATMENT

### GENERAL MEASURES

- Anatomic articular alignment is paramount.
- For nondisplaced and impacted fractures, a splint, cast, or fracture brace is used.
- For extra-articular fractures and medically unstable patients, skeletal traction is an option.
- For severe open fractures, external fixation is used.
  - May be applied across the knee to provide initial fracture stabilization
  - May be converted to internal fixation when soft-tissue injuries are controlled
- Open reduction and internal fixation are used for most closed fractures.
- In pediatric patients with epiphyseal injury, closed reduction with casting can be done if the fracture is stable.

#### *Activity*

- Initial activity should be nonweightbearing on the affected extremity until fracture callus forms.
- Then, weightbearing is advanced gradually.

### SPECIAL THERAPY

#### *Physical Therapy*

- ROM and quadriceps and hamstring strengthening may begin early postoperatively.
- The patient can advance to gait training as tolerated.
  - Some advocate toe-touch weightbearing.
- Progressive weightbearing and resistance exercises when clinical and radiographic evidence of healing occurs (usually 2–3 months)
- Complete union usually takes 4–6 months.

### MEDICATION (DRUGS)

- Analgesics such as narcotics or acetaminophen are given.
- NSAIDs are avoided because they may inhibit bone healing.

### SURGERY

- Goals are anatomic alignment and stable fixation of the fracture to allow early motion of the limb.
- Indications include:
  - Open or displaced fractures
  - Fractures with vascular compromise
  - Irreducible fractures
  - Fractures in the patient with multiple injuries or ipsilateral lower-extremity fractures
- Relative contraindications to surgery include:
  - Infection of the fracture area
  - A medically unstable patient
  - Very osteopenic bone
- Surgical implant options include:
  - Metal plates angled blade plate
  - Condylar buttress plates
  - Locked plates
  - External fixation
  - Intramedullary nails
  - Total knee replacement

- Metal plates (5,6):
  - Come in a variety of shapes
  - Can be used with simple and comminuted fractures
  - Can be applied through small incisions and placed on the bone submuscularly
- External fixation most frequently is used to temporize fractures with extensive soft-tissue damage or in the unstable, polytrauma patient.
- Intramedullary nails work well to stabilize comminuted fractures and can be placed antegrade or retrograde.
- Total knee replacement with distal femoral replacement can be used in patients with severe osteopenia or pre-existing arthrosis (7).
- When fractures occur near a knee prosthesis:
  - Fixation can be achieved through a retrograde intramedullary nail, fixed-angle device, or revision arthroplasty.
  - In general, the best treatment choices are (8):
    - Intramedullary nails for proximal fractures
    - Fixed-angle devices for fractures at the level of the implant
    - Revision arthroplasty for distal fractures or those with implant loosening

### *Pediatric Considerations*

- Closed reduction with percutaneous pinning has been shown to give satisfactory results for displaced pediatric fractures (9).
- If the fracture is unstable, open reduction with internal fixation can be performed.
- Postoperatively, the knee is immobilized in 10° of flexion until radiographic evidence of healing is present (~4 weeks).

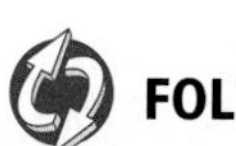

## FOLLOW-UP

### DISPOSITION

Patients should be monitored closely after initial trauma to rule out the development of compartment syndrome of the thigh.

### PROGNOSIS

- The prognosis depends on the type and severity of the fracture; more complex fractures generally have poorer prognoses.
- In general, patients have a good to excellent result with appropriate treatment (10).
- Midterm results of treatment of periprosthetic fractures with intramedullary nails are excellent (11).

### COMPLICATIONS

- Knee stiffness
- Infection
- Nonunion
- Malunion
- Loss of fixation
- Traumatic arthritis
- Compartment syndrome
- Physeal injury can result in an angular deformity or leg-length inequality.
  - Discrepancies >2.5 cm can be managed by contralateral epiphysiodesis, femoral shortening, or ipsilateral femoral lengthening.

### PATIENT MONITORING

- Patients are seen initially a few weeks after definitive fixation and then approximately monthly until the fracture heals and ROM is acceptable.
- Clinical (pain to palpation) and radiographic (callus) monitoring is done until the fracture is healed.
- Limited weightbearing may be started when good callus is evident and the patient is not tender to palpation around the fracture.

### REFERENCES


1. Muller ME, Nazarian S, Koch P, et al. *The Comprehensive Classification of Fractures of Long Bones*. Berlin: Springer-Verlag, 1990.
2. Arneson TJ, Melton LJ, III, Lewallen DG, et al. Epidemiology of diaphyseal and distal femoral fractures in Rochester, Minnesota, 1965–1984. *Clin Orthop Relat Res* 1988;234:188–194.
3. Martinet O, Cordey J, Harder Y, et al. The epidemiology of fractures of the distal femur. *Injury* 2000;31:C62–C63.
4. Salter RB, Harris WR. Injuries involving the epiphyseal plate. *J Bone Joint Surg* 1963;45A: 587–622.
5. Kregor PJ, Stannard JA, Zlowodzki M, et al. Treatment of distal femur fractures using the less invasive stabilization system: surgical experience and early clinical results in 103 fractures. *J Orthop Trauma* 2004;18:509–520.
6. Schutz M, Muller M, Regazzoni P, et al. Use of the less invasive stabilization system (LISS) in patients with distal femoral (AO33) fractures: a prospective multicenter study. *Arch Orthop Trauma Surg* 2005;125:102–108.
7. Rosen AL, Strauss E. Primary total knee arthroplasty for complex distal femur fractures in elderly patients. *Clin Orthop Relat Res* 2004;425: 101–105.
8. Su ET, DeWal H, Di Cesare PE. Periprosthetic femoral fractures above total knee replacements. *J Am Acad Orthop Surg* 2004;12:12–20.
9. Butcher CC, Hoffman EB. Supracondylar fractures of the femur in children: closed reduction and percutaneous pinning of displaced fractures. *J Pediatr Orthop* 2005;25:145–148.
10. Weight M, Collinge C. Early results of the less invasive stabilization system for mechanically unstable fractures of the distal femur (AO/OTA types A2, A3, C2, and C3). *J Orthop Trauma* 2004;18:503–508.
11. Gliatis J, Megas P, Panagiotopoulos E, et al. Midterm results of treatment with a retrograde nail for supracondylar periprosthetic fractures of the femur following total knee arthroplasty. *J Orthop Trauma* 2005;19:164–170.


### ADDITIONAL READING


- Forster MC, Komarsamy B, Davison JN. Distal femoral fractures: a review of fixation methods. *Injury* 2006;37:97–108.
- Papadokostakis G, Papakostidis C, Dimitriou R, et al. The role and efficacy of retrograding nailing for the treatment of diaphyseal and distal femoral fractures: a systematic review of the literature. *Injury* 2005;36:813–822.


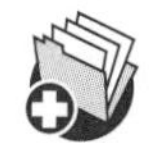

## MISCELLANEOUS

### CODES

#### *ICD9-CM*

821.23 Femur supracondylar fracture

### FAQ

- Q: How should a distal femur fracture be treated?
  - A: Most fractures are treated with surgery using an intramedullary retrograde nail or a percutaneous locking plate. Rigid fixation allows for early motion of the knee to prevent knee stiffness.

K

# KÖHLER DISEASE

*Paul D. Sponseller, MD*

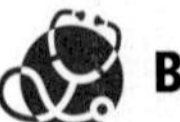

## BASICS

### DESCRIPTION
- Köhler disease is an eponym for osteochondrosis of the tarsal navicular (scaphoid) bone (Figs. 1 and 2).
- Pain in the medial midfoot in a young boy (aged 3–7 years) is the typical clinical presentation.
- The condition usually is worsened with activity and relieved with rest.
- Clinical outcome usually is good after healing.
- Classification:
  - This disorder is 1 of multiple disorders termed "osteochondroses," which are characterized by transient vascular impairment of developing bones.
  - Others in this category include Legg-Calvé-Perthes disease and OSD
- Synonyms: Osteonecrosis; Osteochondrosis; Osteochondritis of the tarsal navicular

### GENERAL PREVENTION
Prevention is not effective or practical in this rare disease.

### EPIDEMIOLOGY
A male predominance exists; it is 2–3 times more common in males than in females (1).

#### *Incidence*
This disease is uncommon.

### RISK FACTORS
- Male gender
- High activity level
- Sports involving running and kicking

#### *Genetics*
No known genetic transmission of this disorder

### ETIOLOGY
- The most likely cause is mechanical compression of the navicular, thus impairing vascularity.
- The navicular, which forms the apex of the longitudinal arch of the foot, is subject to constant compression during walking.
- These forces appear to compromise the circulation within the bone during a critical phase early in the ossification of the navicular.

### ASSOCIATED CONDITIONS
A slight association seems evident with Legg-Calvé-Perthes disease (childhood osteonecrosis of the femoral head) (1).

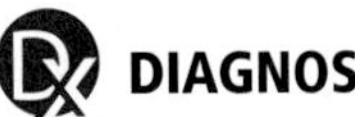

## DIAGNOSIS

### SIGNS AND SYMPTOMS
- Medial midfoot pain worsening with activity
- Tenderness to palpation
- Limp
- Walking on the outside of the foot to avoid stress on the navicular

#### *Physical Exam*
- Look for tenderness over the navicular with soft-tissue swelling about the navicular and an antalgic gait.
- Some patients walk on the outer border of the foot to minimize compression of the navicular.

### TESTS

#### *Imaging*
- Plain films are sufficient to make the diagnosis during the established phase.
  - The normal navicular begins to ossify at age 2–3 years.
  - It may start normally from several small ossification centers that eventually coalesce.
  - In Köhler disease, the navicular is flattened in its AP diameter and may show irregular sclerosis.
  - It may be bilateral.
- If the suspicion is high in spite of normal radiographs, MRI may be used to look for abnormal circulation within the navicular.
- With healing, increased ossification and resumption of normal growth occur.

#### *Pathological Findings*
- Pathologic specimens are not obtained routinely nor are they necessary for diagnosis.
- Some specimens reported in the literature show areas of necrosis, resorption of dead bone, and formation of new bone, which are general findings of healing osteonecrosis.

### DIFFERENTIAL DIAGNOSIS
- Ankle fracture
- Ankle sprain
- Navicular fracture
- Accessory navicular
- Soft-tissue infection

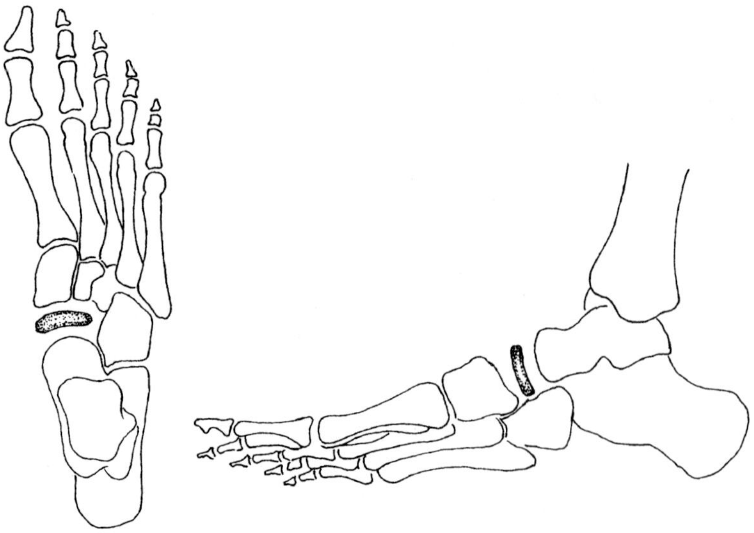

**Fig. 1.** Köhler disease is AVN of the tarsal navicular, which usually produces compression of this bone (*stippled*).

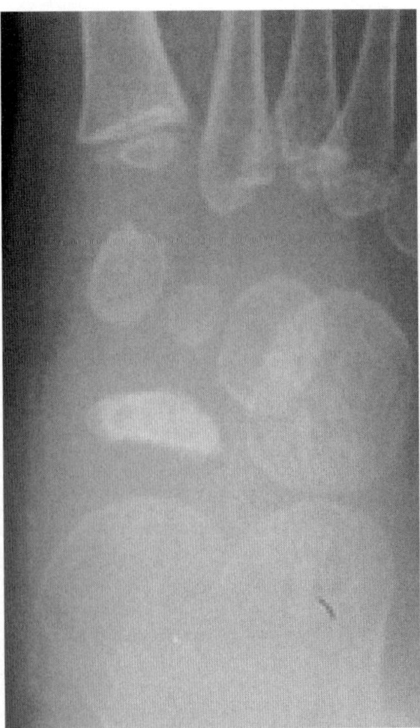

**Fig. 2.** Radiographic appearance of Köhler disease. Note the relative sclerosis and collapse of the navicular.

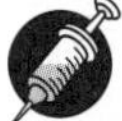

## TREATMENT

### GENERAL MEASURES

- Rest, arch support, and/or casting, depending on the level of symptoms:
  - For minimally symptomatic patients, the use of an arch support or refraining from strenuous activities may be all that is needed.
  - For more pronounced symptoms, a below-the-knee cast with a well-molded arch, worn for 4–8 weeks, usually provides relief.
  - If the symptoms are severe, the patient may need to avoid weightbearing in the cast.
  - After casting, if tenderness is minimal, use of an arch support and gradual resumption of activities are advised.
- Return to activity is based on physical examination.

#### *Activity*

- The patient should avoid activities that produce the pain, including sports involving running, jumping, and kicking.
- After symptoms resolve, the patient may resume those activities gradually, with use of an arch support.

### SPECIAL THERAPY

#### *Physical Therapy*

- Physical therapy is not needed.
- Parents may be put in charge of timing the return to activities, based on the child's symptoms.

### MEDICATION (DRUGS)

Acetaminophen or NSAIDs as needed

### SURGERY

- Surgery rarely is needed.
- Some persistent symptoms after maturity have required fusion of the talonavicular joint (1).

## FOLLOW-UP

### PROGNOSIS

- Prognosis is good.
- In 2–3 years, the radiographic appearance of the navicular usually returns to normal, and the patient's symptoms resolve (2).

### COMPLICATIONS

- Rarely, ache or tenderness may persist.
- These symptoms may be treated in the same fashion, by rest, arch support, or (rarely) surgery.

### PATIENT MONITORING

The course of the disease should be followed by clinical examination (tenderness, limp), rather than by radiography.

### REFERENCES


1. Kasser JR. The foot. Acquired conditions. In: Morrissy RT, Weinstein SL, eds. *Lovell and Winter's Pediatric Orthopaedics*, 6th ed. Philadelphia: Lippincott Williams & Wilkins, 2006:1311–1321.
2. Ippolito E, Ricciardi Pollini PT, Falez F. Kohler's disease of the tarsal navicular: long-term follow-up of 12 cases. *J Pediatr Orthop* 1984;4:416–417.


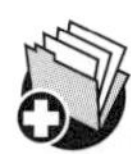

## MISCELLANEOUS

### CODES

#### *ICD9-CM*

732.5 Juvenile osteochondrosis of foot

### PATIENT TEACHING

#### *Activity*

Patients should be counseled about the benign, self-resolving nature of this condition and its relation to activity so they may moderate activities accordingly.

#### *Prevention*

Prevention is not effective or practical in this rare disease.

### FAQ

- Q: Does Köhler disease lead to arthritis of the foot?
  - A: No evidence exists of long-term sequelae after the process heals.

# KYPHOSIS

*Andrew P. Manista, MD*
*Damien Doute, MD*
*A. Jay Khanna, MD*

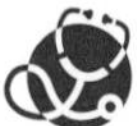

## BASICS

### DESCRIPTION

- Kyphosis, a spine curve in the sagittal plane with an anterior concavity, is normally present in the thoracic and sacral spine.
  - Normal thoracic kyphosis values: 20–40° (1,2).
  - Values >40° in the thoracic spine may be associated with postural kyphosis, congenital kyphosis, Scheuermann kyphosis, osteoporosis, AS, paralytic disorders, myelomeningocele, trauma, infection, surgery, and malignancy.
- Kyphotic deformity (curvature >40°) may lead to increased incidences of back pain, lumbar spondylolysis and, in the case of congenital and infectious kyphosis, neurologic compromise (3).

### GENERAL PREVENTION

- Postural kyphosis ("round back") can be influenced by attention to proper posture.
- Prevention of osteoporosis

### EPIDEMIOLOGY

Kyphotic deformity development is associated with NF, mucopolysaccharidosis, achondroplasia, myelomeningocele, AS, benign and malignant tumors (4).

#### *Incidence*

- Kyphotic deformity secondary to osteoporotic fractures occur in 15% of Caucasian females (5).
- Spinal tuberculosis complicates 3–5% of the 8 million new cases of tuberculosis reported worldwide per year (6).
- In those with HIV, spine involvement may be as high as 60% (6).

#### *Prevalence*

- Postural kyphosis is seen in young girls self-conscious of their breast development and in young patients who are taller than their peers (7).
- Congenital kyphosis is rare.
- Scheuermann kyphosis has been reported in 0.4–8.3% of the general population, and males are affected slightly more often than females (8).
- Osteoporosis is more common in patients who are female, elderly, of Caucasian or Asian descent, or taking steroids chronically.

### RISK FACTORS

- Osteoporosis
- Positive family history of kyphosis
- History of spine fracture
- Heavy loading of the spine during adolescence
- Exposure to tuberculosis
- Malignancy

#### *Genetics*

Some causes of kyphosis may be inherited, including AS (9), osteoporosis (10), and Scheuermann disease (11).

### ETIOLOGY

- Postural kyphosis results from ligament stretching; the vertebrae are formed normally.
- Scheuermann kyphosis is caused by wedging of the vertebrae, which usually develops during early adolescence.
- Congenital kyphosis is present at birth and is characterized by hemivertebrae or by fusion of the vertebrae anteriorly.
- Kyphosis develops in patients with osteoporosis through the anterior wedge vertebral fractures produced by insufficiency fractures of the thoracic or lumbar spine.
- Kyphosis develops in patients with tuberculosis as a result of destruction of the vertebral body.

### ASSOCIATED CONDITIONS

- Congenital kyphosis:
  - Kyphosis progresses rapidly over a short segment, and the resultant stretch of the spinal cord leads to neurologic decline (12).
  - Cardiac, renal, pulmonary, and auditory abnormalities
- Congenital scoliosis or kyphosis presents intraspinal abnormalities in 30% (13,14)
- Scheuermann kyphosis:
  - Increased lumbar lordosis is associated with a 50% incidence of spondylolysis (15).
  - 1/3 of patients have mild to moderate scoliotic curves (10–20°).
- Osteoporosis:
  - Insufficiency fractures of the hip, pelvis, and wrist

## DIAGNOSIS

### SIGNS AND SYMPTOMS

- Congenital kyphosis may be detected on prenatal ultrasound but usually is diagnosed by a pediatrician or parent noticing the initial or increasing deformity.
- "Poor posture" noted by parents, a sharp apex to the curve, and pain at the apex are indicative of Scheuermann kyphosis.
- A loss of height, increasing curvature to the spine, and back pain are associated with kyphosis from osteoporosis.
- Night sweats, weight loss, new deformity, and new neurologic deficit suggest tuberculosis or malignancy as a cause of kyphosis.
- Postsurgical kyphotic deformity may be noted by comparison of the patient's previous examinations, radiographs, and history.

#### *History*

- Other congenital abnormalities
- Family history of kyphosis
- Progression of deformity
- Neurologic deficit (onset and progression)
- Constitutional signs (weight loss, fevers, etc.)
- History of steroid use or insufficiency fractures
- History of trauma

#### *Physical Exam*

- Examine the patient when he or she is in the neutral standing position and bending forward.
- Flexibility of the curve should be assessed by prone hyperextension.
- Complete neurologic examination

### TESTS

#### *Lab*

- If infection is suspected, it should be evaluated by obtaining a complete blood count, ESR, and possibly blood cultures.
- Skin testing if tuberculosis is suspected
- Biopsy may be indicated if the organism is not known.
- Results of routine laboratory studies are normal in most cases of kyphosis, even if osteoporosis is present.
- In AS, patients may have antibodies to HLA-B27, although the diagnosis remains largely clinical.

#### *Imaging*

- Conventional radiographs:
  - For all types of kyphosis, conventional standing AP and lateral views of the entire spine on 1 cassette are required.
  - Additional plain films include focused views of the deformity to assess for bony abnormality and hyperextension views over a bolster to assess curve flexibility.
  - Risser sign usually can be assessed on the AP film.
- MRI is indicated for patients with congenital kyphosis, neurologic deficit, and/or suspicion of malignancy.
- Renal ultrasound to evaluate congenital abnormalities should be performed in children with congenital kyphosis (16).
- DEXA scan to ascertain baseline values of osteoporosis should be considered for patients with osteoporotic kyphosis.

#### *Pathological Findings*

- Scheuermann kyphosis (2 types) (17):
  - Typical: Wedging of 3 or more consecutive vertebrae by ≥5° and an apex between T7–T9
  - Atypical: Vertebral endplate changes, Schomorl nodes, and disc space narrowing, but may lack 3 consecutive vertebrae with 5° of wedging
- Anterior wedging of the superior end plate and loss of bone mass are seen in patients with osteoporosis.
- In patients with AS, the vertebral bodies are wedged into a triangular shape at several levels, the spine is stiff, and eventually the involved vertebrae become fused.
- In patients with kyphosis from infection or tumor, a soft-tissue mass that narrows the spinal cord may be present posterior to the vertebrae.

## DIFFERENTIAL DIAGNOSIS
- Scoliosis may resemble kyphosis because of the rib deformity on the convex side but, in fact, most patients with thoracic scoliosis have less than normal kyphosis.
- The causes of kyphosis must be differentiated because the corresponding treatments differ.
- Neuromuscular disorders may cause kyphosis because of low muscle tone.
- Surgical laminectomy of the spine in a growing child may cause subsequent kyphosis to develop.

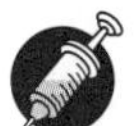

# TREATMENT

## GENERAL MEASURES
- Observation: it is acceptable to use serial radiographs to monitor progression in patients with mild deformity.
- Exercise:
  - For those complaining of pain, exercises and analgesics are the mainstays of treatment
  - Postural exercises for postural kyphosis
- Bracing:
  - Not indicated for congenital kyphosis
  - Indicated for growing adolescents with Scheuermann kyphosis with an apex below the 8th thoracic vertebrae and curves ranging 40–70°.
  - Indicated for acute osteoporotic fractures
- For patients with congenital kyphosis, surgery should be performed if the patient is still growing because a substantial chance exists for neurologic compromise if the curve worsens.

## SPECIAL THERAPY
### *Radiotherapy*
Postirradiation kyphosis can be minimized with careful pretreatment planning to minimize exposure to the growth centers of the spine.

### *Physical Therapy*
- Exercises provide benefit for pain from many types of kyphosis.
- Stretch the hamstrings, the tight structures on the anterior aspect of the kyphosis, and the tight muscles in the lumbar lordosis.
- Strengthening should include abdominal muscles and the back extensors.

## MEDICATION (DRUGS)
### *First Line*
- Analgesics, usually NSAIDs or acetaminophen, may be used if back pain recurs.
- Physical therapy is the mainstay of treatment for Scheuermann kyphosis, but bracing treatment should be considered for curves >60° (18).
- Calcium with vitamin D supplementation for patients at risk of developing osteoporosis
- Diphosphonate or estrogens may be considered as part of a program to prevent or treat osteoporosis in appropriate patients.
- Multidrug therapy is the mainstay of tuberculosis treatment.

## SURGERY
- Surgery is indicated for various types of kyphosis if deformity or pain is unacceptable and unresponsive to nonoperative measures.
  - Congenital kyphosis:
    - Requires surgery in all but rare instances
    - *In situ* fusion or corrective osteotomy with posterior or anterior/posterior instrumentation are current treatments.
  - Scheuermann kyphosis:
    - Requires surgery for pain refractory to nonoperative measures, progression, neurologic compromise, cardiovascular compromise, or deformity
    - Posterior or anterior/posterior fusion after corrective osteotomy are current treatments.
- Osteoporotic fractures can be treated with kyphoplasty to restore height and relieve pain or with vertebroplasty for pain relief alone.
- Decompression, correction of deformity, and stabilization are indicated for infectious or malignant lesions with neurologic compromise.

# FOLLOW-UP

## PROGNOSIS
- Kyphosis tends to progress with age.
  - The back and neck pain it causes may range from minor to persistent.
- Patients usually are able to carry out full-time jobs, although physical work may be limited.

## COMPLICATIONS
- Patients with severe, sharp kyphosis may have neurologic compromise from the apex of the curve.
  - May be triggered by a fall or fracture
- Surgical correction carries an increased risk of neurologic compromise when compared with curves of the same magnitude in scoliotic deformity.
- Pseudarthrosis
- Curve progression

## PATIENT MONITORING
- In growing patients, the curve should be monitored every 4–6 months.
- Adults may be seen as needed.

## REFERENCES

1. Fon GT, Pitt MJ, Thies AC, Jr. Thoracic kyphosis: range in normal subjects. *Am J Roentgenol* 1980;134:979–983.
2. Propst-Proctor SL, Bleck EE. Radiographic determination of lordosis and kyphosis in normal and scoliotic children. *J Pediatr Orthop* 1983;3:344–346.
3. James JIP. Kyphoscoliosis. *J Bone Joint Surg* 1955;37B:414–426.
4. Warner WC, Jr. Kyphosis. In: Morrissy RT, Weinstein SL, eds. *Lovell and Winter's Pediatric Orthopaedics*, 6th ed. Philadelphia: Lippincott Williams & Wilkins, 2006:797–837.
5. Dennison E, Cooper C. Epidemiology of osteoporotic fractures. *Horm Res* 2000;54:58–63.
6. Moon MS. Tuberculosis of the spine. Controversies and a new challenge. *Spine* 1997;22:1791–1797.
7. Pring ME, Wenger DR. Adolescent deformity. In: Bono CM, Garfin SR, Tornetta P, et al., eds. *Spine*. Philadelphia: Lippincott Williams & Wilkins, 2004:163–174.
8. Murray PM, Weinstein SL, Spratt KF. The natural history and long-term follow-up of Scheuermann kyphosis. *J Bone Joint Surg* 1993;75A:236–248.
9. Breban M, Miceli-Richard C, Zinovieva E, et al. The genetics of spondyloarthropathies. *Joint Bone Spine* 2006; 73:355–362.
10. Huang QY, Kung AWC. Genetics of osteoporosis. *Mol Genet Metab* 2006; 88:295–306.
11. Findlay A, Conner AN, Connor JM. Dominant inheritance of Scheuermann's juvenile kyphosis. *J Med Genet* 1989;26:400–403.
12. McMaster MJ, Singh H. Natural history of congenital kyphosis and kyphoscoliosis. A study of one hundred and twelve patients. *J Bone Joint Surg* 1999;81A:1367–1383.
13. Prahinski JR, Polly DW, Jr, McHale KA, et al. Occult intraspinal anomalies in congenital scoliosis. *J Pediatr Orthop* 2000;20:59–63.
14. Suh SW, Sarwark JF, Vora A, et al. Evaluating congenital spine deformities for intraspinal anomalies with magnetic resonance imaging. *J Pediatr Orthop* 2001;21:525–531.
15. Ogilvie JW, Sherman J. Spondylolysis in Scheuermann's disease. *Spine* 1987;12:251–253.
16. MacEwen GD, Winter RB, Hardy JH. Evaluation of kidney anomalies in congenital scoliosis. *J Bone Joint Surg* 1972;54A:1451–1454.
17. Blumenthal SL, Roach J, Herring JA. Lumbar Scheuermann's. A clinical series and classification. *Spine* 1987;12:929–932.
18. Lowe TG. Scheuermann's disease. *Orthop Clin North Am* 1999;30:475–485.


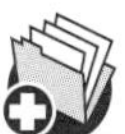

# MISCELLANEOUS

## CODES
### *ICD9-CM*
- 732.0 Scheuermann kyphosis
- 733.0 Congenital kyphosis
- 737.10 Postural kyphosis
- 737.41 Tuberculosis

## PATIENT TEACHING
Stress adequate daily calcium intake because, although osteoporosis may not play a role in the causes of most types of kyphosis, it may affect patients later and may worsen the kyphosis.

## FAQ
- Q: At what point should bracing be considered for Scheuermann kyphosis?
  - A: Approximately ≥60° of curvature.
- Q: What is the most common cause of kyphosis in elderly Caucasian females?
  - A: Osteoporotic vertebral compression fractures.

# LIMB LENGTHENING (ILIZAROV METHOD)

*Paul D. Sponseller, MD*

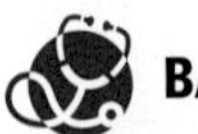

## BASICS

### DESCRIPTION

- The process of forming new bone by slow, gentle stretching is called "distraction osteogenesis."
- 1 method of lengthening was developed in Kurgan, Russia, by G. I. Ilizarov as a means of slowly and completely correcting many congenital and acquired abnormalities.
  - The Ilizarov method uses a versatile external fixator to produce gradual changes in the length and alignment of an extremity.
    - The fixator consists of circular rings attached to bone with wires.
    - These rings are distracted (spread apart) by threaded rods.
    - Each fixator is custom assembled for the given patient and indication.
- Fixators other than the Ilizarov (versatile but tend to be bulky) may be used:
  - Monolateral fixators and spatial frames
  - If complex rotation and angular correction are not needed, fixators with pins in a straight line may be used (many different models are available).
- Nevertheless, the principles described here are general and apply not to the device but, rather, to the concept and procedure.
- The Ilizarov method is applicable to all extremities, but it is used most commonly in the lower extremities where alignment is more critical than in the upper extremities.
- The ideal age for performing the Ilizarov method is in the preteen and teen years.
  - At this time, the skeleton is almost finished growing, so its final shape can be determined, yet the potential for healing and remodeling is that of a child.
  - In addition, the patient has the maturity to undergo an arduous treatment process.
  - Bone healing, however, is slower with advancing age.
- For certain indications, this procedure can be performed in younger patients (with severe congenital abnormalities) or in adults (with nonunions and acquired deformities).
- Classification for types of procedures performed using with Ilizarov method:
  - Extremity lengthening
  - Angular correction
  - Repair of nonunion
  - Restoration of lost bone
  - Correction of contracture
  - Fracture treatment
- Synonyms: Limb lengthening; Callotasis

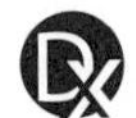

## DIAGNOSIS

### SIGNS AND SYMPTOMS

#### *History*

In deciding whether this treatment method is appropriate for a given individual, the physician should determine the degree of functional impairment, degree of patient adaptation, and degree of patient understanding and motivation to undergo a treatment that lasts for many months.

#### *Physical Exam*

The patient should be checked for pin-tract problems, nerve function, and joint ROM at each visit (1,2).

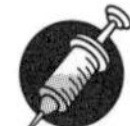

## TREATMENT

### SPECIAL THERAPY

#### *Physical Therapy*

- Patients may benefit from:
  - Instruction on appropriate weightbearing and transfers
  - Maintaining joint ROM
  - Strengthening
  - Monitoring the correction process daily

### MEDICATION (DRUGS)

#### *First Line*

NSAIDs should not be taken for a long period because they may suppress bone healing.

### SURGERY

- Surgery (to create the osteotomy and attach the fixator) is performed with the patient under general anesthesia (bone elongation usually is performed later).
- The external fixator frame is assembled on the patient's limb according to its shape and the goal of treatment.
  - Several pins or rings are needed above and below the site of bone correction.
  - Threaded distraction rods are positioned to provide the needed correction over time (Fig. 1).
- The osteotomy is performed once the bone is stabilized.
  - Use a small incision.
  - Try to limit as much as possible the disruption of the blood supply.
  - Often, the fixator is extended to an adjacent bone for stability.
- If the needed correction is minor, it can be performed while the patient is under anesthesia,

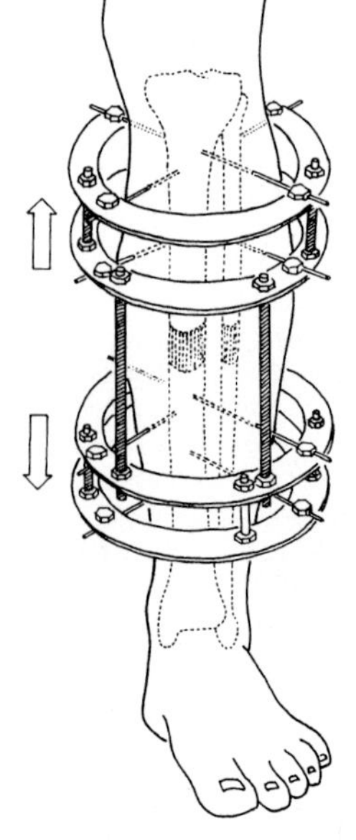

**Fig. 1.** The Ilizarov method may be used to lengthen a limb. Bone regenerates to fill in the gap.

but usually no distraction or lengthening is performed at the time of the surgery.
- Distraction:
  - Started 7–10 days postsurgery (approximately the time the healing callus is 1st seen radiographically)
  - Continued at a rate of 1 mm per day:
    - Usually divided into at least 4 segments so the tissues are not stretched too suddenly
    - In this way, the callus is stretched slowly (distraction osteogenesis).
- Once the desired length is achieved, the new bone is allowed to strengthen, which occurs with time and weightbearing.
- The fixator is removed when the bone appears strong enough.
- The total time spent in the fixator can be estimated by the lengthening index:
  - Time (per centimeter of length gained) needed for the process of lengthening and consolidation
  - Averages 1–1.6 months/cm

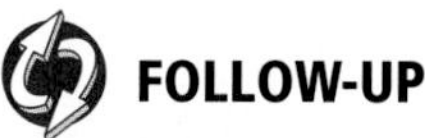

## FOLLOW-UP

### PROGNOSIS
- The results usually are good, although problems and complications may require additional procedures before completion.
- An 80–90% success rate may be expected (1–4), although the healing time often is prolonged.

### COMPLICATIONS
- Nonunion
- Joint stiffness or subluxation
- Fracture
- Nerve injury

### PATIENT MONITORING
- Patients must be seen periodically during the procedure to monitor the correction process and to check on the status of the pin sites.
- Radiographs usually are necessary.

### REFERENCES

1. Paley D, Lamm BM, Katsenis D, et al. Treatment of malunion and nonunion at the site of an ankle fusion with the Ilizarov apparatus. Surgical technique. *J Bone Joint Surg* 2006;88A:119–134.
2. Patil S, Montgomery R. Management of complex tibial and femoral nonunion using the Ilizarov technique, and its cost implications. *J Bone Joint Surg* 2006;88B:928–932.
3. Cho TJ, Choi IH, Chung CY, et al. Isolated congenital pseudarthrosis of the fibula: Clinical course and optimal treatment. *J Pediatr Orthop* 2006;26:449–454.
4. McGarvey WC, Burris MW, Clanton TO, et al. Calcaneal fractures: Indirect reduction and external fixation. *Foot Ankle Int* 2006;27:494–499.


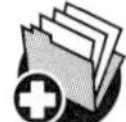

## MISCELLANEOUS

### PATIENT TEACHING
- Patients should be told of the duration of treatment (usually many months).
- They should be helped to make arrangements for school or work and for care after the procedure.
  - Admission to a rehabilitation hospital sometimes is indicated.
- Patients should be assessed to determine whether they have the level of maturity needed for the treatment.
- Patients may be allowed to bear weight and to swim with the device, if the surgeon allows.

### FAQ
- Q: Can young children undergo this process?
  - A: Yes, if the deformity or discrepancy is severe and is limiting them.
- Q: How do I decide whether to undergo limb lengthening versus shortening of the other side?
  - A: The decision depends on the patient's expected stature at adulthood and on the condition of the joints and muscles in each limb.
- Q: Can the Ilizarov procedure be used to make me taller?
  - A: In certain circumstances, yes. However, the treatment time is long and must be applied to both limbs.

# LISFRANC FRACTURE-DISLOCATION

*Simon C. Mears, MD, PhD*
*Clifford L. Jeng, MD*

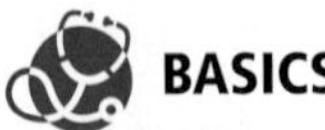

## BASICS

### DESCRIPTION
- Dislocation of the TMT joints of the foot (Fig. 1).
  - Can occur at any age
  - Often accompanied by fractures around the TMT joints
- Classification (1):
  - Type A: Total incongruity of TMT joint
  - Type B: Partial incongruity of TMT joint complex, either medial or lateral
  - Type C: Divergent (1st metatarsal medial, 2nd–5th lateral)

### EPIDEMIOLOGY
#### *Incidence*
Lisfranc injuries account for ~1/3 of midfoot injuries (2).

### RISK FACTORS
- Car accidents
- Motorcycle accidents

### ETIOLOGY
- The mechanism of injury includes a wide spectrum of causes from low-energy compression and twisting to high-energy crush injuries.
- Common cause: Car and motorcycle accidents (3):
  - Pressure on a brake pedal with a plantar flexed foot leads to the Lisfranc pattern of injury (4).
- Sporting events (5)

### ASSOCIATED CONDITIONS
- Comminuted fractures of the metatarsal bases or cuneiforms
- Severe soft-tissue injury
- Compartment syndrome
- Open fractures

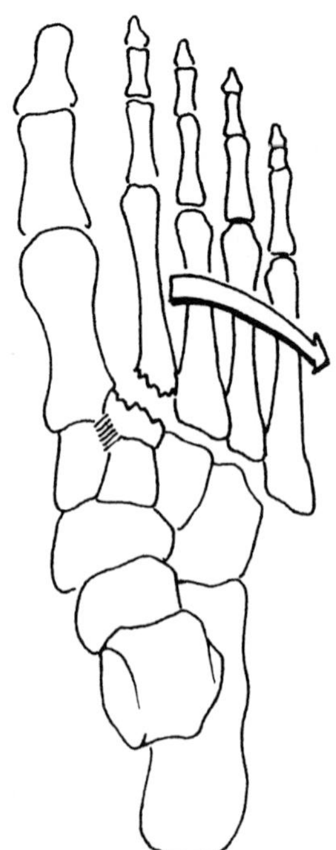

**Fig. 1.** Lisfranc dislocation occurs at the midfoot joints, usually with substantial trauma.

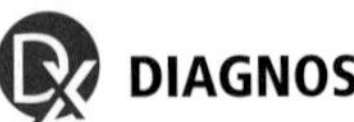

## DIAGNOSIS

### SIGNS AND SYMPTOMS
- Pain
- Swelling
- Deformity
- Ecchymosis
- Difficulty bearing weight
- Tenderness over midfoot
- Possible spontaneous reduction

#### *Physical Exam*
- Rotational stress on the forefoot causes pain at Lisfranc joint.
- Palpation over the 2nd metatarsal base also can cause pain.

### TESTS
#### *Imaging*
- Radiography:
  - Plain films usually are diagnostic.
  - AP, lateral, and oblique projections are mandatory.
    - On the AP view, the medial margin of the 2nd metatarsal base should be aligned with the middle cuneiform.
    - On the oblique view, the medial base of the 4th metatarsal should be aligned with the medial margin of the cuboid.
    - On the lateral view, an unbroken line should run from the dorsum of the 1st and 2nd metatarsals to the corresponding cuneiform.
  - Avulsion fracture of the 2nd metatarsal base ("fleck" fracture) and compression fracture of the cuboid are pathognomonic of this condition (6).
  - If the diagnosis is uncertain on plain film, especially if the Lisfranc joint has reduced spontaneously, stress radiography with fluoroscopy may be helpful in further defining the instability pattern.
- CT is an important adjunct to plain radiographs.
  - Shows small fractures and displacements that are not visible on plain films
  - In 1 study, radiographs missed the Lisfranc injury in 24% of cases and CT scan revealed the injury (7).

### DIFFERENTIAL DIAGNOSIS
- Soft-tissue contusion
- Ligament sprain
- Isolated metatarsal or midfoot fractures

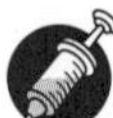

## TREATMENT

### GENERAL MEASURES
- Before the patient is taken to the operating room:
  - Compartment syndrome and neurovascular injury should be assessed.
  - The foot is splinted and kept elevated until surgery.
- The goal of treatment is to achieve and maintain anatomic reduction of the joints while the ligaments heal.
  - Usually requires surgical intervention
- Before and after surgery: Ice, elevation, and a compression dressing
- Foot pumps may help reduce foot swelling.

### SPECIAL THERAPY
#### *Physical Therapy*
- Patients should be referred for gait training on a nonweightbearing basis postoperatively.
- Edema control and ROM of the toes and ankle are important to decrease late stiffness.

### SURGERY
- Open reduction and internal fixation of joints:
  - Through 2–3 dorsal longitudinal incisions
  - Fixation may consist of Kirschner wires or 3.5-mm cortical screws.
    - If Kirschner wires are used as fixation, they can be removed in the office at 6 weeks, and the patient may begin protected weightbearing.
    - If screws are used as fixation, unprotected weightbearing is not permitted until the screws have been removed, at 10–12 weeks after surgery.
- Fusion of the joints with 3.5-mm cortical screws has been advocated by some as primary treatment (8) or as a salvage procedure for later arthritis of the midfoot (9).

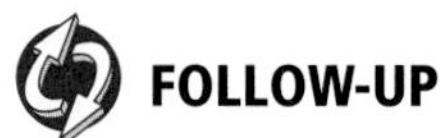

## FOLLOW-UP

### PROGNOSIS

- Patients with anatomic reduction generally have good results.
  - In 1 study, 11 of 24 patients had a good to excellent result (10).
- Outcomes are worse with nonanatomic reduction and extensive joint injury (11).
- Patients with worker compensation claims have poorer outcomes (12).
- The role of joint fusion is controversial.
  - Recently, a randomized study showed that joint fusion gave better results than did reduction and fixation (8).
- Patients with posttraumatic arthritis can undergo salvage procedures with arthrodesis.

### COMPLICATIONS

- Traumatic arthritis
- Fixed deformity
- For injuries diagnosed late (7–8 weeks):
  - Poor prognosis
  - Patients may be candidates for primary arthrodesis (13).

### PATIENT MONITORING

Follow-up radiographs (at 1-month intervals) should be taken to check for maintained alignment of the Lisfranc complex.

### REFERENCES


1. Hardcastle PH, Reschauer R, Kutscha-Lissberg E, et al. Injuries to the tarsometatarsal joint. Incidence, classification and treatment. *J Bone Joint Surg* 1982;64B:349–356.
2. Richter M, Wippermann B, Krettek C, et al. Fractures and fracture dislocations of the midfoot: occurrence, causes and long-term results. *Foot Ankle Int* 2001;22:392–398.
3. Jeffers RF, Tan HB, Nicolopoulos C, et al. Prevalence and patterns of foot injuries following motorcycle trauma. *J Orthop Trauma* 2004;18: 87–91.
4. Smith BR, Begeman PC, Leland R, et al. A mechanism of injury to the forefoot in car crashes. *Traffic Inj Prev* 2005;6:156–169.
5. Nunley JA, Vertullo CJ. Classification, investigation, and management of midfoot sprains: Lisfranc injuries in the athlete. *Am J Sports Med* 2002;30:871–878.
6. Pearse EO, Klass B, Bendall SP. The 'ABC' of examining foot radiographs. *Ann R Coll Surg Engl* 2005;87:449–451.
7. Haapamaki VV, Kiuru MJ, Koskinen SK. Ankle and foot injuries: analysis of MDCT findings. *AJR Am J Roentgenol* 2004;183:615–622.
8. Ly TV, Coetzee JC. Treatment of primarily ligamentous Lisfranc joint injuries: primary arthrodesis compared with open reduction and internal fixation. A prospective, randomized study. *J Bone Joint Surg* 2006;88A:514–520.
9. Komenda GA, Myerson MS, Biddinger KR. Results of arthrodesis of the tarsometatarsal joints after traumatic injury. *J Bone Joint Surg* 1996;78A: 1665–1676.
10. O'Connor PA, Yeap S, Noel J, et al. Lisfranc injuries: patient- and physician-based functional outcomes. *Int Orthop* 2003;27:98–102.
11. Kuo RS, Tejwani NC, Digiovanni CW, et al. Outcome after open reduction and internal fixation of Lisfranc joint injuries. *J Bone Joint Surg* 2000;82A:1609–1618.
12. Calder JDF, Whitehouse SL, Saxby TS. Results of isolated Lisfranc injuries and the effect of compensation claims. *J Bone Joint Surg* 2004; 86B:527–530.
13. Aronow MS. Treatment of the missed Lisfranc injury. *Foot Ankle Clin* 2006;11:127–142.


### ADDITIONAL READING


Sands AK, Grose A. Lisfranc injuries. *Injury* 2004;35:B71–B76.


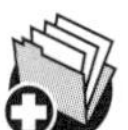

## MISCELLANEOUS

### CODES

#### *ICD9-CM*

825.25 Metatarsal fracture

### PATIENT TEACHING

Patients must be warned about the risks of traumatic arthritis and fixed deformity, which may require later arthrodesis.

### FAQ

- Q: How long will it take to recover from a Lisfranc injury?
  - A: Lisfranc injuries are severe injuries to the midfoot and commonly require surgery. Recovery takes at least a year. Patients may require hardware removal. ~25% develop arthritis and may require later fusion.

L

# LITTLE LEAGUE ELBOW

*Paul D. Sponseller, MD*

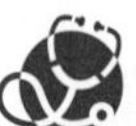

## BASICS

### DESCRIPTION

- "Little League elbow" refers to a group of injuries about the elbow that arise in children and adolescents (ages 7–15 years) from repetitive throwing or use of a racquet or bat (Fig. 1).
  - Younger patients (7–11 years old) in that group often have an injury of the physis, whereas older adolescents (15–19 years old) are subject to avulsion fractures or ligament tears.
- These injuries also are referred to as osteochondroses, or disordered behavior of growing cartilage under load.
- Classification:
  - Medial disease involves the MCL, the medial epicondyle, and the surrounding soft tissues.
  - Lateral disease involves the radial head, the capitellum, the lateral epicondyle, and surrounding soft tissues.
- Synonym: Osteochondritis (or osteochondrosis) of the radial head or capitellum (Panner disease)

### GENERAL PREVENTION

- League guidelines (1,2) on the frequency of pitching for juvenile players exist to minimize this disorder.
- Elbow pain in juvenile athletes should be a guide to slowing down.

### EPIDEMIOLOGY

#### *Incidence*

The incidence increases with the intensity of competition.

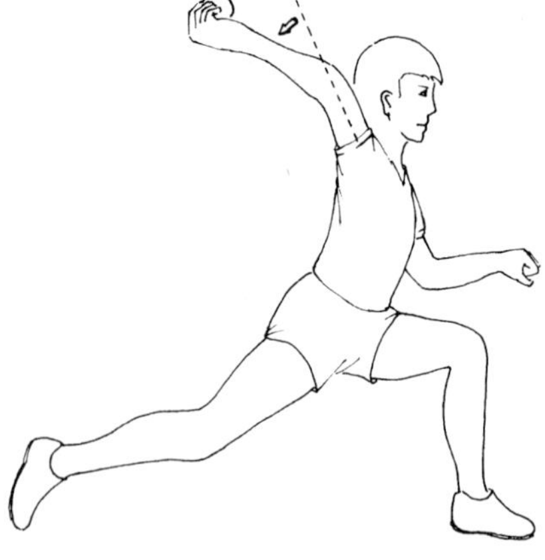

**Fig. 1.** Little League elbow results from valgus strain, which may cause tendinitis medially or osteochondritis laterally in the growing elbow.

### RISK FACTORS

Throwing or serving sports in young children and adolescents (e.g., baseball, football, javelin, and tennis) are risk factors.

#### *Genetics*

No Mendelian inheritance pattern is known.

### ETIOLOGY

- Medial epicondylar fragmentation or avulsion
- Delayed or accelerated growth of the medial epicondyle
- Delayed closure of the medial epicondylar growth plate
- Osteochondritis (irregular ossification) of the capitellum
- Deformation and osteochondritis of the radial head
- Olecranon apophysitis with or without delayed closure of the olecranon apophysis

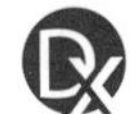

## DIAGNOSIS

### SIGNS AND SYMPTOMS

- Most patients present with medial elbow pain, although some have lateral pain (see later), with diminished throwing distance and decreased throwing effectiveness.
  - The patient may present with vague lateral elbow pain and swelling (capitellar osteonecrosis [Panner disease; ages 7–12 years]) versus osteochondritis dissecans of the capitellum (ages 13–16 years).
- Pain is aggravated by throwing.
- Examination shows point tenderness over the medial epicondyle, swelling, and a flexion contracture often $>30°$.
- The injury most often involves the dominant elbow.
- Nocturnal pain is uncommon.
- Burning around the medial elbow associated with paresthesias or dysesthesias in the ulnar digits signifies ulnar nerve involvement.
- Duration of symptoms can help to differentiate injuries such as UCL ruptures (acute) and medial epicondylitis (chronic).
  - Late-presenting lateral symptoms include locking, catching, and severe pain.
- Posterior abnormalities suggest involvement of the olecranon and surrounding soft tissues.

#### *History*

Obtain detailed frequency of athletic elbow use.

#### *Physical Exam*

- Document the elbow ROM, including flexion, extension, pronation, and supination.
- Look for an effusion, as signified by loss of the normal lateral soft-tissue recess.
- Pinpoint the location of tenderness.
- Perform a neurovascular examination of the extremity.
- Observe the patient performing the causative motion.
- Stability of the elbow to valgus stress with the elbow in 25° of flexion helps assess the collateral ligaments.

### TESTS

#### *Imaging*

- Radiography:
  - Plain radiographs (AP and lateral) are obtained to rule out fractures, loose bodies, or osteochondritis dissecans.
  - Stress radiographs may be helpful.
- Bone scan is useful to assess asymmetrical activity.
- MRI may be useful in evaluating injury to cartilage, physis, tendons, muscles, and ligaments (2).

#### *Pathological Findings*

- Weak physes in growing children make injuries to this area (fracture or osteochondritis) common, whereas young adults with fused physes tend to develop more soft-tissue injuries.
- The pathologic process of Panner disease and osteochondritis dissecans is unknown but thought to arise from repetitive trauma.
- Osteochondritis dissecans may progress to loose bodies with painful locking.

### DIFFERENTIAL DIAGNOSIS

- Elbow fracture (supracondylar humerus, olecranon)
- Ulnar nerve subluxation
- Ulnar nerve entrapment or posterior interosseous nerve entrapment
- Tendinitis of the medial or lateral elbow muscle origin
- Loose bodies in the joint

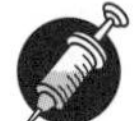

## TREATMENT

### GENERAL MEASURES

- Most injuries resolve with 4–6 weeks of rest.
- With severe pain, a regimen of 1–2 weeks of splint immobilization is helpful, followed by active ROM exercises.
- Loose bodies often require surgical removal.
- Occasionally, large osteochondritis dissecans fragments and avulsion fragments with >2 mm of displacement require surgical fixation.
- Activity should be resumed on a gradual, stepwise basis.
- Stability of the elbow should be assessed before the patient returns to competitive throwing.
- If symptoms resume with activity after 6 weeks of rest, additional investigation into causes should be investigated (via CT, MRI).

### SPECIAL THERAPY

#### *Physical Therapy*

- After 6–8 weeks of rest, when the patient is asymptomatic and has pain-free ROM, begin elbow strengthening exercises with a progressive throwing program.
- The therapist or trainer may be effective in supervising the patient's return to sports more closely than the physician is able to do.

### MEDICATION (DRUGS)

- NSAIDs are the drugs of choice.
- Steroid injections rarely are indicated.

### SURGERY

- Many of these conditions may be treated arthroscopically, including pinning of osteochondritis dissecans fragments, removal of loose bodies, and removal of osteophytes.
- Occasionally, open reconstruction or repair of the UCL is necessary for avulsion injuries.

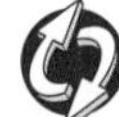

## FOLLOW-UP

### PROGNOSIS

- Overall, most patients do well with rest.
- Occasionally, one may develop slight flexion contractures and valgus deformity of throwing arm, which is rarely symptomatic.

### COMPLICATIONS

- Rare: Panner disease may lead to late deformity and collapse of the capitellum articular surface (3).
- Osteochondritis dissecans fragments may displace and become a loose body in the joint, requiring removal.
- Epicondyle fractures may progress to a nonunion, usually asymptomatic.

### PATIENT MONITORING

Patients with Panner disease should have follow-up radiographs every 3–4 months to assess healing of the capitellum.

### REFERENCES


1. Adirim TA, Cheng TL. Overview of injuries in the young athlete. *Sports Med* 2003;33:75–81.
2. Kocher MS, Waters PM, Micheli LJ. Upper extremity injuries in the paediatric athlete. *Sports Med* 2000;30:117–135.
3. Hang DW, Chao CM, Hang YS. A clinical and roentgenographic study of Little League elbow. *Am J Sports Med* 2004;32:79–84.


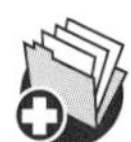

## MISCELLANEOUS

### CODES

#### *ICD9-CM*

726.32 Little League elbow

### PATIENT TEACHING

- Instruct the patient in proper throwing mechanics.
- Recognize symptoms early.
- Rest from throwing activities (6–8 weeks) to avoid additional injury.
- Advise a gradual return to competitive sports when the patient is asymptomatic.
- Recurrence of symptoms often requires longer rest followed by strengthening exercises.

### FAQ

- Q: If a preteen pitcher has Little League elbow, should he be counseled to switch positions?
  - A: Recurrence is likely, and switching should be discussed as an option. However if it is a 1st presentation, a cycle of rest and graduated resumption of pitching may be successful in some cases.

# LUMBAR DISC HERNIATION

*Philip R. Neubauer, MD*
*David B. Cohen, MD*

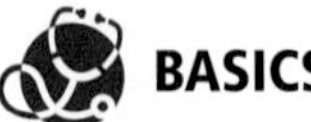

## BASICS

### DESCRIPTION

- Low back pain affects up to 85% of the population at some point in their lives (1).
- Low back pain is one of the leading causes of disability in patients <50 years old.
- Herniation of a lumbar disc:
  - 1 of the major causes of acute and chronic lower back pain
  - May be associated with leg pain, weakness, and numbness, often referred to as "sciatica."
- Classification:
  - By location:
    - Posterolateral are the most common; the posterior longitudinal ligament is the weakest structure.
    - Usually affects the ipsilateral nerve root of the lower lumbar vertebrae.
    - Far lateral herniations may affect the ipsilateral nerve roots of the upper lumbar vertebrae.
    - Central herniations often are associated with back pain only, but they also may lead to cauda equina syndrome.
  - By morphology:
    - Protruded: Eccentric bulge of the nucleus pulposus with intact annulus fibrosis
    - Extruded: The nucleus protrudes through the annulus but remains intact.
    - Sequestered: Nucleus not intact, and a free fragment within the spinal canal
- Synonyms: Herniated nucleus pulposus; Slipped disc; Ruptured disc; Sciatica

### EPIDEMIOLOGY

- Most commonly seen in patients 30–50 years old; rare before age 20 years (1).
- Men are affected more often than women (2).
- The lumbar spine is the spinal level most commonly affected by disc herniation (1).
- The L4–L5 vertebral level is the most commonly affected level, followed by the L5–S1 vertebral level (1).

### RISK FACTORS

- Tobacco smoking
- Jobs that require repetitive lifting
- Obesity

#### *Genetics*

Controversy exists regarding a genetic link to lumbar disc herniation.

### PATHOPHYSIOLOGY

- The intervertebral disc is made of an inner nucleus pulposus and an outer annulus fibrosis.
- Formed primarily of type I and type II collagen, the intervertebral disc's main functions are to absorb axial loads on the spinal column and to allow for fluid movements between vertebrae.
- Vascular and neural elements are found exclusively within the peripheral fibers of the annulus fibrosus.
- Nutrients flow to the intervertebral disc via diffusion from the hyaline cartilage endplates located above and below the disc (3).
- Beginning in a person as young as 20 years old, the nucleus pulposus gradually looses water content.
- With age, the intervertebral discs lose volume, shape, and viscoelastic ability.

### ETIOLOGY

- The cause of lumbar disc herniation appears to be related primarily to the normal degenerative process that occurs with aging.
- It may be secondary to trauma.
- Repetitive stresses on the lower back, as with heavy labor, may accelerate the process.

## DIAGNOSIS

### SIGNS AND SYMPTOMS

- Pain is the usual presenting symptom.
  - May affect the back only, leg only, or both
  - Pain often is aggravated by forward flexion of the lumbar spine and relieved by extension.
- Numbness in the dermatome associated with the affected nerve root may occur.
- Weakness in the muscle associated with the affected nerve root may occur.
- L3–L4 herniation causes an L4 root compression characterized by anterior tibialis weakness, decreased patellar reflex, and medial knee and leg sensory changes.
- L4–L5 herniation results in L5 symptoms, including altered sensation over the lateral aspect of the calf and the 1st dorsal web space; extensor hallucis longus weakness may be evident.
- L5–S1 herniation compresses the S1 nerve root, decreases ankle reflex, and causes decreased plantarflexion strength and diminished sensation over the lateral aspect of the foot.
- Saddle anesthesia and changes in bowel or bladder habits may indicate cauda equina syndrome.
- Cauda equina compression, which can result from a large herniated disc, should be decompressed on an emergency basis.

#### *History*

- A thorough history should include the time course for the onset of pain.
- Risk factors (e.g., occupation, tobacco history)
- Changes in bowel or bladder function, specifically urinary retention, which may indicate cauda equina syndrome.
- History of fall or trauma
- History of constitutional symptoms (e.g., night sweats, fever, weight loss) should be included.

#### *Physical Exam*

- A detailed neurologic evaluation is the most important aspect of examination.
  - Sensation in the lower extremity dermatomes and the strength of all major muscle groups should be documented.
  - All lower extremity reflexes should be tested.
  - Rectal examination:
    - Important for assessing sacral nerve roots; assess rectal tone, perianal light touch and pinprick sensation, and the anal wink reflex
  - A straight-leg-raise test:
    - Replication of symptoms is a result of stretched nerve roots (Fig. 1).
    - The pain is increased by ankle dorsiflexion.
    - A contralateral test with pain radiation below the knee is highly specific for lumbar disc herniation.
- Gait disturbances or foot-drop may be a result of nerve compression and muscular weakness.

### TESTS

#### *Imaging*

- AP and lateral radiographs for patients with symptoms lasting >6 weeks.
- MRI:
  - Used to document the pathologic features if surgery is contemplated or spinal stenosis is suspected
  - Results may be misleading because false-positive findings are common.
  - Can be used to confirm the diagnosis of cauda equina syndrome
- CT myelography may be used to diagnose lumbar disc herniation, but it is more invasive than, and has been replaced by, MRI.
- Discography may help evaluate for discogenic back pain and localize the site of pain generation to the disc complex, but use and acceptance of this technique remains controversial.

#### *Pathological Findings*

- The nucleus pulposus is extruded through defects in the annulus fibrosis, but it usually remains covered by the thick posterior longitudinal ligament.
- Symptoms are secondary to tenting of nerve roots over the herniation.
- The release of inflammatory mediators may exacerbate the mechanical pressure.

### DIFFERENTIAL DIAGNOSIS

- Lumbar spinal stenosis
- Sciatic nerve entrapment below the spine
- Spondylolysis
- Muscular back pain
- Degenerative disc disease

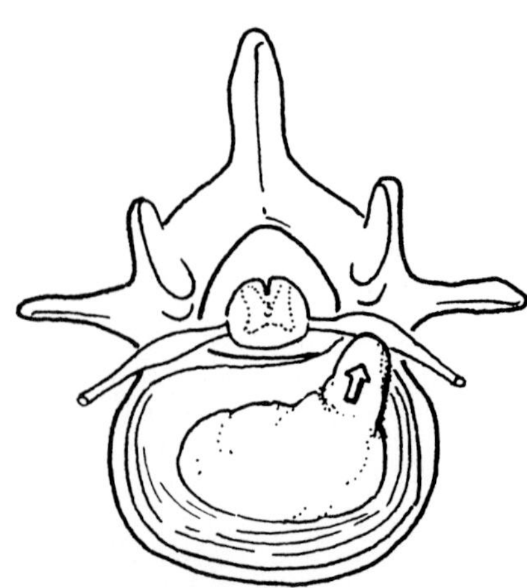

**Fig. 1.** In a herniated disc in the lumbar spine, material from the nucleus pulposus exerts pressure on the nerve root.

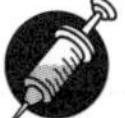

## TREATMENT

### INITIAL STABILIZATION

Bed rest (not >2–3 days), then gradual increase in activity as cardiovascular status allows

### GENERAL MEASURES

- Initial treatment is nonoperative; surgical intervention is reserved for patients for whom nonoperative therapy fails or who present initially with severe symptoms.
- Care is directed toward symptomatic relief.
- Early resumption of activity is important for recovery.
  - Prolonged bed rest should be avoided.
  - Activities that cause exacerbation of symptoms should be avoided.
- NSAIDs or acetaminophen are recommended.
- Diazepam or muscle relaxants have only a limited role for patients with lumbar disc herniations associated with muscle spasms.
- Epidural steroids may be helpful for short- and long-term relief.
- Manipulation, either manually or in traction, also may be beneficial on a short-term basis.
- Narcotics should be reserved for the most severely symptomatic patients.

### SPECIAL THERAPY

#### *Physical Therapy*

- Physical therapy in addition to NSAIDs for most patients with lumbar disc herniations
- Proprioceptive techniques and abdominal and back-strengthening programs are essential.
- The therapy program should include lower extremity stretching and strengthening.

### MEDICATION (DRUGS)

#### *First Line*

- Acetaminophen
- NSAIDs
- Narcotics in the early acute stage

#### *Second Line*

- Oral corticosteroids
- Epidural corticosteroid and anesthetic injections

### SURGERY

- The decision to pursue surgery should be made on an individualized basis with patient input.
- In general, surgical intervention is reserved for patients for whom aggressive nonoperative treatments have failed.
- Operative therapy is more effective in treating symptoms related to the lower extremities than those related to back pain.
- Postoperatively, patients may have recurrent or new onset back pain, with incidence rates up to 14% (4).
- For patients with severe progressive neurologic deficit, or the development of cauda equina syndrome, surgery should be considered the 1st-line intervention.
- Surgical options include:
  - Open discectomy, laminectomy, or laminotomy
  - Microscopic discectomy
  - Endoscopic discectomy
- Invasive nonsurgical options, such as chemonucleolysis, have fallen out of favor because of associated complications (5).

## FOLLOW-UP

- Patients treated nonoperatively should be seen every 6 weeks for 12–18 weeks and then on an as-needed basis.
- After surgery:
  - Monitor patients for signs of nerve injury and postoperative wound infection.
  - Restrict activity for ~6 weeks to decrease the risk of recurrent disc herniation.
  - Request the patient to avoid lifting >10 pounds, bending, stooping, or twisting for 6 weeks after surgery.

### PROGNOSIS

- Prognosis is excellent for complete recovery in most patients.
- Intermittent back pain may persist in some patients.

### COMPLICATIONS

- Degenerative disc disease or persistent pain from other causes
- Repeat herniation at the same or other levels
- Disc infection or arachnoiditis after discectomy

### PATIENT MONITORING

Monitoring of the healing progress is based clinically on patient signs and symptoms, whether nonoperative or surgical treatment was used.

### REFERENCES


1. Andersson GBJ. Epidemiological features of chronic low-back pain. *Lancet* 1999;354:581–585.
2. Battie MC, Videman T, Parent E. Lumbar disc degeneration: epidemiology and genetic influences. *Spine* 2004;29:2679–2690.
3. Urban JPG, Holm S, Maroudas A, et al. Nutrition of the intervertebral disc: effect of fluid flow on solute transport. *Clin Orthop Relat Res* 1982;170: 296–302.
4. Carragee EJ, Han MY, Suen PW, et al. Clinical outcomes after lumbar discectomy for sciatica: the effects of fragment type and anular competence. *J Bone Joint Surg* 2003;85A:102–108.
5. Mathews HH, Long BH. Minimally invasive techniques for the treatment of intervertebral disk herniation. *J Am Acad Orthop Surg* 2002;10: 80–85.


### ADDITIONAL READING


- Biyani A, Andersson GBJ. Low back pain: pathophysiology and management. *J Am Acad Orthop Surg* 2004;12:106–115.
- Buttermann GR. Treatment of lumbar disc herniation: epidural steroid injection compared with discectomy. A prospective, randomized study. *J Bone Joint Surg* 2004;86A:670–679.


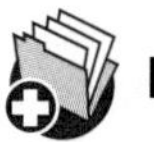

## MISCELLANEOUS

### CODES

#### *ICD9-CM*

722.10 Herniated disc in lower spine

### PATIENT TEACHING

Patients should understand that most herniated discs improve with time and symptomatic treatment.

#### *Activity*

- Patients should be encouraged to pursue activity as tolerated.
- Long periods of bed rest may delay improvement of symptoms.

#### *Prevention*

Patients involved in heavy lifting may benefit from instruction in proper lifting technique by a physical therapist or an occupational medicine specialist.

### FAQ

- Q: Which provocative physical examination maneuvers can be used to help evaluate for a herniated lumbar disc?
  - A: Ipsilateral and contralateral straight-leg-raise tests.
- Q: What are the signs of a herniated disc?
  - A: Pain in both the back and the legs caused by pressure on the nerve from the disc herniation. In severe cases, loss of bowel or bladder function may occur, and these patients should be evaluated emergently.

# LUMBAR SPINE ANATOMY AND EXAMINATION

*Rohit Robert Dhir, BA*
*A. Jay Khanna, MD*

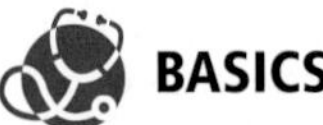

## BASICS

### DESCRIPTION

- The spine is a complex system composed of bony elements, articulations, ligaments, muscles, spinal cord, and peripheral nerves divided into anterior, middle, and posterior columns.
- The vertebral body, lamina, and the spinous process protect the spinal cord.
- The lumbar spine (Fig. 1) contains 5 vertebrae and 5 nerve roots.
  - Most lumbar spines have a lordotic secondary curvature acquired when an infant begins walking (1).
  - The defining characteristics of the lumbar spine include a substantially large, kidney-shaped vertebral body, long and slender transverse processes (with accessory processes on the posterior base), and short and sturdy spinous processes (1).
- The thick intervertebral discs, large articular surfaces, and the lack of rib attachments give the lumbar spine a wide ROM.
  - This freedom of motion allows for lumbar flexion, extension, lateral bending, and trunk rotation.

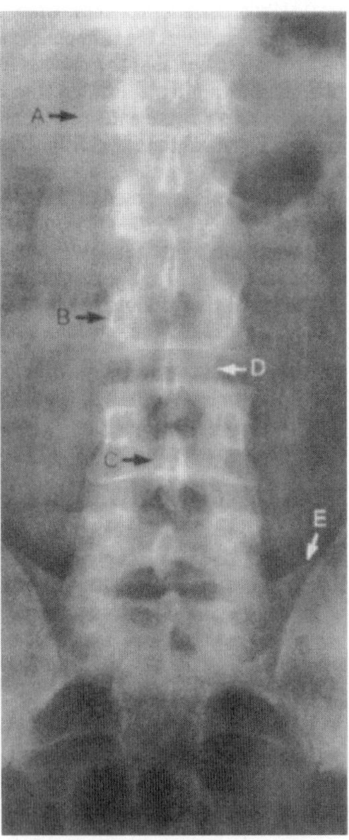


**Fig. 1.** Roentgenogram of normal lumbosacral spine. **A:** Transverse process. **B:** Pedicle. **C:** Posterior spinous process. **D:** Lamina. **E:** Sacrum. (From Steinberg GG, Akins CM, Baran DT. *Orthopaedics in Primary Care*, 3rd ed. Philadelphia: Lippincott Williams & Wilkins, 1999, with permission.)

  - The lumbar spine also functions to support the lumbosacral nerve roots (cauda equina), transmit weight to the pelvis and legs, and support the upper body.

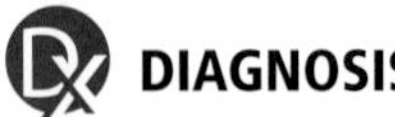

## DIAGNOSIS

### *Physical Exam*

- Gait: Look for:
  - Antalgic (painful) gait
  - Muscle wasting and weakness
  - Signs of hip or knee problems
  - Trendelenburg sign (abductor weakness with an ipsilateral pelvic tilt when the leg is lifted off the ground)
- Inspection:
  - As the patient disrobes, pay attention to fluidity of motion and any associated pain.
  - Inspect the back for clues to underlying bone or neurologic pathology: Areas of redness, hair patches, birthmarks, or skin markings such as café-au-lait spots (2).
  - Analyze the patient's posture and inspect the curvature of the lumbar spine.
  - A slight lordotic curve is normal, but normal lordosis can be absent in cases of paravertebral muscle spasm, and occasionally an extreme kyphosis (Gibbus deformity) is present.
    - A weak anterior abdominal wall generally leads to an exaggerated lordosis (2).
  - Structural scoliosis:
    - A patient's tendency to favor 1 side while standing may indicate structural scoliosis (2), which is characterized by a fixed curve and no change with flexion or recumbency.
  - Sciatic scoliosis:
    - Characterized by a more diffuse curve that worsens with flexion and by limited flexion that disappears with recumbency
  - Spondylolisthesis:
    - A palpable "step" from 1 spinous process to another may indicate spondylolisthesis.
    - May also present with segmental tenderness or nerve root injury (2)
  - NF:
    - May impinge on the spinal cord and roots
    - Often accompanied by café-au-lait spots (2)
  - Spina bifida:
    - Absence of spinous processes, along with birthmarks, excessive port wine marks, or a tuft of hair, may indicate spina bifida (2).
  - AS:
    - Usually begins with pain and stiffness in the SI joints, spreads to the spine, and eventually leads to the ossification of spinal ligaments; eventually, the spine may fuse.
- Palpation:
  - Bony (anterior):
    - Vertebral body and disc: L4, L5, S1 (abdominal palpation: below aortic bifurcation)
    - Sacral promontory: L5–S1 (abdominal palpation through the linea alba below the umbilicus)
  - Bony (posterior):
    - Spinous processes of the lumbar region
    - Spinous processes of the sacral region
    - Iliac crest: L4–L5
    - Posterior superior iliac spine: S2
  - Soft tissue
- ROM evaluation:
  - Substantial motion in the lumbar spine
  - Motion between L5–S1 >motion between L1–L2
  - Flexion:
    - Anterior longitudinal ligament relaxes as the supraspinous and interspinous ligaments, ligamentum flavum, and posterior longitudinal ligament stretch (2).
  - Extension:
    - Posterior ligaments relax as the anterior longitudinal ligament stretches (2).
  - Lateral bending
  - Rotation
  - Resisted movement tests of flexion, lateral bending, and rotation (3)
  - Passive movement tests:
    - Conduct when a patient does not have full ROM.
    - Do not test for passive flexion because of possible aggravation of a disc herniation.
  - Root irritation from disc herniation: Deviation to painful side with spine flexion
- Waddell signs: 3 of the following 5 signs indicate a malingering patient (2):
  - Nonanatomic superficial tenderness
  - Simulation tests (pain with axial loading or rotation of the spine)
  - Nonanatomic weakness and sensory findings
  - Overreaction: "Cogwheeling" or jerky muscle relaxation
  - Inappropriate response to provocative maneuvers with distraction (i.e., supine versus seated straight-leg-raise test)
- Rectal examination checks for:
  - Tone
  - Volition
  - Anal wink (stroke perianal skin, feel anal sphincter contraction around finger)
  - Bulbocavernosus maneuver: Signals end of spinal shock (Pull on Foley catheter in urethra or pull on glans penis; feel anal wink.)
  - Light touch and pin-prick perianal sensation: S2–S4 (If sensation is absent, a mass lesion such as a disc or tumor may be pressing on the nerve roots.)

**Table 1 Motor Examination of the Lumber Spine**

| Root | Muscle Group | Action |
|---|---|---|
| T12, L1–L3 | Iliopsoas | Hip flexion |
| L2–L4 | Quadriceps | Knee extension |
| L4 | Tibialis anterior | Foot dorsiflexion |
| L5 | Extensor hallucis longus | Big toe extension |
| S1 | Gastrocnemius | Foot plantarflexion |

- Upper motor neuron disorders:
  - Hoffman sign:
    - Nip the nail of the patient's middle finger.
    - A positive reaction produces flexion of the terminal phalanx of the thumb and of the 2nd and 3rd phalanx of another finger.
  - Babinski sign:
    - Stroke the plantar lateral foot.
    - A positive test (extended great toe while other toes plantarflex and splay) indicates an upper motor neuron lesion.
    - Use to rule out cervical or thoracic myelopathy (2).
  - Loss of any of the superficial reflexes, such as the abdominal, cremasteric, or anal reflex, suggests an upper motor neuron lesion.
  - Sustained clonus of the patellar or Achilles reflex or hyperreflexia indicates an upper motor neuron lesion (4).

## TESTS

- Motor examination (Table 1):
  - Systematically examines the nerve roots
  - Muscle wasting and weakness suggests nerve root compression.
- Reflex tests (Table 2):
  - Loss of the patellar or Achilles reflex suggests ipsilateral nerve root compression.

**Table 2 Reflex Tests of the Lumbar Spine**

| Disc | Root | Reflex | Muscles |
|---|---|---|---|
| L3–L4 | L4 | Patellar reflex | Anterior tibialis |
| L5–S1 | S1 | Achilles reflex | Peroneus longus and brevis |

**Table 3 Sensation Tests of the Lumbar Spine**

| Nerve Root | Area of Skin Innervation |
|---|---|
| L–1 | Groin, upper anterior thigh, posteromedial leg |
| L–2 | Anterior mid-thigh; lateral groin |
| L–3 | Anterior thigh above knee cap, posterolateral lower leg |
| L–4 | Anteromedial shin |
| L–5 | Dorsum of foot, anterior aspect lower leg |
| S–1 | Lateral foot |
| S2–S5 | Perianal |

- Sensation tests (Table 3):
  - Pin-prick testing compares 2-point discriminatory sensibility on the lower extremities.
  - Vibration sensibility and temperature sense also are tested.
- Nerve root tension tests:
  - Straight-leg-raise test:
    - Raise the leg of the supine patient slowly by supporting the foot slightly above the malleoli and keeping the knee extended (2).
    - Differentiating radiculopathy from tight hamstring pain is important (3).
    - This procedure reproduces the sciatic-type radicular leg pain that is relieved when the knee is bent and is exacerbated by foot dorsiflexion.
    - Cross-leg straight-leg-raise test is less sensitive than the straight-leg-raise test but a more specific physical examination finding for lumbar disc herniation (5).
    - A positive test (flexion of 1 leg with pain in the contralateral leg or buttocks [5]) suggests disc herniation axillary or medial to the root.
  - Femoral nerve stretch test:
    - The patient is prone, and the hip is extended with the knee slightly flexed.
    - Pain radiating down the front of the thigh indicates L3–L4 nerve root irritation.
  - Patrick (FABER) test:
    - Test the SI joint by **F**lexing, **AB**ducting, and **E**xternally **R**otating the hip to reproduce SI joint pain.
    - Pain usually is associated with pelvic trauma or infectious disease (2).
- Muscle strength grading:
  - 5: Normal strength
  - 4: Weakness with resistance, full movement against gravity
  - 3: Full ROM against gravity but marked weakness against resistance
  - 2: Full ROM with gravity eliminated
  - 1: Flicker of tendon unit
  - 0: No movement

### *Imaging*

- Imaging confirms or supports the diagnosis of disorders suspected from the history and physical examination.
- Radiographs should show normal alignment of the vertebrae, the presence of bony landmarks, and maintenance of the disc spaces.
- False-positive MRI scans occur in 35% of patients <40 years old and in 93% of patients >60 years old (6).
- SPECT is more sensitive in detecting isthmic spondylolisthesis than technetium-99m methylene diphosphonate bone scintigraphy, and plain radiographs (7).

## REFERENCES


1. Moore KL, Agur AMR. Back. In: *Essential Clinical Anatomy*. Philadelphia: Lippincott Williams & Wilkins, 2002:275–313.
2. Hoppenfeld S. Physical examination of the lumbar spine. In: *Physical Examination of the Spine and Extremities*. Norwalk, CT: Appleton-Century-Crofts, 1976:237–263.
3. Albert TJ, Vaccaro AR. Physical examination of the lumbosacral spine. In: *Physical Examination of the Spine*. New York: Thieme, 2005:89–121.
4. Kahanovitz N. Physical examination. In: *Diagnosis and Treatment of Low Back Pain*. New York: Raven Press, 1991:31–42.
5. Engstrom JW. Back and neck pain. In: Kasper DL, Fauci AS, Longo DL, et al., eds. *Harrison's Principles of Internal Medicine*, 16th ed. McGraw-Hill Medical Publishing Division, 2005: 94–104.
6. Boden SD, McCowin PR, Davis DO, et al. Abnormal magnetic-resonance scans of the cervical spine in asymptomatic subjects. A prospective investigation. *J Bone Joint Surg* 1990;72A:1178–1184.
7. Logroscino G, Mazza O, Aulisa AG, et al. Spondylolysis and spondylolisthesis in the pediatric and adolescent population. *Childs Nerv Syst* 2001;17:644–655.


## ADDITIONAL READING


McCulloch J, Transfeldt E. Musculoskeletal and neuroanatomy of the lumbar spine. In: *Macnab's Backache*, 3rd ed. Baltimore: Williams & Wilkins, 1997:1–74.


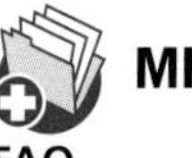

## MISCELLANEOUS

### FAQ

- Q: Which reflex evaluates the L5 nerve root?
  - A: No reflex exists for L5. The patellar reflex evaluates the L4 nerve root, and the Achilles reflex evaluates the S1 nerve root.
- Q: Which test is more specific for a lumbar disc herniation at the L4–L5 level: the straight-leg-raise test or the contralateral straight-leg-raise test?
  - A: The contralateral straight-leg-raise test.

# LYME DISEASE

*Paul D. Sponseller, MD*

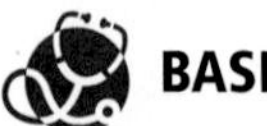

## BASICS

### DESCRIPTION

- Lyme disease is an immune-mediated disorder.
- It may include rash, arthritis, synovitis, carditis, or neurologic manifestations.
- Children and adults are affected equally.
- Classification (1):
  - Acute stage:
    - Rash
    - Early arthritis
  - Chronic stage:
    - Arthritis
    - Carditis
    - Neuritis
- Synonym: Deer tick disease

### GENERAL PREVENTION

- Awareness of endemic areas
- Avoidance of deer tick exposure

### EPIDEMIOLOGY

#### *Incidence*

- The incidence varies with the region of the country, but it has been reported in most states.
- 3 major endemic areas in the United States:
  - Upper mid-Atlantic area from Massachusetts to Maryland
  - Upper Midwest (especially Wisconsin and Minnesota)
  - Western states of Oregon, Utah, Nevada, and California

### RISK FACTORS

- Endemic area
- Deer tick exposure
- HLA-DR4 antigen haplotype

#### *Genetics*

The HLA-DR4 haplotype predicts increased risk of disease.

### ETIOLOGY

- Lyme disease is a reaction to an infection by the spirochete *Borrelia burgdorferi*, which is transmitted by the deer tick, *Ixodes dammini* (1,2).
- The disease was characterized after an epidemic of involvement in Old Lyme, Connecticut, in the mid-1970s (3,4).
  - Since then, other endemic areas have been identified.

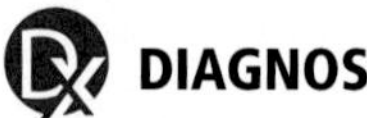

## DIAGNOSIS

### SIGNS AND SYMPTOMS

- Acute:
  - Spreading rash known as *erythema chronicum migrans*, beginning 3–30 days after a tick bite
  - Fever
  - Headache
  - Malaise
  - Migratory arthralgias and myalgias
- Chronic:
  - Swelling of large joints, most commonly the knee
  - Involvement of 1 or more joints
  - Pain, which may be minimal, as in juvenile rheumatoid arthritis, or acute, resembling bacterial arthritis
  - Cardiac involvement, possibly including atrioventricular block or myocarditis
  - Neurologic involvement, possibly including the 7th cranial nerve (facial) palsy, meningoencephalitis, or peripheral neuropathy

#### *Physical Exam*

- Inspect the patient's skin for the spreading, oval rash.
- Question about a rash occurring earlier.
- Examine for cranial nerve or peripheral nerve palsy.
- Examine all joints for effusion, even if painless.
- Listen to the patient's heart.

### TESTS

#### *Lab*

- The ESR usually is elevated (3,5).
- Tests for Lyme disease include 2 methods of antibody detection.
  - Enzyme-linked immunosorbent assay for spirochete:
    - Sensitive but not specific
    - A titer of $>$1:80 is considered positive.
    - If positive, this test should be followed by the Western blot test, a more specific gel electrophoresis technique.
  - Arthrocentesis:
    - Not a specific test for Lyme disease, but often performed to rule out other disorders
    - The white blood cell count is 25,000–90,000 and may include up to 95% polymorphonuclear leukocytes.
    - The spirochete is not recoverable from joint fluid.
- Electrocardiography may be indicated to show atrioventricular block.

#### *Imaging*

- Plain radiographs of the affected area are indicated (6).
- Joint changes may include soft-tissue swelling in early stages, osteopenia if the inflammation has been present for several weeks, and joint space narrowing if it has been chronic.

#### *Pathological Findings*

- Usually, no pathologic specimens are taken or required for diagnosis.
- When the joint lining is examined by biopsy, it shows nonspecific synovitis.

### DIFFERENTIAL DIAGNOSIS

- The diagnosis of juvenile rheumatoid arthritis requires at least 6 weeks of continued arthritis, but the arthritis does not respond to antibiotics, in contrast to Lyme disease.
- Bacterial arthritis usually produces more acute pain and fever and does not have a characteristic prodromal rash.
- Rheumatic fever should be excluded.

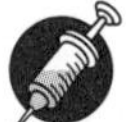

## TREATMENT

### GENERAL MEASURES

- Consult other specialists, such as those in infectious disease, neurology, rheumatology, or cardiology, as appropriate.
- Arrange diagnostic testing.

#### *Activity*

Restrict the patient's activity in the presence of substantial joint, cardiac, or neurologic involvement.

### MEDICATION (DRUGS)

- Start treatment with oral (early stages of disease) penicillin or amoxicillin empirically.
- Administer these drugs intravenously if the disease is treated later.
- Tetracycline is an option for children who are >8 years old.
  - It should not be used in younger children because of potential discoloration of the teeth.

### SURGERY

Synovectomy is a rare option for chronic disease that does not respond to initial antibiotic therapy.

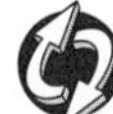

## FOLLOW-UP

### PROGNOSIS

Prognosis usually is good, unless late joint changes or neurologic complications have occurred.

### COMPLICATIONS

- Carditis (conduction block, myocarditis)
- Neurologic involvement (e.g., cranial or peripheral nerve palsy, meningoencephalitis)

### PATIENT MONITORING

- Follow patients daily to weekly to monitor response to therapy.
- Possibly admit patients to the hospital if cardiac or neurologic involvement is severe.

### REFERENCES


1. Steere AC. Lyme disease. *N Engl J Med* 1989;321: 586–596.
2. Phillips SE, Harris NS, Horowitz R, et al. Lyme disease: scratching the surface. *Lancet* 2005;366: 1771.
3. DePietropaolo DL, Powers JH, Gill JM, et al. Lyme disease: what you should know. *Am Fam Physician* 2005;72:309.
4. Kulie T, Vogt K, Sevetson E, et al. Clinical inquiries. When should you order a Lyme titer? *J Fam Pract* 2005;54:1084–1086,1088.
5. Cristofaro RL, Appel MH, Gelb RI, et al. Musculoskeletal manifestations of Lyme disease in children. *J Pediatr Orthop* 1987;7:527–530.
6. Rose CD, Fawcett PT, Eppes SC, et al. Pediatric Lyme arthritis: clinical spectrum and outcome. *J Pediatr Orthop* 1994;14:238–241.


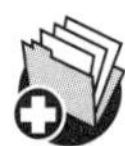

## MISCELLANEOUS

### CODES

#### *ICD9-CM*

- 714.0 Inflammatory arthritis
- 727.0 Synovitis

### PATIENT TEACHING

- Patients should be educated about prevention of re-exposure, and the family should be so counseled.
- They should also be informed about the late signs and symptoms of cardiac and neurologic involvement.

### FAQ

- Q: Should patients with tick bites be treated prophylactically for Lyme disease?
  - A: Because the risk of Lyme disease per exposure is low, this is not recommended generally.
- Q: Does Lyme disease always follow the classic sequence and presentation?
  - A: No. Many atypical forms are seen, so an index of suspicion is needed.

L

# MACRODACTYLY

Paul D. Sponseller, MD

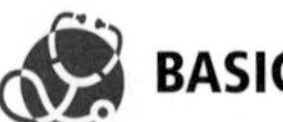

## BASICS

### DESCRIPTION

- Macrodactyly is overgrowth of 1 or several adjacent digits or rays of a hand or foot that produces the appearance of localized gigantism (Fig. 1).
- Virtually all cases are present at birth, although some cases worsen disproportionately.
  - Growth of the enlarged digits ceases when the patient reaches skeletal maturity.
- Classification (1):
  - Static: Enlargement remains proportionate to other digits
  - Dynamic: Enlargement increases with time, even by proportion
- Synonym: Localized gigantism

### EPIDEMIOLOGY

- Upper extremity more commonly affected than lower extremity
- No gender-specific predilection for increased frequency

#### *Incidence*

- <1 per 10,000 (2,3)
- Most cases (95%) are unilateral (3,4).

### RISK FACTORS

- Most cases are isolated (idiopathic).
- Also may occur in:
  - NF
  - Proteus syndrome
  - Klippel-Trenaunay syndrome

#### *Genetics*

- Isolated macrodactyly is not a heritable condition.
- Only if it is associated with NF does a familial tendency exist.

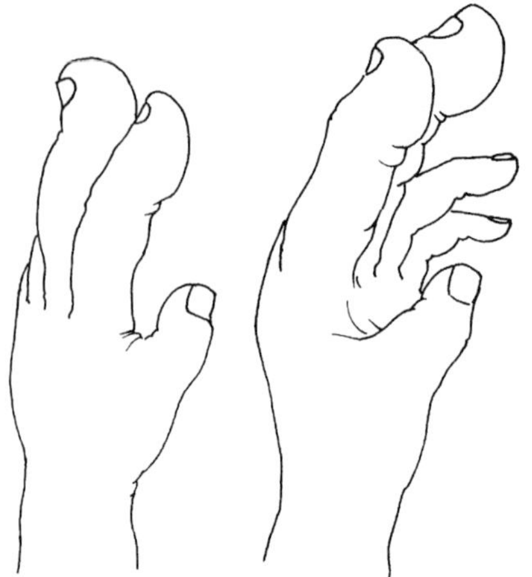

**Fig. 1.** Macrodactyly is generalized enlargement of 1 or 2 digits of the hand or foot.

### ETIOLOGY

- In idiopathic macrodactyly, the cause is unknown; it may be secondary to a localized disturbance of growth factors in the ectodermal ridge.
- Other cases of macrodactyly occur in patients with NF, Proteus syndrome, lymphedema, and hemangiomas.

### ASSOCIATED CONDITIONS

- Proteus syndrome (multiple hamartomatous abnormalities)
- NF
- Klippel-Trenaunay syndrome

## DIAGNOSIS

### SIGNS AND SYMPTOMS

- Generalized overgrowth of all tissues in the affected digits occurs.
- Enlargement is greater distally than proximally.
- The nail is especially enlarged.
- Tissues on the plantar or palmar surface of the digit are more greatly enlarged than those on the dorsal side, thus causing the digit to become hyperextended (dorsiflexed).
- The 2nd ray is affected most commonly, followed by the 3rd, 1st, and 4th.
- Syndactyly may coexist (Fig. 2).

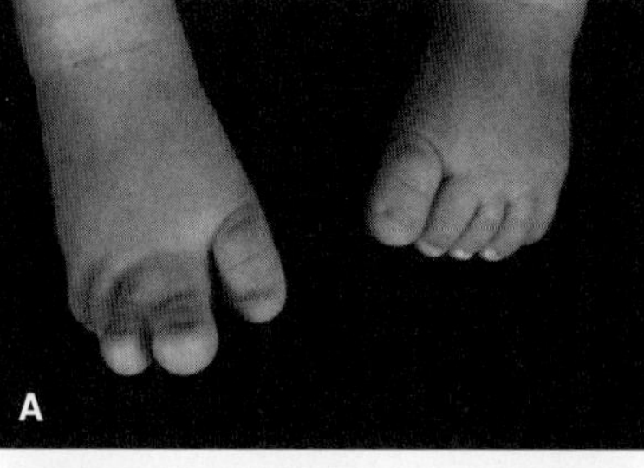


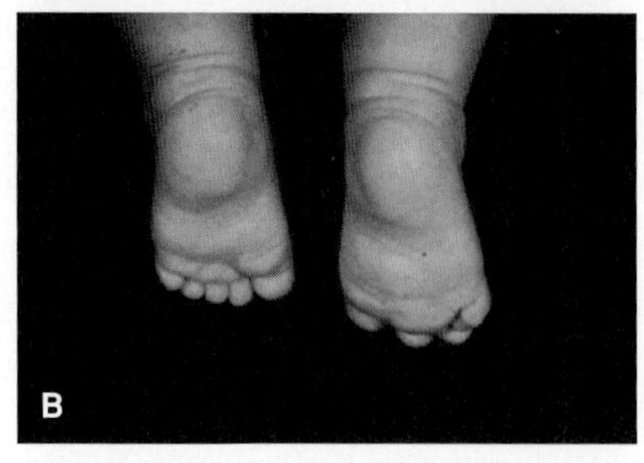


**Fig. 2.** Macrodactyly of the foot in a 2-year-old. Note the central involvement, syndactyly, involvement is greatest plantarly and distally, and contralateral normal foot. **A**: Dorsal view. **B**: Plantar view.

- If 2 digits are involved, they grow away from each other.
- In some cases, the enlargement becomes proportionately greater with time (dynamic type).
- Main clinical symptoms are related to overgrowth, such as clumsiness in the hand or difficulty with shoe wear.
- Pain may occasionally develop in adulthood because degeneration of the involved joints is premature.

#### *Physical Exam*

- Diagnosis is made purely by physical examination.
- Inspect the patient's hands and feet for hemangiomas and other signs of Proteus syndrome and NF.
- Compare limb lengths; they are rarely uneven in idiopathic macrodactyly.
- Check the motion of the affected digits.
- Compare the widths and lengths of the 2 hands or feet.
- Progression of growth of the hand or foot may be tracked clinically by making tracings or prints of both hands or feet over time, so length and width may be measured and compared.

### TESTS

#### *Lab*

Genetic testing is available for Proteus syndrome and NF, if they are suspected.

#### *Imaging*

- Plain films should be obtained to help assess and document the extent of overgrowth and the segments involved.
  - Soft-tissue enlargement also may be quantified from these films.
  - The extent of skeletal maturity also may be judged; it often is advanced in the enlarged rays.
- MRI is rarely necessary.

#### *Pathological Findings*

- All tissue types are overgrown in the affected digit.
- Fibrofatty proliferation accounts for the greatest bulk.
- Vessel, bone, subcutaneous tissue, and dermis are enlarged, and the changes are greatest distally.
- Pathologic changes are greatest in the digital nerves.

### DIFFERENTIAL DIAGNOSIS

- Hemihypertrophy, in which all digits in a hand or foot are uniformly overgrown
- Acrodactyly, in which overgrowth of all digits is greatest distally
- Growth hormone overabundance (hypersecretion), acromegaly

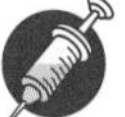

# TREATMENT

## GENERAL MEASURES

- Serial follow-up:
  - The pattern of growth may be determined by serial follow-up.
  - In this way, the static and the progressive types may be distinguished, and the appropriate treatment may be chosen: observation, shoe modification, or surgery.
- Measurements of length and width
- Surgery

## MEDICATION (DRUGS)

No drugs are known to help this condition.

## SURGERY

- Surgery may involve resection of the most enlarged ray, if the width of the hand or foot is greatly increased.
  - Surgery is the fastest way to make an important difference.
- Phalangectomy may make the length more even if the width is not a problem.
  - It also may be performed in addition to ray resection to address excessive length of adjacent digits.
- Epiphysiodesis (closure of the growth plates) is another way of evening length.
  - The correction occurs more gradually with time, and it may not completely correct the length inequality.
- Debulking of fat may improve the appearance, especially of the plantar fat hypertrophy.
- To avoid tissue ischemia, surgeon discretion on staging these multiple procedures is advised.

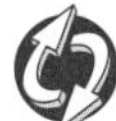

# FOLLOW-UP

## PROGNOSIS

- Most patients are made substantially better by judicious surgery.
- At the same time, it is important to realize that the parts will not be completely normal.

## COMPLICATIONS

- Stiffness and aching in the joints of the enlarged digits often develop in adulthood.
- Persistent enlargement, especially in the width of the involved digits, is the norm.
- Circulatory disturbance may occur if both sides of an involved digit undergo surgery concurrently.

## PATIENT MONITORING

- Serial follow-up appointments every 6–12 months are needed to develop and monitor a treatment plan.
- To keep records, tracings or radiographs should be made at each visit.
- Follow-up should be continued up to, and past, maturity.

## REFERENCES


1. Dennyson WG, Bear JN, Bhoola KD. Macrodactyly in the foot. *J Bone Joint Surg* 1977;59B:355–359.
2. Akinci M, Ay S, Ercetin O. Surgical treatment of macrodactyly in older children and adults. *J Hand Surg* 2004;29A:1010–1019.
3. Barsky AJ. Macrodactyly. *J Bone Joint Surg* 1967;49A:1255–1266.
4. Chang CH, Kumar SJ, Riddle EC, et al. Macrodactyly of the foot. *J Bone Joint Surg* 2002;84A:1189–1194.


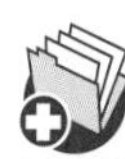

# MISCELLANEOUS

## CODES

### *ICD9-CM*

- 755.57 Macrodactyly of fingers or thumb
- 755.65 Macrodactyly of toes

## PATIENT TEACHING

- Show radiographs to help explain the nature of the condition.
- Advise that macrodactyly often requires several surgical procedures to achieve an optimal result.
- Emphasize the benefits of ray resection, if appropriate.

## FAQ

- Q: When will the affected digits stop their overgrowth?
  - A: Only with maturity will the affected digits stop their overgrowth.
- Q: What is the cause of macrodactyly?
  - A: Currently, it is unknown.

M

# MAGNETIC RESONANCE IMAGING

*Laura M. Fayad, MD*

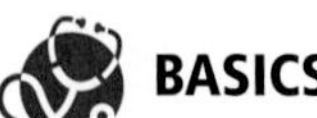

## BASICS

### DESCRIPTION

- MRI is a noninvasive diagnostic technique that uses hydrogen atoms in the body to create an image.
- MRI has several advantages over other imaging techniques:
  - Higher contrast resolution
  - More sensitive than CT in detecting bone marrow/soft-tissue disease
- No exposure to irradiation
- Multiplanar imaging capability

## DIAGNOSIS

- Indications:
  - Evaluation of joints
    - Detection of ligament or tendon pathology; fibrocartilage tears (e.g., menisci, glenoid labrum); hyaline cartilage defects; and associated bone marrow changes of arthritis
    - Detection and characterization of synovial disease (e.g., PVNS, synovial osteochondromatosis)
  - Evaluation of bone marrow:
    - Determination of extent of bone marrow tumors for treatment planning; residual or recurrent bone tumor after treatment (distinction between viable tumor and necrosis, degeneration, hemorrhage, and fibrosis)
    - Detection of osteomyelitis, bone marrow edema, and (occasionally) tumors (although plain radiographs often serve as the 1st line of diagnosis for tumors)
  - Evaluation of soft tissues:
    - Detection and definition of extent of soft-tissue tumors with respect to muscle, compartmental involvement, and extension to neurovascular bundles
    - Determination of residual or recurrent disease after treatment (distinction between viable tumor and necrosis, degeneration, hemorrhage, and fibrosis)
    - Characterization of a limited number of soft-tissue tumors

### TESTS

- Technique:
  - Prescription of MRI sequences varies, depending on the indication.
  - In general, sequences for joint evaluation are designed to depict the anatomy and detect fluid around injured articular structures, whereas for the evaluation of bone and soft-tissue tumors, T1 and T2 properties of the tissue are used to detect and characterize disease.
  - Sequences for joint evaluation:
    - High-resolution noncontrast sequences
    - Intermediate-weighted (proton density)
    - T1-weighted
    - 3D gradient echo
  - Fluid-sensitive noncontrast sequences:
    - Fat-suppressed T2-weighted
    - STIR
  - MRA (postcontrast, T1-weighted):
    - Direct MRA: Contrast directly into the joint
    - Indirect MRA (1): Contrast injected intravenously; imaging shortly thereafter
    - Used for increased specificity for ligament injuries, evaluation of OCDs, detection of intra-articular bodies, and postoperative determination of recurrent injuries
- Sequences for tumor/infection evaluation:
  - T1-weighted
  - Fluid-sensitive sequences (as noted earlier)
  - Gradient echo for detecting calcification or hemosiderin
  - Contrast-enhanced T1-weighted images:
    - For posttreatment evaluation to determine residual or recurrent disease
    - Adds specificity to detection of osteomyelitis and soft-tissue tumor characterization
- Advanced techniques (e.g., diffusion weighted imaging and magnetic resonance spectroscopy) are under investigation and may become useful clinically.

#### *Pathological Findings*

- Internal derangement of joints:
  - Shoulder:
    - Fluid signal in the rotator cuff tendon indicates a tear; partial is distinguished from full-thickness by depth of fluid signal.
    - Fatty atrophy of rotator cuff muscles is seen as increased signal on T1-weighted images.
    - Biceps tendon subluxation or dislocation is well visualized on axial views; tendon splits or complete tears are detected in 3 planes (axial, coronal, sagittal).
    - Glenoid labral tears are identified by abnormal morphology and fluid dissecting deep to or within the labrum; paralabral cysts may be located in the suprascapular or spinoglenoid notch.
    - Acromial shape (flat, curved, hooked) and subacromial spurs are detected on sagittal oblique views.
  - Elbow:
    - Collateral ligament tears are detected by fluid or contrast through the ligament, best seen on coronal oblique views (Fig. 1).
    - Medial and lateral epicondylitis present as flexor or extensor tendinosis (increased T2 signal), partial tear (fluid signal partly dissecting through the tendon), or complete tear (complete disruption of tendon with only fluid at origin); may be accompanied by bone marrow edema at epicondyles.
    - Biceps tendon pathology is best seen on axial views at the insertion on radial tuberosity.
    - Triceps tendon pathology is best seen on sagittal and axial views at the insertion on the olecranon.
    - Bone marrow edema secondary to arthritis or fracture is detected on fluid-sensitive sequences.
    - Intra-articular bodies may have variable signals.
  - Wrist:
    - TFCC normally is dark on all sequences: Degeneration, perforations, and tears are defined by abnormal signal within the fibrocartilage; tears are associated with distal radioulnar joint effusion.
    - Intrinsic ligament (scapholunate and lunotriquetral ligaments) tears are detected by fluid or contrast passage through the ligament.
    - All abnormalities and extrinsic ligaments may be better shown by MRA.
    - Carpal tunnel is assessed on axial views for median nerve enlargement or signal abnormality and flexor tendon pathology.
    - Ulnar nerve and Guyon canal are assessed on axial views for possible mass or ulnar artery aneurysm.
    - Articular cartilage defects may be detected directly or indirectly (the latter through associated bone marrow changes).
    - Kienböck disease typically is accompanied by diffuse decreased signal in the lunate.
    - Hook of hamate fractures: Axial views are best.
  - Hip:
    - Fractures can be identified by linear signal abnormality and surrounding bone marrow edema.
      - MRI is useful for rapid detection of occult hip fractures (2) and AVN, identified by low signal intensity on T1-weighted and "double line sign" on fluid-sensitive sequences.
      - The degree of involvement of weightbearing surface is aided by sagittal views.
    - Acetabular labrum morphology/tears are better identified by direct than indirect MRA.
    - Gluteus and hamstring tendons normally are dark on all sequences, but when torn, the MRI shows fluid signal.

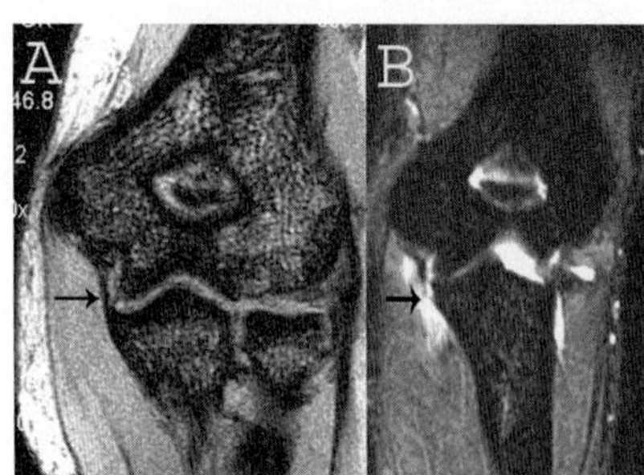


**Fig. 1.** Coronal images of the MCL. **A:** 3D gradient echo showing the normal anterior bundle of the MCL (*arrow*). **B:** Fat-suppressed T2-weighted images showing a completely torn distal attachment.

- Knee:
  - The most sensitive sequence for meniscal tears is the intermediate-weighted sequence, which shows tears as increased signal reaching the meniscal surface.
  - Flipped fragments may be detected as a double PCL sign (sagittal view) or occasionally seen in the medial gutter (coronal view).
  - Postoperative meniscal evaluation may be aided by MRA.
  - Complete ACL tears are detected by frank disruption with abnormal signal, failure to parallel Blumensaat line, and secondary signs (anterior tibial translation, specific contusion pattern).
  - Collateral ligament sprains may be grade 1 (abnormal signal adjacent to ligament), grade 2 (fluid signal within and adjacent to ligament), or grade 3 (complete disruption of ligament) (3).
  - Patellar tendinosis manifests with abnormal thickness and signal, and tendon tears are accompanied by fluid signal.
  - Quadriceps tendon tears should be assessed in all 3 planes (sagittal, coronal, and axial) for width of involvement.
  - Articular cartilage defects may be detected in several ways: T1-weighted 3D gradient echo sequences, as decreased signal; fluid-sensitive sequences, as fluid at the defect site, often accompanied by underlying bone marrow abnormalities; contrast-enhanced T1 sequences, as contrast at site of defect
- Ankle:
  - The Achilles tendon normally is dark on all sequences: Degeneration may be detected by abnormal thickness and internal signal; tears are seen as fluid signal.
  - PTT pathology is seen as abnormal tendon thickness or abnormal signal within the tendon; associated findings are PTT dysfunction (heel valgus deformity, midfoot fault, and os naviculare).
  - Peroneal tendon subluxation is detected by axial views: Presplit condition (boomerang deformity) or actual split of the peroneus brevis tendon is detectable in 3 planes; complex fluid in peroneal sheath suggests tenosynovitis.
  - Lateral ankle ligament (talofibular and tibiofibular) injuries are classified as grade 1 (increased signal), grade 2 (partial tear with fluid signal), or grade 3 (complete disruption) (4).
  - Sinus tarsi normally contains fat and is best evaluated on a sagittal T1-weighted image for loss of fat signal in sinus tarsi syndrome.
  - Plantar fasciitis accompanied by increased signal and abnormal thickness of the plantar fascia may have associated reactive bone marrow edema in the calcaneus.

- Tumors:
  - Bone:
    - A tumor appears as a marrow replacement process on T1-weighted images (5).
    - T2-weighted images are useful for defining extension into adjacent soft tissues.
    - Contrast-enhancement is useful for differentiating posttreatment residual or recurrent disease from fibrosis.
    - Fluid levels may be identified in bone cysts, giant cell tumors, chondroblastomas, telangiectatic osteosarcoma, and any lesion with a fracture (Fig. 2).
  - Soft tissue:
    - Only a small percentage of tumors (including lipomas, cysts, and vascular malformations) can be characterized definitively.
    - Some lesions (e.g., nerve sheath tumors, giant cell tumor of a tendon sheath, some fibrous tumors such as elastofibroma and desmoid tumors) have a few specific MRI characteristics.
    - Contrast enhancement characteristics may help distinguish benign and malignant soft-tissue lesions, but much overlap occurs in enhancement (6).

## DIFFERENTIAL DIAGNOSIS

- Notes on interpretation:
  - An MRI scan should be reviewed in conjunction with a plain radiograph.
  - Magic angle effects occur in cartilage, tendons, and ligaments when they are oriented 55° to the main magnetic field and cause increased signal on short time-to-echo sequences.
  - MRI of the shoulder: Much normal variant anatomy occurs at the anterosuperior labrum and may simulate a labral tear.
  - MRI of the elbow: A pseudodefect of the capitellum occurs posteriorly, whereas OCDs of the capitellum occur anteriorly.
  - MRI of the wrist: Ulnar variance by MRI must be assessed with caution because positioning of the wrist during scan affects apparent variance.
  - MRI of the hip: The sacrum and pubic bones always are evaluated for causes of referred hip pain.
  - MRI of the knee: Menisci should be evaluated in all planes (7).

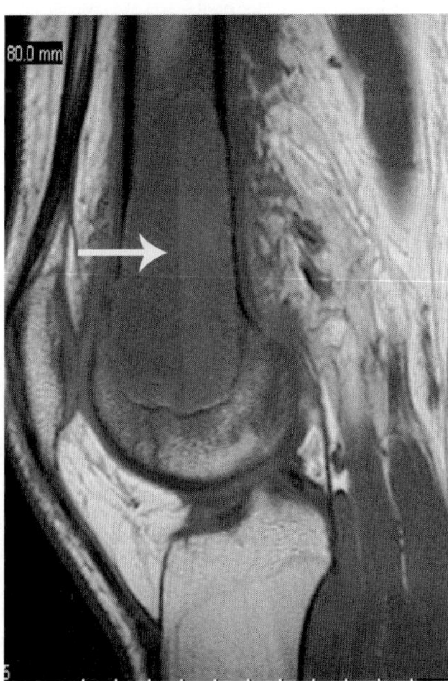


**Fig. 2.** Sagittal T1-weighted image showing distal femur telangiectatic osteosarcoma with fluid-fluid levels (*arrow*).

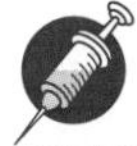

# TREATMENT

## PEDIATRIC CONSIDERATIONS

Pediatric patients, particularly those <5 years old, usually require sedation.

### *Pregnancy Considerations*

MRI is considered safe in pregnancy, although informed consent is obtained before the examination is performed and contrast is administered with great caution.

# FOLLOW-UP

## COMPLICATIONS

Contraindications to MRI include cardiac pacemaker, implanted cardiac defibrillator, aneurysm clips, carotid artery vascular clamp, neurostimulator, insulin or infusion pump, implanted drug infusion device, bone growth/fusion stimulator, and cochlear, otologic, or ear implants.

## REFERENCES


1. Steinbach LS, Palmer WE, Schweitzer ME. Special focus session. MR arthrography. *Radiographics* 2002;22:1223–1246.
2. Quinn SF, McCarthy JL. Prospective evaluation of patients with suspected hip fracture and indeterminate radiographs: use of T1-weighted MR images. *Radiology* 1993;187:469–471.
3. Schweitzer ME, Tran D, Deely DM, et al. Medial collateral ligament injuries: evaluation of multiple signs, prevalence and location of associated bone bruises, and assessment with MR imaging. *Radiology* 1995;194:825–829.
4. Erickson SJ, Smith JW, Ruiz ME, et al. MR imaging of the lateral collateral ligament of the ankle. *AJR Am J Roentgenol* 1991;156:131–136.
5. Nomikos GC, Murphey MD, Kransdorf MJ, et al. Primary bone tumors of the lower extremities. *Radiol Clin North Am* 2002;40:971–990.
6. van der Woude HJ, Verstraete KL, Hogendoorn PCW, et al. Musculoskeletal tumors: does fast dynamic contrast-enhanced subtraction MR imaging contribute to the characterization? *Radiology* 1998;208:821–828.
7. Magee T, Williams D. Detection of meniscal tears and marrow lesions using coronal MRI. *AJR Am J Roentgenol* 2004;183:1469–1473.


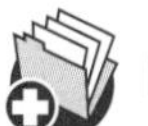

# MISCELLANEOUS

## PATIENT TEACHING

- The patient should expect to be in the MRI scanner, motionless, for 20–40 minutes.
- Intravenous contrast may be administered, depending on the indication.

# MALIGNANT FIBROUS HISTIOCYTOMA

*Frank J. Frassica, MD*

## BASICS

### DESCRIPTION
- MFH is an uncommon, malignant, primary mesenchymal tumor of soft tissue or bone that resembles fibrosarcoma.
- In primary MFH of bone, the long bones are affected most commonly.
- Classification: Several subtypes have been described, but typing has not been shown to have prognostic implications.

### GENERAL PREVENTION
No preventive measures are known.

### EPIDEMIOLOGY
- Individuals can be affected at any age, but the tumor mainly occurs in the 5th–7th decades.
- No real gender predominance, although a slight male predominance may occur (1).

#### *Incidence*
- An uncommon primary bone tumor:
  - The Mayo Clinic (Rochester, MN) has recorded 83 cases of MFH, representing 1% of the primary bone tumors (2).
- In contrast, MFH is the most common soft-tissue sarcoma in adults.

### RISK FACTORS
- This tumor may arise as a complication of pre-existing bone disease (e.g., Paget disease) within a bone infarct, or from irradiation.
- Up to 25% of cases are believed to be secondary (3).

#### *Genetics*
No known correlation exists.

### ETIOLOGY
The cause is unknown.

## DIAGNOSIS

### SIGNS AND SYMPTOMS
- Identical to those of other primary bone tumors
- Symptoms include pain and swelling, which is progressive.
- Patients often are symptomatic for 3–6 months before diagnosis.

#### *Physical Exam*
- The physical examination may be normal or may show only subtle findings.
- When the tumor has penetrated the bone, a soft-tissue mass may be felt.
- Muscle atrophy in the involved extremity is common.

### TESTS

#### *Lab*
The serum alkaline phosphate level may be increased secondary to bone destruction.

#### *Imaging*
- Lytic bone destruction has a moth-eaten or permeative pattern.
  - Reactive bone formation may be present.
- Large lesions may show soft-tissue extension or may be complicated by a pathologic fracture.
- Occasionally, lesions may show focal areas of calcification.

#### *Pathological Findings*
- Grossly, these tumors appear fibrous.
- Light microscopy reveals spindle-cell stroma with a characteristic "storiform pattern" (irregularly whorled).
- Histiocytes with slightly foamy cytoplasm and multinucleated giant cells also are prominent features.
- Any chondroid or osteoid matrix production by the tumor cells excludes the diagnosis of MFH.

### DIFFERENTIAL DIAGNOSIS
- Metastatic disease
- Myeloma
- Lymphoma
- Other primary mesenchymal tumors
- Osteosarcoma
- Fibrosarcoma

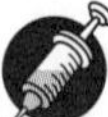

## TREATMENT

### GENERAL MEASURES
- MFH typically is radioresistant, but preoperative chemotherapy may improve the surgical outcome.
- Any patient in whom the diagnosis of MFH is suspected should be referred to a musculoskeletal oncologist for additional evaluation and treatment.

### SPECIAL THERAPY

#### *Physical Therapy*
Physical therapy is used extensively after limb salvage surgery or amputation.

### MEDICATION (DRUGS)
Preoperative and postoperative chemotherapy are used to minimize the risk of systemic metastasis.

### SURGERY
- In the past, amputation was the mainstay of therapy for lesions in the appendicular skeleton.
- With recent refinements in surgical technique, limb salvage surgery with prosthetic or allograft reconstruction frequently is an option.

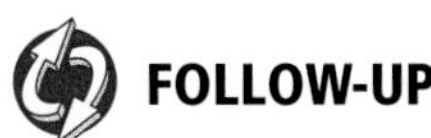

## FOLLOW-UP

### DISPOSITION

#### *Issues for Referral*

- Patients are monitored carefully for the development of pulmonary metastases or local recurrence.
  - Pulmonary surveillance:
    - Patients undergo serial chest CT scans every 3 months for 2 years and then every 6 months for 3 more years.
    - If metastases develop, patients are referred to a medical oncologist and thoracic surgeon.
  - Local control surveillance:
    - Patients are followed with serial radiographs, physical examinations, and sometimes CT/MRI scans (not possible in the presence of metal hardware) at 6-month intervals.
    - If local recurrence develops, patients are referred to a medical oncologist and thoracic surgeon.

### PROGNOSIS

MFH is a high-grade bone sarcoma with a >50% risk of pulmonary metastasis (2).

### COMPLICATIONS

Recurrence and metastasis are the most feared complications.

### REFERENCES


1. Dorfman HD, Czerniak B. Fibrous and fibrohistiocytic lesions. In: *Bone Tumors*. St. Louis: Mosby, 1998:492–558.
2. Nishida J, Sim FH, Wenger DE, et al. Malignant fibrous histiocytoma of bone. A clinicopathologic study of 81 patients. *Cancer* 1997;79:482–493.
3. McCarthy EF, Frassica FJ. Primary bone tumors. In: *Pathology of Bone and Joint Disorders: With Clinical and Radiographic Correlation*. Philadelphia: WB Saunders, 1998:195–275.


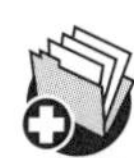

## MISCELLANEOUS

### CODES

#### *ICD9-CM*

171.3 Malignant fibrous histiocytoma

### PATIENT TEACHING

Patients with lower extremity lesions should be limited to partial weightbearing until referral to an oncologist, to avoid the possibility of pathologic fracture.

### FAQ

- Q: Do patients with MFH need surgery?
  - A: MFH of the bone is treated by wide resection of the bone. In addition, most patients are treated with chemotherapy.

# MALLET FINGER

*Dawn M. LaPorte, MD*

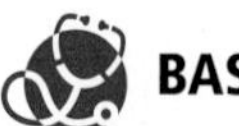

## BASICS

### DESCRIPTION

- Mallet finger is a loss of continuity of the conjoined lateral bands at the DIP joint of the finger that results in a characteristic flexion deformity of the distal joint.
- Mallet finger deformity resulting from the fracture of a child's distal phalanx usually is a transepiphyseal fracture of the phalanx.
- Classification (1) is used as an aid in establishing an appropriate treatment plan.
  - Type I (most common): Closed or blunt trauma with loss of tendon continuity with or without a small avulsion fracture
  - Type II: Laceration at or proximal to the DIP joint with loss of tendon continuity
  - Type III: Deep abrasion with loss of skin, subcutaneous cover, and tendon substance
  - Type IV:
    - a: Transepiphyseal plate fracture in children
    - b: Hyperflexion injury with fracture of the articular surface of 20–50%
    - c: Hyperextension injury with fracture of the articular surface usually >50% and with early or late volar subluxation of the distal phalanx
- Synonyms: Drop finger; Baseball finger

### GENERAL PREVENTION

- No effective means of prevention are known.
- Early detection is associated with a better prognosis.

### EPIDEMIOLOGY

Males are affected more often than females, but the numbers vary with the population studied.

#### *Incidence*

- This injury may occur at any age.
- The highest incidence in males occurs in adolescence and young adulthood (range, 11–40 years), whereas that in females occurs in middle age (range, 41–60 years) (2).
- Incidence increases progressively from the radial to ulnar side of the hand.

### ETIOLOGY

- Mallet finger can occur secondary to a variety of sports, occupational, or home activities.
- Open injuries may be caused by sharp or crush-type lacerations, but closed injuries are more common.
- The usual mechanism of injury is sudden, acute, forceful flexion of the extended digit, which results in rupture of the extensor tendon or avulsion of the tendon with or without a small fragment of bone from its dorsal insertion.
- Forced hyperextension of the distal joint may result in a fracture at the dorsal base of the distal phalanx involving 1/3 or more of the phalanx.
  - Although a mallet deformity is associated with this injury, the lesion should be considered a fracture with a secondary mallet finger deformity.
- The microvascular anatomy of the distal digital extensor tendon reveals an area of deficient blood supply in the region of insertion over the DIP; this vascularity may have implications in the cause of mallet finger.

## DIAGNOSIS

### SIGNS AND SYMPTOMS

- The DIP joint of the involved finger is held in flexion, and active extension is lost; full passive extension usually is present.
- Hyperextension of the PIP joint also may be observed.

#### *Physical Exam*

- Document the integrity of the skin and nail bed.
- Note active and passive extension (and flexion if not acute).
- Observe the status of the proximal joints.
- Diagnosis is based on physical examination with radiographs to assess for fracture.

### TESTS

#### *Lab*

No laboratory tests aid in this diagnosis.

#### *Imaging*

AP and lateral radiographs of the involved finger are mandatory to assess for fracture, because a fracture influences classification and treatment options.

#### *Pathological Findings*

- Normal anatomy:
  - The lateral bands of the extensor tendon from each side of the digit merge and join to form a single tendon on the proximal portion of the middle phalanx.
  - This tendon continues distally to form a wide unit for insertion into the dorsal base of the distal phalanx.
- Loss of continuity of the conjoined lateral bands at the distal joint of the finger results in a characteristic flexion deformity of the distal joint.
- A study of the microvascular anatomy of the distal digital extension tendon noted an area of deficient blood supply here and suggested that this zone of avascularity could have implications in the cause and treatment of mallet finger (3).

### DIFFERENTIAL DIAGNOSIS

- Fracture of the dorsal base of the distal phalanx with secondary mallet finger deformity
- Transepiphyseal plate fracture of the distal phalanx
- Flexion contracture/osteoarthritis

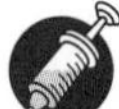

## TREATMENT

### GENERAL MEASURES

- Initial intervention is a minimum of 6 weeks of continuous DIP joint immobilization.
- Partial recurrence of the extension lag is common, and a subsequent regimen of at least 2–3 weeks of night splinting of the DIP joint in extension is mandatory.
- Careful follow-up is required and, if recurrent extension lag is severe, a second course of full-time splinting for 8 weeks may be considered.
- Surgical treatment frequently is recommended for type IV injuries (4), but splinting often is adequate treatment.
- Management of chronic mallet deformities seen late includes arthrodesis or secondary extension tendon reconstruction.
  - Mallet deformities not seen until 2–3 months after injury have been improved with prolonged splinting of the distal joint.
  - If the patient has severe symptoms, surgical options should be considered.
- Medical treatment depends on classification.
- Type I:
  - A dorsal or volar prefabricated splint (e.g., the stack splint)
  - If treated early, excellent to good results in nearly 80% (2,5,6)
  - For patients with delayed treatment or incorrect splint use, fair to poor results (7)
  - Length of treatment:
    - Continuous maintenance of the extended position of the DIP joint must be achieved for a minimum of 6 weeks for the splint to be effective.
    - Some clinicians recommend 8 weeks of splinting, followed by 2 weeks of night splinting.
  - Direct repair is to be avoided because the extensor tendon at this level is extremely thin and has a poor blood supply.
  - Nonoperative treatment yields a more satisfactory result than surgical repair.
  - A transarticular Kirschner wire may be placed in patients who cannot wear a splint for 6 weeks.

- Types II and III:
  - Repair with a simple figure-8 or roll-type suture, which reapproximates the skin and tendon simultaneously.
  - Apply a small dressing, incorporating a splint, which maintains the distal joint in full extension.
  - Remove the suture in 10–12 days.
  - Maintain the distal joint in the extended position by a stack or aluminum foam splint (as for type I injuries) for a minimum of 6 weeks, followed by protective ROM.
  - Reapply the splint if any extension loss is noted after its removal.
  - Type III mallet deformities with loss of tendon substance and soft-tissue coverage require reconstructive surgery to provide skin coverage, with late reconstruction by free tendon graft to restore tendon continuity or with arthrodesis of the joint.
  - Mallet finger resulting from a distal phalanx fracture in a child usually is a transepiphyseal fracture of the phalanx.
    - Closed reduction of the fracture usually results in correction of the deformity.
    - Continuous external splinting of the distal joint in full extension for 3–4 weeks results in fracture union and deformity correction.
- Type IV:
  - In an adult, type IV injuries are associated with major fracture fragments.
  - This type of fracture with an associated mallet finger deformity is a relatively uncommon injury.
  - Treatment:
    - Operative treatment has been recommended for fracture fragments >1/3 of the articular surface.
    - An accurate reduction is advocated to prevent joint deformity with secondary arthritis and stiffness.
    - However, excellent results have been reported with splinting alone, and nonoperative treatment avoids any surgery-related complications.
    - Indications for surgery are controversial and may depend on the amount of volar subluxation of the distal phalanx.
  - After 6–10 weeks of continuous splinting, the patient may begin guarded flexion exercises; splinting is continued at night.

### SPECIAL THERAPY

#### *Physical Therapy*

Occupational therapy may benefit the patient who has a difficult time regaining flexion after the splinting is completed or the surgical Kirschner wire is removed.

### SURGERY

- Indicated for open injuries, for a closed injury in a person who would be unable to work with a splint, and for a large dorsal fragment with volar subluxation of the distal phalanx.
- Reduce the joint, manipulate the fracture fragment into place, and pass a Kirschner wire longitudinally across the joint to hold it in full extension.
- Options for chronic mallet finger include plication or reefing of the scarred tendon, arthrodesis, tenodermodesis, spiral oblique retinacular ligament reconstruction, and even DIP disarticulation.

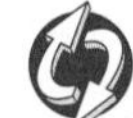

## FOLLOW-UP

### PROGNOSIS

- Poor prognostic factors include:
  - Age >60 years
  - Delay in treatment >4 weeks
  - Initial active extension lag
  - >4 weeks of immobilization without substantial improvement
  - Short, stubby fingers

### COMPLICATIONS

- Skin problems (e.g., dorsal maceration, skin ulceration, tape allergy):
  - Dorsal ulceration and maceration with the use of dorsal aluminum foam splints: Place tubular gauze or moleskin beneath the splint.
  - Full-thickness skin necrosis over the DIP joint after dorsal splint immobilization in hyperextension: Splint the distal joint with minimal hyperextension; do not exceed the amount of hyperextension that produces blanching.
- Transverse nail grooves
- Pain from the splint
- Patients treated surgically for mallet finger have a >50% complication rate, including permanent nail deformities, joint incongruities, infection, pin or pullout wire failure, radial or ulnar prominence, and deviation of the DIP joint.
- Loss of surgical reduction, requiring additional surgery

### PATIENT MONITORING

- Because of the high complication rate (up to 45%; mostly transient skin problems) reported with splinting (7), most patients require 2 visits during the 1st week of treatment, and weekly visits thereafter to monitor their progress and check their skin.
- After 6–10 weeks, the splint is removed, the finger is inspected, and night splinting is begun.
- Careful follow-up is required to monitor for recurrence and to individualize treatment.

### REFERENCES


1. Doyle JR. Extensor tendons–acute injuries. In: Green DP, Hotchkiss RN, Pederson WC, eds. *Green's Operative Hand Surgery*, 4th ed. New York: Churchill Livingstone, 1999:1950–1987.
2. Abouna JM, Brown H. The treatment of mallet finger. The results in a series of 148 consecutive cases and a review of the literature. *Br J Surg* 1968;55:653–667.
3. Warren RA, Kay NRM, Norris SH. The microvascular anatomy of the distal digital extensor tendon. *J Hand Surg* 1988;13B:161–163.
4. Baratz ME, Schmidt CC, Hughes TB. Extensor tendon injuries. In: Green DP, Hotchkiss RN, Pederson WC, et al., eds. *Green's Operative Hand Surgery*, 5th ed. Philadelphia: Elsevier Churchill Livingstone, 2005:187–217.
5. Crawford GP. The molded polythene splint for mallet finger deformities. *J Hand Surg* 1984;9A: 231–237.
6. Garberman SF, Diao E, Peimer CA. Mallet finger: results of early versus delayed closed treatment. *J Hand Surg* 1994;19A:850–852.
7. Doyle JR. Extensor tendon injuries. In: Manske PR, ed. *Hand Surgery Update*. Rosemont, IL: American Society for Surgery of the Hand, 1994:149–159.


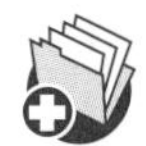

## MISCELLANEOUS

### CODES

#### *ICD9-CM*

736.1 Mallet finger

### PATIENT TEACHING

For the splint to be effective, patients should understand the importance of the continuous maintenance of the extended position of the DIP joint for a minimum of 6 weeks.

### FAQ

- Q: Is treatment of an open mallet injury different from that of closed injury?
  - A: Yes. Open mallet injuries are repaired using suture, with or without pinning the DIP joint in extension for 6 weeks. The preferred treatment for closed mallet injury is DIP extension splinting worn full-time for 6 weeks and then converted to nighttime wear.
- Q: How is a mallet thumb managed?
  - A: Mallet thumb injuries are treated the same as mallet fingers: Closed injuries are splinted and open injuries are managed with direct repair.

# MARFAN SYNDROME

*Paul D. Sponseller, MD*

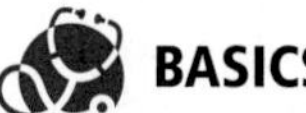

## BASICS

### DESCRIPTION

- Marfan syndrome is a familial disorder of elastic connective tissue that is characterized by aortic root dilatation and dissection, valvular insufficiency, lens dislocation, and arachnodactyly, among other findings.
- It affects the cardiovascular, ocular, skeletal, and neurologic systems and has caused sudden death in many patients, including several prominent basketball and volleyball players.
- Although the disorder is inherited at birth, some of the manifestations, such as aortic dilatation, scoliosis, and sternal deformity, take time to develop.
- This delayed manifestation may cause the diagnosis to be delayed until later in childhood.
- Classification (1):
  - Classic Marfan syndrome (2):
  - MASS (**M**itral prolapse, **A**ortic dilatation, **S**kin and **S**keletal findings) phenotype, which is a *forme fruste* of the syndrome
  - Contractural arachnodactyly (Beals syndrome), disorder of fibrillin-2 (2)

### EPIDEMIOLOGY

#### *Incidence*

Males and females are affected equally.

#### *Prevalence*

~1 in 5,000 persons is affected (2).

### RISK FACTORS

- Positive family history of Marfan syndrome
- Family history of aortic dissection or unexplained sudden death
- Tall, slender habitus

#### *Genetics*

- The syndrome is autosomal dominant with variable expressivity.
- Some patients are affected by a *de novo* mutation, and they are more likely to have severe cases or be diagnosed in the neonatal period.
- Even among families with high penetrance, manifestations may vary from member to member.

### ETIOLOGY

- Marfan syndrome results from a defect in the fibrillin-1 gene, which is found on chromosome 15.
- Multiple different deletions have been found that result in Marfan syndrome and probably explain the condition's heterogeneity.
- Fibrillin is found in the zonules that suspend the lens of the eye, as well as in the arterial walls.
- The explanation for other findings is still being sought, but it may involve molecular signaling and structural differences.

## DIAGNOSIS

### SIGNS AND SYMPTOMS

- The diagnosis is made mainly by clinical (Ghent) criteria (1).
- The patient must have at least 2 systems involved, at least 2 major criteria (ascending aortic enlargement or dissection, ectopia lentis, dural ectasia, positive family history, proven mutation, or 4 skeletal findings), and 1 minor criterion.
- Symptoms:
  - Relatively few; rarely the means for diagnosis
  - Delay in walking or coordination, fatigability, poor vision, chest pain (at aortic dissection)
- Signs:
  - Tendency to tall stature
  - Long limbs in relation to the trunk (3)
  - Scoliosis
  - Kyphosis
  - Multiple foot deformities
  - Pectus excavatum or carinatum
  - Slender cranium
  - Joint hypermobility, which usually is moderate and is considerably less than in Ehlers-Danlos syndrome
  - Often, a positive thumb sign, in which the clenched thumb protrudes beyond the ulnar border of the closed fist (2)

#### *Physical Exam*

- Measure the patient's height: The upper:lower segment ratio (head to symphysis over symphysis to floor) is <0.85.
- Check for kyphosis, scoliosis, and pectus deformity.

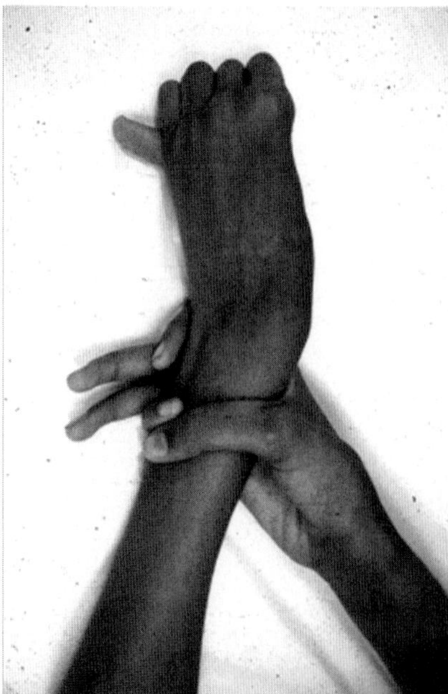

**Fig. 1.** The thumb sign is positive when the entire distal phalanx of the thumb protrudes beyond the ulnar border of the clenched fist. The wrist sign is positive when the thumb can completely overlap the 5th fingernail when wrapped around the wrist.

- Assess thumb and wrist signs (4) (Fig. 1).
- Asses leg-length inequality.
- Slit-lamp examination by an experienced ophthalmologist also is helpful in making the diagnosis and in following the patient's course.

### TESTS

#### *Lab*

- Results of routine laboratory tests are normal, but genetic testing for mutations in fibrillin is available.
- False-negative results are still possible with this test.
- Therefore, genetic testing is not used routinely in clinical practice (2,5).

#### *Imaging*

- Echocardiography is key to assessing main structures at risk in this syndrome, such as the heart valves and the ascending aorta.
  - This test should be performed as a baseline at the time of diagnosis and periodically afterward, according to the judgment of the cardiologist.
- MRI is useful for imaging entire aorta; it also can be used to evaluate the spine for dural ectasia (6–8) (Fig. 2).
- Radiography:
  - Plain radiographs of the spine are used for the diagnosis of scoliosis, if it is suspected.
  - Patients also should have an AP radiograph of the pelvis to evaluate for protrusio acetabulae (Fig. 3), which is an excessive deepening of the hip sockets (9).

#### *Pathological Findings*

- The aortic root shows dissection of the medial layer in some patients.
- The dura of the lower lumbar spine sometimes shows dilatation and saclike protrusions from the sides and front of the spinal canal.

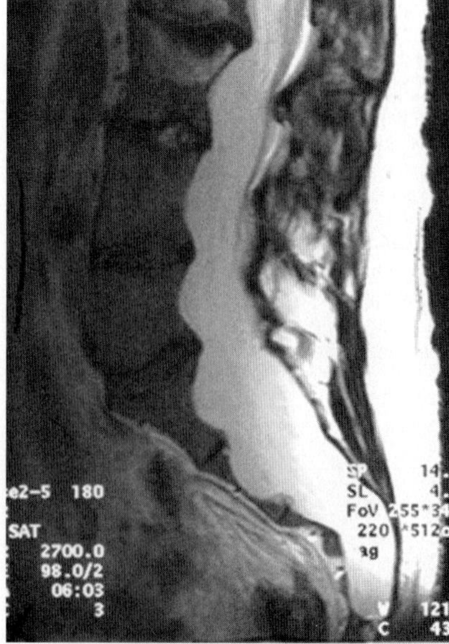


**Fig. 2.** Dural ectasia is enlargement of the dural sac, usually in the lowest portion of the spine.

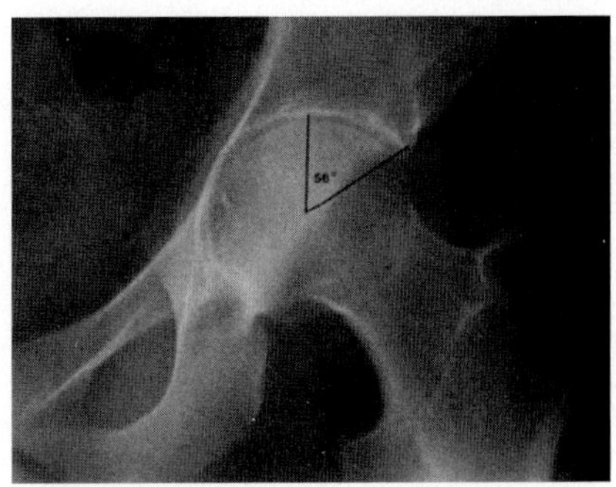

**Fig. 3.** Protrusio acetabulae is considered as a center-edge angle >50°.

## DIFFERENTIAL DIAGNOSIS

- Congenital contractural arachnodactyly (caused by a fibrillin-2 defect coded on chromosome 5), which is distinguished by multiple joint contractures in the presence of arachnodactyly
- Stickler syndrome (hereditary arthro-ophthalmopathy)
- Homocystinuria (characterized by mental delay and inferior dislocation of the lens)
- Ehlers-Danlos syndrome (generalized ligamentous laxity more extreme than in Marfan syndrome, with more cutaneous laxity)
- MASS phenotype
- Familial aortic dissection

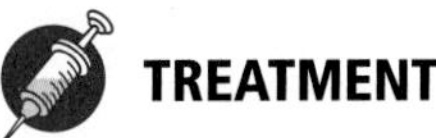

# TREATMENT

## GENERAL MEASURES

- Medication for aortic dilatation
- Genetic counseling
- Periodic cardiology follow-up with ultrasound, as indicated (2)
  - If aortic enlargement is suspected, a $\beta$-2 blocking drug may be started to minimize pressure in the aorta; this medication has been shown to be effective in slowing dilatation in clinical trials.
  - Atenolol is the $\beta$-2 blocker most commonly used for this syndrome.
- Patients should avoid sports that cause high impact or cardiac stress.
- Bracing or surgery for spinal deformities occasionally may be appropriate (10).
- Procedures with which to address a partially dislocated lens or a retinal detachment are available.
- No current drug or therapy can correct the basic defect in fibrillin.

### *Activity*

- Persons with Marfan syndrome should keep active, but they should avoid high-impact or high-stress sports.
- A geneticist or cardiologist should be consulted if specific questions arise.

## SPECIAL THERAPY

### *Physical Therapy*

- May help an infant who is severely delayed in walking or achieving other motor milestones
- Also useful as part of a nonoperative program for back pain

## SURGERY

- Spinal fusion (correction with instrumentation and bone graft for fusion) occasionally is indicated for severe scoliosis or kyphosis (7).
- Spinal fusion sometimes is indicated for severe or symptomatic spondylolisthesis of L5 on S1.
- Hip replacement occasionally is indicated for arthritis related to protrusio acetabuli (9).
- Aortic root and valve repair or replacement with a composite graft are indicated when the dilatation reaches a certain size; this procedure is highly successful and is preferable to waiting for aortic dissection to occur!

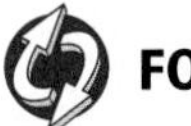

# FOLLOW-UP

## DISPOSITION

### *Issues for Referral*

If Marfan syndrome is suspected, the patient should be referred to a cardiologist or geneticist.

## PROGNOSIS

- Without modern cardiovascular management, the life expectancy for patients with this condition would be <50 years.
- Lifespan can be prolonged substantially, and many patients live into or past the 7th decade.

## COMPLICATIONS

- Aortic dissection
- Valvular insufficiency
- Retinal detachment
- Spontaneous pneumothorax
- Chronic musculoskeletal pain

## PATIENT MONITORING

- Coordinate care by a geneticist and a cardiologist.
- See other specialists as needed.
- Routine checkups may prevent catastrophes.

## REFERENCES


1. De Paepe A, Devereux RB, Dietz HC, et al. Revised diagnostic criteria for the Marfan syndrome. *Am J Med Genet* 1996;62:417–426.
2. Judge DP, Dietz HC. Marfan's syndrome. *Lancet* 2005;366:1965–1976.
3. Jones KB, Sponseller PD, Hobbs W, et al. Leg-length discrepancy and scoliosis in Marfan syndrome. *J Pediatr Orthop* 2002;22:807–812.
4. Pradhan BB, Bhasin M, Otsuka NY. A metatarsal equivalent to the metacarpal index in Marfan syndrome. *Foot Ankle Int* 2005;26:881–885.
5. Dietz HC, Loeys B, Carta L, et al. Recent progress towards a molecular understanding of Marfan syndrome. *Am J Med Genet* 2005;139C:4–9.
6. Foran JRH, Pyeritz RE, Dietz HC, et al. Characterization of the symptoms associated with dural ectasia in the Marfan patient. *Am J Med Genet* 2005;134A:58–65.
7. Jones KB, Erkula G, Sponseller PD, et al. Spine deformity correction in Marfan syndrome. *Spine* 2002;27:2003–2012.
8. Sponseller PD, Ahn NU, Ahn UM, et al. Osseous anatomy of the lumbosacral spine in Marfan syndrome. *Spine* 2000;25:2797–2802.
9. Sponseller PD, Jones KB, Ahn NU, et al. Protrusio acetabulae in Marfan syndrome: age-related prevalence and associated hip function. *J Bone Joint Surg* 2006;88A:486–495.
10. Sponseller PD, Bhimani M, Solacoff D, et al. Results of brace treatment of scoliosis in Marfan syndrome. *Spine* 2000;25:2350–2354.


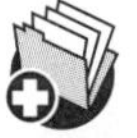

# MISCELLANEOUS

## CODES

### *ICD9-CM*

759.82 Marfan syndrome

## PATIENT TEACHING

- Describe the warning signs of aortic dissection and retinal detachment.
- Stress the importance of taking $\beta$-blockers when prescribed.
- Offer genetic counseling.
- Evidence suggests that the risk of aortic dissection or critical dilatation may be decreased by cardioselective $\beta$-blockade.
- Support group in the United States: National Marfan Foundation, Port Washington NY (tel. 800-4-MARFAN)

## FAQ

- Q: Are braces effective for the scoliosis seen in Marfan syndrome?
  - A: Braces rarely influence the scoliosis seen in Marfan syndrome unless started early.
- Q: Are braces indicated for flat feet in Marfan syndrome?
  - A: They do not change the shape of the feet. In most cases, they are not indicated unless pain is severe.

# MEDIAL COLLATERAL LIGAMENT INJURY

*John H. Wilckens, MD*
*Marc Urquhart, MD*

## BASICS

### DESCRIPTION

- An MCL injury is a sprain of the MCL, which is the primary restraint to valgus stress on the knee.
- It occurs mainly in athletic teenagers and young adults, and equally among males and females.
- Classification (Fig. 1) (1):
  - Grade I (mild): Microscopic sprain with intact fibers
  - Grade II (moderate): Partial tear
  - Grade III (severe): Complete tear

### GENERAL PREVENTION

Prevention is best accomplished through conditioning before sport activities.

### RISK FACTORS

- Contact sports
- Falls

### ETIOLOGY

- Direct blow to the lateral knee
- Valgus load to the knee

### ASSOCIATED CONDITIONS

ACL injuries via a noncontact mechanism

## DIAGNOSIS

### SIGNS AND SYMPTOMS

- Pain along the medial aspect of the knee, typically extending proximally and distally along the course of the MCL
- Possible knee effusion
- Can be associated with an ACL tear and/or a meniscus tear
- Increased pain with valgus loading
- Occasionally, recollection by patient of a "pop" or "snap" at the time of the injury

#### *History*

- Occurs most commonly with a direct blow to the lateral knee, causing the knee to gap open
- If MCL injury occurs with a noncontact mechanism, a high association with ACL injury exists.

#### *Physical Exam*

- MCL ruptures can be associated with other injuries; physical examination and diagnostic workup should reflect a high suspicion.
- Test the stability of the MCL:
  - Flex the patient's knee 30° and apply a valgus force
  - Estimate degree of opening and character of the end point (soft, solid).
  - Valgus laxity of the knee in 0° of flexion suggests an MCL injury in addition to a cruciate ligament injury.
- Perform a complete neurovascular examination distal to the knee.
- Perform the Lachman and posterior drawer tests to rule out associated ACL or PCL injury.
- Compare with the contralateral knee.

### TESTS

#### *Imaging*

- AP and lateral plain radiographs should be obtained initially to rule out fractures.
- MRI is an appropriate study because of its sensitivity to other ligamentous or meniscal disease.

### DIFFERENTIAL DIAGNOSIS

- ACL rupture
- Medial meniscal tears
- PCL rupture
- Tibial plateau fractures
- Tibial spine avulsions
- Patella dislocation

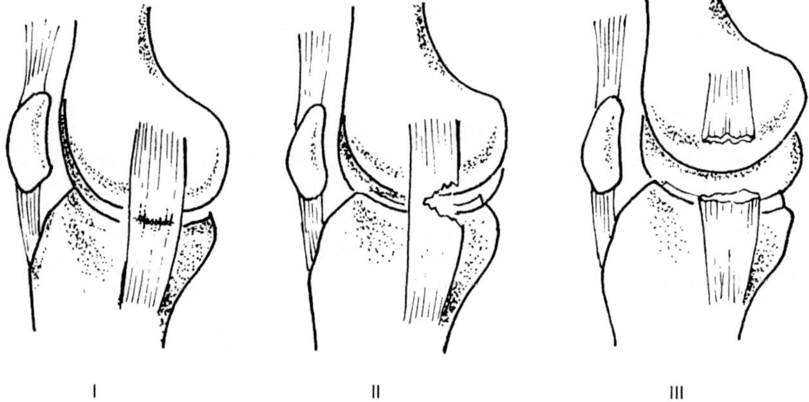


**Fig. 1.** MCL injuries may be graded as follows: I, microscopic strain; II, partial tear; or III, complete tear.

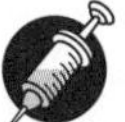

# TREATMENT

## GENERAL MEASURES

- Initially, a patient with an MCL injury is treated with ice, elevation, analgesics, a hinged knee brace, and protected weightbearing as tolerated.
- The patient should be referred to physical therapy.
- If the patient has a suspicion for an associated cruciate ligament injury, early referral to an orthopaedic surgeon is indicated.

## SPECIAL THERAPY

### *Physical Therapy*

- Gentle ROM exercises
- Muscle-strengthening program with emphasis on medial hamstrings (MCL agonists) and core muscles
- Progressive weightbearing in hinged knee brace as tolerated
- Ice, electrical stimulation (2)
- Once pain free, progressive agility and proprioception training

## SURGERY

Chronic MCL tears unresponsive to nonoperative treatment may require surgical repair.

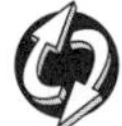

# FOLLOW-UP

## PROGNOSIS

- Most patients with MCL injuries respond to nonoperative treatment (bracing and early ROM).
- Bracing should be considered for patients returning to contact sports.

## PATIENT MONITORING (3,4)

- Patients are followed at 2–6 weeks to check ROM, muscle strength, and joint laxity.
- MRI if examination suggests associated cruciate ligament and/or meniscal injuries.

## REFERENCES


1. O'Donoghue DH. Treatment of acute ligamentous injuries of the knee. *Orthop Clin North Am* 1973;4:617–645.
2. Wilk KE, Andrews JR, Clancy WG. Nonoperative and postoperative rehabilitation of the collateral ligaments of the knee. *Oper Tech Sports Med* 1996;4:192–201.
3. Bergfeld J. Symposium: functional rehabilitation of isolated medial collateral ligament sprains. First-, second-, and third-degree sprains. *Am J Sports Med* 1979;7:207–209.
4. Inoue M, McGurk-Burleson E, Hollis JM, et al. Treatment of the medial collateral ligament injury. I: The importance of anterior cruciate ligament on the varus-valgus knee laxity. *Am J Sports Med* 1987;15:15–21.


## ADDITIONAL READING


- Indelicato PA, Hermansdorfer J, Huegel M. Nonoperative management of complete tears of the MCL of the knee in intercollegiate football players. *Clin Orthop Relat Res* 1990;256:174–177.
- Shelbourne KD, Nitz PA. The O'Donoghue triad revisited. Combined knee injuries involving anterior cruciate and MCL tears. *Am J Sports Med* 1991;19:474–477.


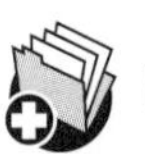

# MISCELLANEOUS

## CODES

### *ICD9-CM*

844.1 Medial collateral ligament

## PATIENT TEACHING

- Most MCL injuries heal without surgery.
- Patients are instructed in ROM and muscle-strengthening exercises.

## FAQ

- Q: How can you tell if someone has had an associated injury with the MCL sprain?
  - A: An MCL injury sustained via a noncontact incident, with a large effusion, or with valgus laxity in full extension suggests that another structure (commonly the ACL) has been injured.

# MENISCUS TEAR

*Carl Wierks, MD*
*Bill Hobbs, MD*

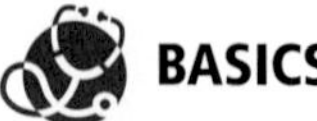

## BASICS

### DESCRIPTION
- A meniscus tear is an acute or degenerative injury to the meniscal fibrocartilage of the knee (Fig. 1).
- Classification:
  - Acute tear:
    - Longitudinal (50–90%)
    - Radial (6%)
    - Flap (4%)
  - Degenerative tear:
    - Mostly horizontal cleavage or complex tears

### EPIDEMIOLOGY
- Acute tears occur mainly in adolescents and young adults, and degenerative tears predominate in the 40–60-year-old population.
- Degenerative medial tears occur more frequently than do degenerative lateral meniscal tears (1).
- Acute lateral meniscus tears occur more frequently than do acute medial tears (2).

#### *Incidence*
- In 1 study of asymptomatic individuals, MRI showed that 13% of those <45 years old and 36% of those >45 years old had a meniscus tear (3).
- Another study showed that 60% of cadavers aged 65 years at time of death had degenerative tears (4).
- Concomitant ACL tear occurs in ~30% of patients with acute meniscus tears (1).

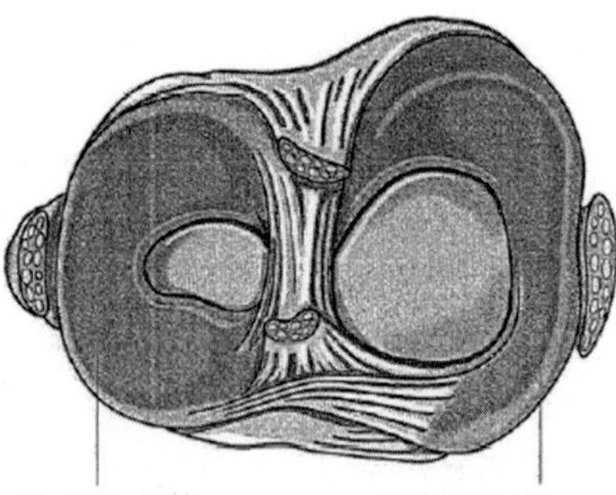


**Fig. 1.** Artist's sketch of a meniscal tear in the right knee. (From: Sports Tips: "Meniscal tears in athletes." Used with permission of the American Orthopaedic Society for Sports Medicine, Rosemont, IL.)

### RISK FACTORS
- Twisting, hyperflexion injury
- Age >40 years
- Chronic ACL deficiency
- Tibial plateau fracture
- Arthritis affecting the knee

#### *Genetics*
No Mendelian inheritance is known.

### ETIOLOGY
- Acute:
  - Often occurs during athletic activities, most commonly football, basketball, and wrestling
  - A common mechanism is a severe twisting at the knee, often during change of direction.
  - Can be associated with ACL injury
- Degenerative:
  - Age-related breakdown of collagen fibers

### ASSOCIATED CONDITIONS
Ligamentous injury (ACL, collateral ligament) in acute tears

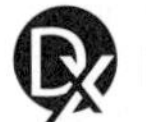

## DIAGNOSIS

### SIGNS AND SYMPTOMS
- Acute pain and swelling
- Tenderness localized to the joint line or popliteal region with the knee flexed
- Popping, locking, catching, or buckling with large, unstable the tears
- Inability of the patient to extend the knee fully in the presence of a displaced bucket-handle tear
- May have chronic mild swelling and joint-line pain in the presence of a degenerative tear

#### *History*
- Acute twisting of the knee while weightbearing
- Chronic knee pain

#### *Physical Exam*
- Assess knee stability.
- Joint-line tenderness is the best clinical sign (74% sensitivity, 50% positive predictive value) (5).
- McMurray test:
  - Hyperflex the knee and gently rotate it internally and externally, applying valgus and varus stress while extending the knee.
  - May feel click, pop, or crepitance
  - Reproduces patient symptoms
- Apley grind test:
  - Position the patient prone.
  - Internally and externally rotate the leg with traction and compression.
  - Pain or mechanical symptoms indicate likely meniscal pathology.

### TESTS

#### *Imaging*
- Plain radiographs: 30° flexed posteroanterior view is best for observing weightbearing surfaces.
- MRI is 90–98% accurate, although it can give false-positive results (6).

#### *Diagnostic Procedures/Surgery*
Arthroscopy is the gold standard for diagnosis.

#### *Pathological Findings*
- Collagen fibers:
  - Oriented circumferentially
  - Resistant to compressive forces
  - May tear under shear stress
- Tears in inner 2/3 heal poorly because of the lack of blood supply.
- Degeneration from repeated microtrauma occurs, with gradual loss of collagen and integrity that leads to tears.

### DIFFERENTIAL DIAGNOSIS
- Chondral lesion
- ACL or collateral ligament tear
- Fibrotic plica
- Fat-pad impingement
- Osteoarthritis
- Patellofemoral chondrosis
- Spontaneous osteonecrosis

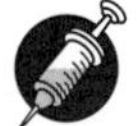

# TREATMENT

## GENERAL MEASURES

- Begin with a trial of rest, protected weightbearing, and modified activity.
- If the patient remains symptomatic, offer MRI or arthroscopic evaluation.

### *Activity*

- Weightbearing as tolerated
- Often return to full activities 2–3 weeks after injury

## MEDICATION (DRUGS)

Drugs of choice are analgesics or NSAIDs.

## SURGERY

- Indications for arthroscopy:
  - Symptoms that affect activities of daily living or work, mechanical symptoms
  - Positive physical findings (joint tenderness, effusion)
  - Failure of nonsurgical treatment
- The following lesions should be repaired:
  - Complete vertical tear >10 mm long
  - Tear within the peripheral 10–30% of the meniscus or 3–4 mm of the meniscocapsular junction
- Better healing of meniscal repairs with concurrent ACL reconstruction
- Complex tears and those in the avascular inner 2/3 are resected.
- Total meniscectomy is not recommended because of the increased risk of degenerative arthritis.

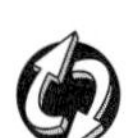

# FOLLOW-UP

- Initiate gradual strengthening and ROM program.
- Return to full activities 6–8 weeks after partial meniscectomy

## COMPLICATIONS

- Complications are uncommon but include:
  - Injury to neurovascular structures (infrapatellar branch of saphenous nerve, causing pain, dysesthesias at the portal site)
  - Infection
  - DVT
  - Arthritis

## REFERENCES


1. Poehling GG, Ruch DS, Chabon SJ. The landscape of meniscal injuries. *Clin Sports Med* 1990;9:539–549.
2. Baker BE, Peckham AC, Pupparo F, et al. Review of meniscal injury and associated sports. *Am J Sports Med* 1985;13:1–4.
3. LaPrade RF, Burnett QM, II, Veenstra MA, et al. The prevalence of abnormal magnetic resonance imaging findings in asymptomatic knees. With correlation of magnetic resonance imaging to arthroscopic findings in symptomatic knees. *Am J Sports Med* 1994;22:739–745.
4. Noble J, Hamblen DL. The pathology of the degenerate meniscus lesion. *J Bone Joint Surg* 1975;57B:180–186.
5. Anderson AF, Lipscomb AB. Clinical diagnosis of meniscal tears. Description of a new manipulative test. *Am J Sports Med* 1986;14:291–293.
6. De Smet AA, Norris MA, Yandow DR, et al. MR diagnosis of meniscal tears of the knee: importance of high signal in the meniscus that extends to the surface. *AJR Am J Roentgenol* 1993;161:101–107.


## ADDITIONAL READING


- Andrish JT. Meniscal injuries in children and adolescents: diagnosis and management. *J Am Acad Orthop Surg* 1996;4:231–237.
- Greis PE, Holmstrom MC, Bardana DD, et al. Meniscal injury: II. Management. *J Am Acad Orthop Surg* 2002;10:177–187.
- Greis PE, Bardana DD, Holmstrom MC, et al. Meniscal injury: I. Basic science and evaluation. *J Am Acad Orthop Surg* 2002;10:168–176.
- Hardin GT, Farr J, Bach BR, Jr. Meniscal tears: diagnosis, evaluation, and treatment. *Orthop Rev* 1992;21:1311–1317.
- Phillips BB. Arthroscopy of lower extremity. In: Canale ST, ed. *Campbell's Operative Orthopaedics*, 10th ed. St. Louis: Mosby, 2003:2515–2612.
- Urquhart MW, O'Leary JA, Giffin JR, et al. Knee. Section D. Meniscal injuries. 1. Meniscal injuries in the adult. In: DeLee JC, Drez D, Jr, Miller MD, eds. *DeLee & Drez's Orthopaedic Sports Medicine: Principles and Practice*, 2nd ed. Philadelphia: WB Saunders, 2003:1668–1686.
- Weiss CB, Lundberg M, Hamberg P, et al. Non-operative treatment of meniscal tears. *J Bone Joint Surg* 1989;71A:811–822.


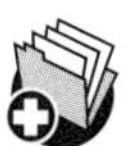

# MISCELLANEOUS

## CODES

### *ICD9-CM*

836.2 Meniscus tear

## FAQ

- Q: When can I walk after an arthroscopic meniscectomy?
  - A: For an isolated arthroscopic partial meniscectomy, weightbearing as tolerated can begin almost immediately.
- Q: What decides if a meniscus tear is repaired?
  - A: The decision is based on the capacity to heal, i.e., the presence of a blood supply. Acute tears, near the periphery, usually are repaired. Less peripheral and degenerative tears are resected.

# METACARPAL FRACTURE

*Emmanuel Hostin, MD*
*Simon C. Mears, MD, PhD*

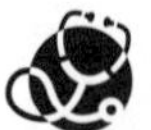

## BASICS

### DESCRIPTION

- A fracture of the metacarpal bone, the small tubular bone in the hand
- A 5th metacarpal neck fracture is called a "boxer fracture."
- Metacarpal fractures are classified according to their anatomic location (at the head, neck, shaft, or base).
- Metacarpal fractures of the thumb are classified into 4 patterns (some eponymous), according to whether they are intra-articular or extra-articular and by the amount of comminution.
  - The Bennett fracture has a volar lip fragment of variable size at the CMC joint, and the remainder of the base is displaced from the joint.
  - The Rolando fracture is a Y-shaped intra-articular fracture.

### EPIDEMIOLOGY

Most common in males 10–29 years old (1)

#### *Incidence*

Hand fractures account for ~19% of all fractures, and the metacarpals are the 2nd most commonly broken bone in the hand (after the phalanges) (2).

#### *Prevalence*

In children, metacarpal fractures account for ~10–40% of all hand injuries and are most common in those 13–16 years old (3).

### RISK FACTORS

- Sports injuries
- Falls
- Bicycle injuries
- Maladaptive personality traits and anxiety symptoms (4)

### ETIOLOGY

- Mechanisms of metacarpal fractures include direct trauma and crush injuries, but most occur from axial loading applied at the metacarpal head.
- A common injury, the boxer fracture, is a fracture of the 5th metacarpal neck sustained while striking the 5th MCP joint of the clenched fist.

## DIAGNOSIS

### SIGNS AND SYMPTOMS

- The combination of history, physical examination, and radiographic views nearly always is diagnostic.
- Pain and swelling mainly occur in the dorsum of the hand.

#### *Physical Exam*

- Patients present with pain, swelling, and deformity at the location of the fracture.
- Assess the shortening and malrotation of the affected digit by looking at the cascade of fingers when a fist is made.
- Document the neurologic examination with 2-point discrimination and capillary refill.
- Examine any break in the skin to ensure that the fracture is not open or that an intra-articular injury did not occur.

### TESTS

There are no laboratory tests to aid in the diagnosis.

#### *Imaging*

- Obtain AP, lateral, and oblique plain radiographic views.
- A true lateral view is necessary to measure fracture angulation.
- Focused views on the involved metacarpal can give better detail of the fracture pattern.

#### *Pathological Findings*

- Disruption of the bone cortex and periosteum
- Hematoma formation
- Later callus formation with eventual healing

### DIFFERENTIAL DIAGNOSIS

- Dislocation of the MCP joint
- Extensor or flexor tendon injury
- Contusion or soft-tissue trauma

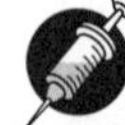

## TREATMENT

### GENERAL MEASURES

- Nonoperative treatment:
  - Most metacarpal fractures can be treated by splinting and casting.
  - An angulated fracture should be reduced and splinted.
  - The role of immobilization for 5th metacarpal fractures has been questioned.
    - 1 study has shown that an Ace wrap is sufficient treatment for displacement of <70° (5).
  - The hand should be splinted in the "position of function," which is thought to lessen later stiffness.
    - Wrist in ~20° of dorsal angulation
    - MCP joints of both the affected and adjacent finger at 70–90° of flexion
    - The PIP and DIP joints in full extension
  - However, a recent study questioned the importance of the splint position and focused on keeping the length of time of immobilization to <5 weeks (6).
  - A recent meta-analysis showed no difference in outcomes among several methods of casting or splinting (7).
  - The patient should be instructed about the possibility of surgery if fracture reduction cannot be maintained with splinting.
  - Ice, elevation, and analgesics are important adjuncts in the initial treatment.
- Operative treatment is indicated for:
  - Unstable, intra-articular, or multiple-digit fracture pattern.
    - Intra-articular fractures must be anatomically reduced.
  - Inability to obtain a satisfactory reduction
  - Malrotation of the digits
  - Open fractures:
    - Common in fight–bite injuries in which the MCP joint is penetrated by a tooth
    - Treated with operative irrigation, débridement, and pin fixation

- Reasonable guidelines for permissible apex–dorsal angulation of the fractures are 10° for the index, 20° for the middle, 30° for the ring, and 40° for the small fingers.
  - Rotatory displacements in general are not acceptable and require additional treatment.
- Most metacarpal fractures heal by 2 months.

### SPECIAL THERAPY

#### *Physical Therapy*

Gentle, active, and passive ROM motion exercises typically can be performed.

### SURGERY

- Treatment of metacarpal fractures includes the use of pins, plates, screws, external fixators, and intramedullary pins.
  - Pins or Kirschner wires may be used in a longitudinal fashion to maintain length and rotation of fractures.
  - Mini-fragment plates may be used to repair fractures.
  - Kirschner wires also may be used as intramedullary pins to maintain fracture reduction.
- Fractures with substantial bone loss, such as from a gunshot wound, occasionally require an external fixator.

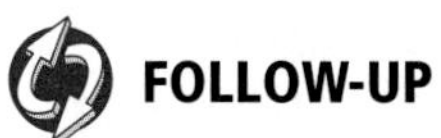

## FOLLOW-UP

### PROGNOSIS

- The prognosis is good to excellent when fractures are treated nonoperatively (6).
- Kirschner wire and intramedullary pin fixation have been shown to have excellent results for metacarpal neck fractures (8).
- Kirschner wire fixation gives excellent results for metacarpal shaft and base fractures (9).
- Plate fixation may have more complications than nonoperative treatment or less invasive surgical techniques but may be necessary for comminuted fractures or those with bone loss (10).
- Intra-articular fractures of the base of the thumb have good results when treated with Kirschner wires (11).
- Comminuted intra-articular fractures have the worst prognosis, with subsequent joint pain and decreased function.

### COMPLICATIONS

- Soft-tissue damage results from the initial injury or is secondary to overzealous reduction attempts.
- Flexor or extensor tendons may be damaged or develop decreased excursion.
- Malunions with angulation and rotational deformity have the worst prognosis.
- MCP stiffness is the result of immobilizing the joint in extension and allowing the collateral ligaments to shorten.
- Surgical complications include infection, delayed wound healing, and sensory nerve injury.
- Septic arthritis of the MCP joint may occur after fight bites or bites from dogs or cats.

### PATIENT MONITORING

- Obtain radiographs 1 week after closed or open reduction, and repeat in another 2–3 weeks.
- Begin early ROM when appropriate.

### REFERENCES


1. de Jonge JJ, Kingma J, van der Lei B, et al. Fractures of the metacarpals. A retrospective analysis of incidence and aetiology and a review of the English-language literature. *Injury* 1994;25:365–369.
2. van Onselen EBH, Karim RB, Hage JJ, et al. Prevalence and distribution of hand fractures. *J Hand Surg* 2003;28B:491–495.
3. Cornwall R. Finger metacarpal fractures and dislocations in children. *Hand Clin* 2006;22:1–10.
4. Mercan S, Uzun M, Ertugrul A, et al. Psychopathology and personality features in orthopedic patients with boxer's fractures. *Gen Hosp Psychiatry* 2005;27:13–17.
5. Statius Muller MG, Poolman RW, van Hoogstraten MJ, et al. Immediate mobilization gives good results in boxer's fractures with volar angulation up to 70 degrees: a prospective randomized trial comparing immediate mobilization with cast immobilization. *Arch Orthop Trauma Surg* 2003;123:534–537.
6. Tavassoli J, Ruland RT, Hogan CJ, et al. Three cast techniques for the treatment of extra-articular metacarpal fractures. Comparison of short-term outcomes and final fracture alignments. *J Bone Joint Surg* 2005;87A:2196–2201.
7. Poolman RW, Goslings JC, Lee JB, et al. Conservative treatment for closed fifth (small finger) metacarpal neck fractures (review). *Cochrane Database Syst Rev* 2006;1–32.
8. Wong TC, Ip FK, Yeung SH. Comparison between percutaneous transverse fixation and intramedullary K-wires in treating closed fractures of the metacarpal neck of the little finger. *J Hand Surg* 2006;31B:61–65.
9. Galanakis I, Aligizakis A, Katonis P, et al. Treatment of closed unstable metacarpal fractures using percutaneous transverse fixation with Kirschner wires. *J Trauma* 2003;55:509–513.
10. Fusetti C, Meyer H, Borisch N, et al. Complications of plate fixation in metacarpal fractures. *J Trauma* 2002;52:535–539.
11. Bruske J, Bednarski M, Niedzwiedz Z, et al. The results of operative treatment of fractures of the thumb metacarpal base. *Acta Orthop Belg* 2001;67:368–373.


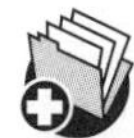

## MISCELLANEOUS

### CODES

#### *ICD9-CM*

- 815.00 Closed metacarpal fracture
- 815.10 Open metacarpal fracture

### PATIENT TEACHING

- Intra-articular fractures have a higher incidence of stiffness and pain after healing.
- Early ROM activities are begun when the fracture is stable.

### FAQ

- Q: How long does a metacarpal fracture take to heal?
  - A: Metacarpal fractures usually heal in ~2–3 months.
- Q: Do metacarpal fractures require surgery?
  - A: Most metacarpal fractures are treated without surgery.

# METASTATIC BONE DISEASE

*Frank J. Frassica, MD*
*Deborah A. Frassica, MD*
*Fariba Asrari, MD*

## BASICS

### DESCRIPTION

- The most common cause of destructive bone lesions in the adult
- The amount of bone destruction varies from small amounts to complete fracture.
- Bone metastases occur less commonly in children than in adults.
- Virtually any malignancy may metastasize to bone.
  - With some cancers (such as breast and prostate cancer), virtually all patients have bone metastases at the time of death.

### ALERT

A patient who has metastatic bone disease with severe back pain and numbness or weakness may be at risk for paralysis and should be evaluated carefully for spinal cord compression.

#### *Geriatric Considerations*

- Metastatic bone disease is common in the geriatric patient.
- This diagnosis should be considered in the older patient with bone pain.

#### *Pediatric Considerations*

- Metastatic bone disease is rare in the pediatric patient.
- Children with rhabdomyosarcoma or neuroblastoma who have bone pain should be evaluated for the presence of metastatic disease.

### EPIDEMIOLOGY

- Some cancers are prone to bone metastases (1):
  - Breast cancer
  - Prostate cancer
  - Kidney cancer
  - Lung cancer

#### *Incidence*

Up to 50% of patients with high-grade cancers may develop bone metastases when they have advanced disease (1).

### RISK FACTORS

- Any cancer
- Advanced disease

#### *Genetics*

No specific genetic associations are known.

### PATHOPHYSIOLOGY

- The bone destruction in metastatic bone disease is directly caused by osteoclasts (2).
- The tumor cells secrete factors that cause osteoclast activation.
  - Breast cancer and parathyroid hormone-related protein:
    - Parathyroid-hormone-related peptide or other factors causes the release of receptor activator of nuclear factor $\kappa$B ligand from the osteoblasts.
    - The receptor activator of nuclear factor $\kappa$B ligand attaches to the receptor activator of nuclear factor $\kappa$B receptor on the osteoclast precursor cells and signals the cell to differentiate into an osteoclast.

### ETIOLOGY

Hematogenous dissemination of cancer cells into the bone marrow

## DIAGNOSIS

### SIGNS AND SYMPTOMS

- Patients present with bone pain.
  - May be dull and occur at rest
  - May be sharp and occur with weightbearing
  - May occur at night and be intense
- Patients may be unable to walk secondary to the pain.

#### *History*

- Patients with a history of cancer should be queried as to whether they have any bone pain.
- Patients >40 years old with bone pain should always be asked about any previous cancer.
- Elicit a careful history of the bone pain:
  - Is the pain constant?
  - Does the pain occur with weightbearing?
  - Does the pain occur at night?
  - Can the patient localize the site of the pain?

#### *Physical Exam*

- The clinician should examine the patient gently (abrupt maneuvers may cause a fracture).
  - Palpate for bone tenderness.
  - Palpate for soft-tissue masses.
  - Check ROM.
  - Perform careful neurologic examination.
  - Evaluate motor weakness.
  - Check sensation.
  - Check deep tendon reflexes.

### TESTS

#### *Lab*

Serum tests to evaluate for anemia, hypercalcemia

#### *Imaging*

- To detect metastases, assess for impending fracture or neurologic compromise, or check the response to treatment.
- Radiography:
  - AP and lateral views to assess the amount of cortical bone destruction
  - Involvement can be categorized as purely lytic, mixed lytic-blastic, or purely blastic.
- Technetium bone scans:
  - Areas of involvement show increased activity.
  - The entire skeleton is imaged.
  - False positives may be caused by degenerative disease or old fractures.
  - False negatives may be caused by rapidly destructive lesions (some lung and kidney cancers).
- CT:
  - Excellent for defining the amount of cortical bone loss
  - Often used for preoperative planning for the pelvis and spine
- MRI:
  - Excellent for detecting marrow involvement when the plain radiographs are normal
  - Often used to determine if positive bone scan findings represent true metastatic involvement
    - Bone metastases are low signal on T1-weighted images and high signal on T2-weighted images.

#### *Diagnostic Procedures/Surgery*

- A systematic approach must be used to evaluate the patient with suspected bone metastases.
  - Imaging studies:
    - Plain radiographs of painful sites
    - CT of the chest and abdomen to detect lung and kidney cancer, adenopathy
    - Technetium bone scan to look for multiple bone sites
  - Blood tests:
    - Complete blood cell count: Low hemoglobin is suggestive of myeloma.
    - ESR: High rate is suggestive of myeloma.
    - Calcium/$PO_4$: Elevated calcium, low $PO_4$ is suggestive of hyperparathyroidism.
  - Biopsy is necessary to establish or confirm the diagnosis.
    - CT-guided needle biopsy is the most commonly performed procedure.

#### *Pathological Findings*

- Marrow is replaced with cancer cells and fibrous tissue (3).
  - Osteoclasts resorb the bone.
  - Tumor cells are characteristically in clumps in an organoid pattern.
  - Special stains (e.g., keratin stain) are used to confirm the epithelial nature of the tumor.

### DIFFERENTIAL DIAGNOSIS

- Metastatic bone disease can be confused with several entities:
  - Multiple myeloma may cause diffuse lytic bone destruction.
  - Lymphoma often causes replacement of the bone marrow in a manner similar to that of metastatic disease.
  - Bone infarcts can cause multiple lesions, especially after chemotherapy, and these may be confused with metastatic disease.
  - Enchondromas (common and inactive) may show increased uptake on the technetium bone scan and be confused with bone metastases.

## TREATMENT

### INITIAL STABILIZATION
- Patients with weightbearing pain are assessed with plain radiographs to determine the fracture risk.
  - If the cortical bone destruction is >25–50%, a walking aid such as crutches or a walker is advised.
  - If the patient has back pain and a neurologic deficit, an emergent MRI is performed to assess the risk of spinal cord compression.
    - If the MRI shows compression of the neural elements, an orthopaedic spine or neurosurgery consultation is obtained.

### GENERAL MEASURES
A systematic treatment plan is developed to halt progression of bone metastases, control pain, and maintain the patient's activity level and independence.

#### *Activity*
- The activity level is modified based on the degree of bone destruction.
  - 25–50% cortical bone destruction (long bone): Activity is restricted to ambulating with a walking aid and avoiding heavy activities (e.g., jumping, twisting, lifting).
  - 25–50% vertebral body destruction: Activity is modified to avoid heavy activities.

#### *Nursing*
Major goal: Control pain, maintain patient independence

### SPECIAL THERAPY
#### *Radiotherapy*
- External beam irradiation often is used to control pain and halt bone destruction.
- Several regimens are efficacious:
  - 3,000 cGy in 10 daily fractions
  - 2,000 cGy in 5 daily fractions
  - 800 cGy in a single fraction:
    - Chosen for the very ill patient who cannot tolerate numerous trips to the radiation oncology unit
    - Used mainly for pain control
  - Systemic radiopharmaceuticals are used occasionally in diffuse blastic disease.
  - Strontium

#### *Physical Therapy*
- To maintain activities of daily living and independence
- Care must be taken not to push patients beyond their capacity or to cause a fracture.
- Manipulation of the limbs or spine should never be performed.

### MEDICATION (DRUGS)
- Medications must be used liberally to control pain (4).
  - Long-acting narcotics are used to achieve basal serum levels.
  - Short-acting narcotics are used to control breakthrough pain.

#### *First Line*
- Diphosphonate therapy has become an integral component of therapy (4).
  - Halts bone destruction and facilitates healing of the defect
  - Skeletal events (e.g., fractures) decrease in patients on diphosphonate therapy (4).
  - Osteonecrosis of the jaw rarely occurs as a side effect of diphosphonates.
  - Patients with poor dentition should be referred to an oral surgeon before beginning diphosphonate therapy.

### SURGERY
- Stabilization of long bones and the spine is important to prevent fracture or spinal cord paralysis.
  - Long bones:
    - Prophylactic fixation is recommended when cortical bone destruction is >50% (3).
    - Internal fixation devices are used when rigid fixation can be achieved.
    - Prosthetic devices are chosen when rigid fixation cannot be achieved or the joint surfaces have been destroyed.
  - Spine:
    - When severe destruction occurs in the vertebral body and/or posterior elements, stabilization is recommended to prevent fracture and neural element compromise.

## FOLLOW-UP

### PROGNOSIS
- Virtually all patients will succumb to their disease.
- The prognosis depends on histologic type.
- Survival after fracture secondary to metastatic bone disease (1):
  - Lung, kidney, melanoma: 6–12 months
  - Breast, prostate: 24–48 months

### COMPLICATIONS
- Systemic complications and complications directly related to the bone metastases may occur.
- Hypercalcemia:
  - Common in lung and breast cancer, myeloma, and lymphoma
  - Treated with hydration and diphosphonates
- Anemia:
  - Common secondary to marrow replacement and chemotherapy/radiation therapy

### PATIENT MONITORING
Patients are followed at 1–6-month intervals depending on the temporal progression of their disease.

### REFERENCES

1. Frassica FJ, Frassica DA. Metastatic bone disease: General considerations. In: Menendez LR, ed. *Orthopaedic Knowledge Update: Musculoskeletal Tumors.* Rosemont, IL: American Academy of Orthopaedic Surgeons, 2002:305–312.
2. Roodman GD. Mechanisms of bone metastasis. *N Engl J Med* 2004;350:1655–1664.
3. McCarthy EF, Frassica FJ. Metastatic carcinoma in bone. In: *Pathology of Bone and Joint Disorders: With Clinical and Radiographic Correlation.* Philadelphia: WB Saunders, 1998:175–183.
4. Galanis E. Supportive measures: Carcinoma metastatic to bone. In: Menendez LR, ed. *Orthopaedic Knowledge Update: Musculoskeletal Tumors.* Rosemont, IL: American Academy of Orthopaedic Surgeons, 2002:331–341.


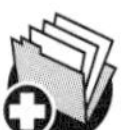

## MISCELLANEOUS

### CODES
#### *ICD9-CM*
198.5 Secondary malignant neoplasm, bone and bone marrow, all sites

### PATIENT TEACHING
- Patients must be taught to recognize the warning signs of spinal cord paralysis and impending fracture of a long bone.
- Paralysis:
  - Numbness/tingling
  - Weakness
  - Change in bowel/bladder habits
- Impending fracture:
  - Lower extremity long bones:
    - Pain with ambulation
    - Inability to stand or bear weight
  - Upper extremity long bones:
    - Pain with activities of daily living
  - Spine:
    - Severe pain
    - Neurologic symptoms/signs

#### *Prevention*
- No methods of preventing bone metastases exist.
- Spinal cord paralysis can be prevented by preventing neurologic compression and stabilizing the unstable spinal segments.
- Long-bone fractures can be prevented by prophylactic internal fixation or prosthetic arthroplasty.

### FAQ
- Q: Can fractures be stabilized so that patients can walk again?
  - A: Because many techniques and devices exist, almost any fracture can be stabilized so that the patient can bear full weight after the surgery.
- Q: Is irradiation necessary after surgery for a fracture?
  - A: Irradiation is always necessary. Up to 15–20% of patients will need additional surgery because of disease progression when postoperative irradiation is not used.
- Q: Will irradiation stop the bone pain?
  - A: External beam irradiation is very effective, controlling pain in 80–90% of patients.

M

# METATARSAL FRACTURE

*Clifford L. Jeng, MD*
*Carl Wierks, MD*

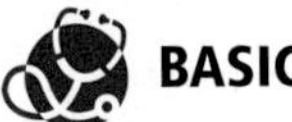

## BASICS

### DESCRIPTION
- Fractures of the forefoot:
- Classification (1):
  - Metatarsal head, neck, or shaft fractures
  - Stress fractures most commonly involve the 2nd metatarsal and result from repetitive overuse.
  - 5th metatarsal fractures can be subdivided:
    - Avulsion fractures, which are proximal to the metaphysis (called "pseudo-Jones" fractures when the 5th metatarsal is involved)
    - Jones fractures are fractures of the 5th metatarsal at the metaphyseal–diaphyseal junction; they are notoriously unstable.
    - Diaphyseal stress fractures
    - Synonyms: Jones fracture; Pseudo-Jones fracture; Stress or marching fracture

### GENERAL PREVENTION
- Avoid foot trauma.
- Modify training regimens to avoid overuse.
  - Gradually increase time and distance when starting or changing a running program.
  - Use new running shoes that are not overly worn.

### EPIDEMIOLOGY
Occurs in both genders at all ages

#### *Incidence*
- These injuries are common, especially 5th metatarsal fractures in athletes.
- Fractures also are common in osteoporotic females (2).

### RISK FACTORS
- Stress fractures of the metatarsals occur with excessive training or repetitive stress in athletes or with a sudden increase in the level of exercise of any person.
- Osteoporosis

### ETIOLOGY
The injury usually is a result of a direct blow, inversion injury, or overuse.

### ASSOCIATED CONDITIONS
- Compartment syndrome (rarely)
- Lisfranc dislocation

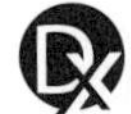

## DIAGNOSIS

### SIGNS AND SYMPTOMS
- Pain
- Swelling
- Deformity
- Ecchymosis
- Difficulty bearing weight
- Tenderness over the affected metatarsals

#### *History*
Direct trauma, inversion injury to foot, or sudden increase in training regimen

#### *Physical Exam*
- Physical examination usually reveals point tenderness over the involved metatarsal.
- Severe swelling of the entire forefoot commonly occurs.

### TESTS

#### *Imaging*
- Plain films usually are diagnostic.
  - AP, lateral, and oblique foot images are mandatory.
  - Alignment in the lateral film is the most important aspect in management of these injuries.
- If plain radiographs are inconclusive, bone scanning or MRI may be helpful in detecting occult fractures (3).

#### *Pathological Findings*
Longstanding fractures may show signs of delayed union or nonunion.

### DIFFERENTIAL DIAGNOSIS
- Soft-tissue contusion
- Sprain
- Lisfranc dislocation

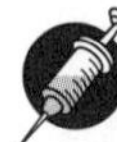

## TREATMENT

### GENERAL MEASURES
- Isolated metatarsal neck or shaft fractures can be treated with a well-fitted below-the-knee cast or postoperative shoe and weightbearing as tolerated for 3–4 weeks, followed by a well-padded shoe.
  - Length of time in a cast should be limited to avoid complications (4).
- If angulation is $>10°$, closed reduction with or without stabilization with percutaneous pins may be required.
- The most important alignment is the sagittal alignment (i.e., apex inferior) because malunion in this plane may cause metatarsalgia or pain on the dorsum of the foot.
  - Displacement in the transverse plane usually is well tolerated in the 2nd–4th metatarsals.
  - Angulation in this plane of the 1st or 5th metatarsal may cause difficulty with shoe wear and should be reduced.
- Injuries with multiple metatarsal fractures often are unstable and require open reduction and internal fixation with small-fragment plates or Kirschner wires.
- Metatarsal head fractures are rare and, if they are unstable after reduction, may require open reduction and internal fixation.
- Closed treatment consists of 4–6 weeks in a below-the-knee walking cast.
- Patients with Jones fractures that are treated closed should remain nonweightbearing for 8 weeks.
  - These fractures have a high rate of subsequent displacement and should be stabilized operatively if they are displaced $>2$ mm.
  - Some authors advocate operative stabilization in all active individuals, even for fractures with $<2$ mm displacement (5).
- Avulsion fractures of the 5th metatarsal need only a postoperative (hard-soled) shoe (6).
- Patients with stress fractures need activity modification for 3–4 weeks and protection in a cast or orthosis.
- Metatarsal head fractures usually result from a direct blow to the foot.
  - Closed reduction usually is successful and stable.
  - If the fracture is unstable, percutaneous pinning with Kirschner wires may be used.

### *Pediatric Considerations*

- Growth plate injuries to the metatarsals are rare but may occur when the chondroepiphysis is avulsed, a fracture extends into the epiphysis, or the condylar surface of the secondary ossification center is avulsed.
- These fractures can be treated in a below-the-knee walking cast for 3–4 weeks.
- Overgrowth is more common than growth inhibition.

## SPECIAL THERAPY

### *Physical Therapy*

- No need for routine physical therapy
- Once healed, patients usually have little difficulty in returning to activities of daily living.

## MEDICATION (DRUGS)

Recommended medications are analgesics other than NSAIDs because the latter may inhibit bone healing.

## SURGERY

- The goal is anatomic reduction to restore the weightbearing complex of the forefoot.
- Indications:
  - 2–4 mm of shortening or elevation of the 2nd–4th metatarsals; less deformity is accepted in the 1st and 5th metatarsals.
  - Other surgical indications are delayed union or nonunion.
- Metatarsal fractures:
  - Open reduction and internal fixation: Dorsal incision with 1/3 tubular plates and 3.5-mm cortical screws on the tension side
  - Intramedullary fixation with Kirschner wires extending out the distal tip of the toe
- Jones fractures:
  - May be treated with open reduction and internal fixation with a long intramedullary malleolar screw because of the increased tendency to nonunion (5)
  - Patients with Jones fractures treated by open reduction and internal fixation can be advanced gradually in weightbearing after 2 weeks.
- Nonunions (usually apex plantar):
  - Should be treated by resection of the edges of the malunion, slight overcorrection of the angular deformity, and stabilization with percutaneous pinning.
  - Bone grafting also may be required.

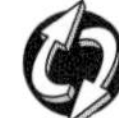

# FOLLOW-UP

## DISPOSITION

Patients generally benefit from walking aides, such as crutches, in the initial postinjury period.

## PROGNOSIS

The prognosis is good if no substantial sagittal displacement occurs at the time of healing.

## COMPLICATIONS

- Transfer metatarsalgia
- Neuroma
- Delayed union
- Nonunion
- Difficulty with shoe wear

## PATIENT MONITORING

- Follow-up radiographs should be obtained 1 week after reduction to ensure satisfactory alignment, and a 2nd set should be obtained 4–5 weeks after injury.
- Follow-up radiographs should show callus and healing of the metatarsal fractures.
- Clinically, the patient should no longer be tender over the healed fracture site.

## REFERENCES


1. Fetzer GB, Wright RW. Metatarsal shaft fractures and fractures of the proximal fifth metatarsal. *Clin Sports Med* 2006;25:139–150.
2. Hasselman CT, Vogt MT, Stone KL, et al. Foot and ankle fractures in elderly white women. Incidence and risk factors. *J Bone Joint Surg* 2003;85A: 820–824.
3. Ashman CJ, Klecker RJ, Yu JS. Forefoot pain involving the metatarsal region: differential diagnosis with MR imaging. *Radiographics* 2001;21:1425–1440.
4. Zenios M, Kim WY, Sampath J, et al. Functional treatment of acute metatarsal fractures: a prospective randomised comparison of management in a cast versus elasticated support bandage. *Injury* 2005;36:832–835.
5. Mologne TS, Lundeen JM, Clapper MF, et al. Early screw fixation versus casting in the treatment of acute Jones fractures. *Am J Sports Med* 2005;33: 970–975.
6. Konkel KF, Menger AG, Retzlaff SA. Nonoperative treatment of fifth metatarsal fractures in an orthopaedic suburban private multispecialty practice. *Foot Ankle Int* 2005;26:704–707.


## ADDITIONAL READING


- Armagan OE, Shereff MJ. Injuries to the toes and metatarsals. *Orthop Clin North Am* 2001;32:1–10.
- Rammelt S, Heineck J, Zwipp H. Metatarsal fractures. *Injury* 2004;35:SB77–SB86.


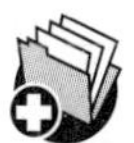

# MISCELLANEOUS

## CODES

### *ICD9-CM*

825.25 Fracture of metatarsal bones

## PATIENT TEACHING

Patients should be warned about the risks of nonunion and possible metatarsalgia.

## FAQ

- Q: Should a cast be applied to all metatarsal fractures?
  - A: Most metatarsal fractures can be treated with a hard-soled shoe. Displaced fractures may be considered for surgery. Jones-type fractures should be treated with a cast or surgery.

# METATARSUS ADDUCTUS

*Paul D. Sponseller, MD*

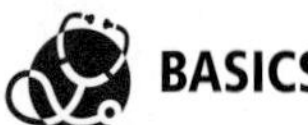

## BASICS

### DESCRIPTION
- Metatarsus adductus is a deformity in which the forepart of the foot is adducted or medially deviated (Fig. 1); the heel is in neutral or mild valgus position.
- The most common foot condition seen by those caring for children
- It appears in the newborn.
- Classification (1) is based on flexibility: Flexible (correctable with manipulation) or rigid (a continuum)
- Degree of deformity:
  - Based on heel bisector method: The line bisecting the heel is drawn by visual examination of the foot's sole; it normally crosses between 2nd and 3rd toes.
    - Mild: Heel bisector crosses the 3rd toe.
    - Moderate: Heel bisector crosses between the 3rd and 4th toes.
    - Severe: Heel bisector crosses between the 4th and 5th toes.
- Synonyms: Metatarsus varus; Pes varus; Metatarsus internus; Hooked forefoot; Z-foot or C-foot

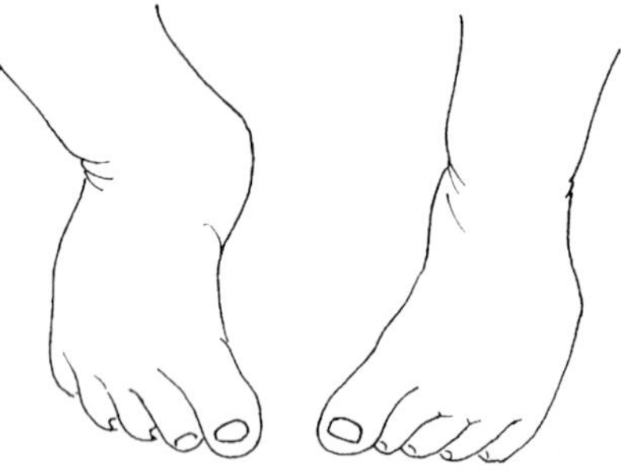

**Fig. 1.** Metatarsus adductus is characterized by a deviated forefoot but a normal hindfoot and ankle.

### GENERAL PREVENTION
No effective means of preventing this deformity exist.

### EPIDEMIOLOGY
#### *Incidence*
- 1–10 per 1,000 infants (2)
- Equally distributed between males and females

### RISK FACTORS
- Family history
- Hip dysplasia

#### *Genetics*
The risk is higher for those with 1st-degree relatives who have metatarsus adductus.

### ETIOLOGY
- Unknown
- No association with birth order, gestational age, or maternal age
- Most accepted theory: Metatarsus adductus is a possible result of tight intrauterine packing.

### ASSOCIATED CONDITIONS
DDH of the hip occurs in 1–5% of patients with metatarsus adductus (2).

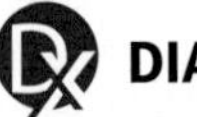

## DIAGNOSIS

### SIGNS AND SYMPTOMS
- Adduction (medial deviation) of the forefoot, with various degrees of supination
  - Concave medial border and convex lateral border of the foot is seen, with prominence at the base of the 5th metatarsal.
- The heel is in neutral or slightly valgus position, but not in equinus (foot-down).
- The flexible deformity may persist until 1–2 years of age.
- Most feet (86% in 1 study) become normal, 10% are mildly adducted, and 4% remain adducted without treatment (2,3).
- In another natural history study (3), no patients had foot problems when treated with observation alone.
- A deep medial crease suggests moderate deformity.

#### *Physical Exam*
- Determine the flexibility of the forefoot adduction by trying to correct it.
- Determine the ankle ROM.
- The forefoot is deviated medially but flexible.
- The hindfoot is normal, and the foot may be dorsiflexed to a flat position.
- Also check the hips for dysplasia.

### TESTS
#### *Imaging*
- Radiographic evaluation is unnecessary for most patients.
- If congenital anomalies are suspected or the foot is stiff, AP and lateral views of foot may be obtained.

#### *Pathological Findings*
All structures of the foot are normal, except for the forefoot, which is deviated medially.

### DIFFERENTIAL DIAGNOSIS
- Clubfoot (heel varus and foot equinus):
  - More rigid
  - Whole foot turned inward

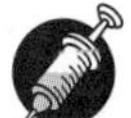

# TREATMENT

## GENERAL MEASURES

- This condition resolves spontaneously in most patients.
- Parents should be educated about this deformity.
- Medical treatment:
  - Most children with metatarsus adductus at birth do not require treatment.
  - For severe unresolving deformity, serial manipulation and casting may be offered.
  - The appropriate age at which to start casting is usually 6–12 months.
  - It is appropriate to wait longer if the parents are willing because most feet will improve spontaneously with time.
  - The duration of cast treatment is several months.
  - Children may be placed in straight- or reverse-last shoes for several months after the foot is straightened by cast treatment.
  - Because most of these feet improve spontaneously, early cast treatment before 6 months is not recommended.

### *Activity*

Patients may participate in weightbearing activity as tolerated.

## SPECIAL THERAPY

### *Physical Therapy*

- Stretching of the foot is recommended for patients with a flexible deformity.
  - Parents may perform this stretching during diaper changes.

## SURGERY

- Surgery is an option, but it is rarely indicated.
  - Only for children >4 years old who have residual metatarsus adductus
- Procedures include the following:
  - Lateral shortening osteotomy
  - Medial cuneiform opening wedge osteotomy

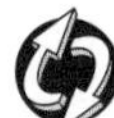

# FOLLOW-UP

## PROGNOSIS

- >95% patients with mild and moderate deformity have done well in long-term, follow-up studies (3).
- It is controversial whether the flexibility of the foot predicts prognosis.

## COMPLICATIONS

- Failure to correct the deformity completely (uncommon)
- AVN of the cuneiform

## PATIENT MONITORING

- Frequency of follow-up varies by the individual.
- It should be more frequent in patients with moderate and severe deformity and in those undergoing treatment.

## REFERENCES

1. Cook DA, Breed AL, Cook T, et al. Observer variability in the radiographic measurement and classification of metatarsus adductus. *J Pediatr Orthop* 1992;12:86–89.
2. Kasser JR. The foot. In: Morrissy RT, Weinstein SL, eds. *Lovell and Winter's Pediatric Orthopaedics*, 6th ed. Philadelphia: Lippincott Williams & Wilkins, 2006:1257–1328.
3. Farsetti P, Weinstein SL, Ponseti IV. The long-term functional and radiographic outcomes of untreated and non-operatively treated metatarsus adductus. *J Bone Joint Surg* 1994;76A:257–265.

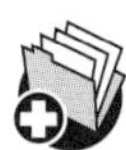

# MISCELLANEOUS

## CODES

### *ICD9-CM*

754.53 Metatarsus adductus

## PATIENT TEACHING

- Stress the benign nature of this condition.
- Even if a mild degree of adduction persists, it has no functionally negative consequences.

## FAQ

- Q: What problems could arise from untreated metatarsus adductus?
  - A: In most patients, the adduction resolves if given enough time. The only possible sequelae relate to the fitting of shoes in a minority of patients.

# MONTEGGIA FRACTURE

*Paul D. Sponseller, MD*
*Simon C. Mears, MD, PhD*

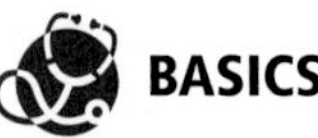

## BASICS

### DESCRIPTION

- Because the radius and ulna are bound by ligaments and an interosseous membrane, a displaced fracture of the ulna often is accompanied by dislocation of the radial head, a combination termed a Monteggia fracture (Fig. 1).
- The diagnosis sometimes is missed because the dislocation can be overlooked.
- Reduction of both the fracture and the dislocation must be achieved.
- Bado (1) classification:
  - Most commonly used system
  - Based on the direction of the dislocation of the radial head, which is the same as the direction of the apex of the ulnar fracture
  - 4 types:
    - I: Anterior dislocation of the radial head (most common type)
    - II: Posterior dislocation of the radial head
    - III: Lateral dislocation of the radial head (2nd most common pattern in childhood)
    - IV: Anterior dislocation of the radial head in combination with a proximal radial fracture

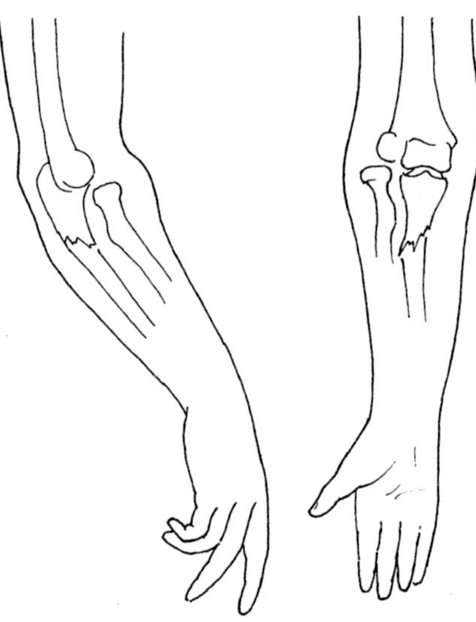

**Fig. 1.** An angulated, isolated ulna fracture causes the radial head to dislocate. This combination is called a Monteggia fracture.

### EPIDEMIOLOGY

Fracture occurrence is distributed evenly between males and females (2).

#### *Incidence*

- Relatively uncommon
- Peak incidence: Ages 4–10 years (3)
- However, this fracture may occur at any age, including adulthood.

#### *Prevalence*

- Most common in children: Bado type-I fractures, with plastic deformation of the ulna (4).
- Most common in adults: Bado type I and type II fractures (5)

### RISK FACTORS

Any child or adult with a fracture of the proximal or middle of the ulnar shaft should be considered at risk for this fracture.

### ETIOLOGY

- The ligamentous connections between the radius and ulna cause the radial head dislocation to occur when the ulna fractures, or vice versa.
- Type I fracture mechanism: Hyperpronation or hyperextension
- Type II fracture mechanism: Axial loading of a partially flexed elbow

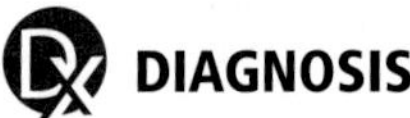

## DIAGNOSIS

### SIGNS AND SYMPTOMS

- Signs:
  - Swelling in the forearm and elbow
  - In cases diagnosed late, a bump may be present over the elbow at the time a cast is removed for treatment of an ulnar fracture, indicating the dislocated radial head.
- Symptoms:
  - Acutely, tenderness over the elbow and deformity
  - If diagnosed late, the unreduced radial head could block the full range of flexion or extension or cause clicking with pronation and supination.

#### *Physical Exam*

- In acute cases, diagnosis should be made primarily by radiography showing both the ulnar fracture and the radial head dislocation.
- In chronic cases, a prominence of the radial head is visible when the arm is out of the cast.
  - This prominence represents the dislocated radial head and may be compared with the opposite side.

### TESTS

#### *Imaging*

- Radiography:
  - Plain radiographs are sufficient for diagnosis.
  - All forearm fractures should include visualization of the elbow and wrist joints.
  - These radiographs should be true AP and lateral views.
    - If they cannot be obtained on the same film, separate films of these regions should be ordered.
    - The physician should be available to help in positioning, if needed.
- MRI is not required for diagnosis.

#### *Pathological Findings*

- At the time of injury, the annular ligament of the radius is torn and becomes infolded.
- If the radial head remains unreduced for several years, it degenerates because the cartilage wears away.

### DIFFERENTIAL DIAGNOSIS

- An isolated ulnar fracture may occur without radial head dislocation.
- The status of the radial head may be determined by drawing a line on the radiograph through the radial shaft.
  - This line should fall in the center of the capitellum of the distal humerus.
- An isolated radial head dislocation may occur, but it is rare.
- Congenital dislocation of the radial head does occur.
  - May be distinguished by changes in the shape of the radial head: Overgrowth and loss of the normal concave reciprocal articular surface

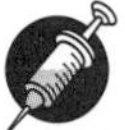

# TREATMENT

## GENERAL MEASURES

- For children, closed reduction usually is successful for treating both the dislocated radial head and the ulnar fracture.
- The mechanism used to reduce the ulnar fracture also is used to maintain reduction of the radial head fracture.
  - Type I fractures: The forearm should be in supination to midposition, and the elbow should be in flexion of >110°.
  - Type II fractures: The elbow should be in extension.
- In both type I and type II fractures, the radial head may require a push to place it properly.
- An above-the-elbow cast should be applied, and a bivalved cast should be used if substantial swelling is present.
- A radiograph should be obtained after reduction to confirm that alignment is satisfactory.
- Unstable or displaced fractures after reduction:
  - In children: Require open reduction and fixation
  - In adults: Require open reduction and internal fixation
- Follow-up in 1 week
- Late detection of a Monteggia fracture:
  - 1–3 weeks after injury, the radial head may require open reduction, even in children.
  - >3 weeks after injury, reconstruction of the annular ligament of the radial head may be necessary.

## SPECIAL THERAPY

### *Physical Therapy*

- Adults often need therapy to regain optimal motion.
- In children, physical therapy is not needed because parents can do the necessary exercises with them.

## SURGERY

- If the ulnar fracture cannot be maintained or reduced, open reduction and internal fixation should be performed, which usually causes the radial head to become and remain reduced.
- If it is not reduced, then an open reduction of the radial head should be performed.
- In a child, internal fixation of the ulna may be done with an intramedullary nail if closed reduction has failed.
- In adults, a Monteggia fracture should be treated directly with open reduction and internal fixation (rigid plate and screws) of the ulna.
  - Radial head reduction only if needed
- Late reconstruction of the annular ligament of the ulna is done using the Bell-Tawse technique (6).
  - A strip of triceps fascia is used to reconstruct the ligament and is anchored to the ulna.

# FOLLOW-UP

- In children, immobilization is continued for 6 weeks.
- In adults, because of a greater risk of stiffness, carefully supervised ROM may be started earlier.

## DISPOSITION

### *Issues for Referral*

Monteggia fractures should be referred to an orthopaedic surgeon promptly to ensure timely and adequate reduction.

## PROGNOSIS

- With careful reduction and follow-up, the prognosis is good (3).
- Stable injuries in children have an excellent prognosis with closed treatment.
- Bado type I injuries are thought to have a worse prognosis (7).
- Injuries that are associated with coronoid or radial head fracture also have poorer outcomes (2).
- Patients with missed injuries have a poorer prognosis.
- Results of late reconstruction are unpredictable (8).

## COMPLICATIONS

- Redislocation
- Stiffness
- Proximal radioulnar synostosis
- Elbow instability
- Nerve injury (usually radial) at time of radial head dislocation (9)

## PATIENT MONITORING

- The patient should be seen 1 week after injury to rule out redisplacement.
- Additional follow-up should be continued until ROM is satisfactory.

## REFERENCES


1. Bado JL. The Monteggia lesion. *Clin Orthop Relat Res* 1967;50:71–86.
2. Ring D, Jupiter JB, Simpson NS. Monteggia fractures in adults. *J Bone Joint Surg* 1998;80A:1733–1744.
3. Wiley JJ, Galey JP. Monteggia injuries in children. *J Bone Joint Surg* 1985;67B:728–731.
4. Ring D, Jupiter JB, Waters PM. Monteggia fractures in children and adults. *J Am Acad Orthop Surg* 1998;6:215–224.
5. Llusa Perez M, Lamas C, Martinez I, et al. Monteggia fractures in adults. Review of 54 cases. *Chir Main* 2002;21:293–297.
6. Bell Tawse AJS. The treatment of malunited anterior Monteggia fractures in children. *J Bone Joint Surg* 1965;47B:718–723.
7. Givon U, Pritsch M, Levy O, et al. Monteggia and equivalent lesions. A study of 41 cases. *Clin Orthop Relat Res* 1997;337:208–215.
8. David-West KS, Wilson NIL, Sherlock DA, et al. Missed Monteggia injuries. *Injury* 2005;36:1206–1209.
9. Ristic S, Strauch RJ, Rosenwasser MP. The assessment and treatment of nerve dysfunction after trauma around the elbow. *Clin Orthop Relat Res* 2000;370:138–153.


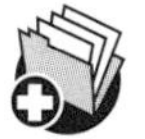

# MISCELLANEOUS

## CODES

### *ICD9-CM*

- 813.03 Closed Monteggia fracture
- 813.13 Open Monteggia fracture

## PATIENT TEACHING

- At the time of initial consultation, patients should be counseled about the risk of redislocation.
- Such counseling helps encourage compliance with follow-up care and exercises.

## FAQ

- Q: What is the prognosis of a Monteggia fracture in a child?
  - A: The prognosis of stable fractures treated without surgery is excellent. Missed fractures that are displaced have a much poorer outcome.

# MULTIPLE MYELOMA

*Frank J. Frassica, MD*

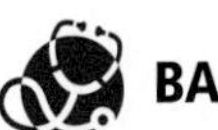

## BASICS

### DESCRIPTION
- The most common of the plasma cell dyscrasias (usually with a monoclonal gammopathy) affecting the hematopoietic, musculoskeletal, and renal systems.
- Classification (plasma cell dyscrasias):
  - Solitary myeloma
  - Multiple myeloma
  - Osteosclerotic myeloma
- Synonyms: Myeloma; Plasmacytoma

### EPIDEMIOLOGY (1)
- Rare in patients <40 years old
- The Male:Female ratio is ~2:1.
- The peak age is the 6th decade of life.

#### *Incidence*
~15,000 new cases (United States) annually (1)

### RISK FACTORS
Age >40 years

### ETIOLOGY
The cause is unknown.

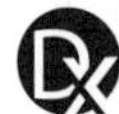

## DIAGNOSIS

### SIGNS AND SYMPTOMS
- Bone pain (usually of 6 months' duration) is the most frequent complaint at diagnosis.
- Constitutional symptoms of weakness, lethargy, and weight loss often occur.
- Back pain and rib pain are the 2 most frequent initial skeletal symptoms at presentation.
- Pathologic fracture usually results in sudden-onset pain.
- Peripheral neuropathy may be present.
- Tendency toward bleeding and fever
- Hypercalcemia is common.
- Monoclonal gammopathy is revealed by serum electrophoresis and urine immunoelectrophoresis.

#### *Physical Exam*
- Local pain and tenderness may be present.
- A palpable mass may be found, secondary to extraosseous extension of the tumor or hemorrhage related to it.
- Peripheral neuropathy may be detected in some patients with osteosclerotic myeloma.

### TESTS

#### *Lab*
- Hypercalcemia is seen in 1/3 of cases (2).
- Serum creatinine levels are elevated in ~50% of patients (2).
- Anemia with hemoglobin is <12 mg/dL in 2/3 of patients (2).
- Elevated ESRs are >50 mm/hour in 2/3 of patients (2).
- Serum electrophoresis and immunoelectrophoresis usually reveal monoclonal gammopathy.
- Bence Jones proteinuria is noted.
- Hypergammaglobulinemia may manifest itself as rouleaux formation appreciable on a peripheral blood smear.

#### *Imaging*
- Radiography:
  - Plain film radiographs reveal multiple small, discrete, lytic lesions most commonly involving the axial skeleton (skull, spine, ribs).
  - The surrounding bone does not show a sclerotic reaction, nor is there a periosteal reaction.
- Because bone scans have a high incidence of false-negative results, they are not used routinely.
  - A skeletal survey to evaluate for distant involvement often is a better study.

#### *Pathological Findings*
Monoclonal plasma cells are found in bone marrow.

### DIFFERENTIAL DIAGNOSIS
- Metastatic bone disease
- Malignant lymphoma
- Fibrosarcoma

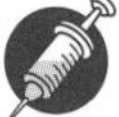

# TREATMENT

## GENERAL MEASURES

- The mainstay of treatment is chemotherapy.
- Surgical stabilization with irradiation is used for impending or complete pathologic fractures.
- External-beam irradiation is used for painful lesions that do not meet the criteria for pathologic fracture.
- Medical treatment:
  - Orthopaedic surgery consultation to consider surgical stabilization
  - Selected patients are treated with bone marrow transplantation.
    - Diphosphonate therapy has become an integral component of medical therapy because these drugs effectively halt osteoclastic bone resorption.
- Bone marrow transplantation commonly is offered.

### *Activity*

Limited activity, according to the level of symptoms and the nature of the bony lesions

## MEDICATION (DRUGS)

- NSAIDs or narcotic analgesics for pain control
- Chemotherapeutics (prednisone, alkylating agents)

## SURGERY

- Mostly internal fixation for stabilization of the long bones
- Decompression with spinal instrumentation may be necessary for patients with pathologic fractures and neurologic deficits.

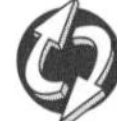

# FOLLOW-UP

## PROGNOSIS

- Prognosis is related to the stage of the disease, with an overall median survival of 18–24 months (1).
  - Virtually all patients eventually die of the disease.
- Bone marrow transplantation currently is being tried in an attempt to cure selected patients.

## COMPLICATIONS

- Pathologic fractures
- Spinal stenosis with compressive myelopathy
- Renal failure
- Amyloidosis (CTS)

## PATIENT MONITORING

- Monitor closely for impending pathologic fractures so that appropriate surgical intervention can occur before completion of pathologic fractures.
- Patients undergoing chemotherapy are monitored for changes in their serum protein levels to assess the response to treatment.

## REFERENCES


1. McCarthy EF, Frassica FJ. Plasma cell dyscrasia. In: *Pathology of Bone and Joint Disorders: With Clinical and Radiographic Correlation*. Philadelphia: WB Saunders, 1998:185–193.
2. Kyle RA. Multiple myeloma: review of 869 cases. *Mayo Clin Proc* 1975;50:29–40.


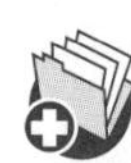

# MISCELLANEOUS

## CODES

### *ICD9-CM*

- 238.6 Solitary myeloma
- 302.0 Multiple myeloma

## FAQ

- Q: What is multiple myeloma?
  - A: Multiple myeloma is a malignant proliferation of plasma cells with end organ damage to bone and the kidneys.
- Q: Do all patients with multiple myeloma need diphosphonate therapy?
  - A: Yes, the diphosphonates are very effective in halting the osteoclastic bone resorption. The number of fractures of the long bones and vertebra are decreased markedly.
- Q: When is surgery necessary in patients with multiple myeloma?
  - A: Patients with impending fractures or those with severe weightbearing pain benefit from prophylactic fixation. Patients with a complete fracture are treated with internal fixation or a prosthetic arthroplasty.

# MUSCULAR DYSTROPHIES

*Paul D. Sponseller, MD*

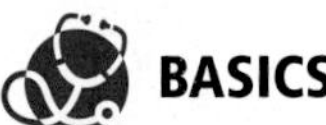

## BASICS

### DESCRIPTION

- Muscular dystrophies are a group of inherited disorders characterized by progressive degeneration and weakness of skeletal muscle without apparent cause in the nervous system.
- Skeletal and cardiac muscles are affected, and secondary effects occur in the lungs, skeleton, and many other systems.
- These conditions have been categorized by clinical distribution, severity of muscle weakness, and pattern of genetic inheritance.
- Because of limited space, only Duchenne muscular dystrophy is described in detail (Fig. 1).
- Classification:
  - Sex-linked muscular dystrophy: Duchenne muscular dystrophy, Becker, Emery-Dreifuss
  - Autosomal-recessive muscular dystrophy: Limb-girdle, infantile fascioscapulohumeral
  - Autosomal-dominant muscular dystrophy: Fascioscapulohumeral, distal, ocular, oculopharyngeal

### EPIDEMIOLOGY

#### *Incidence*

- Duchenne muscular dystrophy occurs in young boys.
- Duchenne muscular dystrophy occurs in 1 in 3,500 live male births (1).
- Becker dystrophy occurs in ~1 in 30,000 live male births (1).

### RISK FACTORS

Male gender

#### *Genetics*

- Duchenne muscular dystrophy is sex-linked, as is Becker-type tardive dystrophy.
- Other dystrophies are autosomal recessive and autosomal dominant.

### ETIOLOGY

- A single gene defect in the short arm of the X chromosome has been identified as being responsible for Duchenne muscular dystrophy and Becker muscular dystrophy.
  - The gene encodes the protein dystrophin, which is a component of the cell membrane cytoskeleton.

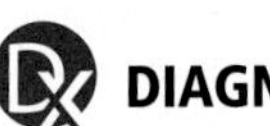

## DIAGNOSIS

### SIGNS AND SYMPTOMS

- Duchenne muscular dystrophy:
  - The disease occurs only in males, and it usually becomes evident at 3–6 years of age.
  - Common presentations include:
    - Delayed walking
    - "Waddling," Trendelenburg gait, or lordotic gait
    - Frequent tripping and falling
    - Inability to hop and jump
  - Progressive weakness occurs in the proximal muscle groups, including the gluteus, quadriceps, abdominal muscles, and shoulder girdle muscles
  - Pseudohypertrophy and contracture of calf muscles is common.
  - Most patients have cardiac involvement, most commonly tachycardia and right ventricular hypertrophy.
  - Many also have static encephalopathy with mental retardation.
  - Death from pulmonary and cardiac failure occurs during the 2nd or 3rd decade of life.
  - Because of hip muscle weakness, patients compensate by carrying the head and shoulders behind the pelvis during gait, thus producing an anterior pelvic tilt and increased lumbar lordosis.
  - Weakness in the shoulder girdle occurs 3–5 years after presentation.
    - It is difficult to lift the patient under the arms because of the weakness.
    - This weakness has been termed the "Meryon" sign.
  - No sensory deficits are detected.
  - Children usually are unable to ambulate effectively beyond 10 years of age.
- Becker muscular dystrophy:
  - Similar to Duchenne muscular dystrophy in clinical appearance and distribution of weakness, but less severe
  - The onset usually occurs after the age of 7 years.
  - The rate of progression is slower than in Duchenne muscular dystrophy
- Many more types of muscular dystrophy exist (not described here).

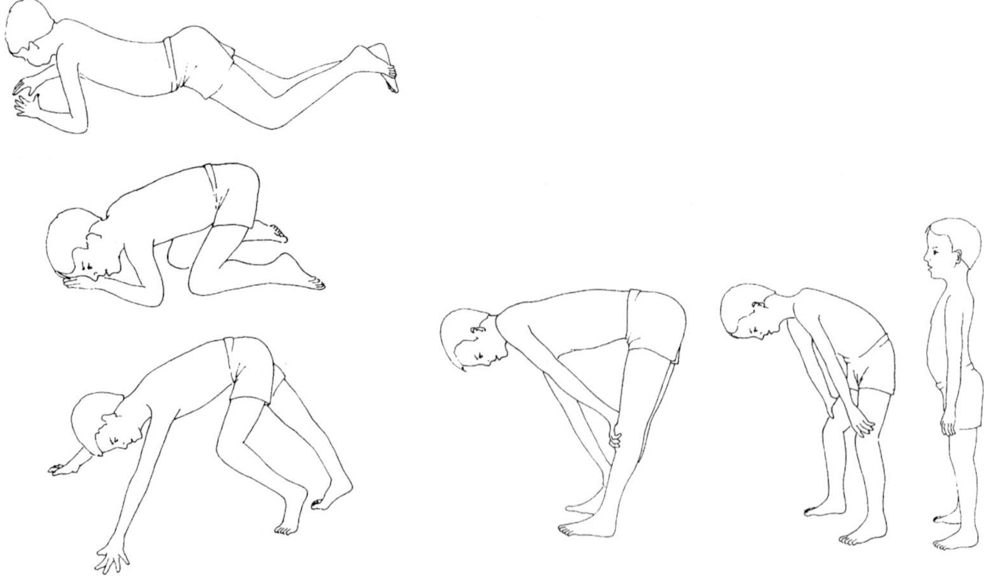

**Fig. 1.** This series of 6 drawings illustrates the Gower maneuver of a 7-year-old child with Duchenne muscular dystrophy.

### *Physical Exam*
- History, physical examination, measurement of creatine phosphokinase and dystrophin, and electromyography help in making the diagnosis.
- Electromyography shows a myopathic pattern, with reduced amplitude, short duration, and polyphasic muscle action potentials.
- Muscle biopsy also may be performed.
- Evaluate muscle bulk to assess for pseudohypertrophy of the calves.
- Observe the patient's gait and look for Trendelenburg gait.
- Starting proximally, look for muscle weakness.
- Evaluate the patient's ability to stabilize the shoulder; test for Meryon sign.
- Note contracture, developing later, followed by scoliosis.

## TESTS
### *Lab*
- Serum creatine phosphokinase markedly is elevated in the early stages of Duchenne muscular dystrophy.
  - It may be 200 times normal, but it later declines as muscle degeneration becomes complete.
- Dystrophin levels are completely absent in Duchenne muscular dystrophy; they are less than normal in Becker dystrophy.

### *Pathological Findings*
- Muscle degeneration, with subsequent loss of fibers
- Variation in fiber size
- Proliferation of connective tissue

## DIFFERENTIAL DIAGNOSIS
- Peripheral neuropathy
- Anterior horn cell disease
- Poliomyelitis

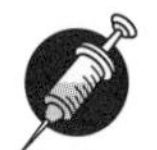

# TREATMENT

## GENERAL MEASURES
Most patients with Duchenne muscular dystrophy die in their 2nd or 3rd decade of life; therefore, orthopaedic treatment should be designed to improve or maintain the functional capacity of the involved adolescent.

### *Activity*
- No restrictions on activity.
- Activity is to be encouraged as much as possible.

## SPECIAL THERAPY
### *Physical Therapy*
- Test muscle strength to assess the rate of deterioration.
- Use ankle-foot orthoses for correctable deformities.
- The best treatment for fractures is closed reduction and immobilization.
- Fractures of the lower extremities occur frequently in children with Duchenne muscular dystrophy, especially in children who are wheelchair bound.
- Contractures of both lower and upper extremities may occur.
  - Surgical release of contractures sometimes is indicated to improve function.
- ~95% of patients with Duchenne muscular dystrophy develop progressive scoliosis (2).
  - Surgical correction of scoliosis improves sitting balance and minimizes pelvic obliquity.
  - Posterior spinal fusion is recommended for curves of $>20$–$30°$.
- Programs of vigorous respiratory therapy and the use of home negative-pressure and positive-pressure ventilators may promote life extension.
- Proper diagnosis and early genetic counseling may help parents to be aware of the risk of additional male infants with Duchenne muscular dystrophy.

## MEDICATION (DRUGS)
- No drugs have been proved effective.
- Steroids have some benefit (delaying scoliosis and prolonging function), but they also are associated with long-term problems, including weight gain and osteoporosis.

## SURGERY
- Contracture release (Achilles, fascia lata) may be indicated.
- Correction of scoliosis involves fusion of nearly the entire thoracic and lumbar spine (T2–L5 or sacrum).
  - Rods are used to straighten and hold the spine.
  - This intervention should be performed for curves of $\geq 30°$.

# FOLLOW-UP

## PROGNOSIS
- Duchenne muscular dystrophy is fatal in the 2nd or 3rd decade of life.
- Becker dystrophy is more slowly progressive, and life expectancy is greater.

## COMPLICATIONS
- Respiratory failure
- Cardiac failure
- Fracture
- Scoliosis

## PATIENT MONITORING
Patients must be followed frequently (every 4–6 months) by a neurologist to assess their progression.

## REFERENCES

1. Alman BA, Raza SN, Biggar WD. Steroid treatment and the development of scoliosis in males with Duchenne muscular dystrophy. *J Bone Joint Surg* 2004;86A:519–524.
2. Biggar WD, Gingras M, Fehlings DL, et al. Deflazacort treatment of Duchenne muscular dystrophy. *J Pediatr* 2001;138:45–50.


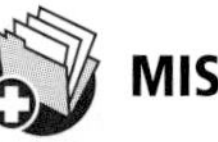

# MISCELLANEOUS

## CODES
### *ICD9-CM*
359.1 Duchenne muscular dystrophy

## PATIENT TEACHING
Genetic counseling is important, to warn of the risk of additional affected infants.

## FAQ
- Q: What is the benefit of scoliosis surgery in patients with Duchenne muscular dystrophy?
  - A: It improves sitting balance and prevents discomfort that develops as the spine collapses.

# MUSCULOSKELETAL RADIOGRAPHY

*William W. Scott, Jr, MD*

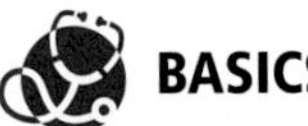

## BASICS

### DESCRIPTION

- Plain radiography has been the primary musculoskeletal imaging technique for >100 years (1).
- X-ray beams generated by an x-ray tube pass through the body part to be imaged, and differential absorption and scattering of the x-ray beams occur.
- The exiting beam carries information about the density of the material traversed.
- This information is captured by:
  - Film (almost always with intensifying screens to reduce radiation dose to the patient) or
  - Another receptor system such as CR or DR, in which the x-ray energy is converted into electrical energy in a pattern reflecting the x-ray absorption of the traversed structure.
- The advantages of digital images such as those produced by CR and DR or by digitizing conventional film images are:
  - They can be transmitted easily and stored electronically.
  - Multiple individuals at multiple locations can view the images simultaneously.
  - The problem of "lost" or misplaced films is lessened.

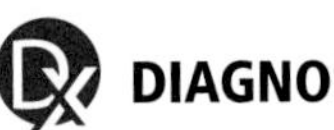

## DIAGNOSIS

### SIGNS AND SYMPTOMS

#### *History*

- The specific reason for obtaining the imaging study and the coexistence of other important illnesses are important factors in the interpretation of imaging studies.
  - This information must be provided to the radiologist interpreting the studies to maximize the possibility of a correct diagnosis.
  - Providing this information also has become a legal requirement in studies of Medicare and Medicaid patients.
- The best practice is for the radiologist to interpret the images 1st without the history and then again with the history.

#### *Physical Examination*

- In musculoskeletal imaging, the exact site of point tenderness is often the most important facet of the clinical information in fracture detection and may help with other types of abnormalities as well.
- Soft-tissue masses easily palpated on physical examination may not be seen on plain radiographs.
  - Absence on radiographs does not mean masses do not exist.
  - MRI should be obtained for suspected soft-tissue masses if additional imaging is necessary.

#### *Diagnostic Procedures/Surgery*

- Cautions
  - 1 view is almost always unsatisfactory.
    - Injured patients may have difficulty moving as requested.
    - Be certain that orthogonal projections were obtained.
  - Complex body parts such as the pelvis, especially when obscured by bowel content, often require CT for satisfactory imaging.
- Sequences
  - For suspected fractures, dislocations, congenital bone abnormalities:
    - Imaging of bony structures is done with relatively low kilovoltage (compared with that used for chest radiography) to provide better contrast between bone and soft tissue.
    - Long bones (femur, tibia and fibula, radius, and ulna, etc.) require 2 radiographs at 90° to one another (orthogonal projections).
    - Joints should be imaged in 3 projections (frontal, lateral, and oblique).
  - For suspected bone tumor:
    - Orthogonal plain radiographs usually provide the diagnosis.
    - MRI provides detailed information on extent of lesion and involvement of neighboring structures.
    - CT may best show calcified tumor matrix.
  - For suspected soft-tissue tumor:
    - Orthogonal radiographs show calcification within the lesion (if present) and effects on neighboring bony structures.
    - Large, fatty lesions may be identified on orthogonal radiographs, but MRI is far better for lesion characterization (except for calcification).
    - MRI also shows the relation of lesion to surrounding structures.
  - For suspected osteomyelitis:
    - Orthogonal radiographs that show definite bone destruction, sequestrum formation, or periosteal reaction without other explanation in the appropriate clinical setting are relatively specific for osteomyelitis, although not sensitive.
    - MRI and radionuclide bone scans provide better sensitivity.
  - For suspected arthritis:
    - 3 views (frontal, lateral, and oblique) of the symptomatic hand and wrist are helpful.
    - Plain radiographic examination can show cartilage narrowing, erosions, osteophytes, soft-tissue calcifications, and pattern of joint involvement and frequently can identify the cause of the arthritis.
    - In long-standing knee arthritis, decision about the appropriate intervention is aided by standing posteroanterior radiographs with the knees flexed 28°, the position in which cartilage wear usually is most marked (Fig. 1).

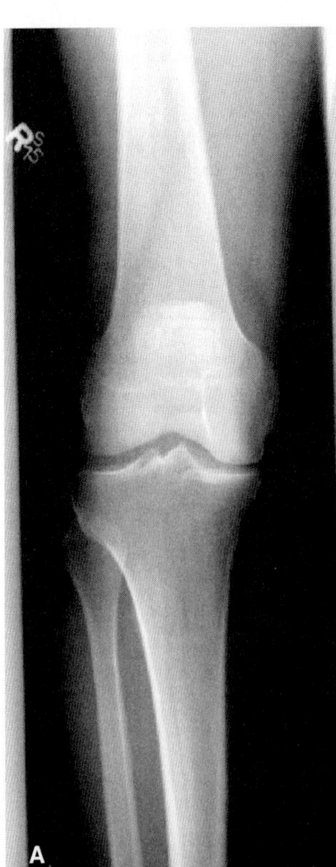


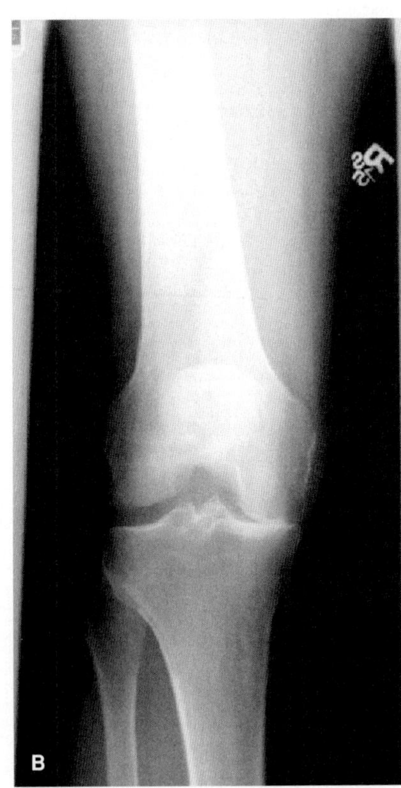


**Fig. 1.** Patient with chronic knee pain believed to be secondary to osteoarthritis. **A**: Standing AP view does not show substantial medial compartment narrowing. **B**: Standing posterior flexed view shows marked medial compartment narrowing and articular cartilage loss.

- For suspected osteonecrosis:
  - Plain radiographs of the hips should include frontal and lateral views; frequently, deformity of the articular surface of the femoral head is better seen on the lateral view.
  - MRI is the most sensitive imaging study for early detection of AVN, but plain radiographs, when positive, are quite specific for the diagnosis.
  - When articular surface collapse is shown, the joint will eventually need prosthetic replacement, so the expense of MRI can be avoided.

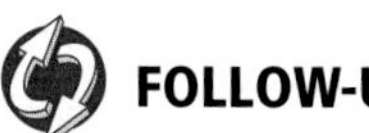

## FOLLOW-UP

- A fat-fluid level in a joint after trauma is a strong indication of the presence of intra-articular fracture, and identification or documentation of a fracture should be pursued aggressively.
  - This situation most commonly involves the knee.
  - If frontal and lateral views are negative, obtain oblique views.
  - If oblique views are negative, obtain a CT scan.
  - Joint effusion in the elbow after trauma, as indicated by a positive "fat pad" sign, is highly correlated with the presence of fracture, especially in adult patients (2).
  - Follow-up imaging after 10–14 days of treatment is advised.
- Suspected scaphoid fracture with initial negative radiographs should be reimaged after 10–14 days of treatment.
- For rare circumstances in which 10–14 days of treatment causes logistic difficulty, as for the professional athlete, an MRI scan can provide an immediate answer at greater expense.
- For a suspected hip fracture, especially in elderly individuals, negative plain radiographs and even negative CT cannot rule out the possibility of fracture.
  - Only a negative MRI exam can exclude the possibility of fracture immediately postinjury.
  - Although MRI is expensive, overall care may cost less because the patient will not have to be kept nonweightbearing for a prolonged period.

### *Pediatric Considerations*

- Ionizing radiation used in imaging has the potential to cause tumors, an especially important consideration in pediatric patients.
- Effort should be made to use the least radiation and number of exposures consistent with obtaining the necessary diagnostic information.
- Most experienced pediatric radiologists only rarely obtain comparison views of the contralateral extremity in cases of suspected fracture.
- Scoliosis views can be obtained in the posteroanterior rather than the AP projection to limit radiation exposure to the breast in young female patients who may need multiple follow-up studies.
- To limit the radiation dose to tiny pediatric patients, CT scans can be performed with exposure factors different than those used in adults.

### *Pregnancy Considerations*

- Female patients should always be questioned directly about the possibility of pregnancy.
- Radiation to the pregnant patient, especially during the 1st trimester, can cause fetal abnormalities (3).
- Exposure of the developing fetus to the direct x-ray beam is the most damaging, so exposures of the pelvic region should be limited as much as possible (3).
- Extremity examinations usually pose little hazard to the fetus.
- Studies sometimes can be delayed without compromising care.
- Alternative studies, such as MRI and ultrasound, should be considered if they can provide the needed information.
- Should a pregnant patient receive a number of examinations to the pelvic region (lumbar spine, multiple views of pelvis, CT, etc.), a medical physicist should be consulted.
  - The radiation dose to the fetus can be estimated, and appropriate counseling can be given to the patient.

### REFERENCES


1. Kotzur IM. W. C. Rontgen: a new type of ray. *Radiology* 1994;193:329–332.
2. O'Dwyer H, O'Sullivan P, Fitzgerald D, et al. The fat pad sign following elbow trauma in adults: its usefulness and reliability in suspecting occult fracture. *J Comput Assist Tomogr* 2004;28: 562–565.
3. Janower ML, Linton OW, eds. *Radiation Risk: A Prime*. Reston, VA: American College of Radiology, 1996.


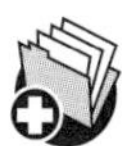

## MISCELLANEOUS

### FAQ

- Q: What is the most important piece of clinical information in the evaluation of bony structures for possible trauma?
  - A: The location of point tenderness indicates where to examine the images most carefully.
- Q: When should one obtain flexed posteroanterior standing views of the knees?
  - A: These views are always valuable in patients with relatively severe disease to show "bone on bone" narrowing, which indicates that arthroscopy is unlikely to be of benefit. Patients with severe symptoms that do not correlate with the apparent degree of joint cartilage narrowing on AP standing views are also likely to benefit from the flexed posteroanterior standing views.
- Q: Will CT "rule out" a hip fracture?
  - A: No. There is a temptation to use CT to look for hip fractures in elderly fall victims. However, if CT shows a fracture, it is diagnostic, but a negative CT does not exclude fracture. MRI should be obtained to exclude fracture.
- Q: What imaging modality is most specific for diagnosing the specific types of bone neoplasm?
  - A: Plain radiographs should always be obtained when evaluating a possible bone neoplasm because they are the most specific for identifying the type of tumor.

# NECK PAIN

*Karl A. Soderlund, BS*
*Sanjog Mathur, MD*
*A. Jay Khanna, MD*

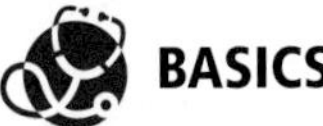

## BASICS

### DESCRIPTION

- In adults:
  - Common
  - Usually secondary to degenerative disc disease and arthritis
- In children and adolescents:
  - Less common
  - When it does occur, the pain often is secondary to a neoplasm or infection.
- Neck pain also occurs after trauma and is extremely common after motor vehicle accidents.

### GENERAL PREVENTION

- No definite methods of prevention are known.
- General measures such as the use of seat belts and avoidance of motorcycles are recommended.

### EPIDEMIOLOGY

#### *Incidence*

- Neck pain occurs in 10% of the population at any given time (1).
- In a 1994 survey of Norwegian adults, nearly 35% of respondents reported experiencing neck pain within the last year (2).
- A 1991 study of adults in Finland showed that 9.5% of males and 13.5% of females suffer chronic neck pain (3).

### RISK FACTORS

Congenital fusions of the spine (Klippel-Feil syndrome) are risk factors.

### ETIOLOGY

- The many different causes can be divided broadly into atraumatic and traumatic types.
  - Atraumatic neck pain usually is a secondary symptom of inflammation, degenerative disc disease, arthritis, infection, or a neoplasm.
  - Traumatic neck pain often is caused by soft-tissue sprains, fractures, subluxations, dislocations, and herniated discs—conditions that can exist in elderly patients without any occurrence of trauma.

## DIAGNOSIS

### SIGNS AND SYMPTOMS

- Pain well localized to the neck
- Stiffness
- Cervical radiculopathy

#### *Physical Exam*

- Routine cervical spine examination differs from examination of cervical spine trauma patients.
- Routine examinations should focus on ROM, regions of tenderness, and neurologic assessment.
  - Note loss of flexion, extension, and rotation.
  - Palpate the posterior ligamentous structures to detect tenderness and the paraspinal muscles for spasm.
  - Perform a careful neurologic examination, including motor testing, deep tendon reflexes, and sensation.
  - Look for upper motor neuron signs and assess muscle strength.
- Examination of a trauma patient must include the following:
  - Immobilization until neurologic testing rules out neurologic deficit
  - A full neurologic examination, including the anal wink and bulbocavernosus reflex tests
  - Radiographic studies to evaluate the extent of cervical spine trauma

### TESTS

The Spurling maneuver tests for cervical radiculopathy.

#### *Lab*

- Laboratory studies are indicated if spine abnormality is not present.
- For suspected infection, white blood cell count and ESR should be obtained.

#### *Imaging*

- Conventional radiographs:
  - Indicated in patients with history of neck trauma and those >50 years old
  - AP and lateral radiographs are the 1st step in imaging.
  - Other useful views include:
    - Oblique views to evaluate the neural foramen if osteophytic nerve root impingement or facet dislocation/subluxation is suspected
    - Open mouth view to evaluate for C1 fractures (atlas) or odontoid fractures
    - Flexion/extension views to evaluate for segmental instability
- MRI and CT are indicated in the presence of neurologic abnormalities and to evaluate for occult fractures and ligamentous injuries.
  - Both are sensitive and specific modalities with which to detect structural abnormalities.
  - May be used independently or in combination
  - CT is the most useful for detecting osseous abnormalities such as fractures, facet dislocations, and osteoid osteomas.
  - MRI is useful for detecting abnormalities in the marrow or soft-tissue structures, such as nerve root impingement or spinal cord compression, as well as disc herniation and foraminal stenosis.

### DIFFERENTIAL DIAGNOSIS

- Adults:
  - Atraumatic:
    - Degenerative disc disease
    - Inflammatory arthritis (rheumatoid arthritis, AS)
    - Infection (discitis, vertebral osteomyelitis, meningitis)
    - Herniated disc
    - Neoplasm
  - Traumatic:
    - Ligament sprain
    - Fracture
    - Subluxation and dislocation
    - Herniated disc
- Children:
  - Atraumatic:
    - Rotatory subluxation
    - Abscess
    - Osteomyelitis
    - Neoplasm
  - Traumatic:
    - Ligament disruption
    - Fracture
    - SCIWORA
  - SCIWORA:
    - Occurs in 19–34% of pediatric spinal cord injuries (4)
    - Neurologic deficits after trauma may be delayed up to 4 days in young children, and a 2nd such injury may occur as many as 10 weeks after the trauma (5).
    - Transient posttraumatic neurologic symptoms in the arms or legs should be evaluated carefully.

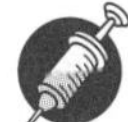

# TREATMENT

## GENERAL MEASURES

- Most patients with neck pain suffer from an inflammatory process.
- Rest and NSAIDs are the mainstays of treatment.
- Soft cervical collars are useful for support and to prevent additional injury, but the clinician should avoid prolonged immobilization to prevent deconditioning of the cervical paraspinal musculature (6).
- Posture modification and changes in sleep position are important nonsurgical treatments that may be beneficial in treating neck pain.
- Exercise can be important in maintaining ROM and strength of the cervical paraspinal musculature.

## SPECIAL THERAPY

### *Physical Therapy*

- Physical therapy is useful for regaining ROM and strength of the paraspinal muscles.
- Gentle traction of the spine can be useful for decreasing nerve root irritation.

## MEDICATION (DRUGS)

- NSAIDs are the drug of choice for decreasing inflammation.
  - Usually prescribed initially for 4–6 weeks
  - If the pain has resolved at that time, the medication may be discontinued.

## SURGERY

- All efforts should be made to treat axial neck pain nonoperatively because surgery for isolated axial neck pain has worse outcomes than surgery for other causes (e.g., cervical spinal stenosis).
- Most commonly, surgery is performed to remove nerve root or spinal cord compression from degenerative disease, trauma, and neoplastic disorders.

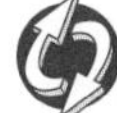

# FOLLOW-UP

## PROGNOSIS

- Relieving localized neck pain often is a difficult task because of the diversity of its causes, including idiopathic origins.
- A combination of physical therapy, occupational therapy, and NSAIDs is the best course of treatment for neck pain not caused by a tumor or an infection or not associated with neurologic deficits.
- The prognosis for nonoperative treatment usually is good unless the cause is a malignant bone tumor.

## COMPLICATIONS

- The major complication is progressive neural deficit from nerve root or spinal cord compression.
- Symptoms of nerve root or spinal cord compression include:
  - Weakness in the arms and hands
  - Sensory deficits in the upper extremities
  - Difficulty in walking
  - Bladder and bowel abnormalities

## PATIENT MONITORING

Patients are followed at 4–6-week intervals until the discomfort resolves.

## REFERENCES


1. Hadler NM. Illness in the workplace: the challenge of musculoskeletal symptoms. *J Hand Surg* 1985;10A:451–456.
2. Bovim G, Schrader H, Sand T. Neck pain in the general population. *Spine* 1994;19:1307–1309.
3. Makela M, Heliovaara M, Sievers K, et al. Prevalence, determinants, and consequences of chronic neck pain in Finland. *Am J Epidemiol* 1991;134:1356–1367.
4. Launay F, Leet AI, Sponseller PD. Pediatric spinal cord injury without radiographic abnormality: a meta analysis. *Clin Orthop Relat Res* 2005;433: 166–170.
5. Pang D, Pollack IF. Spinal cord injury without radiographic abnormality in children—the SCIWORA syndrome. *J Trauma* 1989;29:654–664.
6. Rosenfeld M, Gunnarsson R, Borenstein P. Early intervention in whiplash-associated disorders: a comparison of two treatment protocols. *Spine* 2000;25:1782–1787.


## ADDITIONAL READING


Hardin JG, Halla JT. Cervical spine syndromes. In: McCarty DJ, Koopman WJ, eds. *Arthritis and Allied Conditions. A Textbook of Rheumatology*, 4th ed. Malvern, PA: Lea & Febiger, 1993:1563–1572.


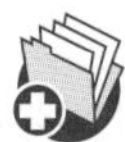

# MISCELLANEOUS

## CODES

### *ICD9-CM*

723.1 Cervicalgia

## PATIENT TEACHING

- Patients with neck strains (whiplash injuries) are counseled that full recovery can be expected in the motivated patient.
- Patients with severe cervical degenerative disease generally improve but may have chronic, mild to moderate symptoms after treatment.
- Patients who spend a substantial amount of time using a computer should be counseled to take breaks often and to attempt to maintain appropriate posture.

## FAQ

- Q: What is SCIWORA, and in which patient population is it most commonly seen?
  - A: SCIWORA is an acronym for spinal cord injury without radiographic abnormality, and it is usually seen after trauma in children.
- Q: In which infectious disease is neck stiffness a common symptom?
  - A: Meningitis.

N

# NEUROFIBROMATOSIS

*Paul D. Sponseller, MD*

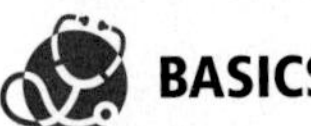

## BASICS

### DESCRIPTION

- Most common single gene disorder in humans
- The disease involves multiple organ systems; the skeletal and nervous systems account for the greatest number of clinical features.
- The most common form is NF1 (addressed here); NF2 refers to bilateral acoustic neuromas.
- The manifestations of NF1 may not develop until late childhood.
  - Some signs may be present at birth, but neurofibromas may take years to become apparent, and diagnosis usually is made in later childhood.
- Synonym: von Recklinghausen disease

### EPIDEMIOLOGY

#### *Incidence*

- ~1 in 3,000 newborns (1,2)
- Males and females are affected equally.

### RISK FACTORS

Advanced paternal age has been associated with an increased incidence of NF.

#### *Genetics*

- Inherited in an autosomal-dominant pattern
- Presents in ~1/2 of the patients as new mutations
- Thought to occur with complete penetrance

### ETIOLOGY

- Genetic disorder
- Secondary to a defect in the protein neurofibromin

### ASSOCIATED CONDITIONS

- Nearly 50% of people have cognitive delays ranging from severe retardation to slight learning disabilities (2).
- A few patients develop metabolic bone disease that results in a type of osteomalacia.
- Hypertension on the basis of renal artery stenosis or pheochromocytoma may be found.

## DIAGNOSIS

### SIGNS AND SYMPTOMS

- To establish the diagnosis, 2 of the following National Institutes of Health diagnostic criteria must be met (Fig. 1):
  - 6 café-au-lait spots measuring ≥5 mm in children and ≥15 mm in adults
  - 1 optic glioma
  - ≥2 Lisch nodules on the iris
  - 1 osseous lesion typically seen in NF, including vertebral scalloping, dystrophic scoliosis, rib penciling, or pseudarthrosis of a long bone
  - A 1st-degree relative with the disease
  - Axillary or inguinal freckling
  - Cutaneous or plexiform neurofibromas
- Symptoms vary, depending on the criteria:
  - Plexiform neurofibromas often are associated with pain and neurologic deficit in the distribution of the particular nerve.
  - Cutaneous neurofibromas usually cause few symptoms.

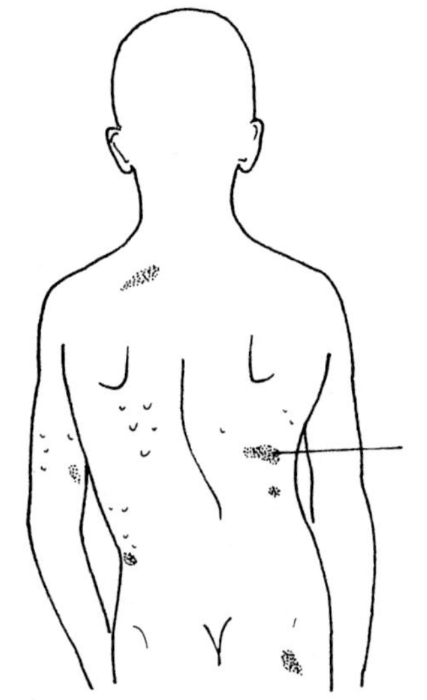

**Fig. 1.** This patient displays multiple café-au-lait spots, subcutaneous neurofibromas, and scoliosis characteristic of NF.

#### *Physical Exam*

- Examine the neck and spine for deformity.
- Inspect all the skin, including the axillae.
- Ophthalmologic referral should be made so that the eyes can be examined with a slit lamp for Lisch nodules and optic glioma.
- Limb lengths should be measured and checked for angulation (Fig. 2).

### TESTS

#### *Lab*

No laboratory tests reveal abnormalities specific for NF.

#### *Imaging*

- The skeletal manifestations usually can be identified on plain radiographs:
  - May show posterior vertebral body scalloping
  - The dystrophic type of scoliosis is characterized by penciling of the ribs, severe apical rotation, short, segmented curves, and malformed vertebrae (3,4) (Figs. 3 and 4).
  - The features of the pseudarthrosis that can occur in long bones can range from a cystic appearance to severely thinned and pointed pseudarthrosis, which fractures at birth.
  - Sclerosis and constriction also can be found at the pseudarthrosis site.
  - Dural ectasia and pseudomeningocele also can affect the spine.

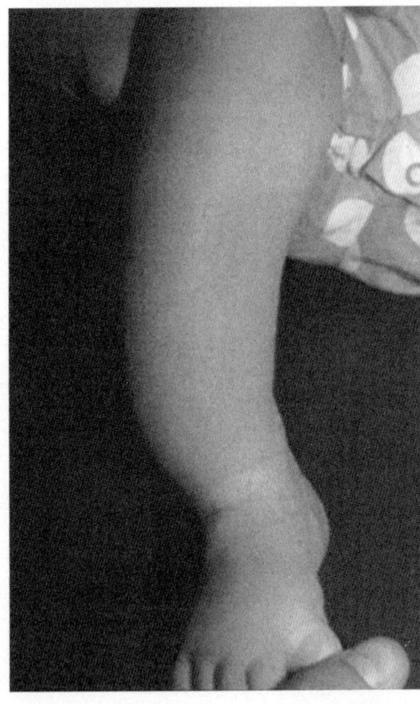

**Fig. 2.** Distal anterolateral bow associated with NF1.

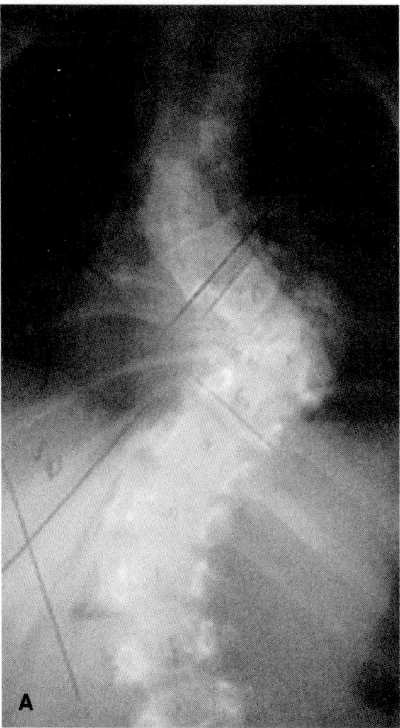
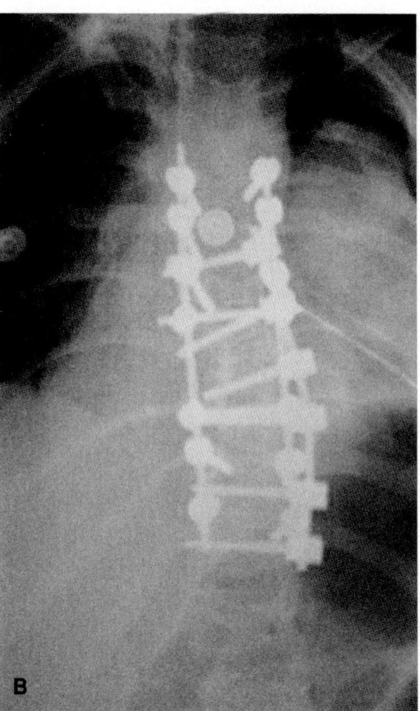

**Fig. 3.** Dystrophic scoliosis with NF1. **A**: Dystrophic scoliosis has short, sharp curves with penciling of the ribs. **B**: After surgical correction.

- When instrumentation is planned to correct a spinal deformity, MRI should be obtained to evaluate the spinal canal for these changes.
- CT scanning may be helpful in assessing the laminae and pedicles for fixation.
- Characteristic long-bone lesions can include anything from benign scalloping of cortices to permeative lesions that resemble malignant disease radiographically.

### *Pathological Findings*

- The disorder is 1 of cells of neural crest origin: The cells of the embryonic neural crest are destined to form tissue in many different organ systems, accounting for the diverse manifestations of the disease.
- Lisch nodules of the iris are hamartomatous deposits.

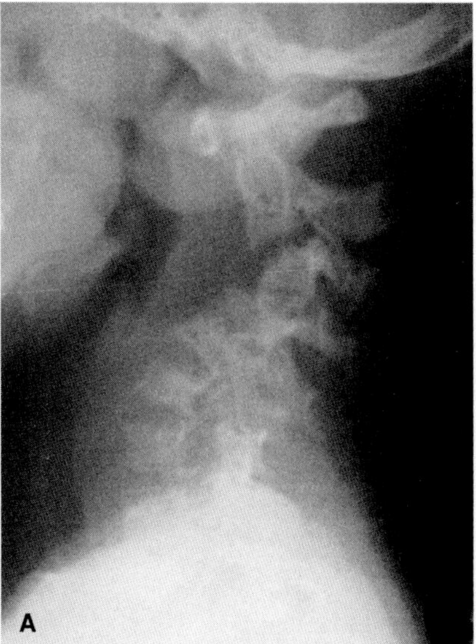
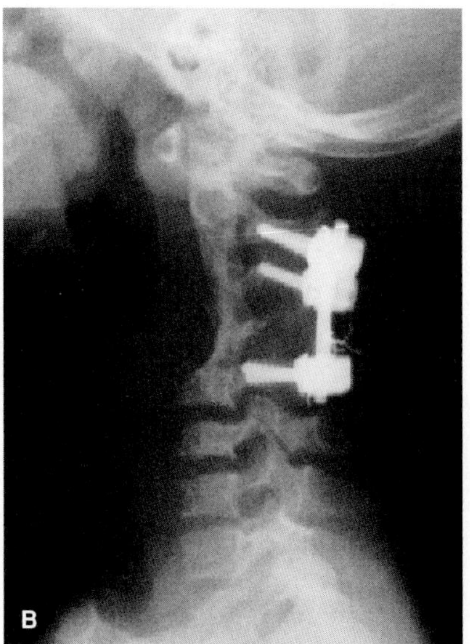

**Fig. 4.** Dystrophic cervical changes. **A:** Dystrophic change in NF1 may involve the neck. **B:** After surgery.

- The bone in pseudarthrosis typically is fibrotic, with few osteoblasts.
- Cutaneous neurofibromas are composed of Schwann cells and connective tissue.

### DIFFERENTIAL DIAGNOSIS

- Proteus syndrome most closely resembles NF in its manifestations.
- Patients with isolated congenital pseudarthrosis of the tibia must be monitored for NF because the café-au-lait spots may develop later NF.
- NF2 consists of only bilateral acoustic neuromas.

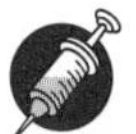

## TREATMENT

### GENERAL MEASURES

- Patients should be seen regularly by a geneticist or primary physician to rule out developmental delay, growth disturbance, scoliosis, or neurologic deterioration.
- Patients usually are functional, except those who are severely mentally handicapped.
- No specific dietary requirements exist.

### *Activity*

- Bracing for prepseudarthrosis of the tibia, especially during activities, is recommended.
- Otherwise, activity should not be restricted unnecessarily.

### MEDICATION (DRUGS)

Although speculative, angiogenesis inhibitors may be used to decrease the vascularity of plexiform neurofibromas and allow easier surgical removal.

### SURGERY
- Dystrophic scoliosis should be treated surgically if any evidence of progression is seen.
- Anterior and posterior fusions usually are recommended if focal kyphosis or a curve >50–60° is present in a skeletally immature patient.
- When diagnosed, patients with dystrophic tibial changes should be braced, and the bracing should be continued until skeletal maturity.
- If fracture occurs, use intramedullary nails (with bone grafting or vascularized fibula bone grafting) or compression and distraction (Ilizarov) treatment with ring fixators.
  - All treatment should be protected after union occurs until the end of growth.
- Plexiform neurofibromas should not be treated surgically because total removal is nearly impossible and neurologic deficits typically occur.
- Leg-length inequality should be charted and followed with serial scanograms to ascertain the timing of contralateral leg epiphysiodesis or limb lengthening.

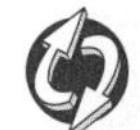

## FOLLOW-UP

### PROGNOSIS
Life expectancy may be compromised by severe mental retardation and malignant disease.

### COMPLICATIONS
- Patients with NF1 have a high incidence of malignancy.
- Usually, these tumors are of the central nervous system.
- Plexiform neurofibromas also can degenerate into neurofibrosarcomas.
- Amputation of a leg may be necessary in a patient with severe pseudarthrosis because correction of the nonunion is not always successful.
- In rare instances, the function of the patient may be best served with amputation.
- Some patients with dystrophic scoliosis have malformed vertebrae.
- If substantial kyphosis exists, correction can cause neurologic compromise.
- Spinal cord monitoring should be performed during all spinal procedures.

### PATIENT MONITORING
- Annual scanograms are indicated for limb-length discrepancy.
- Physical examinations for detection of scoliosis should be performed on a yearly basis while the child is growing.
- Hypertension is a common finding in patients with NF and should be monitored regularly.

### REFERENCES

1. Akbarnia BA, Gabriel KR, Beckman E, et al. Prevalence of scoliosis in neurofibromatosis. *Spine* 1992;17:S244–S248.
2. Alman BA, Goldberg MJ. Syndromes of orthopaedic importance. In: Morrissy RT, Weinstein SL, eds. *Lovell and Winter's Pediatric Orthopaedics*, 6th ed. Philadelphia: Lippincott Williams & Wilkins, 2006:251–313.
3. Crawford AH, Jr, Bagamery N. Osseous manifestations of neurofibromatosis in childhood. *J Pediatr Orthop* 1986;6:72–88.
4. Vitale MG, Guha A, Skaggs DL. Orthopaedic manifestations of neurofibromatosis in children: an update. *Clin Orthop Relat Res* 2002;401:107–118.

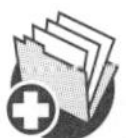

## MISCELLANEOUS

### CODES

#### *ICD9-CM*

237.7 Neurofibromatosis

### PATIENT TEACHING

- The incidence of tumors (especially those of the nervous system), including optic gliomas, astrocytomas, and acoustic neuromas, is increased.
  - Education about the early signs of auditory, visual, or motor disturbances should be discussed with patients.
- Educate the patient regarding the need to protect against pseudarthrosis of the tibia until skeletal maturity.
- Discuss the potential for limb-length discrepancy when pseudarthrosis of the lower extremity or limb gigantism is present.
  - Typical discrepancy in both disorders rarely exceeds 6 cm.
- If possible, bracing of pseudarthrosis in the tibia should be attempted.
- Bracing for dystrophic scoliosis is not effective.
- Bracing for the more commonly encountered idiopathic type of scoliosis should be instituted when the regular indications for idiopathic scoliosis are met.

### FAQ

- Q: Should soft-tissue neurofibromas be removed?
  - A: Only if they are growing excessively or are causing symptoms.

# NONUNION OF FRACTURES

*Simon C. Mears, MD, PhD*
*Melanie Kinchen, MD*

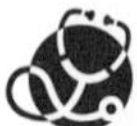

## BASICS

### DESCRIPTION

- Presence of a postfracture defect in a long bone beyond a reasonable expected healing date, or if no radiographic progression of healing is noted
- If internal fixation is used to stabilize a fracture, a race exists between fracture healing and hardware failure.
- Children, because of their active healing potential, rarely develop a nonunion unless other predisposing conditions are present (1).
- Classification (2):
  - Atrophic nonunion:
    - Often poor blood supply
    - When visualized on radiographs, often show poor bone quality with tapered edges
    - Often occur in osteoporotic bone
  - Hypertrophic nonunions:
    - Good blood supply
    - Most go on to heal if adequate stabilization can be achieved.

### EPIDEMIOLOGY

#### *Incidence*

- The incidence depends on the fracture type.
  - 13% of tibial fractures (3)
  - 4–11% of clavicle fractures, depending on location (4)
  - Tibial shaft, femoral neck, and scaphoid fractures are at high risk for nonunion because they have a more tenuous blood supply than other bones, which often is damaged with the injury.

### RISK FACTORS

- Poor nutritional status
- Poor bone quantity and quality
- Suppressed immune system
- Presence of bone infection may contribute to development of a nonunion.
- Smoking (5)
- Poor soft-tissue envelope
- Vascular compromise
- NSAID use
- Open fractures
- Poor fracture reduction
- Distal tibia fractures

### ETIOLOGY

- Injury-related causes include segmental bone loss, extensive soft-tissue damage, and loss of adequate blood supply.
- Treatment-related factors include quality of reduction, amount of distraction, and length of immobilization.
- Inadequate fracture stabilization is a common cause of fracture nonunion.

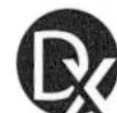

## DIAGNOSIS

### SIGNS AND SYMPTOMS

#### *History*

- Patients have a history of a fracture that continues to be painful.
- The patient may have broken hardware.
- Pain often occurs after use of the limb.

#### *Physical Exam*

- Patients have continued tenderness at the fracture site.
- Motion of the bony fragments may or may not be evident.

### TESTS

#### *Imaging*

- Radiography:
  - Plain AP and lateral radiographs, to determine the presence of callus formation
  - Serial radiographs, to ensure callus progression
- CT:
  - Excellent at revealing nonunion
  - In many fractures, the fracture plane is difficult to see on plain radiographs because of overlap of the bone fragments.
- Bone scans, to help determine whether increased blood flow and subsequently increased bone turnover is present at the fracture site
- MRI is useful when hardware is not present.

#### *Pathological Findings*

- Thick fibrous tissue with areas of uncalcified callus formation
- A synovial pseudarthrosis or false joint may develop with excessive motion.

### DIFFERENTIAL DIAGNOSIS

- Delayed union, characterized by some tenderness and motion at the fracture site with variable amounts of callus present after a period in which most fractures would be healed clinically
- Painful hardware
- Posttraumatic arthritis

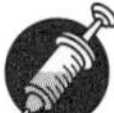

## TREATMENT

### GENERAL MEASURES

- Most nonunions are treated with surgical intervention.
- Aggressive treatment of delayed union can help prevent nonunion and hardware breakage.
- Nonoperative interventions:
  - Bone stimulators (electrical or ultrasound)
  - Smoking cessation
  - Discontinuation of NSAIDs
  - Use of weightbearing casts or functional braces

### SURGERY

- Surgical treatment of nonunions is determined by type of host, soft-tissue coverage, precise location of the nonunion, type of nonunion, and previous fracture treatment.
- Patients with severe medical compromise, poor soft-tissue coverage, or poor vascular supply may be candidates for amputation.
- Hypertrophic nonunion should be treated with rigid fixation of the nonunion, which may require revision of the internal fixation.
- Nonunion of long-bone fractures with intramedullary nails may be treated with nail dynamization or exchange nailing.
  - Reaming the canal provides local bone graft and allows for placement of a larger diameter nail (6).
- Bypass or wave plating allows for fixation and bone grafting (7).
- For tibial nonunions, bracing may be combined with fibular osteotomy (8).
- Well-stabilized atrophic nonunions are treated with bone grafting.
  - Bone graft may be autograft, allograft, or synthetic.
  - The fracture nonunion should be exposed and curetted, and the bone ends should be burred back to bleeding, viable bone.
  - Bone graft material then is packed into the nonunion.

- The use of bone morphogenic protein 2 recently has been approved for tibial nonunion treatment (9).
- The optimal bone graft material or bone morphogenic protein is unknown.
  - Factors to consider with the use of autograft include the need for a 2nd incision and the relative quality of the patient's bone.
  - Some patients may not want to have a 2nd incision with its risk of pain or infection (10).
- Femoral neck nonunions may be treated with realignment osteotomy or joint replacement.
- Infected nonunion:
  - Treatment is challenging and requires débridement of the infection, fracture stabilization, removal of dead space, and soft-tissue coverage.
  - Plastic surgery reconstruction may be necessary, and multiple surgeries often are necessary (11).
- Large bone defects may be managed with bone transport via an external fixation and the Ilizarov method (12).

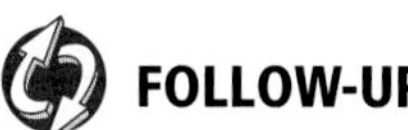

## FOLLOW-UP

### PROGNOSIS

- 90% of nonunions are treated successfully with 1 surgery (13).
- In 80% of nonunions, limb length and alignment are restored (13).
- If infection is present, often >1 surgery is required.

### COMPLICATIONS

- Infection and osteomyelitis
- Hardware failure
- Continued nonunion
- Pain
- Malunion
- Joint stiffness
- Pain and infection at the bone graft donor site

### PATIENT MONITORING

Serial radiographs are obtained once a month, to assess the development of callus.

### REFERENCES

1. Arslan H, Subasy M, Kesemenli C, et al. Occurrence and treatment of nonunion in long bone fractures in children. *Arch Orthop Trauma Surg* 2002;122:494–498.
2. McKee MD. Aseptic non-union. In: Ruedi TP, Murphy WM, eds. *AO Principles of Fracture Management*. New York: Thieme, 2000: 749–762.
3. Audige L, Griffin D, Bhandari M, et al. Path analysis of factors for delayed healing and nonunion in 416 operatively treated tibial shaft fractures. *Clin Orthop Relat Res* 2005;438: 221–232.
4. Robinson CM, Court-Brown CM, McQueen MM, et al. Estimating the risk of nonunion following nonoperative treatment of a clavicular fracture. *J Bone Joint Surg* 2004;86A:1359–1365.
5. Adams CI, Keating JF, Court-Brown CM. Cigarette smoking and open tibial fractures. *Injury* 2001;32:61–65.
6. Pihlajamaki HK, Salminen ST, Bostman OM. The treatment of nonunions following intramedullary nailing of femoral shaft fractures. *J Orthop Trauma* 2002;16:394–402.
7. Ring D, Jupiter JB, Quintero J, et al. Atrophic ununited diaphyseal fractures of the humerus with a bony defect: treatment by wave-plate osteosynthesis. *J Bone Joint Surg* 2000;82B: 867–871.
8. Sarmiento A, Burkhalter WE, Latta LL. Functional bracing in the treatment of delayed union and nonunion of the tibia. *Int Orthop* 2003;27:26–29.
9. Friedlaender GE, Perry CR, Cole JD, et al. Osteogenic protein-1 (bone morphogenetic protein-7) in the treatment of tibial nonunions. *J Bone Joint Surg* 2001;83A:S1-151–S1-158.
10. Giannoudis PV, Dinopoulos H, Tsiridis E. Bone substitutes: an update. *Injury* 2005;36:S20–S27.
11. Patzakis MJ, Zalavras CG. Chronic posttraumatic osteomyelitis and infected nonunion of the tibia: current management concepts. *J Am Acad Orthop Surg* 2005;13:417–427.
12. Rozbruch SR, Weitzman AM, Watson JT, et al. Simultaneous treatment of tibial bone and soft-tissue defects with the Ilizarov method. *J Orthop Trauma* 2006;20:197–205.
13. Rodriguez-Merchan EC, Forriol F. Nonunion: general principles and experimental data. *Clin Orthop Relat Res* 2004;419:4–12.

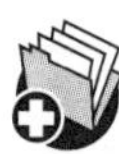

## MISCELLANEOUS

### CODES

#### *ICD9-CM*

733.82 Nonunion fracture

### PATIENT TEACHING

Strict adherence to the recommendations of the orthopaedic surgeon regarding activity and care of the fracture may reduce the likelihood of developing a nonunion, particularly with problematic fractures.

#### *Prevention*

Excellent reduction of fractures, smoking cessation, and aggressive treatment of delayed unions decrease nonunion rates.

### FAQ

- Q: How long does a nonunion take to heal?
  - A: 90% of nonunions are treated successfully with 1 surgical intervention, and healing occurs over a 3–4-month period. Full rehabilitation with muscle strengthening takes longer, because the patient often is debilitated before treatment.

# NURSEMAID'S ELBOW

*Paul D. Sponseller, MD*

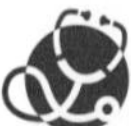

## BASICS

### DESCRIPTION

- Nursemaid's elbow results from injury to the annular ligament that surrounds the radial head at the elbow in a young child (Fig. 1).
- The injury causes guarding and failure to use the elbow.
- It is not a subluxation or dislocation.
- Synonyms: Pulled elbow; Annular ligament entrapment

### GENERAL PREVENTION

Care should be taken to avoid traction on the arm of a young child.

### EPIDEMIOLOGY

- It usually affects children 1–5 years old (1).
- Boys and girls are affected equally.

#### *Incidence*

This is 1 of the most common elbow injuries in young children.

### RISK FACTORS

- Ages 1–5 years
- Stubborn behavior (pulling away)

#### *Genetics*

No genetic predisposition is known.

### ETIOLOGY

- With traction, a small part of the annular ligament that surrounds the radial head is pulled toward the joint and may be partially torn, causing painful rotation of the radius.
- This injury usually does not result from a fall on the outstretched hand, which typically produces a buckle fracture of the distal radius or an elbow injury.

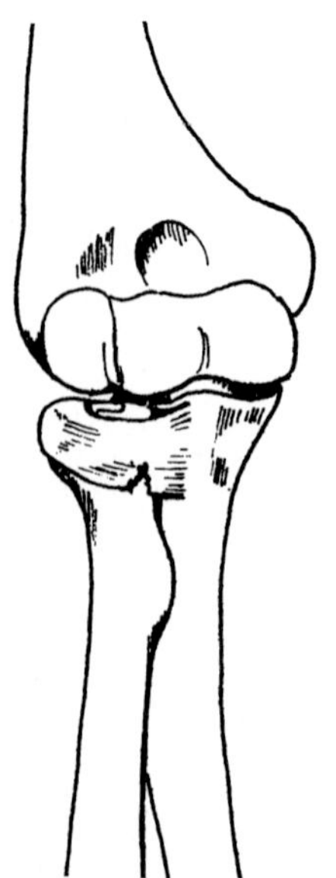

**Fig. 1.** Nursemaid's elbow is a strain or a tear in the annular ligament around the radial neck.

## DIAGNOSIS

### SIGNS AND SYMPTOMS

- Pain in the elbow after a traction injury, such as pulling on the arm by a parent or sibling (Fig. 2)
- Usually, minimal pain to palpation
- No substantial swelling
- Resistance by the patient to use the elbow
- The response to reduction of the displaced ligament is the most diagnostic feature of all: The child starts using the elbow again shortly, and no residual tenderness is present.

#### *Physical Exam*

The child usually holds the elbow at the side and refuses to use the extremity.

### TESTS

#### *Lab*

No laboratory tests aid in the diagnosis.

#### *Imaging*

- Radiographs are not required if the diagnosis is clear.
- If in doubt, order AP and lateral films of the elbow to rule out fracture.
- If it is a true nursemaid's elbow, the radiograph should be normal.

#### *Pathological Findings*

- The ligament surrounding the radial head is partially, but not totally, torn.
- Few specimens have been examined because the natural history of the condition is benign.

### DIFFERENTIAL DIAGNOSIS

- Buckle or greenstick fracture of the distal humerus
- Growth plate injury of the distal humerus or proximal radius
- Infection, juvenile rheumatoid arthritis, and Lyme disease, which are all possibilities but which occur much less frequently than nursemaid's elbow

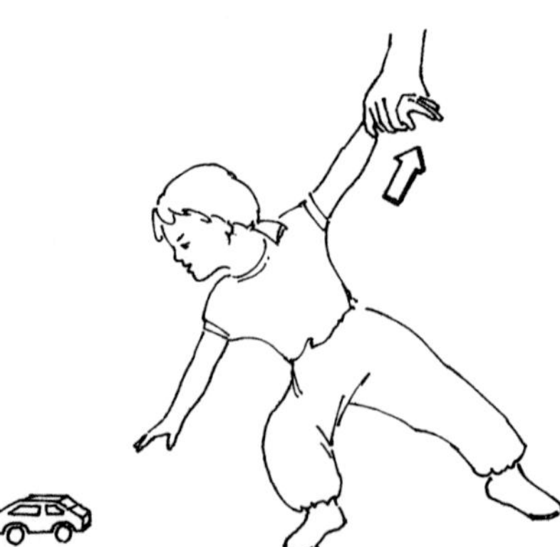

**Fig. 2.** The mechanism of nursemaid's elbow is traction, not a fall.

## TREATMENT

### GENERAL MEASURES

- Rule out other conditions (usually by physical examination).
- Reduce the displaced annular ligament by flexing the child's elbow fully, bringing the child's hand up to touch the shoulder, while supinating the forearm (Fig. 3).
  - Usually, no sedation is needed.
  - A slight "pop" often is felt.
  - The maneuver may be resisted initially by the child, but then the child begins to use the arm again.
- A sling or splint usually is not needed unless the episode is a recurrence.

#### *Activity*

The child should be allowed to return to activities as tolerated.

### SPECIAL THERAPY

#### *Physical Therapy*

In children in this age group, physical therapy is not needed for this injury.

### MEDICATION (DRUGS)

- Medications usually are not needed once the injury is reduced, but acetaminophen may be given.
- If stronger medication is needed, suspect another diagnosis.

### SURGERY

- Not needed
- Closed manipulation is always successful.

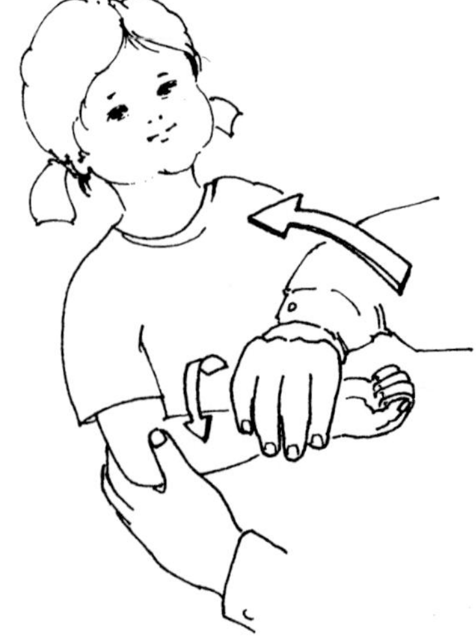

**Fig. 3.** Nursemaid's elbow usually is reduced by flexion and supination.

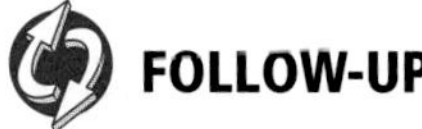

## FOLLOW-UP

### PROGNOSIS
- The prognosis usually is excellent; there should be no sequelae.
- A few children suffer a recurrence, which can be reduced and splinted for 1–2 weeks.
- Sometimes several recurrences may happen within a year, but the child will eventually "grow out" of this predisposition.

### COMPLICATIONS
- None are known, except misdiagnosis, such as missing a fracture about the elbow.
- This condition can be distinguished from a fracture by the latter's different mechanism and greater swelling and tenderness.

### PATIENT MONITORING
Monitoring is not needed unless problems persist.

### REFERENCE
1. Sponseller PD. Disorders of bone, joint, and muscle problems. In: McMillan JA, Feigin RD, DeAngelis CD, et al., eds. *Oski's Pediatrics: Principles and Practice*, 4th ed. Philadelphia: Lippincott Williams & Wilkins, 2006:2470–2505.

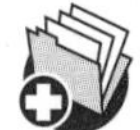

## MISCELLANEOUS

### CODES
#### *ICD9-CM*
832.0 Annular ligament disruption

### PATIENT TEACHING
- Educate parents about the traction mechanism of the injury and the need to avoid pulling on the child's elbow.
- If a child has had several recurrences, it is appropriate for a parent to learn the reduction maneuver so that it can be handled at home.

#### *Prevention*
Avoid strong traction on the arm of a young child.

### FAQ
- Q: When should a radiograph be taken for a presumed nursemaid elbow?
  - A: When the swelling is excessive or the mechanism is atypical, such that a fracture may be suspected.

N

# OLECRANON FRACTURE

*Andrew M. Richards, MD*
*Jinsong Wang, MD*

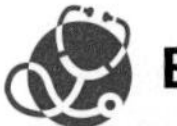

## BASICS

### DESCRIPTION

- The olecranon:
  - Is the proximal bony projection of the ulna at the elbow
  - Articulates with the trochlea of the distal humerus to form the ulnohumeral portion of the elbow joint:
    - This articulation is responsible for flexion and extension of the elbow joint.
  - Is the insertion site of the triceps tendon
- Contraction of the triceps pulling on the olecranon produces extension of the elbow.
- Fracture of the olecranon disrupts the extensor mechanism of the elbow, which is critical to arm function (Fig. 1).
- If these intra-articular fractures are not repaired anatomically, posttraumatic arthritis will develop.
- Classification:
  - By characteristic
    - Nondisplaced or displaced
    - Transverse or oblique
    - Simple or comminuted
  - By the amount of involvement of the articular surface in the olecranon notch (1)
    - Type 1: Proximal 1/3 of the notch
    - Type 2: Middle 1/3
    - Type 3: Distal 1/3

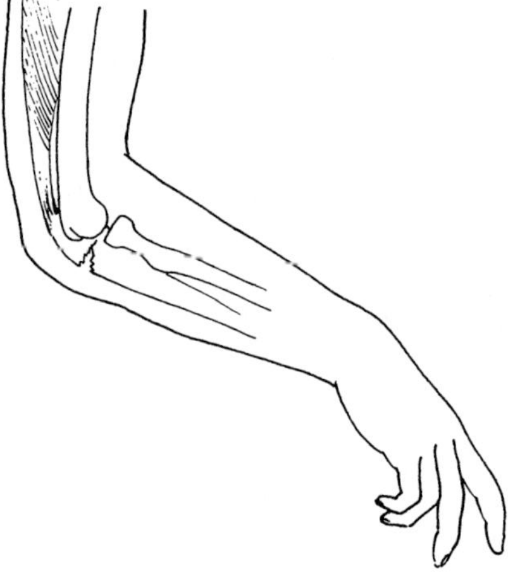

**Fig. 1.** Olecranon fractures involve the proximal ulna and enter the elbow joint.

### GENERAL PREVENTION

Elbow pads should be used for contact sports and skating (2).

### EPIDEMIOLOGY

- Olecranon fracture may occur after a fall, sports injury, or motor vehicle accident.
- Elderly or osteoporotic patients may sustain an olecranon fracture after a low-energy fall.
- Olecranon fractures occur less frequently in children than in adults because in children, this type of force is more likely to produce a fracture of the distal humerus (supracondylar) (3).

### RISK FACTORS

Activities with high fall rates, such as inline skating, have a high risk of elbow fractures.

### ETIOLOGY

- The most common mechanisms of injury are:
  - Fall on the outstretched hand with the elbow in flexion
  - Direct blow to the tip of the elbow

### ASSOCIATED CONDITIONS

- Elbow dislocation
- Radial head fracture
- Triceps avulsion
- Elbow instability
- Neurologic damage (ulnar, median, and radial nerves)

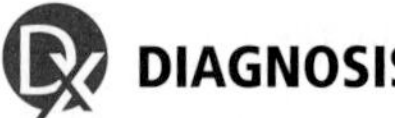

## DIAGNOSIS

### SIGNS AND SYMPTOMS

- Pain, swelling, ecchymosis, and deformity of the elbow
- Inability to extend the elbow
- These injuries often are associated with radial head fractures and elbow dislocations.

#### *History*

History should be obtained to determine the mechanism of injury.

#### *Physical Exam*

- Initial evaluation should include particular attention to the function of the triceps muscle, the function of the radial and ulnar nerves, and the vascular status of the upper extremity.
- Palpable defect often detected on posterior elbow
- Test for triceps mechanism integrity by asking the patient to actively extend the elbow against gravity.
- Examine the degree of soft-tissue injury and determine whether the fracture is open or closed.

### TESTS

#### *Lab*

Before surgery, routine preoperative laboratory tests are performed, depending on the age and medical condition of the patient.

#### *Imaging*

- Radiography:
  - Obtain AP and lateral radiographs of the elbow.
  - A radiocapitellar view may be helpful if there appears to be an associated radial head injury.
- Obtain a CT scan of the elbow to evaluate complex fracture dislocations of the elbow.

### DIFFERENTIAL DIAGNOSIS

- Distal humerus fracture
- Elbow dislocation
- Radial head fracture

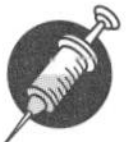

# TREATMENT

## GENERAL MEASURES

- Nondisplaced fractures are treated with immobilization in an above-the-elbow splint or cast with the elbow in 90° of flexion for 4 weeks.
- Follow-up radiography is necessary 7–10 days after injury to ensure that the fracture has not displaced.
- Displaced fractures usually require surgical fixation to restore extensor mechanism function.

### *Activity*

- After fracture, the arm should be splinted comfortably at 90° of flexion, and a sling should be offered.
- Patients should be encouraged to move the hand and shoulder to prevent stiffness.

### *Nursing*

- Patients in a sling should be helped with personal hygiene in the armpit area.
- Care should be taken that the splint is comfortable and does not rub.

## SPECIAL THERAPY

### *Physical Therapy*

- Initially, strengthening and gentle passive ROM exercises to address the common sequelae (decreased ROM and muscle strength) of elbow immobilization after olecranon fractures
- Gradually progress to active ROM exercises when radiographic evidence shows callus formation and fracture healing.
- Motion of the ipsilateral shoulder and hand should be encouraged.

## MEDICATION (DRUGS)

### *First Line*

Narcotic medicines may be necessary for pain relief after fracture.

## SURGERY

- Most olecranon fractures are treated surgically because they disrupt the extensor mechanism.
- Fractures must be repaired anatomically to restore the joint surface.
- Choice of repair technique depends on the size of the fragment, the direction of the fracture line, and the amount of fracture comminution.
  - Stable, nondisplaced fractures may be treated nonoperatively.
  - Displaced fractures require open reduction and fixation.
  - Open fractures should be treated with surgical débridement and fixation.
  - Small avulsion fractures are treated with excision and repair.
    - The triceps tendon is sutured back to the olecranon.
    - Bone removal does increase joint pressures and, if possible, bony fixation should be attempted (4).
  - Transverse fractures are repaired using 2 Kirschner wires and a tension band wire to resist the pull of the triceps muscle.
  - Oblique fractures may be repaired using interfragmentary screw fixation and an accompanying tension band wire.
    - Fixation with screws has been shown to be stronger than that with tension band wires (5).
  - Severely comminuted fractures are not amenable to tension wiring and require fixation with plating.
    - A 3.5-mm reconstruction plate can be bent to fit the olecranon, or a precontoured plate can be used.
  - Fractures with bone loss may require bone grafting to repair defects (6).

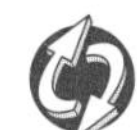

# FOLLOW-UP

## DISPOSITION

After surgery, the arm is splinted until skin healing occurs, and then early ROM exercises are started.

## PROGNOSIS

- The prognosis is good for >90% of patients (7).
- Fractures with more articular involvement and more severity have been shown to have worse outcomes (8).

## COMPLICATIONS

- Painful hardware requiring removal occurs in 20–80% of patients (9,10).
- Radial neuropathy
- Ulnar neuropathy
- Flexion contracture
- Elbow arthritis
- Malunion
- Nonunion

## PATIENT MONITORING

- Patients should be monitored until fracture healing is observed radiographically.
- ROM of the elbow and strength of the arm should be monitored.

## REFERENCES


1. Crenshaw AH, Jr. Fractures of the shoulder, arm, and forearm. In: Canale ST, ed. *Campbell's Operative Orthopaedics*, 10th ed. St. Louis: Mosby, 2003:2985–3069.
2. Jerosch J, Heidjann J, Thorwesten L, et al. Injury pattern and acceptance of passive and active injury prophylaxis for inline skating. *Knee Surg Sports Traumatol Arthrosc* 1998;6:44–49.
3. Carson S, Woolridge DP, Colletti J, et al. Pediatric upper extremity injuries. *Pediatr Clin North Am* 2006;53:41–67.
4. Moed BR, Ede DE, Brown TD. Fractures of the olecranon: an in vitro study of elbow joint stresses after tension-band wire fixation versus proximal fracture fragment excision. *J Trauma* 2002;53:1088–1093.
5. Hutchinson DT, Horwitz DS, Ha G, et al. Cyclic loading of olecranon fracture fixation constructs. *J Bone Joint Surg* 2003;85A:831–837.
6. Ikeda M, Fukushima Y, Kobayashi Y, et al. Comminuted fractures of the olecranon. Management by bone graft from the iliac crest and multiple tension-band wiring. *J Bone Joint Surg* 2001;83B:805–808.
7. Karlsson MK, Hasserius R, Karlsson C, et al. Fractures of the olecranon: a 15- to 25-year followup of 73 patients. *Clin Orthop Relat Res* 2002;403:205–212.
8. Rommens PM, Kuchle R, Schneider RU, et al. Olecranon fractures in adults: factors influencing outcome. *Injury* 2004;35:1149–1157.
9. Bailey CS, MacDermid J, Patterson SD, et al. Outcome of plate fixation of olecranon fractures. *J Orthop Trauma* 2001;15:542–548.
10. Karlsson MK, Hasserius R, Besjakov J, et al. Comparison of tension-band and figure-of-eight wiring techniques for treatment of olecranon fractures. *J Shoulder Elbow Surg* 2002;11: 377–382.


## ADDITIONAL READING


- Hak DJ, Golladay GJ. Olecranon fractures: treatment options. *J Am Acad Orthop Surg* 2000;8:266–275.
- Nork SE, Jones CB, Henley MB. Surgical treatment of olecranon fractures. *Am J Orthop* 2001;30:577–586.


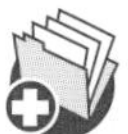

# MISCELLANEOUS

## CODES

### *ICD9-CM*

- 813.01 Closed olecranon fracture
- 813.11 Open olecranon fracture

## PATIENT TEACHING

- Even with a perfect reduction, patients may still have decreased ROM.
- Patients often lose 5–10° of extension.

### *Activity*

Until fracture healing, patients should limit lifting with the arm.

### *Prevention*

individuals involved in sports with high risks of falls, such as skating or rollerblading, should use elbow pads (2).

## FAQ

- Q: How long do olecranon fractures take to heal?
  - A: Fracture healing usually occurs in 2–3 months. Additional therapy is required to strengthen the arm over the next 3 months.

# OPEN FRACTURES

*Theodore T. Manson, MD*

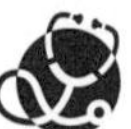

## BASICS

### DESCRIPTION

- Open fractures are defined as situations in which the fracture site communicates with the outside environment.
  - The bone does not need to protrude from the skin for the injury to be an open fracture.
  - Any full-thickness skin laceration in the zone of fracture injury is considered an open fracture.
- Open fractures can be classified by the Gustilo-Anderson system (1).
  - Type I: Low-energy fracture with a clean wound <1 cm long
  - Type II: Low- to medium-energy fracture with a laceration >1 cm long but without extensive soft-tissue damage
  - Type III:
    - High-energy fracture
    - Segmental fractures, gunshot injuries
    - More extensive soft-tissue devitalization than in type II
    - Type IIIA: Adequate soft-tissue coverage of bone
    - Type IIIB: Inadequate soft-tissue coverage of bone, fractures that need rotational or free flap coverage
    - Type IIIC: Fracture with an arterial injury

### RISK FACTORS

Bones with thin soft-tissue envelopes (such as the tibia) are more likely to present with open fracture than bones well-protected with soft tissue (such as the femur).

### PATHOPHYSIOLOGY

- Treatment of open fractures is based on preventing infection and stabilizing the injured bone.
  - Infection is promoted by:
    - Bacterial contamination of wound
    - Devitalized muscle and bone
    - Dead space
    - Foreign material

### ASSOCIATED CONDITIONS

- Many open injuries occur in the setting of multitrauma.
  - Follow ATLS protocol (2):
  - Palpate and examine every joint and the spine to assess for additional injury.

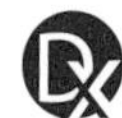

## DIAGNOSIS

### SIGNS AND SYMPTOMS

- Patients often are involved in high-energy trauma, although open fractures can occur via low-energy mechanisms.
- Follow ATLS protocols.

#### *History*

- When did the injury occur?
- What was the mechanism (i.e., high or low energy)?
- Was the limb exposed to:
  - Barnyard contamination?
  - Marine or freshwater contamination?
  - Oil or grease?

#### *Physical Exam*

- The physician must 1) diagnose the open fracture and then 2) follow a general fracture physical examination.
- Diagnosing an open fracture:
  - Bone protruding from skin (not required)
  - Fat or blood oozing from a laceration
  - Laceration in the zone of injury, which can be large in high-energy fractures
- General examination for fractures:
  - Palpate joint above and below injury as well as every other joint in body.
  - Assess vascular viability of limb and damaged soft tissues.
    - Pulses or arterial brachial indices
    - Color and capillary refill of contused skin and muscle
  - Presence or absence of:
    - Periosteal stripping
    - Gross contamination with foreign material
    - Compartment syndrome
  - Neurologic motor and sensory examinations

### TESTS

#### *Lab*

Most patients with open fractures require operative treatment and should have a full set of preoperative labs.

#### *Imaging*

- Imaging should be appropriate for the fracture site.
  - Usually AP and lateral radiographs of the bone in question and of the joints proximal and distal to the injury
  - CT scan is indicated for some fracture patterns but should not delay surgical débridement and stabilization.

#### *Diagnostic Procedures/Surgery*

If the limb is swollen or if the neurologic examination is not intact, compartment pressures should be monitored.

### DIFFERENTIAL DIAGNOSIS

- Sometimes a laceration is present on a fractured extremity that does not communicate with the fracture.
- However, it is always prudent to assume that a laceration in the zone of fracture injury indicates an open fracture.

## TREATMENT

### INITIAL STABILIZATION

- After being stabilized according to ATLS guidelines, patients should have:
  - The wound covered with a sterile dressing
  - The extremity splinted
  - Antibiotics administered (see "Medication" section)
  - Tetanus prophylaxis as indicated
- The clinician should ensure that exposures of the wound to viewing are kept to a minimum.

### GENERAL MEASURES

- The goals of treatment are to prevent infection and restore musculoskeletal function.
- Antibiotic therapy and prompt débridement and stabilization are the hallmarks of open fracture treatment.
  - Antibiotics as prophylaxis to infection is indicated in all cases.
  - Operative débridement is indicated in almost all cases.
  - Stabilization by fracture-specific implants is indicated in most cases.

#### *Activity*

Patient activity levels are governed by the fracture type.

#### *Nursing*

Fractured extremities should be elevated on pillows.

### SPECIAL THERAPY

#### *Physical Therapy*

Physical therapy after fracture repair is individualized to attain joint ROM and muscular strength.

### MEDICATION (DRUGS)

- Parenteral and oral narcotics are used for pain control.
- Parenteral antibiotics are essential on presentation to the emergency room (3).

#### *First Line*

- Antibiotics should be used to limit infection.
  - In general, antibiotics are continued 24–72 hours after the last surgical procedure, depending on the severity of the fracture.
  - Parenteral 1st-generation cephalosporin or clindamycin for all open fractures
  - Add aminoglycosides for type III fractures.
  - Ampicillin or penicillin should be used when anaerobes may be present.
    - Farm injuries
    - Vascular injuries
    - Extensive muscle necrosis

#### *Second Line*

- Other antibiotics are used on a situational basis:
  - Quinolones, aztreonam, or 3rd-generation cephalosporins can be used as substitutes for aminoglycosides for type III fractures, but they are not as effective.
  - Culture-specific antibiotics are used for documented postoperative infections.

### SURGERY

- The key to effective treatment is meticulous débridement.
- The goal is a clean wound with viable tissues and no infection.
  - Irrigate the wound (usually 6–10 L of saline) to decrease bacterial load and remove foreign material.
  - Débride skin and subcutaneous tissues back to bleeding edges.
  - Débride nonviable muscle based on assessment of muscle color, circulation, contraction, and consistency.
  - Débride cortical bone fragments that are devoid of soft-tissue attachments.
  - Most open fracture wounds should not be closed initially (4).
  - The timing of the closure of open-fracture wounds is controversial.
    - Many type I and some type II wounds can be closed primarily after débridement.
    - A repeat débridement in 24–48 hours with delayed wound closure is in general a safe practice.
    - Larger, devitalized wounds may require the assistance of plastic surgeons for soft-tissue coverage, including rotational and free flaps.
  - Fracture stabilization helps minimize infection risk and maximizes functional recovery.
    - Implant choice depends on fracture location and severity.
    - Staged treatment with an initial external fixator may reduce tissue inflammation in the early injury phase (5).
    - Later, definitive fixation may involve intramedullary nailing or plate fixation (6).

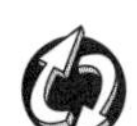

## FOLLOW-UP

- Follow-up depends on the type of fracture and the severity of the wound.
- Wounds should be assessed for advancing erythema and drainage.

### DISPOSITION

- Most open fractures are treated operatively.
  - Adults: Typically within 6–24 hours of injury
  - Pediatric patients: Within 6–24 hours of injury (7)

#### *Issues for Referral*

All open fractures should be seen by an orthopaedic surgeon on presentation.

### COMPLICATIONS

- Complications and prognosis are related to fracture type and location but include (1):
  - Infection:
    - Type I: 2%
    - Type II: 2–10%
    - Type III: 10–50% depending on the subtype and location
  - Osteomyelitis
  - The occurrence of nonunion increases with the amount of periosteal stripping.
  - Malunion
  - Arthritis

### REFERENCES


1. Gustilo RB, Anderson JT. Prevention of infection in the treatment of one thousand and twenty-five open fractures of long bones: retrospective and prospective analysis. *J Bone Joint Surg* 1976;58A: 453–458.
2. American College of Surgeons Committee on Trauma. *Advanced Trauma Life Support Program for Doctors*, 6th ed. Chicago: American College of Surgeons, 1997.
3. Zalavras CG, Patzakis MJ. Open fractures: evaluation and management. *J Am Acad Orthop Surg* 2003;11:212–219.
4. Weitz-Marshall AD, Bosse MJ. Timing of closure of open fractures. *J Am Acad Orthop Surg* 2002;10: 379–384.
5. Roberts CS, Pape HC, Jones AL, et al. Damage control orthopaedics: evolving concepts in the treatment of patients who have sustained orthopaedic trauma. *Instr Course Lect* 2005;54: 447–462.
6. Nowotarski PJ, Turen CH, Brumback RJ, et al. Conversion of external fixation to intramedullary nailing for fractures of the shaft of the femur in multiply injured patients. *J Bone Joint Surg* 2000;82A:781–788.
7. Skaggs DL, Friend L, Alman B, et al. The effect of surgical delay on acute infection following 554 open fractures in children. *J Bone Joint Surg* 2005;87A:8–12.


### ADDITIONAL READING


- Castillo RC, Bosse MJ, MacKenzie EJ, et al. Impact of smoking on fracture healing and risk of complications in limb-threatening open tibia fractures. *J Orthop Trauma* 2005;19:151–157.
- Norris BL, Kellam JF. Soft-tissue injuries associated with high-energy extremity trauma: principles of management. *J Am Acad Orthop Surg* 1997;5: 37–46.


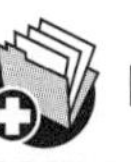

## MISCELLANEOUS

### CODES

#### *ICD9-CM*

Depends on fracture location

### PATIENT TEACHING

- Compared with closed fractures, open fractures:
  - Take longer to heal
  - Have higher rates of nonunion
  - Have higher rates of infection and osteomyelitis
- Limbs with open fractures may develop compartment syndrome.
- Treatment may require staged interventions.
- Multiple surgeries may be needed to clean a dirty wound.
- Wound closure may require rotational or free muscle flaps.

### FAQ

- Q: What is the risk of infection after open fracture?
  - A: The risk depends on the grade of injury. Patients who smoke or have chronic illnesses have higher infection rates.
- Q: How long do open fractures take to heal?
  - A: Although a closed long-bone fracture generally heals in 10–14 weeks, time to healing for an open fracture can be much longer and depends on the amount of soft-tissue damage and bone loss.

# OSTEOARTHRITIS

*Tariq A. Nayfeh, MD, PhD*
*Tung B. Le, MD*

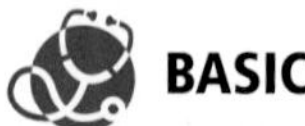

## BASICS

### DESCRIPTION

- The most prevalent form of arthritis
- May occur in virtually any joint of the body
- Has no cure and leads to pain and joint dysfunction
- The end result is loss of articular cartilage with secondary bone changes, including osteophytes, subchondral sclerosis, and subchondral cysts.
- Classification is by single or multiple joint involvement.
- Synonyms: Degenerative joint disease; Wear-and-tear arthritis

### EPIDEMIOLOGY

#### Incidence

- The knee is the most commonly affected joint, followed by the hand and hip (1).
- In a study of 697 females >65 years old, knee arthritis occurred in 30%, hand arthritis in 15%, and hip arthritis in 8% (2).

#### Prevalence

- Osteoarthritis, the most common form of arthritis, affects females more often than males (3).
- In contrast to inflammatory arthritis, osteoarthritis occurs principally in individuals >60 years old.
- In 1 study (4):
  - Hand osteoarthritis occurred in 23% of females >65 years old.
  - The most commonly affected joints were the DIP and 1st CMC joints.

### RISK FACTORS

- Obesity
- AVN
- Septic arthritis
- Advancing age
- Female gender

#### Genetics

A genetic predisposition is thought to exist, but genes have not yet been identified.

### ETIOLOGY

- No known cause of osteoarthritis (idiopathic osteoarthritis):
  - The common pathway is loss of the articular cartilage with progressive overloading of the joint.
- Many conditions that injure the joint may lead to secondary arthritis.
  - Trauma: Posttraumatic arthritis
  - Infection: Postinfectious arthritis
  - AVN: Arthritis associated with the condition

### ASSOCIATED CONDITIONS

No conditions are associated with osteoarthritis.

## DIAGNOSIS

### SIGNS AND SYMPTOMS

- Discomfort with weightbearing and joint motion
- Stiffness
- Loss of function:
  - Inability to do heavy work
  - Inability to tie or put on shoes
  - Limitation to short distance walking

#### History

Pain and swelling that increase with activity or prolonged inactivity

#### Physical Exam

- The principal features are:
  - Stiffness and loss of ROM
  - Joint effusion
  - Limb deformity
  - Painful joint motion
  - Gait disorder

### TESTS

#### Lab

No specific laboratory features

#### Imaging

- Radiography:
  - AP and lateral radiographs are the main imaging modalities.
  - In the knee, foot, and ankle, weightbearing radiographs are obtained.
- MRI can be used to exclude other diagnoses such as AVN, stress fractures, and neoplasms.

#### Pathological Findings

Loss of the thickness and organization of the articular cartilage

### DIFFERENTIAL DIAGNOSIS

- The diagnosis of osteoarthritis is not difficult when the disease is in the moderate or advanced stage.
- Early arthritis can be confused with the following conditions:
  - Tendinitis or bursitis
  - Stress fractures
  - Synovial proliferative disorders

## TREATMENT

### GENERAL MEASURES

Rest, activity modification, weight loss, and NSAIDs

### SPECIAL THERAPY

#### Physical Therapy

- Patients should begin a program to preserve muscle strength and ROM and to avoid contractures (5).
- Heavy-impact activity (such as running, contact sports, and heavy work) exacerbates symptoms.
- A cane used in the opposite hand substantially reduces the forces across the hip joint and will relieve discomfort and improve gait.

#### Complementary and Alternative Therapies

- Acupuncture may provide pain relief for knee arthritis in the short term (6).
- Many herbal medicines are used for the treatment of osteoarthritis.
  - Evidence to support their use is limited (7).

### MEDICATION (DRUGS)

#### First Line

- NSAIDs, including COX-2 inhibitors, are mainstays in the nonoperative treatment of arthritis.
  - Meta-analysis shows these medications to be slightly more effective than a placebo in the short term (8).
  - NSAIDS have a high rate of side effects, including gastrointestinal bleeding.
- Acetaminophen is widely used for pain relief (9).

#### Second Line

- The use of nutraceuticals, such as glucosamine and chondroitin sulfate, is controversial, with a recent study showing no benefit (10).
- Intra-articular injection:
  - With corticosteroids, decreases pain for short periods (11)
  - With hyaluronic acid, may have a small effect on knee pain (12)
- Opioid pain medicine may be used for severe pain in patients who are not operative candidates (13).

### SURGERY

- 2 main types of surgery: Realignment osteotomy and joint replacement
  - Realignment osteotomy:
    - The joint surfaces are repositioned by cutting the bone and changing the axis of weightbearing.
    - Purpose: Allows the healthiest articular cartilage to bear the most weight
    - May be combined with ligament or meniscal repair
  - Arthroplasty:
    - The arthritic joint surfaces are removed, and a new joint surface is implanted.
    - The bearing surface is typically metal on high-density polyethylene.
    - Examples are total hip arthroplasty, total knee arthroplasty, and total shoulder arthroplasty.

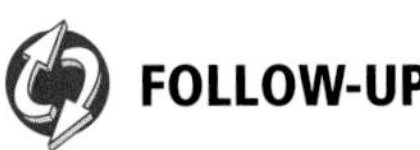

## FOLLOW-UP

### DISPOSITION

#### *Issues for Referral*

Patients with end-stage arthritis or severe pain from arthritis should be referred to an orthopaedic surgeon for consideration of surgical treatment.

### PROGNOSIS

- Osteoarthritis progressively worsens with time.
- No cure exists.
- Modern methods of joint replacement provide excellent function and pain relief.

### COMPLICATIONS

- Progressive arthritis leads to worsening deformity and stiffness.
  - In the lower extremity, patients may stop walking and rely on wheelchairs
  - In the upper extremity, prevents activities and leads to lack of function
- Treatment also may lead to complications.
  - The side effects of NSAIDs include gastritis and gastrointestinal bleeding.
  - Surgical intervention may lead to infection, DVT, or failure of the replacement mechanical joint.

### PATIENT MONITORING

- Patients are followed at 3–12-month intervals, depending on the severity of their symptoms.
- Plain radiographs are taken every 6–12 months.

### REFERENCES


1. Felson DT, Lawrence RC, Dieppe PA, et al. Osteoarthritis: new insights. Part 1: the disease and its risk factors. *Ann Intern Med* 2000;133: 635–646.
2. Mannoni A, Briganti MP, Di Bari M, et al. Epidemiological profile of symptomatic osteoarthritis in older adults: a population based study in Dicomano, Italy. *Ann Rheum Dis* 2003; 62:576–578.
3. Sharma L, Kapoor D, Issa S. Epidemiology of osteoarthritis: an update. *Curr Opin Rheumatol* 2006;18:147–156.
4. Hirsch R, Guralnik JM, Ling SM, et al. The patterns and prevalence of hand osteoarthritis in a population of disabled older women: The Women's Health and Aging Study. *Osteoarthritis Cartilage* 2000;8:S16–S21.
5. Devos-Comby L, Cronan T, Roesch SC. Do exercise and self-management interventions benefit patients with osteoarthritis of the knee? A meta-analytic review. *J Rheumatol* 2006;33: 744–756.
6. Witt C, Brinkhaus B, Jena S, et al. Acupuncture in patients with osteoarthritis of the knee: a randomised trial. *Lancet* 2005;366:136–143.
7. Ernst E. Musculoskeletal conditions and complementary/alternative medicine. *Best Pract Res Clin Rheumatol* 2004;18:539–556.
8. Bjordal JM, Ljunggren AE, Klovning A, et al. Non-steroidal anti-inflammatory drugs, including cyclo-oxygenase-2 inhibitors, in osteoarthritic knee pain: meta-analysis of randomised placebo controlled trials. *Br Med J* 2004;Epub. (DOI:10.1136/bmj.38273.626655.63):1–6.
9. Towheed TE, Maxwell L, Judd MG, et al. Acetaminophen for osteoarthritis. *Cochrane Database Syst Rev* 2006;1(CD004257):1–56.
10. Clegg DO, Reda DJ, Harris CL, et al. Glucosamine, chondroitin sulfate, and the two in combination for painful knee osteoarthritis. *N Engl J Med* 2006;354:795–808.
11. Bellamy N, Campbell J, Robinson V, et al. Intraarticular corticosteroid for treatment of osteoarthritis of the knee. *Cochrane Database Syst Rev* 2006;2(CD005328):1–186.
12. Lo GH, LaValley M, McAlindon T, et al. Intra-articular hyaluronic acid in treatment of knee osteoarthritis: a meta-analysis. *JAMA* 2003; 290:3115–3121.
13. Dieppe PA, Lohmander LS. Pathogenesis and management of pain in osteoarthritis. *Lancet* 2005;365:965–973.


### ADDITIONAL READING


Hunter DJ, Felson DT. Osteoarthritis. *Br Med J* 2006; 332:639–642.


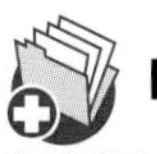

## MISCELLANEOUS

### CODES

#### *ICD9-CM*

715.9 Osteoarthritis, unspecified whether generalized or localized

### PATIENT TEACHING

- Patients are:
  - Taught to avoid activities that worsen the pain
  - Shown how to prevent contractures
  - Encouraged to lose weight

#### *Activity*

- Patients should be encouraged to maintain muscle strength and joint mobility.
- Exercises that do not cause pain are best.
- Activities with little or no impact include elliptical trainers, bicycling, swimming, and water aerobics or running.

#### *Prevention*

Weight loss may help prevent joint degeneration.

### FAQ

- Q: What can be done to prevent osteoarthritis?
  - A: In general, interventions have not been found to prevent osteoarthritis. However, osteoarthritis is associated with obesity, and weight loss may help prevent joint degeneration.
- Q: When is surgery indicated for the treatment of osteoarthritis?
  - A: Surgery is the final treatment after nonoperative measures (such as muscle strengthening, ambulatory aids, and medications) have been tried. The most commonly performed surgery is total knee replacement.

# OSTEOCHONDRAL DEFECT OF THE TALUS

*Marc D. Chodos, MD*

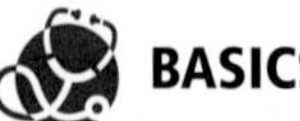

## BASICS

### DESCRIPTION

- OCDs of the talus represent damage to the articular surface of the talar dome in the ankle joint.
- The talus is the 3rd most common site (after the knee and elbow) of osteochondral lesions.
- The most common sites are the posteromedial (53%) (Fig. 1) and anterolateral (46%) talar dome (1).
- Most classification systems are based on lesion descriptions by Berndt and Harty (2):
  - Stage 1: Subchondral bone compression
  - Stage 2: Partially detached osteochondral fragment
  - Stage 3: Detached but stable/nondisplaced osteochondral fragment
  - Stage 4: Detached and displaced fragment
  - Stage 5: Subchondral cyst (added by Loomer et al.) (1)

### GENERAL PREVENTION

No clear method is available for preventing this disorder, although early surgical treatment of chronic ankle instability may prevent the development of OCD attributable to instability.

### EPIDEMIOLOGY

- Most patients who develop OCDs are in their 2nd–4th decades, with a mean age of 26.9 years (3).
- 65% are male (3).

#### *Incidence*

- 0.09% of all fractures (4)
- 0.1% of all talus fractures (4)
- 4% of all osteochondral lesions (5)

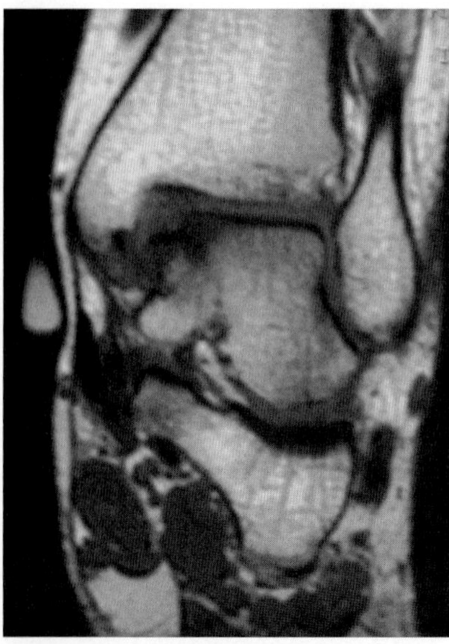

**Fig. 1.** Coronal T1-weighted image of the ankle, showing a medial talar OCD.

### RISK FACTORS

- Most OCDs are traumatic in origin.
- Therefore, ankle fracture, sprain, and chronic ankle instability are risk factors.

#### *Genetics*

Weak evidence suggests that a genetic component might be involved in some OCDs (5).

### PATHOPHYSIOLOGY

OCDs can be produced in cadaveric models by shear and compression forces (2).

### ETIOLOGY

- Most commonly caused by trauma:
  - Acute: Ankle fracture or sprain
  - Chronic: Recurrent injury from chronic ankle instability
  - Lateral OCD is associated with a recognized traumatic episode in 93% of cases (3).
  - Medial OCD is associated with a recognized traumatic episode in 61% of cases (3).
- Other possible causes include ischemic events (AVN).

### ASSOCIATED CONDITIONS

- Ankle fracture
- Ankle sprain
- Chronic ankle instability

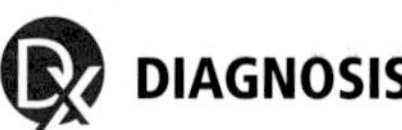

## DIAGNOSIS

### SIGNS AND SYMPTOMS

#### *History*

- Assess for:
  - History of previous ankle injury
  - History of ankle instability or sprains
  - Mechanical symptoms (locking, catching)

#### *Physical Exam*

- Perform general foot and ankle examination.
- Specific areas for concentration:
  - Palpate for ankle swelling or effusion.
  - Evaluate for tenderness over the talar dome.
  - Examine for ankle instability (anterior drawer test, talar tilt test) or evidence of general ligamentous laxity.
  - Examine for crepitus or mechanical signs with ankle ROM.
- Make sure the patient does not have other abnormalities that explain chronic ankle pain, including peroneal tendon subluxation, fracture of the lateral process of the talus, 5th metatarsal fracture, syndesmosis sprain, or tarsal coalition.

### TESTS

The diagnosis of OCD most frequently depends on obtaining an imaging study: Plain radiographs or CT, MRI, or bone scans.

#### *Imaging*

- Weightbearing radiographs should be obtained initially.
  - Sensitivity = 0.70, specificity = 0.94 (6)
  - Although OCDs frequently are not well visualized on plain radiographs, this modality is inexpensive, easy to obtain, and can help rule out other abnormalities.
- CT:
  - Sensitivity = 0.81, specificity = 0.99 (6)
  - If a lesion is seen on plain radiographs, then a CT scan provides the greatest certainty of all imaging modalities that the lesion is real and an OCD (i.e., best positive predictive value).
  - Best method for accurately characterizing the size and extent of a defect
- MRI:
  - Sensitivity = 0.96, specificity = 0.99 (6)
  - A negative MRI provides the greatest certainty of all imaging modalities that no lesion exists (i.e., best negative predictive value).
  - Tends to overestimate the size of a lesion because of bone marrow edema
  - Metal artifact can make MRI difficult to interpret in certain cases.
  - Best modality for finding associated soft-tissue abnormalities
- No difference in the effectiveness of CT and MRI in diagnosing an OCD (6)

#### *Diagnostic Procedures/Surgery*

- Arthroscopy provides the best and most direct method for evaluating the articular surface and treating the abnormality.
- Problems with arthroscopy include:
  - Surgeon-dependent
  - Cannot evaluate subchondral abnormalities
  - Invasive

#### *Pathological Findings*

- When not displaced, a chronic osteochondral fragment often is attached to the defect by fibrous tissue.
  - If the subchondral bone is violated, the defect attempts to heal with fibrous tissue or fibrocartilage.
  - If the subchondral bone is not violated, no healing occurs.
  - Although the cartilage cap remains viable (7), the osseous component of a displaced OCD is avascular and has a low potential to heal in chronic cases.

### DIFFERENTIAL DIAGNOSIS

- The differential diagnosis includes any cause of chronic pain in the region of the ankle joint:
  - Occult fracture (5th metatarsal, lateral process of talus, medial or lateral malleolus)
  - Ankle or syndesmosis sprain
  - Chronic ankle instability
  - Peroneal tendon subluxation
  - Anterior ankle impingement
  - Tarsal coalition
  - Ankle or subtalar joint synovitis
  - Posterior tibialis tendinitis

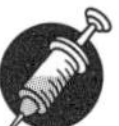

# TREATMENT

## GENERAL MEASURES

- Nonoperative management consisting of cast or boot immobilization can be attempted for stage 1, stage 2, and some stage 3 lesions.
  - Success rate is ~50% (3).
  - Delaying surgical intervention for chronic OCD does not appear to alter results of later surgery.

### *Pediatric Considerations*

- Children are thought to have better healing potential than adults.
- Although nonoperative management is recommended more often for children, the results are not necessarily better than those for adults.
- Letts et al. (8) found that only 9 of 24 (37.5%) pediatric patients with an OCD managed without surgery had a good or excellent result.

### *Activity*

- Nonoperative management recommendations range from activity modification alone to nonweightbearing in a cast.
- Microfracture or drilling: 4–6 weeks of nonweightbearing is recommended to allow the defect to heal, with ankle ROM encouraged.
- Any procedure that requires an osteotomy necessitates nonweightbearing until the osteotomy heals (4–8 weeks).
  - ROM usually is started 2–6 weeks after surgery, depending on the quality of the osteotomy fixation.

## SPECIAL THERAPY

### *Physical Therapy*

Ankle ROM exercises, peroneal strengthening, progressive ambulation, and proprioception training

## SURGERY

- Several surgical options exist, but the indications for 1 procedure over another are not well defined by evidence-based medicine.
- Procedures that reduce and stabilize the displaced fragment:
  - Usually recommended only for lesions that are large enough to be amenable to internal fixation
  - Acute fractures do better than chronic lesions.
- Procedures that stimulate fibrocartilage formation include débridement, curettage, and microfracture or drilling of the subchondral bone.
  - Generally recommended as the initial method of surgical treatment because it can be done arthroscopically with minimal morbidity and is associated with an 85% success rate (3).
  - Loose bodies, fibrous tissue, and unstable cartilage are débrided.
  - Subchondral bone is penetrated to allow bleeding and fibrin clot formation.
    - It is thought that mesenchymal stem cells in the clot lead to the formation of fibrocartilage.
  - Although biomechanically inferior to hyaline cartilage, fibrocartilage formation appears to be sufficient for smaller lesions.
  - Defects with a surface area <1 cm$^2$ seem to have better results than larger lesions.
- Procedures that transfer hyaline cartilage to the defect: OATS/mosaicplasty, allograft transfer
  - Generally recommended for large lesions or lesions that fail other forms of treatment
  - Osteotomy usually is required as part of the surgical approach.
  - OATS/mosaicplasty:
    - Osteochondral tissue harvested from a remote nonloadbearing site (usually the ipsilateral knee) and transplanted into talar defect
    - Limited by the amount of donor tissue that can be harvested
    - 94% good to excellent results (9)
  - Allograft transfer:
    - Osteochondral tissue harvested from fresh allograft talus and transplanted into the defect
    - Best for large (>3 cm$^2$) lesions, as an alternative to arthrodesis (10)
    - 66% success rate (11)
- Procedures that regrow hyaline cartilage, such as autologous chondrocyte transfer:
  - Cartilage is harvested (usually from the knee) and grown in culture.
  - Once enough cells are available, the chondrocytes are reimplanted into the defect.
    - Because cells are grown *in vitro*, defect size is not limited with this procedure.
    - Osteotomy usually is required as part of the surgical approach.
  - 1st- and 2nd-generation techniques rely on injection of the cell suspension under a periosteal flap or collagen membrane that is sewn and glued over the defect (12).
  - 3rd-generation techniques rely on a 3D bioscaffold to contain the cells instead of a periosteal flap (7).
  - Short-term clinical results generally are good, although biopsies of treated lesions often show fibrocartilage, not hyaline cartilage.
  - In the future:
    - More complex scaffolds that better replicate the microarchitecture of articular cartilage may become available.
    - Growth factors and the use of mesenchymal stem cells also will be important in refining the procedure and improving results.
- Other surgical options: Concurrent chronic ankle instability should be addressed with ligament reconstruction.

# FOLLOW-UP

## PROGNOSIS

With proper treatment, the prognosis generally is good.

## COMPLICATIONS

Complications include malunion or nonunion of an osteotomy, persistent pain, stiffness, and arthritis.

## PATIENT MONITORING

The patient is followed regularly to make sure that ROM is regained, any osteotomies heal, and clinical resolution of symptoms occurs.

## REFERENCES

1. Loomer R, Fisher C, Lloyd-Smith R, et al. Osteochondral lesions of the talus. *Am J Sports Med* 1993;21:13–19.
2. Berndt AL, Harty M. Transchondral fractures (osteochondritis dissecans) of the talus. *J Bone Joint Surg* 1959;41A:988–1020.
3. Verhagen RAW, Struijs PAA, Bossuyt PMM, et al. Systematic review of treatment strategies for osteochondral defects of the talar dome. *Foot Ankle Clin* 2003;8:233–242.
4. Giannini S, Vannini F. Operative treatment of osteochondral lesions of the talar dome: current concepts review. *Foot Ankle Int* 2004;25: 168–175.
5. Santrock RD, Buchanan MM, Lee TH, et al. Osteochondral lesions of the talus. *Foot Ankle Clin* 2003;8:73–90.
6. Verhagen RAW, Maas M, Dijkgraaf MGW, et al. Prospective study on diagnostic strategies in osteochondral lesions of the talus. Is MRI superior to helical CT? *J Bone Joint Surg* 2005;87B:41–46.
7. Giannini S, Buda R, Grigolo B, et al. The detached osteochondral fragment as a source of cells for autologous chondrocyte implantation (ACI) in the ankle joint. *Osteoarthritis Cartilage* 2005;13: 601–607.
8. Letts M, Davidson D, Ahmer A. Osteochondritis dissecans of the talus in children. *J Pediatr Orthop* 2003;23:617–625.
9. Hangody L, Kish G, Modis L, et al. Mosaicplasty for the treatment of osteochondritis dissecans of the talus: two to seven year results in 36 patients. *Foot Ankle Int* 2001;22:552–558.
10. Raikin SM. Stage VI: massive osteochondral defects of the talus. *Foot Ankle Clin* 2004;9: 737–744.
11. Gross AE, Agnidis Z, Hutchison CR. Osteochondral defects of the talus treated with fresh osteochondral allograft transplantation. *Foot Ankle Int* 2001;22:385–391.
12. Giannini S, Buda R, Grigolo B, et al. Autologous chondrocyte transplantation in osteochondral lesions of the ankle joint. *Foot Ankle Int* 2001; 22:513–517.

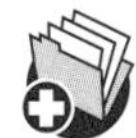

# MISCELLANEOUS

## CODES

### *ICD9-CM*

732.7 Osteochondritis dissecans

## PATIENT TEACHING

The patient should be actively involved in the decision-making process, with a clear understanding of the risks and benefits of surgical and nonsurgical treatments.

## FAQ

- Q: How are unstable OCD lesions of the ankle treated?
  - A: A patient with an unstable, displaced OCD of the talus typically presents with mechanical symptoms, including locking or giving way of the ankle because of the loose body. Such lesions have poor prognoses with nonoperative treatment and typically are addressed with arthroscopic surgery. Stable OCDs may respond to a short trial of rest, immobilization, and physical therapy; failures are treated surgically.

# OSTEOCHONDRITIS DISSECANS OF THE KNEE

*Dennis E. Kramer, MD*
*John H. Wilckens, MD*

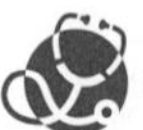

## BASICS

### DESCRIPTION

- A pathologic joint entity of localized bone necrosis with overlying cartilage injury
- Osteochondritis dissecans primarily affects the knee, but it is also seen in the hip (in late Legg-Calvé-Perthes disease), elbow, and ankle.
- Osteochondritis dissecans occurs primarily in the 2nd decade of life, but it also is seen in children and older adults.
- Older adolescents, after physeal closure, have less ability to heal these lesions with nonoperative treatment.
- Several forms of "Little League elbow" are types of osteochondritis dissecans of the radial head and capitellum.
- Also called "osteochondral fracture"
- Most common locations (1–3):
  - Posterolateral medial femoral condyle: 70%
  - Inferocentral lateral femoral condyle: 20%
  - Patella: 10%
  - Trochlea: 1%

### EPIDEMIOLOGY

- Juvenile and adult forms
- More common in males
- 25% bilateral (3,4)

#### *Incidence*

More frequent in active sports participants

### RISK FACTORS

Patients susceptible to trauma (i.e., those with increased joint laxity, genu valgum, obesity, or intraosseous vascular anomalies)

#### *Genetics*

- Increased predilection in some families
- No known Mendelian pattern

### ETIOLOGY

- Unknown and controversial
- Repetitive trauma versus inflammatory versus ischemic cause

## DIAGNOSIS

### SIGNS AND SYMPTOMS

#### *History*

- Knee pain: Insidious and activity related
- Occasionally locking or catching of the knee if the fragment becomes loose

#### *Physical Exam*

- Check knee ROM.
- Tenderness over the lesion
- Knee effusion:
  - Graded as mild, moderate, large
  - Mostly seen in unstable lesions
- McMurray test (for meniscal pathology)
- Lachman test (for ACL pathology)
- Antalgic gait
- Thigh atrophy
- Examine the contralateral knee: 25% of these injuries are bilateral (3,4)

### TESTS

#### *Imaging*

- Radiography:
  - AP, lateral, and tunnel needed
  - Radiographs may be negative.
  - Bilateral views often obtained for comparison and to look for contralateral lesions
  - Tunnel radiographs are taken with knee in 45° of flexion, which allows improved visualization of areas of the femoral condyle commonly involved in osteochondritis dissecans
- MRI:
  - Often required for diagnosis if radiographs are negative
  - Look for:
    - Bone marrow edema
    - Lesion size
    - Loose bodies
  - MRI classification of lesions (5):
    - Stage I: Small signal change, no clear margins
    - Stage II: Osteochondritis dissecans fragment with clear margins without fluid between fragment and bone
    - Stage III: Fluid partially visible between fragment and bone
    - Stage IV: Fluid completely surrounds fragment
    - Stage V: Fragment displaced
  - Unstable lesion: 4 criteria on T2-weighted images (6):
    - Line of high signal intensity >5 mm in length between the osteochondritis dissecans lesion and underlying bone
    - Area of increased homogenous signal >5 mm in diameter beneath the lesion
    - Focal defect >5 mm in articular surface
    - High signal line traversing the subchondral plate into the lesion
  - Lesion size may be main determinant of healing
  - High signal line behind the fragment is most predictive of unstable lesions:
    - Found in 72% of unstable lesions (6)
    - Most common sign in patients for whom nonoperative management fails
- Bone scans:
  - Outdated
  - Can be used to predict potential for healing of osteochondral lesions
  - Increased uptake = More likely to heal

#### *Pediatric Considerations*

In children <7 years old, irregularities of the distal femoral epiphyseal ossification center may mimic osteochondritis dissecans.

#### *Pathological Findings*

A separated articular fragment with attached necrotic bone is noted.

### DIFFERENTIAL DIAGNOSIS

- Stress fracture: Pain is of acute onset.
- ACL injury: Positive Lachman test
- Physiologic ossification abnormalities in children <7 years old (see earlier)
- Meniscal injury: Patients have mechanical symptoms of locking and clicking and may have a positive McMurray test
- Spontaneous osteonecrosis of the knee:
  - History of steroid use

## TREATMENT

### GENERAL MEASURES

- Treatment principles:
  - Small, stable lesions with intact cartilage in skeletally immature patients are most likely to heal with nonoperative management.
  - Unstable lesions warrant arthroscopic evaluation.
  - Treatment is based on:
    - Patient's age
    - Lesion size and location
    - Lesion's radiographic stage
    - Whether the lesion is unstable
- Nonoperative treatment:
  - Best for lesions presenting before physeal closure (best prognosis)
  - Lesions <5 mm often can be managed with observation alone (no surgery, just follow-up).
  - Recent recommendations: 3-phase nonoperative management protocol (3)
    - Phase 1: 6 weeks of knee immobilizer and crutch-protected gait; child should be pain free at the end; repeat radiographs at the end.
    - Phase 2 (weeks 6–12): Weightbearing as tolerated without immobilization; physical therapy for knee ROM; quadriceps strengthening
    - Phase 3 (begins at 3 months): Supervised increase in activities, high-impact and shear activities restricted until patient is pain free for several months; consider repeat MRI; repeat immobilization for lesion progression.

### SURGERY

- Consider for:
  - All patients with detached or unstable lesions
  - Symptomatic patients approaching physeal closure and unresponsive to nonoperative treatment
  - Stable lesions that have not healed in 6–9 months
  - Large lesions (>5 mm)
- Techniques:
  - Arthroscopic drilling:
    - Stable lesions with intact articular surfaces
    - Creates channels for revascularization
    - Can be transarticular or through epiphysis (very difficult)
    - Transarticular drilling is effective for osteochondritis dissecans lesions in skeletally immature patients (7).
    - Curative in 85% with open physes and 75% with closed physes (3)
    - Factors associated with failure of treatment include nonclassic lesion location, multiple lesions, and underlying medical problems.
  - Reduction and fixation of fragment:
    - For unstable and partially unstable lesions
    - Can pack autogenous bone graft into crater if subchondral bone loss is present
    - Headless screws
    - Titanium screws are MRI compatible.
    - Long-established loose fragments are difficult to stabilize and have poor healing potential.
  - Large, unsalvageable fragments:
    - Drilling
    - Abrasion arthroplasty
    - Microfracture
    - Recruited cells form fibrocartilage.
    - Autologous osteochondral plug transplantation for lesions <2 mm in diameter
    - Autologous chondrocyte implantation for large defects and skeletally mature patients

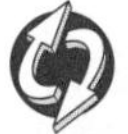

## FOLLOW-UP

### PROGNOSIS

- Small nondisplaced fragments or those occurring before physeal closure usually heal.
- Large, unstable lesions may lead to early osteoarthritis.

### COMPLICATIONS

- Nonunion of the reduced fragment
- Displacement of a nondisplaced lesion, creating a loose body

### PATIENT MONITORING

- Nondisplaced fragments treated nonoperatively should be followed closely for evidence of displacement.
- Serial radiographs or MRI every 3–6 months to follow healing or lack thereof

### REFERENCES


1. Aichroth P. Osteochondritis dissecans of the knee. A clinical survey. *J Bone Joint Surg* 1971;53B: 440–447.
2. Desai SS, Patel MR, Michelli LJ, et al. Osteochondritis dissecans of the patella. *J Bone Joint Surg* 1987;69B:320–325.
3. Flynn JM, Kocher MS, Ganley TJ. Osteochondritis dissecans of the knee. *J Pediatr Orthop* 2004;24: 434–443.
4. Schenck RC, Jr, Goodnight JM. *Osteochondritis dissecans. J Bone Joint Surg* 1996;78A:439–456.
5. Hefti F, Beguiristain J, Krauspe R, et al. Osteochondritis dissecans: a multicenter study of the European Pediatric Orthopedic Society. *J Pediatr Orthop B* 1999;8:231–245.
6. De Smet AA, Ilahi OA, Graf BK. Untreated osteochondritis dissecans of the femoral condyles: prediction of patient outcome using radiographic and MR findings. *Skeletal Radiol* 1997;26: 463–467.
7. Kocher MS, Micheli LJ, Yaniv M, et al. Functional and radiographic outcome of juvenile osteochondritis dissecans of the knee treated with transarticular arthroscopic drilling. *Am J Sports Med* 2001;29:562–566.


### ADDITIONAL READING


- Cahill B. Treatment of juvenile osteochondritis dissecans and osteochondritis dissecans of the knee. *Clin Sports Med* 1985;4:367–384.
- Makino A, Muscolo DL, Puigdevall M, et al. Arthroscopic fixation of osteochondritis dissecans of the knee: clinical, MRI, and arthroscopic follow-up. *Am J Sports Med* 2005;33: 1499–1504.
- Peterson L, Minas T, Brittberg M, et al. Treatment of osteochondritis dissecans of the knee with autologous chondrocyte transplantation: results at two to ten years. *J Bone Joint Surg* 2003;85A: 17–24.
- Willis RB. Sports medicine in the growing child. Overuse injuries. In: Morrissy RT, Weinstein SL, eds. *Lovell and Winter's Pediatric Orthopaedics*, 6th ed. Philadelphia: Lippincott Williams & Wilkins, 2006: 1414–1421.


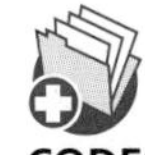

## MISCELLANEOUS

### CODES

#### *ICD9-CM*

732.7 Osteochondritis dissecans

### PATIENT TEACHING

Stress the importance of avoiding the offending activities to allow time for the lesion to heal.

### FAQ

- Q: What is the best initial treatment of a large, unstable osteochondritis dissecans lesion in a skeletally mature patient?
  - A: This lesion has a poor prognosis with nonoperative management. Therefore, the best treatment is débridement of the dead bone on the fragment and in the crater, subchondral drilling with or without bone grafting, and fragment fixation with a headless titanium screw to allow MRI follow-up studies. Postoperatively, the patient is treated nonweightbearing for 6–8 weeks with early motion.

# OSTEOCHONDROMA

*Frank J. Frassica, MD*

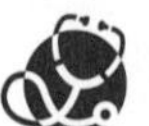

## BASICS

### DESCRIPTION

- An osteochondroma is a common developmental abnormality of the peripheral growth plate that results in a lobulated outgrowth of cartilage and bone from the metaphysis.
  - Appears as a cartilage-capped bony projection from the metaphysis of long bones
  - Can occur in any bone that develops from enchondral ossification
  - Most commonly occurs in:
    - Long bones, usually the proximal or distal femur, proximal tibia, pelvis, or scapula
    - 10–25-year-old persons (stops growing at skeletal maturity)
- Growth of the lesions parallels that of the patient.
- Classification:
  - Solitary osteochondroma (nonheritable)
  - Multiple hereditary exostoses (autosomal dominant):
    - Osteochondromatosis
    - Diaphyseal aclasis
- Synonym: Osteocartilaginous exostosis

### EPIDEMIOLOGY

#### *Incidence*

No substantial difference in frequency between males and females

#### *Prevalence*

This most common benign bone lesion comprises 40% of all benign bone tumors (1,2).

### RISK FACTORS

#### *Genetics*

- Multiple hereditary exostoses often is inherited in an autosomal dominant manner.
- To date, 3 different genetic mutations have been isolated:
  - EXT 1
  - EXT 2
  - EXT 3

### ETIOLOGY

The cause of an osteochondroma most likely is a detached portion of the growth plate that grows on the surface of the bone.

## DIAGNOSIS

### SIGNS AND SYMPTOMS

- Symptoms result from pressure on adjacent nerves and muscle and from local irritation.
  - Hard, painless, fixed mass
  - Associated symptoms of tissue or nerve irritation
- The skeletal deformity is secondary to undergrowth of the affected bones, with narrower bones being affected more seriously.
  - Therefore, the tibia and radius grow longer than the ulna and fibula.
  - This phenomenon produces valgus at the knee, ankle, and elbow in some patients.

#### *Physical Exam*

- Note any hard, painless, fixed mass in the metaphyseal region of the fastest growing bones; the region around the knee is the most common.
- Height in most patients falls in the low-normal range.
- Group findings occur in 4 major categories:
  - Local impingement, which may include peroneal palsy and soreness of the muscles about the knee
  - Valgus at knee, ankle, elbow, and wrist (variable)
  - Limb-length inequality
  - ROM may be limited secondary to the presence of the osteochondroma.
- Physical examination and radiography should confirm the diagnosis.

### TESTS

#### *Lab*

Blood tests are not altered by this condition.

#### *Imaging*

- Radiography:
  - Plain films typically depict a compact pedunculated or sessile protuberance of bone.
  - The well-defined lesion projects from the metaphysis.
- CT scans are helpful in locations that are difficult to image, such as the scapula, pelvis, and proximal femur.
- MRI scans can be used when a suspicion of malignancy is present.
  - The size of the cartilage cap can be measured (a cap >1 cm is worrisome for malignancy).
  - Symptomatic bursae can be detected with MRI.
  - MRI can detect soft-tissue masses.

#### *Pathological Findings*

Normal hyaline cartilage undergoes normal enchondral ossification, occurring on the end of a stalk or ridge of bone.

### DIFFERENTIAL DIAGNOSIS

- Surface chondrosarcoma
- Parosteal osteosarcoma
- Periosteal chondroma

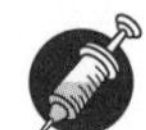

## TREATMENT

### GENERAL MEASURES

- Local measures or analgesics are indicated for minor aches.
- Medical treatment:
  - The lesion may be left untreated unless it is symptomatic.
  - It should be followed clinically, because a 1–10% risk of malignant transformation to chondrosarcoma is present in persons with multiple hereditary exostoses (1,2).

#### *Activity*

Activity is allowed as tolerated.

### SPECIAL THERAPY

#### *Physical Therapy*

Not usually necessary

### MEDICATION (DRUGS)

Tylenol or NSAIDs may be used by the patient with occasional symptoms.

### SURGERY

- Surgical resection of symptomatic lesions is successful with minimal morbidity.
- In patients with the multiple hereditary exostoses form of the disorder, new lesions may form in multiple areas, and they may grow.
- Osteotomies and physeal stapling may be done for angular disturbances.

## FOLLOW-UP

### PROGNOSIS

- The prognosis is good.
- The chance of recurrence after excision of a solitary lesion is very small.
- The risk of malignant transformation of isolated osteochondromas is even lower.
- Patients with multiple hereditary exostoses have a 1–10% risk of malignant transformation (1,2).

### COMPLICATIONS

- Fracture may occur during the first 3 months after removal of an osteochondroma.
- Vascular or neurologic injury during surgery may occur if the osteochondroma is associated closely with these structures.
- Occasionally, the stalk may fracture.

### PATIENT MONITORING

Patients should be followed regularly (for 1–2 years) for angular disturbances, limb-length inequality, or serious problems from pressure of lesion so they can be treated in a timely fashion before more complex intervention is needed.

### REFERENCES


1. Dorfman HD, Czerniak B. Benign cartilage lesions. In: *Bone Tumors*. St. Louis: Mosby, 1998:253–352.
2. McCarthy EF, Frassica FJ. Primary bone tumors. In: *Pathology of Bone and Joint Disorders: With Clinical and Radiographic Correlation*. Philadelphia: WB Saunders, 1998:195–275.


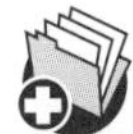

## MISCELLANEOUS

### CODES

#### *ICD9-CM*

756.4 Osteochondroma

### PATIENT TEACHING

- Reassure the patient about the benign nature of the lesions.
- Teach adults to be alert for growth or new onset of pain in osteochondroma, which may be a sign of a malignant transformation.

### FAQ

- Q: Is it necessary to remove all osteochondromas?
  - A: In general, if the patient is asymptomatic, surgical removal is not necessary.
- Q: What is the risk of malignant degeneration, and are the resultant cancers treatable?
  - A: The risk of malignancy in an isolated osteochondroma is extremely low, and the prognosis for the resulting low-grade chondrosarcomas is excellent.
- Q: How are patients with multiple hereditary exostoses followed to check for malignant degeneration?
  - A: Patients are queried about new masses or pain. Plain radiographs, CTs, or MRIs can be used to monitor exostosis in the axial skeleton or large lesions in the extremities.

# OSTEOGENESIS IMPERFECTA

*Paul D. Sponseller, MD*

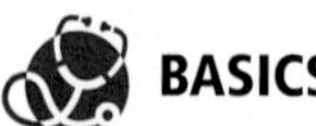

## BASICS

### DESCRIPTION
- OI is a collagen disorder causing osseous fragility.
- May affect bones, teeth, eyes, hearing, and soft tissue
- The Sillence classification (1,2) is the most widely accepted.
  - Type I: Mild, common form:
    - Fractures occur in later childhood and decrease toward adolescence.
    - Patients with type IA do not have dentinogenesis imperfecta; those with type IB do.
  - Type II: Lethal in the perinatal period
  - Type III (Fig. 1): Most severe survivable form
  - Type IV: Moderately severe
  - Type V: Moderately severe, with dislocated radial heads and hyperplastic callus

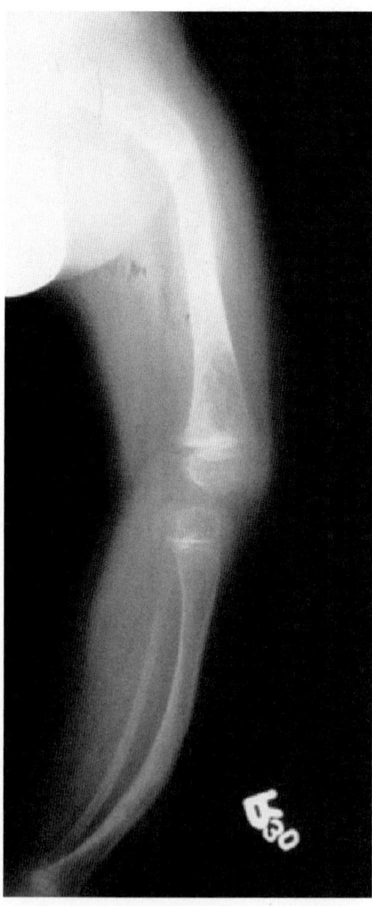

**Fig. 1.** Typical features of type III OI include long, thin, bowed, osteopenic bones.

#### *Pediatric Considerations*
- Types II and III are diagnosed at birth with perinatal death or intrauterine fractures, respectively.
- Types I and IV may be diagnosed after birth, but generally in early childhood.
- In the milder forms, the incidence of fractures decreases with age.

### EPIDEMIOLOGY
#### *Prevalence*
Overall, affects ~1 per 10,000 persons (1)

### RISK FACTORS
None, other than heredity

#### *Genetics*
- All types have a moderately high rate of spontaneous mutation.
- Type I: Autosomal dominant with variable penetrance and expressivity
- Type II: Autosomal recessive or dominant
- Type III: Autosomal recessive
- Type IV: Autosomal dominant with variable penetrance and expressivity
- Type V: Autosomal dominant

### ETIOLOGY
- Defects in type I collagen
- Type I collagen:
  - Is the main collagen in bone matrix
  - Is a triple helix
  - Has glycine as every 3rd amino acid:
    - Substitutions of this amino acid impair coiling of the nonmutated product and exert a dominant negative effect.

### ASSOCIATED CONDITIONS
- Platybasia, potential brainstem compression
- Dentinogenesis imperfecta
- Hypermobile joints with increased incidence of joint dislocation
- Inguinal, umbilical, and diaphragmatic hernias

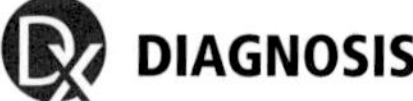

## DIAGNOSIS

### SIGNS AND SYMPTOMS
- Fragility of bone
- Short stature
- Scoliosis, back pain
- Defective dentinogenesis of deciduous or permanent teeth, or both, resulting in soft, translucent, and brownish teeth
- Middle-ear deafness
- Laxity of ligaments, which results in hypermobile joints and potential ankle instability
- Blue sclerae
- Skull: Patients may have a widened cranium and small, triangular faces.
- Increased incidence of musculoskeletal pain in adulthood
- Symptoms of basilar invagination may include respiratory depression, dyscoordination, spasticity, weakness, contracture, and changes in voice.

#### *Physical Exam*
- OI is diagnosed by fractures of unusual frequency or mechanism.
- A positive family history and signs such as abnormal dentition, blue sclerae, ligament laxity, scoliosis, or bone bowing/fragility are helpful.

### TESTS
#### *Lab*
- Cultures of dermal fibroblasts for characterization of type I collagen may be part of the workup; absence of matching may not exclude diagnosis.
- DNA mutation analysis (blood test) is available through specialized labs.

### *Imaging*

- Radiography may reveal systemic osteopenia.
- Other radiographic findings may include long bones with narrow diaphyses and bowing, protrusio acetabuli, vertebral or other fractures, scoliosis, and a "concertina" femur.
- Bones are gracile and osteopenic.
- The pelvis may have a trefoil shape, and protrusio acetabuli is common.
- The osteopenic vertebrae may fracture easily, resulting in a flattened or biconcave shape; severe scoliosis and kyphosis may develop.
- The skull may exhibit wormian bones (inclusions in the suture lines).
- Severe cases: Metaphyses may appear cystic.

### *Diagnostic Procedures/Surgery*

- Dermal punch biopsy to analyze collagen if routine diagnostic criteria are inconclusive (1)
- The synthesis and structure of type I collagen produced by the cultured fibroblasts obtained from biopsy then can be analyzed.
- The mutation can be characterized by specialized lab tests, from DNA in a blood test.

### *Pathological Findings*

- The bone often appears woven and only occasionally has a normal lamellar pattern.
- The cortices are thin, and the trabeculae in the metaphyses are markedly attenuated.
- The collagen fibers of the cornea and skin have a looser arrangement than normal (1).

## DIFFERENTIAL DIAGNOSIS

- Infant with very low birth weight
- Primary hyperparathyroidism
- Scurvy
- Hypophosphatasia
- Achondrogenesis
- Chondroectodermal dysplasia
- Juvenile osteoporosis
- Nonaccidental injury (child abuse)
- Congenital syphilis
- Malignancy (e.g., leukemia)
- Rickets
- It may be difficult to discern child abuse from OI (1,3).
  - Fractures from child abuse occur most frequently in children <1 year old (3).
  - Multiple fractures at different stages of healing, posterior rib fractures, and metaphyseal corner fractures are highly specific for nonaccidental injury.
- A positive family history and signs such as abnormal dentition, blue sclerae, or systemic osteopenia revealed by radiographs may be helpful in the diagnosis of OI.

# TREATMENT

## GENERAL MEASURES

- Treatment depends on the type of OI.
  - Type I may have little impact on the patient.
  - Type II: Lethal perinatal OI:
    - Has some degree of variability
    - In the most severe cases, early death
  - Types III and IV:
    - Greatest therapeutic challenges (3–8).
    - Treatment with growth hormone, calcium, and calcitonin has shown little benefit (1,4).
- Diphosphonates treatment (pamidronate, alendronate, etc.) may improve (but will not normalize) bone density, decrease fracture frequency, and improve quality of life in children but not adults (1,4,8).
- Molecular treatments are a goal for the future.
- Exercise: A physical therapist should be involved with most children to assess their abilities and plan realistic goals, working to develop ambulatory potential and proceeding with appropriate seating, including a wheelchair if required (3).
- Fractures:
  - Usually treated nonoperatively:
    - Fractures heal readily.
    - A fracture is less likely to heal well if substantial angulation develops (1,5).
    - Use of lightweight splints or braces may help in getting the child to bear weight quickly.
  - Internal fixation may be used if management by closed treatment proves difficult (5,8,9).
    - Intramedullary fixation is superior to plates and screws because screws tend to dislodge from the weakened bone.
    - A new fracture is more likely to occur at the end of a plate ("stress riser" effect).

## SPECIAL THERAPY

### *Physical Therapy*

- Important component of treatment plan (3):
  - Goals for physical therapy: Muscle and bone strengthening, standing, and ambulation
  - Hydrotherapy for extremities allows active motion and strengthens musculature (3).
  - Orthotics are an important adjunct (3).
  - Braces should be lightweight and total contact in design, with joint hinges (3).

## MEDICATION (DRUGS)

### *First Line*

Diphosphonates

### SURGERY

- Anesthesia:
  - Patients with OI are at high risk for many reasons: Restricted neck and jaw mobility, pulmonary function abnormalities from thoracic cage distortion, dentinogenesis imperfecta, and valvular heart disease
  - Avoid anticholinergic agents because they can cause malignant hyperthermia.
- Osteotomy:
  - At ~5 years of age, corrective osteotomies of larger bones with intramedullary fixation may be performed if indicated (5).
  - The Bailey-Dubow or Fassier elongating rod (Fig. 2) diminishes the reoperation rate (5).
  - Intramedullary nail placement is optimal for children with the potential to stand who have severe bowing or repeated fractures.
  - No absolute rule exists for when intramedullary nail placement should be performed; risk-to-benefit analysis should consider recurrent fracture and deformity versus infection, pain, and the need for nail replacement (5).
- Scoliosis:
  - Curves tend to advance relentlessly; bracing has little effect on deformity progression.
  - New instrumentation methods are changing the approach to scoliosis in OI (7) (Fig. 3).
  - Curves may be fused early (at 40°) to halt the relentless progression; this procedure is important in maintaining function and in preventing respiratory complications.
- A less obvious area of spinal involvement is at the craniocervical junction.
  - Basilar invagination may result and present with neurologic signs resulting from brainstem compression (7).
  - Once diagnosed, decompression and spinal stabilization are recommended.

## FOLLOW-UP

Because of multiple potential deformities, patients with OI are best managed in a specialized clinic.

### PROGNOSIS

- Type II disease is lethal perinatally.
- Type III (next most severe form) patients often require multiple orthopaedic procedures.
- Types I and IV are milder forms of OI, with type I being the mildest.
- The fracture rate in all types decreases around puberty.
- Presenile hearing loss may be the most severe long-term handicap in patients with type I disease.

### COMPLICATIONS

A softened base of the skull may lead to platybasia and potential neurologic sequelae (7).

### PATIENT MONITORING

- Scoliosis:
  - Patients with OI must be followed closely from an early age to monitor the development and progression of scoliosis.
  - Continue to monitor patients as adults.
- Neurologic signs: Patients must be followed for neurologic signs of brainstem compression that may be caused by basilar invagination (7).

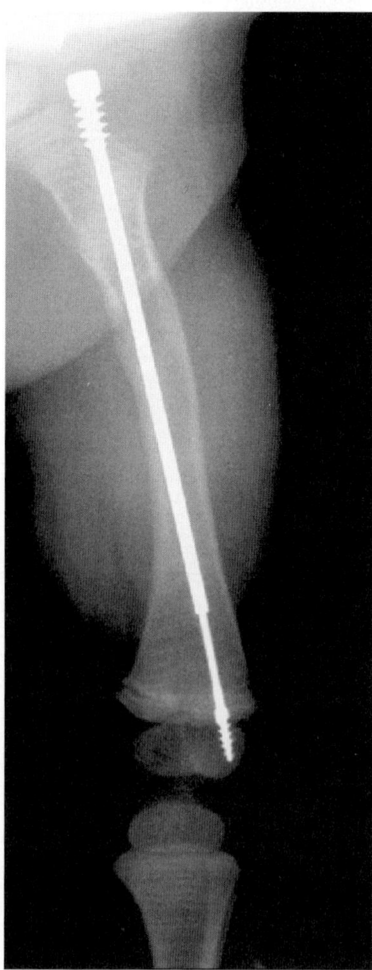

**Fig. 2.** The Fassier rods are telescoping and expand with growth. Also note multiple transverse lines in bone from diphosphonate administration.

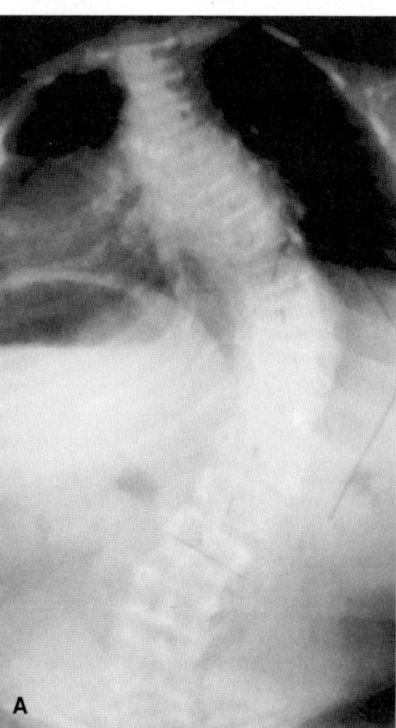

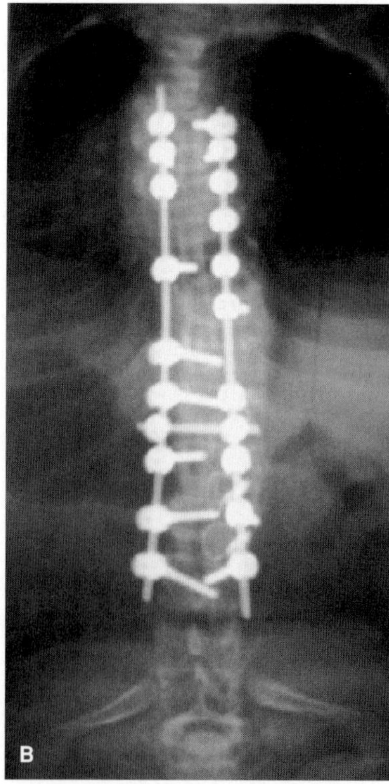

**Fig. 3.** Scoliosis in osteogenesis before **(A)** and after **(B)** surgical correction with rods and screws.

## REFERENCES


1. Cole WG. Advances in osteogenesis imperfecta. *Clin Orthop Relat Res* 2002;401:6–16.
2. Sillence DO, Rimoin DL, Danks DM. Clinical variability in osteogenesis imperfecta–variable expressivity or genetic heterogeneity. *Birth Defects Orig Artic Ser* 1979;15:113–129.
3. Marini JC, Gerber NL. Osteogenesis imperfecta. Rehabilitation and prospects for gene therapy. *JAMA* 1997;277:746–750.
4. Glorieux FH, Bishop NJ, Plotkin H, et al. Cyclic administration of pamidronate in children with severe osteogenesis imperfecta. *N Engl J Med* 1998;339:947–952.
5. Luhmann SJ, Sheridan JJ, Capelli AM, et al. Management of lower-extremity deformities in osteogenesis imperfecta with extensible intramedullary rod technique: a 20-year experience. *J Pediatr Orthop* 1998;18:88–94.
6. Ring D, Jupiter JB, Labropoulos PK, et al. Treatment of deformity of the lower limb in adults who have osteogenesis imperfecta. *J Bone Joint Surg* 1996;78A:220–225.
7. Sawin PD, Menezes AH. Basilar invagination in osteogenesis imperfecta and related osteochondrodysplasias: medical and surgical management. *J Neurosurg* 1997;86:950–960.
8. Seikaly MG, Kopanati S, Salhab N, et al. Impact of alendronate on quality of life in children with osteogenesis imperfecta. *J Pediatr Orthop* 2005;25:786–791.
9. Stott NS, Zionts LE. Displaced fractures of the apophysis of the olecranon in children who have osteogenesis imperfecta. *J Bone Joint Surg* 1993;75A:1026–1033.


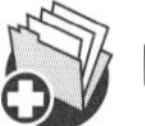

## MISCELLANEOUS

### CODES

#### *ICD9-CM*

756.51 Osteogenesis imperfecta

### PATIENT TEACHING

- Understanding the necessity of muscle strengthening and ROM exercises is important.
- Family members must monitor the skin around braces and casts.
- They must also try to recognize when fractures occur and be compliant with frequent follow-up.

### FAQ

- Q: Does exercise improve bone density in OI?
  - A: It improves it, but not to a normal degree.
- Q: When, if ever, should patients with OI be treated with intramedullary nails?
  - A: If they have repeated fractures, the bowing interferes with function, and the age and size allows durable correction. Some patients have such severe OI that surgery is not successful.

# OSTEOID OSTEOMA

*Frank J. Frassica, MD*

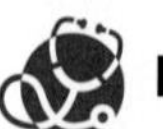

## BASICS

### DESCRIPTION

- A small, benign bone tumor that causes intense pain and marked sclerosis
- The lucent nidus in the bone is 0.5–1.5 cm in diameter.
- Although the proximal femur is the most common site, followed by the tibia, almost any bone may be affected, including the phalanges.

### EPIDEMIOLOGY

#### *Incidence (1,2)*

- Comprises 10% of all benign bone tumors
- Occurs primarily in persons 5–25 years old
- Male:Female ratio, 3:1 (reason unknown)

### RISK FACTORS

#### *Genetics*

No genetic predisposition is known.

### ETIOLOGY

The cause is unknown.

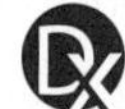

## DIAGNOSIS

### SIGNS AND SYMPTOMS

- Pain is more severe at night and often is relieved by aspirin or other NSAIDs.
- A limp is common.
- Mild atrophy or wasting of muscles in the area may occur.
- The region is tender to palpation.
- If the osteoid osteoma is near a joint, it may cause stiffness.
  - If it involves the spine, scoliosis may be seen.
- The presence of osteoid osteoma in >1 site in a patient is unusual.

#### *Physical Exam*

- Mild swelling, erythema, and occasional muscle wasting in the involved area
- Absence of fever
- Tenderness and stiffness in the region of the osteoid osteoma

### TESTS

#### *Lab*

No laboratory findings aid in the diagnosis.

#### *Imaging*

- In many areas, because the bone is not seen in cross-section, the diagnosis may not be apparent with plain films.
- CT is the best imaging modality for confirming the lesion, but the lesion's location must be known to obtain the correct position on the CT scan.
  - Characteristic "target" appearance of the nidus and its sclerotic rim:
    - An oval radiolucent nidus of ~5–10 mm surrounded by a dense reactive zone
    - Nidus often visible in the bone's cortex
- Bone scanning is useful for confirming or localizing an osteoid osteoma if the lesion's location cannot be determined by plain radiographs.
  - The bone scan is always focally positive.

#### *Pathological Findings*

- On cross-section, the nidus appears as a haphazard arrangement of osteoblasts and trabeculae, which is surrounded by a dense shell of cortical bone.
- On microscopic examination:
  - The nidus is composed of dense, normally woven bone with osteoblastic rimming, and the reactive shell around it is composed of dense cortical bone.
  - The cells have a normal, benign appearance.

### DIFFERENTIAL DIAGNOSIS

- Osteomyelitis
- Stress fracture
- Buckle fracture

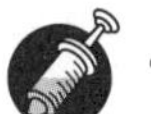

## TREATMENT

### GENERAL MEASURES

- Osteoid osteomas may resolve spontaneously in 2–6 years.
- NSAIDs may be used during this time to control the pain.
- Because of pain or intolerance to analgesics, many patients request treatment of the lesion.

#### *Activity*

- For patients treated nonoperatively, activity may be allowed as tolerated.
- Return to normal activity is allowed within 2–4 weeks of radiofrequency ablation.
- After surgical excision, partial weightbearing should be recommended for 6–8 weeks until the bone has had time to remodel and gain strength.

### MEDICATION (DRUGS)

- Aspirin, regular or enteric-coated
- Ibuprofen
- Naproxen

### SURGERY

- Radiofrequency ablation is the preferred method of treatment.
  - Patients are given general anesthesia.
  - The radiofrequency probe is placed into the nidus under CT guidance.
    - The radiofrequency probe must be insulated to prevent soft-tissue necrosis.
  - The nidus is heated to ~80°C for 4–6 minutes.
  - Effective in 90% of patients with 1 or 2 treatments (3,4)
- Surgical resection may be necessary after failed radiofrequency ablation or in sites where the risk of thermal injury is high.
  - *En bloc* resection is not necessary.
  - Removal of the cortical bone over the lesion and curettage of the nidus is effective.

## FOLLOW-UP

### PROGNOSIS

- The prognosis is excellent.
- No risk of malignant transformation exists.

### COMPLICATIONS

- Fracture after surgical excision may occur.
- Gastritis or ulcers from NSAIDs

### PATIENT MONITORING

Frequent monitoring is not needed because these lesions have no malignant potential.

### REFERENCES


1. McCarthy EF, Frassica FJ. Primary bone tumors. In: *Pathology of Bone and Joint Disorders: With Clinical and Radiographic Correlation.* Philadelphia: WB Saunders, 1998:195–275.
2. Frassica FJ, Waltrip RL, Sponseller PD, et al. Clinicopathologic features and treatment of osteoid osteoma and osteoblastoma in children and adolescents. *Orthop Clin North Am* 1996;27:559–574.
3. Rosenthal DI, Hornicek FJ, Torriani M, et al. Osteoid osteoma: Percutaneous treatment with radiofrequency energy. *Radiology* 2003;229:171–175.
4. Venbrux AC, Montague BJ, Murphy KP, et al. Image-guided percutaneous radiofrequency ablation for osteoid osteomas. *J Vasc Interv Radiol* 2003;14:375–380.


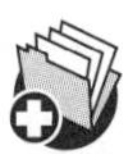

## MISCELLANEOUS

### CODES

#### *ICD9-CM*

213.9 Osteoid osteoma

### PATIENT TEACHING

- Patients should be counseled about the benign nature of the lesion and its tendency to resolve spontaneously over the years.
- Patients may be offered medical or surgical treatment and allowed to choose between them.
- For intensely painful or disabling lesions, or in patients unable to tolerate NSAIDs, an intervention such as radiofrequency ablation or surgical excision often is selected.

### FAQ

- Q: Is protected weightbearing necessary after radiofrequency ablation?
  - A: In general, protected weightbearing is not necessary, and the patient may resume normal activities quickly.
- Q: Who performs radiofrequency ablation of osteoid osteomas?
  - A: Patients should be seen by an orthopaedic oncologist first and then be referred to an interventional radiologist for the procedure.
- Q: What is the best imaging modality for detecting an osteoid osteoma?
  - A: CT scanning (thin cuts, 1 mm) is the best method.

# OSTEOMYELITIS

*Frank J. Frassica, MD*

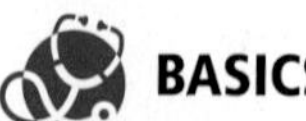

## BASICS

### DESCRIPTION

- Osteomyelitis is inflammation or infection of bone.
- Classification is most commonly based on the timing of onset:
  - Acute: Most often from hematogenous spread:
    - The most common organism in neonates is *Staphylococcus aureus,* followed by *Streptococcus* or Gram-negative organisms.
    - In older infants and children, it usually is *S. aureus*.
  - Subacute:
    - Accounts for 1/3 of primary bone infections
    - Is characterized by insidious onset, mild symptoms, longer duration of infection, and inconclusive laboratory data.
    - The most common organism is *Staphylococcus* species.
    - It usually requires longer duration of antibiotic treatment than the acute condition.
  - Chronic:
    - *S. aureus* is the most common organism.
    - Usually, these patients have sequestra and multiple cavities that require curettage and occasionally bone grafting.
  - Other classification schemes focus on factors such as patient age (neonatal, child, or adult), causative organism (pyogenic or granulomatous), or route of infection (hematogenous, direct inoculation, or contiguous spread).
- Synonym: Bone infection

### EPIDEMIOLOGY

A seasonal variation in acute hematogenous osteomyelitis may occur, with more cases in late summer and early autumn.

#### *Incidence*

The incidence is higher in children than in adults, with a peak occurring in the later years of the 1st decade.

#### *Prevalence*

- A male predilection appears, which is not clearly understood.
- It affects <1% of children (1).

### RISK FACTORS

- Deficient immune systems as a result of viral illness, trauma, anesthesia, or malnutrition also may play a role in the development of osteomyelitis.
- Children and adults may have a history of antecedent trauma.
- Sickle cell disease:
  - In this population, hematogenous osteomyelitis is more common secondary to bone infarcts than to other causes.
  - Although *S. aureus* is the most common organism, *Salmonella* infections may occur.

### ETIOLOGY

- Although the causes remain unknown, factors suspected of having an association with infection include trauma and an altered immune system (especially in adults).
- Most children who develop osteomyelitis are otherwise completely healthy.

### ASSOCIATED CONDITIONS

Nearly 1/2 of these patients have a history of a recent or a concurrent infection such as a viral or upper respiratory infection.

## DIAGNOSIS

### SIGNS AND SYMPTOMS

- Pain is the most common symptom, followed by swelling, erythema, warmth, and limited ROM of the adjacent joints.
- Fever is not always present.
- Because children may not be able to verbalize symptoms, refusal to bear weight, inability to walk or move a limb, and development of a limp all suggest infection.
- The index of suspicion must be highest in the neonate.
- Consider a firm diagnosis when 2 of these 4 criteria are present:
  - Pus aspirated from bone
  - Positive bone or blood culture
  - Symptoms of pain, swelling, warmth, and decreased ROM
  - Typical radiographic changes consistent with osteomyelitis

#### *Physical Exam*

- The goal of the examination is to localize the area of involvement and to identify any possible source.
- The appearance of the child may vary from cranky to lethargic, depending on the extent and duration of infection.
- Before palpation, visually assess the amount of limb movement or usage.
- Tenderness to palpation may need to be elicited by the parent, with instructions to differentiate the cry of a frightened child from a cry of true pain.
- Tenderness, warmth, and erythema usually are present in the bone's metaphyseal region.

### TESTS

#### *Lab*

- A white blood cell count is not a reliable indicator of infection, but if it is elevated, it is suggestive of infection.
- Blood cultures also should be obtained with the initial diagnostic blood sample.
  - ~1/2 of cases are positive.
  - If a case is positive, it may eliminate the need to aspirate bone to obtain the organism.
- The ESR rate is a nonspecific acute-phase reactant that is elevated in many cases and is a reliable indicator of inflammation.
  - It begins to elevate at 48–72 hours and returns to normal after 2–3 weeks if the infection has resolved.
  - Because of the lag time of the ESR, it is not helpful in assessing resolution of infection.
- An elevated level of C-reactive protein resulting from inflammation also is useful.
  - This test is more reliable than ESR in assessing infection because it not only peaks earlier (50 hours versus 3–5 days) but also returns to normal earlier (7 days).
- Aspiration of the site may be performed to identify the causative organism.
  - The specimen should be sent for Gram stain, aerobic and anaerobic cultures, acid-fast bacilli, and tests for fungi.
  - Bone cultures often are positive.
  - Some clinicians suggest fine-needle biopsy with an 11-gauge bone biopsy (or bone marrow) needle for histologic examination.
    - Heavy sedation usually is required to allow the patient to be comfortable and to obtain a specimen from the proper area reliably.
    - The site of involvement usually is metaphyseal bone rather than hard cortical bone, so it is possible to penetrate the bone for a sample.
    - If the site of involvement is not clear, it should be localized via bone scanning or MRI.
- All cultures and laboratory tests should be obtained before starting antibiotic treatment.

### *Imaging*

- Radiography:
  - Soft-tissue swelling is the earliest radiographic change.
  - Classic radiographic bony changes, such as osteopenia, bone resorption, and new periosteal bone formation, may not occur until 14–21 days after symptom onset.
- Bone scan:
  - May be used to localize the area of involvement
  - Results may be falsely negative in the 1st month of life.
  - Bone aspiration will not affect bone scan results if the scan is performed within 48 hours of aspiration.
  - A bone scan is not needed if the area of involvement is already known.
- CT:
  - Not useful in diagnosing acute osteomyelitis, but it may assist in differentiating other lucent lesions such as osteoid osteoma or chondroblastoma.
- MRI:
  - Excellent sensitivity and specificity
  - T1-weighted images give excellent anatomic detail of the site of infection.
  - T2-weighted images show high signal in areas of inflammation and periosteal reaction.
- Ultrasound may help to identify a subperiosteal fluid collection, but because it does not penetrate bone well, it is not useful in assessing metaphyseal fluid collections.

### *Pathological Findings*

- Infection begins in the sinusoids of the metaphysis, usually near the end of a long bone.
- As the infection spreads, the medullary vessels thrombose and cause a mechanical blockage of inflammatory cells.
  - Results in inflammatory cell migration into the medullary cavity, with consequent intraosseous pressure buildup and development of pus
  - The pus then takes the path of least resistance and exits through the metaphyseal cortex, thereby elevating the periosteum.
  - A subperiosteal abscess subsequently forms under the elevated periosteum.
- The elevated periosteum manifests ~10–14 days later as a periosteal reaction.

### DIFFERENTIAL DIAGNOSIS

- Trauma
- Septic arthritis
- Cellulitis
- Malignancy (leukemia or Ewing sarcoma)
- Thrombophlebitis
- Sickle cell crisis
- Toxic synovitis
- EOG
- Osteoid osteoma

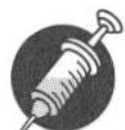

## TREATMENT

### GENERAL MEASURES

- Principles of treatment include identification of the organism, selection of an appropriate antibiotic, surgical débridement if necessary, and sufficient duration of treatment to allow complete resolution.
- Surgery is not indicated if the condition is detected early and no devascularized bone is present.

### MEDICATION (DRUGS)

- Antibiotic selection (guided by cultures and sensitivities):
  - Oxacillin in combination with cefotaxime or gentamicin in neonates and oxacillin alone in infants and children
  - Cefazolin is recommended for patients allergic to penicillin.
  - Clindamycin or vancomycin is recommended for patients allergic to both penicillin and cephalosporin.
- The duration of antibiotic treatment is debatable.
  - It typically involves intravenous antibiotics for 5 days until symptoms resolve and antibiotic sensitivities are identified.
  - Thereafter, a regimen of 4–6 weeks of oral therapy is indicated, provided an appropriate oral antibiotic is available.

### SURGERY

- Indications for surgery are controversial but usually include the following:
  - Aspiration of frank pus initially
  - Presence of substantial bone resorption
  - Failure of symptom resolution after 36–48 hours of antibiotic treatment
- Surgical treatment consists of opening the periosteum, drilling the cortex, and débriding any devascularized bone.

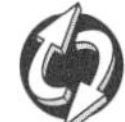

## FOLLOW-UP

### PROGNOSIS

- Most children do extremely well with appropriate treatment, and they suffer no long-term effects.
- Problems arise usually when infection is not recognized or treated in a timely manner, with the possible development of chronic osteomyelitis.

### COMPLICATIONS

- Growth plate arrest may occur, if the infection crosses the growth plate.
- A pathologic fracture may develop if the bone is excessively loaded before healing and remodeling.

### REFERENCES

1. McCarthy EF, Frassica FJ. Infections of bones and joints. In: *Pathology of Bone and Joint Disorders: With Clinical and Radiographic Correlation.* Philadelphia: WB Saunders, 1998:153–164.

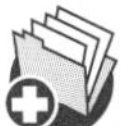

## MISCELLANEOUS

### CODES

#### *ICD9-CM*

- 730.0 Acute or subacute osteomyelitis
- 730.1 Chronic osteomyelitis

### FAQ

- Q: When do patients with osteomyelitis need surgery?
  - A: Surgery often is necessary if there is lytic bone destruction or extension of the infection into the soft tissue with abscess formation.
- Q: Can bone infection be confused with bone cancer?
  - A: Yes, it can. Ewing tumor and blood malignancies, such as lymphoma and leukemia, can be confused with osteomyelitis.

# OSTEOPOROSIS

*Anirudh Sridharan, MD*

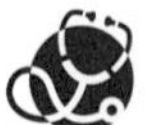

## BASICS

### DESCRIPTION
- Osteoporosis is characterized by low bone mass and microarchitectural deterioration of bone tissue, leading to enhanced bone fragility and an increase in fracture risk.
- The World Health Organization defines osteoporosis as a bone mineral density score 2.5 standard deviations less than the mean value for a young person of the same gender (1).

### GENERAL PREVENTION
Prevention of bone loss in asymptomatic females is achieved through behavior modification, including alterations in nutrition and lifestyle.

### EPIDEMIOLOGY
- Osteoporosis is responsible for 1.3 million fractures yearly: 1/2 are vertebral fractures, 1/4 are hip fractures, and 1/4 are wrist fractures (2).
- The fracture rate increases with age, especially after age 75 (2).
- After age 50, females are 3 times more likely than males to sustain a fragility fracture (40% versus 13%, respectively) (2).

### RISK FACTORS
- Caucasian (Northern European descent) and Asian ethnicity
- Female gender
- Late menarche, nulliparity, early menopause, excessive exercise (producing amenorrhea)
- Increasing age
- Positive family history
- Small body frame (<127 lb)

#### *Genetics*
The genetic component of this disease is not known.

### ETIOLOGY
- Idiopathic secondary
- Nutritional: Milk intolerance, vegetarian dieting, low dietary calcium, excessive alcohol intake
- Lifestyle: Smoking, inactivity
- Medical: Type I diabetes, Cushing syndrome, chronic renal disease, inflammatory bowel disease, cystic fibrosis, hyperparathyroidism, hyperthyroidism, anorexia nervosa, celiac disease, idiopathic hypercalciuria, premature ovarian failure
- Medications: Glucocorticoid drugs, long-term lithium therapy, chemotherapy, anticonvulsants (phenytoin, phenobarbital, valproate, and carbamazepine), long-term phosphate-binding antacid use, thyroid replacement drugs, methotrexate, FK-506

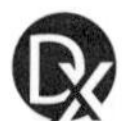

## DIAGNOSIS

### SIGNS AND SYMPTOMS

#### *History*
High suspicion of osteoporosis in any patient with a fracture caused by minimal trauma

#### *Physical Exam*
Vertebral fractures are associated with loss of stature caused by a progressive increase in the degree of kyphosis and lordotic curve flattening.

### TESTS
- DEXA:
  - Measures bone density at the femoral neck, spine, and distal radius
  - Results are related as T scores: The number of standard deviations the bone mineral density measurement is above or below the young normal mean bone mineral density.

#### *Lab*
- A comprehensive metabolic panel, complete blood count, and thyroid stimulating hormone level
- A normal calcium, thyroid stimulating hormone, and creatinine rule out hyperparathyroidism, hyperthyroidism, and chronic renal disease.
- Normal blood count, a normal serum protein, and normal calcium virtually exclude multiple myeloma.
- Serum 25-hydroxyvitamin D and parathyroid hormone if the patient is elderly or if a history of renal disease, gastrointestinal malabsorption, liver disease, or anticonvulsant drug therapy is present

#### *Imaging*
- Radiography:
  - Plain radiographs are unremarkable until bone loss has reached 30%.
  - Moderate osteoporosis of the thoracic and lumbar spine causes signs of overall loss of bone density (osteopenia).
  - Widening of the medullary canal with thinning of the cortices can be seen in long bones.
- Fractures may not be seen on initial radiographs, and may require bone scintigraphy, CT, MRI, or repeat plain radiographs.

#### *Pathological Findings*
- Excessive bone loss results from abnormalities in the bone remodeling cycle.
- The cycle involves resorption of old bone by osteoclasts, recruitment of osteoblasts to deposit new matrix, and mineralization of that newly deposited matrix.
- In osteoporosis, a loss of a small amount of bone mass occurs with each cycle.
- Hyperparathyroidism increases the rate of activation of bone remodeling.

### DIFFERENTIAL DIAGNOSIS
- Osteomalacia
- Neoplasm (myeloma, leukemia)
- Paget disease of the bone
- OI

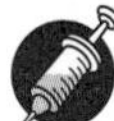

## TREATMENT

### GENERAL MEASURES

#### *Activity*
Weightbearing exercise regimens cause modest increases in bone mineral density.

### MEDICATION (DRUGS)

#### *First Line*
- Calcium supplements: 1,200 mg per day.
- Vitamin D: 800 IU per day.
- Diphosphonates:
  - Cause decreased osteoclast activity.
  - Decreases fracture rate at hip, spine, and wrist by 50% (3)
  - Patients require calcium and vitamin D for maximal benefit.
  - Weekly (alendronate, risedronate) and monthly dosing (ibandronate) is available (4).

#### *Second Line*
- Selective estrogen receptor modulators:
  - Reduce the vertebral fracture rate by 50%, but have no effect on the hip fracture rate (5)
  - Raloxifene is the only FDA-approved selective estrogen receptor modulator for treating osteoporosis.
- Estrogen replacement reduces the risk of fracture but is associated with an increase in cardiovascular and thromboembolic events (6).
- Calcitonin:
  - Inhibits bone resorption by acting on osteoclasts
  - Its ability to reduce fracture rates has been questioned (7).
- Recombinant parathyroid hormone:
  - Results in stimulation of new bone formation
  - It is expensive and should be prescribed only by specialists (8).

### SURGERY
- Surgical treatment is related to the management of impending or completed fractures.
- Vertebroplasty and kyphoplasty, procedures in which methacrylate bone cement is injected percutaneously into osteoporotic vertebrae that have collapsed, show promise but await long-term study.

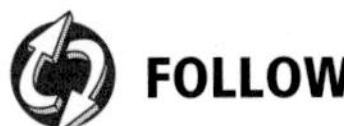

## FOLLOW-UP

### DISPOSITION

#### *Issues for Referral*

Patients with severe osteoporosis (T-score <3) should be referred to an endocrinologist to evaluate for secondary causes of osteoporosis.

### PROGNOSIS

The earlier therapy is instituted, the better the prognosis.

### COMPLICATIONS

Fractures may occur.

### REFERENCES

1. Kanis JA, WHO Study Group. Assessment of fracture risk and its application to screening for postmenopausal osteoporosis: synopsis of a WHO report. *Osteoporos Int* 1994;4:368–381.
2. US Department of Health and Human Services. *Bone Health and Osteoporosis: A Report of the Surgeon General*. Rockville, MD: U.S. Department of Health and Human Services, Office of the Surgeon General, 2004.
3. Papapoulos SE, Quandt SA, Liberman UA, et al. Meta-analysis of the efficacy of alendronate for the prevention of hip fractures in postmenopausal women. *Osteoporos Int* 2005;16:468–474.
4. Fleisch H. Development of bisphosphonates. *Breast Cancer Res* 2002;4:30–34.
5. Ettinger B, Black DM, Mitlak BH, et al. Reduction of vertebral fracture risk in postmenopausal women with osteoporosis treated with raloxifene: results from a 3-year randomized clinical trial. *JAMA* 1999;282:637–645.
6. Rossouw JE, Anderson GL, Prentice RL, et al. Risks and benefits of estrogen plus progestin in healthy postmenopausal women: principal results from the Women's Health Initiative randomized controlled trial. *JAMA* 2002;288:321–333.
7. Chesnut CH, III, Silverman S, Andriano K, et al. A randomized trial of nasal spray salmon calcitonin in postmenopausal women with established osteoporosis: the prevent recurrence of osteoporotic fractures study. *Am J Med* 2000;109: 267–276.
8. Rosen CJ, Rackoff PJ. Emerging anabolic treatments for osteoporosis. *Rheum Dis Clin North Am* 2001;27:215–233.

### ADDITIONAL READING

Favus MJ, ed. *Primer on the Metabolic Bone Diseases and Disorders of Mineral Metabolism*, 5th ed. Washington, DC: American Society for Bone and Mineral Research, 2003.

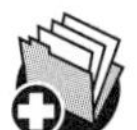

## MISCELLANEOUS

### CODES

#### *ICD9-CM*

- 733.0 Generalized osteoporosis
- 733.01 Senile osteoporosis/postmenopausal osteoporosis
- 733.7 Posttraumatic osteoporosis

### PATIENT TEACHING

#### *Activity*

Exercise programs should focus on compliance through recreational therapy.

#### *Prevention*

Patients should take the daily recommended amounts of calcium and vitamin D and perform daily exercise.

### FAQ

- Q: What is the correct way to take a diphosphonate?
  - A: After getting up for the day and before taking food, beverage, or other medication, the individual should swallow the tablet whole with a full glass of plain water. Stay fully upright for at least 30 minutes and do not lie down until after the 1st food of the day. Wait at least 30 minutes before you eat or drink anything other than plain water.
- Q: How soon after starting treatment of osteoporosis should you check a DEXA scan?
  - A: A DEXA scan will not show substantial changes in bone mineral density any sooner than 1 year after the initiation of therapy.

# OSTEOSARCOMA

*Frank J. Frassica, MD*

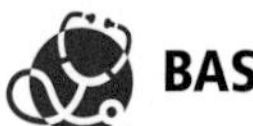

## BASICS

### DESCRIPTION

- The most common primary malignant bone tumor in children and young adolescents
- May occur occasionally in older adults but is much less common than chondrosarcoma and MFH
- May occur within other lesions (secondary sarcoma) such as Paget disease, bone infarcts, and irradiated bone
- A highly malignant tumor with invasive local growth and early pulmonary metastasis
  - Bones most commonly affected include those that grow most rapidly (1):
    - Femur: 41.5%
    - Tibia: 16.5%
    - Humerus: 15%
- Classification: The many different types of osteosarcoma often are classified by their location and degree of differentiation.
  - High-grade intramedullary: Most common type
  - Well-differentiated intramedullary: Very rare
  - Surface osteosarcomas:
    - Parosteal osteosarcoma: Most common surface osteosarcoma; well differentiated; occurs most commonly on the distal femoral or proximal tibial metaphysis
    - Periosteal osteosarcoma: Intermediate grade, predominantly cartilage with bone formation
    - High-grade: Very rare
  - Osteosarcoma of the jaw: Behaves in a less malignant fashion than high-grade intramedullary osteosarcoma
  - Lesions usually are staged according to the Enneking staging system (2), most commonly:
    - Stage IIB: High-grade, soft-tissue extension (80–90%)
    - Stage III: Metastatic disease (~10–15%)
- Synonym: Osteogenic sarcoma

### EPIDEMIOLOGY

- Adolescents in their 2nd decade are the most commonly affected group.
- The median age range at presentation is 13–17 years (1).
- Some authors report a slight male predominance (1.3:1) (1).

#### *Incidence*

- Primary sarcomas of bone are rare, with only ~2,500 new cases per year in the United States (1).
- Osteosarcoma is one of the most common primary bone sarcomas, representing up to 40% (1).

### RISK FACTORS

- Osteosarcomas may occur (rarely) in abnormal bone.
  - After irradiation
  - Paget disease
  - Bone infarcts

### ETIOLOGY

- The cause of classic high-grade osteosarcoma is unknown.
- A relationship between incidence and high rates of growth has been noted.
- Osteosarcoma occasionally develops in areas of pre-existing bone lesions such as Paget disease, fibrous dysplasia, bone infarcts, or OI.
- The retinoblastoma often is present.

### ASSOCIATED CONDITION

Retinoblastoma (high incidence of osteosarcoma)

## DIAGNOSIS

### SIGNS AND SYMPTOMS

- Pain and swelling are the most consistent symptoms of osteosarcoma.
- Onset usually is gradual and progressive.
- Pain is aching and persistent.
- Many patients report night pain, which awakens them.

#### *Physical Exam*

- A soft-tissue mass often is palpable and tender.
- The mass frequently is warm and may limit ROM of the adjacent joint.
- Once diagnosed, patients:
  - Usually undergo a staging workup, including chest CT, MRI of the lesion, and technetium bone scan
  - Should undergo a staging biopsy

### TESTS

#### *Lab*

- Alkaline phosphatase is elevated in many patients.
- In patients with a high pretherapeutic alkaline phosphatase level, serial measurements may be used to monitor therapeutic response and tumor recurrence.
- Serum lactate dehydrogenase also may be elevated.

#### *Imaging*

- The location of osteosarcoma usually is the metaphysis of a long bone.
- Lesions typically show features of bone destruction, bone formation, periosteal reaction, and a mineralized soft-tissue mass.
- The classic radiographic appearance is that of a destructive lesion of bone that is itself forming bone.
- Rapid cortical destruction and periosteal reaction at the proximal or distal margin may produce the classic "Codman triangle."
  - Alternatively, radial reactive trabeculation may produce a sunburst appearance.
- Lesions rarely involve the joint.

#### *Pathological Findings*

- Many subtypes of osteosarcoma have been identified.
  - All osteosarcoma types have a malignant fibrous stroma forming bone as a least common denominator.
  - Broad histologic subtypes are as follows:
    - Fibrogenic
    - Chondrogenic
    - Osteogenic

### DIFFERENTIAL DIAGNOSIS

- Infection
- Ewing sarcoma
- Giant cell tumor
- Metastatic disease
- EOG

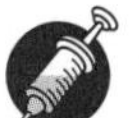

# TREATMENT

## GENERAL MEASURES

Any patient with a destructive lesion of a long bone that is forming bone should be referred immediately to an experienced musculoskeletal oncologist.

### *Activity*

- Once the diagnosis has been made, activity should be restricted to prevent fracture, which could necessitate an amputation.
- Patients with lower-extremity tumors are placed on crutches.

## SPECIAL THERAPY

### *Physical Therapy*

- Most patients with local extremity lesions begin gait training with crutches to prevent pathologic fracture.
- In the upper extremity, function of the hand and elbow must be maintained.

## MEDICATION (DRUGS)

- Multiple chemotherapy regimens are being developed, refined, and evaluated (3).
- Current regimens include 3–6 different cytotoxic agents given for 10–12 weeks preoperatively and 6 months postoperatively (see "Prognosis" section).

## SURGERY

- Historically, treatment generally consisted of amputation.
- Newer surgical techniques and chemotherapeutic regimens allow limb salvage in most cases.
- Resected bone segments may be replaced by allografts or large-segment metal prostheses, depending on the situation.
- Limb salvage surgery can be accomplished in up to 90% of patients (4).

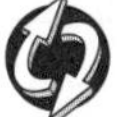

# FOLLOW-UP

## PROGNOSIS

- Historically, patients with primary osteosarcoma had a 5-year survival rate of only 20–30% (1).
- Newer chemotherapeutic regimens are effective in killing occult metastases.
  - With preoperative and postoperative multiagent chemotherapy and wide resection, long-term disease-free survival is 60–70% (3).

## COMPLICATIONS

- Development of lung and bone metastases is the most feared complication.
  - Metastasis may occur years after diagnosis and treatment, but most occur within the first 2 years.
- Other complications secondary to limb salvage surgery are relatively common and include:
  - Local recurrence in ~5–10% of patients, usually within 2 years (4)
  - Pulmonary metastases in ~1/3 of patients, usually found within 3 years (1)
  - Infection
  - Pathologic fracture
  - Loosening of prosthetic components
  - Wound breakdown

## PATIENT MONITORING

- After definitive treatment, patients should be followed to detect recurrence or metastasis.
- Patients are monitored closely for the first 2 years with CT scans of the chest every 3–4 months to detect pulmonary metastases.
- Plain radiographs of the limb are performed to detect local recurrences.

## REFERENCES

1. Dorfman HD, Czerniak B. Osteosarcoma. In: *Bone Tumors*. St. Louis: Mosby, 1998:128–252.
2. Enneking WF, Spanier SS, Goodman MA. A system for the surgical staging of musculoskeletal sarcoma. *Clin Orthop Relat Res* 1980;153: 106–120.
3. Gebhardt MC, Hornicek FJ. Osteosarcoma. In: Menendez LR, ed. *Orthopaedic Knowledge Update: Musculoskeletal Tumors*. Rosemont, IL: American Academy of Orthopaedic Surgeons, 2002:175–186.
4. McCarthy EF, Frassica FJ. Primary bone tumors. In: *Pathology of Bone and Joint Disorders: With Clinical and Radiographic Correlation*. Philadelphia: WB Saunders, 1998:195–275.

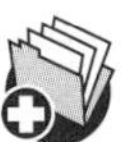

# MISCELLANEOUS

## CODES

### *ICD9-CM*

170.9 Osteogenic sarcoma

## PATIENT TEACHING

Patients who have been treated successfully must be alert for any new areas of bone pain that could herald a bone metastasis.

## FAQ

- Q: Do all children with osteosarcoma need chemotherapy?
  - A: Chemotherapy is essential to improve the prognosis from only 20–30% to 65–75% long-term disease-free survival.
- Q: Does limb salvage increase the risk of systemic spread?
  - A: Several studies have shown that limb salvage surgery does not increase the risk of pulmonary or bone metastases.
- Q: Are there poor prognostic findings?
  - A: Yes, several: Pulmonary metastases at initial presentation, location in the pelvis or spine, increased serum alkaline phosphatase or lactate dehydrogenase, and (very importantly) a poor response to chemotherapy.
- Q: What are the greatest risks of limb salvage surgery?
  - A: Local recurrence and deep infection. Both these complications often necessitate amputation.

# PAGET DISEASE

*Frank J. Frassica, MD*

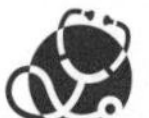

## BASICS

### DESCRIPTION

- First described by Sir James Paget in 1877 (1), Paget disease (osteitis deformans) is a bone disorder commonly seen in the geriatric population.
- As implied by the name "osteitis deformans", the involved bone may be severely deformed and enlarged, features that suggest an inflammatory origin.
- A chronic and slowly progressive disease of disorganized bone remodeling
- Can affect any bone
- Often asymmetric process
- May involve one bone (monostotic) or multiple bones (polyostotic)
- Classification:
  - Active phase:
    - Early (lytic) phase: Purely bone destruction
    - Mixed phase: Both bone destruction and formation
    - Late (sclerotic) phase: Predominantly bone formation
  - Inactive phase (patients 60–90 years old):
    - Many patients have inactive disease with no radiographic progression, symptoms, or laboratory abnormalities.

### EPIDEMIOLOGY

This disease of late adulthood is rarely seen before the 4th decade of life.

#### *Incidence*

- It affects 3–4% of the population >50 years old and is slightly more common in males (2).
- It is more common in Caucasians of Anglo-Saxon descent (2).

#### *Prevalence*

Its prevalence increases with advancing age, up to 5–15% by the 9th decade (2).

### RISK FACTORS

- 1st-degree relatives of affected persons
- Advancing age

#### *Genetics*

Ample evidence exists to suggest that 1st-degree relatives of affected persons carry a higher risk (up to 7 times higher) of developing the disease than those without family history of the disease.

### ETIOLOGY

- Genetic associations have been identified.
- Infectious (one of the paramyxoviruses): Some investigators believe that the cause is a slow virus because of the long incubation periods, absence of fevers, and involvement of a single organ system.

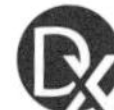

## DIAGNOSIS

### SIGNS AND SYMPTOMS

- Clinical manifestations depend on the severity of the disease and the site of involvement.
  - Pain:
    - Many patients are asymptomatic, but others have mild to severe bone pain.
    - Acute bone pain suggests pathologic fracture or malignant degeneration.
    - Usually constant and unrelated to activity
  - Frontal bossing and conductive hearing loss may be present.
  - If the spine is involved, the patient may develop spinal stenosis with or without radiculopathy.
  - Arthritis:
    - Pagetic arthritis is common in the hip and knee.
    - Patients have severe pain and difficulty in ambulating.

#### *Physical Exam*

- The most common findings are bowing of the extremity and local warmth if the bone is subcutaneous, such as the tibia.
- Restricted ROM is common in the hip in patients with pagetic arthritis.

### TESTS

- The basic components of the diagnostic evaluation are:
  - History and physical examination:
    - The involved area is warm to the touch because of the increased vascularity of the underlying bone.
  - Laboratory tests
  - Plain radiographs
  - Bone scan to evaluate the extent of skeletal involvement

#### *Lab*

- Increased serum alkaline phosphatase levels are noted.
- The 24-hour urine may show an increase in collagen breakdown products (N-telopeptide or hydroxyl proline, pyridinoline cross links; normal in 5% of patients [2]).
- Serum calcium usually is normal unless concurrent generalized inactivity, hyperparathyroidism, hyperthyroidism, or malignancy is present.

#### *Imaging*

- Radiography:
  - Plain films show enlarged bone with thick, coarsened trabeculae and sclerotic and lytic changes in the affected bone.
  - A flamed-shaped area of radiolucency strongly suggests an advancing edge of a pagetic lesion.
- A "hot" technetium-99m methylene diphosphonate bone scan also is observed.
- The bone scan will quantify the number of bones involved.

#### *Pathological Findings*

- Highly vascular bone resulting from high turnover rate
- Multiple pathologic fractures resulting from structurally weaker bone
- Histologically, more numerous osteoclasts and less mature (but fully mineralized) bone

### DIFFERENTIAL DIAGNOSIS

- Metastatic cancer
- Fibrous dysplasia
- Paget sarcoma

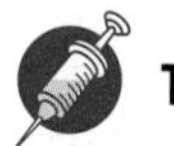

## TREATMENT

### GENERAL MEASURES

- Therapy depends on the severity of the disease: Not all patients require treatment.
- Indications for treatment include bone pain, high-output cardiac failure, and prevention of pathologic fracture.
- Pain from associated arthritis can be treated with NSAIDs.
- A cane or walker may be used for gait stabilization.
- Surgery is indicated for patients with severe arthritis who are refractory to medical management or for patients with impending pathologic fractures.
  - Preoperatively, medical therapy should be initiated to reduce disease activity, to minimize blood loss, and to optimize surgical outcome.

### SPECIAL THERAPY

#### *Physical Therapy*

Physical therapy may be used to improve the patient's ambulatory ability before or after surgery.

### MEDICATION (DRUGS)

- Medical treatment should be initiated for symptomatic patients or in preparation for orthopaedic surgery to prevent perioperative hypercalcemia or excessive bleeding.
  - Calcitonin:
    - Inhibits bone resorption by direct action on osteoclasts
    - Side effects include nausea, facial flushing, and polyuria.
- Diphosphonates (commonly used):
  - Potent inhibitors of bone resorption
  - Bind to hydroxyapatite crystals in bone and thereby prevent osteolysis
  - Also may function as metabolic poisons for osteoclasts
  - Common side effects include nausea, vomiting, and loose bowel movements.

### SURGERY

- Surgery usually is undertaken for 1 of 3 reasons:
  - Replacement of an arthritic joint
  - Internal fixation of a long-bone fracture
  - Correction of a long-bone deformity
- Total hip and knee arthroplasty is extremely effective in relieving pain and improving function.
- Intramedullary nails are the main modality for fixing long-bone diaphyseal fractures.
  - Multiple osteotomies may be necessary to correct the deformities.

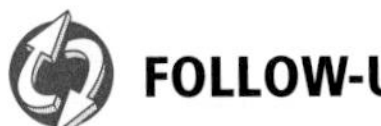

## FOLLOW-UP

### PROGNOSIS

- Most patients with Paget disease are asymptomatic and have a normal life expectancy.
- Long-term survival for patients with Paget sarcoma (<1% of patients with Paget disease) is poor: ~20% survival in 5 years (3).

### COMPLICATIONS

- Pathologic fractures
- High-output cardiac failure
- Malignant degeneration (Paget sarcoma)

### PATIENT MONITORING

- Patients usually are followed once a year.
- Usually, plain radiographs are obtained.

### REFERENCES


1. Paget J. On a form of chronic inflammation of bones (osteitis deformans). *Med Chir Trans* 1877; 60:37–63.
2. Siris ES, Roodman GD. Paget's disease of bone. In: Favus MJ, ed. *Primer on the Metabolic Bone Diseases and Disorders of Mineral Metabolism*, 6th ed. Washington, D.C.: American Society for Bone and Mineral Research, 2006:320–330.
3. McCarthy EF, Frassica FJ. Paget's disease. In: *Pathology of Bone and Joint Disorders: With Clinical and Radiographic Correlation*. Philadelphia: WB Saunders, 1998:165–173.


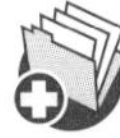

## MISCELLANEOUS

### CODES

#### *ICD9-CM*

731.0 Paget disease of bone

### PATIENT TEACHING

- Patients should be well informed about their disease and the goals of treatment.
- Treatment should be aimed at slowing or arresting disease progression, providing pain relief, or restoring function.
- Appropriate consultations should be made to address any extraskeletal abnormalities (e.g., deafness).
- The need for long-term follow-up should be emphasized.
- Resources for patient education in the United States can be obtained from the Paget Foundation, 200 Varick Street, New York, NY 10014 (Telephone: 212-229-1502).

### FAQ

- Q: Are there effective treatments for Paget disease?
  - A: Diphosphonate therapy is very effective in halting bone resorption in Paget disease.
- Q: Is hip replacement successful in patients with Pagetic arthritis of the hip?
  - A: Joint replacement surgery is an excellent method of relieving pain and improving function in patients with Paget disease of the hip.
- Q: What are the warning signs of cancer in Paget disease?
  - A: Bone pain or the development of a soft-tissue mass are the earliest signs. Cortical bone destruction and a soft-tissue mass can be detected with CT or MRI.

# PARONYCHIA (NAIL INFECTION)

*Dawn M. LaPorte, MD*
*Marc Urquhart, MD*

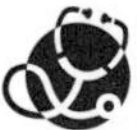

## BASICS

### DESCRIPTION

Paronychia is an infection of the radial or ulnar margins of the nails (lateral fold) of the hand (Fig. 1).

### GENERAL PREVENTION

- Keep the nail clean and appropriately trimmed.
- Use gloves for work and washing.
- Avoid nail biting.

### EPIDEMIOLOGY

#### *Incidence*

- It is the most common infection in the hand (1–3).
- Affects all ages

### RISK FACTORS

- Nail-biting
- Manicures
- Diabetes

### ETIOLOGY

- Typically secondary to the introduction of *Staphylococcus aureus* under the nail fold
- May be related to a hangnail, biting the nail edge, or manicure instrumentation

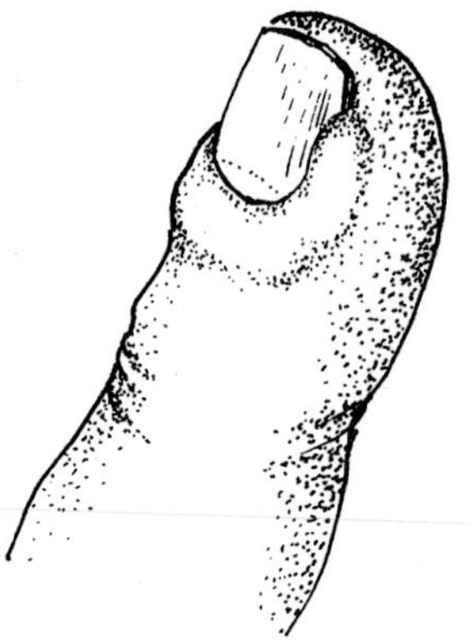

**Fig. 1.** Swelling along the nail. There may or may not be pus coming from the involved area.

### ASSOCIATED CONDITIONS

- Eponychia:
  - Location: In the periungual tissue at the proximal nail bed (Fig. 2)
  - Treatment (similar to that of paronychia):
    - Incise with a scalpel.
    - Insert small clamp into the abscess and open the inflammatory pocket.
    - Gram stain, culture, and antibiotics.
- Felons:
  - Location: Pulp of the finger
  - Treatment:
    - Incise and drain with a lateral incision down to the bone.
    - Spread the tissues with a clamp to disrupt the fibrous septa.
    - Gram stain, culture, and antibiotics
- Subungual abscess:
  - Location: Beneath the nail
  - Treatment:
    - Administer an adequate digital block.
    - Remove the nail plate and nail.
    - Obtain a specimen for Gram stain and culture.
    - Irrigate and gently débride any purulent material.
    - Replace the nail and nail fold with nonadherent gauze.
    - 1 dose of intravenous antistaphylococcal antibiotics, followed by a 10–14-day course of penicillin or erythromycin.
    - Follow-up as in paronychia is indicated.

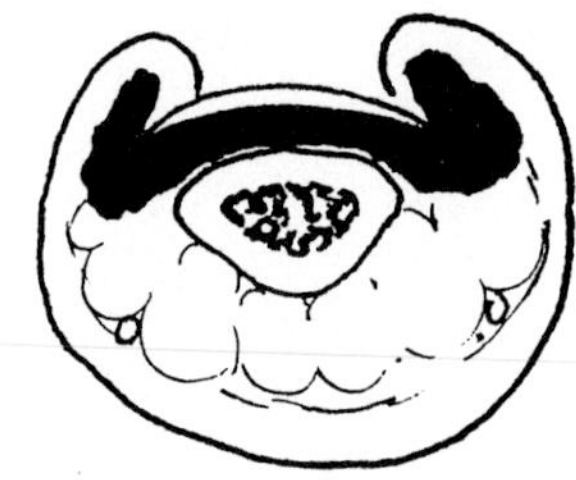

**Fig. 2.** Infection spreading along the nail bed.

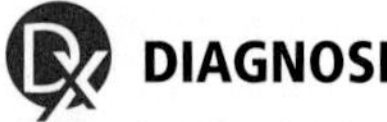

## DIAGNOSIS

### SIGNS AND SYMPTOMS

- Redness and swelling on the side of the nail fold with pain
- Possibly becoming fluctuant with discharge

#### *Physical Exam*

Examine for infection below the nail plate or in the finger pulp.

### TESTS

#### *Lab*

Lab tests are not needed unless the infection is aggressive and is spreading.

#### *Imaging*

Imaging is not necessary unless the nail infection is chronic, aggressive, unresponsive to treatment, or related to trauma.

#### *Pathological Findings*

- Typically, these infections are caused by *S. aureus*.
- Changes consistent with acute inflammation are noted.

### DIFFERENTIAL DIAGNOSIS

- Eponychia
- Felons
- Subungual abscess
- Tumor or cyst

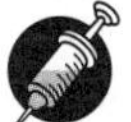

## TREATMENT

### GENERAL MEASURES

- Early diagnosis: If there is erythema without an abscess, then treat with oral antibiotics and warm, soapy soaks.
- Abscess:
  - If an abscess has formed:
    - Use a digital block with local anesthetic.
    - Immediately drain with a scalpel.
    - Send purulent material for Gram stain and culture.
    - Remove the lateral 1/5 of the nail if necessary.
    - Irrigate the wound copiously with saline solution through an angiocatheter or needle
    - Pack the wound with nonadherent sterile gauze.
    - Initiate a 10–14-day course of empiric antibiotics: Synthetic penicillin is the drug of choice, or erythromycin for penicillin-allergic patients because *S. aureus* is the most common causative organism.
- Chronic paronychia:
  - Often occurs in patient populations exposed to water.
    - These patients often have concomitant fungal infections and should have a topical antifungal ointment or possibly an oral antifungal agent added to the regimen.

### MEDICATION (DRUGS)

#### *First Line*

Synthetic penicillins are the drugs of choice.

### SURGERY

- Eponychial marsupialization is the most common surgical treatment for chronic paronychia (4,5).
- Consideration should be given to nail removal, particularly in the presence of a nail deformity.

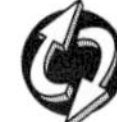

## FOLLOW-UP

### PROGNOSIS

The prognosis is good, with appropriate care.

### COMPLICATIONS

Progressive infection may require more aggressive treatment if it involves the pulp of the finger or extends into the bone.

### PATIENT MONITORING

Reevaluate within 48 hours of initial treatment to ensure that treatment is effective.

### REFERENCES


1. Brown DM, Young VL. Hand infections. *South Med J* 1993;86:56–66.
2. Canales FL, Newmeyer WL, III, Kilgore ES, Jr. The treatment of felons and paronychias. *Hand Clin* 1989;5:515–523.
3. Flynn JE. Modern considerations of major hand infections. *N Engl J Med* 1955;252:605–612.
4. Baran R, Bureau H. Surgical treatment of recalcitrant chronic paronychias of the fingers. *J Dermatol Surg Oncol* 1981;7:106–107.
5. Bednar MS, Lane LB. Eponychial marsupialization and nail removal for surgical treatment of chronic paronychia. *J Hand Surg* 1991;16A:314–317.


### ADDITIONAL READING


Stevanovic MV, Sharpe F. Acute infections in the hand. In: Green DP, Hotchkiss RN, Pederson WC, et al., eds. *Green's Operative Hand Surgery*, 5th ed. Philadelphia: Elsevier Churchill Livingstone, 2005:55–93.

## MISCELLANEOUS

### CODES

#### *ICD9-CM*

- 681.02 Paronychia (finger)
- 681.9 Paronychia with lymphangitis
- 681.9 Subungual abscess
- 757.5 Eponychia

### PATIENT TEACHING

#### *Prevention*

- Avoid nail-biting
- Appropriate care of hang-nails

### FAQ

- Q: What is the treatment for early presentation of a paronychia?
  - A: Early infections can be addressed nonsurgically with oral antibiotics and soaks 2–3 times daily in warm water and dilute Betadine.
- Q: Is chronic paronychia treated in the same way as an acute infection?
  - A: No. Chronic paronychia is a distinctly different clinical problem and is best managed with surgery with eponychial marsupialization in conjunction with oral antibiotics (if cultures are positive) and possibly antifungal medication.

# PATELLAR DISLOCATION

*Simon C. Mears, MD, PhD*
*Bill Hobbs, MD*

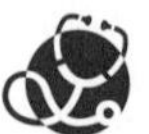

## BASICS

### DESCRIPTION

- Patellar dislocation usually refers to lateral displacement of the patella out of its normal alignment in the trochlear groove of the femur.
- The patella is held stable by ligamentous forces, muscular forces, and bony anatomy.
  - Disruption of any of these 3 components can lead to recurrent patellar instability.
- Classification:
  - Subluxation: Patella sits on the edge of the femoral groove, but not out of the track.
  - Dislocation: Patella is completely displaced out of the patellofemoral groove, usually laterally.

### EPIDEMIOLOGY

- Seen primarily in young patients (10–17 years old)
- Occurs more often in females than in males

#### *Incidence*

- The incidence is difficult to quantitate because many knees relocate spontaneously and are misdiagnosed.
- A 9% incidence of a positive family history (1) is noted.

### RISK FACTORS

- Positive family history
- Participation in football, basketball, baseball, gymnastics, or dancing
- Age 10–17 years (2)
- High level of activity or competition in a youth
- Mechanism other than a direct blow
- Hypermobility of the patella
- Previous dislocations (49% of patients with a dislocation have a history of a previous dislocation) (2)
- Patella alta (50% of patients) (1)
- Shallow patellofemoral groove
- Excessive Q angle
- Ligamentous laxity
- Excessive femoral anteversion
- Vastus medialis dysplasia
- Excessive genu valgus

#### *Genetics*

A congenital predisposition to knee malalignment and propensity to patellar dislocation is thought to exist.

### PATHOPHYSIOLOGY

- Patellar dislocation can disrupt the medial patellofemoral ligament.
- Chondral injury or fracture can occur from the impact of the patella on the trochlea (3).

### ETIOLOGY

- A direct blow to the medial aspect of the patella
- Severe valgus injury to the knee
- Twisting injury or other minor trauma, usually associated with congenital deficiencies

### ASSOCIATED CONDITIONS

- Connective tissue disease with ligamentous laxity, such as Ehlers-Danlos and Marfan syndromes
- Femoral anteversion and pes planus

## DIAGNOSIS

### SIGNS AND SYMPTOMS

- Patients with acute dislocation may present with the knee held in a flexed position as a result of hamstring spasms.
- The femoral condyles may be prominent medially.
- Often, the patella has spontaneously reduced, with the following findings:
  - Diffuse parapatellar tenderness
  - Positive apprehension test
  - Palpable defect at the insertion of the vastus medialis muscle
  - Hemarthrosis

#### *History*

- Direct blow to the knee
- Twisting injury to the leg

#### *Physical Exam*

- After the acute symptoms subside, examine the knee for the following:
  - Effusion
  - Apprehension, with patellar translation both medially and laterally
  - Lateral tracking of the patella (in the shape of a "J") with the knee extended from a flexed position (Fig. 1)
  - Injury to the medial, collateral, or cruciate knee ligaments
  - Lateral tilt

### TESTS

#### *Imaging*

- Radiography:
  - Postreduction plain radiographs are obtained for evidence of osteochondral fragments.
  - Axial views of the bilateral patella may show substantial lateral tracking.
- MRI or CT can reveal osteochondral injury and rupture of the medial patellofemoral ligament.

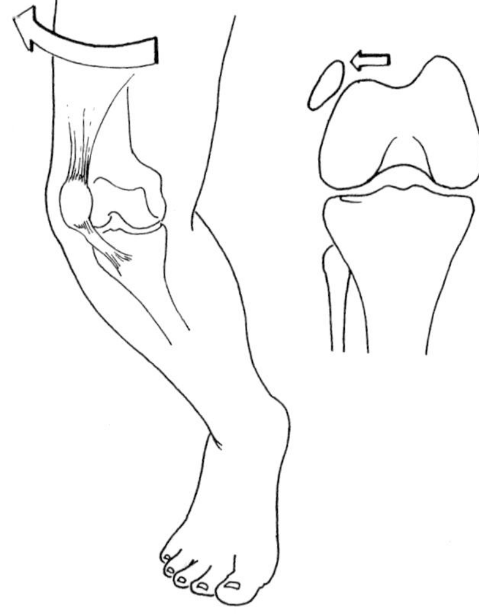

**Fig. 1.** Patellofemoral dislocation is almost always lateral.

#### *Pathological Findings*

- Abnormalities in the patellofemoral articulation allow the pull of the vastus lateralis and lateral retinaculum muscles to overcome that of the vastus medialis, even during minor trauma.
- This unbalanced pulling often tears the medial retinaculum and vastus medialis insertion.

### DIFFERENTIAL DIAGNOSIS

- Cruciate ligament injury
- Patellar fracture
- Patellofemoral pain syndrome
- Osteochondral fracture

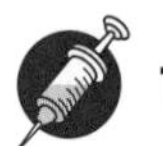

## TREATMENT

### GENERAL MEASURES

- Reduce acute dislocations and then immobilize the knee.
  - Reduce acute dislocation by gentle, steady extension of the knee, facilitated with the patient prone and the patient's hip extended to relax the hamstrings.
  - Avoid forceful manipulation.
  - Once the knee is reduced, immobilize it in extension with a compression dressing.
  - Evaluate the medial retinacular structure for tenderness every 2 weeks for up to 6 weeks.
  - When the patient is comfortable, apply a Neoprene sleeve with a laterally based felt pad.
- Surgical stabilization is recommended for the following:
  - Recurrent dislocations
  - Dislocations in carefully selected, highly active, competitive athletes
  - Acute dislocations with avulsive detachment of the vastus medialis muscle by bony fragment, seen on radiographs

#### *Activity*

- Patients may bear weight after relocation.
- Crutches should be supplied to facilitate weightbearing as tolerated.
- Twisting motions should be avoided.

### SPECIAL THERAPY

#### *Physical Therapy*

- The main goal of therapy is to strengthen the injured extensor mechanism and to improve patellofemoral tracking.
  - Straight-leg raises may begin immediately with appropriate support.
- Patients with recurrent dislocations often advance more quickly with physical therapy for quadriceps strengthening.

### MEDICATION (DRUGS)

Advise the patient that analgesics may be taken in the acute phase.

### SURGERY

- Several procedures have been attempted for treatment of patellar dislocation (4).
- Patients with acute dislocations and disruption of the medial patellofemoral ligament have been treated with acute repair (5).
- Lateral release for patellar instability has poor results (6).
- Patients with excessive Q angles (>150°) and recurrent dislocation may benefit from distal realignment via the Elmslie-Trillat or Fulkerson procedure.
- To prevent distal migration of the tibial tubercle, procedures that involve the tibial physis should be avoided in children with open physeal plates.
- Arthroscopy does not have a place in the treatment of patellar dislocation other than for intra-articular assessment of patellofemoral tracking or the treatment of associated injuries.

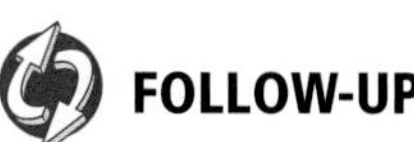

## FOLLOW-UP

### PROGNOSIS

- Overall, 75% of patients are treated successfully with nonoperative means (2).
- The key is to identify patients at risk for recurrence and to treat them more aggressively early in the course.
- Long-term results after surgical treatment do not seem to be better than those after nonoperative treatment (7,8).
- Long-term results of the Elmslie-Trillat osteotomy show improvement of instability, but results deteriorate over time (9).

### COMPLICATIONS

- Recurrent dislocations
- Chronic anterior knee pain
- Reflex sympathetic dystrophy
- Hemarthrosis with a lateral release
- Patellofemoral arthritis
- Osteochondral fractures

### PATIENT MONITORING

Patients are followed at 2–4-week intervals to monitor the progress of quadriceps rehabilitation.

### REFERENCES

1. Atkin DM, Fithian DC, Marangi KS, et al. Characteristics of patients with primary acute lateral patellar dislocation and their recovery within the first 6 months of injury. *Am J Sports Med* 2000;28:472–479.
2. Fithian DC, Paxton EW, Stone ML, et al. Epidemiology and natural history of acute patellar dislocation. *Am J Sports Med* 2004;32:1114–1121.
3. Nomura E, Inoue M, Kurimura M. Chondral and osteochondral injuries associated with acute patellar dislocation. *Arthroscopy* 2003;19:717–721.
4. Fithian DC, Paxton EW, Cohen AB. Indications in the treatment of patellar instability. *J Knee Surg* 2004;17:47–56.
5. Mikashima Y, Kimura M, Kobayashi Y, et al. Clinical results of isolated reconstruction of the medial patellofemoral ligament for recurrent dislocation and subluxation of the patella. *Acta Orthop Belg* 2006;72:65–71.
6. Panni AS, Tartarone M, Patricola A, et al. Long-term results of lateral retinacular release. *Arthroscopy* 2005;21:526–531.
7. Buchner M, Baudendistel B, Sabo D, et al. Acute traumatic primary patellar dislocation: long-term results comparing conservative and surgical treatment. *Clin J Sport Med* 2005;15:62–66.
8. Nikku R, Nietosvaara Y, Aalto K, et al. Operative treatment of primary patellar dislocation does not improve medium-term outcome: a 7-year follow-up report and risk analysis of 127 randomized patients. *Acta Orthop* 2005;76:699–704.
9. Carney JR, Mologne TS, Muldoon M, et al. Long-term evaluation of the Roux-Elmslie-Trillat procedure for patellar instability: a 26-year follow-up. *Am J Sports Med* 2005;33:1220–1223.

### ADDITIONAL READING

Hinton RY, Sharma KM. Acute and recurrent patellar instability in the young athlete. *Orthop Clin North Am* 2003;34:385–396.

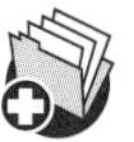

## MISCELLANEOUS

### CODES

#### *ICD9-CM*

836.3 Patellar dislocation

### PATIENT TEACHING

Discuss the risk factors for recurrent dislocation with a possible recommendation that the patient avoid high-risk activities or sports.

#### *Prevention*

Patients who are at high risk or have had previous instability should keep their quadriceps strong and consider bracing or taping.

### FAQ

- Q: What is the treatment for a 1st-time patellar dislocation?
  - A: Treatment is nonsurgical with relocation, quadriceps strengthening, and gentle return to activity. Surgical intervention should be considered with care and only if specific indications are present.

# PATELLAR FRACTURE

*John H. Wilckens, MD*

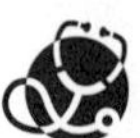

## BASICS

### DESCRIPTION
- Fracture of the patella (knee cap)
- Loss of extensor mechanism
- Classification: by pattern of fracture (1):
  - Vertical
  - Transverse
  - Stellate
  - Polar
- In children, the most common fracture pattern is the "sleeve" fracture (2).
  - The sleeve of periosteum is pulled off the bone.
  - Radiographs reveal patella alta, and the injury may be missed.

### EPIDEMIOLOGY
Affects all ages and both genders

#### *Incidence*
1% of all fractures (3)

### RISK FACTORS
- Blunt trauma
- Dashboard injury
- ACL reconstruction with patellar graft (4)

### ETIOLOGY
- Direct blow to the patella of a flexed knee, as occurs during a traffic accident in which the flexed knee hits the dashboard
- The exact angle of the applied force directly influences the pattern of injury to the patella (5).
- Sudden powerful quadriceps muscle eccentric contracture
- Fractures may happen after knee replacement secondary to osteolysis of the bone or direct trauma (6).

### ASSOCIATED CONDITIONS
- Femoral shaft fracture
- Knee ligament injury

## DIAGNOSIS

### SIGNS AND SYMPTOMS
- Acute knee pain and swelling after trauma
- Inability to extend or straighten the injured knee

#### *Physical Exam*
- Localized pain or swelling in the injured knee
- Patient inability to perform a straight-leg raise
- Visible or palpable defect of the extensor mechanism

### TESTS

#### *Imaging*
- Radiography:
  - AP and lateral views
  - Axial and tangential ("sunrise") views are helpful with longitudinal fractures.
- CT/MRI are rarely indicated for isolated patellar fractures.

#### *Pathological Findings*
- Hemarthrosis
- Interruption of extensor mechanism

### DIFFERENTIAL DIAGNOSIS
- Distal femoral or tibial plateau fracture
- Collateral ligament tear
- PCL tear
- Quadriceps tendon or patellar ligament rupture

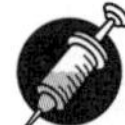

## TREATMENT

### GENERAL MEASURES
- Nondisplaced fractures:
  - Only patellar fractures amenable to nonoperative treatment (casting or splinting the knee in full extension)
  - Close follow-up is required because nondisplaced fractures may displace.
- Displaced fractures:
  - Best managed with open reduction and internal fixation:
    - Allows for anatomic reduction
    - Allows early ROM and reduced immobilization

### SPECIAL THERAPY

#### *Physical Therapy*
- Nonsurgical patients may bear weight as tolerated in the cast or splint.
- Patients may resume active ROM exercises once the cast is removed.

### MEDICATION (DRUGS)

#### *First Line*
- Acetaminophen
- NSAIDs after 6 weeks (healed fracture)

#### *Second Line*
Narcotics

### SURGERY (7)
- All displaced fractures should undergo open reduction and internal fixation.
  - Parallel Kirschner wires with tension band wiring is adequate for most transverse fractures (8).
  - Tension band wiring also can be accomplished using parallel cannulated screws (9).
- Stellate fractures may require additional cerclage wiring.
- Distal pole fractures can be excised, and the patellar tendon can be repaired to the proximal fragment (10).
- Patellectomy is used only for the most comminuted fractures that cannot be stabilized.

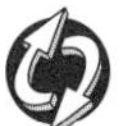

## FOLLOW-UP

### PROGNOSIS

- Nondisplaced patellar fractures have a good prognosis with nonoperative treatment.
- Well-aligned and stabilized fractures have a good prognosis.
- Even in elderly patients, surgery gives better results than nonsurgical treatment of displaced fractures (11).
- Open fractures should be managed with débridement and fixation, with an attempt to preserve as much bone as possible (12).

### COMPLICATIONS

- Fracture nonunion/malunion (13)
- Refracture
- Need for hardware removal (14)
- Arthritis
- Extensor mechanism weakness:
  - As comminution and loss of articular surface of the patella increase and as more of the patella is excised, extensor mechanism strength decreases.

### PATIENT MONITORING

Serial radiographs are obtained at 4-week intervals until healing.

### REFERENCES


1. Carpenter JE, Kasman R, Matthews LS. Fractures of the patella. *J Bone Joint Surg* 1993;75A: 1550–1561.
2. Hunt DM, Somashekar N. A review of sleeve fractures of the patella in children. *Knee* 2005; 12:3–7.
3. Bostrom A. Fracture of the patella. A study of 422 patellar fractures. *Acta Orthop Scand Suppl* 1972;143:1–80.
4. Stein DA, Hunt SA, Rosen JE, et al. The incidence and outcome of patella fractures after anterior cruciate ligament reconstruction. *Arthroscopy* 2002;18:578–583.
5. Atkinson PJ, Haut RC. Injuries produced by blunt trauma to the human patellofemoral joint vary with flexion angle of the knee. *J Orthop Res* 2001;19:827–833.
6. Ortiguera CJ, Berry DJ. Patellar fracture after total knee arthroplasty. *J Bone Joint Surg* 2002;84A: 532–540.
7. Cramer KE, Moed BR. Patellar fractures: contemporary approach to treatment. *J Am Acad Orthop Surg* 1997;5:323–331.
8. Chen A, Hou C, Bao J, et al. Comparison of biodegradable and metallic tension-band fixation for patella fractures. 38 patients followed for 2 years. *Acta Orthop Scand* 1998;69:39–42.
9. Berg EE. Open reduction internal fixation of displaced transverse patella fractures with figure-eight wiring through parallel cannulated compression screws. *J Orthop Trauma* 1997;11: 573–576.
10. Kastelec M, Veselko M. Inferior patellar pole avulsion fractures: osteosynthesis compared with pole resection. *J Bone Joint Surg* 2004;86A: 696–701.
11. Shabat S, Mann G, Kish B, et al. Functional results after patellar fractures in elderly patients. *Arch Gerontol Geriatr* 2003;37:93–98.
12. Catalano JB, Iannacone WM, Marczyk S, et al. Open fractures of the patella: long-term functional outcome. *J Trauma* 1995;39:439–444.
13. Klassen JF, Trousdale RT. Treatment of delayed and nonunion of the patella. *J Orthop Trauma* 1997;11:188–194.
14. Smith ST, Cramer KE, Karges DE, et al. Early complications in the operative treatment of patella fractures. *J Orthop Trauma* 1997;11: 183–187.


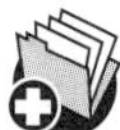

## MISCELLANEOUS

### CODES

#### *ICD9-CM*

822.2 Patellar fracture

### PATIENT TEACHING

- Injury to the cartilage and bone is typical in patellar fractures.
- The risk of future knee pain and arthritis exists.
- Full recovery can take up to 1 year.

### FAQ

- Q: How soon can a patient walk after open reduction and internal fixation of the patella?
  - A; If the fracture is well reduced and stabilized, the patient can begin weightbearing as tolerated with the leg locked straight. The patient also may begin early ROM.
- Q: Does the hardware (screws, pins, and wires) need to be removed after fracture healing?
  - A: If the hardware is asymptomatic, it usually does not need to be removed. However, because little soft tissue covers the patella, the hardware usually irritates the quadriceps and patellar tendons and should be removed.

# PATELLAR TENDON RUPTURE

*John H. Wilckens, MD*
*Jamil Jacobs-El, MD*

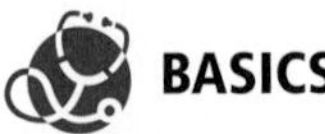

## BASICS

### DESCRIPTION

Patellar tendon rupture is a disruption of the segment of the extensor mechanism extending from the inferior aspect of the patella to the tibial tubercle.

### EPIDEMIOLOGY

- Patients usually <40 years old
- Affects males more than females

### RISK FACTORS

- History of patellar tendinitis
- Steroid injections around the patellar tendon
- Dialysis
- Anabolic steroid use
- Corticosteroid use

### ETIOLOGY

Ruptures usually result from trauma in which a violent quadriceps muscle contraction occurs against resistance in the flexed knee.

## DIAGNOSIS

### SIGNS AND SYMPTOMS

- Defect in the patellar tendon
- Inability to extend the knee from the flexed position
- Injured patella resting more proximally than the uninjured knee and migrating proximally with active quadriceps contraction
- Acute injuries usually are associated with substantial knee effusion and pain on active or passive ROM.

#### *Physical Exam*

- Check for pain or swelling in the affected knee.
- Patient is unable to perform a straight-leg raise.
- Perform an active knee extension test to identify loss of integrity to the extensor mechanism.
- Palpate for a defect in the patellar tendon.

### TESTS

#### *Imaging*

- Radiography:
  - Obtain plain AP and lateral radiographs of the knee to rule out patellar fracture and tibial plateau fractures.
    - Usually, the patella has migrated proximally.
- MRI is diagnostic.

#### *Pathological Findings*

- Complete rupture of the patellar tendon with degenerative changes noted in the tendon (1)
- The patellar tendon may avulse from the inferior pole of the patella or from the tibial tubercle, or it may sustain an intrasubstance rupture.

### DIFFERENTIAL DIAGNOSIS

- Extensor mechanism injuries (2):
  - Quadriceps tendon rupture
  - Patellar dislocation
  - Patellar fracture
- Intra-articular disorders:
  - Ligament tears
  - Occult tibial plateau fractures
  - With the previously listed 2 disorders, extensor mechanism function may shut down with a large effusion.

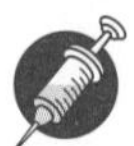

## TREATMENT

### GENERAL MEASURES

- Patellar tendon ruptures require operative repair.
- Patients with acute ruptures should be placed in a knee immobilizer for comfort and referred to an orthopaedist for surgical treatment.
- Patients may bear weight as tolerated as long as the knee is locked in extension.

### SPECIAL THERAPY

#### *Physical Therapy*

- Patients may require physical therapy for quadriceps strengthening and ROM exercises.
  - Begin with straight-leg raises and quadriceps sets.
  - Allow early ROM within the limits of tension of surgical repair.
  - May bear weight as tolerated with the knee locked in extension
- Core strengthening:
- After 6 weeks, advanced ROM and strength training as tolerated

### MEDICATION (DRUGS)
Analgesics can be given for pain management acutely and after surgery.

### SURGERY
- Acute ruptures must be repaired surgically.
- Early repair allows for maintenance of patellar tendon length and better functional results.
- Chronic patellar tendon tears usually require some type of reconstructive procedure and/or augmentation (3).
- Patients usually are treated with an above-the-knee cast or a knee brace locked in extension for ~6 weeks after surgery.

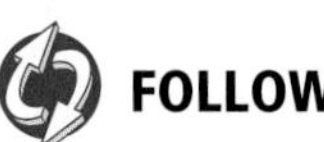

## FOLLOW-UP

### PROGNOSIS
- Most patients treated with early patellar tendon repair have good or excellent results.
- Chronic tendon ruptures are more difficult to repair, but repair provides better results than nonoperative treatment.

### COMPLICATIONS
- Knee loss of motion
- Extensor weakness

### PATIENT MONITORING
- See patients 7–14 days after surgery for removal of stitches.
- Follow-up every 4–6 weeks until full ROM and strength are achieved.

### REFERENCES

1. Kannus P, Jozsa L. Histopathological changes preceding spontaneous rupture of a tendon. A controlled study of 891 patients. *J Bone Joint Surg* 1991;73A:1507–1525.
2. Wilckens JH, Mears SC, Byank RP. Knee, lower leg, and ankle pain. In: Barker LR, Burton JR, Zieve PD, eds. *Principles of Ambulatory Medicine*, 7th ed. Philadelphia: Lippincott Williams & Wilkins, in press, 2006.
3. Matava MJ. Patellar tendon ruptures. *J Am Acad Orthop Surg* 1996;4:287–296.


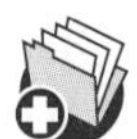

## MISCELLANEOUS

### CODES
#### *ICD9-CM*
844.8 Patellar tendon rupture

### FAQ
- Q: How can a quadriceps tendon rupture, a patellar tendon rupture, and a patellar fracture be differentiated?
  - A: All 3 result in extensor mechanism weakness and inability to perform a straight-leg raise. All of them also have a palpable defect. With a patellar fracture, the proximal fragment is retracted proximally and the distal fragment is retracted distally, creating a gap between the fracture fragments. A quadriceps tendon rupture results in the distal migration of the patella with the defect above the patella. A patellar tendon rupture results in the proximal migration of the patella and a defect distal to the patella.
- Q: Can you rupture a healthy patellar tendon?
  - A: Although some patients may not report a prodromal period of patellar tendinitis, all ruptured patellar tendons reveal evidence of tendon degeneration. However, it is possible to lacerate a healthy tendon.

# PATELLOFEMORAL SYNDROME

*Henry Boateng, MD*
*John H. Wilckens, MD*

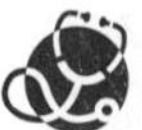

## BASICS

### DESCRIPTION

- Patellofemoral syndrome:
  - Disorder of the patellofemoral joint presenting with anterior knee pain.
  - Insidious in onset
  - Exacerbated by activity involving strenuous or continuous flexion

### GENERAL PREVENTION

- Quadriceps muscle strengthening
- Avoidance of overuse in activities requiring repetitive knee flexion
- Improvement in training protocols
- Avoidance of open-chain quadriceps exercise

### EPIDEMIOLOGY

- More common in females than in males (1)
- Seen especially in the adolescent athlete (1)
- Most common cause of knee pain in runners (1)

#### *Incidence*

Common, but true incidence is unknown.

#### *Prevalence*

Prevalence is unknown.

### RISK FACTORS

- Training errors (e.g., rapidly increased mileage)
- Female gender
- Poor quadriceps strength
- Dysplastic vastus medialis obliquus
- Generalized ligamentous laxity
- Heel cord and hamstring tightness
- Patella alta
- Extensor mechanism malalignment (increased femoral anteversion, increased Q angle (Fig. 1), genu varum/valgus, external tibial torsion, pronated feet)

#### *Genetics*

No known inheritance pattern

### PATHOPHYSIOLOGY

Biomechanical malalignment of the patella, causing uneven pressure and wear on the patellofemoral joint, leading to anterior knee pain

### ETIOLOGY

- Extensor mechanism malalignment
- Contracted lateral retinaculum (also may be result)

### ASSOCIATED CONDITIONS

- Quadriceps dysplasia/weakness
- Extensor mechanism malalignment
- Patellar instability

## DIAGNOSIS

### SIGNS AND SYMPTOMS

#### *History*

- Pain in the anterior knee, worse after strenuous and bent-knee activities
- Pain with stair climbing, worse with going down
- Pain after prolonged knee flexion, such as at theatres ("movie-goer's knee") or during long car rides
- Pain with squatting and rising from squatted position
- Pseudo giving-way of the knee

#### *Physical Exam*

- Extensor mechanism alignment:
  - Q angle
  - Femoral anteversion
  - Tibial torsion
  - Pronated feet
- Tender medial and lateral patella retinaculum
- Patellar laxity/instability (lateral displacement with apprehension) (Fig. 2)
- Tight quadriceps, hamstrings, Achilles tendon
- $\pm$ Effusion
- Pain with patellar loading

### TESTS

#### *Imaging*

- Plain radiographs:
  - AP
  - Lateral: Look for patella alta
  - Axial:
    - Merchant standardized tangential view of the patella with 30° of flexion
    - "Sunrise" views require more knee flexion and do not show subtle malalignment and instability.
- CT and MRI are useful for recalcitrant cases (>6 months of symptoms).

#### *Diagnostic Procedures/Surgery*

Arthroscopy may show patella maltracking and patella chondromalacia.

#### *Pathological Findings*

- Extensor mechanism malalignment
- Patella chondromalacia
- Instability

### DIFFERENTIAL DIAGNOSIS

- Quadriceps tendinitis
- Patellar tendinitis
- Patellofemoral arthritis
- Osteochondritis desiccans
- Symptomatic plica
- Patellofemoral instability
- Fat pad impingement

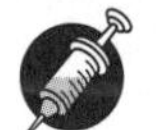

## TREATMENT

### INITIAL STABILIZATION

- Initial stage of treatment is reduction of symptoms.
- NSAIDs
- Ice
- Activity modification
- Isometric quadriceps and core strengthening
- Quadriceps, hamstring, and Achilles stretching

### GENERAL MEASURES

- The overall goal in treatment is to reduce pain.
- Nonoperative measures include physical therapy, activity modification, and NSAIDs.
- NSAIDs and ice may help with pain reduction in acute exacerbations.

#### *Activity*

- Activity modification, such as avoidance of open-chain leg extensions and uphill running
- Graduated training protocols to avoid acute increase in activities
- Quadriceps and hamstring stretching before and after running

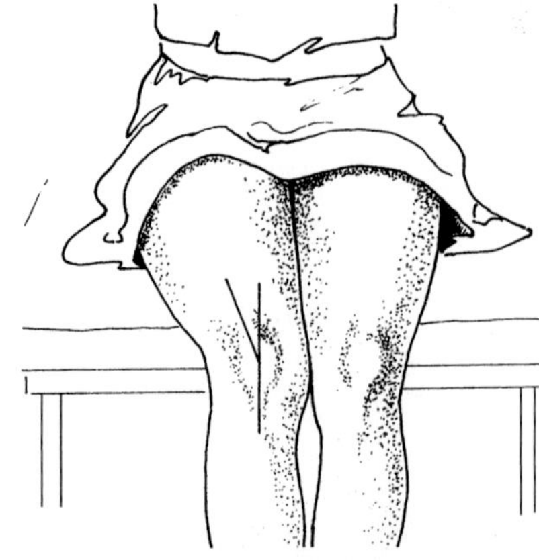

**Fig. 1.** The Q angle is the angle formed between the tibial tubercle, the patella, and the femur. The greater the angle, the more likely the development of patellofemoral syndrome.

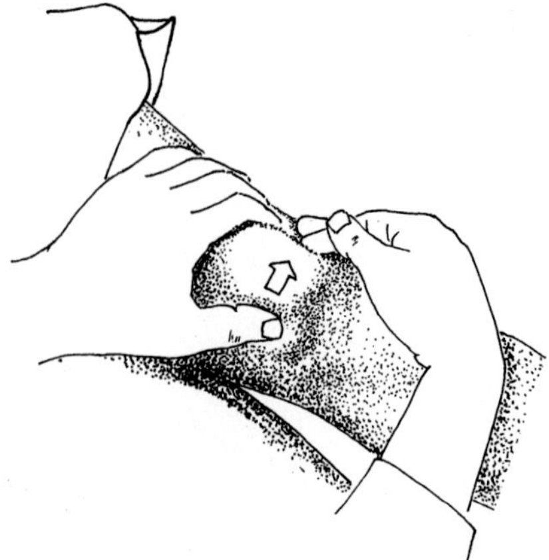

**Fig. 2.** Patients who previously experienced patellofemoral subluxation or dislocation exhibit a positive apprehension sign when the patella is pushed laterally.

## SPECIAL THERAPY
Bracing during activity, such as using a patellar sleeve, may help with patella tracking and improve muscle proprioception (muscle responsiveness).

### *Physical Therapy*
- Physical therapy for quadriceps strengthening and stretching is the initial line of treatment.
- Alternative exercises (swimming)
- Reconditioning:
  - Eccentric quadriceps strengthening
  - Modalities such as iontophoresis
  - Hamstring and Achilles stretching
  - Core strengthening

## MEDICATION (DRUGS)
NSAIDs

## SURGERY
- Only when symptomatic and after an exhaustive and documented course of physical therapy (6 months)
- Lateral release for contracted, tight lateral retinaculum:
  - Too vigorous a release can lead to medial instability.
- Realignment (proximal and/or distal), depending on type of malalignment
- Chondroplasty for extensive chondromalacia

# FOLLOW-UP

- Early quadriceps activation
- Early ROM

## DISPOSITION
### *Issues for Referral*
Anterior knee pain associated with patellar instability or malalignment should be referred.

## PROGNOSIS
- Most patients improve with physical therapy and nonoperative measures.
- Surgery is successful for patients with identified mechanical causes of pain such as instability or malalignment of the patella.

## COMPLICATIONS
Hemarthrosis is the most common complication after lateral release (2).

## REFERENCES

1. DeHaven KE, Dolan WA, Mayer PJ. Chondromalacia patellae in athletes. Clinical presentation and conservative management. *Am J Sports Med* 1979;7:5–11.
2. Small NC. An analysis of complications in lateral retinacular release procedures. *Arthroscopy* 1989;5:282–286.


## ADDITIONAL READING

- Carson WG, Jr, James SL, Larson RL, et al. Patellofemoral disorders: physical and radiographic evaluation. Part I: physical examination. *Clin Orthop Relat Res* 1984;185:165–177.
- Carson WG, Jr, James SL, Larson RL, et al. Patellofemoral disorders: physical and radiographic evaluation. Part II: Radiographic examination. *Clin Orthop Relat Res* 1984;185:178–186.
- Fox JM, Del Pizzo W, eds. *The Patellofemoral Joint*. New York: McGraw-Hill, 1993.
- Fulkerson JP, Shea KP. Disorders of patellofemoral alignment. *J Bone Joint Surg* 1990;72A:1424–1429.
- Hungerford DS, Lennox DW. Rehabilitation of the knee in disorders of the patellofemoral joint: relevant biomechanics. *Orthop Clin North Am* 1983;14:397–402.
- Kujala UM, Kvist M, Osterman K, et al. Factors predisposing army conscripts to knee exertion injuries incurred in a physical training program. *Clin Orthop Relat Res* 1986;210:203–212.
- Theur PC, Fulkerson JP. Knee. Section E: Patellofemoral joint. Part 6: Anterior knee pain and patellar subluxation in the adult. In: DeLee JC, Drez D, Jr, Miller MD, eds. *DeLee & Drez's Orthopaedic Sports Medicine: Principles and Practice*, 2nd ed. Philadelphia: WB Saunders Co, 2003:1772–1815.


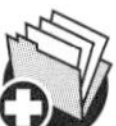

# MISCELLANEOUS

## CODES
### *ICD9-CM*
- 717.7 Chondromalacia patella
- 719.46 Patellofemoral pain syndrome

## PATIENT TEACHING
- It is important to stress that surgery may improve patellar tracking and prevent dislocation or subluxation, but it is not guaranteed to relieve pain.
- Proper conditioning
- Avoid training errors such as too rapid increase in mileage/intensity.

## FAQ
- Q: What radiographs are helpful for evaluating the knee with patellofemoral pain syndrome?
  - A: In addition to AP and lateral radiographs of the knee, a standardized axial or tangential view of the patella (Merchant view) is helpful to evaluate alignment, tilt, and stability.
- Q: What should be emphasized in the rehabilitation of patellofemoral pain syndrome?
  - A: In addition to identifying and correcting training errors, therapy should emphasize quadriceps, hamstring, and hip flexor stretching and strengthening and core strengthening. Patellar taping may help reduce pain during therapy.
- Q: When would surgery be considered for anterior knee pain?
  - A: Patients with demonstrated patellar malalignment and/or instability for whom a rigorous rehabilitation program has failed may be candidates for surgery.

# PATHOLOGIC FRACTURE

*Frank J. Frassica, MD*

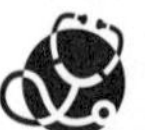

## BASICS

### DESCRIPTION

- A pathologic fracture occurs through diseased bone rather than through normal bone.
  - The normal bone is replaced by abnormal bone or no bone at all.
    - The involved bone is no longer able to withstand normal physiologic forces.
    - Fracture often occurs with activities of daily living.
    - The weakened state may be caused by a benign or malignant process.

#### *Geriatric Considerations*

- Pathologic fractures in the geriatric patient are most likely secondary to bone metastases, multiple myeloma, and lymphoma.
- Occasionally, a destructive lesion such as a chondrosarcoma or malignant fibrous histiocytoma is the cause of the fracture.

#### *Pediatric Considerations*

- In children and adolescents, the most common benign cause of a pathologic fracture is a unicameral bone cyst or a NOF.
- The 2 malignancies that may cause a pathologic fracture are osteosarcoma and Ewing sarcoma.

### GENERAL PREVENTION

- No preventative measures if the patient is unaware of the pathologic process
- Many patients do have antecedent pain with activity.
  - The pain usually is directly referable to the involved bone.

### EPIDEMIOLOGY

- Pathologic fractures usually are caused by well-recognized conditions in children, adolescents, and adults.
  - Children and adolescents:
    - Benign: Unicameral bone cysts (proximal humerus and femur), NOF, fibrous dysplasia
    - Malignant: Osteosarcoma, Ewing sarcoma
  - Adults:
    - Benign: Giant cell tumor, fibrous dysplasia
    - Malignant: Metastases, myeloma, lymphoma, malignant fibrous histiocytoma
  - Geriatric patients:
    - Benign: Hyperparathyroidism (rare)
    - Malignant: Metastases, myeloma, lymphoma, chondrosarcoma, malignant fibrous histiocytoma

### RISK FACTORS

- Bone strength is weakened substantially when >50% cortical bone destruction occurs.
  - Measure on AP and lateral radiographs.
  - CT scans are excellent for defining bone loss if it is not apparent on radiographs.

#### *Genetics*

No specific genetic associations are known.

### PATHOPHYSIOLOGY

- Any defect in the cortex of a long bone results in diminished capacity to withstand forces.
  - 50% symmetric cortical involvement results in a 60% reduction in bending strength (1).
  - 50% asymmetric cortical involvement results in 90% reduction in strength (1).
  - Long lytic defects (length longer than the diameter of the bone) result in up to 90% reductions in torsional strength (1).

### ASSOCIATED CONDITIONS

Any condition that substantially weakens the bone by replacing normal bone tissue

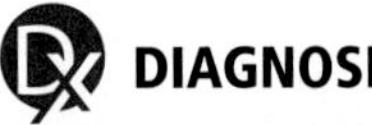

## DIAGNOSIS

### SIGNS AND SYMPTOMS

- Pain and bone tenderness are the 2 dominant findings
  - Bone pain: Before fracture, patients may note moderate or severe pain with ambulation.
  - Bone tenderness: Palpation often will cause severe pain.
  - Once complete fracture has occurred, patients will note severe pain that is excruciating with any motion or palpation.

#### *History*

- Bone pain:
  - Begins intermittently and then occurs with all activities
  - Characteristically occurs before fracture

#### *Physical Exam*

- Before pathologic fracture, physical examination findings may be few or nonexistent.
  - Palpate for bone tenderness.
  - Palpate for a soft-tissue mass that sometimes is present in malignancies.
  - Check ROM gently so as not to cause a pathologic fracture.

### TESTS

Imaging studies are the major modalities.

#### *Lab*

Serum tests are not helpful.

#### *Imaging*

- Radiography:
  - Once a pathologic fracture has occurred, plain radiographs are the major diagnostic modality.
  - AP/lateral plain radiographs are used to look for the cause.
    - Look for lytic bone destruction.
    - Look for host bone reaction: Sclerotic rim, thickening of cortex
- CT:
  - Once a pathologic fracture has occurred, CT can be used on a limited basis to aid in the diagnostic evaluation.
  - Can show the pattern of bone destruction and an approximate assessment of a soft-tissue mass
- MRI:
  - Once a pathologic fracture has occurred, MRI can be used on a limited basis to aid the diagnostic evaluation.
  - Can be used to evaluate for soft-tissue masses and extent of marrow involvement

#### *Diagnostic Procedures/Surgery*

- The evaluation strategy is based on the assessment of the plain radiographs.
  - If the radiographs suggest a malignant process:
    - Chest radiograph, chest CT, and abdominal CT to look for a carcinoma or metastases from the lesion causing the pathologic fracture
    - Needle or open biopsy after the staging evaluation is complete
  - If the radiographs suggest a benign process:
    - If the plain radiographs are diagnostic (unicameral bone cyst, NOF, fibrous dysplasia), treatment can be planned and initiated without a biopsy.
    - If plain radiographs are not diagnostic, a biopsy is necessary.

#### *Pathological Findings*

Depend on the nature of the underlying lesion

## DIFFERENTIAL DIAGNOSIS
- The differential diagnosis varies based on the age of the patient and the plain radiographs.
  - Young patient, benign appearance:
    - Unicameral bone cyst
    - NOF
    - Fibrous dysplasia
  - Young patient, malignant appearance:
    - Osteosarcoma
    - Ewing sarcoma
  - Adult patient, malignant appearance:
    - Metastatic disease
    - Myeloma
    - Lymphoma

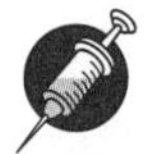

# TREATMENT

## INITIAL STABILIZATION
- Many patients have bone pain with activity, and it may occur weeks to months before pathologic fracture.
  - When activity-related pain exists with a radiographically documented destructive lesion, an ambulatory support to reduce loading should be recommended.
    - Walker
    - 2 crutches
    - Single cane

## GENERAL MEASURES
- Control pain.
- Reduce forces with walking aid or by placing patient at bed rest.

### *Activity*
- Reduce activity.
  - Recommend ambulatory aid.
  - If patient is unable to walk, recommend a wheelchair.
  - If unable to control pain, recommend bed rest.

### *Nursing*
- Assess patient and recommend general measures:
  - Walking aid
  - Activity reduction

## SPECIAL THERAPY
### *Radiotherapy*
- Often used after pathologic fractures are treated surgically.
- Specific indications include:
  - Metastatic bone disease
  - Multiple myeloma
  - Lymphoma

### *Physical Therapy*
- Used before and after surgery:
  - Before surgical stabilization:
    - Instruct patient on protected weightbearing with walking aid.
  - After stabilization:
    - Instruct patient on use of walking aid.
    - Begin program to regain strength.

## MEDICATION (DRUGS)
- Pain medications used as necessary
- Diphosphonates for metastatic bone disease and multiple myeloma

## SURGERY
- Pathologic fractures usually are treated with an internal fixation device such as an intramedullary nail.
  - Hip replacement is used for femoral neck fractures.
  - Patients with pathologic fractures secondary to sarcomas, such as osteosarcoma, usually are treated with a cast and then wide resection after several cycles of chemotherapy.

# FOLLOW-UP

- Patients are followed at 1-month intervals until the fracture heals.
  - Plain radiographs are used to assess healing.

## DISPOSITION
### *Issues for Referral*
Patients are referred to an orthopaedic oncologist for management.

## PROGNOSIS
- The prognosis depends entirely on the underlying process.
- Benign diagnoses: Excellent
- Malignant diagnoses:
  - Metastases (uniformly fatal, median survival)
  - Lung, kidney: 6–12 months
  - Breast, prostate: 24–48 months
  - Myeloma: Median survival, 3–5 years (2)
  - Lymphoma: 60–80% survival at 5 years (3)
  - Osteosarcoma: 60–70% survival at 5 years (4)

## COMPLICATIONS
- Related to the surgery:
  - Infection
  - Delayed wound healing
  - Failure to heal

## PATIENT MONITORING
1-month intervals until the fracture heals

## REFERENCES

1. Hipp JA, Springfield DS, Hayes WC. Predicting pathologic fracture risk in the management of metastatic bone defects. *Clin Orthop Relat Res* 1995;312:120–135.
2. McCarthy EF, Frassica FJ. Plasma cell dyscrasia. In: *Pathology of Bone and Joint Disorders: With Clinical and Radiographic Correlation.* Philadelphia: WB Saunders, 1998:185–193.
3. McCarthy EF, Frassica FJ. Primary bone tumors. In: *Pathology of Bone and Joint Disorders: With Clinical and Radiographic Correlation.* Philadelphia: WB Saunders, 1998:195–275.
4. Hornicek FJ. Ewing's sarcoma. In: Menendez LR, ed. *Orthopaedic Knowledge Update: Musculoskeletal Tumors.* Rosemont, IL: American Academy of Orthopaedic Surgeons, 2002:195–202.


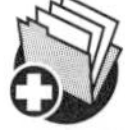

# MISCELLANEOUS

## CODES
### *ICD9-CM*
733.10 Pathologic fracture

## PATIENT TEACHING
Patients are instructed on the nature of the underlying lesion.

### *Activity*
Protected weightbearing until fracture union occurs

### *Prevention*
Prophylactic fixation often is recommended if the weakened bone state is detected before the fracture occurs.

## FAQ
- Q: What is the most common cause of a pathologic fracture in the adult patient?
  - A: Bone metastases and myeloma are the most common causes.
- Q: How long does it take for a pathologic fracture to heal?
  - A: In general, ~6–10 weeks, depending on the fracture pattern and the amount of bone loss.

# PECTORALIS MAJOR TENDON RUPTURE

*Mark Clough, MD*
*John H. Wilckens, MD*

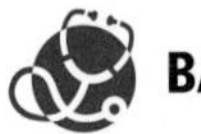

## BASICS

### DESCRIPTION

- The pectoralis major is an adductor, flexor, and internal rotator of the humerus.
- Muscular origins are on the clavicle, sternum, ribs, and external oblique fascia.
- The insertion is on the crest of the lateral aspect of the midhumerus.
- The muscle twists so that the lower fibers insert highest on the humerus.
- Anatomic classification system (1):
  - Type I: Muscle strain, microscopic tear
  - Type II: Partial tear
  - Type III: Complete tear

### GENERAL PREVENTION

- Avoid extreme weightlifting, including bench press and butterfly curls.
- Avoid anabolic steroid use.

### EPIDEMIOLOGY

- Usually occurs in male power athletes 20–40 years old (2)
- Can occur in the elderly (>65 years old) (3)

#### *Incidence*

Unknown

#### *Prevalence*

Unknown

### RISK FACTORS

- Anabolic steroid use
- Power lifting, weightlifting

### PATHOPHYSIOLOGY

Depends on the location of the rupture

### ETIOLOGY

- Strains and partial tears:
  - Most common forms of injury
  - Involve the muscle belly
  - Partial ruptures generally occur at the musculotendinous junction or are intramuscular.
- Total rupture:
  - Rare injury
  - The mechanism of injury is usually a sudden forceful overload of an eccentrically contracted muscle, such as during a weightlifter's bench press.
  - Usually occurs as avulsion at or near the muscular insertion on the humerus

## DIAGNOSIS

### SIGNS AND SYMPTOMS

#### *History*

- Patients often present with a history of sudden onset of severe arm and shoulder pain associated with the time of injury.
  - Audible "snap" or "pop" during injury
  - Limited ROM
  - Local swelling
  - Ecchymosis

#### *Physical Exam*

- Disruption in the anterior axillary contour
- A thin anterior axillary fold or a sulcus may be seen at the deltopectoral groove
- A defect may be palpable.
- A bulging may be seen at the muscular origins when a patient is asked to tension the muscle.

### TESTS

Manual muscle testing of adduction and internal rotation will show weakness.

#### *Imaging*

- Plain radiographs:
  - Always start with plain radiographs to rule out any bony pathology.
  - Bony avulsions also may appear on plain radiographs.
- Ultrasonography:
  - Can help locate tears and help define diagnosis when diagnosis is unclear clinically
  - Safe and cost-effective, but user-dependent
- MRI:
  - Has been used to diagnose and localize muscle tears
  - Can be helpful in the acute setting when physical examination is limited by swelling and pain
  - Is now the imaging modality of choice because it can distinguish acute and chronic tears and can determine the exact location and size of the tear

#### *Diagnostic Procedures/Surgery*

- The diagnosis of a pectoralis major muscle tear is generally a clinical one.
- For purposes of surgical planning, the location of the tear should be localized with MRI.

#### *Pathological Findings*

- Torn muscle and tendon fibers may be visualized at time of surgery.
- Muscle attenuation and atrophy can be seen in the elderly population.

### DIFFERENTIAL DIAGNOSIS

- Pectoralis major tendon rupture
- Pectoralis major tendon strain
- Proximal humerus fracture
- Coracoid avulsion fracture

## TREATMENT

Treatment options include operative and nonoperative management.

### INITIAL STABILIZATION

The patient should be stabilized initially in a sling and/or swath.

### GENERAL MEASURES

- Nonoperative treatment:
  - Includes rest, immobilization, analgesia, and ice.
  - Can lead to a functional result but will not restore full preinjury strength or cosmetic appearance
  - Regard the patient as an individual when considering treatment options.
    - An elderly patient of limited functional status may prefer nonoperative treatment
    - A professional athlete may require surgery to have the best chance of returning to the preinjury level of activity.

#### *Activity*

The patient's activity status is dictated by whether nonoperative or operative therapy is chosen.

### SPECIAL THERAPY

#### *Physical Therapy*

- After the acute injury, patients may begin physical therapy.
- Strengthening exercises may start once painless ROM is achieved and the hematoma has resolved.

### MEDICATION (DRUGS)

- NSAIDs
- Narcotics may be necessary for severe pain or postsurgical pain.

### SURGERY

- Surgical treatment is based on anatomic repair of the muscle.
- The literature supports anatomic surgical repair as resulting in the best outcomes (as measured by return of strength, regaining preinjury activity status, and return to work).
  - In a review article (4), patients who underwent surgical repair had decreased pain and a higher rate of return to preinjury strength and activity than did those treated nonoperatively.
  - Hanna et al. (5) compared measures of strength and subjective functional outcomes in complete tears treated surgically or nonsurgically.
    - Surgical treatment resulted in greater return of muscular strength than did nonoperative treatment.
    - Delays in surgery make surgical repair more difficult, but a good outcome is still possible.
- The specific type of surgical repair depends on the classification of the tear (6).
  - Tears at the musculotendinous junction require direct suturing of the ruptured ends.
  - Ruptures at the tendon or at the insertion site require reapproximation of the remaining tendon to the bony insertion via drill holes, direct suture, or bone anchors.
  - Contracted tendon tears may require interpositional tendon grafting.

## FOLLOW-UP

### DISPOSITION

- The patient is immobilized for 4–6 weeks with the shoulder adducted, internally rotated, and slightly flexed, allowing Codman exercises only.
- ROM exercises are initiated after the immobilization period.
- Once full ROM has been achieved, usually 12–14 weeks after surgery, patients may begin active strengthening.

### PROGNOSIS

- Generally good
- Patients can expect to regain motion and strength, but the degree depends on the type of treatment.
  - Nonoperative treatment often leads to loss of adduction strength, shoulder flexion, and internal rotation (7).

### COMPLICATIONS

- Complications from pectoralis major tendon ruptures are rare.
  - Rerupture
  - Hematoma infection
  - Heterotopic ossification
  - Unable to return to prerupture strength

### PATIENT MONITORING

- Patients should be seen 10–14 days after surgery for wound check and suture removal.
- As therapy progresses, patients should be seen every 2–3 weeks to monitor strength and ROM.

### REFERENCES


1. Tietjen R. Closed injuries of the pectoralis major muscle. *J Trauma* 1980;20:262–264.
2. Petilon J, Carr DR, Sekiya JK, et al. Pectoralis major muscle injuries: evaluation and management. *J Am Acad Orthop Surg* 2005;13:59–68.
3. Beloosesky Y, Hendel D, Weiss A, et al. Rupture of the pectoralis major muscle in nursing home residents. *Am J Med* 2001;111:233–235.
4. Bak K, Cameron EA, Henderson IJP. Rupture of the pectoralis major: a meta-analysis of 112 cases. *Knee Surg Sports Traumatol Arthrosc* 2000;8:113–119.
5. Hanna CM, Glenny AB, Stanley SN, et al. Pectoralis major tears: comparison of surgical and conservative treatment. *Br J Sports Med* 2001;35: 202–206.
6. Dodds SD, Wolfe SW. Injuries to the pectoralis major. *Sports Med* 2002;32:945–952.
7. Aarimaa V, Rantanen J, Heikkila J, et al. Rupture of the pectoralis major muscle. *Am J Sports Med* 2004;32:1256–1262.


### ADDITIONAL READING


Quinlan JF, Molloy M, Hurson BJ. Pectoralis major tendon ruptures: when to operate. *Br J Sports Med* 2002;36:226–228.


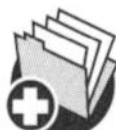

## MISCELLANEOUS

### CODES

#### *ICD9-CM*

840.8 Sprains and strains of joints and adjacent muscles, other specified sites of shoulder and upper arm

### FAQ

- Q: How long after pectoralis tendon rupture can it be repaired successfully?
  - A: Generally, repair in the 1st few weeks to months allows for a simple repair of the ruptured tendon without much difficulty. After 6 months, considerable scarring around the tendon and retraction of the muscle has occurred, making a primary repair difficult. In those cases, an Interpositional tendon graft can bridge the gap with good clinical results.

# PERONEAL TENDON SUBLUXATION

*Brett M. Cascio, MD*

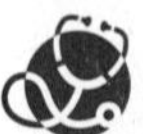

## BASICS

### DESCRIPTION

- The 2 main peroneal tendons include the peroneal longus and brevis.
  - The accessory peroneus quartus muscle is variably present in up to 21% of people (1).
- The peroneal longus and brevis share a common tenosynovial sheath as they course posterior to the lateral malleolus.
- The tendons are held in their groove by the superior and inferior peroneal retinacula.
- The peroneal tendons can sublux or dislocate out of the groove with ankle motion, which can be associated with pain and a palpable or audible snap (Fig. 1).
- Subluxation can be secondary to acute trauma or chronic in nature.

### EPIDEMIOLOGY

Most common in adults

#### *Incidence*

Rare

### RISK FACTORS

Athletic patients are at risk.

#### *Genetics*

No known Mendelian predisposition exists.

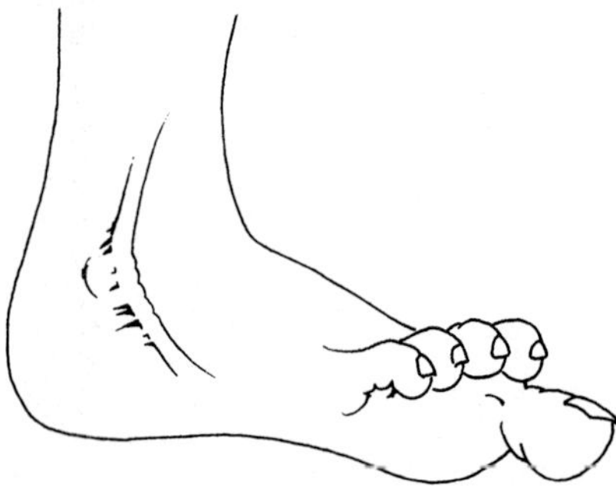

**Fig. 1.** The peroneal tendons may subluxate anteriorly over the fibular head if the retinaculum is torn or stretched.

### ETIOLOGY

- Classically occurs in persons participating in sports, such as skiing, in which the ankle is dorsiflexed forcefully with the foot in eversion, tearing the superior peroneal retinaculum
- May develop spontaneously in predisposed persons, resulting from a shallow groove behind the fibula or generalized ligamentous laxity

### ASSOCIATED CONDITION

- Ligamentous laxity
- Shallow peroneal groove
- Ankle instability
- Varus hindfoot alignment

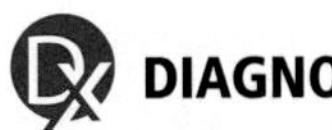

## DIAGNOSIS

### SIGNS AND SYMPTOMS

- Lateral ankle pain with activity that does not resolve
- Snapping of the peroneal tendons over the fibula
- Tenderness behind the lateral malleolus along the peroneus brevis muscle; subluxation elicited with the patient attempting to dorsiflex the affected foot from a plantarflexed, everted position

#### *History*

- Running athlete or skier with lateral, painful snapping of the ankle
- Recurrent ankle instability

#### *Physical Exam*

- Acutely, ecchymosis and swelling are present posterior to the fibula.
- Assess the neurovascular status of the ankle and foot.
- Assess lateral ligament stability, including anterior drawer and inversion tilt tests.
- Have the patient dorsiflex the ankle from a plantarflexed and everted position to reproduce posterolateral symptoms.
- Have the patient invert and evert the foot while the examiner palpates behind the lateral malleolus muscle.
  - The peroneal tendons may palpably subluxate out of their groove and over the fibula.
- Peroneal tendons normally snap or click while in place within their sheath; only subluxation with reproduction of symptoms or pain is diagnostic.

### TESTS

#### *Lab*

No laboratory tests for this condition

#### *Imaging*

- Ankle radiographs are used to evaluate for fracture: An avulsion fracture of lateral malleolus occurs in ~10% of cases (2).
- CT shows the shape of the peroneal groove.
- MRI may show attenuation or tearing of retinaculum, fluid in the peroneal sheath, or a longitudinal tear of the peroneus brevis.

#### *Diagnostic Procedures/Surgery*

Diagnostic injection of the peroneal sheath with local anesthetic may help confirm tendon abnormality.

#### *Pathological Findings*

- Possible shallow groove for the peroneal tendons behind the fibula
- Attenuated superior peroneal retinaculum
- Patients with chronic subluxation may have longitudinal tearing of the peroneus brevis tendon.

### DIFFERENTIAL DIAGNOSIS

- Ankle sprain
- Chronic ankle instability
- Lateral malleolar fracture
- Posterolateral ankle impingement
- Osteochondral talar dome fracture

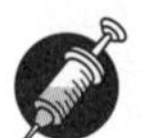

## TREATMENT

### GENERAL MEASURES

- Attempt nonoperative treatment initially.
  - After an acute injury, cast or boot immobilization may help relieve the patient's symptoms and reduce inflammation.
  - Cast treatment is unlikely to be successful in chronic cases.
  - NSAIDs, ice, and rest
  - An ankle brace may limit the excursion of the foot and may decrease the episodes of painful subluxation.
  - Taping or lateral crescent- or J-shaped pads also can be used to stabilize tendons in athletes.

- Surgical intervention:
  - Competitive athletes usually require operative treatment early to expedite return to play.
  - If nonoperative treatment fails, surgery commonly is necessary to resolve symptoms in patients with recurrent subluxation.

### *Activity*
Activity modification may reduce the occurrence of subluxation in certain patients if the subluxation is activity-specific.

## SPECIAL THERAPY
### *Physical Therapy*
- Physical therapy alone is not an effective treatment.
- Usually used postoperatively for functional rehabilitation of the ankle

## MEDICATION (DRUGS)
NSAIDs can be used acutely and during rehabilitation to relieve pain and to facilitate physical therapy.

## SURGERY
- Surgical treatment (3,4) addresses all pathologic elements present; options include:
  - Tendon repair
  - Retinacular repair
  - Peroneal groove deepening or bone block procedures
  - Rerouting procedures deep to the CFL

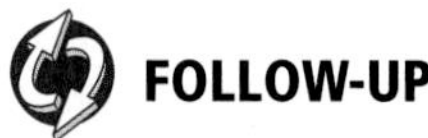

# FOLLOW-UP

## PROGNOSIS
- Few cases are successfully managed nonsurgically (5).
- Athletic individuals who require surgery usually can return to their sporting activity, but possibly not to their previous performance levels.
- Patients can return to activity gradually after a 2–3-month postoperative rehabilitation regimen, but return to full sports activity often requires 5–6 months.

## COMPLICATIONS
Complications of surgery include recurrence, sural nerve entrapment, and sural neuroma.

## PATIENT MONITORING
Re-education in ankle strengthening exercises is sometimes necessary.

## REFERENCES

1. Sobel M, Levy ME, Bohne WHO. Congenital variations of the peroneus quartus muscle: an anatomic study. *Foot Ankle* 1990;11:81–89.
2. Alm A, Lamke LO, Liljedahl SO. Surgical treatment of dislocation of the peroneal tendons. *Injury* 1975;7:14–19.
3. Kollias SL, Ferkel RD. Fibular grooving for recurrent peroneal tendon subluxation. *Am J Sports Med* 1997;25:329–335.
4. Zoellner G, Clancy W, Jr. Recurrent dislocation of the peroneal tendon. *J Bone Joint Surg* 1979; 61A:292–294.
5. Eckert WR, Davis EA, Jr. Acute rupture of the peroneal retinaculum. *J Bone Joint Surg* 1976; 58A:670–672.


## ADDITIONAL READING

- Brage ME, Hansen ST, Jr. Traumatic subluxation/dislocation of the peroneal tendons. *Foot Ankle* 1992;13:423–431.
- Keene JS. Foot and ankle. Section G: Tendon injuries of the foot and ankle. In: DeLee JC, Drez D, Jr, Miller MD, eds. *DeLee & Drez's Orthopaedic Sports Medicine: Principles and Practice*, 2nd ed. Philadelphia: WB Saunders, 2003:2409–2446.


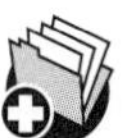

# MISCELLANEOUS

## CODES
### *ICD9-CM*
718.3 Peroneal tendon subluxation

## PATIENT TEACHING
- Educate the patient about the anatomy of the lower limb and which positions of eversion and dorsiflexion of the ankle are most likely to reproduce the subluxation.
- The condition does not lead to degenerative joint disease, but it may:
  - Cause the ankle to give way unexpectedly
  - Lead to peroneal tendinopathy or partial tearing of the peroneus brevis

### *Activity*
- For some patients, activity modification can provide symptomatic relief.
- Protected weightbearing after surgery in a cast or boot brace for 6 weeks, followed by a stirrup brace for 6 additional weeks

## FAQ
- Q: What is the typical mechanism of injury of the superior peroneal retinaculum?
  - A: Dorsiflexion and eversion.
- Q: What examination finding is pathognomonic for peroneal subluxation?
  - A: Painful snapping and subluxation of tendons with dorsiflexion and eversion.
- Q: How are most athletes treated for symptomatic peroneal subluxation?
  - A: Surgically.

# PERTHES DISEASE

*Kris J. Alden, MD, PhD*
*Simon C. Mears, MD, PhD*

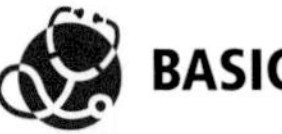

## BASICS

### DESCRIPTION

- Perthes disease is a self-limited, idiopathic disorder of the hip in young children.
  - Stages include ischemia, resorption, repair, and ultimately collapse of the femoral head.
  - Although most patients do well after healing in childhood, it may lead to collapse of the femoral articular surface and subsequent degenerative joint disease.
  - Up to 50% of affected patients develop disabling arthritis in their mid-50s (1).
- All classification systems are based on radiographs showing femoral head involvement.
  - Catterall staging system (2):
    - Stage I: Involvement of the anterior femoral head alone
    - Stage II: Involvement of the entire medial dome
    - Stage III: Progression into the lateral column of the head
    - Stage IV: Involvement of the whole head
  - Lateral pillar staging system (3):
    - Group A: <10% involvement of the lateral pillar with incongruent joint; evaluates appearance of the hip at maturity to forecast the potential for hip arthrosis; uses several radiographic parameters (femoral head sphericity, femoral neck length, acetabular slope, and presence of coxa magna)
    - Group B: >50% of the lateral pillar is maintained.
    - Group C: <50% of the lateral pillar is maintained.
  - Stulberg classification (used to predict onset of degenerative changes) (4):
    - Class 1: Normal hip
    - Class 2: Spherical femoral head short neck
    - Class 3: Ovoid or mushroom-shaped head
    - Class 4: Flat femoral head with congruous acetabulum
    - Class 5: Flat femoral head ion
- Synonyms: Legg-Calvé-Perthes disease; Osteochondritis deformans juvenilia

### EPIDEMIOLOGY

- Most common in children 4–10 years old, but reported from 2 years old to teens (5)
- Males affected 4–5 times more often than females
- More common in Caucasians and Asians than in African Americans and Native Americans
- Bilateral involvement is present in 10% of cases, but rarely is it synchronous (5).
- Symmetric involvement suggests a more general disorder (e.g., hypothyroidism or multiple epiphyseal dysplasia).

#### *Incidence*

<1% of the population (2)

### RISK FACTORS

- Small stature
- Low socioeconomic level
- Increased parental age
- Living in urban areas
- Ethnicity (Asian, Inuit, Central European)

#### *Genetics*

A positive family history is noted in 2–10% of cases (5).

### ETIOLOGY

- The cause is unknown, but most current theories are based on vascular compromise of the femoral head.
- Proposed causes of the limited blood supply:
  - Trauma
  - Intraosseous venous hypertension or obstruction
  - Hypercoagulable disorders
- Perthes disease in an African American child should prompt a hypercoagulability workup.
- Minor trauma may have role in initiating events in any of these theories.

### ASSOCIATED CONDITIONS

- Short stature
- AVN of the tarsal navicular vessels (Köhler disease)

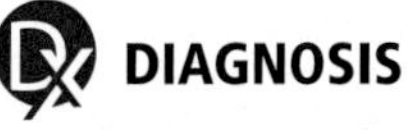

## DIAGNOSIS

### SIGNS AND SYMPTOMS

- Limited abduction and internal rotation
- Child often leaning the trunk over the affected limb while walking (Trendelenburg sign)
- In long-standing disease, mild atrophy of the thigh, calf, and buttock
- Leg-length inequality (late finding)

#### *History*

- Insidious onset of a limp (most common presentation)
- Pain either absent or mild
- When pain is present, usually related to activity and relieved by rest
- Pain usually in the groin area, but can be referred to the anteromedial thigh or knee

#### *Physical Exam*

- Observe the child's gait for indications of pain: Short, quick steps or shift of the shoulders with each stride.
- Check for limitation of internal or external rotation compared with contralateral side.
- Check abduction while holding the child's pelvis still.

### TESTS

#### *Lab*

- No diagnostic lab tests
- On occasion, laboratory studies may be indicated to rule out hyperthyroidism, septic arthritis, or sickle cell disease.

#### *Imaging*

- Radiographs of the hip are the most useful imaging study and show several stages of disease:
  - Initial phase:
    - Affected epiphysis is smaller than that on the contralateral side, with widening of the medial joint space.
    - Physeal irregularity and subchondral radiolucency also may be present.
  - Fragmentation phase:
    - The bony epiphysis begins to fragment.
    - Mixed lucent and dense areas appear in the epiphysis.
  - Reparative phase:
    - Normal bone density returns.
    - Alterations in the shape of the femoral head and neck become obvious.
  - Healed phase:
    - Residual deformity is revealed.
  - 4 head-at-risk signs:
    - Gage sign: A radiolucent "v" in the lateral portion of the epiphysis
    - Calcification lateral to the epiphysis
    - Lateral subluxation of the femoral head
    - Horizontal physis
- MRI detects infarction but does not give information on the stage of the disease (no specific indication for this test).
- Arthrography is useful for assessing femoral head deformity and congruency.

#### *Pathological Findings*

- The physeal plate shows the formation of histologic clefts.
- Cartilage clusters are present, extending into the metaphysis.

### DIFFERENTIAL DIAGNOSIS

- Fracture
- Gaucher disease
- Glycogen storage diseases
- Hypothyroidism
- Juvenile rheumatoid arthritis
- Multiple epiphyseal dysplasia
- Multiple or spondyloepiphyseal dysplasia
- Osteoid osteoma
- PVNS
- Septic arthritis
- Septic hip
- Sickle cell disease
- SCFE
- Steroid arthropathy
- Transient synovitis of the hip
- Traumatic AVN node
- Tuberculous arthritis
- Tumors

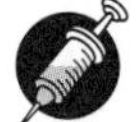

## TREATMENT

### GENERAL MEASURES

- The position of best containment of the femoral head within the acetabulum is determined by plain radiographs or arthrography.
- Containment of the femoral head:
  - If containable, it is maintained in this position by abduction orthosis or casts or by femoral or acetabular osteotomy.
  - If not containable, salvage procedures can reduce pain, equalize leg length, and improve movement.
- Surgery is not recommended for children <6 years old unless substantial subluxation is shown.
- Restoration of joint motion is critical to maintaining synovial and, therefore, cartilage nutrition.
- Containment of the femoral head in the acetabulum prevents deformity.
- A cast or brace may be used to abduct the leg and contain the femoral head.

#### *Activity*

- If weightbearing is painful, protect the child with the use of crutches.
- If marked stiffness occurs, the patient should rest until stiffness resolves.

### SPECIAL THERAPY

#### *Physical Therapy*

- May be helpful for maintaining ROM of the hip.
- Most critical for maintaining abduction motion.

### MEDICATION (DRUGS)

#### *First Line*

Pain should be treated with medications such as acetaminophen or NSAIDs based on the child's age and weight.

### SURGERY

- Osteotomy of the femur or acetabulum (or both) repositions the femoral head into a contained place within the acetabulum and allows growth and remodeling to occur in a spheric, congruous fashion.
- Internal fixation (e.g., a plate) is used to stabilize the osteotomy so early motion may be started.
  - Hardware should be removed because future procedures are likely.
- Up to 50% of patients develop end-stage arthritis in their mid-50s and are treated with total hip arthroplasty.

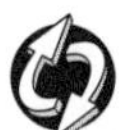

## FOLLOW-UP

### DISPOSITION

#### *Issues for Referral*

Patients with Perthes disease should be followed by an orthopaedic surgeon or pediatric orthopaedic surgeon.

### PROGNOSIS

- The younger the child is at the healing stage, the better the potential for remodeling of the femoral head.
- Poor results are rare in children <6 years old.
- Almost always, symptoms resolve after the healing phase, and patients have freedom from pain during the teenage years.
- Factors for a poorer prognosis (6):
  - Children present at ≥8 years old.
  - Involvement of the lateral column of the femoral head
  - Poor ROM
  - Nonconcentric or noncontained femoral head after healing
- ~50% of patients with Perthes disease as a child will need hip replacement by later adulthood (50–60 years old) (1).

### COMPLICATIONS

- Loss of sphericity or collapse causes the following:
  - Early degenerative joint disease
  - Leg-length discrepancy
  - Loss of ROM with flexion and adduction contractures

### PATIENT MONITORING

- Brace or cast containment usually averages 6–18 months or until the reossification stage occurs and the risk of femoral head collapse has passed.
- Examine the child out of the brace to check ROM.
- Take radiographs with the child in the brace.
- See the patient every 4–8 weeks until reossification occurs.

### REFERENCES


1. McAndrew MP, Weinstein SL. A long-term follow-up of Legg-Calvé-Perthes disease. *J Bone Joint Surg* 1984;66A:860–869.
2. Weinstein SL. Legg-Calvé-Perthes disease. In: Morrissy RT, Weinstein SL, eds. *Lovell and Winter's Pediatric Orthopaedics*, 6th ed. Philadelphia: Lippincott-Raven, 2006:1039–1083.
3. Herring JA, Neustadt JB, Williams JJ, et al. The lateral pillar classification of Legg-Calvé-Perthes disease. *J Pediatr Orthop* 1992;12:143–150.
4. Stulberg SD, Cooperman DR, Wallensten R. The natural history of Legg-Calvé-Perthes disease. *J Bone Joint Surg* 1981;63A:1095–1108.
5. Wynne-Davies R, Gormley J. The aetiology of Perthes' disease. Genetic, epidemiological and growth factors in 310 Edinburgh and Glasgow patients. *J Bone Joint Surg* 1978;60B:6–14.
6. Herring JA, Kim HT, Browne R. Legg-Calvé-Perthes disease. Part II: Prospective multicenter study of the effect of treatment on outcome. *J Bone Joint Surg* 2004;86A:2121–2134.


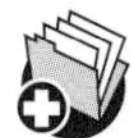

## MISCELLANEOUS

### CODES

#### *ICD9-CM*

732.1 Perthes disease

### PATIENT TEACHING

- Maintaining ROM is important.
- Parents should be told that the disease often takes ~2 years to heal.
- Patients usually have a largely pain-free childhood after healing, even though problems may develop later in adulthood.
- Healing of the disorder cannot be accelerated.
- No effective means of prevention exists.
- Early detection is important, so containment can be achieved before substantial deformity of the femoral head occurs.

#### *Activity*

Activity should be restricted if the hip is painful.

#### *Prevention*

Surgery may be helpful in increasing the containment of the femoral head, which can lessen or prevent later arthritic changes in the hip.

### FAQ

- Q: How likely is the development of later arthritis?
  - A: Children who develop Perthes disease by 6 years of age have a better prognosis than those who present at ≥8 years old. ~50% of patients develop arthritis in their 50s.

# PHALANGEAL JOINT ARTHRITIS

*Tung B. Le, MD*
*Dawn M. LaPorte, MD*

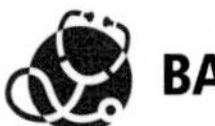

## BASICS

### DESCRIPTION
- Phalangeal joint arthritis is a degenerative "wear and tear" process involving articular tissues that leads to the destruction of cartilage, local bone loss, and the formation of osteophytes.
- Most commonly affected joints are:
  - DIP joints of the fingers
  - PIP joints of the fingers
  - CMC joint of the thumb
- Classification:
  - Primary: No preexisting joint problem
  - Secondary: History of trauma or other joint conditions:
    - Infection
    - Hemophilia

### EPIDEMIOLOGY
#### *Incidence*
- This condition occurs in 37.4% of people 18–79 years old (1).
- It is estimated that, after the age of 65 years, 99% of females and 78% of males will have radiographic evidence of arthritis in the hand (2).

#### *Prevalence*
- Osteoarthritis of the hand increases in prevalence with advancing age (2), and the average age of onset is 58 years (1).
- Males are affected more commonly than females until menopause (2).

### RISK FACTORS
- Increasing age
- Trauma

#### *Genetics*
- A single gene mutation is implicated in the development of osteoarthritis.
- For example, primary generalized osteoarthritis, a disease commonly affecting middle-aged females and characterized by nodular arthritis involving the DIP joint of the hand and occasionally the knees and other joints, is thought to be the result of a single gene mutation that substitutes cysteine for arginine in position 519 of the type II procollagen gene (3).

### ETIOLOGY
- Genetic changes in cartilage
- Mechanical changes in cartilage
- Chemical changes in cartilage

### ASSOCIATED CONDITIONS
Arthritis of the hip and knee

## DIAGNOSIS

### SIGNS AND SYMPTOMS
- Rapid onset of pain in the digital joints with no specific history of trauma
- Progressive deformity of the DIP and PIP joints of the hand
- Rare involvement of the MCP joints
- Most common complaints are pain and morning stiffness
- Finger deformity in osteoarthritis in a lateral deviation pattern shown during physical examination and on radiography
- Decrease in ROM and stiffness from joint space incongruity and osteophytes that block flexion and extension
- Eventual periarticular soft-tissue contracture, further limiting joint motion

#### *Physical Exam*
- Reduced ROM
- Ankylosis
- Osteophytes

### TESTS
#### *Lab*
- When appropriate:
  - Rheumatoid factor
  - HLA-B27
  - Antinuclear antibody
  - ESR

#### *Imaging*
- Plain film radiographs show the following:
  - Narrowing of joint spaces
  - Subchondral sclerosis
  - Osteophyte formation
  - Cyst formation

#### *Pathological Findings*
- Early disease:
  - Increased water content in the cartilage
  - Increased proteoglycan level
- Progressive disease:
  - Decrease in both cartilaginous water and proteoglycan levels
  - Increased friction with motion
  - Decreased shock-absorbing capability of cartilage
  - Eventual progressive cartilage fissuring and destruction
- End-stage disease:
  - Abnormal joint loading
  - Subchondral microfractures
  - Cyst formation

### DIFFERENTIAL DIAGNOSIS
- Gout
- Inflammatory arthropathies
- Pseudogout
- Rheumatoid arthritis
- Septic arthritis
- Trauma

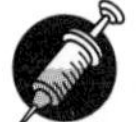

## TREATMENT

### GENERAL MEASURES

Splinting of the involved joints with well-padded splints to decrease pain and swelling

#### *Activity*

- Rest
- Avoidance of aggravating activity

### SPECIAL THERAPY

#### *Physical Therapy*

- Active isometric and passive ROM exercises to maintain motion
- Ultrasound and diathermy therapy to decrease the inflammation

### MEDICATION (DRUGS)

- Analgesics (acetaminophen, aspirin)
- NSAIDs
- Local steroid injections

### SURGERY

- PIP joints: Arthrodesis or arthroplasty
- DIP joints: Arthrodesis
- Thumb CMC joint: Arthroplasty with tendon interposition

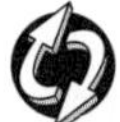

## FOLLOW-UP

### PROGNOSIS

Excellent pain control and restoration of function may be achieved in most patients with analgesics, splinting, exercise, or surgical management, or a combination thereof.

### COMPLICATIONS

- Articular deformity
- Infection
- Malunion in attempted joint fusion
- Nonunion in attempted joint fusion
- Prosthetic dislocation or fracture
- Wear of prosthesis

### PATIENT MONITORING

Patients are checked at 6–12-month intervals.

### REFERENCES


1. Swanson AB, Swanson GD. Osteoarthritis in the hand. *J Hand Surg* 1983;8A:669–675.
2. Naidu S, Temple JD. Arthritis. In: Beredjiklian PK, Bozentka DJ, eds. *Review of Hand Surgery*. Philadelphia: WB Saunders, 2004:171–187.
3. Mankin HJ, Mow VC, Buckwalter JA, et al. Articular cartilage structure, composition, and function. In: Buckwalter JA, Einhorn TA, Simon SR, eds. *Orthopaedic Basic Science. Biology and Biomechanics of the Musculoskeletal System*, 2nd ed. Rosemont, IL: American Academy of Orthopaedic Surgeons, 2000:443–470.


### ADDITIONAL READING


Shin AY, Amadio PC. Stiff finger joints. In: Green DP, Hotchkiss RN, Pederson WC, et al., eds. *Green's Operative Hand Surgery*, 5th ed. Philadelphia: Elsevier Churchill Livingstone, 2005;417–459.


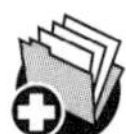

## MISCELLANEOUS

### CODES

#### *ICD9-CM*

716.94 Arthritis of hand/fingers

### PATIENT TEACHING

- Reassure patients about the relatively benign natural course of the disease.
- Treatments often are effective in relieving pain and in preventing progressive deformity.
- Control additional articular damage by minimizing joint loading.

### FAQ

- Q: How is phalangeal joint arthritis diagnosed?
  - A: Patients typically present with complaints of pain and bony prominence or deformity at the affected joints. The diagnosis is made with radiographs showing joint space narrowing and possibly osteophyte formation.
- Q: How is phalangeal arthritis treated?
  - A: The 1st line of treatment is anti-inflammatory medication unless contraindicated secondary to medical comorbidity. Therapy with modalities may be a helpful adjunct as well as activity modification. Splint immobilization may be helpful for an isolated digit or joint. Persistent symptoms at the PIP joints can be treated with corticosteroid injection. Recurrent or persistent symptoms may be addressed surgically with fusion at the DIP joints and arthroplasty versus fusion at the PIP joints.

# PHALANX DISLOCATION

*Tung B. Le, MD*
*Andrew M. Richards, MD*

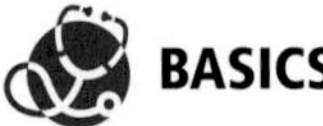

## BASICS

### DESCRIPTION

- Dislocations involve the following joints of the hand
  - MCP joint
  - PIP joint
  - DIP joint
- Dislocations can be associated with fractures, ligament, tendon, or joint capsule injury.
- Classification is by the joint and the direction of dislocation:
  - PIP dislocations:
    - Dorsal: Most common, resulting from volar plate injury
    - Volar: Rare, associated with central slip disruption
    - Rotatory: Rare, from "buttonholing" of 1 condyle of the head of proximal phalanx through the space between the central slip and the lateral band
  - MCP dislocations:
    - Lateral: Collateral ligament injuries
    - Dorsal: Volar plate injury, may be irreducible closed
  - DIP dislocations:
    - Simple: Reducible
    - Complex: Irreducible closed because of entrapment of the volar plate between 2 dislocated middle and proximal phalanges
- Synonym (MCP joint dislocation): Skier's thumb

### GENERAL PREVENTION

Simple changes have been proposed to decrease hand injuries in children's sports, including softening the ball, increasing awareness of parents and coaches, and having weight categories (1).

### EPIDEMIOLOGY

- Joint dislocation usually occurs in skeletally mature patients.
- In the pediatric population, the physes are weaker than the capsular structures.
  - Therefore, physeal fractures or separations are more common than joint dislocations in children.
- Thumb MCP dislocations are common among skiers (2).

#### *Incidence*

A study of pediatric hand injuries showed that 68% were fractures, 26% were soft-tissue injuries, and 11% were dislocations (3).

#### *Prevalence*

- Common
- In 1 study, 28% of all visits to an emergency department were secondary to hand injury (4).

### RISK FACTORS

- Basketball
- Skiing

#### *Genetics*

No known Mendelian pattern exists.

### ETIOLOGY

- Trauma is the cause of phalanx dislocations.
  - Dorsal dislocation is caused by a hyperextension force.
  - Volar dislocation is caused by a hyperflexion force.

### ASSOCIATED CONDITIONS

- Phalangeal fractures:
  - Look carefully for small fracture fragments because they usually are indicators of a soft-tissue avulsion injury.
- Injuries of the periarticular structures of the involved joints (especially volar plate, ligaments)

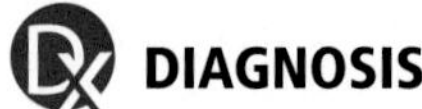

## DIAGNOSIS

### SIGNS AND SYMPTOMS

- Pain
- Deformity (Fig. 1)
- Ecchymosis
- Loss of motion
- Altered sensation or perfusion (or both) from neurovascular compression

#### *History*

- Mechanism of injury
- Time and events since injury
- Dominant hand of the patient

#### *Physical Exam*

- Assess the neurovascular status of the hand.
- Examine the skin for open wounds.
- Clinical assessment for instability and tenderness should be performed a few days after injury to allow the worst of the swelling to resolve.

### TESTS

#### *Imaging*

- To evaluate adequately the phalangeal bones and joints, initial radiographs include true lateral, AP, and oblique views.
- Stress views of the relocated joint may be important in assessing dislocations when ligamentous disruptions are possible.

#### *Pathological Findings*

- Dislocations of the phalangeal joints often result in injuries to surrounding soft-tissue structures.
- Lateral dislocations of these joints lead to collateral ligament tears.
- The volar plate is at risk in hyperextension injuries and dorsal dislocations.
- In skier's thumb (dislocation of the thumb MCP joint with or without avulsion fracture of the metacarpal base), both the collateral ligament and the volar plate are torn.

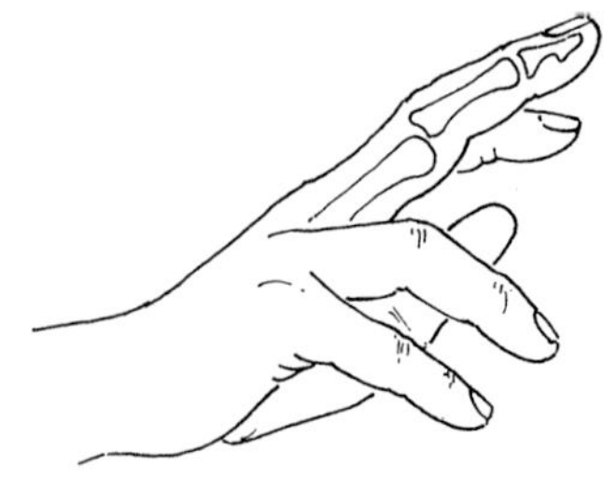

**Fig. 1.** IP joint dislocations are almost always dorsal because of hyperextension injuries.

P

## DIFFERENTIAL DIAGNOSIS
- Fracture dislocation
- Chronic dislocation
- Collateral ligament injury
- Associated volar plate injury
- Rheumatoid arthritis
- Septic arthritis

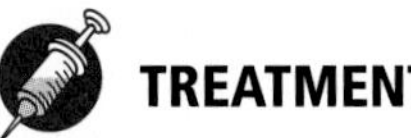

# TREATMENT

## GENERAL MEASURES
- Phalangeal dislocations:
  - Attempt closed reduction (Fig. 2).
  - Once reduced, minimize swelling with RICE protocol.
- Joint reduction:
  - Gentle traction coupled with additional hyperextension/flexion to disimpact the dislocation
  - Gradually reduce the phalanx to its anatomic position.
- Dislocations that are not reducible require surgical intervention.
- Ligamentous tears:
  - Protective immobilization with "buddy" taping for collateral injuries.
- Volar plate disruption:
  - Extension block splint
- Complete ruptures of the collateral ligaments, volar plates, or central slips:
  - Immobilize for 3–6 weeks.
- PIP joints:
  - Splint in 15° of flexion after reduction of dorsal dislocations.
- MCP joints:
  - Immobilize in 50–70° of flexion.
- Central slip disruptions:
  - Use an extension splint for 3 weeks, followed by dynamic splinting.

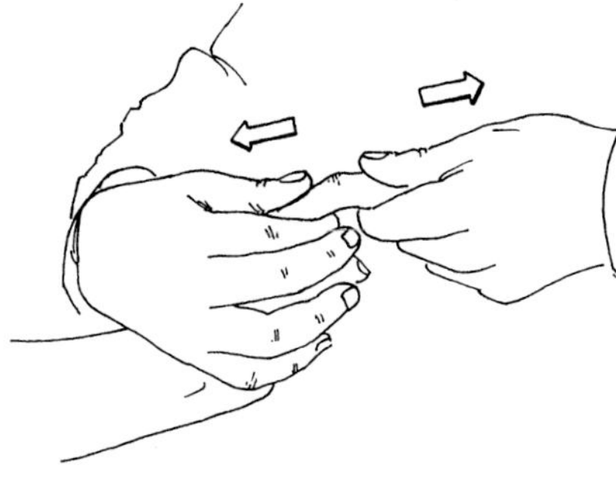

**Fig. 2.** IP dislocation is reduced by longitudinal traction and gentle flexion.

## SPECIAL THERAPY
### *Physical Therapy*
- Active and gentle passive ROM exercises are begun once stability of the joint is confirmed.
- Therapy to reduce swelling and prevent stiffness is extremely important after surgical repair (5).

## MEDICATION (DRUGS)
### *First Line*
Analgesics or NSAIDs are used as needed.

## SURGERY
- Surgery is indicated when closed reduction fails.
  - Failure occurs when:
    - A blockage of a bone fragment or soft tissue occurs within the joint.
    - A buttonholed fragment is present.
- Volar or dorsal approach both allow the joint to be cleared and reduced.
- Surgery also may be required to stabilize associated fractures or attend to wounds.
- Dislocations of the thumb MCP joint:
  - May lead to interposition of the UCL of the thumb (the Stener lesion)
  - Requires open repair (6)

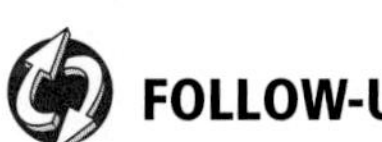

# FOLLOW-UP

## DISPOSITION
### *Issues for Referral*
Injuries to the MCP joint of the thumb, fracture dislocations, open injuries, and irreducible dislocations should be referred to an orthopedic surgeon.

## PROGNOSIS
Some loss of motion can be expected.

## COMPLICATIONS
- Persistent pain and swelling (up to 12 months)
- Instability with recurrent dislocation
- Stiffness
- Associated neurovascular injuries (rare)

## PATIENT MONITORING
- Patients are followed at 3–6-week intervals to ensure that they maintain adequate ROM.
- After reduction (with or without surgery), patients should be followed by a hand therapist.

## REFERENCES

1. Macgregor DM. Don't save the ball! *Br J Sports Med* 2003;37:351–353.
2. Deibert MC, Aronsson DD, Johnson RJ, et al. Skiing injuries in children, adolescents, and adults. *J Bone Joint Surg* 1998;80A:25–32.
3. Choyce MQ, Potts M, Maitra AK. A profile of sports hand injuries in an accident and emergency department. *J Accid Emerg Med* 1998;15:35–38.
4. Packer GJ, Shaheen MA. Patterns of hand fractures and dislocations in a district general hospital. *J Hand Surg* 1993;18B:511–514.
5. Chinchalkar SJ, Gan BS. Management of proximal interphalangeal joint fractures and dislocations. *J Hand Ther* 2003;16:117–128.
6. Catalano LW, III, Cardon L, Patenaude N, et al. Results of surgical treatment of acute and chronic grade III [corrected] tears of the radial collateral ligament of the thumb metacarpophalangeal joint. *J Hand Surg* 2006;31A:68–75.


## ADDITIONAL READING

- Glickel SZ, Barron OA, Catalano LW, III. Dislocations and ligament injuries in the digits. In Green DP, Hotchkiss RN, Pederson WC, et al., eds. Green's *Operative Hand Surgery,* 5th ed. Philadelphia: Elsevier Churchill Livingstone, 2005:343–388.
- Freiberg A, Pollard BA, Macdonald MR, et al. Management of proximal IP joint injuries. *J Trauma* 1999;46:523–528.
- Glickel SZ, Barron OA. PIP joint fracture dislocations. *Hand Clin* 2000;16: 333–344.
- Green DP, Butler TE, Jr. Fractures and dislocations in the hand. In: Rockwood CA, Jr, Green DP, Bucholz RW, et al., eds. *Rockwood and Green's Fractures in Adults*, 4th ed. Philadelphia: Lippincott-Raven, 1996:607–744.


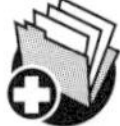

# MISCELLANEOUS

## CODES
### *ICD9-CM*
834.0 Dislocation, phalanx

## PATIENT TEACHING
- Advise patients that recovery up to 12 months depends on continuing rehabilitation.
- Prescribe strict initial immobilization of the involved joint to achieve stability and healing.
- Advise patients to use protective hand wear or finger taping during sports.

### *Prevention*
- Be aware of the risk of injury, particularly in children's sporting events.
- Use the lightest ball possible in sporting events.

## FAQ
- Q: How long does a finger dislocation take to heal?
  - A: Continued swelling of the finger and knuckle often is seen for at least 1 year after injury. In some cases, finger size does not return to normal.

# PHALANX FRACTURE

*Dawn M. LaPorte, MD*
*Mark Clough, MD*

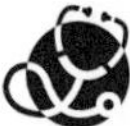

## BASICS

### DESCRIPTION
- A phalanx fracture is a break in 1 or more phalanges in the fingers.
- Finger fractures are classified by:
  - Which phalanx is involved
  - Location within the phalanx
  - Pattern
  - Complexity
  - Open or closed
  - Stable or unstable to motion

### EPIDEMIOLOGY
- Fractures of the metacarpals and the phalanges are common (1).
- Occur among all ages
- Common causes vary substantially with age.

#### *Incidence*
The reported incidence varies because patients with phalanx fractures present to a variety of medical practitioners.

### RISK FACTORS
Involvement in a sport, job, or hobby that involves power tools or machinery.

### ETIOLOGY
- The specific cause depends on patient age (2,3).
  - Children >10 years old: Compression
  - Adolescents and young adults 10–39 years old: Sports
  - Adults 30–69 years old: Machinery
  - Elderly persons (≥60 years old): Falls
- Other causes include crush injury and motor vehicle accidents.
- The most common cause of a distal phalanx fracture is a crush injury.
- The most likely cause of a transverse or comminuted fracture is a direct blow.
- The most common cause of an oblique or spiral fracture is a twisting injury.

### ASSOCIATED CONDITIONS
Possible additional fractures in the hand and upper extremity

## DIAGNOSIS

### SIGNS AND SYMPTOMS
- Pain, swelling, or deformity after some trauma to the finger
- Laceration
- Decreased ROM
- Numbness of the affected digit

#### *History*
- Determine the mechanism of injury and where it occurred (whether in a clean or dirty environment).
- Determine how much time has elapsed since the injury.
- Ascertain the patient's age, hand dominance, occupation, and hobbies.

#### *Physical Exam*
- Assess and document the patient's neurovascular status.
- Determine the precise area of tenderness and whether any lacerations and possible open fractures are present.
- Evaluate for injury to soft tissues, including tendons, ligaments, nerves, and blood vessels.
- Evaluate the digit for length, rotation, and angular alignment by comparing the appearance of the injured digit with that of adjacent digits.
- Assess the nail plate by comparing with those of the surrounding digits.

### TESTS

#### *Imaging*
- Radiography:
  - AP and lateral views of the finger should be obtained.
  - Oblique views assess intra-articular fractures.
- Low-kilovolt mammography film is recommended as an initial screening test for a foreign body (e.g., wood splinter, glass) because many foreign bodies are not visible on plain film.
- CT is the preferred method for detecting wood and thorns.
- MRI detects all types of foreign bodies except gravel.

#### *Pathological Findings*
- Proximal shaft fractures are angulated palmarly.
  - The proximal fragment is flexed because of interossei pull and the distal fragment is extended because of central slip insertion.
- Digital function is impaired not only by fracture stability or deformity, but also by concomitant injury to soft tissues, including tendons, ligaments, blood vessels, and nerves.
- Injury to soft-tissue structures is common.

### DIFFERENTIAL DIAGNOSIS
Pathologic fracture, most commonly with an enchondroma (benign cartilage tumor)

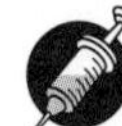

## TREATMENT

### GENERAL MEASURES
- Most fractures can be treated nonsurgically with closed reduction, splinting, and early motion.
- Surgery is indicated for:
  - All displaced intra-articular fractures
  - Unstable fractures associated with severe soft-tissue injury
  - A fracture that remains unstable after closed reduction
  - A rotational deformity
- >25° of palmar angulation causes functional deficits and cosmetic deformity and should be corrected surgically.
- Nondisplaced and impacted transverse fractures of the phalanges are managed ideally with "buddy" taping, in which 2 fingers are taped together so that 1 acts as a splint for the other.
  - The fracture must truly be stable with minimal angulation in any plane.
- Closed reduction and splinting:
  - Use digital nerve block for anesthesia.
  - Manipulate the distal fragment to align with the proximal fragment.
  - Place the splint.
  - The fracture must be stable after reduction for the splint to maintain reduction.
  - Splint the hand in the "intrinsic plus" position, with the MCP joints at 90° of flexion and the IP joints in full extension.
  - Use a gutter splint for the involved fingers.

#### *Activity*
- Immobilize unstable closed fractures for 3–4 weeks.
- Children tolerate immobilization better than adults, and adults will likely have more joint stiffness.

### SPECIAL THERAPY

#### *Physical Therapy*
- To prevent stiffness, the patient is encouraged to perform ROM exercises as soon as possible for all fingers not included in the splint.
- Digital performance deteriorates when active ROM is delayed >3 weeks.
- Soft-tissue mobilization with active motion is initiated once clinical healing is achieved (as evidenced by minimally tender fracture site that is not painful when manipulated), usually at 3–4 weeks.
- The radiographic appearance of union lags behind clinical union.
- ROM exercises for the involved fingers usually are initiated at 2–4 weeks after surgery.

## MEDICATION (DRUGS)

### *First Line*

- NSAIDs or acetaminophen usually are sufficient for finger fractures.
- Opioid medicines may be necessary for severe pain.

## SURGERY

- Indications:
  - Failure of closed reduction to maintain rotation, length, or angular alignment
  - Intra-articular fracture in which joint congruity is lost, resulting in small joint dysfunction
  - Unstable fractures associated with severe soft-tissue injury in which fracture instability precludes a normal soft-tissue rehabilitation program
  - Rotational deformity
- Distal tuft fractures may be treated with nail repair.
  - Pinning may be necessary.
- Shaft fractures may be stabilized with Kirschner wires, lag screws, miniplates, or intramedullary devices (4).
- The direct visualization afforded by an open approach permits more accurate reduction and adequate implant application (5).
- Intra-articular volar fractures may be pinned or treated with volar plate arthroplasty (6).
- Tension banding can supplement fixation, especially for small, less stable fragments.
- Segmental defects should be treated with open reduction and internal fixation to preserve digital length and later with bone grafting.
- Arthroplasty (constrained silicone or nonconstrained bicondylar implants) may be used as a salvage procedure in irreparable IP fractures or after failure for up to 2 years after injury.
- Arthrodesis may be considered as an alternative to arthroplasty.

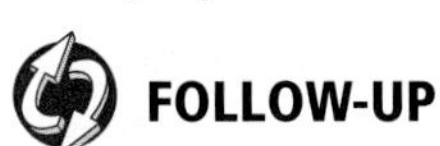

# FOLLOW-UP

## PROGNOSIS

- A poor prognosis is more likely with:
  - Age >50 years
  - Associated tendon injuries (especially extension)
  - Associated joint injury
  - >1 fracture in a finger
  - Crush injury
  - Skin loss

## COMPLICATIONS

- Malunion:
  - Malrotation requiring rotational osteotomy
  - Lateral deviation requiring closing wedge osteotomy
  - Volar angulation requiring volar closing wedge osteotomy
  - Intra-articular realignment osteotomy
- Tendon adherence:
  - Common, especially in crush injuries
  - Intensive hand rehabilitation is needed.
  - Surgical treatment should be considered only after maximum passive joint motion is regained.
- Nonunion:
  - Rare, but more common with open than with closed fractures
- Soft-tissue interposition
- Infections
- Stiffness:
  - Immobilization for >3 weeks can result in permanent loss of motion.
  - Comminuted and open fractures treated with internal fixation have a higher rate of stiffness and poor outcomes (5).

## PATIENT MONITORING

- Obtain postreduction radiographs immediately and in 3–7 days to check for displacement.
- Obtain subsequent radiographs every 4 weeks to monitor for displacement and to assess for healing.
- Monitor the patient until the fracture has healed clinically and finger function is acceptable.

## REFERENCES


1. van Onselen EBH, Karim RB, Hage JJ, et al. Prevalence and distribution of hand fractures. *J Hand Surg* 2003;28B:491–495.
2. Larsen CF, Mulder S, Johansen AMT, et al. The epidemiology of hand injuries in The Netherlands and Denmark. *Eur J Epidemiol* 2004;19:323–327.
3. Vadivelu R, Dias JJ, Burke FD, et al. Hand injuries in children: a prospective study. *J Pediatr Orthop* 2006;26:29–35.
4. Horton TC, Hatton M, Davis TRC. A prospective randomized controlled study of fixation of long oblique and spiral shaft fractures of the proximal phalanx: closed reduction and percutaneous Kirschner wiring versus open reduction and lag screw fixation. *J Hand Surg* 2003;28B:5–9.
5. Tan V, Beredjiklian PK, Weiland AJ. Intra-articular fractures of the hand: treatment by open reduction and internal fixation. *J Orthop Trauma* 2005;19:518–523.
6. Rettig ME, Dassa G, Raskin KB. Volar plate arthroplasty of the distal interphalangeal joint. *J Hand Surg* 2001;26A:940–944.


## ADDITIONAL READING


- Blazar PE, Steinberg DR. Fractures of the proximal IP joint. *J Am Acad Orthop Surg* 2000;8:383–390.
- Freeland AE, Geissler WB, Weiss APC. Surgical treatment of common displaced and unstable fractures of the hand. *Instr Course Lect* 2002;51:185–201.


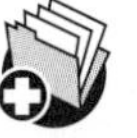

# MISCELLANEOUS

## CODES

### *ICD9-CM*

- 816.0 Closed phalanx fracture
- 816.1 Open phalanx fracture

## PATIENT TEACHING

- Underscore the importance of performing ROM exercises to prevent stiffness in affected and surrounding digits.
- Emphasize the importance of maintaining therapy and ROM exercises to ensure functional outcome.

### *Prevention*

- Attention to prevention in sports and leisure activities.
- Machine-related injuries should be prevented by attention to specific safety precautions.

## FAQ

- Q: How long should a phalanx fracture be splinted?
  - A: To prevent stiffness, a fracture should not be splinted for >3 weeks.

# PIGMENTED VILLONODULAR SYNOVITIS

*Dennis E. Kramer, MD*
*Frank J. Frassica, MD*

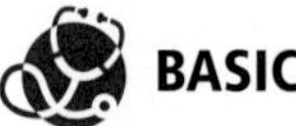

## BASICS

### DESCRIPTION

- PVNS is an uncommon lesion characterized by diffuse proliferation of the synovium to form yellow-brown villous projections.
- The knee is the most commonly affected joint, followed by the hip and shoulders (1).
- Lesions almost always are unilateral.
- Synonyms: Giant cell tumor of the tendon sheaths and joints; Hemorrhagic villous synovitis

### EPIDEMIOLOGY

#### *Incidence*

Uncommon

#### *Prevalence*

- Usually found in young to middle-aged adults
- No definite gender correlation; may have slight female predominance (2)

### RISK FACTORS

PVNS may have a slight association with recurrent hemarthrosis, but it has not been established definitively.

#### *Genetics*

No known correlation exists.

### ETIOLOGY

- The cause is unknown.
- Studies in animals have produced similar lesions in response to recurrent hemarthroses, but lesions resolve when the inciting stimulus is removed (3).
- In humans, slow progression of PVNS is the rule.

### ASSOCIATED CONDITIONS

None are known.

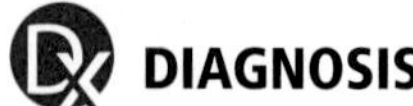

## DIAGNOSIS

### SIGNS AND SYMPTOMS

- Insidious onset
- Slow progression
- Recurrent nontraumatic effusions
- Symptoms:
  - Pain
  - Swelling
  - Limitation of ROM
- Joint possibly warm to the touch
- Mild to moderate effusion
- Tender mass occasionally palpated (especially in the suprapatellar pouch of the knee)

#### *Physical Exam*

- Perform a complete examination of the knee, looking for the following:
  - Ligamentous and meniscal status
  - Possible effusion
  - Warmth at the joint
  - Pain
  - Swelling
  - Tender mass
- Determine the ROM of the affected joint.
- Assess for muscle atrophy.
- With shoulder, ankle, and hip involvement, no physical findings or only subtle findings may be present, such as muscle atrophy or decreased ROM.

### TESTS

#### *Lab*

Joint aspiration reveals reddish brown fluid.

#### *Imaging*

- Radiography:
  - Early findings:
    - Frequently no abnormalities
    - Subtle erosions or periosteal reaction in nonweightbearing regions
  - Late findings:
    - Erosive lesions on both sides of the joint
    - Possible diffuse joint space narrowing seen in late cases
- MRI:
  - Increasingly helpful in establishing the diagnosis and directing treatment
  - Areas of extremely low signal are seen in the synovial lining on both T1- and T2-weighted images ("signal dropout") (4).
  - Characteristically, joint effusion and irregularity of the synovial lining are seen.

#### *Pathological Findings*

- Lesions may be large and diffuse or more discrete.
- Grossly, PVNS is characterized by villous projections or matted nodules stained with hemosiderin.
- Microscopically, elongated villi or nodules contain inflammatory infiltrates, foamy histiocytes, and hemosiderin deposits.

### DIFFERENTIAL DIAGNOSIS

- Inflammatory arthritis
- Traumatic effusions
- Infection
- Synovial sarcoma
- Hemosiderosis
- Hemochromatosis

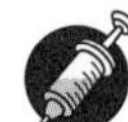

## TREATMENT

### GENERAL MEASURES

- PVNS is a benign lesion.
  - The potential for malignant degeneration has been reported but is extremely rare (5).
- In diffuse lesions:
  - It is almost impossible to remove the entire lesion without injuring important ligaments and capsular structure.
  - Therefore, the recurrence rate is high.
- In severe or recurrent cases, radiotherapy has been effective (6,7).
- Make appropriate referrals to establish the diagnosis and consider treatment options.
- Treat patients symptomatically with:
  - Immobilization
  - Splinting
  - NSAIDs
  - Analgesics

### SPECIAL THERAPY

#### *Radiotherapy*

- External beam irradiation is commonly used for recurrent PVNS (6, 7).
- Radiation synovectomy with an intra-articular injection of radioactive isotope also has been used (8).

### MEDICATION (DRUGS)

- NSAIDS
- Analgesics

### SURGERY
- Arthroscopic synovectomy through multiple portals is the 1st line of treatment for diffuse PVNS.
  - An open posterior synovectomy may be necessary with extensive posterior extra-articular extension (2,10).
- Some surgeons prefer both open anterior and posterior synovectomies for diffuse PVNS (8).
- Localized, nodular PVNS responds well to simple excision (open or arthroscopic) (11).

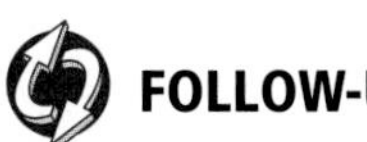

## FOLLOW-UP

Patients are followed every 6–12 months with MRI scans and physical examination (8).

### PROGNOSIS
The prognosis is good.

### COMPLICATIONS
- Recurrence is common.
- Articular damage and bone loss may occur in long-standing disease.
- Joint replacement may be necessary.

### PATIENT MONITORING
- MRI is effective in detecting early local recurrences (8).
- Patients with asymptomatic local recurrences are treated with observation.

### REFERENCES

1. Dorwart RH, Genant HK, Johnston WH, et al. Pigmented villonodular synovitis of synovial joints: clinical, pathologic, and radiologic features. *AJR Am J Roentgenol* 1984;143:877–885.
2. Ogilvie-Harris DJ, McLean J, Zarnett ME. Pigmented villonodular synovitis of the knee. The results of total arthroscopic synovectomy, partial, arthroscopic synovectomy, and arthroscopic local excision. *J Bone Joint Surg* 1992;74A:119–123.
3. Granowitz SP, D'Antonio J, Mankin HL. The pathogenesis and long-term end results of pigmented villonodular synovitis. *Clin Orthop Relat Res* 1976;114:335–351.
4. Goldman AB, Dicarlo EF. Pigmented villonodular synovitis. Diagnosis and differential diagnosis. *Radiol Clin North Am* 1988;26:1327–1347.
5. Bertoni F, Unni KK, Beabout JW, et al. Malignant giant cell tumor of the tendon sheaths and joints (malignant pigmented villonodular synovitis). *Am J Surg Pathol* 1997;21:153–163.
6. O'Sullivan B, Cummings B, Catton C, et al. Outcome following radiation treatment for high-risk pigmented villonodular synovitis. *Int J Radiat Oncol Biol Phys* 1995;32:777–786.
7. Rodriguez Blanco CE, Leon HO, Guthrie TB. Combined partial arthroscopic synovectomy and radiation therapy for diffuse pigmented villonodular synovitis of the knee. *Arthroscopy* 2001;17:527–531.
8. Chin KR, Barr SJ, Winalski C, et al. Treatment of advanced primary and recurrent diffuse pigmented villonodular synovitis of the knee. *J Bone Joint Surg* 2002;84A:2192–2202.
9. de Ponti A, Sansone V, da Gama Malcher M. Result of arthroscopic treatment of pigmented villonodular synovitis of the knee. *Arthroscopy* 2003;19:602–607.
10. Zvijac JE, Lau AC, Hechtman KS, et al. Arthroscopic treatment of pigmented villonodular synovitis of the knee. *Arthroscopy* 1999;15:613–617.
11. Lee BI, Yoo JE, Lee SH, et al. Localized pigmented villonodular synovitis of the knee: arthroscopic treatment. *Arthroscopy* 1998;14:764–768.


### ADDITIONAL READING

- Cotten A, Flipo RM, Chastanet P, et al. PVNS of the hip: review of radiographic features in 58 patients. *Skeletal Radiol* 1995;24:1–6.
- Granowitz SP, D'Antonio J, Mankin HL. The pathogenesis and long-term end results of PVNS. *Clin Orthop Relat Res* 1976;114:335–351.
- Spjut HJ, Dorfman HD, Fechner RE, et al. Lesions of synovial origin. In: *Tumors of Bone and Cartilage.* Washington, DC: Armed Forces Institute of Pathology, 1971:391–410.


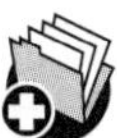

## MISCELLANEOUS

### CODES
#### *ICD9-CM*
215.3 Benign neoplasm, knee

### PATIENT TEACHING
Even with appropriate care, the recurrence rate is high, especially in diffuse PVNS (2,8).

#### *Activity*
After surgery, ROM exercises are important to prevent contractures.

### FAQ
- Q: Is irradiation effective in controlling recurrent disease?
  - A: External beam irradiation, when combined with repeat surgery, can be very effective.
- Q: How do patients know if they have PVNS in 1 of their joints?
  - A: Patients most commonly present with severe joint pain and palpable swelling in superficial joints.
- Q: When do patients with PVNS need a joint replacement?
  - A: Joint replacement surgery is needed when the joint surfaces have been destroyed or the bone involvement is so severe that curettage and grafting is not feasible.

# POLYDACTYLY

*Dawn M. LaPorte, MD*
*John J. Hwang, MD*

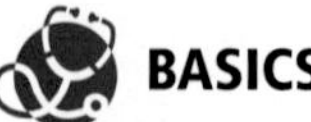

## BASICS

### DESCRIPTION

- Polydactyly is a duplication of the fingers or toes that is detected at birth (Fig. 1).
- Classification:
  - Preaxial (involving thumb or great toe, Fig. 2): Wassel classification (1):
    - I: Bifid distal phalanx
    - II: Duplicated distal phalanx
    - III: Bifid proximal phalanx
    - IV: Duplicated proximal phalanx
    - V: Bifid metacarpal
    - VI: Duplicated metacarpal
  - Central
  - Postaxial (involving small finger or toe) (2):
    - Type A: Complete duplication with bony attachment to an adjacent digit
    - Type B: Rudimentary, incomplete duplication of the phalanges
- Synonyms: Accessory digits, Split thumb

### EPIDEMIOLOGY

- Postaxial form occurs at a rate of 1 per 150 in African Americans versus 1 per 1,500 in Caucasians (3,4).
- Preaxial form is more common in whites than in other races (3,4), and most cases are sporadic.
- Central polydactyly is uncommon compared with border polydactyly.
- No significant difference in reported occurrence between the genders (3,4)

### RISK FACTORS

African heritage is a risk factor.

#### *Genetics*

- Postaxial polydactyly frequently is inherited as an autosomal dominant pattern but with variable penetrance.
- Polydactyly of the index finger and polysyndactyly of the ring and long fingers probably are autosomal dominant conditions.

### ETIOLOGY

The cause is unknown, unless the condition is associated with a syndrome.

### ASSOCIATED CONDITIONS

- Holt-Oram syndrome
- Fanconi syndrome
- Trisomy 13
- Ellis-van Creveld syndrome
- Grebe chondrodysplasia

## DIAGNOSIS

### SIGNS AND SYMPTOMS

Duplicated fingers or toes

#### *Physical Exam*

- Check for active and passive movement at each joint.
- Assess the stability of the digit.
- Look for an angular deformity at each joint.
- Look at the skin coverage and webbing.
- All these factors are important in determining surgical treatment.

### TESTS

#### *Imaging*

Plain film radiography of the hand is indicated.

#### *Pathological Findings*

The digits may vary in the extent of development of the phalanges and tendons.

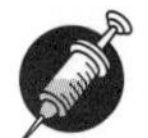

## TREATMENT

### GENERAL MEASURES

- Mild, type B postaxial polydactyly:
  - Treatment in the newborn:
    - Tie off the digit if it has no underlying skeletal connection.
    - In the presence of a skeletal connection, the "extra digit" should be electively removed surgically after 6 months of age.
  - This method is:
    - Safe
    - Not associated with bleeding complications
    - Associated with a satisfactory appearance
  - The rudimentary digit falls off in ~10 days.
- Type A:
  - Requires operative ablation with transfer of any important parts to the adjacent finger.
  - Cosmetic concerns: Surgery is indicated to restore a normal appearance.
  - Polydactyly of the foot: Surgery often is needed to make normal shoe wear possible.

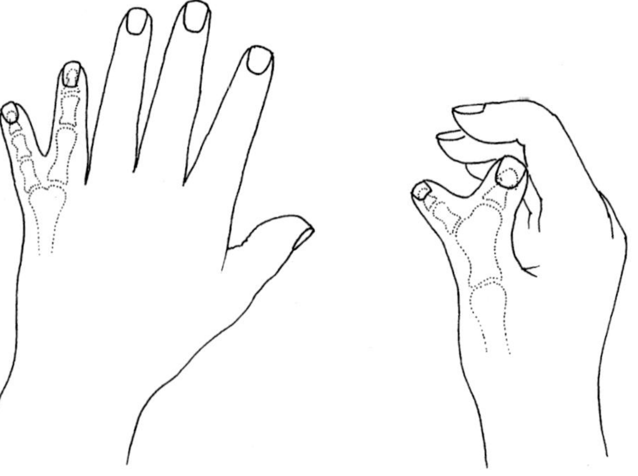

**Fig. 1.** Polydactyly involves variable skeletal duplications.

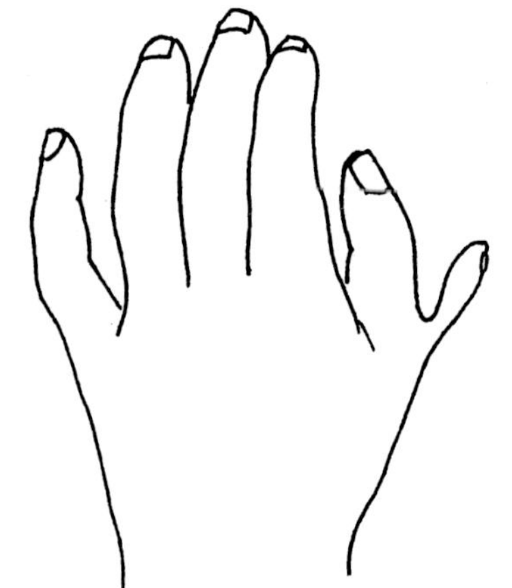

**Fig. 2.** Polydactyly is termed preaxial if it involves the thumb.

### SURGERY

Excision of the least developed digit, with preservation of the UCL and osteotomy, if indicated

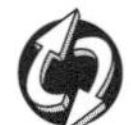

## FOLLOW-UP

### PROGNOSIS

- Rudimentary, type-B postaxial polydactyly: Good
- Other types of polydactyly (type A, duplicated thumb): Possible risk of angular growth of the adjoining digit or stiffness, but such problems rarely are symptomatic.

### COMPLICATIONS

- Small skin tag at the site of the polydactyly removal (rare)
- Angular deformity possible after complex polydactyly reconstructions; possible "Z deformity" after thumb reconstruction

### PATIENT MONITORING

For complex polydactyly, follow periodically with yearly checkups during growth.

### REFERENCES

1. Wassel HD. The results of surgery for polydactyly of the thumb. *A review. Clin Orthop Relat Res* 1969; 64:175–193.
2. Trumble TE. Congenital hand deformities. In: Trumble TE, ed. *Principles of Hand Surgery and Therapy*. Philadelphia: WB Saunders, 2000: 579–601.
3. Frazier TM. A note on race-specific congenital malformation rates. *Am J Obstet Gynecol* 1960;80: 184–185.
4. Watson BT, Hennrikus WL. Postaxial type-B polydactyly. Prevalence and treatment. *J Bone Joint Surg* 1997;79A:65–68.

### ADDITIONAL READING

- Kozin SH. Deformities of the hand and fingers. Central polydactyly. In: Green DP, Hotchkiss RN, Pederson WC, et al., eds. *Green's Operative Hand Surgery*, 5th ed. Philadelphia: Elsevier Churchill Livingstone, 2005:1393–1394.
- Kozin SH. Deformities of the thumb. In: Green DP, Hotchkiss RN, Pederson WC, et al., eds. *Green's Operative Hand Surgery*, 5th ed. Philadelphia: Elsevier Churchill Livingstone, 2005:1445–1468.
- Kozin SH. Deformities of the hand and fingers. Ulnar polydactyly. In: Green DP, Hotchkiss RN, Pederson WC, et al., eds. *Green's Operative Hand Surgery*, 5th ed. Philadelphia: Elsevier Churchill Livingstone, 2005:1392–1393.

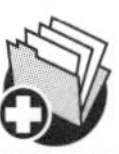

## MISCELLANEOUS

### CODES

***ICD9-CM***

- 755.0 Polydactyly (general)
- 755.01 Polydactyly (fingers)
- 755.20 Polydactyly (toes)

### PATIENT TEACHING

Inform patients with complex or preaxial polydactyly about the possibility of angular deformity of the thumb during growth.

### FAQ

- Q: If 1 child is born with polydactyly, is there an increased risk of it occurring in additional children?
  - A: Postaxial polydactyly (ulnar side) frequently is inherited in an autosomal-dominant pattern, but it has a variable penetrance pattern.
- Q: Is the treatment for ulnar and radial polydactyly the same?
  - A: No. Ulnar polydactyly frequently can be treated with surgical ablation, whereas a duplicated thumb most often requires a more technical reconstructive procedure with creation of a new ligament and possible osteotomy.

# POPLITEAL CYST IN THE ADULT

*Carl Wierks, MD*
*Bill Hobbs, MD*

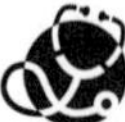

## BASICS

### DESCRIPTION

- Popliteal cyst in an adult is a distended cyst in the posterior fossa of the knee that often is connected directly to the joint space.
- Synonym: Baker cyst

### EPIDEMIOLOGY

- Bimodal distribution: 1 subset in children, 1 in adults >55 years old:
  - In adults, cysts usually are the result of intra-articular abnormalities.
  - In children, the cyst is the primary disorder.
- Males and females are affected equally.

### RISK FACTORS

Intra-articular knee disease (meniscus tear or arthritis)

#### *Genetics*

No known Mendelian pattern

### ETIOLOGY

- Herniation of the synovial membrane through a weak point of the medial posterior capsule between 2 expansions of the semimembranosus tendon
- Formation of a 1-way valve between the joint and the bursa

### ASSOCIATED CONDITIONS

- Rheumatoid arthritis (1)
- Osteoarthritis
- Chronic ACL tear
- Medial or lateral meniscal tears

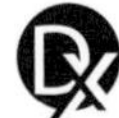

## DIAGNOSIS

### SIGNS AND SYMPTOMS

- Mass or fullness in the popliteal fossa of the knee
- Knee effusion
- Symptoms of ruptured cyst are warmth, tenderness, and erythema of the calf, or isolated calf swelling, mimicking DVT.
- Large cysts can produce posterior tibial nerve compression neuropathy.

#### *History*

Acute or chronic history of pain and/or mass behind knee

#### *Physical Exam*

- Fullness and tenderness posteriorly in the popliteal fossa
- Calf tenderness and swelling in the case of ruptured cyst
- Presence of other potential causes of knee swelling, such as meniscal injury (joint line tenderness) or chronic ligamentous tear

### TESTS

#### *Lab*

Rheumatoid factor

#### *Imaging*

- Standing flexed posteroanterior and lateral radiographs
- MRI to evaluate the size of the cyst, differentiate it from a soft-tissue tumor, and identify intra-articular abnormalities
- Duplex ultrasound is the most cost-effective imaging study for diagnosis and can help rule out DVT as the cause of a ruptured cyst (2).

#### *Pathological Findings*

- Swelling in the popliteal fossa bursae, usually secondary to intra-articular disease
- Herniation of the synovial membrane through a weakened area in the posterior joint capsule
- Differentiating from DVT:
  - Important because anticoagulation in the presence of a ruptured cyst could lead to hematoma or compartment syndrome
  - Physical examination can be unreliable.
  - MRA provides the best resolution, but duplex ultrasound is the best test because of its availability and low cost.

### DIFFERENTIAL DIAGNOSIS

- Semimembranosus bursa
- Ruptured cyst
- Soft-tissue tumor
- Lipoma in the popliteal fossa
- Synovial cell sarcoma
- Pseudoaneurysm (usually pulsatile)
- Primary bone malignancy (e.g., parosteal osteosarcoma)
- DVT

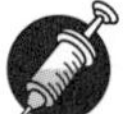

## TREATMENT

### GENERAL MEASURES

- Symptomatic: Needle aspiration with or without steroid injection:
  - Observation with symptomatic care is acceptable if pain is tolerable.
  - Address intra-articular pathology (e.g., arthroscopic meniscectomy for meniscus tear)
- Asymptomatic cyst requires no treatment.
- >90% of popliteal cysts have associated intra-articular abnormalities; these must be addressed to prevent recurrence of the cyst (3).
- Cysts often resolve spontaneously after treatment of the intra-articular abnormality.

#### *Activity*

The patient may continue all activities, limited only by pain.

### SPECIAL THERAPY

#### *Physical Therapy*

- General knee and core strengthening program
- Postoperative therapy as dictated by the surgical procedure; early ROM and weightbearing usually allowed

### MEDICATION (DRUGS)

Resolution of symptoms in most cysts with nonoperative care and reassurance

#### *First Line*

Analgesics and NSAIDs are treatment mainstays.

#### *Second Line*

Narcotic analgesics rarely needed

### SURGERY

- Arthroscopic evaluation and treatment of any intra-articular abnormalities are indicated.
- A cyst that persists after treatment of the joint disorder can be removed via a posteromedial incision, but it has a high rate of recurrence unless intra-articular abnormalities are addressed.

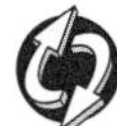

## FOLLOW-UP

### PROGNOSIS

- Most cysts resolve once the intra-articular disorder is treated.
- Untreated cysts may increase in size, but they often reach a stable, constant size.

### COMPLICATIONS

- Recurrence
- Rupture, causing a painful, swollen calf and lower extremity (simulating DVT)
- Popliteal artery or vein occlusion, posterior tibial nerve entrapment, and compartment syndrome are rare.

### PATIENT MONITORING

Patients are followed at 4–6-week intervals after surgery until ROM and function return.

### REFERENCES


1. Wilson PD, Eyre-Brook AL, Francis JD. A clinical and anatomical study of the semimembranosus bursa in relation to popliteal cyst. *J Bone Joint Surg* 1938;20:963–984.
2. Volteas SK, Labropoulos N, Leon M, et al. Incidence of ruptured Baker's cyst among patients with symptoms of deep vein thrombosis. *Br J Surg* 1997;84:342.
3. Hughston JC, Baker CL, Mello W. Popliteal cyst: a surgical approach. *Orthopedics* 1991;14:147–150.


### ADDITIONAL READING


- Childress HM. Popliteal cysts associated with undiagnosed posterior lesions of the medial meniscus. *J Bone Joint Surg* 1954;36A:1233–1237.
- Gristina AG, Wilson PD. Popliteal cysts in adults and children: a review of 90 cases. *Arch Surg* 1964;88: 357–363.
- Sansone V, de Ponti A, Paluello GM, et al. Popliteal cysts and associated disorders of the knee. Critical review with MR imaging. *Int Orthop* 1995;19: 275–279.


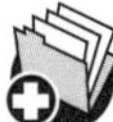

## MISCELLANEOUS

### CODES

#### *ICD9-CM*

727.51 Popliteal cyst

### PATIENT TEACHING

Reassure the patient that the cyst is benign and will not damage the knee.

### FAQ

- Q: How can a popliteal cyst be differentiated from a soft-tissue tumor such as a synovial cell sarcoma?
  - A: Popliteal cysts usually are asymptomatic with incidental findings on MRI evaluation for knee conditions. If the lesion is getting larger and is painful, particularly at night, synovial cell sarcoma should be considered as a diagnosis. MRI and needle aspiration are required to make the diagnosis.
- Q: How does a ruptured popliteal cyst present?
  - A: Patients complain of acute pain and swelling in the calf. Symptoms mimic DVT, which must be ruled out with duplex sonography.

# POPLITEAL CYST IN THE CHILD

*Paul D. Sponseller, MD*

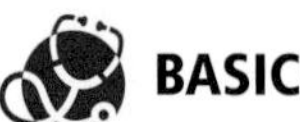

## BASICS

### DESCRIPTION

Popliteal cyst is a painless soft-tissue mass in the medial popliteal fossa behind the knee.

### EPIDEMIOLOGY

- Most common soft-tissue lesion about the knee in children
- Affects children 2–14 years old

#### *Incidence*

Incidence decreases after 9 years of age (1,2).

#### *Prevalence*

Twice as common in males (2)

### RISK FACTORS

- Most are isolated cases.
- Juvenile rheumatoid arthritis
- Other chronic inflammation of the knee

#### *Genetics*

No Mendelian pattern is known.

### ETIOLOGY

- Likely resulting from weakness in the posterior knee joint capsule between the semimembranosus muscle and the medial head of the gastrocnemius
- Rarely related to intra-articular lesions

## DIAGNOSIS

### SIGNS AND SYMPTOMS

- Protrusion between the medial gastrocnemius and semitendinosus muscles
- Swelling of the medial side of the popliteal space just lateral to the semitendinosus muscle
- Usually asymptomatic, but can cause discomfort and restrict ROM of knee if excessively enlarged
- Usually waxes and wanes in size, depending on the child's activity level
- Typically present for some time before the child is brought to the physician

#### *Physical Exam*

- Examine the affected lower limb for swelling of the medial side of the popliteal space just medial to the semimembranosus muscle.
- Compress the cyst to check for pain.
  - Usually painless
  - The remainder of the knee examination usually is normal.
- Examine the gait.
  - No limp should be evident.
- Transilluminate the cyst in a darkened room with a point light source (e.g., strong penlight) (Figs. 1 and 2).
  - With the patient prone, place the light source on the skin next to the area of swelling.
  - If the mass illuminates more strongly and evenly than the surrounding fatty tissue, the fluid-filled nature of cyst is confirmed, and a diagnosis of solid tumor is excluded.

### TESTS

#### *Lab*

- Aspiration is not commonly performed.
- However, if the cyst is aspirated, the cyst fluid is clear and gelatinous.
  - If the cyst fluid is not clear and gelatinous, send the aspirate for the following tests to rule out septic arthritis or soft-tissue abscess:
    - Cell count
    - Gram stain
    - Culture

#### *Imaging*

- Plain-film radiography is optional to rule out bony disorder.
- Duplex ultrasound and MRI (rarely indicated) characterize a questionable cyst further and rule out malignancy (3).

#### *Pathological Findings*

- Synovial fluid–filled sac in the semimembranosus-gastrocnemius interval
- Rarely related to intra-articular lesions

### DIFFERENTIAL DIAGNOSIS

- Malignant disease
- Vascular anomaly
- Soft-tissue abscess

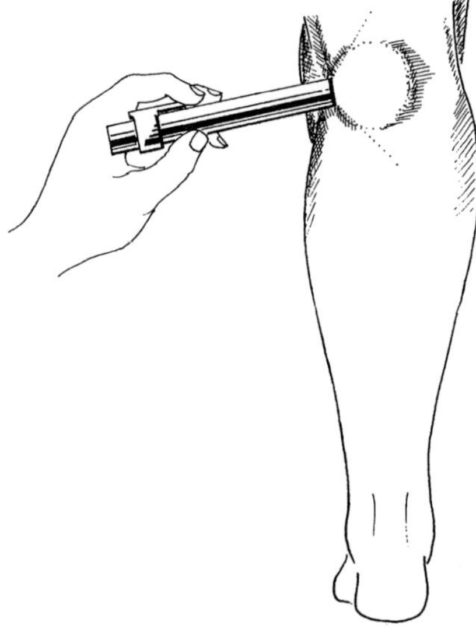

**Fig. 1.** A diagnosis of popliteal cyst in a child may be confirmed by transillumination.

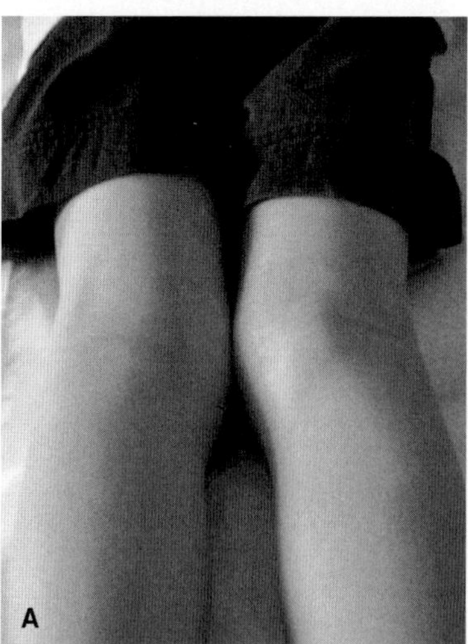


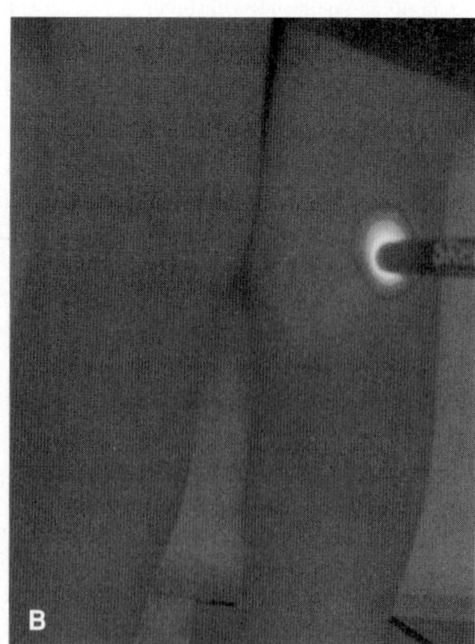


**Fig. 2.** Prone 7-year-old with popliteal cyst. **A**: External appearance of cyst. **B**: After transillumination. Note that the cyst picks up light remote from the source in comparison with surrounding tissues.

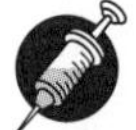

# TREATMENT

## GENERAL MEASURES

- The patient's activity may be restricted when the cyst is large.
- Surgical excision may be necessary if the cyst is symptomatic (rare).
  - The recurrence rate after surgical excision is 20–40% (2).
- No treatment is required if no intra-articular lesion is present.
  - Left untreated, 70% of cysts disappear spontaneously after months to years (they may wax and wane in size) (3,4).
- If it is desired to confirm the diagnosis and increase the chance of resolution, the cysts may be aspirated with a large-bore needle, followed by immobilization for immediate decompression.
  - However, the recurrence rate is high.

## SURGERY

- Excision of the cyst through a transverse incision in the posterior popliteal region:
  - May be done as an outpatient procedure
- Immobilization for several weeks postoperatively

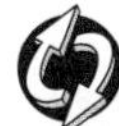

# FOLLOW-UP

## COMPLICATIONS

The rate of recurrence of the cyst after surgical treatment is ~20–40% (2).

## PATIENT MONITORING

- No routine follow-up is needed.
- Instruct the parent to return if the lesion changes in symptoms or in character.

## REFERENCES


1. De Greef I, Molenaers G, Fabry G. Popliteal cysts in children: a retrospective study of 62 cases. *Acta Orthop Belg* 1998;64:180–183.
2. Willis RB. Sports medicine in the growing child. Overuse injuries. In: Morrissy RT, Weinstein SL, eds. *Lovell and Winter's Pediatric Orthopaedics*, 6th ed. Philadelphia: Lippincott Williams & Wilkins, 2006:1414–1421.
3. De Maeseneer M, Debaere C, Desprechins B, et al. Popliteal cysts in children: prevalence, appearance and associated findings at MR imaging. *Pediatr Radiol* 1999;29:605–609.
4. Seil R, Rupp S, Jochum P, et al. Prevalence of popliteal cysts in children. A sonographic study and review of the literature. *Arch Orthop Trauma Surg* 1999;119:73–75.


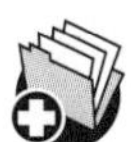

# MISCELLANEOUS

## CODES

### *ICD9-CM*

727.51 Popliteal cyst

## PATIENT TEACHING

- Inform parents about the benign nature of the condition.
- Explain the similarity of the pathologic process to that of the Baker cyst in adults.
- Mention the lack of underlying knee disease and the absence of increased synovial fluid production.

## FAQ

- Q: Is MRI indicated for a popliteal cyst in a child?
  - A: Not unless the cyst is atypical and does not transilluminate, or separate symptoms are referable to the knee.
- Q: Is follow-up needed?
  - A: If it is a typical cyst, no follow-up is needed unless symptoms develop.

# POSTERIOR CRUCIATE LIGAMENT INJURY

*Marc Urquhart, MD*
*John H. Wilckens, MD*

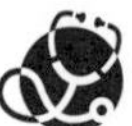

## BASICS

### DESCRIPTION

- Injury to the PCL, the primary stabilizer to posterior translation of the tibia on the femur at the knee (1)
- Classification (see "Posterior drawer test" under "Physical Exam") (2):
  - Grade 1: Tibial plateau is anterior to the femoral condyles.
  - Grade 2: Tibial plateau is level with the femoral condyles.
  - Grade 3: Tibial plateau is posterior to the femoral condyles.

### EPIDEMIOLOGY

- Young adults
- Males affected more than females

#### *Incidence*

Uncommon

### RISK FACTORS

- Motor vehicle accident
- Participation in collision sports
- Hyperextension injury to the knee

#### *Genetics*

No Mendelian pattern is known.

### ETIOLOGY

- Direct blow to the anterior tibia with the knee flexed and the foot plantarflexed
- Hyperflexion without a blow
- Hyperextension

### ASSOCIATED CONDITIONS

Popliteal artery injury

## DIAGNOSIS

### SIGNS AND SYMPTOMS

- Knee pain and swelling after the injury with gradual improvement in generalized pain symptoms
- Minimal symptomatic instability, usually when climbing stairs
- Recurrent effusion
- Posterior knee pain
- Knee recurvatum (late finding)

#### *Physical Exam*

- Perform a complete neurovascular examination.
- Tests for ligamentous stability:
  - Posterior drawer test:
    - Position the patient supine with the knee flexed 90° and the foot stabilized on the examination table.
    - Apply posterior force to the anterior tibia.
    - Note the excursion of the tibia underneath the femoral condyles.
    - Note the quality of the end point.
    - Compare the involved and contralateral sides.
    - The position of the affected knee can reveal a posterior sag of the tibia when the patient is supine with hips flexed 45°, knees flexed 90°, and feet flat on the examination table.
  - Lachman test:
    - Anterior drawer test at 30° of flexion
    - To rule out associated ACL rupture
  - Rule out collateral ligament injury

### TESTS

#### *Lab*

None indicated

#### *Imaging*

- Radiography:
  - Plain film AP and lateral views of the knee:
    - To evaluate for fracture about the knee
    - May reveal an avulsion fracture off the proximal posterior tibia
  - Stress radiography
- MRI is very sensitive for identifying PCL injury and associated injuries

#### *Pathological Findings*

Either midsubstance rupture or proximal or distal bony avulsion is noted.

### DIFFERENTIAL DIAGNOSIS

- ACL injury
- Tibial plateau fracture
- Meniscal tear

## TREATMENT

### GENERAL MEASURES

- Patients may be partial weightbearing as tolerated.
- History and physical examination for a provisional diagnosis
- Radiography and MRI to confirm the diagnosis
- Nonoperative treatment initially, except for high-grade injuries/knee dislocations
- Knee immobilizer and crutch ambulation as tolerated until comfortable
- Early ROM and strengthening
- Knee braces are of questionable use.

## SPECIAL THERAPY

### *Physical Therapy*

A specific PCL-insufficiency knee program is initiated.

## MEDICATION (DRUGS)

### *First Line*

- NSAIDs
- Acetaminophen

### *Second Line*

Mild, as-needed narcotics for acute/severe pain

## SURGERY

- Relative indications for surgery:
  - Grade 3 PCL injuries
  - Posterolateral corner injuries
  - Associated ligamentous, meniscal, or articular surface injuries
  - Giving-way of the knee
  - Pain
  - Radiographically documented progressive articular deterioration
- Reduction and internal fixation of avulsion fractures
- Reconstruction is reserved for patients with symptomatic swelling and activity-related pain (3).
  - The procedure entails reconstruction of the ligament with an autograft or allograft.
  - Arthroscopically assisted reconstructions are demanding technically but obviate wide surgical exposure.

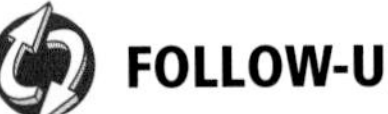

# FOLLOW-UP

## PROGNOSIS

- Extremely good
- Most patients do not require surgery (4).

## COMPLICATIONS

- Recurrent symptomatic giving-way of the knee
- Failure of reconstruction
- Progressive medial compartment arthrosis, followed by patellofemoral compartment arthrosis

## PATIENT MONITORING

Patients are followed at 3–6-month intervals to check on their prognosis with ROM, muscle strength, and function.

## REFERENCES


1. Miller MD, Bergfeld JA, Fowler PJ, et al. The posterior cruciate ligament injured knee: principles of evaluation and treatment. *Instr Course Lect* 1999;48:199–207.
2. Shelbourne KD, Rubinstein RA, Jr. Methodist Sports Medicine Center's experience with acute and chronic isolated posterior cruciate ligament injuries. *Clin Sports Med* 1994;13:531–543.
3. Johnson TS, Cosgarea AJ. Posterior cruciate ligament injuries. In: Garrick JG, ed. *Orthopaedic Knowledge Update: Sports Medicine 3*. Rosemont, IL: American Academy of Orthopaedic Surgeons, 2004:155–168.
4. Shelbourne KD, Davis TJ, Patel DV. The natural history of acute, isolated, nonoperatively treated posterior cruciate ligament injuries. A prospective study. *Am J Sports Med* 1999;27:276–283.


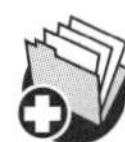

# MISCELLANEOUS

## CODES

### *ICD9-CM*

717.84 Disruption of the posterior cruciate ligament

## PATIENT TEACHING

Isolated PCL injuries often are treated nonoperatively.

## FAQ

- Q: What is the natural history of nonoperatively treated isolated PCL injuries?
  - A: Most patients are able to return to functional activity in 6–8 weeks. Although progressive laxity is uncommon, patients can develop medial and patellofemoral compartment changes over the ensuing years of PCL laxity.
- Q: Are other injuries associated with PCL injury?
  - A: Low-energy PCL injuries usually are isolated. However, high-energy PCL injuries usually are accompanied by collateral ligament injury and/or ACL injury. A patient with a high-energy PCL tear should be evaluated for concomitant vascular and neurologic injury.

# POSTERIOR INTEROSSEOUS NERVE ENTRAPMENT

*Paul D. Sponseller, MD*
*Dawn M. LaPorte, MD*

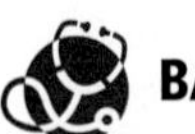

## BASICS

### DESCRIPTION

- PINS occurs when muscles innervated by the posterior interosseous nerve are affected secondary to entrapment of the posterior interosseous nerve by 1 of several structures (Fig. 1).
- The related, but separate, radial tunnel syndrome is characterized by pain and weakness on the lateral side of the elbow after activities with forceful elbow extension or forearm rotation.

### EPIDEMIOLOGY

- Most common in individuals 20–50 years old
- Male and females are affected approximately equally.

#### *Incidence*

Uncommon

### RISK FACTORS

Repetitive supinating or gripping motions are risk factors.

#### *Genetics*

No Mendelian pattern is known.

### ETIOLOGY

- Typically, involvement of ≥1 of the following structures:
  - Fibrous edge of the supinator muscle (most common cause), known as the "arcade of Frohse"
  - Fibrous bands over the radial head
  - Radial recurrent vessels to the elbow, known as the "leash of Henry"
  - Fibrous edge of the extensor radialis brevis muscle
  - Distal edge of the supinator (1)

### ASSOCIATED CONDITIONS

Lateral epicondylitis

## DIAGNOSIS

### SIGNS AND SYMPTOMS

- Aching pain in the muscles of the lateral forearm, just distal to the elbow (the extensor-supinator mass)
- Symptoms usually occur after muscular effort.
- Numbness is rare in PINS because the course of the sensory nerve is separate from that of the motor nerve.

#### *Physical Exam*

- Complete neurovascular examination of the affected limb:
  - The area of tenderness in PINS is ~4 fingerbreadths distal to the lateral epicondyle of the elbow.
  - Pain is worsened by active supination of the forearm (turning the palm up) or extension of the wrist.
  - Pain is worsened by pressing down on the extended long finger.
  - Sensation of the forearm and hand is normal.
  - Motor strength may be diminished in chronic cases because of longstanding compression.
- Diagnostic local anesthetic injection:
  - Inject local anesthetic into the extensor-supinator mass and lateral side of the elbow, on separate days, to determine where pain relief occurs.

### TESTS

#### *Lab*

Laboratory tests are not helpful for this diagnosis.

#### *Imaging*

Imaging studies are not needed unless an unusual mass is felt in the area.

#### *Pathological Findings*

- On surgical exploration, compression of the radial nerve
- Nerve possibly having constricted area from long-standing pressure

### DIFFERENTIAL DIAGNOSIS

- Lateral epicondylitis (tennis elbow): Usually a more proximal pain, directly over the lateral epicondyle or radial head (i.e., over the elbow itself)
- Cervical radiculopathy (nerve compression in the neck): Usually associated with a more radiating pain
- Cheiralgia paresthetica (Wartenberg symptom): Entrapment of the radial sensory nerve, producing numbness

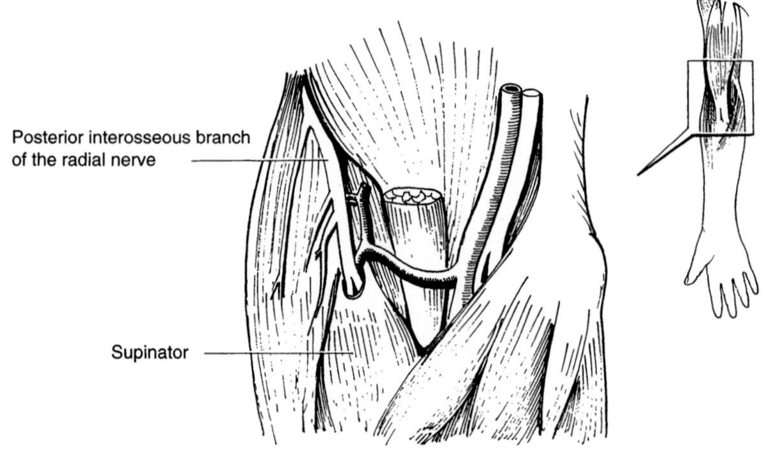


**Fig. 1.** The posterior interosseous branch of the radial nerve may become entrapped in the arcade around the supinator muscle.

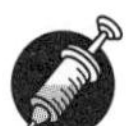

## TREATMENT

### GENERAL MEASURES

- Rest from the causative activity, if one can be identified
- If no cause identified, immobilization of the elbow and forearm in a splint
- Surgery if nonoperative measures are not successful
- After nonoperative or surgical cure, slow resumption of activity
- Repetitive supination or gripping activities limited to the extent that they do not cause discomfort

### SPECIAL THERAPY

#### *Physical Therapy*

- Occupational therapy for gradual mobilization and strengthening of the elbow is begun when the splint is removed.
- Therapy should be performed by an experienced hand therapist.

### MEDICATION (DRUGS)

NSAIDs

### SURGERY

- Surgical exploration of the path of the posterior interosseous nerve in this region, which may be an outpatient procedure (2)
- Release of constricting structures
- Usually satisfactory results
- No permanent deficit resulting from release

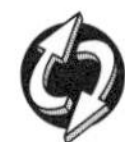

## FOLLOW-UP

### PROGNOSIS

- Most patients have a good result after nonoperative or surgical cure.
- Causative activities should be modified or eliminated, if possible.

### COMPLICATIONS

Recurrence is possible.

### PATIENT MONITORING

Patients are followed every 3 months until the symptoms resolve.

### REFERENCES


1. Gupta R. Nerve. In: Beredjiklian PK, Bozentka DJ, eds. *Review of Hand Surgery.* Philadelphia: WB Saunders, 2004:79–100.
2. Arle JE, Zager EL. Surgical treatment of common entrapment neuropathies in the upper limbs. *Muscle Nerve* 2000;23:1160–1174.


### ADDITIONAL READING


- Lister GD, Belsole RB, Kleinert HE. The radial tunnel syndrome. *J Hand Surg* 1979;4A:52–59.
- MacKinnon SE, Novak CB. Compression neuropathies. In: Green DP, Hotchkiss RN, Pederson WC, et al., eds. *Green's Operative Hand Surgery*, 5th ed. Philadelphia: Elsevier Churchill Livingstone, 2005;999–1045.


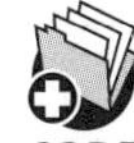

## MISCELLANEOUS

### CODES

#### *ICD9-CM*

723.4 Brachial neuritis or radiculitis not otherwise specified

### PATIENT TEACHING

- Demonstrate motions that constrict the nerve.
- Explain the dosing and side effects of analgesics.
- Explain that changing manual jobs or repetitive motions may prevent the development of full-blown PINS.

### FAQ

- Q: How do patients with PINS present?
  - A: Patients present with pain at the proximal lateral forearm and weakness in the extensor muscles of the digits and wrist.
- Q: Is radial tunnel syndrome different from PINS entrapment?
  - A: Yes. Radial tunnel syndrome affects only the sensory component of the radial nerve, and patients present with pain but not motor weakness.

# POSTERIOR TIBIAL TENDON RUPTURE

*Kris J. Alden, MD, PhD*

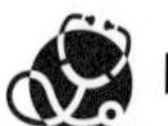

## BASICS

### DESCRIPTION

- PTT dysfunction or rupture is the most common cause of adult acquired flatfoot deformity.
- A working knowledge of the anatomy and function of the PTTin the normal foot is necessary to understand the pathophysiology that results from dysfunction.
  - Origin:
    - Posterior aspect of the tibia, the fibula, and the interosseous membrane
  - Course:
    - Runs medially and posteriorly adjacent to the medial malleolus
    - Runs posterior to the ankle joint's axis and medial to the axis of the subtalar joint
  - Insertion:
    - Navicular tuberosity, plantar aspect of the cuneiforms and 2nd, 3rd, and 4th metatarsal bases
  - Function:
    - Plantarflexion of the ankle
    - Inversion of the subtalar joint and locking of the transverse tarsal joints during push-off phase of gait
    - Stabilizer of the medial longitudinal arch
- Insufficient PTT function results in secondary attenuation of the medial arch joint capsules and ligaments, producing a progressive flatfoot deformity.
- Loss of function also hampers efficient gastrocnemius action so that gait is impaired.
- Overt rupture of the PTT may be posttraumatic in nature and produce substantial pain in the medial aspect of the foot.
- Classification (1):
  - Stage I: Tendinitis with normal alignment of the foot, characterized by pain along the route of the tendon and local inflammatory changes
  - Stage II: Presents with dynamic hindfoot deformity as seen by increased valgus of the hindfoot, midfoot abduction and supination, and weakness of the PTT
    - Subtalar motion is passively correctible.
  - Stage III: Fixed valgus deformity of the hindfoot or abduction-supination of talonavicular joint, or hindfoot arthritis
  - Stage IV (2): Long-standing disease with fixed deformities of the hindfoot and either severe ankle arthritis or valgus angulation of the talus secondary to laxity of the deltoid ligament complex
- Synonym: Adult acquired flatfoot

### EPIDEMIOLOGY

#### *Incidence*

Most common cause of adult acquired flatfoot

#### *Prevalence*

- Affects adults 40–60 years old
- Common in middle-aged females
- Prevalence increases with age

### RISK FACTORS

- Obesity
- Pes planus (flatfoot)
- Diabetes mellitus
- Steroid injection around the tendon
- Seronegative arthropathies
- Inflammatory arthropathy
- Fractures/trauma to ankle
- Accessory navicular

#### *Genetics*

No Mendelian pattern is known.

### ETIOLOGY

- Tendinitis(tendon inflammation) and tendinosis (tendon degeneration) causes subsequent fibrosis as a result of repeated microtrauma.
- Most cases represent chronic tendon degeneration, although acute tendinitis may occur with overuse or inflammatory arthropathy.
- Posterior to the medial malleolus, the tendon has a poor blood supply, which may exacerbate its degeneration and contribute to inadequate healing.
- Underlying flatfoot deformity or presence of accessory navicular may produce abnormal mechanical demands on the PTT.
- Ankle fracture, sprain, or a direct blow to the tendon may cause (but rarely) concomitant tendon rupture.

### ASSOCIATED CONDITIONS

Valgus hindfoot deformity may lead to secondary contracture of the gastrocnemius-soleus or Achilles tendon.

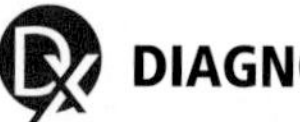

## DIAGNOSIS

### SIGNS AND SYMPTOMS

- Progressive flatfoot deformity
- Pain at medial arch or lateral hindfoot secondary to subfibular impingement.
- Unilateral swelling, particularly medially at ankle
- Pain or weakness while walking

#### *History*

Some patients may recall a specific traumatic episode, but most cases present in an insidious manner with progressive swelling and flattening of the arch.

#### *Physical Exam*

- Conduct a neurovascular examination of the affected foot.
- Assess the patient's gait, identifying asymmetric external rotation or eversion.
- Pain, weakness, or inability to invert the foot from a plantarflexed-everted position against manual resistance (a position that isolates the PTT).
- Tenderness is present at the insertion of the PTT into the navicular, or along the tendon itself as it curves around the medial malleolus.
- "Too-many-toes" sign (Fig. 1): When the patient is viewed from behind, more toes are visible lateral to the ankle on the affected than on the contralateral foot.
- Inability to perform multiple single-limb heel rises or insufficient heel inversion during heel rise

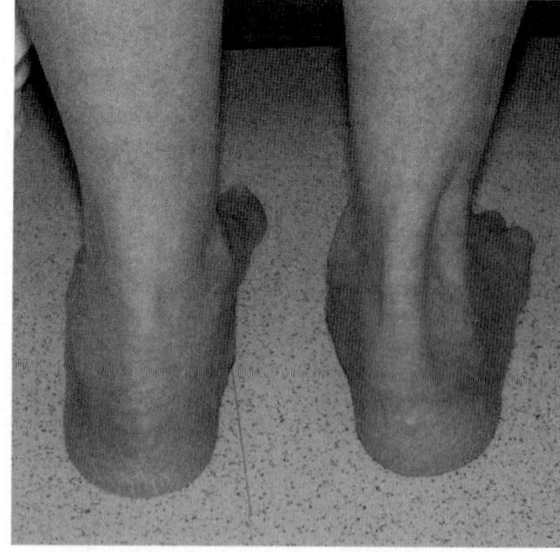

**Fig. 1.** Clinical photograph showing increased valgus and the too-many-toes sign on the right foot.

## TESTS
### *Lab*
None is needed.

### *Imaging*
- Radiography:
  - Weightbearing foot radiographs to assess the deformity and identify hindfoot arthritis
    - AP view: Lateral navicular subluxation with uncovering of talar head
    - Lateral view: Loss of medial arch height and decreased calcaneal pitch
  - Weightbearing ankle radiographs to assess alignment and identify arthritis:
    - Rule out valgus tilt of the talus on the mortise view.
- If the diagnosis is in question, use MRI.
  - The PTT may show hypertrophy, thickening, splitting, attenuation, or frank rupture.

### *Pathological Findings*
- Tenosynovitis in an early stage
- Progressive tendinosis with degeneration and attenuation
- Continued strain on the tendon can lead to complete rupture.

## DIFFERENTIAL DIAGNOSIS
- Benign flatfoot
- Tarsal tunnel syndrome
- Inflammatory arthritis of the hindfoot
- Charcot arthropathy

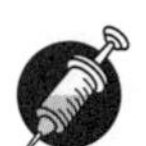

# TREATMENT

## GENERAL MEASURES
- Ankle stirrup brace, cast, or boot brace immobilization until acute symptoms subside
- Rest and assistive devices, such as a cane
- Patients with tenosynovitis or partial tear may benefit from NSAIDs.
- Once severe pain improves with immobilization, patients may transition to a semirigid orthotic arch support.
- More severe deformity may necessitate the use of an ankle-foot orthosis.

## SPECIAL THERAPY
### *Physical Therapy*
Physical therapy is used for muscle strengthening, motion exercises, ultrasound therapy, proprioception training, and gait mechanics.

## MEDICATION (DRUGS)
NSAIDs

## SURGERY
- Surgery is indicated for persistent pain, worsening deformity, or failure of nonsurgical treatments.
  - Stage I: Tenosynovectomy, possible flexor digitorum longus transfer ± medial sliding calcaneal osteotomy
  - Stage II: Multiple components needed, including:
    - ± Flexor digitorum longus tendon transfer and medial sliding calcaneal osteotomy *or* lateral column distraction arthrodesis *or* subtalar arthrodesis
    - ± Plantarflexion cuneiform osteotomy or first tarsometatarsal arthrodesis
    - Achilles lengthening or gastrocnemius recession
  - Stage III: Triple arthrodesis ± Achilles lengthening or gastrocnemius recession
  - Stage IV: Pantalar arthrodesis

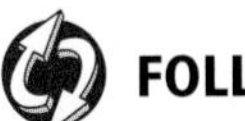

# FOLLOW-UP

## DISPOSITION
### *Issues for Referral*
- May be treated by general orthopaedist with experience in foot reconstructive surgery
- Often results in referral to orthopaedic foot and ankle specialist

## PROGNOSIS
- Nonoperative treatment (brace, orthotics) may be sufficient in sedentary or elderly patients, but if the condition is left untreated because the patient cannot tolerate the devices, a high risk of progression of hindfoot and ankle arthritis occurs (3,4).
- The prognosis is good with various surgical reconstructions, yielding high rates of patient satisfaction and functional recovery (5,6).

## COMPLICATIONS
- Weakness
- Recurrent deformity
- Arthritis

## PATIENT MONITORING
Patients are followed every 2–3 months until symptoms resolve.

## REFERENCES

1. Johnson KA, Strom DE. Tibialis posterior tendon dysfunction. *Clin Orthop Relat Res* 1989;239: 196–206.
2. Myerson MS. Adult acquired flatfoot deformity. Treatment of dysfunction of the posterior tibial tendon. *J Bone Joint Surg* 1996;78A:780–792.
3. Chao W, Wapner KL, Lee TH, et al. Nonoperative management of posterior tibial tendon dysfunction [see comments]. *Foot Ankle Int* 1996;17:736–741.
4. Friedman MA, Draganich LF, Toolan B, et al. The effects of adult acquired flatfoot deformity on tibiotalar joint contact characteristics. *Foot Ankle Int* 2001;22:241–246.
5. Myerson MS, Corrigan J, Thompson F, et al. Tendon transfer combined with calcaneal osteotomy for treatment of posterior tibial tendon insufficiency: a radiological investigation. *Foot Ankle Int* 1995;16:712–718.
6. Toolan BC, Sangeorzan BJ, Hansen ST, Jr. Complex reconstruction for the treatment of dorsolateral peritalar subluxation of the foot. Early results after distraction arthrodesis of the calcaneocuboid joint in conjunction with stabilization of, and transfer of the flexor digitorum longus tendon to, the midfoot to treat acquired pes planovalgus in adults. *J Bone Joint Surg* 1999;81A:1545–1560.


## ADDITIONAL READING

- Anderson RB, Davis WH. Management of the adult flatfoot deformity. In: Myerson MS, ed. *Foot and Ankle Disorders*. Philadelphia: WB Saunders, 2000:1017–1039.
- Basmajian JV, Stecko G. The role of muscles in arch support of the foot. *J Bone Joint Surg* 1963;45A: 1184–1190.
- Frey C, Shereff M, Greenidge N. Vascularity of the PTT. *J Bone Joint Surg* 1990; 72A:884–888.
- Holmes GB, Jr, Mann RA. Possible epidemiological factors associated with rupture of the PTT. *Foot Ankle* 1992;13:70–79.
- Mann RA, Thompson FM. Rupture of the PTT causing flat foot. Surgical treatment. *J Bone Joint Surg* 1985;67A:556–561.
- Pomeroy GC, Pike RH, Beals TC, et al. Acquired flatfoot in adults due to dysfunction of the PTT. *J Bone Joint Surg* 1999;81A: 1173–1182.


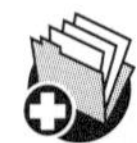

# MISCELLANEOUS

## CODES
### *ICD9-CM*
- 726.72 Posterior tibialis tendinitis
- 727.68 Posterior tibial tendon rupture
- 734 Acquired pes planus (flatfoot)

## PATIENT TEACHING
Inform the patient that the disorder is degenerative in nature and may progress to worsened deformity, arthritis, and pain.

## FAQ
- Q: What are the typical foot deformities seen with PTT dysfunction?
  - A: Progressive collapse of the medial longitudinal arch occurs with abduction and supination of the midfoot and valgus of the heel.
- Q: What is the most common underlying pathology of PTT dysfunction?
  - A: The tendon shows chronic degenerative changes, with splitting, attenuation, or frank tearing.
- Q: What is the pathognomonic physical finding suggestive of PTT dysfunction?
  - A: The too many toes sign, indicating abduction of the midfoot with arch collapse. The patient is viewed from behind, and the involved side shows more toes lateral to the fibula than does the uninvolved foot.

# POSTEROMEDIAL BOW OF THE TIBIA

*Paul D. Sponseller, MD*

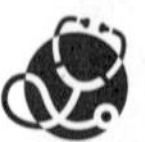

## BASICS

### DESCRIPTION

- Posteromedial bowing of the tibia is an angulation of the lower leg noticed at birth (Fig. 1).
- The foot typically is in a calcaneovalgus position.
- The angulation of leg is secondary to a deformity in the tibia.
- In most children, the angle gradually corrects itself during growth.
- The limb-length discrepancy persists and increases proportionately during growth.

### EPIDEMIOLOGY

- This condition is rare.
- Noticed at birth
- Occurs equally in males and females (1,2)

### RISK FACTORS

No risk factors are known.

#### *Genetics*

No Mendelian pattern is known.

### ETIOLOGY

- Unknown, but thought to be secondary to intrauterine positioning
- May also represent an inborn error in physeal growth
- Unlikely to be the result of fracture because of the proportionate shortening that follows

### ASSOCIATED CONDITIONS

No known associated conditions

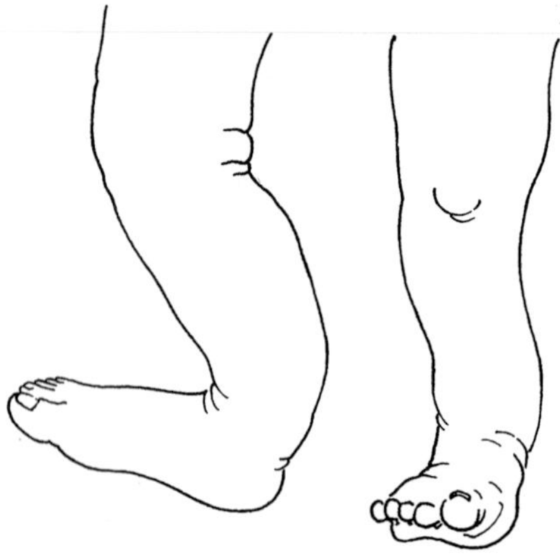

**Fig. 1.** Posteromedial bow of the tibia occurs just above the ankle of infants.

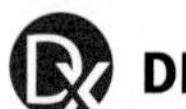

## DIAGNOSIS

### SIGNS AND SYMPTOMS

- At birth, the ankle is dorsiflexed, and the foot is in the calcaneovalgus position.
  - An obvious bow is present in the distal part of the tibia posteromedially.
- The condition is painless.
- The condition is almost always unilateral.

#### *History*

No history of gestational abnormality or birth trauma

#### *Physical Exam*

- Perform a complete examination of the lower extremity.
  - The leg appears shortened below the knee.
- Measure the leg length bilaterally.
- Measure the range of foot dorsiflexion, plantarflexion, inversion, and eversion.
- The foot is calcaneovalgus.
- Check for active function of all ankle muscles.

### TESTS

#### *Lab*

None is needed.

#### *Imaging*

- Plain radiographs reveal the deformity.
- Angulation of the tibia may be up to 60°.
- Tibial bone may be normal or thickened.
- No internal cystic change is seen.

#### *Pathological Findings*

- All muscles, tendons, and tissues are within normal limits, although the anterolateral muscles are underdeveloped.
- Only the bone is abnormal, with thickening and bowing.

### DIFFERENTIAL DIAGNOSIS

- Tibial fracture (3)
- Fibular hemimelia
- Calcaneovalgus foot (similar foot position)
- Congenital pseudarthrosis and NF, which are associated with anterolateral bow

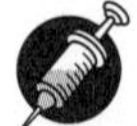

## TREATMENT

### GENERAL MEASURES

- This condition often resolves spontaneously with growth (Fig. 2), so initial treatment is watchful waiting.
- Residual deformity may be up to 6–8° of angulation and limb length inequality of up to 5 cm at maturity.
  - Usually, it is much less.
- Patients with a projected limb-length inequality of >2 cm at skeletal maturity should be candidates for epiphysiodesis or limb lengthening, depending on the degree of discrepancy and their preference for a major versus minor procedure.
- Casting, bracing, and stretching provide no benefit in most cases (2).
- In some extreme cases, a splint may be helpful in placing the foot flat to allow walking.
- No activity restrictions are necessary.
- A heel lift may benefit some patients with large limb-length inequalities.

### SPECIAL THERAPY

#### *Physical Therapy*

Physical therapy is not indicated.

### SURGERY

- Epiphysiodesis of the contralateral tibial epiphysis is the most common procedure.
  - Performed near adolescence, long after the bow has straightened
- Residual angulation of the tibia is sometimes problematic (5–10% of patients) (2).
- Osteotomy of the tibia is used to correct the angulation.
- Tibial lengthening procedures are used rarely.

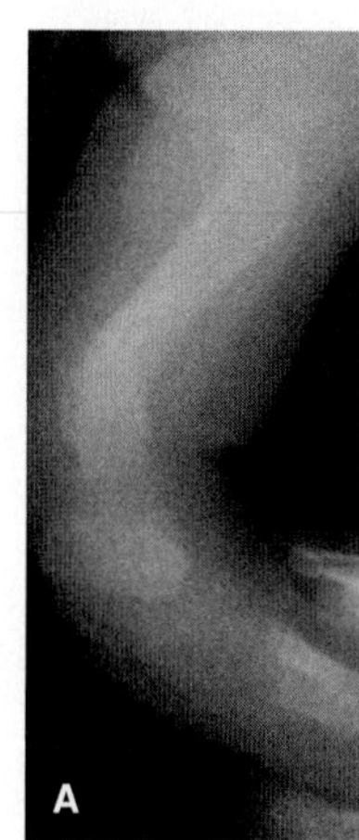


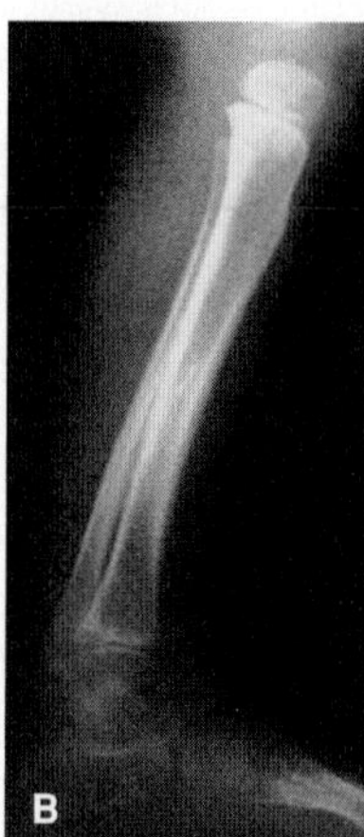


**Fig. 2.** Spontaneous resolution in a child.
**A:** Lateral radiograph of 1-year-old patient.
**B:** Lateral radiograph of same patient at 6 years of age.

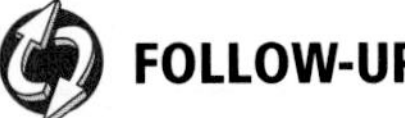

## FOLLOW-UP

### PROGNOSIS
- Prognosis is generally good.
- No long-term sequelae occur as long as lengths are corrected.

### COMPLICATIONS
- Limb-length inequality:
  - The main complication
  - Thought to be secondary to damage to physis by asymmetric forces as a result of bowing
  - Is correctable by surgery

### PATIENT MONITORING
- Obtain radiographic measurements of limb lengths (scanogram) by age 5 years, so they can be plotted onto a growth curve.
- Usually, growth inhibition remains proportionate.
- Radiographic measurement allows for prediction of final discrepancy and determination of the need for future surgery.

### REFERENCES

1. Pappas AM. Congenital posteromedial bowing of the tibia and fibula. *J Pediatr Orthop* 1984;4: 525–531.
2. Schoenecker PL, Rich MM. The lower extremity. Bowing of the tibia. In: Morrissy RT, Weinstein SL, eds. *Lovell and Winter's Pediatric Orthopaedics*, 6th ed Philadelphia: Lippincott Williams & Wilkins, 2006:1189–1200.
3. Hofmann A, Wenger DR. Posteromedial bowing of the tibia. Progression of discrepancy in leg lengths. *J Bone Joint Surg* 1981;63A:384–388.


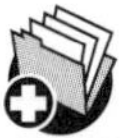

## MISCELLANEOUS

### CODES
#### *ICD9-CM*
736.89 Posteromedial bowing of the tibia

### PATIENT TEACHING
- Educate the family about the benign course of the disease.
- Bowing should correct itself over the 1st few years.
- Impress on the family that the patient must be followed throughout growth to assess limb lengths, angulation, and the need for surgery.

### FAQ
- Q: Could posteromedial bow be the result of a fracture in utero?
  - A: No, because the discrepancy in length increases proportionately in patients with posteromedial bow, whereas in patients with fracture, the discrepancy decreases slightly because of the overgrowth phenomenon.
- Q: Is casting or bracing helpful in speeding resolution?
  - A: No evidence suggests that it does. The only role for bracing is in children who have such malposition of the foot that a brace improves function.
- Q: What percentage of children with posteromedial bow require surgery?
  - A: More than 1/2 of children require epiphysiodesis near maturity for leg-length equalization. Fewer than 1/4 require treatment of the angulation.

# PREPATELLAR BURSITIS

*John J. Carbone, MD*
*John H. Wilckens, MD*

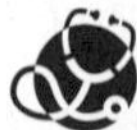

## BASICS

### DESCRIPTION

- Prepatellar bursitis is an inflammation of the bursa in front of the patella.
  - Bursae are located between structures to reduce friction.
  - These sacs are lined with a membranous synovium that produces and absorbs fluid; they are subject to acute or chronic trauma or infection and to low-grade inflammatory conditions such as gout, syphilis, tuberculosis, and rheumatoid arthritis (1).
- Classification:
  - Traumatic
  - Septic
  - Inflammatory
- Synonyms: Housemaid knee; Carpenter knee; Carpet-layer knee

### EPIDEMIOLOGY

- Particularly common in middle and old age
- Occurs equally in males and females

#### *Incidence*

Common

### RISK FACTORS

Occupations that create repetitive pressure and trauma to the anterior aspect of the knee

#### *Genetics*

No known Mendelian pattern

### ETIOLOGY

- Acute injury such as from a fall or motor vehicle accident (2)
- Repetitive minor trauma (2)

## DIAGNOSIS

### SIGNS AND SYMPTOMS

- Pain, worse with motion of and pressure over the knee
- Erythema
- Obvious swelling over the anterior patella (Fig. 1)

#### *Physical Exam*

- Examine the knee carefully and compare the affected with the contralateral side.
- Check for joint effusion.
- Palpate the quadriceps and patellar tendons and check for knee extension with the knee flexed 90°.
- Palpate the patella for tenderness.
- Check for erythema and local warmth.

### TESTS

#### *Lab*

- Routine tests:
  - Complete blood cell count
  - ESR
- If the bursa is aspirated:
  - Culture
  - Cell count
  - Gram stain
  - Crystal analysis

#### *Imaging*

AP and lateral radiographs to rule out an intra-articular or bony process

#### *Pathological Findings*

Usually, Gram-positive organisms (*Staphylococcus aureus*) (3)

### DIFFERENTIAL DIAGNOSIS

- Intra-articular disorders of a similar nature:
  - Sepsis
  - Low-grade inflammatory process
  - Trauma
- Cellulitis

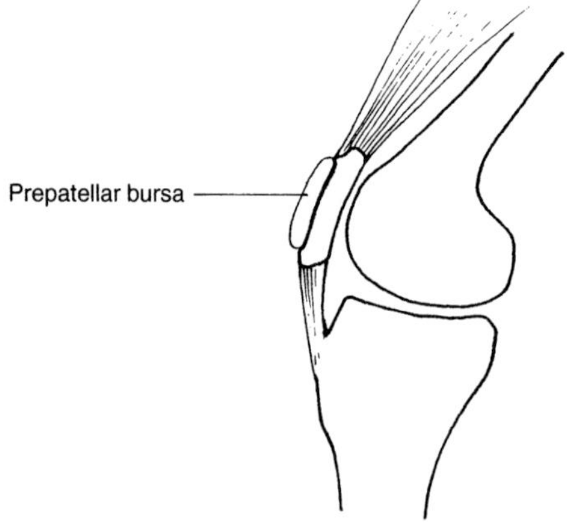


**Fig. 1.** Prepatellar bursitis produces swelling in the bursa directly over the kneecap.

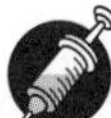

## TREATMENT

### GENERAL MEASURES

- Immobilize the joint in extension (knee immobilizer).
- Treat traumatic and inflammatory bursitis symptomatically with NSAIDs.
- Aspirate the bursa if a septic process is suspected.
- Traumatic injuries often heal spontaneously with:
  - Immobilization
  - NSAIDs
  - Heat or ice for symptomatic relief
- Septic injuries:
  - Immobilize the joint.
  - Aspirate the bursa to identify the infectious organism.
  - Administer parenteral antibiotics.
  - Begin with empiric gram-positive coverage while awaiting culture and sensitivity results.
- Perform incision and drainage of bursa if no improvement occurs in 36–48 hours.

### SPECIAL THERAPY

#### *Physical Therapy*

Therapy is given as needed to regain ROM lost as a result of immobilization and to restore quadriceps strength.

### MEDICATION (DRUGS)

- NSAIDS (traumatic injuries)
- Parenteral antibiotics (septic injuries)

### SURGERY

- Indicated for fibrosis or synovial thickening with painful nodules that fails to respond to medical treatment
- Indicated for septic prepatellar bursitis that does not respond to antibiotics

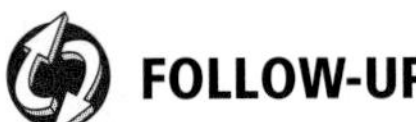

## FOLLOW-UP

### DISPOSITION

#### *Issues for Referral*

Ascending lymphangitis requires hospitalization and intravenous antibiotics.

### PROGNOSIS

Most patients do well with immobilization and NSAIDs.

### COMPLICATIONS

Infection and chronic drainage may occur after repeated aspirations.

### REFERENCES

1. Dlabach JA. Nontraumatic soft tissue disorders. In: Canale ST, ed. *Campbell's Operative Orthopaedics*, 10th ed. St. Louis: Mosby, 2003:885–904.
2. Safran MR, Fu FH. Uncommon causes of knee pain in the athlete. *Orthop Clin North Am* 1995;26: 547–559.
3. McAfee JH, Smith DL. Olecranon and prepatellar bursitis. Diagnosis and treatment. *West J Med* 1988;149:607–610.

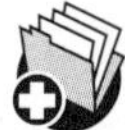

## MISCELLANEOUS

### CODES

#### *ICD9-CM*

726.65 Prepatellar bursitis

### PATIENT TEACHING

- Patients are instructed to avoid provocative activities such as prolonged kneeling.
- Protective coverings over the knee are helpful for patients with occupational exposures.

### FAQ

- Q: How can you differentiate bursal swelling and knee joint effusion?
  - A: Prepatellar bursitis has swelling on top of the patella, making it difficult to palpate the patella. With even a large knee joint effusion, the patella is palpated easily and is ballottable; direct pressure on the patella makes it "bob" on the effusion.
- Q: How can you tell if a prepatellar bursitis is septic?
  - A: The bursa is fluctuant with overlying cellulitis, and it usually is more painful than traumatic or inflammatory bursitis. Definitive diagnosis is made with aspiration of the bursa and analysis of the fluid.

# PUNCTURE WOUNDS OF THE FOOT

*Gregory Gebauer, MD, MS*

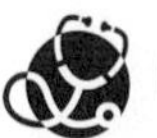

## BASICS

### DESCRIPTION

- Puncture injuries of the foot typically occur on the plantar surface of the forefoot or heel.
- The injuring object usually is a nail, needle, or pin, but it can be anything that punctures the soft tissue, including thorns, glass, and splinters.
- Classification:
  - Early presentation: Day of injury
  - Late presentation: At least 3–5 days after puncture, when deep infection develops

### GENERAL PREVENTION

Avoid going barefoot outdoors or in areas with debris such as wood fragments or nails.

### EPIDEMIOLOGY

- Anecdotally, this injury is more common in children.
- Males are affected more often than females.

#### *Incidence*

- Puncture wounds of the foot constitute 0.5–1% of all emergency room visits by children (1).
- Only 0.6% of children with puncture wounds develop deep infection (1).

### RISK FACTORS

- Walking barefoot
- Construction work

### ETIOLOGY

- The penetrating object carries with it organisms from the soil, the skin, or a sock or shoe sole, if these are worn.
  - *Pseudomonas* and other atypical infections are common.
- Many times, the flora is polymicrobial.
- Usually, the site developing infection is a synovial-lined space such as a tendon sheath, joint, plantar bursa, or bone.

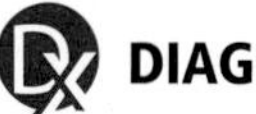

## DIAGNOSIS

### SIGNS AND SYMPTOMS

- Acute phase:
  - Pain
  - Swelling
  - Bleeding
- Late presentation:
  - Redness
  - Tenderness
  - Cellulitis
  - Fluctuance or drainage (purulent or serous)
  - Patient may limp, refuse to bear weight, or walk on the heel to avoid pressure on the forefoot.

#### *History*

- Timing of injury
- Location of injury, degree of environmental contamination
- Absence or presence of shoe wear at time of puncture wound

#### *Physical Exam*

- Early presentation:
  - Inspect to assess the depth, severity, and contamination of the soft tissue.
  - Palpate the area to determine if any evidence of a retained foreign body is present.
  - Evaluate for joint involvement by proximity of the puncture wound and examination of joint ROM.
  - Examine shoe wear for evidence of penetration.
- Late presentation:
  - Evaluate for local and systemic evidence of infection.
    - Erythema
    - Swelling
    - Cellulitis
    - Fluctuance
    - Enlargement of lymph nodes (popliteal, inguinal)
  - Check for pain with ROM of the adjacent joints.
    - MTP joint
    - IP joint
    - Midfoot joint
  - Circumferential or dorsal swelling likely indicates a deep infection.

### TESTS

- Late presentation:
  - Area of infection (joint, bursa or tendon sheath) may be aspirated to obtain Gram stain and culture to identify an organism, which may guide treatment.

#### *Lab*

- Early presentation: Usually not needed
- Late presentation (infection suspected): The following can be helpful, although not specific.
  - White blood cell count with differential
  - ESR
  - C-reactive protein

#### *Imaging*

- Plain radiography:
  - To rule out associated fracture, bony involvement, or retained foreign body
  - In late presentations, also may evaluate for osteomyelitis or gas in tissue
- MRI:
  - May be reserved for difficult cases with deep involvement
  - Can identify abscess, osteomyelitis, and in some cases, retained foreign body
- Ultrasound:
  - Can diagnose abscess
  - Can identify foreign body retained in foot
- Nuclear medicine imaging:
  - Alternative to MRI
  - May help differentiate local inflammation from osteomyelitis

#### *Diagnostic Procedures/Surgery*

Local wound exploration should be performed to determine the extent of the wound and assess for any contamination.

### DIFFERENTIAL DIAGNOSIS

- Osteomyelitis
- Septic arthritis
- Tenosynovitis
- Septic bursitis of the foot
- Cellulitis

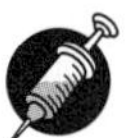

# TREATMENT

## GENERAL MEASURES

- Acute presentation:
  - Local irrigation and débridement are indicated.
  - Debate arises whether prophylactic antibiotics are necessary for patients with acute puncture.
  - Tetanus prophylaxis booster should be given.
  - Instruct the patient to return if signs of deep infection develop.
- Late presentation:
  - Deep infections require surgical irrigation and débridement, and tissue cultures should be obtained.
  - Soft-tissue infections are often Gram-positive *Staphylococcus* or *Streptococcus*, but *Pseudomonas* is not uncommon.
  - If the patient presents with cellulitis, aspiration should be attempted, and the patient should be treated empirically with oral or intravenous therapy for 24 hours with clinical evaluation.
    - If the condition improves, the patient should complete a 5-day course of oral antibiotics.
    - If the condition does not improve, or if *Pseudomonas* is recovered from the aspirate, surgical drainage is preferred.
  - Areas of fluctuance should be incised and drained.
  - For patients with a small, localized abscess that has been drained adequately with no other evidence of infection:
    - Broad-spectrum oral antibiotic coverage probably is adequate initially, but it should be changed to a culture-specific treatment as soon as possible.
    - Weightbearing activity may be resumed as tenderness resolves.

## MEDICATION (DRUGS)

- Acute puncture:
  - Antibiotic treatment remains controversial: It may not be indicated, but a short course may be prudent.
- Late presentation:
  - After aspiration, administer antibiotics that are effective against Gram-positive organisms.
  - Add an antibiotic effective against *Pseudomonas* if this organism is recovered from cultures or if symptoms do not resolve.

## SURGERY

- If needed, the site of infection should be localized by physical examination or plain radiography.
  - Occasionally, MRI is needed.
- The approach should be the most direct to the pathologic features and should follow the tract of the puncture wound, if possible.
- Plantar incisions are acceptable, although they should be positioned to avoid pressure points such as the heel or ball of the foot.
- Thorough débridement should be performed.
- Cultures should be sent for identification, including *Mycobacterium,* if clinically indicated.

# FOLLOW-UP

## PROGNOSIS

- Generally good
- Complications include cellulitis, abscess, osteomyelitis, and septic arthritis.
- The rate of subsequent osteomyelitis is ~0.6–1.8% (1).

## COMPLICATIONS

- Rate of complications in 1 study was 3.2% (1).
- Osteomyelitis (rare)
- Septic arthritis (rare)

## PATIENT MONITORING

Follow-up examination is performed by a primary care physician or a specialist if symptoms persist.

## REFERENCE

1. Fitzgerald RH, Jr, Cowan JD. Puncture wounds of the foot. *Orthop Clin North Am* 1975;6:965–972.

## ADDITIONAL READING

- Fisher MC, Goldsmith JF, Gilligan PH. Sneakers as a source of *Pseudomonas aeruginosa* in children with osteomyelitis following puncture wounds. *J Pediatr* 1985;106:607–609.
- Green NE. Musculoskeletal infections in children. Part IV. *Pseudomonas* infections of the foot following puncture wounds. *Instr Course Lect* 1983; 32:43–46.
- Reichl M. Septic arthritis following puncture wound of the foot. *Arch Emerg Med* 1989;6:277–279.

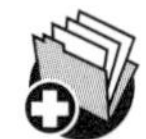

# MISCELLANEOUS

## CODES

### *ICD9-CM*

- 682.7 Cellulitis/abscess foot
- 711.07 Pyogenic arthritis ankle and foot
- 730.07 Acute osteomyelitis ankle and foot

## PATIENT TEACHING

After an acute puncture wound, patients should be instructed about the signs and symptoms of infection and told to return if these occur.

## FAQ

- Q: How should an acute puncture wound be treated?
  - A: Puncture wounds that present early should be thoroughly cleaned and irrigated. Foreign bodies should be removed. Antibiotics are not necessarily required. Wounds that present late with signs of infection require aggressive irrigation and débridement and antibiotic therapy.
- Q: What are the most common pathogens?
  - A: The most common organisms in infected puncture wounds are skin flora, commonly Gram-positive cocci. *Pseudomonas* is not an uncommon pathogen and should be suspected in wounds that fail to respond to initial treatment or that show signs typical of this organism (blue-green tinted, foul-smelling, or musty discharge).

# QUADRICEPS TENDON RUPTURE

*Carl Wierks, MD*
*Michelle Cameron, MD*

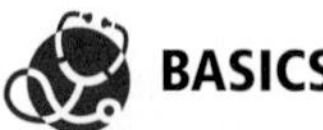

## BASICS

### DESCRIPTION
- Rupture of the quadriceps tendon (knee extensor mechanism) results in an inability to extend the leg.
  - In patients >40 years old, rupture may be secondary to tendon degeneration.
- Classification:
  - Complete versus incomplete

### GENERAL PREVENTION
Stretching before athletics and thigh-strengthening exercises in patients with chronic tendinitis could provide some protection.

### EPIDEMIOLOGY
- A rare occurrence
- Can occur in any age group
- Affects males more than females

### RISK FACTORS
- Trauma, usually in the setting of an underlying chronic tendinitis
- Medical conditions such as renal disease, diabetes mellitus, gout, rheumatoid arthritis, chronic steroid use, obesity, lupus, hyperparathyroidism, and dialysis
- Previous total knee arthroplasty

#### *Genetics*
No known inheritance of predisposition to quadriceps tendon rupture

### ETIOLOGY
- Tendon rupture can occur:
  - During attempts to regain balance to avoid a fall; maximum force can be placed across the quadriceps tendon when eccentric loading is placed on a semiflexed of knee.
  - Secondary to direct or penetrating knee trauma

### ASSOCIATED CONDITIONS
Meniscal or knee ligament damage

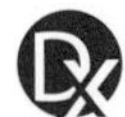

## DIAGNOSIS

### SIGNS AND SYMPTOMS
- Inability to extend the knee actively
- Acute pain
- Suprapatellar gap
- Weak leg extension with partial rupture

#### *History*
- Acute trauma
- Attempt to regain balance before a fall, with a history of a chronic condition or tendinitis

#### *Physical Exam*
- Inability to perform a straight-leg raise
- Inability to actively extend the leg
- Holding the knee in full extension may be possible if the knee retinaculum is intact; patients should be asked to extend the knee from the flexed position.
- Palpation of a gap 1–2 cm proximal to the superior pole of the patellar; examination of the contralateral knee is important.
- Nearly full passive ROM is possible.
- Routine knee ligament examination is performed to ensure that no other damage has occurred.

### TESTS

#### *Imaging*
- Routine AP and lateral radiographs:
  - The patella is displaced distally on lateral radiographs.
  - May see calcifications in the presence of chronic tendinitis
- MRI or ultrasound may be useful when the physical examination is inconclusive.

#### *Pathological Findings*
Degenerative changes are seen in the quadriceps tendon in patients with collagen vascular disease and in persons >40 years.

### DIFFERENTIAL DIAGNOSIS
- Patellar fracture
- Patellar tendon rupture
- Knee ligament injury
- Quadriceps muscle rupture

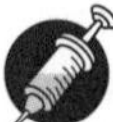

## TREATMENT

### GENERAL MEASURES
- Partial tears with an intact extensor mechanism are rare.
  - Treated nonoperatively
  - The knee is immobilized in full extension with a brace or cast.
  - Protected ROM and strength training is begun after 6 weeks.
  - Weightbearing as tolerated with the knee braced
- Complete tears:
  - Repaired surgically
  - Ideally, operative repair should be performed as soon as possible.
  - Quadriceps ruptures also may require quadriceps lengthening and augmentation because muscle retraction can occur and the muscle can adhere to the femur (tendon cannot be mobilized) (1).
  - Quadriceps sets and straight-leg raises in a knee immobilizer are begun immediately after surgery.

#### *Physical Therapy*
- Therapy is best begun early, 1–2 weeks after repair.
- Passive ROM and active flexion exercises are emphasized.
- May wean from use of the knee brace with improved quadriceps strength (6–8 weeks)

### MEDICATION (DRUGS)
- NSAIDs are helpful for reducing swelling and pain.
- Narcotics may be added for analgesia.

### SURGERY
- Primary end-to-patella repair:
  - Results are better with early intervention.
  - Delayed repairs may require augmentation or interpositional tendon graft.

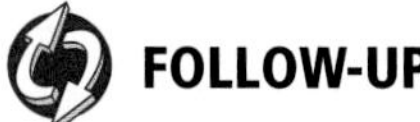

## FOLLOW-UP

### PROGNOSIS
- Results are excellent with appropriate treatment.
- ~90% of patients achieve full or near-full ROM and full or near-full return of preinjury strength (2).

### COMPLICATIONS
- Extensor lag
- Extension weakness
- Tendon rerupture

### PATIENT MONITORING
Patients are followed at 1-month intervals until they attain full ROM and strength, and normal gait and function.

### REFERENCES

1. Scuderi C. Ruptures of the quadriceps tendon: study of twenty tendon ruptures. *Am J Surg* 1958;95:626–634; discussion 634–635.
2. Ilan DI, Tejwani N, Keschner M, et al. Quadriceps tendon rupture. *J Am Acad Orthop Surg* 2003;11: 192–200.


### ADDITIONAL READING

Dobbs RE, Hanssen AD, Lewallen DG, et al. Quadriceps tendon rupture after total knee arthroplasty. Prevalence, complications, and outcomes. *J Bone Joint Surg* 2005;87A:37–45.


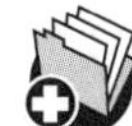

## MISCELLANEOUS

### CODES
***ICD9-CM***

844.8 Quadriceps tendon rupture

### PATIENT TEACHING
- Chronic quadriceps tendinitis should not be ignored because it puts the tendon at risk for rupture with a sudden misstep.
- After surgical repair, patients can recover full motion, strength, and function with an intensive physical therapy program.

### FAQ
- Q: Is quadriceps tendon rupture the only mechanism for losing the ability to extend a flexed knee?
  - A: The extensor mechanism includes the quadriceps muscles, quadriceps tendon, patella, and patellar tendon. All are required to extend the knee forcefully or to perform a straight-leg raise. A rupture of the quadriceps or patellar tendon or a fracture of the patella will make extending the knee difficult.

# RADIAL HEAD DISLOCATION

*Paul D. Sponseller, MD*

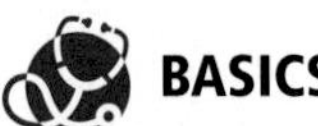

## BASICS

### DESCRIPTION

- Isolated traumatic dislocation of the radial head is a rare injury seen mainly in children, although several reports have described this injury in adults (1–3).
- Congenital and developmental radial head dislocations are seen more commonly, although they rarely are seen in the absence of other congenital abnormalities of the elbow or forearm.
- The radial head may be dislocated anteriorly, anterolaterally, posteriorly, or posterolaterally.
- Classification:
  - Direction of radial head displacement: Anterior, posterior, or lateral
  - Pathogenesis: Traumatic, congenital, or pathologic

### EPIDEMIOLOGY

Radial head dislocations are uncommon injuries, usually occurring with an associated ulna fracture.

### RISK FACTORS

- OI
- Fibrous dysplasia
- Osteochondromas
- Achondroplasia
- Congenital forearm synostosis

#### *Genetics*

No genetic inheritance pattern for radial head dislocation is known, but because the main restraints to radial head dislocation in the normal elbow are ligamentous, children with ligamentous laxity (e.g., achondroplasia) may have a predisposition to such conditions without associated fractures.

### PATHOPHYSIOLOGY

- In the normal elbow, the critical restraint to radial head dislocation is the annular ligament.
  - This ligament usually is torn or severely stretched in the case of a dislocation.
- In the congenitally dislocated radial head, a hypoplastic capitellum and an ovoid radial head are essentially pathognomonic.
- Proximal ulnar bowing also is evident on radiographs, although this finding is not unique to the congenital dislocation.

### ETIOLOGY

The mechanism of injury is believed to be a fall onto the outstretched hand with the elbow extended and the forearm pronated, resulting in a varus stress on the elbow.

### ASSOCIATED CONDITIONS

- In the setting of trauma, this injury may be associated with a proximal ulna fracture, a radial neck fracture, or an elbow dislocation.
- Isolated radial head dislocations, particularly posterior dislocations, may be associated with radial nerve or posterior interosseous nerve stretch injuries.

## DIAGNOSIS

### SIGNS AND SYMPTOMS

- Pain, swelling, and decreased supination or pronation of the forearm are the main symptoms of the traumatic dislocation.
- The congenitally dislocated radial head:
  - Normally is painless in childhood, although it usually is discovered in the young child after elbow trauma
  - Also may come to attention secondary to a painless lateral prominence in the setting of a posterolateral dislocation

#### *Physical Exam*

- Perform a complete neurovascular examination at presentation and before undertaking any manipulations.
- Examine the function of the radial nerve because it may have undergone traction injury.
- Perform an examination of the contralateral elbow to rule out bilateral radial head dislocations, which may suggest a congenital dislocation and pre-existing disease in the affected elbow.
- On physical examination, hold the elbow immobile and flexed with the forearm in pronation.
  - The child often refuses to use the injured arm.
  - The radial head usually can be palpated, particularly with posterior and posterolateral dislocations, in which there is little overlying soft tissue.
  - Nearly full flexion and extension usually are noted, although some limitation often exists at 1 extreme, depending on the direction of the dislocation (mildly limited flexion if anteriorly dislocated and extension if posteriorly dislocated).
  - Supination and pronation are markedly limited and cause pain.

### TESTS

#### *Imaging*

- Radiography:
  - AP and lateral radiographs of the elbow usually are sufficient for making the diagnosis and for assessing reduction.
  - A separate film of the forearm usually is helpful to look for ulnar bowing or shortening, which may contribute to the dislocation.
  - Abnormalities of the capitellum and radial head may suggest a congenital dislocation.
  - Radiographs of the contralateral elbow should be obtained to rule out bilateral involvement, which also would indicate a congenital dislocation.
  - Congenital dislocations may be associated with a dysplastic capitellum, a bowed ulna, a relatively long radius, or an ovoid radial head, but a long-standing traumatic dislocation may have similar radiographic findings unilaterally.
  - Heterotopic ossification in the soft tissues about the radial head may suggest an old, unreduced traumatic dislocation.
- Some authors advocate elbow arthrograms if it is difficult in young children to distinguish between congenital and traumatic causes (4,5).
  - A congenital dislocation would show an ovoid radial head within the joint capsule.
  - A traumatic dislocation would be associated with a normally shaped radial head.
  - In the acute situation, extravasation of the arthrogram's contrast agent occurs.

### DIFFERENTIAL DIAGNOSIS

- Subluxated elbow
- Congenital dislocation
- Monteggia fracture with an occult fracture
- Radial neck fracture
- Generalized disorder (OI, fibrous dysplasia, osteochondromas)

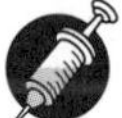

## TREATMENT

### GENERAL MEASURES

- It is important to distinguish a traumatic from a congenital dislocation because the latter does not require treatment.
- If the condition is judged to be an acute, traumatic dislocation, closed reduction usually can be performed in the acute setting.
  - With gentle traction and the elbow in full extension, varus stress is applied to the elbow joint.
  - The forearm is supinated while direct pressure is applied to the radial head to reduce it.
  - The reduction then is held in 120° of flexion for children (90° and in supination for adults).
  - A posterior splint usually suffices, although a bivalved cast may be necessary in the young child who may remove the splint.
- If the injury is >7 days old, open reduction may be necessary if closed reduction is unsuccessful.
  - After 3 weeks, a successful closed reduction is impossible, and open technique is universally required.
  - For long-standing traumatic dislocations (>2–3 years), deformation of the radial head and capitellum may occur, which would preclude a stable reduction.

### SPECIAL THERAPY

#### *Physical Therapy*

- Full, pain-free ROM of the elbow (flexion, extension, supination, and pronation) are the goals of treatment of this injury.
- Elbow ROM exercises are begun as early as possible without compromising the stability of the joint.
- The pediatric elbow is more forgiving than the adult's with respect to regaining full ROM after prolonged immobilization.

### MEDICATION (DRUGS)

#### *First Line*

- Symptomatic treatment for pain is suggested.
- Analgesia is a necessary part of rehabilitation after surgery or cast immobilization.
- In a patient with a history of heterotopic ossification or neurologic injury (which may predispose to heterotopic ossification), prophylaxis with indomethacin may decrease the incidence of heterotopic ossification of the elbow (1,6).

### SURGERY

- In the unstable reduction, a prolonged period of immobilization may be necessary to allow for fibrous tissue to confer stability.
  - Occasionally, the immobilization may be augmented by a Kirschner wire across the radiocapitellar joint.
- When elbow contractures are of concern (in patients >30 years old, particularly the elderly) or in patients with long-standing dislocations, a radial head resection may be performed to begin early ROM of the elbow.
- With open reduction of the radiocapitellar joint, most surgeons advocate repair or reconstruction of the annular ligament.
  - May be performed successfully up to 2 years or more after traumatic dislocation
  - Any ulnar bowing should be addressed at the same time.

## FOLLOW-UP

### PROGNOSIS

- The prognosis is excellent for a functional ROM of the elbow, forearm, and wrist, particularly in patients <30 years old.
- Mild ROM restrictions may be present compared with the contralateral side but usually none that would be noted by the patient.

### COMPLICATIONS

- Recurrent dislocations
- Decreased ROM secondary to contracture or heterotopic ossification
- Radial or posterior interosseous nerve palsies and degenerative changes of the radiohumeral joint

### PATIENT MONITORING

Patients are followed at 1-month intervals until they regain their ROM.

### REFERENCES


1. Belangero WD, Livani B, Zogaib RK. Treatment of chronic radial head dislocations in children. *Int Orthop* 2006; Epub (DOI: 10.1007/s00264-006-0153-4):1–4.
2. Burgess RC, Sprague HH. Post-traumatic posterior radial head subluxation. Two case reports. *Clin Orthop Relat Res* 1984;186:192–194.
3. Salama R, Wientroub S, Weissman SL. Recurrent dislocation of the head of the radius. *Clin Orthop Relat Res* 1977;125:156–158.
4. Thompson GH. Dislocations of the elbow. In: Beaty JH, Kasser JR, eds. *Rockwood and Wilkins' Fractures in Children*, 5th ed. Philadelphia: Lippincott-Raven, 2001:705–739.
5. Beaty JH, Kasser JR. The elbow: Physeal fractures, apophyseal injuries of the distal humerus, avascular necrosis of the trochlea, and T-condylar fractures. In: Beaty JH, Kasser JR, eds. *Rockwood and Wilkins' Fractures in Children*, 5th ed. Philadelphia: Lippincott Williams & Wilkins, 2001:625–703.
6. Kim HT, Park BG, Suh JT, et al. Chronic radial head dislocation in children, Part 2: Results of open treatment and factors affecting final outcome. *J Pediatr Orthop* 2002;22:591–597.


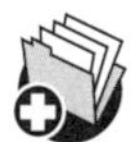

## MISCELLANEOUS

### CODES

#### *ICD9-CM*

832.9 Dislocation of radial head

### PATIENT TEACHING

- Patients are instructed on the need for home ROM exercises.
- Patients also are told that they may lose 10° of elbow extension.

### FAQ

- Q: What are the signs of a radial head dislocation?
  - A: A bony prominence anteriorly (with block to full flexion) or posteriorly (with block to full extension).
- Q: Is surgery indicated for a radial head dislocation?
  - A: Usually a closed reduction can be undertaken within the 1st few weeks after injury. If closed reduction fails, or the dislocation is detected late, then surgery is indicated.

# RADIAL HEAD FRACTURE

*John H. Wilckens, MD*
*Michelle Cameron, MD*

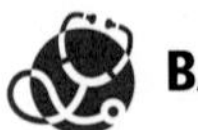

## BASICS

### DESCRIPTION
- Radial head fractures:
  - Occur in the proximal 2–3 cm of the radius
  - Are intra-articular fractures (The radial head articulates with capitellum.)
- Classification (1):
  - Type 1: Nondisplaced fractures
  - Type 2: Partial head fractures
  - Type 3: Complete head fractures
- Radial head fractures often are associated with other injuries to the elbow or the forearm.

### EPIDEMIOLOGY
#### *Incidence*
- Fractures can occur in any age group.
- In 1 series of 333 fractures (2):
  - 67% of fractures were Mason type 1, 14% were type 2, and 19% were type 3.
  - Ligamentous injuries requiring repair were found in 13% of patients.

### ETIOLOGY
- This fracture generally results from a fall on the outstretched hand with the forearm in pronation.
- The position of the elbow and forearm at the time of injury directly affects the injury pattern (3).

### ASSOCIATED CONDITIONS
- Elbow dislocation
- Carpal fractures
- Wrist fractures
- Olecranon fracture dislocation (the posterior Monteggia lesion)
- Radial head dislocation
- Rupture of the MCL
- Elbow instability secondary to extensive damage to soft-tissue restraints

## DIAGNOSIS

### SIGNS AND SYMPTOMS
- Tenderness or swelling over the lateral surface of the elbow
- Painful ROM of the elbow
- Elbow hemarthrosis

#### *Physical Exam*
- Examine for range of supination and pronation and for elbow flexion and extension.
- Because of the mechanism of injury, include examination of the wrist and hand.
- Assess carefully the neurovascular status of the forearm and hand.
- If the patient has tenderness of the interosseous membrane and distal radioulnar joint, an Essex-Lopresti injury should be considered.
  - This injury involves a radial head fracture combined with an intraosseous membrane disruption and distal radial ulnar joint dislocation.
  - The radius pull test may help diagnose ligamentous injury (4).
- If a fracture occurs with an elbow dislocation, determine the ROM at which the elbow is stable.

### TESTS
#### *Imaging*
- Radiography:
  - Obtain routine AP and lateral radiographs of the elbow.
    - Occult or nondisplaced radial neck fractures may have no bony findings.
    - A "posterior fat pad sign" and "anterior sail sign" suggest a hemarthrosis and radial head/neck injury (5).
  - A radiocapitellar view may be necessary to identify nondisplaced fractures or to characterize additionally displaced or comminuted fractures.
- Comminuted fractures with associated injury may require a CT or MRI scan for identification of the abnormality and for preoperative planning.

#### *Diagnostic Procedures/Surgery*
- It is important to determine whether the fracture blocks motion of the elbow.
- Aspiration of the joint with injection of lidocaine gives pain relief and allows for examination.
  - For aspiration, insert a needle on the lateral side of the elbow in the center of a triangle formed by the radial head, the tip of the olecranon, and the lateral epicondyle.

### DIFFERENTIAL DIAGNOSIS
- Distal humerus fracture
- Radial head dislocation

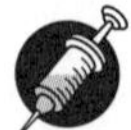

## TREATMENT

### GENERAL MEASURES
- For nondisplaced or minimally displaced fractures: Early mobilization (6)
- Fractures involving >1/3 of the articular surface: Splint for 1–2 weeks, followed by protected ROM for 7–10 days.
- Moderately displaced or comminuted fractures or those with fragments blocking ROM at the elbow: Surgical repair (open reduction with internal fixation or excision of the radial head)

#### *Activity*
- For nondisplaced or minimally displaced fractures, active and passive ROM should begin shortly after injury.
- Patients with moderately displaced or severely comminuted fractures should begin active and passive ROM as soon as tolerated.

### SPECIAL THERAPY
#### *Physical Therapy*
- Decreased ROM and muscle strength are common sequelae of elbow immobilization after radial head fractures.
- Therefore, it is important to begin active and passive ROM exercises as soon as tolerated.

### MEDICATION (DRUGS)
#### *First Line*
NSAIDs and acetaminophen

#### *Second Line*
Narcotics

### SURGERY
- Fixation of moderately displaced fractures usually is accomplished with the use of small-diameter screws.
- Comminuted fractures are treated with internal fixation, if possible.
  - Results after internal fixation have been shown to be better than those after resection (7).
  - With >4 fracture fragments, fracture fixation is more difficult and results are poorer (8).
- If resection is necessary, it may be performed early or late (9).
  - In general, results of resection are good except when other injuries or elbow dislocation have occurred.
  - A prosthetic head may be placed in the presence of an elbow fracture/dislocation.
- Complex elbow dislocations with ligamentous injury and radial head fracture should be treated with ligament repair, coronoid repair, and either repair or replacement of the radial head fracture so that early mobilization can be achieved (10).

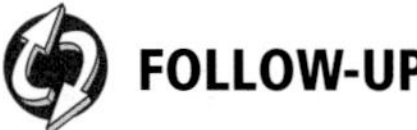

# FOLLOW-UP

## PROGNOSIS

- Nondisplaced fractures treated with mobilization have a good prognosis (11).
- Displaced fractures:
  - Results usually are good.
  - Excellent results have been reported with mobilization and no surgery if fracture displacement is <4 mm (12).
  - Long-term results after fixation of displaced fractures with few fracture fragments are good (13).
- The prognosis for recovery of full elbow function is inversely proportional to the degree of comminution and the extent of associated ligamentous injuries.
- In patients treated with radial head excision, the more severe injuries had a worse prognosis (14).
- Radial head replacement also gives good results (15).
  - The exact sizing of the replacement is important for reconstruction of the radiohumeral joint (16).
- Long-term results in children after radial head fracture treatment are good (17).

## COMPLICATIONS

- Decreased elbow ROM
- Elbow arthritis
- Malunion
- Nonunion
- Elbow instability

## PATIENT MONITORING

It is important to document preoperative and postoperative neurovascular status and ROM.

## REFERENCES


1. Mason ML. Some observations on fractures of the head of the radius with a review of one hundred cases. *Br J Surg* 1954;42:123–132.
2. van Riet RP, Morrey BF, O'Driscoll SW, et al. Associated injuries complicating radial head fractures: a demographic study. *Clin Orthop Relat Res* 2005;441:351–355.
3. McGinley JC, Hopgood BC, Gaughan JP, et al. Forearm and elbow injury: the influence of rotational position. *J Bone Joint Surg* 2003;85A: 2403–2409.
4. Smith AM, Urbanosky LR, Castle JA, et al. Radius pull test: predictor of longitudinal forearm instability. *J Bone Joint Surg* 2002;84A: 1970–1976.
5. O'Dwyer H, O'Sullivan P, Fitzgerald D, et al. The fat pad sign following elbow trauma in adults: its usefulness and reliability in suspecting occult fracture. *J Comput Assist Tomogr* 2004;28: 562–565.
6. Unsworth-White J, Koka R, Churchill M, et al. The non-operative management of radial head fractures: a randomized trial of three treatments. *Injury* 1994;25:165–167.
7. Ikeda M, Sugiyama K, Kang C, et al. Comminuted fractures of the radial head. Comparison of resection and internal fixation. *J Bone Joint Surg* 2005;87:76–84.
8. Ring D, Quintero J, Jupiter JB. Open reduction and internal fixation of fractures of the radial head. *J Bone Joint Surg* 2002;84A:1811–1815.
9. Broberg MA, Morrey BF. Results of delayed excision of the radial head after fracture. *J Bone Joint Surg* 1986;68A:669–674.
10. Pugh DMW, Wild LM, Schemitsch EH, et al. Standard surgical protocol to treat elbow dislocations with radial head and coronoid fractures. *J Bone Joint Surg* 2004;86A: 1122–1130.
11. Herbertsson P, Josefsson PO, Hasserius R, et al. Displaced Mason type I fractures of the radial head and neck in adults: a fifteen- to thirty-three-year follow-up study. *J Shoulder Elbow Surg* 2005;14:73–77.
12. Akesson T, Herbertsson P, Josefsson PO, et al. Displaced fractures of the neck of the radius in adults: an excellent long-term outcome. *J Bone Joint Surg* 2006;88B:642–644.
13. Herbertsson P, Josefsson PO, Hasserius R, et al. Uncomplicated Mason type-II and III fractures of the radial head and neck in adults. A long-term follow-up study. *J Bone Joint Surg* 2004;86A: 569–574.
14. Herbertsson P, Josefsson PO, Hasserius R, et al. Fractures of the radial head and neck treated with radial head excision. *J Bone Joint Surg* 2004;86A:1925–1930.
15. Ashwood N, Bain GI, Unni R. Management of Mason type-III radial head fractures with a titanium prosthesis, ligament repair, and early mobilization. *J Bone Joint Surg* 2004;86A: 274–280.
16. Van Glabbeek F, van Riet RP, Baumfeld JA, et al. Detrimental effects of overstuffing or understuffing with a radial head replacement in the medial collateral-ligament deficient elbow. *J Bone Joint Surg* 2004;86A:2629–2635.
17. Malmvik J, Herbertsson P, Josefsson PO, et al. Fracture of the radial head and neck of Mason types II and III during growth: a 14–25 year follow-up. *J Pediatr Orthop B* 2003;12:63–68.


## ADDITIONAL READING


- McKee MD, Jupiter JB. Trauma to the adult elbow and fractures of the distal humerus. In: Browner BD, Jupiter JB, Levine AM, et al., eds. *Skeletal Trauma: Basic Science, Management, and Reconstruction*, 3rd ed. Philadelphia: WB Saunders, 2003: 1404–1480.
- Tashjian RZ, Katarincic JA. Complex elbow instability. *J Am Acad Orthop Surg* 2006;14: 278–286.


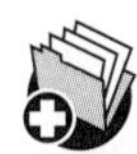

# MISCELLANEOUS

## CODES

### *ICD9-CM*

- 813.05 Radial head fracture
- 832.00 Elbow dislocation

## PATIENT TEACHING

Elbow stiffness can occur even with a perfect surgical result.

### *Activity*

- Early ROM should be used.
- Care should be taken to mobilize the shoulder, wrist, and hand to avoid stiffness.

### *Prevention*

The use of protective elbow pads is encouraged with skating and other sports in which falls are likely.

## FAQ

- Q: How long should patients with a nominally displaced radial head be immobilized?
  - A: In general, if the elbow is stable, early ROM as tolerated is advocated with the use of a sling and/or posterior splint for early pain control.
- Q: If a patient has a comminuted radial head fracture that cannot be stabilized with internal fixation, when should head excision be considered?
  - A: Such a patient may have associated elbow instability or an Essex-Lopresti injury. Early head excision may complicate these 2 conditions. Because the results of late radial head excision are superior to those of early excision, delay in excision is recommended. In the context of a grossly unstable elbow or Essex-Lopresti lesion in a patient for whom early excision is indicated because of motion problems, a radial head prosthesis should be inserted.

# REACTIVE ARTHRITIS

*Chris Hutchins, MD*
*Derek F. Papp, MD*

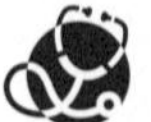

## BASICS

### DESCRIPTION

- Reactive arthritis (previously called Reiter syndrome) is a form of reactive, inflammatory arthritis classically associated with urogenital, ocular, mucocutaneous, and musculoskeletal involvement.
- This syndrome is categorized with the group of seronegative arthritides, along with AS, psoriatic arthritis, and enteropathic arthritis.
- Diagnosis often is overlooked because of its variable presentation and the similarities with other seronegative arthritides and with gonococcal arthritis.
- At examination, the classic triad of symptoms—urethritis (or cervicitis in females), conjunctivitis, and arthritis—often is not present or the symptoms of the urethritis or conjunctivitis are mild and not recognized or described by the patient.
- Moreover, cervicitis often is asymptomatic, thus making the probability of missing the diagnosis in females even greater.

### GENERAL PREVENTION

- Barrier methods of contraception to prevent transmission of venereal disease
- Proper food handling and preparation to prevent food-borne infection

### EPIDEMIOLOGY

Mean age of onset in 1 study was 38 years (1).

#### *Incidence*

- The incidence of reactive arthritis is unknown and appears to depend on the population studied.
- Affects whites more than other racial groups because of the former's higher frequency of the HLA-B27 gene.
- In Rochester, MN, the incidence in males <50 years old was 3.5 per 100,000 (2).

### RISK FACTORS

- HIV
- HLA-B27 haplotype
- Poor hygiene with associated exposure to enteric pathogens
- Increased sexual activity and thus wider exposure to sexually transmitted pathogens
- Geographic location, although this may be related to hygienic conditions and sexual behavior of the population

#### *Genetics*

- HLA-B27 gene: 60% of patients (3):
  - Persons with this gene are thought to be more susceptible to the disease.
  - 80% of affected individuals have this haplotype (4).

### ETIOLOGY

- The cause of the disease is thought to be an immune response to a sexually transmitted bacterial infection or to bacterial gastroenteritis.
- Most cases are transmitted sexually, as opposed to enterically.
- Organisms that have been associated with the disease include the following:
  - *Chlamydia:*
    - *Chlamydia trachomatis* and *Chlamydia psittaci*
    - Recent evidence shows that *Chlamydia pneumoniae* may be implicated (5).
  - *Campylobacter fetus or Campylobacter fetus jejuni*
  - *Salmonella enteritidis, Salmonella heidelberg, or Salmonella paratyphi*
  - *Shigella flexneri*
  - *Ureaplasma urealyticum*
  - *Yersinia enterocolitica* or *Yersinia pseudotuberculosis*
  - *Giardia lamblia*
  - *Cryptosporidium*

### ASSOCIATED CONDITIONS

HIV syndromes

## DIAGNOSIS

### SIGNS AND SYMPTOMS

- The onset of the disease process generally occurs 2–4 weeks after enteric or sexually transmitted infection.
- Urethritis (classic presentation):
  - Often the initial feature of the disease
  - Males experience mild dysuria and/or a mucopurulent urethral discharge.
  - Females may have dysuria, vaginal discharge, with or without purulent cervicitis/vaginitis.
  - Genitourinary symptoms may evolve after sexual or enteric exposure.
- Conjunctivitis in 30–50% of patients (4):
  - Usually bilateral and can be as mild as onset of crusting of the eyelids each morning
  - As such, often unnoticed by patient and physician
  - Ocular involvement occurs along with urethral involvement, or within a few days of onset.
  - Less commonly seen but much more serious is unilateral, acute uveitis with associated severe ocular erythema and photophobia (6).
- Articular involvement:
  - Most commonly includes acute oligoarticular arthritis with effusion, marked tenderness, and overlying erythema; a marked blue discoloration also appears sometimes.
  - Pain on active and passive ROM
  - The average number of joints involved is 4:
    - 1 or 2 joints have more severe involvement than do the others.
  - Typically involves lower extremities (knees, ankles, feet) asymmetrically, although upper extremity involvement may be present.
  - Axial involvement, with spondylitis or sacroiliitis:
    - Much more common in the chronic form
  - Rarely involves hip
  - Back pain and buttock pain are common.
- Enthesopathies:
  - An enthesis is an insertion of a tendon or ligament into bone.
  - Very commonly involves the insertion of the Achilles tendon into the calcaneus or the plantar aponeurosis, causing characteristic heel pain
  - Involvement of the extensor hallucis longus or extensor digitorum longus tendons gives rise to "sausage toes," a characteristic of reactive or psoriatic arthritis.
  - Although severe, the condition usually lasts only days to weeks before resolving.
- Skin and mucous membrane involvement occur weeks after the inciting infection in 1 of several typical lesions.
  - In keratoderma blennorrhagica, clear vesicles erupt on the palms and soles, then crust, forming hyperkeratotic lesions that look similar to psoriasis.
  - Circinate balanitis is marked by small vesicles about the margins of the glans penis that are painless and self-limited.
  - Small, painless, shallow erosions occur in the buccal mucosa.
  - Fingernails and toenails are opaque and thickened, and can crumble and resemble mycotic infection.

#### *History*

- The triad of urethritis, conjunctivitis, and arthritis is present in <1/3 of affected persons on examination.
- Therefore, emphasis on the history—especially sexual history—is crucial!

#### *Physical Exam*

- Given the often mild presentation, a thorough urogenital examination is important, especially in females.
- All involved joints should be examined for the presence of effusion, surrounding erythema, and pain on passive and/or active ROM.
- ROM of the lumbar spine

### TESTS

#### *Lab*

- Positive HLA-B27 haplotype
- Elevated ESR
- Elevated C-reactive protein
- Elevated C3 and C4 complement levels
- Moderate leukocytosis with left shift
- Mild anemia
- Negative antinuclear antibody and rheumatoid factor
- Joint fluid aspirate generally reveals an elevated white blood cell count with values from 500–50,000 with predominantly neutrophils.
- Normal glucose and negative cultures, despite increased protein levels in the synovial fluid
- Urethral swabs, cervical brushings, or fecal samples may be analyzed for chlamydial ribonucleic acid.
- Sterile pyuria can be seen on 1st-voided morning urine sample.

#### *Imaging*

- Radiographs are essential for documenting joint destruction: Obtain AP and lateral films.
- Look for joint destruction, which may manifest as degenerative changes on either side of the involved joint and deformity.
- Periosteal reactions indicating enthesitis can be seen at tendon insertions.

### DIFFERENTIAL DIAGNOSIS

- The differential diagnosis must include the other seronegative spondyloarthropathies: Psoriatic arthritis; AS; enteropathic arthritis
- Psoriatic arthritis often presents with sausage digits, and enteropathic arthritis may be associated with gastrointestinal symptoms.
- The differential diagnosis also must include gonococcal arthritis, which may present with urethritis and is associated with a positive sexual history.

## TREATMENT

### GENERAL MEASURES

Treatment is 2-fold, aimed at relieving the symptoms and eradicating the infection to prevent chronic reactive arthritis.

#### *Activity*

- To prevent muscle atrophy or contractures, prolonged bed rest should be avoided.
- Activity should be advanced as tolerated.

### SPECIAL THERAPY

#### *Physical Therapy*

A physical therapy program aimed at maintaining ROM should be instituted gradually.

### MEDICATION (DRUGS)

#### *First Line*

- NSAIDs:
  - Indomethacin (25–50 mg orally 4 times daily)
  - Sulfasalazine (2 g/day)
- Steroids:
  - Intra-articular injection of steroids may be helpful.
  - Cutaneous lesions can be controlled with topical corticosteroids.
  - Limited scientific evidence suggests that long-term treatment with antibiotics is effective in shortening the acute course of the disease or in preventing chronic disease.
- Antibiotics: Treatment of bacterial infections such as *Chlamydia* may help lessen chronic sequelae (7).

#### *Second Line*

- Immunosuppressive agents:
  - Drugs such as methotrexate should be reserved for patients with severe, unremitting symptoms.
  - Disease-modifying agents such as TNF inhibitors may offer hope in the future for those affected with chronic disease.

### SURGERY

Occasionally, arthroplasty is necessary.

## FOLLOW-UP

Patients are followed-up at 3–6-month intervals, depending on the severity of their symptoms.

### DISPOSITION

#### *Issues for Referral*

Joint destruction

### PROGNOSIS

- The arthritis typically resolves over several months to a year and leaves no disability.
- 15% of patients have chronic disease, typically marked by chronic joint discomfort with occasional exacerbations that are less severe than the initial presentation (8).
  - Chronic arthritis may lead to permanent joint destruction and deformity.

### COMPLICATIONS

Chronic arthritis may occur.

### REFERENCES


1. Savolainen E, Kaipiainen-Seppanen O, Kroger L, et al. Total incidence and distribution of inflammatory joint diseases in a defined population: results from the Kuopio 2000 arthritis survey. *J Rheumatol* 2003;30:2460–2468.
2. Michet CJ, Machado EBV, Ballard DJ, et al. Epidemiology of Reiter's syndrome in Rochester, Minnesota: 1950–1980. *Arthritis Rheum* 1988; 31:428–431.
3. Ozgul A, Dede I, Taskaynatan MA, et al. Clinical presentations of chlamydial and non-chlamydial reactive arthritis. *Rheumatol Int* 2006;24:1–7.
4. Kataria RK, Brent LH. Spondyloarthropathies. *Am Fam Physician* 2004;69:2853–2860.
5. Reveille JD, Arnett FC, Keat A, et al. Seronegative spondyloarthropathies. In: Klippel JH, ed. *Primer on the Rheumatic Diseases*, 12th ed. Atlanta: Arthritis Foundation, 2001:239–258.
6. Kiss S, Letko E, Qamruddin S, et al. Long-term progression, prognosis, and treatment of patients with recurrent ocular manifestations of Reiter's syndrome. *Ophthalmology* 2003;110:1764–1769.
7. Carter JD, Valeriano J, Vasey FB. Doxycycline versus doxycycline and rifampin in undifferentiated spondyloarthropathy, with special reference to chlamydia-induced arthritis. A prospective, randomized 9-month comparison. *J Rheumatol* 2004;31:1973–1980.
8. Colmegna I, Espinoza LR. Recent advances in reactive arthritis. *Curr Rheumatol Rep* 2005;7: 201–207.


### ADDITIONAL READING


Petersel DL, Sigal LH. Reactive arthritis. *Infect Dis Clin North Am* 2005;19:863–883.


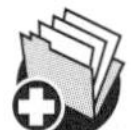

## MISCELLANEOUS

### CODES

#### *ICD9-CM*

099.3 Reiter syndrome

### PATIENT TEACHING

#### *Prevention*

- Prevent sexually acquired disease by using condoms.
- Prevent food-borne infection by following proper food-preparation techniques.

### FAQ

- Q: How often does reactive arthritis lead to chronic problems?
  - A: ~15% of people develop chronic disease; only 20% of those develop chronic arthritis.

R

# RHEUMATOID ARTHRITIS

*Gregory Gebauer, MD, MS*
*John J. Hwang, MD*

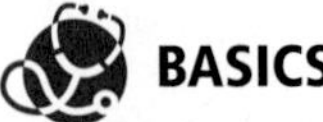

## BASICS

### DESCRIPTION
Rheumatoid arthritis is a chronic, systemic, autoimmune inflammatory disease affecting synovial joints and extra-articular systems, including the skin, eyes, cardiovascular system, bronchopulmonary system, spleen, and nervous system.

### EPIDEMIOLOGY
#### *Incidence*
Affects 1% of the population (1)

#### *Prevalence*
- Variable onset, but most frequently between the ages of 35 and 50 years
- Females are affected 2–3 times more frequently than are males (1).

### RISK FACTORS
- Genetic predisposition is a risk factor.
- A higher risk also exists among certain Native American populations.

#### *Genetics*
Family studies indicate a genetic predisposition, although it is multifactorial.

### ETIOLOGY
- T-cell–mediated disease of unknown origin
- Probably a combination of genetic predisposition and environmental factors causing a systemic autoimmune disorder

### ASSOCIATED CONDITIONS
- Felty syndrome
- Chronic rheumatoid arthritis
- Splenomegaly
- Neutropenia
- On occasion, anemia and thrombocytopenia

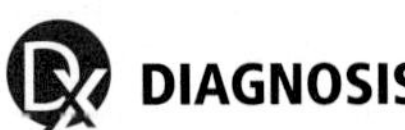

## DIAGNOSIS

The diagnosis of rheumatoid arthritis is often complex and requires the integration of history, physical examination, and laboratory studies.

### SIGNS AND SYMPTOMS
- Rheumatoid arthritis is characteristically bilateral and symmetric.
- Initial symptoms include swelling and morning stiffness lasting up to 1 hour or more.
- In 2/3 of patients, symptoms begin with fatigue, anorexia, generalized weakness, and vague musculoskeletal symptoms until synovitis becomes apparent.
- Pain, swelling, and tenderness are localized to the joints; pain is aggravated by movement.
- Typically, the wrist and MCP joints are affected 1st, followed by PIP and then DIP involvement.
- Synovitis of the wrist is an almost uniform feature.
- An isolated foot problem, such as nonspecific inflammation of forefoot or hind foot, may be the only symptom in early stages of the disease.
- Extra-articular manifestations include:
  - Rheumatoid nodules
  - Rheumatoid vasculitis
  - Pleuropulmonary disease
  - Neuropathy
  - Pericarditis
  - Osteoporosis
  - Congestive heart failure
- Deformities of the wrists and hand occur late, after the hypertrophic synovium has destroyed the capsuloligamentous structures.
- Chronic, progressive deformities of ulnar subluxation occur at the MCP joints.
- The deformities in the digits are caused by displacement or rupture of the normal tendon anatomy.

#### *History*
The disease often is insidious in onset, with the gradual development of generalized symptoms and joint aches and stiffness.

#### *Physical Exam*
- The presentation of patients with rheumatoid arthritis and other inflammatory arthropathies is variable and subtle.
- Important aspects on the physical examination include:
  - Joint effusion
  - Boggy synovium
  - Ulnar drift of the fingers (Fig. 1)
  - Subluxation of the MCP joint
  - Painful, restricted ROM of joints

### TESTS
#### *Lab*
- No test is specific for the diagnosis, although serum rheumatoid factor is present in 2/3 of patients.
- Normochromic, normocytic anemia occurs.
- Increased ESR and C-reactive protein are seen in nearly all patients.
  - These levels can be followed as a marker of disease progression and the efficacy of therapy.
- Synovial fluid analysis confirms an inflammatory arthritis, but it is nonspecific.
- Additional rheumatologic studies, including hepatitis profile, antinucleic antibodies, anti-double-stranded DNA, anti-Smith (and anti-Jo-1 antibodies), also should be analyzed to exclude the possibility of other rheumatologic processes.

#### *Imaging*
- Imaging is not helpful early in the disease, but, as the disease progresses, loss of articular cartilage, bone erosions, and juxtaarticular osteopenia are seen on roentgenograms of the affected joints.
- Plain radiographs show subluxed or dislocated MCP or PIP joints.

#### *Pathological Findings*
Chronic inflammation of the synovial tissue with subsequent bone and cartilage destruction.

### DIFFERENTIAL DIAGNOSIS
- Osteoarthritis
- Acute rheumatic fever
- Ochronosis
- Systemic lupus erythematosus
- Polymyalgia rheumatica
- Juvenile rheumatoid arthritis
- Spondyloarthropathies
- Psoriatic arthritis
- Infectious arthritis

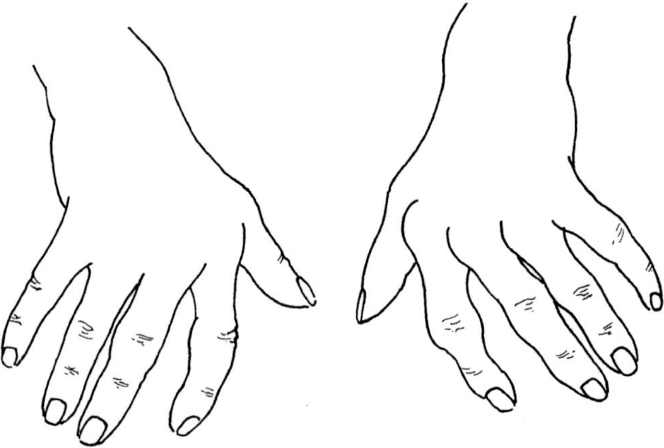

**Fig. 1.** The hand in rheumatoid arthritis is characterized by MCP fullness and ulnar deviation.

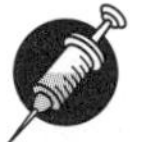

# TREATMENT

## GENERAL MEASURES
- Early involvement of a rheumatologist can be helpful in making the diagnosis and managing the patient.
- Management involves an interdisciplinary approach to relieve pain, reduce inflammation, and maintain function.
- Multiple classes of medication may be used alone or in combination to decrease inflammation and help control pain.
- Surgical treatment should be considered at any time to maximize the treatment.
- Any patient who may need surgery must have a thorough examination of the cervical spine (2).
  - The cervical spine is involved in up to 90% of patients with rheumatoid arthritis.
  - Instability of the cervical spine, including atlantoaxial subluxation and basilar invagination, is a common result of pannus formation, with bone erosion and ligament attenuation.

### *Activity*
The patient's activities should be as-tolerated, and patients are encouraged to have as active a lifestyle as possible.

## SPECIAL THERAPY
### *Physical Therapy*
- To maintain strength and ROM of affected joints
- Does not modify the natural history of the disease process

### *Complementary and Alternative Therapies*
Additional research is needed to determine if complementary approaches are effective in the treatment of rheumatoid arthritis (3).

## MEDICATION (DRUGS) (4)
- The goal of medication is to decrease inflammation, preserve joint function, and reduce pain.
- Many of these medications require careful monitoring of the patient.

### *First Line*
- NSAIDs
- Glucocorticoids
- Methotrexate

### *Second Line*
- Anti-TNF agents
- Immunosuppressive medications, such as azathioprine and cyclophosphamide
- Disease-modifying drugs, such as gold compounds, d-penicillamine, antimalarial agents, and sulfasalazine

## SURGERY
- Synovectomy has been useful in some patients with persistent pain secondary to severe synovitis when no substantial joint destruction is present.
- Early tenosynovectomy of certain joints prevents tendon rupture.
- In patients with severely destroyed joints, arthroplasties and total joint replacements have been successful in relieving pain, especially in the hips and knees.
- Selected fusion in the foot and ankle also is effective in relieving pain and in improving walking ability (5).
- Treatment of rheumatoid hand disorders is complex and involves realignment, arthroplasty, tendon repair, and fusion (6).

# FOLLOW-UP

## DISPOSITION
### *Issues for Referral*
- A multidisciplinary approach to the patient should be used.
  - In addition to the patient's primary physician, rheumatology and orthopaedics should be involved, as well as other specialties as needed.

## PROGNOSIS
- No cure exists for rheumatoid arthritis; the goal is management and delay of disease progression.
- Some surgical treatment (e.g., synovectomy in the upper extremity) can slow the progression of disease.
- Fluctuating disease activity makes prediction of disease behavior difficult.
- At 10–12 years after diagnosis, <20% of patients have no evidence of disability or deformity (7)
- Median life expectancy is shortened by 3–7 years (1).

## COMPLICATIONS
- Variable, depending on the treatment chosen
- A complication of newer TNF inhibitors is serious infection (8).

## PATIENT MONITORING
- Monitoring occurs on an individual basis and also depends on treatment.
- Several medications used in the treatment of rheumatoid arthritis require close monitoring.

## REFERENCES

1. Alamanos Y, Drosos AA. Epidemiology of adult rheumatoid arthritis. *Autoimmun Rev* 2005;4: 130–136.
2. Kim DH, Hilibrand AS. Rheumatoid arthritis in the cervical spine. *J Am Acad Orthop Surg* 2005;13: 463–474.
3. Ernst E. Musculoskeletal conditions and complementary/alternative medicine. *Best Pract Res Clin Rheumatol* 2004;18:539–556.
4. American College of Rheumatology Subcommittee on Rheumatoid Arthritis Guidelines. Guidelines for the management of rheumatoid arthritis: 2002 update. *Arthritis Rheum* 2002;46:328–346.
5. Jaakkola JI, Mann RA. A review of rheumatoid arthritis affecting the foot and ankle. *Foot Ankle Int* 2004;25:866–874.
6. Ghattas L, Mascella F, Pomponio G. Hand surgery in rheumatoid arthritis: state of the art and suggestions for research. *Rheumatology* 2005;44: 834–845.
7. Goronzy JJ, Weyand CM, Anderson RJ, et al. Rheumatoid arthritis. In: Klippel JH, ed. *Primer on the Rheumatic Diseases*, 12th ed. Atlanta: Arthritis Foundation, 2001:209–232.
8. Bongartz T, Sutton AJ, Sweeting MJ, et al. Anti-TNF antibody therapy in rheumatoid arthritis and the risk of serious infections and malignancies: systematic review and meta-analysis of rare harmful effects in randomized controlled trials. *JAMA* 2006;295:2275–2285.


## ADDITIONAL READING

- Firestein GS. Etiology and pathogenesis of rheumatoid arthritis. In: Harris ED, Jr, Budd RC, Genovese MC, et al., eds. *Kelley's Textbook of Rheumatology*, 7th ed. Philadelphia: WB Saunders, 2005:996–1042.
- Genovese MC, Harris ED, Jr. Treatment of rheumatoid arthritis. In: Harris ED, Jr, Budd RC, Genovese MC, et al., eds. *Kelley's Textbook of Rheumatology*, 7th ed. Philadelphia: WB Saunders, 2005:1079–1100.
- Harris ED, Jr. Clinical features of rheumatoid arthritis. In: Harris ED, Jr, Budd RC, Genovese MC, et al., eds. *Kelley's Textbook of Rheumatology*, 7th ed. Philadelphia: WB Saunders, 2005:1043–1078.
- Sayah A, English JC, III. Rheumatoid arthritis: a review of the cutaneous manifestations. *J Am Acad Dermatol* 2005;53:191–209.


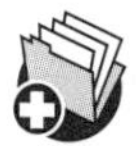

# MISCELLANEOUS

## CODES
### *ICD9-CM*
714.0 Rheumatoid arthritis

## PATIENT TEACHING
It is important for the patient to understand the nature of this disease and the treatment options.

### *Activity*
Patients should continue with their normal activities as much as can be tolerated.

### *Prevention*
Careful observation of symptoms and adherence to treatment regimens can help prevent flare-ups.

## FAQ
- Q: Is there a cure for rheumatoid arthritis?
  - A: No, but disease progression can be controlled with medications.
- Q: What medications will I be taking?
  - A: Anti-inflammatory medications are the mainstay of treatment. Glucocorticoids and methotrexate also are commonly used. Additional medications may be used as indicated.
- Q: What can I do to help prevent progression of the disease?
  - A: Compliance with prescribed medications helps to reduce inflammation and prevent disease progression. Physical therapy and exercise help preserve joint motion and overall health.
- Q: Is my family at increased risk of the disease?
  - A: An increased incidence of rheumatoid arthritis occurs in families, but this fact does not guarantee that individual family members will develop the disease.
- Q: My rheumatoid factor is negative. What does that mean?
  - A: Although a positive rheumatoid factor is common, it is absent in 10–15% of patients with rheumatoid arthritis. In such patients, the diagnosis is made on the basis of the clinical examination.

# ROTATOR CUFF INJURIES

*Kevin W. Farmer, MD*
*John H. Wilckens, MD*
*Bill Hobbs, MD*

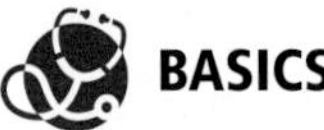

## BASICS

### DESCRIPTION
- Comprises 4 musculotendinous structures (the supraspinatus, infraspinatus, teres minor, and subscapularis) (1,2) that:
  - Compress the humeral head into the glenoid, allowing the larger muscle groups to function properly
  - Provide muscular balance to the glenohumeral joint
- Injuries to the cuff can occur at any age, but injuries to people >60 years old are likely to occur secondary to degenerative changes, whereas injuries in younger patients are less common and tend to follow trauma.
- Injuries affect males slightly more often than females, but females have statistically significant lower shoulder function scores than males (3,4).
  - Full-thickness tears are more common in patients >60 years old.
- Classification:
  - Degenerative tear versus traumatic tear
  - Full-thickness versus partial-thickness tear
  - Size

### GENERAL PREVENTION
- Correct mechanics with overhead athletes
- Overall body conditioning, flexibility, and strengthening are important.

### EPIDEMIOLOGY
- 60% of cuff tears occur in those >60 years old (5).
- Partial-thickness tears are likely to progress to full-thickness tears over time (6).
- The incidence is higher in workers with increased overheard activities, throwing athletes, and swimmers (2).

### RISK FACTORS
- Age >60 years
- Occupations with overhead activity
- Overhead athletics
- Dislocations

#### *Genetics*
No known inheritance patterns

### PATHOPHYSIOLOGY
- Tendon degeneration
- Impingement of the rotator cuff onto the acromion
- An eccentric load that exceeds the strength of the cuff insertion or musculotendinous junction
- Acute traumatic injury/dislocation

### ASSOCIATED CONDITIONS
- Subacromial impingement/bursitis
- Proximal biceps tendinitis/rupture
- Rotator cuff arthropathy
- Glenohumeral arthritis

## DIAGNOSIS

### SIGNS AND SYMPTOMS
- Shoulder pain:
  - Especially over the superolateral shoulder
  - Typically, pain is increased with shoulder motion, especially with attempts at overhead activity.
- Pain at night:
  - Patients describe difficulty with sleeping on the affected side.
  - Pain often wakes patients up at night.
- Shoulder stiffness limiting internal rotation, external rotation, flexion, and abduction is common.
- Weakness:
  - On manual muscle testing of supraspinatus (abduction in the plane of the scapula) and infraspinatus (external rotation with arms at the side); common with full-thickness tears
  - May be secondary to pain inhibition in partial cuff tears
- Instability (2):
  - Loss of compressive forces may lead to increased glenohumeral instability.
  - Subscapularis tears may lead to anterior glenohumeral instability.
  - Anterior-superior subluxation of the humeral head is seen with massive cuff tears.
- Subacromial crepitus with passive ROM

#### *History*
- Acute shoulder pain and weakness after trauma/activity
- Chronic shoulder pain/weakness that may be progressive over time

#### *Physical Exam*
- Evaluate the shoulder for:
  - Muscle atrophy
  - Points of tenderness
  - Active and passive ROM; patients with cuff tears typically have greater passive than active ROM.
  - Muscle strength:
    - Active abduction in the plane of the scapula (supraspinatus)
    - Active external rotation with arms at the side (infraspinatus)
    - Gerber lift-off test (lift the hand off the lower back) and belly press (pressing the hand into the belly while trying to keep the elbow from falling posteriorly) (subscapularis)
- Rule out cervical spine pathology.
  - Thorough neurovascular examination
  - Neck ROM
  - Any pain past the elbow and along the medial border of the scapula should increase suspicion for cervical spine abnormalities.

### TESTS
- Tests for impingement:
  - Positive Hawkins test produces pain with passive internal rotation of shoulder with arm in 90° of flexion.
  - Positive Neer test produces pain with passive flexion of shoulder while scapula is stabilized.
  - Positive impingement test: Pain improves with injection of lidocaine into the subacromial space.

#### *Lab*
None specific

#### *Imaging*
- Radiography:
  - May see avulsion fragment from greater tuberosity in acute tears
  - Chronic cuff disease may show:
    - Sclerosis of undersurface of acromion (or eyebrow sign)
    - Traction spurs of the coracoacromial ligament
    - Cystic changes at the greater tuberosity
    - Calcification in the subacromial space
  - Larger tears may show superior migration of the humeral head.
  - Cuff tear arthropathy:
    - Superior migration of the humeral head with "femoralization" of the humeral head and "acetabularization" of the coracoacromial arch (2)
  - Glenohumeral or AC arthritis
- Arthrography:
  - Of historical interest only
  - Replaced by noninvasive MRI
- Ultrasonography:
  - >90% sensitivity and specificity for full- and partial-thickness tears (7)
  - Efficient and cost-effective method for examining cuff, but is user-dependent
  - Also helpful in evaluation of the biceps tendon
  - Useful after rotator cuff repair (2)
- MRI:
  - 90% sensitivity and 100% specificity (8)
  - Helpful for determining size of tear for preoperative planning
  - Less useful after rotator cuff repair

#### *Diagnostic Procedures/Surgery*
Diagnostic shoulder arthroscopy for definitive diagnosis

#### *Pathological Findings*
- Thinning and degeneration of the rotator cuff with frayed edges at the tear
- Subacromial bone spur
- Cystic change at the cuff insertion site into the greater tuberosity
- Calcific changes of rotator cuff
- Glenohumeral arthritis

### DIFFERENTIAL DIAGNOSIS
- Glenohumeral instability
- Proximal biceps tendinitis
- Subacromial impingement/bursitis
- Cervical radiculopathy
- Snapping scapula
- Adhesive capsulitis
- AC arthritis
- Suprascapular neuropathy
- SLAP lesion

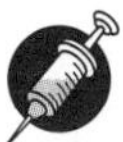

## TREATMENT

### INITIAL STABILIZATION
- May use a sling temporarily for comfort, but immobilization not for more than a few days
- Ice is helpful for the associated inflammation.

### GENERAL MEASURES
- Determine the effect on the patient's daily life.
- For the acute traumatic full-thickness tear in the athlete or young patient, typically operative treatment
- For degenerative tears, a trial of nonoperative management before surgical intervention

#### *Activity*
No activities with >60° of flexion or abduction during the acute period

### SPECIAL THERAPY
#### *Physical Therapy*
- Rotator cuff program:
  - Gradually increase strength and ROM
  - No active movements with >60° of flexion or abduction while painful
- Strengthen cuff muscles, deltoid, biceps, scapular stabilizers.
- Improve scapulothoracic motion.
- Ice, ultrasound, electrical stimulation

#### *Complementary and Alternative Therapies*
None described

### MEDICATION (DRUGS)
- Medications are the initial choice for managing the pain and inflammation associated with rotator cuff injuries.
  - NSAIDs are beneficial during pain exacerbations.
  - Acetaminophen

### SURGERY
- Repair of rotator cuff:
  - Side-to-side repair of tendons
  - Repair of tendon to bone
- Open, mini-open, arthroscopic repair:
  - Arthroscopic repair allows for complete evaluation of the shoulder but is technically challenging.
  - Tear type and pattern may dictate procedure.
- Almost always accompanied by subacromial decompression and acromioplasty

## FOLLOW-UP
- Follow the patient to check progression of the physical therapy regimen and to watch for complications such as stiffness.
- Take care to avoid overly aggressive therapy, which could put the repair at risk.

#### *Issues for Referral*
Almost all patients benefit from a referral to physical therapy.

### PROGNOSIS
- Most patients respond well to nonoperative intervention.
- Surgical intervention usually is successful in patients for whom nonoperative intervention fails.
- Chronic rotator cuff tears with rotator cuff arthropathy have a poor prognosis.

### COMPLICATIONS
- Stiff shoulder:
  - May occur secondary to postoperative scarring
  - Early postoperative pendulum or Codman exercises and passive ROM exercises minimize the risk.
- Repair failure is higher in those who smoke, have diabetes, or undergo too-aggressive rehabilitation.
- Postoperative infection
- Deltoid avulsion: Releasing the deltoid during an open procedure requires a secure reattachment.

### PATIENT MONITORING
Closely monitor ROM; preserving shoulder ROM is critical, but care should be taken to avoid stressing the repair in the postoperative period.

### REFERENCES

1. Krishnan SG, Hawkins RJ. Shoulder. Section L: Rotator cuff and impingement lesions in adult and adolescent athletes. In: DeLee JC, Drez D, Jr, eds. *Orthopaedic Sports Medicine: Principles and Practice*, 2nd ed. Philadelphia: WB Saunders, 2003:1065–1095.
2. Matsen FA, III, Titelman RM, Lippitt SB, et al. Rotator cuff. In: Rockwood CA, Jr, Matsen FA, III, Wirth MA, et al., eds. *The Shoulder*, 3rd ed Philadelphia: WB Saunders, 2004:795–878.
3. Fealy S, April EW, Khazzam M, et al. The coracoacromial ligament: morphology and study of acromial enthesopathy. *J Shoulder Elbow Surg* 2005;14:542–548.
4. Nicholson GP, Goodman DA, Flatow EL, et al. The acromion: morphologic condition and age-related changes. A study of 420 scapulas. *J Shoulder Elbow Surg* 1996;5:1–11.
5. Sher JS, Uribe JW, Posada A, et al. Abnormal findings on magnetic resonance images of asymptomatic shoulders [see comments]. *J Bone Joint Surg* 1995;77A:10–15.
6. Yamanaka K, Matsumoto T. The joint side tear of the rotator cuff. A followup study by arthrography. *Clin Orthop Relat Res* 1994;304:68–73.
7. Mack LA, Matsen FA, III, Kilcoyne RF, et al. US evaluation of the rotator cuff. *Radiology* 1985;157: 205–209.
8. Shellock FG, Bert JM, Fritts HM, et al. Evaluation of the rotator cuff and glenoid labrum using a 0.2-Tesla extremity magnetic resonance (MR) system: MR results compared to surgical findings. *J Magn Reson Imaging* 2001;14:763–770.


### ADDITIONAL READING

- Cofield RH. Rotator cuff disease of the shoulder. *J Bone Joint Surg* 1985;67A:974–979.
- Lehman C, Cuomo F, Kummer FJ, et al. The incidence of full thickness rotator cuff tears in a large cadaveric population. *Bull Hosp Joint Dis* 1995;54:30–31.
- Smith KL, Harryman DT, II, Antoniou J, et al. A prospective, multipractice study of shoulder function and health status in patients with documented rotator cuff tears. *J Shoulder Elbow Surg* 2000;9: 395–402.


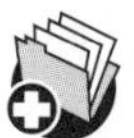

## MISCELLANEOUS

### CODES
#### *ICD9-CM*
- 726.11 Rotator cuff tendinitis
- 840.4 Rotator cuff tear

### PATIENT TEACHING
#### *Activity*
- Avoidance of strenuous overhead activities
- Proper throwing mechanics in throwing athletes

### FAQ
- Q: Do patients with small, full-thickness rotator cuff tears need surgery?
  - A: Most patients with rotator cuff tears, small or large, will improve with an appropriate rotator cuff rehabilitation program. If pain persists or function is still limited thereafter, such patients will benefit from rotator cuff repair and postoperative rehabilitation.

# SACRAL INSUFFICIENCY FRACTURE

*Matthew D. Waites, AFRCS (Ed)*
*Simon C. Mears, MD, PhD*

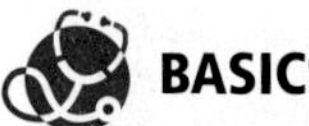

## BASICS

### DESCRIPTION

- Sacral Insufficiency fractures occur in the sacral ala between the SI joints and the neural foramina (Denis Zone 1) (1).
  - The fracture pattern adopts a characteristic H-shape, which is pathonemonic of the condition.
  - It is postulated that the vertical limbs of the H occur 1st, followed by the transverse fracture line.
  - In ~50% of cases, the fracture results from low-energy trauma such as a fall (2).
- Sacral insufficiency fractures often are associated with other insufficiency fractures around the pelvic girdle, most commonly the pubic rami.

### GENERAL PREVENTION

Maintenance of adequate bone mineral density in patients with osteoporosis, including bone density monitoring and treatment with calcium, vitamin D, and bisphosphonates

### EPIDEMIOLOGY

- >90% occur in postmenopausal females (3)
- Predominantly Caucasian females (2)

#### *Incidence*

- Currently, the true incidence is unknown, but based on the fact that plain radiographs do not diagnose the injury, they may be grossly underreported.
- It is estimated that 1–2% of patients attending a rheumatology clinic with lumbar pain have an insufficiency fracture of the pelvic girdle (3).

### RISK FACTORS

- Osteoporosis
- Inflammatory arthritis
- Primary bone or metastatic neoplasms
- Radiotherapy (4)
- Metabolic bone disease
- Corticosteroids
- Total hip replacement (5–7)

### PATHOPHYSIOLOGY

- The mechanism of injury has yet to be defined, but theoretically:
  - During ambulation, load is transmitted from the spine through the sacrum around the pelvic rim to the lower limbs.
  - In people with osteoporosis, the tilting and rotation of the pelvis during ambulation or sudden load transmission during a fall creates shear forces that generate microfractures vertically in the sacral ala.
  - These fractures may be unilateral initially before progressing bilaterally.
  - Continued tilting and rotation of the pelvis around 2 cross-axes lead to microfracture transversely between the 2 vertical fracture lines (2,8,9).
- This theory explains the characteristic H or butterfly appearance on bone scintigraphy and why, in some sacral insufficiency fractures, only 1 or 2 vertical fractures are apparent, depending on how far the fracture has propagated before the diagnosis is made.

### ETIOLOGY

- Sometimes no antecedent trauma is apparent.
- Low-energy fall in up to 50% (2)

### ASSOCIATED CONDITIONS

- Other insufficiency fractures around the pelvic girdle
- Vertebral compression fractures
- Osteoporosis

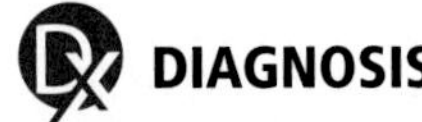

## DIAGNOSIS

### SIGNS AND SYMPTOMS

- No clear set of symptoms that pinpoints the diagnosis
- Suspicion of a sacral insufficiency fracture should be raised in the presence of mechanical low back and buttock pain.
- Pain is exacerbated by sitting or mobilizing.

#### *History*

- Low back and buttock pain of gradual onset that is relieved by lying down.
- Sometimes a fall is recalled on questioning.
- Diagnosis of cancer
- Recent radiotherapy
- Previous or concurrent insufficiency fracture of the pelvic girdle
- Corticosteroids

#### *Physical Exam*

- Pain on palpation of sacrum
- Pain with weightbearing

### TESTS

#### *Lab*

Alkaline phosphatase may be elevated.

#### *Imaging*

- Plain radiographs are unhelpful (rarely show fracture).
- Bone scintigraphy is the test of choice (shows characteristic H-shape).
- CT can outline the fracture accurately.
- MRI signs are sensitive but not specific:
  - Band of low signal on T1-weighted images
  - High-signal associated with edema on T2-weighted images

#### *Diagnostic Procedures/Surgery*

DEXA scan to determine bone density

### DIFFERENTIAL DIAGNOSIS

- Malignancy
- Infection

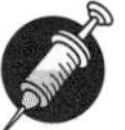

## TREATMENT

### INITIAL STABILIZATION
- Pain relief
- Bed rest

### GENERAL MEASURES
#### *Activity*
- Sacral insufficiency fractures are stable.
- Once pain is controlled, the patient should be mobilized to avoid complications associated with prolonged recumbency.
- Early mobilization reduces additional bone demineralization.

#### *Nursing*
- Patients at rest should be monitored carefully for decubitus ulcers.
- Patients on narcotics should be given stool softeners.

### SPECIAL THERAPY
#### *Physical Therapy*
Therapy may help in strengthening after the fracture is healed.

### MEDICATION (DRUGS)
#### *First Line*
- Acetaminophen
- Oral narcotic analgesics

#### *Second Line*
- Calcium
- Vitamin D
- Calcitonin
- Diphosphonates

### SURGERY
- In cases of prolonged and persistent pain resistant to analgesics, sacroplasty may be considered (8,10,11).
  - Percutaneous injection of small aliquots of bone cement into the fracture site to prevent micromotion at the fracture
  - Performed under regional or general anesthetic using CT guidance
  - The use of bone cement in this manner is not FDA approved.
- Operative internal fixation can improve pain in patients with established nonunion of the sacrum (12).

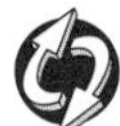

## FOLLOW-UP

Patients should be monitored with radiographs of the pelvis at 6–8-week intervals until pain free.

### DISPOSITION
#### *Issues for Referral*
- Awareness of these insufficiency fractures is key.
- Patients whose fractures do not heal should be referred to an orthopaedist.
- Patients with severe osteoporosis may need referral to an osteoporosis specialist for metabolic workup.

### PROGNOSIS
Most reported cases treated nonoperatively heal in 3–4 months (3).

### COMPLICATIONS
- Nonoperative treatment:
  - Delayed union
  - Recurrent Insufficiency fracture
- Operative treatment:
  - Damage to iliac vessels
  - Damage to lumbosacral nerve roots
  - Chronic pain

### REFERENCES

1. Denis F, Davis S, Comfort T. Sacral fractures: An important problem. Retrospective analysis of 236 cases. *Clin Orthop Relat Res* 1988;227:67–81.
2. Leroux JL, Denat B, Thomas E, et al. Sacral insufficiency fractures presenting as acute low-back pain. Biomechanical aspects. *Spine* 1993;18:2502–2506.
3. Weber M, Hasler P, Gerber H. Insufficiency fractures of the sacrum. Twenty cases and review of the literature. *Spine* 1993;18:2507–2512.
4. Baxter NN, Habermann EB, Tepper JE, et al. Risk of pelvic fractures in older females following pelvic irradiation. *JAMA* 2005;294:2587–2593.
5. Carter SR. Stress fracture of the sacrum: brief report. *J Bone Joint Surg* 1987;69B:843–844.
6. Davies AM. Stress lesions of bone. *Current Imag* 1990;2:209–216.
7. Launder WJ, Hungerford DS. Stress fracture of the pubis after total hip arthroplasty. *Clin Orthop Relat Res* 1981;159:183–185.
8. Cooper KL, Beabout JW, Swee RG. Insufficiency fractures of the sacrum. *Radiology* 1985;156: 15–20.
9. Ries T. Detection of osteoporotic sacral fractures with radionuclides. *Radiology* 1983;146: 783–785.
10. Garant M. Sacroplasty: a new treatment for sacral insufficiency fracture. *J Vasc Interv Radiol* 2002;13:1265–1267.
11. Pommersheim W, Huang-Hellinger F, Baker M, et al. Sacroplasty: A treatment for sacral insufficiency fractures. *Am J Neuroradiol* 2003;24:1003–1007.
12. Mears DC, Velyvis JH. In situ fixation of pelvic nonunions following pathologic and insufficiency fractures. *J Bone Joint Surg* 2002;84A:721–728.


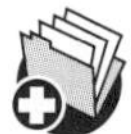

## MISCELLANEOUS

### CODES
#### *ICD9-CM*
- 805.6 Fracture sacrum, closed
- 808.2 Fracture pubis, closed
- 808.43 Multiple pelvic fractures, closed

### PATIENT TEACHING
#### *Activity*
- Activity should be restricted to a level that does not cause pain.
- Assistive devices, such as a walker or a cane, should be used during healing.

#### *Prevention*
- Maintain mobility.
- Adequate daily calcium in diet
- Osteoporosis prevention and treatment

### FAQ
- Q: How are sacral insufficiency fractures treated?
  - A: With activity modification, ambulatory aids, and oral pain medicines. Osteoporosis should be treated.

# SARCOMA (EPITHELOID AND SYNOVIAL)

*Frank J. Frassica, MD*

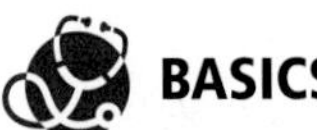

## BASICS

### DESCRIPTION
- Epithelioid sarcoma:
  - A high-grade soft-tissue sarcoma that is prone to local recurrence, lymph node invasion, and pulmonary metastases (1).
  - Most common soft-tissue sarcoma of the upper extremity
  - Often confused with granulomatous processes
  - Occurs often in young patients (15–40 years old)
- Synovial sarcoma:
  - A high-grade malignancy on the soft tissue
  - Occurs in para-articular regions
  - Rarely occurs inside a joint
  - Locations (1):
    - Lower extremity: 60%
    - Upper extremity: 25%
    - Trunk: 10%
    - Head/neck: 10%

### GENERAL PREVENTION
No preventive means are known.

### EPIDEMIOLOGY
No causes are known, but a genetic connection for synovial sarcoma exists.

#### *Incidence*
- No data available for epithelioid sarcoma:
  - Young patients
  - Upper extremity
- Synovial sarcoma:
  - Occurs in young patients: 15–40 years old (1)
  - Male:Female ratio is 1.2:1 (1).

### RISK FACTORS
No risk factors are known.

#### *Genetics*
- Epithelioid: No genetic factors are known.
- Synovial:
  - A characteristic chromosomal abnormality is found in all cases.
  - Balanced reciprocal translocation: t(X;18)(p11.2;q11.2):
    - SYT gene on chromosome 18
    - SSX1 or SSX2 on the X chromosome
    - Gene fusion products: SYT-SSX1, SYT-SSX2

### PATHOPHYSIOLOGY
- Epithelioid and synovial sarcoma:
  - Unregulated growth of the soft-tissue mass
  - Hematologic spread to the lungs
  - Lymphatic spread to the lymph nodes
- Epithelioid sarcoma can arise in the superficial or deep tissues (1).
  - When superficial, it grows in the subcutaneous tissues as a nodule and may ulcerate through the skin.
  - In the deep tissues, it often is firmly attached to muscles, tendons, or fascial structures.

### ETIOLOGY
No etiologic factors are known.

### ASSOCIATED CONDITIONS
No associated conditions are known.

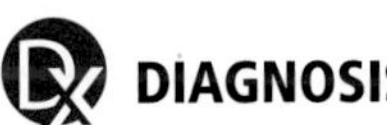

## DIAGNOSIS

### SIGNS AND SYMPTOMS
- Patients present with a soft-tissue mass.
  - Pain is present in ∼50%.
  - Some patients note a long-term presence of the mass.
  - May be slow or rapid growth

#### *History*
Patients may note that the mass has been present for a short time and is growing or that it has existed for a long time with little or no growth.

#### *Physical Exam*
- Carefully examine the extremity and note the following features of the mass:
  - Size
  - Depth: Above or below the fascia (attached to skin or deep tissues?)
  - Mobility: Fixed or movable?
- Also note any overlying skin changes, such as erythema.
- Check for lymphadenopathy.

### TESTS
Imaging studies are the main modality for defining the anatomic parameters of the mass.

#### *Lab*
No specific laboratory studies

#### *Imaging*
- Radiography:
  - Plain films are used to evaluate the primary lesion.
  - Look for:
    - Cortical bone destruction
    - Periosteal reaction
    - In synovial sarcoma only: Mineralization within the mass (occurs in ∼20% of patients)
- MRI:
  - The most useful imaging study
  - Used to define lesion's size, depth, and relationship to important structures such as nerves and blood vessels
- CT:
  - Used to look for pulmonary metastases and lymphadenopathy
  - Chest in all patients
  - Pelvis/abdomen, axilla to evaluate lymph node chains from the primary site

#### *Diagnostic Procedures/Surgery*
- Needle biopsy is necessary to differentiate synovial sarcoma from other sarcomas and the many benign causes of soft-tissue tumors.
- Because of the propensity for lymph node involvement, sentinel-node biopsy sometimes is necessary.

#### *Pathological Findings*
- Characteristic morphologic findings for epithelioid sarcoma (1):
  - Nodular growth pattern
  - Central necrosis
  - Epithelial appearance of the cells
- For synovial sarcoma, several types (listed in order of occurrence):
  - Biphasic (epithelial and fibrous cells)
  - Monophasic fibrous
  - Poorly differentiated
  - Monophasic epithelial

### DIFFERENTIAL DIAGNOSIS
- Soft-tissue masses have a long list of benign and malignant differential diagnoses.
- Epithelioid sarcoma can be confused with a number of entities, both clinically and pathologically (1):
  - Granuloma annulare
  - Rheumatoid nodule
  - Squamous cell carcinoma
  - Necrotizing infectious granuloma
  - Necrobiosis lipoidica

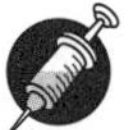

## TREATMENT

### SPECIAL THERAPY

#### *Radiotherapy*

- Virtually all patients are treated with a combination of wide surgical resection and radiation therapy.
- Radiation therapy can be delivered in a number of different ways:
  - Preoperative external beam
  - Postoperative external beam
  - Brachytherapy tubes

#### *Physical Therapy*

Physical therapy often is used after surgery to regain ROM and strength.

### MEDICATION (DRUGS)

- Chemotherapy often is used to reduce the risk of pulmonary metastases.
  - Multiagent intensive therapy

### SURGERY

- Wide surgical resection with as large a margin as possible is the cornerstone of treatment and necessary to reduce the risk of local recurrence.
  - Lymph node dissection is necessary if abnormal nodes are found on physical examination or after imaging.
  - Limb preservation in >90% of patients
  - Amputation occasionally is necessary.
    - Involvement of major nerves and blood vessels
    - Inability to remove the entire tumor with negative margins

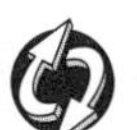

## FOLLOW-UP

- Patients are followed at close intervals to monitor for pulmonary metastases and local recurrence.
  - CT of the chest every 3–4 months for 2–3 years, then every 6 months until 5 years posttreatment, and then annually thereafter
  - MRI with contrast of the limb every 6 months for 2–3 years to monitor for local recurrence

### DISPOSITION

- Patients with epithelioid and synovial sarcoma should be referred to a multidisciplinary team:
  - Orthopedic oncologist
  - Radiation oncologist
  - Medical oncologist
  - Plastic surgeon

### PROGNOSIS

- The prognosis for epithelioid sarcoma is fair with adequate local control.
  - ~40–50% disease-free survival (1)
  - Metastases to lymph nodes, lungs, and other soft-tissue sites
  - Poor prognostic findings (1):
    - Male gender
    - Nondistal extremity tumors
    - Size >5 cm
    - Increased tumor depth
    - High mitotic index
    - Necrosis
    - Vascular invasion
    - Inadequate initial excision
- The prognosis for synovial sarcoma is excellent if local control can be achieved and pulmonary metastases do not develop.
  - 5-year survival rates have been reported to be 50–80% (1).
  - Favorable variables:
    - Age <25 years
    - Size <5 cm
    - Absence of poorly differentiated areas
  - Unfavorable variables:
    - Age >40 years
    - Size >5 cm
    - Poorly differentiated areas

### COMPLICATIONS

- The major complications of surgery and irradiation are:
  - Delayed wound healing
  - Arthrofibrosis (stiffness in joints)
  - Infection

### PATIENT MONITORING

Patients are followed closely after surgery to monitor wound healing, ROM, local recurrence, and pulmonary metastases.

### REFERENCE

1. Weiss SW, Goldblum JR. Malignant soft tissue tumors of uncertain type. In: Weiss SW, Goldblum JR, eds. *Enzinger and Weiss's Soft Tissue Tumors*, 4th ed. St. Louis: Mosby, 2001:1483–1571.

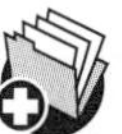

## MISCELLANEOUS

### CODES

#### *ICD9-CM*

171.__Neoplasm, malignant, connective tissue

### PATIENT TEACHING

- Patients must be taught the essential features of this tumor and the principles of treatment.
  - Wide surgical resection is necessary.
  - Irradiation often is necessary to reduce the risk of local recurrence.
  - Careful monitoring with imaging studies and physical examination is necessary after surgery.

#### *Activity*

Unrestricted activity after full wound healing

#### *Prevention*

No preventive methods

### FAQ

- Q: Is surgery necessary for all patients?
  - A. Surgery with as wide a margin as possible is necessary to reduce the risk of local recurrence.
- Q: What is the risk of pulmonary metastases?
  - A: Metastasis to the lungs occurs in ~50% of patients.
- Q: How often can the limb be saved?
  - A: Limb preservation can be achieved in ~90% of patients.
- Q: Is chemotherapy necessary for all patients?
  - A: Patients at high risk for pulmonary metastases, especially those with large tumors (>10 cm), should consider chemotherapy.

S

# SCAPHOID FRACTURE

*Simon C. Mears, MD, PhD*
*John J. Hwang, MD*

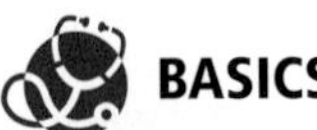

## BASICS

### DESCRIPTION

- Fracture of the most radial (thumb side) of the carpal bones, usually as a result of a dorsiflexion injury to the wrist
- The most common of the carpal fractures, estimated at 60% (1)
- Frequent problems include delayed diagnosis and nonunion.
- Classification:
  - Chronologically: Acute or chronic
  - Anatomically: In the proximal, middle, or distal third
- Displaced or nondisplaced
- Direction: Transverse or oblique
- By mechanism: High-energy (e.g., motor vehicle accident) or simple, low-energy fall
- Simple fracture or complicated fracture with associated ligament injury or dislocation.
- Synonym: Navicular fracture

### GENERAL PREVENTION

Wear wrist protectors during high-risk activities such as rollerblading and in-line skating (2).

### EPIDEMIOLOGY

#### *Incidence*

- In 1 study, the annual fracture rate was 4.3 per 10,000 people, the average age was 25 years, and 82% occurred in males (1).
- Scaphoid fractures account for ~2% of all fractures and 11% of hand fractures (1).
- 2nd most common fracture of the wrist area after the distal radius
- Rare in children (3)

#### *Prevalence*

Usually an injury of young adults (males more commonly than females, probably because of activity level) after a fall, athletic injury, or motor vehicle accident.

### RISK FACTORS

- Contact sports
- Rollerblading and in-line skating (2)
- Risk factors for nonunion:
  - Proximal pole fracture
  - Distal oblique or vertical fracture
  - Large displacement of the fracture
  - High-energy injury

### PATHOPHYSIOLOGY

- The major blood supply to the proximal pole enters the bone through the distal 1/3 of the bone.
- Vessel disruption causes compromise of the blood supply to the proximal pole (4).

### ETIOLOGY

- An axial force impacting on an outstretched hand
- The scaphoid acts as a bridge between the proximal and distal rows of the carpus, making it vulnerable to fracture.

## DIAGNOSIS

### SIGNS AND SYMPTOMS

#### *History*

- Pain or clicking with wrist motion
- The clinician must have a high index of suspicion to avoid missing the injury.
- Patients occasionally present late (months or even years after the injury) with persistent ache, weakness, or clicking.

#### *Physical Exam*

- Pain with wrist motion is common.
- Swelling is variable because the fracture may or may not produce much bleeding.
- Typically, palpate the snuffbox region (between the short and long extensor tendons to the thumb) (Fig. 1) and compare the findings with those of the uninjured side.
  - If tenderness is found here, presume that the patient has a fracture until proven otherwise.

### TESTS

#### *Lab*

No laboratory tests aid in the diagnosis.

#### *Imaging*

- Radiography:
  - Posteroanterior, lateral, pronated oblique, and ulnar deviated posteroanterior radiographs of the wrist (scaphoid views)
  - Displacement of the normal fat plane on the volar surface of the navicular is suggestive of injury.
  - Carefully scrutinize radiographs for signs of ligament disruption and carpal dislocation.

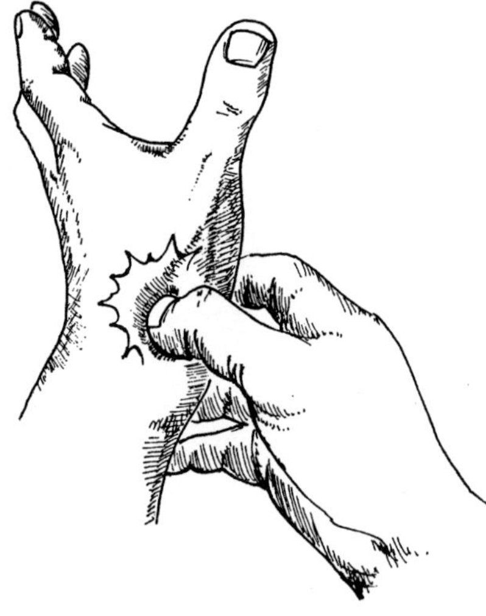

**Fig. 1.** Tenderness in the snuffbox should produce suspicion of a scaphoid fracture.

- If plain radiographs are negative but examination is suggestive of fracture, additional imaging is indicated, including:
  - Bone scan (in acute phase)
  - CT scan with 3D reconstruction
  - MRI, which is becoming the standard test because results are obtained quickly (5)

### DIFFERENTIAL DIAGNOSIS

- Ligament injury or sprain
- Perilunate dislocation
- Distal radius fracture
- Wrist instability

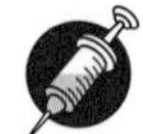

## TREATMENT

### GENERAL MEASURES

- Immobilize the wrist in a thumb spica splint for 2 weeks if clinical suspicion of a fracture exists, even if a fracture is not seen on initial radiographs.
- The type of splint or cast used is controversial; recommendations range from an above-the-elbow thumb spica cast to a below-the-elbow cast that does not immobilize the thumb (6).
- Radiographs should be repeated at 10–14 days, at which time the fracture edges may be better seen.
- For nondisplaced fractures, the patient should be placed in a below-the-elbow thumb-spica cast for 6–8 weeks and then reassessed clinically and radiographically.
- Displaced fractures and proximal pole fractures require surgery.
- Fractures in competitive athletes may be treated surgically to allow for earlier return to activity.

#### *Activity*

Heavy lifting or sports activities should be avoided until the fracture is healed and the patient is pain free.

### SPECIAL THERAPY

#### *Physical Therapy*

Physical therapy maintains finger ROM during immobilization and helps regain wrist motion after immobilization.

### SURGERY

- Displaced fractures should be treated with reduction and screw fixation.
  - Cannulated screws that are headless and have variable threads currently are used for fixation.
  - These screws can gain compression of the fracture site without protrusion of the screw from the edge of the bone.
  - The use of a cannulated screw with a guide wire aids in correct screw placement.
  - Cannulated screws may be placed percutaneously.
- Chronic fractures or nonunions should be treated with reduction and fixation plus bone grafting.
- Salvage procedures for late-stage arthritis seen after untreated fractures include excision of the proximal row of carpal bones or partial wrist fusion.

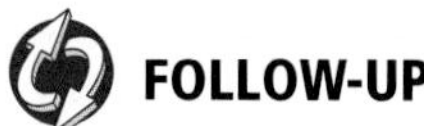

## FOLLOW-UP

### DISPOSITION

#### *Issues for Referral*

- Displaced fractures
- Associated fractures and dislocations
- High-energy injuries

### PROGNOSIS

- >90% of nondisplaced fractures heal (6)
- No benefit has been found for treating nondisplaced fractures with surgery (7).
- No differences have been found between the dorsal and volar approach to scaphoid fixation (8).
- Displaced fractures:
  - Higher nonunion rate if treated closed (9)
  - Good outcomes with surgical reduction and fixation (10)
- Treatment of scaphoid nonunions with vascularized bone grafting and internal fixation seems to have the highest rate of healing (11).

### COMPLICATIONS

- Nonunion
- AVN of the proximal pole
- Reflex sympathetic dystrophy
- Arthritis
- Wrist instability

### PATIENT MONITORING

Patients with acute fractures are reviewed clinically and radiographically every 2–4 weeks until the fracture is healed and rehabilitation has been completed.

### REFERENCES


1. Hove LM. Epidemiology of scaphoid fractures in Bergen, Norway. *Scand J Plast Reconstr Surg Hand Surg* 1999;33:423–426.
2. Brudvik C, Hove LM. Childhood fractures in Bergen, Norway: Identifying high-risk groups and activities. *J Pediatr Orthop* 2003;23:629–634.
3. Elhassan BT, Shin AY. Scaphoid fracture in children. *Hand Clin* 2006;22:31–41.
4. Gelberman RH, Menon J. The vascularity of the scaphoid bone. *J Hand Surg* 1980;5A:508–513.
5. Kumar S, O'Connor A, Despois M, et al. Use of early magnetic resonance imaging in the diagnosis of occult scaphoid fractures: The CAST Study (Canberra Area Scaphoid Trial). *N Z Med J* 2005;118:U1296.
6. Burge P. Closed cast treatment of scaphoid fractures. *Hand Clin* 2001;17:541–552.
7. Dias JJ, Wildin CJ, Bhowal B, et al. Should acute scaphoid fractures be fixed? A randomized controlled trial. *J Bone Joint Surg* 2005;87A: 2160–2168.
8. Polsky MB, Kozin SH, Porter ST, et al. Scaphoid fractures: Dorsal versus volar approach. *Orthopaedics* 2002;25:817–819.
9. Ring D, Jupiter JB, Herndon JH. Acute fractures of the scaphoid. *J Am Acad Orthop Surg* 2000;8: 225–231.
10. Rettig ME, Kozin SH, Cooney WP. Open reduction and internal fixation of acute displaced scaphoid wrist fractures. *J Hand Surg* 2001;26A:271–276.
11. Munk B, Larsen CF. Bone grafting the scaphoid nonunion: A systematic review of 147 publications including 5,246 cases of scaphoid nonunion. *Acta Orthop Scand* 2004;75:618–629.


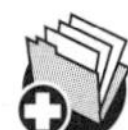

## MISCELLANEOUS

### CODES

#### *ICD9-CM*

814.01 Scaphoid fracture

### PATIENT TEACHING

- Patients should be informed of the difficulty of making the diagnosis of an acute fracture and the need for prophylactic immobilization if snuffbox tenderness is present.
- The risk of delayed union or nonunion should be discussed.

#### *Activity*

Patients should be advised not to attempt pushing or lifting while wearing a cast.

#### *Prevention*

Wrist protectors are thought to prevent wrist injury and should be used for rollerblading or in-line skating (2).

### FAQ

- Q: How is a scaphoid fracture diagnosed?
  - A: Patients with traumatic wrist pain should be assessed carefully for fracture. Good-quality radiographs should be taken acutely. If negative, the patient should be immobilized and then reassessed in 2 weeks or assessed with MRI scanning.
- Q: Why is it important that nondisplaced scaphoid fractures be diagnosed?
  - A: If untreated, nondisplaced fractures may become displaced and lead to scaphoid nonunion, requiring surgery. When nondisplaced fractures are treated with immobilization, results are excellent.

# SCHMORL NODES

*Andrew P. Manista, MD*

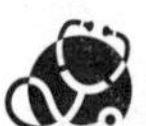

## BASICS

### DESCRIPTION

- Schmorl nodes are intraosseous vertebral lesions that are common incidental findings on plain radiographs and CT and MRI scans of the spine.
  - These nodes represent disc material that has herniated through weak areas in the adjacent vertebral endplates into the vertebral body.
  - In some cases, these weak areas may be the physiologic sequelae of the regression of vascular canals near the end of vertebral growth (particularly in young patients), whereas in other cases they represent a weakened endplate or subchondral bone.
  - Such herniations also may occur through pathologically weakened bone, and they usually are found in the thoracic or lumbar spine, although there have been reports of Schmorl nodes of the cervical spine.
- These lesions were first described by Christian Georg Schmorl (1,2) as the cause of *Scheuermann kyphosis*, which results from decreased growth of the anterior portion of the endplates of at least 3 adjacent vertebral bodies.
  - Although the origin of Scheuermann kyphosis remains unclear, Schmorl nodes are unlikely to be the cause because they are not universally present.
- Synonyms: Vertebral endplate irregularities; Intraosseous disc herniations

### EPIDEMIOLOGY

#### *Incidence*

- ~10% of the general population (3)
- No gender predilection
- Age ranging from childhood to old age, depending on the predisposing condition

### RISK FACTORS

#### *Genetics*

- No specific genetic correlation has been made (4,5).
- Metabolic bone diseases with genetic predispositions may predispose persons to an increased incidence of intraosseous disc herniation secondary to decreased bone density or defective bony matrix of the vertebral bodies.

### ETIOLOGY

- Degenerative or acute rupture of the disc endplate and extrusion of the nucleus pulposus occur with sufficient force to penetrate the vertebral body superior or inferior to it.
- Penetration may be secondary to acute trauma in the case of a normal vertebra and disc.
- In the degenerative setting, penetration may occur slowly over time because of a weakened vertebral body.
- Often, no obvious cause is found.

### ASSOCIATED CONDITIONS (6)

- Scheuermann (juvenile) kyphosis
- Trauma
- Osteoporosis and other metabolic disorders
- Neoplastic disorders
- Degenerative disc disease

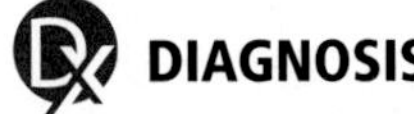

## DIAGNOSIS

### SIGNS AND SYMPTOMS

- Patients may be asymptomatic or may have pain secondary to Schmorl nodes.
- Symptoms prompting radiographs may not necessarily be caused by this lesion.
- Symptoms usually relate to the degenerative change or insufficiency of the particular disc and consist of axial backache or back pain.
- Pain may radiate laterally around the trunk, but not distally down the extremities.

#### *Physical Exam*

- Tenderness may or may not be elicited by deep palpation or percussion over the spine.
- The degrees of kyphosis in the spine should be estimated.
- A complete neurologic exam should be performed, but a neurologic deficit is unlikely.
  - If present, other causes should be sought.

### TESTS

#### *Imaging*

- Conventional radiographs show indentations or "pits" in the vertebral body, with radiolucencies within the body surrounded by varying degrees of sclerosis.
  - Variable degrees of disc thinning may be present as a result of the displaced nucleus.
  - Benign-appearing lesions
- MRI may show low signal on T1-weighted and high signal on T2-weighted images in the setting of acute intraosseous herniation, which is more likely to be symptomatic (7).
  - Old, usually asymptomatic lesions show the opposite findings on T1- weighted and T2-weighted images.
  - MRI is more sensitive than plain radiographs in detecting the lesion.
- Bone scanning may be useful in differentiating an acute lesion from an older lesion, although MRI is the standard.

### DIFFERENTIAL DIAGNOSIS

- Degenerative subchondral cyst
- Bone neoplasm: Osteoid osteoma, metastatic cancer to bone, aneurysmal bone cyst, early EOG, lymphoma, multiple myeloma

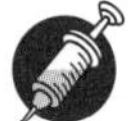

## TREATMENT

### GENERAL MEASURES

- Treatment is symptomatic.
  - In the presence of an acute intraosseous herniation, NSAIDs and rest are the mainstay of care until the patient is able to resume normal activity.
  - Bracing may be initiated for comfort if needed.

### SPECIAL THERAPY

***Physical Therapy***

- Physical therapy may help with persistent backaches.
- Should consist of extensor strengthening and flexibility and endurance training

### MEDICATION (DRUGS)

***First Line***

NSAIDs

### SURGERY

This condition is not a surgical entity.

## FOLLOW-UP

### PROGNOSIS

Prognosis is generally good (8).

### COMPLICATIONS

In the presence of loss of substantial disc space, degenerative joint disease of the facet joints may result, with additional symptoms.

### PATIENT MONITORING

- If the diagnosis is unclear, or if pain does not resolve within 6–8 weeks, serial radiographs should be taken to ensure that the lesion does not grow or change in character.
- An MRI scan also may help rule out a malignant disease.

### REFERENCES


1. Schmorl GC. Die pathologische Anatomie der Wirbelsaule. *Verh Dtsch Ges Orthop* 1927;21: 3–41.
2. Vernon-Roberts B. Christian Georg Schmorl. Pioneer of spinal pathology and radiology. *Spine* 1994;19:2724–2727.
3. Hamanishi C, Kawabata T, Yosii T, et al. Schmorl's nodes on magnetic resonance imaging. Their incidence and clinical relevance. *Spine* 1994;19: 450–453.
4. Hurxthal LM. Schmorl's nodes in identical twins. Their probable genetic origin. *Lahey Clin Found Bull* 1966;15:89–92.
5. Karppinen J, Paakko E, Raina S, et al. Magnetic resonance imaging findings in relation to the COL9A2 tryptophan allele among patients with sciatica. *Spine* 2002;27:78–83.
6. Warner WC, Jr. Kyphosis. In: Morrissy RT, Weinstein SL, eds. *Lovell and Winter's Pediatric Orthopaedics*, 6th ed. Philadelphia: Lippincott Williams & Wilkins, 2006:797–837.
7. Seymour R, Williams LA, Rees JI, et al. Magnetic resonance imaging of acute intraosseous disc herniation. *Clin Radiol* 1998;53:363–368.
8. Murray PM, Weinstein SL, Spratt KF. The natural history and long-term follow-up of Scheuermann kyphosis. *J Bone Joint Surg* 1993;75A:236–248.


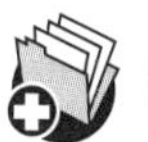

## MISCELLANEOUS

### CODES

***ICD9-CM***

722.30 Schmorl node

### PATIENT TEACHING

**FAQ**

- Q: With what spine condition are Schmorl nodes most commonly associated?
  - A: Scheuermann kyphosis.
- Q: What is the recommended treatment for most patients with Schmorl nodes?
  - A: Observation and nonoperative management.

# SCOLIOSIS

*Paul D. Sponseller, MD*

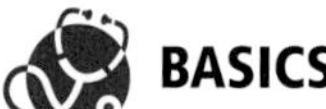

## BASICS

### DESCRIPTION

- Scoliosis is a 3D curvature of the spine, best appreciated on an AP radiograph and physical examination.
- Both thoracic and lumbar segments of the spine may be affected.
- It is defined as a curve >10°.
- Classification (1–3):
  - Etiology:
    - Idiopathic
    - Congenital
    - Neuromuscular
    - Connective tissue
    - Degenerative
  - Location (of the apex or middle of the curve):
    - Thoracic
    - Thoracolumbar
    - Lumbar
  - Subclassification of idiopathic scoliosis by age:
    - Infantile (<3 years)
    - Juvenile (3–10 years)
    - Adolescent (≥11 years)

### EPIDEMIOLOGY

- The most common type is idiopathic scoliosis.
- Scoliosis may occur at any age.
- The most common age at diagnosis of idiopathic scoliosis is 11–13 years (3).

#### *Prevalence*

- Small curves of idiopathic scoliosis are almost equally prevalent in males and females.
- Females, however, are 3–4 times more likely to develop progression of the curve.
- In scoliosis other than the idiopathic type, less difference in gender-related prevalence is noted.
- Prevalence of curves >10° is ~2–3% (3).
- Prevalence of curves requiring bracing (>25°) is ~0.3% (3).
- Prevalence of curves requiring surgery is ~1 in 1,000 (3).

### RISK FACTORS

- Progressive idiopathic scoliosis
- Positive family history
- Female gender
- Premenarchal status
- Paralytic scoliosis
- Severe spinal cord injury before adolescence
- Scoliosis in cerebral palsy, including total involvement

#### *Genetics*

Idiopathic scoliosis is transmitted as autosomal dominant, with incomplete penetrance and variable expressivity.

### ETIOLOGY

- Idiopathic scoliosis:
  - Theories about the cause of idiopathic scoliosis include a subtle connective-tissue abnormality or neurohormonal defect.
  - Causes of congenital scoliosis include hemivertebrae and fusions between vertebrae.
- Neuromuscular scoliosis:
  - Cerebral palsy
  - Traumatic paralysis
  - Spina bifida
  - Poliomyelitis
  - Friedreich ataxia
  - Virtually any systemic neurologic condition that affects the trunk
- Connective tissue-associated scoliosis:
  - Marfan syndrome
  - Ehlers-Danlos syndrome
  - NF
  - Down syndrome

### ASSOCIATED CONDITIONS

- Almost any systemic neurologic disorder that affects the trunk
- Most connective-tissue disorders

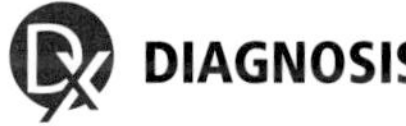

## DIAGNOSIS

### SIGNS AND SYMPTOMS

- Varied, depending on the location of the spine affected (Fig. 1)
- For thoracic curves, the ribs are rotated on the convex side, producing a "rib hump" and a more prominent scapula on the same side.
- With thoracolumbar and lumbar curves, 1 side of the pelvis becomes more prominent, giving the appearance of a "high hip."
- Many, but not all, teens develop increased pain in the area of the curve.
- Symptoms are few until adulthood, when back pain and nerve root pain may develop.

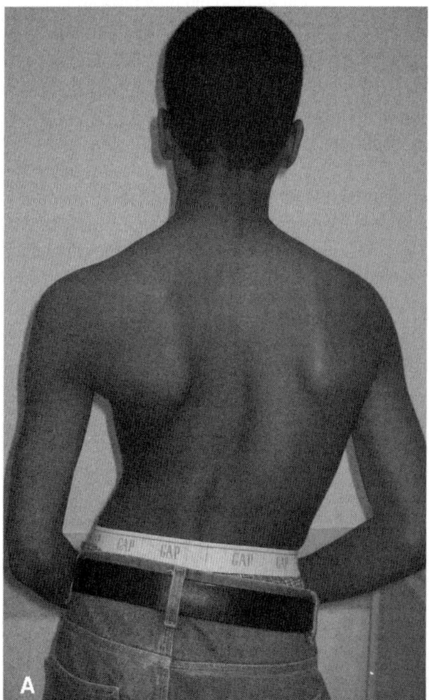

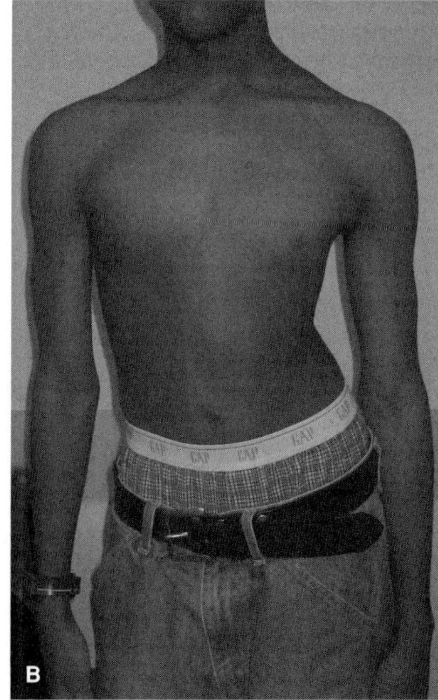

**Fig. 1.** Clinical appearance of severe scoliosis. **A:** Posterior view. **B:** Anterior view.

### *Physical Exam*

- Examine the patient, while he or she is standing, to see shoulder, rib, and hip asymmetry.
- Measure leg lengths.
- Perform the forward bend test with the patient's legs straight and observe the entire spine for asymmetry between the right and left sides (Fig. 2).
  - This test is most useful and highly sensitive, and it is used in school screening programs.
  - If asymmetry is present, measure the slope between the right and left sides of the rib cage.
  - Some patients with a positive forward bend test do not have severe scoliosis.
  - Follow-up a positive test with a radiograph if the rib slope is >6°.
  - Repeat the test if an abnormality is found.
- Quantify rib prominence or a hump by a scoliometer.
- Observe any kyphosis and lordosis.
- Inspect the skin over the entire spine for dimples, hair, or vascular markings, which may signal an underlying congenital anomaly.
- Rule out ligamentous laxity.
- Examine for café-au-lait spots or neurofibromas.
- Perform a careful neurologic examination, which can be practically done by observing gait and 1-legged hop and by testing reflexes.
- Assess the patient's physical maturity by checking for secondary sexual characteristics such as axillary and facial hair, skin changes, breast development.
- Measure the height for serial comparison.

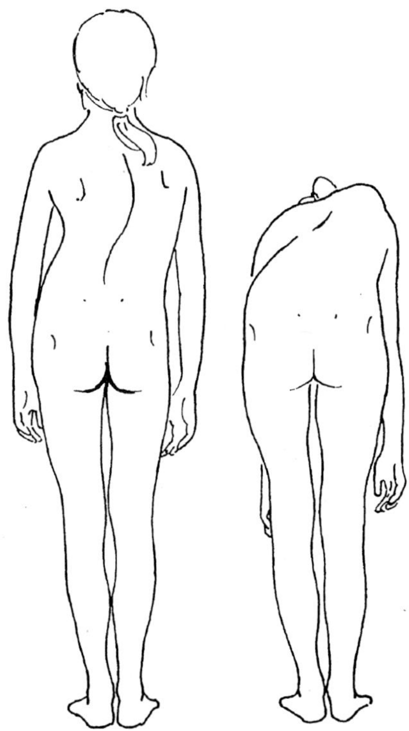

**Fig. 2.** The forward bend test exaggerates the rib deformity in scoliosis and allows sensitive diagnosis.

## TESTS

### *Imaging*

- Radiography:
  - Standing posteroanterior radiography of the entire spine is indicated.
  - Lateral films should be obtained if associated abnormal kyphosis is present.
  - Spine films usually show the iliac crests and allow determination of the Risser stage (3) for skeletal maturity.
    - The Risser stage is the amount of ossification of the iliac growth cartilage.
    - Risser 0, unossified, skeletally immature; Risser V, fully ossified, mature.
  - Presence of an open triradiate cartilage of the hip indicates that the growth spurt has not been completed.
- MRI is indicated only if spinal cord disease is possible.

### *Pathological Findings*

- The vertebrae are rotated toward the convexity of the curve.
- In addition, individual vertebrae are misshapen because of growth while curved.

## DIFFERENTIAL DIAGNOSIS

- Isolated rib rotation may occur without scoliosis.
- Kyphosis (a curvature in the sagittal plane only, which may be confused with scoliosis), clavicle fracture, or Sprengel deformity may give the appearance of a "high shoulder."
- Leg-length inequality may cause the appearance of a "high hip."

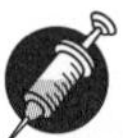

# TREATMENT

## GENERAL MEASURES

- The spine in patients with scoliosis is not unstable.
- Encourage patients to be as active as possible.
- Physical therapy and exercise if pain or stiffness is present
- Patients with minor curves (<25°) should be observed if they are still growing, but they can be discharged if skeletal maturity has been reached.
- Patients with moderate curves (25–40°) should be braced if substantial growth remains.
- Patients with large curves (>45°):
  - See an orthopaedic surgeon to determine whether correction is indicated.
  - Surgery offered.

## SPECIAL THERAPY

### *Physical Therapy*

- Strengthening and stretching of abdominal and extensor muscles if pain exists
- Not indicated for routine cases of scoliosis
- Does not help correct the curves

### *Complementary and Alternative Therapies*

Yoga may be helpful for back discomfort.

## SURGERY
- If a curve is to be fused, 1 or 2 rods (Fig. 3) are used to correct the curve, and a bone graft is placed along the rod to cause the vertebrae to fuse.
  - Only the curved region is fused.
  - The neurologic risk is currently <1% (2).

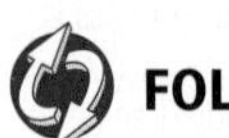

# FOLLOW-UP

Patients should be followed at least until maturity.

## PROGNOSIS
- Pulmonary compromise, including cor pulmonale in congenital or neuromuscular curves, occurs mainly in patients with curves >100° (4).
- Most untreated curves >40–50° in adulthood slowly become worse (3).

## COMPLICATIONS
- Severe curves (>70°) occasionally may progress to the point where they compromise pulmonary function.
- Curves >40° pose an increased risk of back pain in adulthood (3).
- Surgical complications include neurologic injury (<1%), infection, and failure of the vertebrae to fuse (3).

## PATIENT MONITORING
- Growing children should be seen every 4–6 months, usually with radiographs.
- Adults should be seen every 1–5 years.
- Patients with congenital scoliosis should be monitored for associated anomalies.

## REFERENCES

1. Hedequist D, Emans J. Congenital scoliosis. *J Am Acad Orthop Surg* 2004;12:266–275.
2. Lenke LG, Edwards CC, II, Bridwell KH. The Lenke classification of adolescent idiopathic scoliosis: How it organizes curve patterns as a template to perform selective fusions of the spine. *Spine* 2003;28:S199–S207.
3. Newton PO, Wenger DR. Idiopathic scoliosis. In: Morrissy RT, Weinstein SL, eds. *Lovell and Winter's Pediatric Orthopaedics*, 6th ed. Philadelphia: Lippincott Williams & Wilkins, 2006:693–762.
4. Weinstein SL, Dolan LA, Spratt KF, et al. Health and function of patients with untreated idiopathic scoliosis: A 50-year natural history study. *JAMA* 2003;289:559–567.


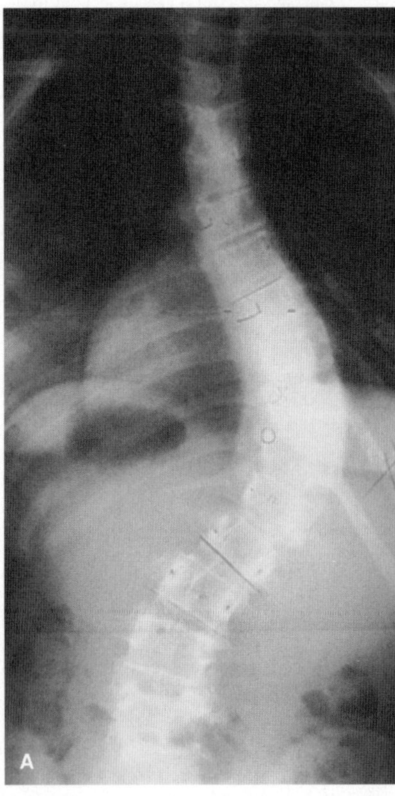


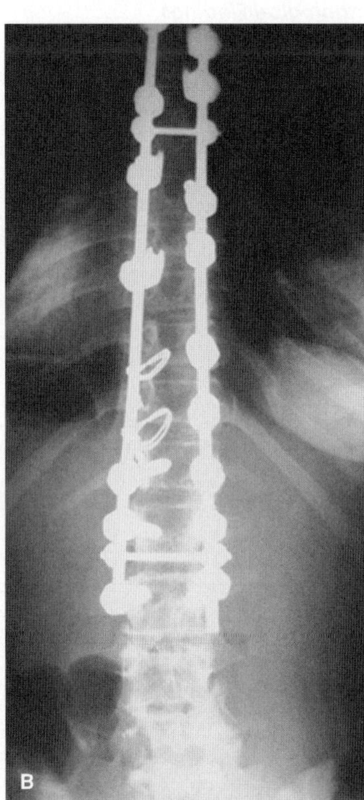


**Fig. 3.** Patient with severe scoliosis before (**A**) and after (**B**) posterior instrumentation and fusion.

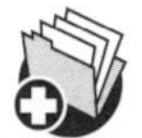

## MISCELLANEOUS

### CODES

#### *ICD9-CM*

- 737.30 Idiopathic scoliosis
- 754.2 Congenital scoliosis

### PATIENT TEACHING

- Instruct patients in the general guidelines and treatment options.
- Remind parents of the genetic nature of the condition so that relatives and young siblings with scoliosis may be detected while bracing is still an option.

#### *Prevention*

- Curve worsening may be effectively prevented in growing children by use of a brace.
  - It must be worn 18–23 hours per day.
  - This intervention is effective in ∼75% of patients (2).
  - Bracing does not correct curves.

### FAQ

- Q: What is the cause of scoliosis?
  - A: It is not known. It often is passed along in families. It may be a subtle disorder of balance or spinal growth.
- Q: Can physical therapy or exercises slow or halt the worsening of the curve?
  - A: No evidence suggests that it can.
- Q: Can bracing correct scoliosis?
  - A: It rarely produces any permanent correction.
- Q: Does scoliosis affect internal organs?
  - A: It is associated with decreased pulmonary function in curves ≥70°. There is little documentation of effects on cardiac, gastrointestinal, or genitourinary function.

S

# SEPTIC ARTHRITIS

*Jason W. Hammond, MD*
*Paul D. Sponseller, MD*

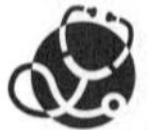

## BASICS

### DESCRIPTION

- Septic arthritis is an infection of the joint.
  - In infants, the capillaries penetrating the physeal plate into the epiphysis persist until age 18 months, so spread of infection may occur from the metaphysis indirectly to the epiphysis and then to the joint.
  - Possible irreparable damage to growth plate occurs.
- Classification: Polyarticular septic arthritis is seen in ~5% of all patients with septic arthritis (1,2).

### GENERAL PREVENTION

- Treatment of systemic infections and prevention of gonorrhea may decrease the risk of septic arthritis (1).
- Most important to recognize and treat the condition early, to avoid complications

### EPIDEMIOLOGY

- It can affect any joint, at any age.
- No gender preference in monarticular septic arthritis
- Gonococcal septic arthritis is 4 times more common in females than in males (1).

#### *Incidence*

- Occurs in <0.5% of infants (1)
- Variable in children and adults

### RISK FACTORS

- Neonates with multiple potential sources of infection
- Concurrent rheumatologic disease, joint prostheses, HIV infection, diabetes mellitus, hemophilia, sickle cell anemia (*Staphylococcus aureus* or *Salmonella*), or intravenous drug abuse (Gram-negative organisms)

### ETIOLOGY

- *S. aureus* causes 80% of cases of septic arthritis in the first 6 months of life (1,3).
- Neonatal septic arthritis also is caused by group B streptococci, *Candida,* and Gram-negative enteric bacteria.
- In children <2 years old, *Haemophilus influenzae* is a cause. (Since 1989, vaccination against *H. influenzae* has become nearly universal and is protective against this source.)
- In children, Gram-negative bacilli, *Streptococcus*, or *Neisseria meningitidis* is the most common cause.
- Young adults:
  - *Neisseria gonorrhoeae* is the most common cause.
  - *S. aureus* is the next most common cause.
  - Other causes include Gram-negative bacilli, *Pseudomonas,* and *Streptococcus.*
- In patients with sickle cell anemia, *Salmonella* is the cause in 50% of infections (4).
- Lyme disease is not a cause of septic arthritis; it is a reactive arthritis.

### ASSOCIATED CONDITIONS

Osteomyelitis

## DIAGNOSIS

### SIGNS AND SYMPTOMS

- Children generally are febrile, irritable, and apprehensive; they may be lethargic and have decreased appetite.
- However, some children may appear healthy with fever of unknown origin and findings localized to a given extremity.
- In the neonate, 75% of patients may not be acutely sick, but symptoms may include failure to eat or to gain weight, and 25% may have signs of sepsis (2,5,6).
- Tenderness to palpation or joint motion is the earliest physical sign in children and adults.
- Swelling, warmth, muscular spasm, and decreased ROM may appear later.
- Joint effusion usually is present.
- Erythema usually is not seen with septic arthritis because the inflammation is contained within the joint capsule.

#### *Physical Exam*

- Tenderness with movement is the earliest physical sign.
- Other signs include fevers, irritability, swelling, warmth, muscle spasm, limited ROM, and joint effusion.

### TESTS

#### *Lab*

- Gram stain is positive in only 30–40% of patients (5,6).
- Cell count and differential
  - A white blood cell count in the aspirate of >50,000 cells/mL in an immunocompetent patient suggests the presence of infection.
  - >90% of the cells are polymorphonuclear.
- Culture of the synovial fluid aspirate; ESR
  - Useful when it is elevated to 50–100 mm per hour unless the patient has had previous antibiotic therapy
  - May be helpful for assessing patient's response to treatment
  - Unreliable in neonates, in children with sickle cell disease, and in patients taking steroids
- C-reactive protein becomes elevated early in the disease process and returns to normal quickly.
- White blood cell count:
  - A high systemic white blood cell count with left shift is nonspecific.
  - 40–75% of patients with septic arthritis have a normal white blood cell count at the time of initial diagnosis (6).
- Urate crystal determination
- Culture and sensitivity:
  - Blood culture always should be obtained before treatment is started because, in 40% of cases, the organism can be identified with blood cultures (3).
  - Fewer cultures are positive after antibiotics.
  - Joint fluid cultures are negative in up to 25% of patients with bacterial septic arthritis, for unknown reasons (2).

#### *Imaging*

- Radiographs may show periarticular soft-tissue swelling and distention of the joint capsule. In neonates; a lateral shift of the femoral neck with respect to the acetabulum is evidence of septic arthritis of the hip.
- Neither MRI nor CT is used in diagnosis of joint infection within the first 24–36 hours.
- Bone scintigraphy can detect alterations in bone much earlier than plain radiographs, but these scans usually are unnecessary because of greater reliability of aspiration.
  - Bone scanning is recommended only when poor localization of clinical findings is present.

#### *Pathological Findings*

- Characterized by purulent synovial fluid, often with >90% polymorphonuclear cells
- The synovium becomes thickened.
- If infection persists for more than a few days without treatment, destruction of joint cartilage may begin.

### DIFFERENTIAL DIAGNOSIS

- Osteomyelitis
- Rheumatologic disease
- Inflammatory arthropathy
- Transient synovitis of the hip:
  - Suggested by inability to bear weight on the limb, temperature <101°, normal white blood count, and normal sedimentation rate.

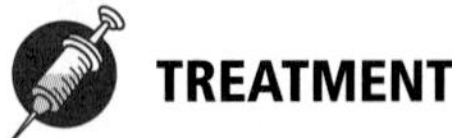

## TREATMENT

### GENERAL MEASURES

- Consider septic arthritis an orthopaedic emergency; initial treatment should include hospitalization.
- Principles of treatment include adequate administration of bactericidal antibiotics, drainage, and early immobilization (3,4).
  - Antibiotics/aspiration:
    - Begin intravenous antibiotics immediately after obtaining samples for culture.
    - 3–6 weeks of antibiotic treatment are needed.
    - Intravenous antibiotic treatment is indicated until clinical improvement is seen.
    - Oral antibiotics may be used if: Patient shows a clinical response to intravenous antibiotics; organism causing infection is known; organism is susceptible to orally administered antibiotics; patient tolerates oral antibiotics.
    - Aspiration and intravenous antibiotics may be sufficient for treating some organisms in small joints.
    - When septic arthritis is diagnosed early in a superficial joint (e.g., ankle, elbow), it is reasonable to aspirate the joint, begin appropriate antibiotics, and carefully monitor the patient for 24–48 hours.
    - Aspiration may be repeated as needed.
  - Drainage:
    - Surgical drainage is necessary for all infections that do not respond to aspiration or antibiotics within 72 hours, have loculated synovial fluid, or involve the hip.
    - Arthroscopic drainage may be a good treatment option for certain joints such as the knee, elbow, ankle, and shoulder.

- Immobilization:
  - Splint in a position of comfort until clinical signs show a decrease in swelling and tenderness, and the patient has a comfortable ROM.
  - Begin muscle strengthening and ROM exercises (see "Physical Therapy").

## SPECIAL THERAPY

### *Physical Therapy*

- Once clinical improvement is noted, deformity should be prevented and function should be re-established gradually.
- Muscle-strengthening exercises with isometric regimens should be instituted in adults, and active ROM exercises are started.
- Some studies have shown that continuous passive motion may inhibit the formation of adhesions and pannus, and promote better nutrition of the cartilage during the healing phase (3,5).

## MEDICATION (DRUGS)

- Antibiotics, which must be started immediately after aspiration and obtaining blood cultures, may be divided into initial and definitive categories.
  - Initial diagnosis:
    - A combination of agents administered parenterally until the identity and susceptibility of the bacteria are known.
    - Initial antibiotic choices are based on broad coverage and knowledge of common causative organisms.
  - Definitive diagnosis:
    - Specific antibiotics given to which the organism is sensitive

### *First Line*

- Except in children <4 years old, the most common causative organism is *Staphylococcus*.
- Because most infections are caused by penicillin-resistant strains, a $\beta$-lactamase–resistant cephalosporin, such as ceftriaxone or cefazolin, is usually a 1st-line drug.
- After local signs of infection have subsided, an oral antibiotic, such as amoxicillin with clavulanic acid, may be substituted.

## SURGERY

- Open irrigation and débridement is the most dependable way to sterilize the joint and remove all inflamed cells, enzymes, and debris; leave an opening in the joint capsule to allow drainage.
- Consider arthroscopic irrigation and débridement in the knee, shoulder, elbow, and ankle.
- Exception: Gonococcal arthritis usually does not need surgical drainage.

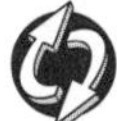

# FOLLOW-UP

## PROGNOSIS

- With prompt diagnosis and appropriate treatment, the prognosis usually is good for complete recovery.
- Prognosis is worse in immunocompromised or premature patients.
- Delay in diagnosis in patients with a generalized septic condition is associated with a poor prognosis, and aggressive surgical débridement and antibiotic therapy are critical.

## COMPLICATIONS

- Delay in diagnosis and treatment >5 days from the onset of symptoms plays an important role in the incidence of complications.
- Pathologic dislocation associated with septic arthritis of the hip occurs in children who are treated late; it is seen rarely in adults.
- Destruction of articular cartilage can lead to restricted joint motion or ankylosis of the joint.
  - Damage to the cartilaginous epiphysis and growth plate in children leads to joint deformity and leg-length discrepancy.
  - Septic necrosis of the femoral head, in hip infections, can cause growth disturbance and later degenerative joint disease.
- Patients with prostheses in joints other than the site of principal infection may experience seeding to the prosthetic joints hematogenously.

## PATIENT MONITORING

- The patient should be monitored in a hospital setting initially until the following occur:
  - The patient is clinically stable.
  - Appropriate antibiotics are instituted.
  - Patient response is noted (patient afebrile in 48–72 hours, decreased swelling and tenderness, return of white blood cell count to normal, and decreasing ESR).
- Then the patient may be discharged home; improvement may be monitored by physical examination, ESR, and possibly C-reactive protein and radiographs.
- Worsening clinical status may indicate a need for repeat aspiration.

## REFERENCES


1. Goergens ED, McEvoy A, Watson M, et al. Acute osteomyelitis and septic arthritis in children. *J Paediatr Child Health* 2005;41:59–62.
2. Kocher MS, Mandiga R, Murphy JM, et al. A clinical practice guideline for treatment of septic arthritis in children. Efficacy in improving process of care and effect on outcome of septic arthritis of the hip. *J Bone Joint Surg* 2003;85A:994–999.
3. McCarthy JJ, Dormans JP, Kozin SH, et al. Musculoskeletal infections in children: Basic treatment principles and recent advancements. *Instr Course Lect* 2005;54:515–528.
4. Stans A. Osteomyelitis and septic arthritis. In: Morrissy RT, Weinstein SL, eds. *Lovell and Winter's Pediatric Orthopaedics*, 6th ed. Philadelphia: Lippincott Williams & Wilkins, 2006:439–491.
5. Sucato DJ, Schwend RM, Gillespie R. Septic arthritis of the hip in children. *J Am Acad Orthop Surg* 1997;5:249–260.
6. Warner WC, Jr. Infectious arthritis. In: Crenshaw AH, ed. *Campbell's Operative Orthopaedics*, 8th ed. St. Louis: Mosby-Year Book, 1992:151–176.


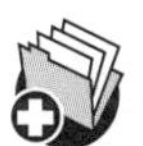

# MISCELLANEOUS

## CODES

### *ICD9-CM*

711.00 Septic arthritis

## PATIENT TEACHING

- Patients must understand the need for compliance with antibiotics and the necessity of preventing deformity and re-establishing function through physical therapy.
- If the organism is gonococcal, patient education and treatment of sexual partners is key to preventing recurrence.

## FAQ

- Q: What is the role of aspiration alone in septic arthritis?
  - A: It is an option for accessible small- to moderate-sized joints in mature patients who show no signs of sepsis. It is not indicated for a septic hip.

# SEPTIC ARTHRITIS OF THE FOOT

*John T. Campbell, MD*

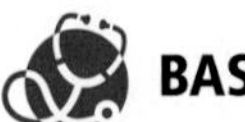

## BASICS

### DESCRIPTION

Septic arthritis is a bacterial or fungal infection of the joints of the foot.

### GENERAL PREVENTION

- Appropriate shoe wear and avoidance of going barefoot to prevent puncture wounds
- Treatment of diabetic or neuropathic ulcers

### RISK FACTORS (1)

- Previous joint trauma or arthritis
- Inflammatory arthropathy
- Diabetes or immunocompromise
- Skin disease
- Peripheral vascular disease
- Intravenous drug abuse

### PATHOPHYSIOLOGY

- Damage to joint cartilage occurs from (1):
  - Bacterial enzymes and toxins
  - Neutrophil-derived proteases and cytokines
  - Ischemia from impaired oxygen diffusion from synovial fluid in presence of purulence

### ETIOLOGY

- Bacteremia to synovium
- Trauma or puncture wound with direct joint seeding
- Iatrogenic seeding after arthroscopy or arthrocentesis
- Patients with diabetes, peripheral neuropathy, or peripheral vascular disease may develop septic arthritis from direct extension of infected foot ulcers.

### ASSOCIATED CONDITIONS

Osteomyelitis

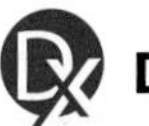

## DIAGNOSIS

### SIGNS AND SYMPTOMS

- Warmth and swelling usually are present at the infection site.
- The affected joint is painful and has decreased ROM.
- The patient may complain of difficulty in bearing weight on the affected extremity.
- Systemic symptoms such as fever, chills, and sweats may be present.

#### *Physical Exam*

- Try to localize the affected joint by careful palpation.
- Note erythema, swelling, and tenderness of the involved joint.
- Assess joint ROM and pain with passive motion.

### TESTS

#### *Lab*

- Aspirate the affected joint.
- Analyze the synovial fluid from the affected joint for cell count, differential, Gram stain, and urate crystals.
- Culture synovial fluid and blood.

#### *Imaging*

- Radiographs may show adjacent osteomyelitis or soft-tissue swelling.
- CT and MRI show fluid in the joint.

#### *Pathological Findings*

- Infections of the foot joints can arise by adjacent spread, direct inoculation, or hematogenous seeding.
- The most common organism infecting the joints is *Staphylococcus aureus*.
- *Haemophilus influenzae* infection is seen in children <6 years old.
- *Pseudomonas* species may infect foot joints from puncture wounds, particularly through the sole of shoe wear.
- Gram-positive organisms are the most common cause of septic arthritis in adults (1).
- Patients with diabetes, foot ulcers, or peripheral vascular disease are likely to have polymicrobial infections with Gram-negative organisms and anaerobes.

### DIFFERENTIAL DIAGNOSIS

- Fracture
- Soft-tissue abscess
- Osteomyelitis
- Gout
- Tumor
- Reactive arthritis (formerly Reiter syndrome)
- Charcot arthropathy

## TREATMENT

### GENERAL MEASURES

- Acute joint infections can be treated with parenteral antibiotics and repeated aspiration of the affected joint.
- If purulence does not improve, if effusions continue to form beyond 5–6 days, or if the infection is chronic, the joint should be opened surgically, irrigated, and débrided.
- In both acute and chronic infections, the patient should be splinted to immobilize the infected joint and should be nonweightbearing on the affected extremity.

### SPECIAL THERAPY

#### *Physical Therapy*

- May assist with recovery of ROM, strength, and gait mechanics after resolution of infection
- Attempt early ROM to prevent contracture.

### MEDICATION (DRUGS)

#### *First Line*

- Initial antibiotic treatment is selected based on patient risk factors and suspected organism.
- Antibiotic regimen is refined based on culture results.

### SURGERY

- Acute infections that respond to aspiration and antibiotics may be observed.
  - Repeat aspiration is indicated until effusions resolve.
- Surgical débridement is indicated for patients with:
  - Sepsis
  - Immunocompromise or systemic disease (e.g., diabetes or rheumatoid arthritis)
  - Chronic infection or delayed presentation
  - Adjacent soft-tissue abscess
  - Infection with necrotizing *Streptococcus* or Gram-negative species
  - Failure to respond clinically to repeat aspirations
- Uncomplicated infection of the ankle can be addressed with arthroscopic débridement, whereas other joints of foot typically are treated with open arthrotomy and débridement.
- Necrotic tissue or associated osteomyelitis also is débrided.

## FOLLOW-UP

### PROGNOSIS

Most infections resolve with aggressive treatment, including antibiotics and surgical débridement.

### COMPLICATIONS

Progressive infections can require amputation.

### PATIENT MONITORING

The patient should be followed closely, and the joint should be reaspirated as the effusion reaccumulates.

### REFERENCE

1. Ross JJ. Septic arthritis. *Infect Dis Clin North Am* 2005;19:799–817.

### ADDITIONAL READING

Frierson JG, Pfeffinger LL. Infections of the foot. In: Coughlin MJ, Mann RA, eds. *Surgery of the Foot and Ankle*, 7th ed. St. Louis: Mosby, 1999.

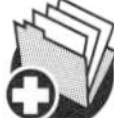

## MISCELLANEOUS

### CODES

#### *ICD9-CM*

741.00 Septic arthritis

### FAQ

- Q: What organism is most commonly involved in septic arthritis?
  - A: *S. aureus*.
- Q: What are common causes of septic arthritis of the foot?
  - A: Bacteremic seeding, infection from adjacent foot ulcer, seeding from trauma or puncture wound.
- Q: What type of antibiotic regimen is most appropriate for patients with diabetes or foot ulceration?
  - A: Infections in these patients usually are polymicrobial, so the initial antibiotic regimen should be broad spectrum and include coverage for Gram-positive, Gram-negative, and anaerobic species.

# SEPTIC HIP

*Tariq A. Nayfeh, MD, PhD*
*Simon C. Mears, MD, PhD*

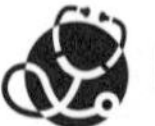

## BASICS

### DESCRIPTION
- The incidence of septic hip is increasing, especially in elderly and immunosuppressed individuals.
- This condition may occur in infants, children, adults, and the elderly, but it is more common in the pediatric population.
- Risks factors include hip surgery (most common cause), intravenous drug abuse, alcoholism, and steroid use.

### EPIDEMIOLOGY
#### *Incidence*
- In children, the hip may be the most common site of joint infection (1).
- In adults, infected knees are more common than infected hips (2).
- The rate of infection after total hip replacement is ~2% (3).

### RISK FACTORS
- Local factors:
  - Previous surgery
  - Previous hip replacement
  - Intra-articular hip injection
  - Osteoarthritis
  - AVN
  - Previous trauma
- Systemic factors:
  - Immunosuppression
  - Intravenous drug abuse
  - Hemophilia
  - Seronegative arthritides
  - Sickle cell disease

### PATHOPHYSIOLOGY
- Direct inoculation secondary to surgery is a common cause of infection in the adult hip.
- Hematogenous spread is more common in the pediatric population than in the adult.
- Sources include:
  - Urinary tract
  - Lung
  - Skin Infections

### ETIOLOGY
- Bacteria in the blood lodge in the vascular synovial membrane or enter directly through a damaged joint capsule or diseased synovium.
- Common organisms:
  - *Staphylococcus aureus:*
    - The most common organism in both children (1) and adults (4).
- *Streptococcus* species
- *Gonococcus*
- *Pseudomonas* species
- *Escherichia coli*
- *Salmonella*
- *Klebsiella*
- *Myobacterium tuberculosis*
- *Brucella*

### ASSOCIATED CONDITIONS
- Hemophilia
- Sickle cell disease
- Intravenous drug abuse
- Immunosuppression

## DIAGNOSIS

### SIGNS AND SYMPTOMS
- Pain in the groin and/or inner thigh
- Fever and occasionally chills
- Concurrent source of infection

#### *History*
- Pain in the affected hip is the most common complaint.
- Occasionally patients present with isolated pain in the ipsilateral knee.

#### *Physical Exam*
- Fever
- Skin changes such as a rash or decubitus ulcer
- Gait disturbances such as antalgic gait or the inability to ambulate
- Hip examination:
  - Tenderness
  - Hip held in flexion, external rotation
  - Restricted and painful ROM

### TESTS
#### *Lab*
- Laboratory tests are unreliable, especially in the immunocompromised patient.
- Elevated ESR
- Elevated C-reactive protein
- White blood cell count may or may not be elevated.
  - Usually an elevated percentage of polymorphonuclear leukocytes is present.
- Hip aspiration
- Blood cultures

#### *Pediatric Considerations*
- Diagnosis in the neonatal and pediatric population is difficult.
- The most sensitive factors are thought to be fever >38.5°C, inability to bear weight, elevated ESR, and C-reactive protein >2.0 mg/dL (5).

#### *Imaging*
- Plain radiography:
  - May remain normal for up to 2 weeks
  - Early findings include widening of the teardrop interval.
  - Late findings include erosive and absorptive changes of surrounding bone and destruction of the femoral head.
- Nuclear scans
- MRI:
  - May show soft-tissue abnormality, pelvic fracture, or osteomyelitis or retroperitoneal fluid
  - No studies show its usefulness in the diagnosis of septic arthritis.
- Ultrasound:
  - Valuable to show effusion in the neonatal and pediatric age groups
  - Used to guide aspiration

#### *Diagnostic Procedures/Surgery*
- Hip aspiration is the most important test in diagnosis.
  - Elevated white blood cell count (100,000–250,000)
- Positive joint fluid culture
- Occasionally a positive Gram stain

#### *Pathological Findings*
- Rapid destruction of the femoral head and acetabulum
- Late findings include septicemia, subluxation, deformity, and ankylosis.

### DIFFERENTIAL DIAGNOSIS
- Crystalline arthropathy
- Inflammatory arthritis
- Rheumatoid arthritis
- Hemophilia
- Transient synovitis of the hip

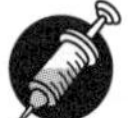

# TREATMENT

## INITIAL STABILIZATION
- Early diagnosis is the key to joint preservation and possibly to patient survival.
- Initiation of empiric antibiotics after joint fluid is obtained
- Diagnosis in neonates and children is particularly difficult, and the use of regimented guidelines has been found to be helpful (6).
- Diagnosis in the presence of a prosthetic joint also may be difficult because cultures may be negative even in the presence of infection (7).

## MEDICATION (DRUGS)
- After obtaining fluid for cultures and sensitivities, antibiotics based on history and Gram stain should be started immediately.
- The antibiotics can be tailored after obtaining identification of the infecting organism.

## SURGERY
- Open surgical drainage and débridement are the mainstays of treatment.
- Case series have reported on using hip arthroscopy to débride the hip (8).
- If the patient is too ill to undergo surgery, serial aspirations can be performed.
- Treatment of the infected prosthetic joint (9):
  - Suppressive antibiotics alone: Used only in patients who cannot tolerate surgery
  - Washout and retention of the components: Useful if the infection is not chronic and the components are stable
  - 1-stage revision surgery:
    - Only 1 surgery for both débridement and revision of the prosthesis
    - Controversial, but may have higher failure rates than 2-stage treatment
  - 2-stage revision surgery is the most reliable method for eradicating infection.
- Treatment of the late sequelae of hip infection is difficult.
  - In children, may include pelvic osteotomy, hip fusion, or hip resection (10)
  - In the adult, may include hip resection or 2-stage hip replacement (11)

# FOLLOW-UP

## DISPOSITION
### *Issues for Referral*
- All patients with painful hips should be referred quickly to an orthopaedic surgeon to rule out sepsis.
- The importance of a quick diagnosis cannot be overemphasized.
- Antibiotics should not be started until cultures are obtained.

## PROGNOSIS
- If diagnosis and treatment are initiated early, prognosis usually is good.
- Outcomes usually are poor if treatment is delayed.
- Infection and osteomyelitis with methicillin-resistant *S. aureus* is thought to have a worse prognosis than that from methicillin-sensitive organisms (1).

## COMPLICATIONS
- Osteomyelitis
- Septicemia
- Degenerative joint disease
- Deformity

## REFERENCES

1. Wang CL, Wang SM, Yang YJ, et al. Septic arthritis in children: Relationship of causative pathogens, complications, and outcome. *J Microbiol Immunol Infect* 2003;36:41–46.
2. Abid N, Bhatti M, Azharuddin M, et al. Septic arthritis in a tertiary care hospital. *J Pak Med Assoc* 2006;56:95–98.
3. Ridgeway S, Wilson J, Charlet A, et al. Infection of the surgical site after arthroplasty of the hip. *J Bone Joint Surg* 2005;87B:844–850.
4. Eder L, Zisman D, Rozenbaum M, et al. Clinical features and aetiology of septic arthritis in northern Israel. *Rheumatology* 2005;44: 1559–1563.
5. Caird MS, Flynn JM, Leung YL, et al. Factors distinguishing septic arthritis from transient synovitis of the hip in children. A prospective study. *J Bone Joint Surg* 2006;88A:1251–1257.
6. Kocher MS, Mandiga R, Murphy JM, et al. A clinical practice guideline for treatment of septic arthritis in children. Efficacy in improving process of care and effect on outcome of septic arthritis of the hip. *J Bone Joint Surg* 2003;85A:994–999.
7. Della Valle CJ, Zuckerman JD, Di Cesare PE. Periprosthetic sepsis. *Clin Orthop Relat Res* 2004;420:26–31.
8. Kim SJ, Choi NH, Ko SH, et al. Arthroscopic treatment of septic arthritis of the hip. *Clin Orthop Relat Res* 2003;407:211–214.
9. Hanssen AD, Spangehl MJ. Treatment of the infected hip replacement. *Clin Orthop Relat Res* 2004;420:63–71.
10. Choi IH, Shin YW, Chung CY, et al. Surgical treatment of the severe sequelae of infantile septic arthritis of the hip. *Clin Orthop Relat Res* 2005;434:102–109.
11. Cherney DL, Amstutz HC. Total hip replacement in the previously septic hip. *J Bone Joint Surg* 1983;65A:1256–1265.


## ADDITIONAL READING

Zacher J, Gursche A. 'Hip' pain. *Best Pract Res Clin Rheumatol* 2003;17:71–85.


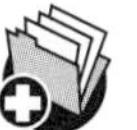

# MISCELLANEOUS

## CODES
### *ICD9-CM*
711.95 Septic arthritis, hip

## FAQ
- Q: How is a septic hip diagnosed and treated in a child?
  - A: The clinical signs are pain and swelling in the hip, inability to walk, and fever. ESR and C-reactive protein tests should be checked. If levels are elevated, the suspicion for sepsis is high. The joint should be aspirated and antibiotics should be started. If infection is found, the hip should be treated surgically with arthrotomy.

# SEPTIC KNEE

*Michelle Cameron, MD*
*John H. Wilckens, MD*

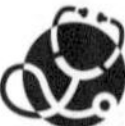

## BASICS

### DESCRIPTION

- A septic knee is an infection of the synovial lining of the knee joint.
- Predisposing factors include arthritis, intravenous drug abuse and alcoholism, steroid use, and any form of immunosuppression (1).

### EPIDEMIOLOGY

#### *Incidence*

- Common
- May occur in infants, children, adults, and the geriatric population

### RISK FACTORS

- Intravenous drug abuse and alcoholism
- Trauma, surgery
- HIV disease
- Steroids
- Immunocompromised hosts (e.g., those with diabetes, HIV)

### ETIOLOGY

- *Staphylococcus aureus* is the most common cause.
- Other common organisms:
  - Hemolytic *Streptococcus*
  - *Pneumococcus*
  - *Gonococcus*
  - *Meningococcus*
  - *Salmonella*
  - *Brucella*
  - *Haemophilus influenzae* (infants)

## DIAGNOSIS

### SIGNS AND SYMPTOMS

- Monarticular erythema
- Swelling
- Fluctuant joint capsule
- Pain on ROM or weightbearing
- Possible fever and leukocytosis

#### *Physical Exam*

- The key findings are:
  - Joint effusion
  - Painful ROM
  - Erythema

### TESTS

#### *Lab*

- The complete blood count may show leukocytosis with a left shift, and the ESR is always almost elevated.
- C-reactive protein also is helpful.
- The primary test is analysis of fluid aspirated from the knee joint.
  - Opinions vary on the leukocyte count that is diagnostic of a septic joint.
  - Most authors agree that an aspirate with >100,000 white cells with >90% polymorphonuclear cells is strongly suggestive.
  - The fluid will have low glucose and high protein levels.
  - The aspirate should be sent for Gram stain and culture.
- The fluid also should be sent for crystal evaluation to rule out gout or pseudogout.
- Any patient suspected of having septic arthritis should have 2–3 blood cultures drawn before administration of antibiotics.
- The ESR also is elevated and may be helpful in following the disease course.

#### *Imaging*

- Chronic, low-grade septic arthritis can be difficult to diagnose.
- MRI scans may show osteomyelitis and a Baker cyst in addition to a large effusion and hypertrophy of the synovium.

#### *Pathological Findings*

- If the infection is not recognized and treated early, destruction of articular cartilage will occur.
- Cartilage erosion leads to degenerative changes in the joint.
  - The amount of bone destruction depends on the virulence of the organism and the length of time infection has been present.
- Long-standing septic arthritis can progress to fibrous or bony ankylosis and septicemia.

### DIFFERENTIAL DIAGNOSIS

- Acute osteomyelitis
- Periarticular cellulitis
- Prepatellar bursitis
- Gout
- Pseudogout
- Acute rheumatoid arthritis
- Hemophilia
- Lyme disease

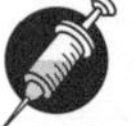

# TREATMENT

## GENERAL MEASURES

- In general, management usually is surgical: Open or arthroscopic débridement (2).
  - If the infection is discovered early, 1 nonoperative treatment can be tried, using intravenous antibiotics and serial aspirations.
- Early diagnosis and prompt treatment are indicated to prevent severe and permanent damage.
- The joint should be irrigated and débrided urgently; multiple débridements may be necessary.
- If present, a popliteal cyst may need to be excised because it can reinoculate the knee joint.
- Immobilization of the leg in a knee immobilizer also is recommended throughout the acute episode.
- Once the infection has subsided, gentle active and passive ROM exercises can be started.

## SPECIAL THERAPY

### *Physical Therapy*

Gentle active and passive ROM exercises of the knee should be initiated after the acute episode has cleared.

## MEDICATION (DRUGS)

### *First Line*

- Institute antibiotic therapy as soon as appropriate specimens are obtained for culture.
- Empiric antibiotic therapy should cover Gram-positive organisms.
- Antibiotic coverage should be modified appropriately when Gram stain and culture results are available.

## SURGERY

- Irrigation and débridement consist of opening the knee arthroscopically or through a standard knee approach and washing the joint with multiple liters of normal saline (3).
- All loculations are found and broken to allow complete drainage.

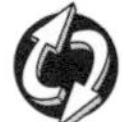

# FOLLOW-UP

## PROGNOSIS

- With early treatment, prognosis usually is good.
- Outcomes are poor if the diagnosis is delayed substantially.

## COMPLICATIONS

- Fibrous or bony ankylosis of the knee
- Osteomyelitis
- Septicemia
- Degenerative joint disease

## REFERENCES


1. Brashear HR, Jr, Raney, RB Sr. Infections of bones and joints. In: *Handbook of Orthopaedic Surgery*, 10th ed. St. Louis: CV Mosby, 1986:110–139.
2. Thiery JA. Arthroscopic drainage in septic arthritides of the knee: A multicenter study. *Arthroscopy* 1989;5:65–69.
3. Ivey M, Clark R. Arthroscopic debridement of the knee for septic arthritis. *Clin Orthop Relat Res* 1985;199:201–206.


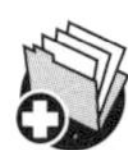

# MISCELLANEOUS

## CODES

### *ICD9-CM*

711.96 Septic arthritis, knee

## PATIENT TEACHING

- Patients are encouraged to work on early ROM.
- Stiffness will occur and can be permanent without ROM exercises.

## FAQ

- Q: What laboratory studies should be requested on an aspirate suspicious for septic knee?
  - A: In addition to culture and sensitivity studies, the aspirate should be sent for Gram stain, cell count, and analysis for crystals. White cell counts >50,000 with a "left shift" are strongly suspicious for infection; counts >100,000 essentially are diagnostic for infection.
- Q: Does a septic knee always require surgical irrigation and débridement?
  - A: Early surgery is recommended for all septic knees. In rare instances, repeat aspirations may be considered in some pediatric patients and when surgical evaluation is delayed.

# SERONEGATIVE SPONDYLOARTHROPATHIES

*Andrew P. Manista, MD*

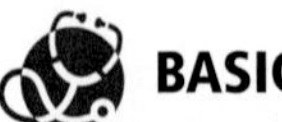

## BASICS

### DESCRIPTION

- Also called "enthesopathies," these inflammatory diseases are associated with a negative rheumatoid factor or antinuclear antibody titer that affects the spine and multiple peripheral joints.
- Included in the seronegative spondyloarthropathies are AS, reactive arthritis (formerly known as Reiter syndrome), psoriatic arthritis, and enteropathic arthritis.
- Synonym: Reactive arthritis

### GENERAL PREVENTION

Although the disease cannot be prevented, careful treatment and follow-up can prevent contractures and pulmonary and cardiac complications.

### EPIDEMIOLOGY

- Onset is usually before 40 years of age and may occur during adolescence.
- Males are clinically affected 2–3 times more often than females (1).

#### *Incidence*

- HLA-B27 gene frequency varies with race (2).
  - Up to 10% of Caucasians
  - 3% of African Americans
  - 0.1% of black Africans
  - Up to 25% of some groups of Native Americans

### RISK FACTORS

- Male gender
- HLA-B27 positive (relative risk)
- Jewish descent (enteropathic arthritis)

#### *Genetics*

>50–90% are HLA-B27 positive (AS, 90%; other enthesopathies, 50–70%), although, as in AS, only 2% of HLA-B27-positive persons develop AS (2).

### ETIOLOGY

- Patients have a genetic predisposition with an environmental influence.
- Many of these patients develop high levels of antibodies directed against *Chlamydia, Yersinia, Salmonella,* and *Campylobacter*.
- Triggering bacteria may share a similar antigenic amino acid sequence with a sequence on the B27 molecules, rendering these "self" proteins foreign in appearance and therefore vulnerable to immunogenic attacks.

### ASSOCIATED CONDITIONS

- Iritis
- Aortitis
- Colitis
- Arachnoiditis
- Amyloidosis
- Pulmonary fibrosis
- Sarcoidosis

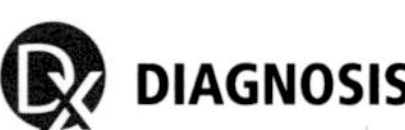

## DIAGNOSIS

### SIGNS AND SYMPTOMS

- AS: Findings include bilateral sacroiliitis with acute uveitis, insidious onset of back or hip pain, and enthesitis.
- Reactive arthritis:
  - The classic clinical picture is a young male presenting with the triad of urethritis, conjunctivitis, and arthritis.
  - Other common presenting symptoms include plantar heel pain, oral ulcers, and genital lesions.
- Psoriatic arthropathies:
  - Affects up to 70% of patients with psoriasis (3).
  - Small joints of the hands (DIP) and feet are most commonly involved, with nail pitting, sausage-like digits, and "pencil in cup" deformities of these small joints on radiographs.
- Enteropathic arthritis:
  - Affects up to 20% of patients with Crohn disease or ulcerative colitis (4)
  - Presentation can be similar to that of AS.
  - Asymmetric involvement of large, weightbearing joints (hips and knees) is common.
  - Abdominal manifestations include cramping, abdominal pain, bloody diarrhea (ulcerative colitis), and dehydration.

### TESTS

#### *Lab*

- Rheumatoid factor and antinuclear antibody titers
- HLA-B27 (poor yield because 2% of HLA-B27-positive patients develop seronegative spondyloarthropathies [2])
- ESR

#### *Imaging*

- Radiography:
  - Obtain AP pelvis, AP lumbar spine, and lateral lumbar spine radiographs.
  - Additional imaging of symptomatic joints may be indicated.
- CT or MRI may afford earlier detection of sacroiliitis (5).
- AS: Findings include symmetric SI joint narrowing, squaring of the vertebral bodies, ascending spinal syndesmophytes seen with time, and protrusio acetabuli.
- Reactive arthritis: Findings include SI joint narrowing (can be asymmetric) and variable regions of spinal involvement.
- Psoriatic arthritis: Findings include small joint involvement, commonly the DIP joints of the hands, with a "pencil in cup" deformity and autofusion of the joints; bony resorption in the hand can be severe.
- Enteropathic arthritis: Findings are similar to those of AS.
- Caution should be exercised when evaluating the patient with AS and "minor" trauma.
  - Conventional radiographs may appear normal.
  - MRI scans to evaluate for nondisplaced fractures and epidural hematomas

#### *Pathological Findings*

- Enthesopathy (inflammation at ligament-bone insertion sites)
- Synovitis
- Pulmonary fibrosis
- Colitis
- Aortitis

### DIFFERENTIAL DIAGNOSIS

- AS
- Reactive arthritis
- Psoriatic arthritis
- Enteropathic arthritis
- Rheumatoid arthritis (seropositive)
- Infection (Lyme disease)

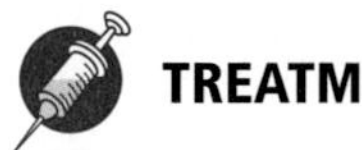

## TREATMENT

### GENERAL MEASURES

- Postural training
- Strengthening and ROM exercises
- Sleeping on a firm mattress (AS)
- Avoidance of contact sports (AS)
- Low impact exercises
- No dietary restrictions

### SPECIAL THERAPY

#### *Physical Therapy*

Physical therapy often is necessary to maintain joint ROM and to prevent contractures.

### MEDICATION (DRUGS)

#### *First Line*

- NSAIDs
- Disease-modifying agents such as sulfasalazine or methotrexate
- Eyedrops for uveitis

### SURGERY

- Hip arthritis may be severe, resulting in the need for hip replacement.
- Cervical, thoracic, and lumbar spinal deformities may occur, necessitating a corrective osteotomy.

## FOLLOW-UP

### PROGNOSIS

- In general, prognosis is better for pediatric-onset than for adult-onset spondyloarthropathies.
- In patients with AS, the prognosis is determined by the rate of disease progression.

### COMPLICATIONS

Cardiac involvement such as aortic insufficiency, pulmonary fibrosis, gastrointestinal complications such as perforations or fistulas, and vertebral (cervical) fractures (AS) may occur.

### PATIENT MONITORING

- Close follow-up with rheumatologists and orthopaedic surgeons is indicated.
- Depending on the severity of the disease, patients are seen every 3–6 months.

### REFERENCES


1. van der Linden SM, Valkenburg HA, de Jongh BM, et al. The risk of developing ankylosing spondylitis in HLA-B27 positive individuals. A comparison of relatives of spondylitis patients with the general population. *Arthritis Rheum* 1984;27:241–249.
2. Liu NYN, Weinstein BR. Seronegative spondyloarthropathies. In: Noble J, ed. *Textbook of Primary Care Medicine*, 3rd ed. St. Louis: Mosby, 2001:1279–1293.
3. Battistone MJ, Manaster BJ, Reda DJ, et al. The prevalence of sacroiliitis in psoriatic arthritis: New perspectives from a large, multicenter cohort. A Department of Veterans Affairs Cooperative Study. *Skeletal Radiol* 1999;28:196–201.
4. Sands BE. Crohn's disease. In: Feldman M, Tschumy WO, Jr, Friedman LS, et al., eds. *Sleisenger & Fordtran's Gastrointestinal and Liver Disease*, 7th ed. St. Louis: Saunders, 2002: 2005–2038.
5. Resnick D, Niwayama G. Ankylosing spondylitis. In: Resnick D, ed. *Diagnosis of Bone and Joint Disorders*, 3rd ed. Philadelphia: WB Saunders, 1995:1008–1074.


### ADDITIONAL READING


- Brinker MR, Miller MD. Basic sciences. In: Miller MD, ed. *Review of Orthopaedics*, 2nd ed. Philadelphia: WB Saunders, 1996:1–122.
- Brown CR, Jr. Medical treatment of arthritis. In: Callaghan JJ, Dennis DA, Paprosky WG, et al., eds. *Orthopaedic Knowledge Update: Hip and Knee Reconstruction*. Rosemont, IL: American Academy of Orthopaedic Surgeons, 1995:69–78.
- Kredich D, Patrone NA. Pediatric spondyloarthropathies. *Clin Orthop Relat Res* 1990;259:18–22.
- Miller-Blair DJ, Tsuchiya N, Yamaguchi A, et al. Immunologic mechanisms in common rheumatologic diseases. *Clin Orthop Relat Res* 1996;326:43–54.
- Reveille JD, Arnett FC, Keat A, et al. Seronegative spondyloarthropathies. In: Klippel JH, ed. *Primer on the Rheumatic Diseases*, 12th ed. Atlanta: Arthritis Foundation, 2001:239–258.


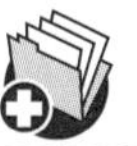

## MISCELLANEOUS

### CODES

#### *ICD9-CM*

721.90 AS

### PATIENT TEACHING

- Explain the genetic aspects of the disease.
- Patients with AS with a sudden onset of neck or back pain must be evaluated for acute fractures.

### FAQ

- Q: Does HAL-B27-positive status confer a diagnosis of AS?
  - A: No. Although patients with HLA-B27 positive status appear to be at increased risk of developing reactive arthritis, only 2%of patients with HLA-B27 status develop AS.
- Q: What are some of the systemic involvements, other than the musculoskeletal system, that can be seen in patients with AS?
  - Iritis, aortitis, colitis, arachnoiditis, amyloidosis, pulmonary fibrosis, sarcoidosis.

# SHIN SPLINTS

*John H. Wilckens, MD*
*Marc Urquhart, MD*

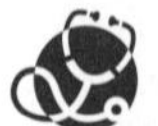

## BASICS

### DESCRIPTION
- Shin splints present with pain and discomfort in the leg from repetitive running on hard surfaces or forceful excessive use of foot plantarflexors.
- Synonyms: Medial tibia stress syndrome; Periostitis of the tibia; Runner's leg

### EPIDEMIOLOGY
Shin splints occur commonly in teens and young adults.

### RISK FACTORS
- Running or jogging, especially a recent increase in distance or speed (1)
- Pronated feet
- Training errors

### ETIOLOGY
Periostitis at the origin of the posterior tibialis muscle or the soleus muscle at the medial tibia or the soleus muscle (2)

### ASSOCIATED CONDITIONS
- Usually affects conditioning athletes
- Any deformity of the leg (e.g., pes planus) that increases stress on the leg may predispose.

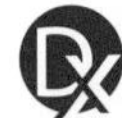

## DIAGNOSIS

### SIGNS AND SYMPTOMS
- Exercise-induced pain occurs along the posteromedial border of the distal tibia.
- Pain usually is dull, but can be intense, and is present at the onset of the workout.
- Pain may persist after the workout but eventually dissipates.

#### *Physical Exam*
- Tenderness to palpation along the medial border of the tibia (Fig. 1)
- Pain with resisted plantarflexion and inversion
- The clinical presentation of medial tibia stress syndrome may closely resemble that of stress fractures and exertional compartment syndrome, which can carry a far worse prognosis if undiagnosed (3).
- Exertional compartment syndrome has characteristic physical findings of anterolateral leg pain, commonly over the anterior compartment; fascial hernias may be present.

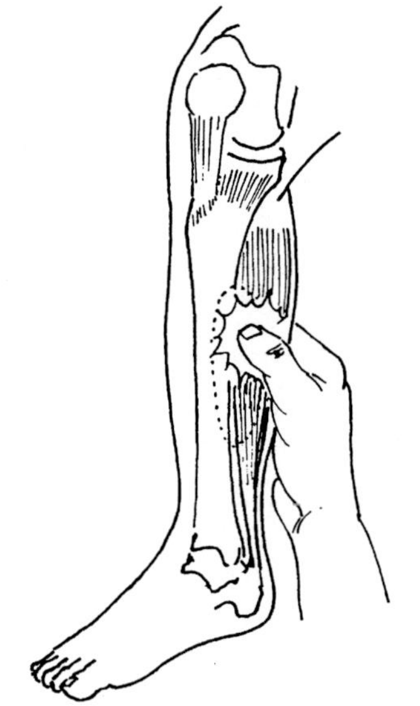

**Fig. 1.** Shin splints produce pain in the anterior or posterior border of the tibia over a long segment.

### TESTS

#### *Imaging*
- Serial plain radiographs are normal but are needed to rule out stress fractures, which usually are positive after 2 weeks of symptoms.
- A bone scan may reveal diffuse longitudinal uptake along the posteromedial border of the tibia, whereas a stress fracture is a localized or transverse uptake on bone scan.
- MRI also can be used to identify a stress fracture earlier.

#### *Diagnostic Procedures/Surgery*
Compartment pressure measurement with exercise may be needed to diagnose exertional compartment syndrome if pain is anterolateral.

#### *Pathological Findings*
Inflammation at the origin of the soleus or PTT on the tibia

### DIFFERENTIAL DIAGNOSIS
- Stress fractures (4)
- Chronic exertional compartment syndrome (5)

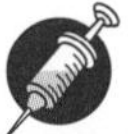

# TREATMENT

## GENERAL MEASURES

- Reduce training activity below symptom level
- Ice on the area of injury

## SPECIAL THERAPY

### *Physical Therapy*

- Therapist-determined modalities
- Strengthening and stretching exercises after acute symptoms disappear
- Core strengthening

### *Complementary and Alternative Therapies*

Orthotic or shoe modification to decrease pronation

## MEDICATION (DRUGS)

### *First Line*

- NSAIDs
- Analgesics

## SURGERY

Only after a documented trial of maximal nonoperative treatment has failed should posterior medial fascia release be considered.

# FOLLOW-UP

## PROGNOSIS

- Most cases respond well to nonoperative treatment.
- Gradual return to activity can be expected.
- Variation of the causative regimen of training and identification of training errors will help prevent recurrence.

## COMPLICATIONS

Undiagnosed stress fracture can lead to complete fracture and displacement.

## REFERENCES


1. Pell RFI, Khanuja HS, Cooley GR. Leg pain in the running athlete. *J Am Acad Orthop Surg* 2004;12: 396–404.
2. Michael RH, Holder LE. The soleus syndrome. A cause of medial tibial stress (shin splints). *Am J Sports Med* 1985;13:87–94.
3. Glorioso JE, Jr, Wilckens JH. Exertional leg pain. In: O'Connor FG, Wilder RP, eds. *Textbook of Running Medicine*. New York: McGraw-Hill, 2001:181–197.
4. Rettig AC, Shelbourne KD, McCarroll, Jr, et al. The natural history and treatment of delayed union stress fractures of the anterior cortex of the tibia. *Am J Sports Med* 1988;16:250–255.
5. Eisele SA, Sammarco GJ. Chronic exertional compartment syndrome. *Instr Course Lect* 1993; 42:213–217.


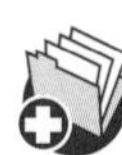

# MISCELLANEOUS

## CODES

### *ICD9-CM*

844.9 Shin splints

## PATIENT TEACHING

- Identify training errors.
- Emphasize the importance of modified activity followed by stretching and strengthening exercises.
- Resumption of activity should be done gradually, below the level of the symptoms.

## FAQ

- Q: Do patients with shin splints need physical therapy?
  - A: Although shin splints usually are self-limiting with rest, identification of training errors, and gradual return to activity, physical therapy can be helpful. Physical therapy can use modalities to reduce the acute symptoms while identifying training errors, flexibility, and limb alignment issues. Concentric and eccentric strengthening of the lower extremity in addition to core strengthening may reduce the risk of recurrence.

# SHORT STATURE

*Paul D. Sponseller, MD*

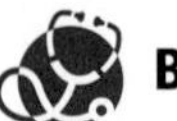

## BASICS

### DESCRIPTION

- Short stature is defined as height under the 3rd percentile for age of the general population.
- Many causes for short stature exist; orthopaedic causes are addressed here.
  - Most common cause overall is familial or constitutional short stature
  - The most common orthopaedic cause is osteochondrodysplasia, a group of skeletal disorders (>600 types) characterized by an intrinsic abnormality in the growth and remodeling of cartilage and bone
- Diagnosis usually is apparent from birth or early childhood.
- Classification:
  - International Classification of Osteochondrodysplasia (1) most widely accepted
  - According to body segment most severely affected: Short limb, short trunk (2)
  - According to area of extremity involved: Epiphyseal, metaphyseal, diaphyseal (1)
    - Patients with epiphyseal involvement are most likely to have contractures and arthritis because of involved joint surfaces.
    - The term "rhizomelic" often is used when extremity shortening is greatest in proximal segments, as in achondroplasia.
- Synonym: Dwarfism, defined as disproportionate short stature

### EPIDEMIOLOGY

#### *Incidence*

~1 per 3,000–1 per 5,000 live births (2).

### RISK FACTORS

- Family history
- Consanguinity
- Regionally concentrated dysplasias (e.g., diastrophic dysplasia in Finland, metaphyseal dysplasia in Amish communities)

#### *Genetics*

- Most dysplasias are transmitted autosomally as dominant or recessive traits.
- However, many affected persons acquire the disorder as a new mutation and may pass it on to their children.
- Genetic testing is becoming available for many disorders and may be useful in family planning when the history is positive.

### ETIOLOGY

- A defect in the locus for the fibroblast growth factor receptor accounts for achondroplasia.
- The gene for the cellular sulfate transporter accounts for diastrophic dysplasia.
- Mucopolysaccharidoses are the result of enzyme deficiencies in the pathway of mucopolysaccharide metabolism.
- Not all causes are identified.

### ASSOCIATED CONDITIONS

- Neurologic and respiratory symptoms, owing to spinal deformity
- Mental retardation in Hurler syndrome
- Hip dysplasia
- Clubfeet in diastrophic dysplasia and spondyloepiphyseal dysplasia
- Scoliosis

## DIAGNOSIS

### SIGNS AND SYMPTOMS

- Achondroplasia:
  - Most common skeletal dysplasia
  - Midface hypoplasia
  - Rhizomelic dwarfism
  - Frontal bossing
  - Delay in motor milestones
  - Thoracolumbar kyphosis
  - Spinal stenosis (mostly lumbar)
  - Overweight
  - Narrowed foramen magnum
  - Height usually <50 inches
- Multiple epiphyseal dysplasia is 1 of the most common dysplasias.
  - Autosomal dominant with disturbed ossification in many epiphyses
  - Mild short stature, so may not present until later in childhood
  - Short limbs
  - Irregular epiphyseal ossification with deformity
  - Hips, knees, and ankles most severely involved
  - Joint pain
  - Decreased ROM
  - Prominent joints
  - Extremity angular deformities
  - Final height: 57–67 inches
- Hypochondroplasia is an autosomal-dominant, mild, short-limb dwarfism.
  - Severe cases share many features with achondroplasia.
  - Mild frontal bossing
  - No midface hypoplasia
  - Symmetric shortening of extremities
  - Mild kyphosis and lordosis
- Diastrophic dysplasia is a rhizomelic dwarfism.
  - Autosomal recessive transmission
  - Cauliflower ear
  - Major joint contracture
  - Hitchhiker (abducted) thumb
  - Foot deformity
  - Scoliosis
  - Cervical spina bifida with kyphosis
- Mucopolysaccharidoses:
  - Joint contractures
  - Organomegaly
  - Often cataracts
  - Sometimes developmental delay
- Multiple osteocartilaginous exostoses:
  - Autosomal dominant
  - Mild short stature
  - Local impingement on tendons, nerves, spinal canal
  - Deformity of extremities
  - Leg-length discrepancy
  - Risk of malignant degeneration in 1% (2)
- Spondyloepiphyseal dysplasia:
  - Cervical spine instability
  - Scoliosis
  - Joint contractures
  - Stiffness at hip and knee
- Down syndrome:
  - Simian crease
  - Pes planus
  - Typical facies
  - Developmental delay
  - Ligamentous laxity
- Turner syndrome:
  - Single X-chromosome
  - Females only
  - Cubitus valgus
  - Webbed neck
  - Delayed sexual development

### *Physical Exam*

- The patient should be examined for proportionality and physical maturity.
- To make the diagnosis of skeletal dysplasia, it is important to know the following patient information:
  - Length at birth
  - Current height and percentile
  - Body proportion by comparing limb and trunk length ratio
  - Dysmorphism (morphologic variations of bone and soft tissue that may characterize disorder)
  - Complete neurologic examination to rule out stenosis or instability
  - Quantitated ROM and contractures
  - Examination for angular disturbances of the limbs and for scoliosis and kyphosis of the spine

## TESTS

### *Lab*

- The following tests usually are not indicated, but they can be useful to rule out other conditions if suspected:
  - Chemistry profile
  - Endocrine evaluation
  - Urine workup for storage disorder

### *Imaging*

- Radiographic evaluation should include:
  - Lateral skull and cervical spine
  - Lateral lumbar spine
  - AP film of the pelvis
  - AP film of the hand and wrist

### *Pathological Findings*

- Vary with the different types of disorder.
- Most dysplasias show alterations in cartilage, ligament, and tendon.

## DIFFERENTIAL DIAGNOSIS

- Consult with a geneticist or endocrinologist.
- Consider other alternatives:
  - Constitutional short stature
  - Malnutrition
  - Hormonal disorder
  - Chronic illness
  - Chronic steroid use

# TREATMENT

## GENERAL MEASURES

- Orthopaedic management of patients with osteochondrodysplasia is mainly symptomatic, correcting and achieving alignment and stability.
  - Evaluate and treat cervical spine instability with collar or fusion, if indicated.
  - Decompress neurologic claudication from spinal stenosis, if indicated.
  - Document and follow scoliosis and kyphosis.
  - Accurate genetic counseling is indicated.
  - Recognition and treatment of musculoskeletal abnormalities and intrinsic medical problems are needed.
  - With age, many patients need powered devices for transport because arthritis or spinal disorder decreases mobility.
  - Growth hormone is not useful for increasing stature.
  - Limb lengthening may gain up to 1 additional foot of height in those with achondroplasia.

## SPECIAL THERAPY

### *Physical Therapy*

Physical therapy will not correct skeletal deformity, but it may improve the patient's function.

## MEDICATION (DRUGS)

### *First Line*

No medications are available for skeletal dysplasia at this time.

## SURGERY

- Spinal fusion, decompression, and instrumentation are used to correct spinal disorders.
- Osteotomy is used to correct extremity deformities.
- Patients with early osteoarthritis from epiphyseal deformity may benefit from joint replacement.

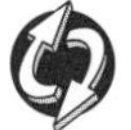

# FOLLOW-UP

## PROGNOSIS

Spinal instability, stenosis, and arthritis frequently are associated with many of the dysplasias.

## COMPLICATIONS

- Degenerative disease of the hips and knees is common.
- Cervical instability is seen in spondyloepiphyseal dysplasia and mucopolysaccharidoses.
- Complications vary with the different types of disorder.

## PATIENT MONITORING

Patients should be followed approximately every 6 months to monitor developmental milestones and skeletal deformities.

## REFERENCES


1. Beighton P, Giedion A, Gorlin R, et al. International classification of osteochondrodysplasias. *Am J Med Genet* 1992;44:223–229.
2. Sponseller PD, Ain MC. The skeletal dysplasias. In: Morrissy RT, Weinstein SL, eds. *Lovell and Winter's Pediatric Orthopaedics*, 6th ed. Philadelphia: Lippincott Williams & Wilkins, 2006:205–250.


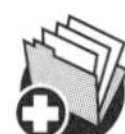

# MISCELLANEOUS

## CODES

### *ICD9-CM*

- 259.4 Dwarfism, nonspecific
- 756.4 Achondroplasia
- 756.56 Multiple epiphyseal dysplasia
- 756.59 Other (Spondyloepiphyseal dysplasia)

## PATIENT TEACHING

- Genetic counseling is indicated.
- Refer families when a positive history becomes known.

## FAQ

- Q: How do I make the diagnosis of short stature?
  - A: It is a statistical definition: Height below 2 standard deviations from the mean for the age. The cause may be determined by physical examination, skeletal survey, and consultation by a geneticist or endocrinologist.
- Q: What is the role of growth hormone in short stature?
  - A: The role varies with the cause. For all skeletal dysplasias, little gain in height occurs. For constitutional short stature, more benefit may accrue. An endocrinologist is best qualified to make recommendations.

# SHOULDER ANATOMY AND EXAMINATION

*Constantine A. Demetracopoulos, BS*
*Timothy S. Johnson, MD*

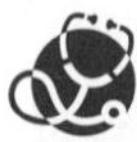

## BASICS

### DESCRIPTION

- Bones:
  - Glenohumeral joint:
    - The humeral head articulates with the glenoid fossa of the scapula.
    - Stabilized by the glenohumeral ligaments (1) capsule and rotator cuff muscles
    - The labrum of the glenoid deepens the joint and enhances stability.
  - AC joint:
    - The acromion process of the scapula articulates with the distal clavicle.
    - Suspends the arm and scapula
  - Sternoclavicular joint:
    - The sternum articulates with the proximal end of clavicle.
    - Suspends the arm and scapula
  - Scapulothoracic joint:
    - Consists of the body of the scapula and the muscles covering the posterior chest wall
    - Contributes to shoulder flexion and rotation
- Muscles:
  - The trapezius, levator, rhomboids, and serratus anterior stabilize the scapula to aid motion at the glenohumeral joint.
  - Deltoid: Flexor, abductor, and extensor
  - Rotator cuff:
    - Supraspinatus: Abductor and external rotator
    - Infraspinatus: External rotator
    - Teres minor: External rotator
    - Subscapularis: Internal rotator and adductor
  - Pectoralis major: Adductor
  - Coracobrachialis and biceps: Flexors
- Nerves:
  - Brachial plexus:
    - Passes through the axilla
    - Branches originate in the neck from C5–T1
  - Axillary nerve:
    - Innervates the deltoid
    - May be injured in anterior shoulder dislocations
  - Musculocutaneous nerve: Innervates the biceps and coracobrachialis

## DIAGNOSIS

### SIGNS AND SYMPTOMS

#### *History*

Thorough history of the mechanism of injury and the nature of pain

#### *Physical Exam*

- Initial assessment:
  - Assess the cervical spine and elbow.
  - Perform a complete neurovascular examination of the extremities.
  - Assess the contralateral shoulder for comparison.
- Inspection:
  - Expose both upper extremities from the shoulder girdle to the hand, inspecting for asymmetry, atrophy, and scapular winging.
- Palpation:
  - Palpate the sternoclavicular joint, clavicle, AC joint, coracoid, acromion, glenohumeral joint, bicipital groove, and the greater and lesser tuberosities of the humerus.
  - Localize the pain.
- ROM:
  - Compare active and passive ROM.
    - Forward flexion: 180°
    - Extension: 50–60°
  - Motion:
    - Assess in adduction and abduction.
    - Distinguish glenohumeral motion from combined glenohumeral and scapulothoracic motion (combined values).
    - External rotation: 80–90°
    - Internal rotation: 60–80°
    - Abduction: 160–180°

### TESTS

- Biceps tendinitis:
  - Pain to palpation in the bicipital groove, found anteriorly on the shoulder with the arm at 10° of internal rotation
  - Yergason test:
    - Test resisted forearm supination with the elbow flexed at 90°.
    - Test is positive when pain is reproduced in the bicipital groove.
  - Speed test:
    - With the elbow extended, the forearm supinated, and the shoulder flexed at 60°, ask the patient to resist additional forward flexion of shoulder.
    - The test is positive when pain is reproduced in the bicipital groove.
- Subacromial bursitis:
  - Presentation is very similar to that of rotator cuff tendinitis.
  - Patient may present with subacromial crepitus.
- Rotator cuff tear (2) (Fig. 1):
  - Diffuse, dull, aching pain localized over the deltoid and upper arm
  - Pain with overhead activities
  - Tenderness to palpation over the greater tuberosity of the humerus
  - Test individual rotator cuff muscles for weakness and or pain.
    - Supraspinatus: Test the patient's strength in active arm elevation in the plane of the scapula with the patient's thumb pointing down.
    - Infraspinatus and teres minor: Test the patient's strength in active external rotation with the patient's arm at the side and the elbow flexed at 90°.
    - Subscapularis ("belly press" test): Place both of the patient's hands on his/her belly; have the patient press the belly inward while thrusting elbows forward; the test is positive if the elbow cannot be actively moved forward.

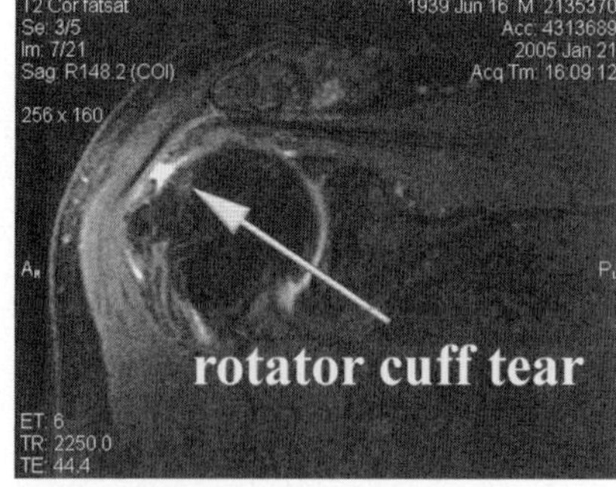


**Fig. 1.** MRI image of a supraspinatus tendon tear.

- Neer sign:
  - Elevate the arm while stabilizing the scapula.
  - Positive sign: Pain at maximal elevation
- Hawkins test:
  - With the patient's elbow flexed at 90°, forward flex the shoulder to 90° and internally rotate the humerus.
  - The test is positive if pain is reproduced on contact of the greater tuberosity with the acromion.
- Painful arc:
  - Active abduction in the coronal plane
  - The test is positive with pain at 60–100° of abduction.
  - Pain is common in tendinitis and small rotator cuff tears
- Drop-arm test:
  - Inability to hold arm up when passively positioned into an elevated position
  - Suggests a large tear
- Weakness, inability to elevate, and passive ROM that exceeds active ROM also suggest rotator cuff tear.
- Popeye sign:
  - The biceps resembles a "Popeye" muscle when resisted elbow flexion is tested.
  - Indicates a proximal rupture of the biceps tendon
  - Note: Also occurs with distal biceps tendon rupture

- Shoulder instability (3):
  - History of previous dislocations
  - Patient complains of instability with or without pain.
  - Anterior instability: Apprehension with 90/90 positioning (90° of abduction and 90° of external rotation)
  - Posterior instability: Apprehension with humeral forward flexion in internal rotation
  - Load and shift test:
    - With the humerus in a neutral position on the glenoid, axially load the humerus and shift the head anteriorly and posteriorly.
    - Excessive translation resulting in palpable subluxation and/or dislocation is a positive finding.
  - Sulcus sign:
    - With the affected elbow flexed, apply inferior traction to the arm and look for skin dimpling near the lateral acromion.
    - Dimpling indicates inferior instability.
- AC joint arthritis/AC separation (4):
  - Palpable point tenderness at the AC joint
  - Palpable step-off at the AC joint in the presence of a separation (Fig. 2)
  - Joint effusion may be present.
  - Cross-body adduction test:
    - With the shoulder at 90° of flexion, passively adduct the arm.
    - The test is positive when pain is reproduced at the AC joint.
- Labrum abnormality (Fig. 3):
  - Patient describes pain as "deep" in the shoulder and occurring with overhead activities.
  - Patient may have anterior or posterior joint line tenderness.
  - Active compression test:
    - Position the affected arm as for the cross-body adduction test.
    - With the elbow extended, and the humerus internally rotated (thumb down), test resisted humeral elevation.
    - Positive test: Pain is elicited when in internal rotation but relieved when the test is repeated in external rotation (thumb up).
    - Pain localized deep in the shoulder is indicative of biceps or labral abnormality.
    - Pain at the top of the shoulder indicates AC abnormality.
    - Pain elsewhere is equivocal.
- Glenohumeral joint arthritis:
  - Start-up pain on initiation of activity
  - Palpable joint-line tenderness
  - Decreased active and passive ROM
  - Active and passive ROM are equal.
  - Pain at the extremes of motion in all planes
  - Glenohumeral crepitus with motion
- Adhesive capsulitis:
  - Palpable joint line tenderness
  - Severely decreased ROM
  - Active and passive ROM are equal.
  - Pain with motion in all planes

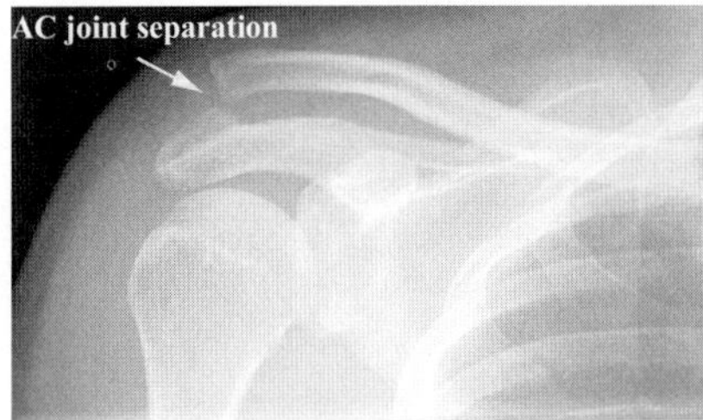


**Fig. 2.** Radiograph of an AC joint separation.

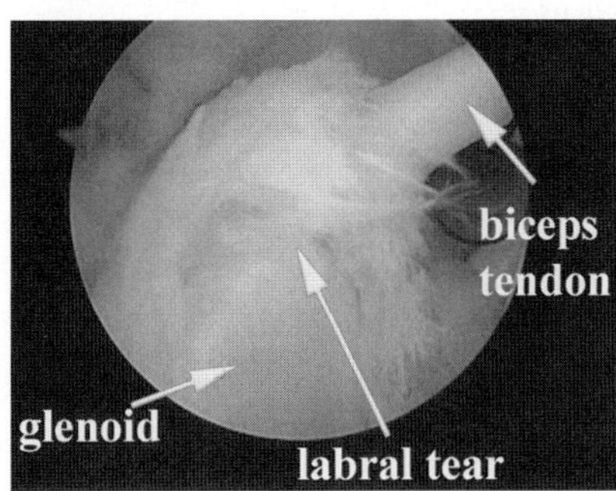


**Fig. 3.** Arthroscopic image of a SLAP tear.

## REFERENCES


1. Curl LA, Warren RF. Glenohumeral joint stability. Selective cutting studies on the static capsular restraints. *Clin Orthop Relat Res* 1996;330:54–65.
2. Tennent TD, Beach WR, Meyers JF. A review of the special tests associated with shoulder examination. Part I: the rotator cuff tests. *Am J Sports Med* 2003;31:154–160.
3. Tennent TD, Beach WR, Meyers JF. A review of the special tests associated with shoulder examination. Part II: laxity, instability, and superior labral anterior and posterior (SLAP) lesions. *Am J Sports Med* 2003;31:301–307.
4. Chronopoulos E, Kim TK, Park HB, et al. Diagnostic value of physical tests for isolated chronic AC lesions. *Am J Sports Med* 2004;32:655–661.


## ADDITIONAL READING


- Hoppenfeld S. Physical examination of the shoulder. In: *Physical Examination of the Spine & Extremities*. Norwalk, CT: Appleton & Lange, 1976:1–34.
- Hoppenfeld S, deBoer P. The shoulder. In: *Surgical Exposures in Orthopaedics: The Anatomical Approach*, 3rd ed. Philadelphia: Lippincott, Williams & Wilkins, 2003:1–66.


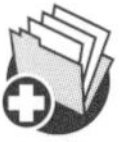

## MISCELLANEOUS

### FAQ

- Q: What are the most common causes of atraumatic shoulder pain?
  - A: Rotator cuff disease, AC joint arthritis, cervical radiculopathy.
- Q: What is the difference between a shoulder separation and a shoulder dislocation?
  - A: A shoulder separation is a dislocation of the AC joint. A shoulder dislocation is a dislocation of the glenohumeral joint.

# SHOULDER DISLOCATION

*Adam J. Farber, MD*

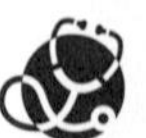

## BASICS

### DESCRIPTION

- The shoulder joint has the greatest ROM of all joints in the body and, thus, is at high risk for dislocations.
- Shoulder joint stability depends on various dynamic and static anatomical restraints.
  - Dynamic restraints include:
    - Tendon of the long head of the biceps
    - Scapular stabilizers
    - Rotator cuff muscles and tendons
  - Static restraints include:
    - Osseous anatomy (the glenoid fossa and humeral head)
    - Joint capsule
    - Glenohumeral ligaments (superior, middle, and inferior)
    - Glenoid labrum
- Shoulder dislocations are classified by:
  - Direction of dislocation (anterior, posterior, inferior, or superior)
  - Chronology (acute versus chronic)
  - Force (traumatic versus atraumatic)
  - Patient contribution (voluntary versus involuntary)

### EPIDEMIOLOGY

- The shoulder is the most commonly dislocated joint in the body, accounting for up to 45% of all dislocations (1).
- Anterior shoulder dislocations account for ~85% of all shoulder dislocations and are 8–9 times more common than posterior dislocations (2).
- Inferior and superior dislocations are rare (2).

### ETIOLOGY

- Trauma (direct or indirect) is the most common mechanism of injury for all shoulder dislocations, and the direction of dislocation depends on direction of force.
- Anterior shoulder dislocation:
  - Most common mechanism is indirect trauma to the upper extremity with the shoulder in abduction, external rotation, and extension
  - An anteriorly directed force to the posterior shoulder
- Posterior shoulder dislocation:
  - Direct trauma, which leads to a posterior shoulder dislocation when a posteriorly directed force is applied to the anterior shoulder
  - Indirect trauma:
    - Axial loading to the upper extremity with the shoulder in a position of flexion, adduction, and internal rotation
    - Common causes: Seizures and electrocution. These causes produce a violent muscular contraction during which the internal rotators overwhelm the external rotators.
- Inferior dislocations (also known as "luxatio erecta") typically result from a hyperabduction force that levers the humeral head out inferiorly as the humeral neck impinges on the acromion.
- Superior shoulder dislocations occur as extreme anterior and superior force is applied to the adducted arm, such as during a fall from a height.

### ASSOCIATED CONDITIONS

- Anterior shoulder dislocations can be associated with:
  - Greater tuberosity humeral fractures, glenoid rim fractures, coracoid or acromion fractures, posttraumatic degenerative changes and, in patients >40 years old, rotator cuff tears
  - Nerve injuries (typically neurapraxias of the axillary or musculocutaneous nerves)
  - Rarely, vascular injuries (usually in elderly atherosclerotic patients).
- Posterior shoulder dislocations can be associated with:
  - Lesser tuberosity fractures of the humerus, glenoid rim fractures, humeral head and shaft fractures, and recurrent instability
  - Rarely, neurovascular injury
- Inferior shoulder dislocations can be associated with:
  - Rotator cuff tears, proximal humerus fractures, neurovascular injuries, compressive neuropathy, and thrombosis of the axillary artery
- Superior shoulder dislocations can be associated with:
  - Fractures of the coracoid, acromion, clavicle, and humeral tuberosities
  - Injury to the AC joint
  - Biceps tendon and rotator cuff injuries

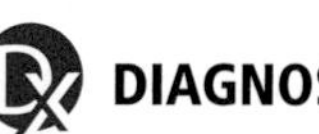

## DIAGNOSIS

### SIGNS AND SYMPTOMS

- Anterior dislocations, commonly associated with trauma, are difficult to overlook on patient evaluation.
- However, posterior dislocations frequently can be missed; they often are diagnosed late.
  - Detection of posterior dislocations is facilitated by heightened clinical suspicion of the injury in high-risk individuals and by appropriate radiographic investigation.

#### *History*

- Patients most commonly present complaining of shoulder pain and limited ROM after direct or indirect trauma to the shoulder.
- Patients with posterior dislocations can present after a seizure or electrocution event.

#### *Physical Exam*

- The position of the arm typically gives the examiner a clue about the direction of dislocation.
  - Anterior dislocation: Affected shoulder is held in slight abduction and external rotation.
  - Posterior dislocation: Affected shoulder is held in adduction and internal rotation.
  - Inferior dislocations: Affected shoulder is held in characteristic "salute" fashion, with the humerus locked in 110–160° of flexion and abduction.
  - Superior dislocation: Foreshortened upper extremity held in adduction.
- Inspection often reveals deformity in the shoulder region that varies with the direction of dislocation.
  - Anterior dislocations:
    - Squaring of the shoulder secondary to a relative prominence of the acromion anteriorly
    - A palpable mass (the humeral head) anteriorly
    - A hollow beneath the acromion posteriorly
  - Posterior dislocation:
    - A flattening of the shoulder anteriorly
    - A palpable mass (the humeral head) posteriorly
    - A prominent coracoid anteriorly
    - Mechanical block to external rotation (often <0°)
  - Inferior dislocations:
    - Humeral head is palpable on the lateral chest wall and axilla.
    - Do not confuse this dislocation with a step-off between the distal clavicle and the acromion in a shoulder separation.
  - Superior dislocations:
    - The humeral head rides above the level of the acromion.
    - The arm is shortened compared with the contralateral side.
    - Shoulder movement is restricted.
- Neurovascular examination:
  - Assess radial and ulnar pulses and capillary refill.
  - Focus on the integrity of the axillary nerve (which provides sensation to the lateral shoulder) is essential.
  - A sensory examination is critical because deltoid motor function often is limited secondary to pain and accompanying muscle spasm.

### TESTS

#### *Imaging*

- Plain radiographs typically are the only imaging studies necessary in the diagnostic workup of acute shoulder dislocations.
  - AP view of the shoulder is diagnostic for superior and inferior dislocations.
  - The axillary view of the shoulder is definitive determination of the direction of the dislocation as anterior or posterior.
  - Radiographic findings may include:
    - A Hill-Sachs lesion of the posterior aspect of the humeral head
    - Bony Bankart lesion
    - Fracture of the anterior-inferior glenoid
- CT scans:
  - May be useful in defining humeral head or glenoid impression fractures, loose bodies, and anterior labral bony injuries
  - Seldom are necessary for the diagnosis of acute shoulder dislocations.

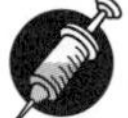

# TREATMENT

## GENERAL MEASURES

- Treatment consists of closed reduction of the dislocation followed by a period of immobilization.
  - Sufficient muscle relaxation for a successful outcome may require analgesia and/or sedation, or occasionally general anesthesia.
  - Anterior dislocation: Traction-countertraction, Hippocratic technique, Stimson technique, Milch technique, and scapular manipulation (2,3)
  - Posterior dislocation:
    - Requires traction to the adducted arm as the humeral head is lifted into the glenoid fossa
    - Because of frequent late presentation, may become locked and difficult, if not impossible, to reduce
  - Inferior or superior dislocation: Traction–countertraction maneuvers
- Repeat neurovascular examination and radiographs (including an axillary view) should be obtained to verify the reduction.

### *Activity*

- The duration of immobilization after successful closed and postoperative reduction depends on patient age and dislocation direction.
  - Reduced anterior dislocation:
    - Patients <40 years old: Immobilization in neutral or external rotation for 3–4 weeks
    - Patients ≥40 years old: Immobilization in neutral or external rotation for ~1–2 weeks
  - Reduced posterior dislocation: Immobilization in neutral rotation for ~4 weeks
  - Reduced superior or inferior dislocation: Immobilization in neutral rotation for 3–6 weeks
- During the immobilization period, daily elbow ROM exercises should be performed.

## SPECIAL THERAPY

### *Physical Therapy*

Aggressive physical therapy should be instituted after immobilization to restore ROM not only to the affected shoulder but also to the ipsilateral hand, wrist, and elbow.

## SURGERY

- The irreducible or open acute shoulder dislocation requires urgent open reduction.
- Nonurgent surgical indications relate to associated injuries and include:
  - Tuberosity fractures displaced >5 mm
  - Lesser tuberosity fractures displaced >1 cm
  - Humeral impaction fractures involving >20% of the humeral head
  - Glenoid rim fractures >5 mm.
- In addition, recurrent shoulder instability may be an indication for surgery (see "Shoulder Instability" chapter).

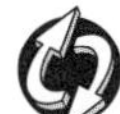

# FOLLOW-UP

## PROGNOSIS

- The prognosis after shoulder dislocation depends on the age of the patient and direction of dislocation.
  - Anterior dislocation:
    - The risk of recurrence is ~85% in patients who 1st dislocate at the age of ≤20 years and decreases to 10–15% in patients who 1st dislocate at the age of ≥40 years (4).
    - If no associated injuries or recurrent instability episodes occur, the outcome is good to excellent in most patients.

## REFERENCES


1. Kazar B, Relovszky E. Prognosis of primary dislocation of the shoulder. *Acta Orthop Scand* 1969;40:216–224.
2. Matsen FA, III, Thomas SC, Rockwood CA, Jr, et al. Glenohumeral instability. In: Rockwood CA, Jr, Matsen FA, III, eds. *The Shoulder*, 2nd ed. Philadelphia: WB Saunders, 1998:611–754.
3. Riebel GD, McCabe JB. Anterior shoulder dislocation: A review of reduction techniques. *Am J Emerg Med* 1991;9:180–188.
4. Simonet WT, Cofield RH. Prognosis in anterior shoulder dislocation. *Am J Sports Med* 1984;12: 19–24.


## ADDITIONAL READING


- Pollock RG, Bigliani LU. Glenohumeral instability: Evaluation and treatment. *J Am Acad Orthop Surg* 1993;1:24–32.
- Robinson CM, Aderinto J. Posterior shoulder dislocations and fracture-dislocations. *J Bone Joint Surg* 2005;87A:639–650.
- Robinson CM, Dobson RJ. Anterior instability of the shoulder after trauma. *J Bone Joint Surg* 2004;86B:469–479.


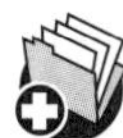

# MISCELLANEOUS

## CODES

### *ICD9-CM*

- 831.01 Anterior dislocation of humerus
- 831.02 Posterior dislocation of humerus
- 831.03 Inferior dislocation of humerus

## FAQ

- Q: Is an axillary radiograph necessary for the evaluation of suspected shoulder dislocation?
  - A: Yes. The axillary view is essential to determine definitively the direction of the dislocation as anterior or posterior. It also provides an excellent view of the glenoid rim to assess for possible fractures. After a reduction maneuver, it is the best view with which to confirm appropriate reduction.
- Q: What is the best method for reducing an anterior dislocation?
  - A: No single best method exists. Several methods (traction–countertraction, Hippocratic technique, Stimson technique, scapular manipulation, Milch technique) have proved successful. Familiarity with >1 method is useful in the event of a difficult reduction. The Kocher maneuver is not recommended because it is associated with a higher rate of fracture than other reduction methods.
- Q: What is the risk of recurrent instability after a first-time dislocation?
  - A: The risk of recurrent instability varies with the age of the patient. The rate is ~85% in patients who 1st dislocate at the age of ≤20 years, and it decreases steadily to a rate of 10–15% in patients who 1st dislocate at the age of ≥40 years.

# SHOULDER IMPINGEMENT SYNDROME

*Kevin W. Farmer, MD*
*John H. Wilckens, MD*
*James F. Wenz, Sr, MD*

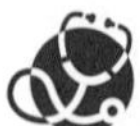

## BASICS

### DESCRIPTION

- Shoulder pain with overhead activities is a common musculoskeletal complaint.
- Impingement syndrome:
  - Inflammatory condition of the soft tissues of the subacromial space
  - Most common cause of presentation for shoulder complaints to a physician's office (>50% of all shoulder complaints) (1)
- Represents a continuum, progressing from acute bursitis, to chronic bursitis, to partial-thickness tears of the rotator cuff, to full-thickness rotator cuff tears, to rotator cuff arthropathy with degenerative changes
- The subacromial space is defined as the humeral head inferiorly, the anterior edge and undersurface of the anterior 1/3 of the acromion, and the coracoacromial ligament and AC joint superiorly.
- The soft tissues of the subacromial space include the subacromial bursa, supraspinatus and infraspinatus tendons, tendon of the long head of the biceps, and capsule of shoulder, all of which are susceptible to inflammation.
- External impingement:
  - The most common type of impingement
  - With overhead elevation of the arm, the rotator cuff "impinges" on the coracoacromial arch.
- Neer classification (2):
  - Stage I:
    - Acute inflammation, edema, and hemorrhage
    - Usually reversible with nonoperative treatment
  - Stage II:
    - Continuum from stage I
    - Progression of rotator cuff abnormalities to fibrosis and tendinitis
    - Less likely than stage I impingement to respond to nonoperative management
  - Stage III:
    - Rotator cuff tears and changes to the coracoacromial arch
    - Spurs form along the anterior–inferior acromion ("hooked acromion")
- Internal impingement:
  - Occurs primarily in overhead and throwing athletes
  - The posterior supraspinatus and infraspinatus tendons are pinched between the humeral head and posterior glenoid during maximum abduction and external rotation, as seen in throwing.
- Secondary impingement: Dynamic impingement, seen with scapular muscle fatigue, occult shoulder instability, and rotator cuff dysfunction (Improper shoulder mechanics leads to dynamic impingement of an intact rotator cuff under an otherwise normal coracoacromial arch.)
- Synonyms: Subacromial bursitis, Subacromial impingement, Rotator cuff tendinitis

### GENERAL PREVENTION

Proper overhead mechanics

### EPIDEMIOLOGY

- Common after the age of 50 years
- Equally as common in males as in females

#### *Incidence*

- May occur at any age
- Increasing incidence with increasing age, likely secondary to degenerative changes in the rotator cuff (3)
- Bone spurring of the acromion, which is associated with impingement syndrome, is 4 times more likely in patients >50 years old (3).
- Internal impingement and secondary impingement from glenohumeral instability can cause shoulder pain in the younger patient (<40 years old), especially in overhead athletes (pitchers, tennis players, swimmers, etc.).

#### *Prevalence*

Very common

### RISK FACTORS

- Increasing age (>50 years)
- Overhead athletics and occupations
- Instability
- Hooked acromion
- Os acromiale (failure of the acromion to fuse after birth)
- Trauma

#### *Genetics*

No known inheritance patterns

### ETIOLOGY

- The pinching of the subacromial soft tissues between the humeral head and coracoacromial arch is the primary cause of the inflammation.
  - Commonly seen in patients with a type III hooked acromion
  - In addition to a congenital type III hooked acromion, the hook may be secondary to calcification at the coracoacromial ligament from repetitive impingement.
  - Mild glenohumeral instability (acquired or congenital) can predispose patients to secondary and internal impingement.
  - Overhead activities: Athletics and occupations that require overhead activities (electricians, builders, shelf stockers, etc.)
  - Rotator cuff dysfunction or weak cuff muscles allow superior migration of the humeral head, narrowing the subacromial space with overhead activities.

### ASSOCIATED CONDITIONS

- Rotator cuff tears (partial thickness and the continuum to full thickness)
- Calcific tendinitis:
  - Calcification in rotator cuff tendons from unknown cause
  - Typically undergoes spontaneous resorption and healing with time
  - Acutely painful during calcium resorption
- Biceps tendinitis:
  - Inflammation of the tendon of the long head on the biceps
  - Incidence increases with rotator cuff disease.
- AC arthritis:
  - Pain at the AC joint
- Adhesive capsulitis:
  - Stiff shoulder secondary to capsular fibrosis
- Labral tears:
  - SLAP tears are common in overhead athletes with internal impingement and in patients with rotator cuff tears

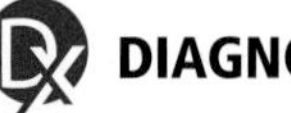

## DIAGNOSIS

### SIGNS AND SYMPTOMS

Pain with overhead activity of the arm

#### *History*

History of pain with overhead activities (combing hair, putting dishes away, etc.)

#### *Physical Exam*

- Tenderness to palpation over anterior and lateral acromion and rotator cuff
- Positive Hawkins sign: Pain with passive flexion and internal rotation
- Positive Neer sign: Pain with passive flexion of shoulder while scapula is stabilized
- Painful arc: Arc where pain occurs with active abduction
- Decreased active and passive forward flexion and abduction secondary to pain
- Pain with infraspinatus and supraspinatus muscle testing

### TESTS

- Impingement test:
  - Inject 10 mL of 1% lidocaine into the subacromial space with sterile technique.
  - Wait 5–10 minutes and repeat the shoulder examination.
  - Positive test: Improvement in symptoms

#### *Imaging*

- AP or 30° caudad angled AP view (Grashey view):
  - Subacromial sclerosis (eyebrow sign)
  - Greater tuberosity cyst
  - Superior migration of humeral head
- Supraspinatus outlet views:
  - Acromial morphology (hooked acromion)
- MRI:
  - Helpful in delineating injury to rotator cuff

#### *Pathological Findings*

- Degenerative changes in rotator cuff tendons
- Inflammation and fibrosis of the subacromial bursa

## DIFFERENTIAL DIAGNOSIS
- Rotator cuff tears:
  - May be partial or full thickness
  - Weakness and pain with supraspinatus and infraspinatus muscle testing
  - Drop arm test: Inability to hold arm abducted
  - MRI >1.5 tesla magnetic and shoulder coil is the best diagnostic test.
- Calcific tendinitis: Calcification of cuff tendons seen on radiographs
- Biceps tendinitis:
  - Tender to palpation along the biceps tendon
  - Positive Speed (resisted shoulder flexion with palm up) and Yergason (pain with resisted supination) tests
- Cervical spine:
  - Any pain that is distal to elbow should raise concern for a cervical spine cause.
  - Always perform a thorough neurovascular examination.
  - Cervical spine imaging
- AC arthritis:
  - Localized pain at AC joint
  - Pain with passive cross-body arm adduction
  - Degenerative changes seen on radiographs
  - Pain improved with injection of lidocaine into the AC joint
- Glenohumeral instability:
  - Apprehension and relocation tests
  - Sulcus sign (passive inferior subluxation of humeral head)
- Glenohumeral arthritis:
  - Decreased active and passive ROM with crepitance and pain
  - Degenerative changes in glenoid and humeral head on radiographs
- Adhesive capsulitis:
  - Decreased ROM, especially external rotation
  - Decreased ROM (active, passive)
  - Pain at extremes of motion
- SLAP lesion:
  - Tear at superior labrum at insertion of biceps tendon
  - Positive O'Brien test
  - MRA is the best diagnostic test.

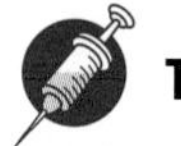

# TREATMENT

## GENERAL MEASURES
Initial nonoperative management trial before surgical intervention is successful in ~70% (4).

### *Activity*
No shoulder abduction or flexion >60° during early inflammatory stage

## SPECIAL THERAPY
### *Physical Therapy*
- Improves ROM, particularly internal rotation
- Rotator cuff program
- Strengthening:
  - Work in pain-free ROM
  - Scapular stabilizers
  - Rotator cuff muscles
  - Help keep humeral head within glenoid
- Ice, ultrasound, electrical stimulation

## MEDICATION (DRUGS)
### *First Line*
NSAIDs

### *Second Line*
Subacromial corticosteroid injections

## SURGERY
- Indicated if symptoms continue after 6 months of a well-designed and monitored nonoperative regimen
- Open or arthroscopic acromioplasty and subacromial decompression:
  - Successful in ~75–90% of cases (5,6)
  - Currently, an arthroscopic procedure is the most common technique:
    - Remove inflamed subacromial bursa.
    - Resect undersurface of acromion and acromial hook.
    - Can resect distal clavicle for AC arthritis
    - Affords visualization of the glenohumeral joint to determine if additional intervention is needed
  - Open acromioplasty:
    - Less commonly used, unless used with an open rotator cuff repair
    - If the deltoid attachment is mobilized, care must be taken to repair it adequately
  - Early ROM is critical for avoiding a stiff shoulder.

# FOLLOW-UP

## PROGNOSIS
- Success rate with nonoperative treatment: ~70% (4)
- Success rate of acromioplasty in those for whom nonoperative treatment fails: ~75–90% (5,6)

## COMPLICATIONS
- Surgical:
  - Failure to resolve symptoms:
    - Inadequate resection of acromion
    - Incorrect diagnosis: AC arthritis, glenohumeral arthritis
  - Stiff shoulder:
    - Postoperative adhesions
    - Inadequate postoperative arm mobilization
  - Infection
  - Hematoma
- Progression of impingement:
  - Rotator cuff tear
  - Cuff arthropathy
  - Tearing of proximal tendon of long head of the biceps ("Popeye arm")

## PATIENT MONITORING
Close outpatient follow-up to monitor ROM

## REFERENCES
1. Vecchio P, Kavanagh R, Hazleman BL, et al. Shoulder pain in a community-based rheumatology clinic. *Br J Rheumatol* 1995;34:440–442.
2. Neer CS, II. Impingement lesions. *Clin Orthop Relat Res* 1983;173:70–77.
3. Nicholson GP, Goodman DA, Flatow EL, et al. The acromion: Morphologic condition and age-related changes. A study of 420 scapulas. *J Shoulder Elbow Surg* 1996;5:1–11.
4. Morrison DS, Frogameni AD, Woodworth P. Non-operative treatment of subacromial impingement syndrome. *J Bone Joint Surg* 1997;79A:732–737.
5. Hawkins RJ, Plancher KD, Saddemi SR, et al. Arthroscopic subacromial decompression. *J Shoulder Elbow Surg* 2001;10:225–230.
6. Patel VR, Singh D, Calvert PT, et al. Arthroscopic subacromial decompression: Results and factors affecting outcome. *J Shoulder Elbow Surg* 1999;8:231–237.

## ADDITIONAL READING
- Gomoll AH, Katz JN, Warner JJP, et al. Rotator cuff disorders: Recognition and management among patients with shoulder pain. *Arthritis Rheum* 2004;50:3751–3761.
- Matsen FA, III, Titelman RM, Lippitt SB, et al. Rotator cuff. In: Rockwood CA, Jr, Matsen FA, III, Wirth MA, et al., eds. *The Shoulder*, 3rd ed. Philadelphia: WB Saunders, 2004:795–878.
- Michener LA, McClure PW, Karduna AR. Anatomical and biomechanical mechanisms of subacromial impingement syndrome. *Clin Biomech (Bristol, Avon)* 2003;18:369–379.

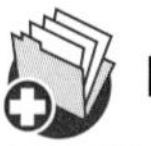

# MISCELLANEOUS

## CODES
### *ICD9-CM*
726.2 Impingement syndrome, shoulder

## PATIENT TEACHING
### *Activity*
Proper overhead technique

## FAQ
- Q: Does shoulder impingement require surgery?
  - A: No. Most impingement symptoms improve with a good rotator cuff rehabilitation program. Subacromial decompression to relieve impingement is recommended only for shoulders unresponsive to 6 months of physical therapy.
- Q: What are some of the causes of shoulder impingement in patients <40 years old?
  - A: Common causes in a young patient are occult instability, rotator cuff dysfunction, and os acromiale.

# SHOULDER INSTABILITY

*Adam J. Farber, MD*

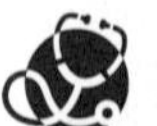

## BASICS

### DESCRIPTION

- Because of the shoulder's extensive ROM, it is prone to instability.
- The term encompasses a spectrum of disorders of varying degree, direction, and cause.
- Instability should be distinguished from laxity.
  - "Laxity" is the symmetric translation of the humeral head over the surface of the glenoid without symptoms.
  - "Instability" occurs when the degree of translation becomes excessive and leads to symptoms.
- Shoulder joint stability depends on various static and dynamic anatomic restraints.
  - Static restraints: Osseous anatomy (glenoid fossa and humeral head), joint capsule, glenohumeral ligaments (superior, middle, and inferior), and glenoid labrum
  - Dynamic restraints: The muscles and tendons of the rotator cuff, the scapular stabilizers
- Shoulder instability is classified by:
  - Direction of dislocation: Anterior, posterior, or multidirectional
  - Degree: Dislocation, subluxation, microinstability
  - Force: Traumatic versus atraumatic
  - Patient contribution: Voluntary versus involuntary

### RISK FACTORS

- Anterior shoulder instability is common.
  - Risk of recurrence after a traumatic anterior shoulder dislocation varies with patient age:
    - 50–85% risk in those initially affected when <20 years old (1,2)
    - 20% risk in those initially affected when >40 years old (1)
- Recurrent posterior shoulder instability most commonly presents with repeated episodes of subluxation with no history of shoulder injury.
  - Usually affects active males (<30 years old)
  - Many patients can demonstrate voluntary posterior shoulder instability.
- MDI:
  - Usually atraumatic
  - Is poorly understood and typically results from a combination of excessive tissue laxity and muscular discoordination
  - Frequently, history of incidental or no trauma

### PATHOPHYSIOLOGY

- Shoulder instability is associated with injury to the capsuloligamentous labral complex.
  - The Bankart lesion is a detachment of the anterior glenoid labrum and capsuloligamentous attachments.
  - Patients with recurrent anterior instability also often have anterior capsular redundancy.
- Recurrent posterior instability may have a detached posteroinferior labrum (reverse Bankart lesion), a patulous posteroinferior capsule, and excessive glenoid retroversion.
- Patients with MDI usually have a generalized increase in joint laxity and redundant capsule.

### ETIOLOGY

Mechanisms of "shoulder dislocation" are addressed elsewhere (see "Shoulder Dislocation" chapter).

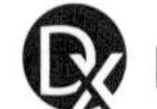

## DIAGNOSIS

### SIGNS AND SYMPTOMS

Keys to accurate diagnosis of shoulder instability are a thorough history and physical examination.

#### *History*

- Key information for the clinician to identify:
  - Initial episode of major, minor, or no trauma
  - Arm position at the time of the initial event (for determining direction of instability) but, more importantly, which arm positions reproduce symptoms
  - The necessity of a formal reduction maneuver for a dislocation and the presence of radiographs documenting a dislocation
  - Symptoms, pain location, exacerbating activities, and any voluntary component to the instability episodes
- Patients with *anterior* instability typically:
  - Have a history of traumatic anterior shoulder dislocation (see "Shoulder Dislocation" chapter).
  - Report symptoms, such as pain or apprehension, during arm abduction, extension, and external rotation.
- Patients with *posterior* instability:
  - Present with a sense of shoulder instability and looseness or episodes of recurrent subluxation, seldom dislocation
  - Experience symptoms with the arm flexed, adducted, and internally rotated (e.g., when pushing a heavy cart or during a seizure)
- Patients with *inferior* instability may become symptomatic when carrying heavy objects, such as a suitcase, at the side.
- Patients with MDI (3):
  - May have a family history of similar findings and personal history of other joint problems
  - Typically have history of minimal or no trauma
  - Commonly complain of pain, rather than episodes of subluxation or dislocation
  - Experience most symptoms in midrange rather than extreme shoulder motions

#### *Physical Exam*

- Examine and compare both shoulders: Laxity, strength, and ROM.
- Include inspection, palpation, ROM, and a thorough neurovascular examination.
  - Inspection may reveal atrophy or mild scapular dyskinesis.
  - Palpation may reveal focal tenderness.
- Ask the patient to demonstrate the positions and actions that produce the symptoms.
  - Symptoms in extension, abduction, and external rotation suggest anterior instability
  - Symptoms in flexion, adduction, and internal rotation suggest posterior instability.
- Patients with MDI often have generalized ligamentous laxity.
- Evaluate shoulder laxity with the load-and-shift test (assesses amount of humeral head translation on the glenoid fossa in the anterior or posterior direction).
  - Patients with instability often have excessive translation and pain.
  - Patients with MDI may have excessive laxity bilaterally.
- Assess inferior laxity with the sulcus test: Pull downward on the neutrally positioned arm, assess amount of inferior translation and presence of an anterior dimple (or sulcus) beneath the acromion.
  - Often increases translation or reproduces symptoms in patients with MDI
- Reproduction of symptoms by provocative tests helps confirm the diagnosis of instability.
  - For anterior instability: Apprehension test:
    - Place the patient supine and abduct the shoulder 90°, flex the elbow 90°, and gradually externally rotate the arm until the patient reports pain or apprehension.
    - Relief of symptoms with the application of a posteriorly directed force on the anterior humeral head constitutes a positive relocation test, another sign of anterior instability.
  - For posterior instability:
    - Arm in 90° of elevation and internal rotation
    - Move the arm from the coronal to the sagittal plane and back while applying an axial load to the humerus.
    - Positive test: Humeral head subluxates over the glenoid rim, reproducing symptoms.

### TESTS

#### *Imaging*

- Radiographic evaluation should include AP and axillary views of the shoulder.
  - Plain radiographs frequently are negative, especially in subtle forms of instability.
  - Findings suggestive of anterior instability:
    - A posterolateral impression defect of the humeral head (Hill-Sachs lesion) suggests traumatic anterior dislocation.
    - An anterior-inferior glenoid rim fracture (a bony Bankart lesion)
  - Findings suggestive of posterior instability:
    - An anterior impression defect of the humeral head (reverse Hill-Sachs lesion)
    - Posterior lesions of the glenoid rim
- CT scanning can help define humeral or glenoid abnormalities.
- MRI is useful in identifying labral or capsuloligamentous pathology.

#### *Diagnostic Procedures/Surgery*

Examination under anesthesia and diagnostic arthroscopy are not routinely necessary, but they can be helpful in selected cases.

### DIFFERENTIAL DIAGNOSIS

Conditions such as internal impingement syndrome or SLAP lesions may be confused with subtle forms of instability, especially in overhead athletes.

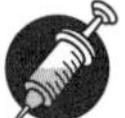

# TREATMENT

## GENERAL MEASURES

- Nonsurgical treatment is recommended for most 1st-time anterior dislocations (see "Shoulder Dislocation" chapter) and for posterior shoulder instability, MDI, and voluntary dislocators.
  - Modalities: Joint reduction (in the case of shoulder dislocation), followed by a period of activity restriction, immobilization, and rehabilitative exercises
  - The duration of immobilization is controversial.
- Surgery may be recommended for recurrent traumatic anterior shoulder instability and for posterior instability or MDI after unsuccessful nonoperative treatment (6 months).

## SPECIAL THERAPY

Psychologic evaluation and treatment for patients with habitual voluntary shoulder instability

### *Physical Therapy*

- Rehabilitative programs emphasize strengthening of the shoulder's dynamic stabilizers (particularly rotator cuff muscles and scapular stabilizers), regaining full ROM, restoring normal shoulder mechanics, improving proprioception, and avoiding provocative arm activities.
  - Progression of the rehabilitation protocol varies with the direction of instability, quality of the tissue, type of repair, and requirements of the patient.
  - In general, return to sports is restricted for 6–9 months after surgery for anterior instability and 9–12 months after surgery for posterior instability and MDI.

## MEDICATION (DRUGS)

Patients with posterior instability from seizures should be treated with medication adjustment to reduce the seizure frequency.

## SURGERY

- The key concept in surgical treatment is the anatomic repair of the capsuloligamentous or labral abnormality rather than nonanatomic reconstructions.
- Capsulorrhaphy (capsular tightening) enhances correction of instability by reducing capsular laxity and excessive joint volume.
- Arthroscopic surgery:
  - For traumatic anterior instability:
    - Treatment of choice is Bankart repair (reattachment of capsulolabral structures to the glenoid rim) with suture anchors and supplemental anterior capsulorrhaphy.
    - Capsular tightening achieved with capsular plication or thermal shrinkage
  - For posterior shoulder instability: Arthroscopic capsulolabral repair and posterior capsulorrhaphy
  - For MDI: Arthroscopic plication or capsular shift procedures
- Nonanatomic open reconstructive procedures:
  - Result in failure, loss of motion, and arthritis
  - Exception is the Bristow procedure (transfer of the coracoid process to the antero-inferior glenoid rim) for patients with large bony defects in the glenoid rim
- Anatomic open reconstructive procedures:
  - For anterior shoulder instability, the classic is the open Bankart procedure.
    - Most commonly used surgical technique
    - Reattaches capsulolabral structures to the glenoid rim
    - Often combined with open capsulorrhaphy to reduce capsular redundancy
  - For symptomatic recurrent posterior instability:
    - Posterior capsulorrhaphy
    - Posterior bone block procedures (glenoid bone stock deficiency)
    - Rotational osteotomy of the proximal humerus (excessive retrotorsion of the proximal humerus)
    - Posterior glenoid osteotomy (abnormal glenoid retroversion)
  - For MDI:
    - Most common procedure is inferior capsular shift with associated closure of the rotator interval defect.
    - Postoperative immobilization with the arm in neutral rotation and 10–15° of abduction
- Because of psychologic problems, surgery is contraindicated for patients with voluntary instability.

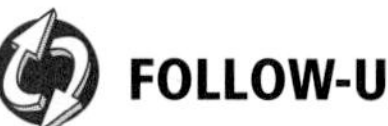

# FOLLOW-UP

## PROGNOSIS

- Prognosis is excellent after surgical treatment of recurrent anterior shoulder instability.
- Posterior shoulder instability and MDI that fail to respond to nonoperative treatment have a good prognosis with surgical treatment.

## COMPLICATIONS

- The risk of recurrent instability after surgical treatment is ~3–10% (4).
- The risk of recurrence is lower after open than after arthroscopic surgical procedures, particularly in contact athletes with recurrent instability (5).
- Complications of open procedures include pain, decreased ROM, infection, neurovascular injury, late degenerative arthritis, subscapularis over tightening or rupture, and hardware-related problems (breakage, loosening, migration, and intra-articular penetration).
- Complications of arthroscopic procedures include neurovascular injury, adhesive capsulitis, synovial fistula, and hardware-related problems.

## REFERENCES


1. Hovelius L, Eriksson K, Fredin H, et al. Recurrences after initial dislocation of the shoulder. Results of a prospective study of treatment. *J Bone Joint Surg* 1983;65A:343–349.
2. Simonet WT, Cofield RH. Prognosis in anterior shoulder dislocation. *Am J Sports Med* 1984;12: 19–24.
3. Schenk TJ, Brems JJ. Multidirectional instability of the shoulder: Pathophysiology, diagnosis, and management. *J Am Acad Orthop Surg* 1998;6: 65–72.
4. Freedman KB, Smith AP, Romeo AA, et al. Open Bankart repair versus arthroscopic repair with transglenoid sutures or bioabsorbable tacks for recurrent anterior instability of the shoulder: A meta-analysis. *Am J Sports Med* 2004;32: 1520–1527.
5. Pagnani MJ, Dome DC. Surgical treatment of traumatic anterior shoulder instability in American football players. *J Bone Joint Surg* 2002;84A: 711–715.


## ADDITIONAL READING


- Matsen FA, III, Thomas SC, Rockwood CA, Jr, et al. Glenohumeral instability. In: Rockwood CA, Jr, Matsen FA, III, eds. *The Shoulder*, 2nd ed. Philadelphia: WB Saunders, 1998:611–754.
- Robinson CM, Dobson RJ. Anterior instability of the shoulder after trauma. *J Bone Joint Surg* 2004;86B:469–479.
- Robinson CM, Aderinto J. Recurrent posterior shoulder instability. *J Bone Joint Surg* 2005;87A:883–892.




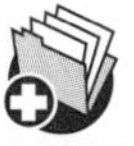

# MISCELLANEOUS

## CODES

### *ICD9-CM*

- 718.81 Shoulder instability
- 831.1 Shoulder dislocation, anterior
- 831.2 Shoulder dislocation, posterior
- 831.3 Shoulder dislocation, inferior

## FAQ

- Q: Should patients with voluntary instability undergo surgery?
  - A: Generally, no. Most patients with voluntary instability have underlying psychologic problems that the surgery cannot help and, thus, make poor surgical candidates.
- Q: What are the indications for arthroscopic anterior shoulder stabilization?
  - A: Patients with acute traumatic anterior dislocation, without multiple dislocations, who have a Bankart lesion are the ideal candidates for arthroscopic stabilization. Assessing capsular laxity arthroscopically requires advanced surgical skills. Arthroscopic stabilization is preferred in overhead athletes (e.g., pitchers), but it has a higher failure rate than open repairs in contact athletes (e.g., football players).

# SHOULDER/GLENOHUMERAL ARTHRITIS

*Jason W. Hammond, MD*

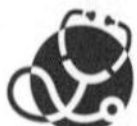

## BASICS

### DESCRIPTION

Progressive loss of glenohumeral joint space with thinning of articular cartilage, formation of osteophytes, and progressive deformity

### EPIDEMIOLOGY

- Females are more likely than males to have primary glenohumeral osteoarthritis.
- Patients >60 years old are more likely to have it than are younger patients.

#### *Incidence*

- ~0.4% in the general population (1)
- Can reach 4.6% in patients with concomitant shoulder diseases (1)

### RISK FACTORS

- Age >60 years
- Excessive joint loading (e.g., throwing athletes and manual laborers)
- Joint injury
- Excessively tight capsulorrhaphy

#### *Genetics*

No known genetic component

### ETIOLOGY (2)

- Osteoarthritis
- Rheumatoid arthritis
- Secondary degenerative joint disease
  - Repetitive and major trauma
  - End-stage AVN
  - Rotator cuff tear arthropathy
  - Capsulorrhaphy arthritis

### ASSOCIATED CONDITIONS

- Rotator cuff tear
- Biceps tendinitis

## DIAGNOSIS

### SIGNS AND SYMPTOMS

- Activity-related pain in the shoulder
- Decreased ROM

#### *History*

- Progressive shoulder pain and stiffness
- Previous shoulder surgery
- Previous diagnosis of rheumatoid arthritis
- Shoulder trauma
- Osteonecrosis
- Cuff tear arthropathy

#### *Physical Exam*

- Assess ROM of the glenohumeral joint, scapulothoracic motion, and cervical spine.
- Test muscle strength, especially of deltoid, rotator cuff, and biceps.
- Perform a full neurologic examination of the upper extremity to differentiate cervical disc or brachial plexus disease.
- Palpate the surrounding structures, including the AC joint and biceps tendon.
- In active rheumatoid arthritis of the glenohumeral joint, an adduction and internal rotation deformity of the joint is produced by protective muscle spasm.

### TESTS

#### *Lab*

- If clinically indicated, the workup for rheumatoid arthritis should include:
  - ESR, C-reactive protein, serum rheumatoid factor
  - Complete blood count, ESR, and C-reactive protein to be obtained if septic arthritis is suspected
- Joint fluid analysis may help with diagnoses other than osteoarthritis.

#### *Imaging*

- Radiography (1):
  - AP and axillary radiographs of the affected shoulder are essential.
  - Joint space narrowing, osteophytes, subchondral sclerosis, and cyst formation are hallmark signs of osteoarthritis.
  - Posterior wear of the glenoid may be seen in osteoarthritis, and symmetric joint space narrowing may be seen in rheumatoid arthritis.
  - Superior subluxation of the humeral head may indicate an associated rotator cuff tear.
  - Athletes also may have a thrower's exostosis on the posterior inferior glenoid, visualized on the Stryker notch view.
- MRI, arthrography, and ultrasound can be used to assess rotator cuff integrity.
  - Mild cartilage loss and other lesions may be visualized on MRI if not seen on plain films.
- CT can be used to assess bone stock for surgical planning.

#### *Diagnostic Procedures*

Lidocaine injection of the subacromial space or joint may help with the diagnosis.

### DIFFERENTIAL DIAGNOSIS

- Rotator cuff tear
- AC joint arthritis
- Isolated chondral lesion
- PVNS
- Synovial chondromatosis
- AVN
- Septic arthritis
- Lyme disease
- Inflammatory arthropathies
- Posttraumatic conditions
- Metastatic disease
- Cervical radiculopathy

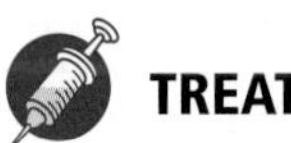

## TREATMENT

### GENERAL MEASURES

- Nonoperative treatments should aim to optimize shoulder flexibility, maintain muscle function, and reduce inflammation and pain.
- Activity modification is helpful but often difficult in the active patient.

### SPECIAL THERAPY

#### *Physical Therapy*

An exercise program to maintain ROM and to strengthen the rotator cuff is an important 1st step in management (3).

### MEDICATION (DRUGS)

#### *First Line*

NSAIDs, acetaminophen, aspirin

#### *Second Line*

- Joint injection with corticosteroid should be considered after other therapeutic interventions (such as NSAIDs, physical therapy, and activity modification) have failed.
  - Indications for glenohumeral joint injection include osteoarthritis, adhesive capsulitis, and rheumatoid arthritis.

### SURGERY

- Arthroscopy with associated débridement and synovectomy can relieve pain, improve function, and delay progression of the disease for inflammatory arthropathies.
- Arthroscopic procedures addressing osteoarthritis consist of débridement, loose body removal, chondroplasty or abrasion of the glenoid and humeral head, and capsular release (4).
- An inferior humeral osteophyte that blocks motion in athletes may be removed arthroscopically.
- Arthroscopic glenoidplasty allows the humeral head to be centered in the glenoid by reestablishing a more normal radius of curvature of the glenoid (4).
  - This procedure has been recommended for severe posterior glenoid wear that may cause posterior subluxation of the humeral head.
- Prosthetic shoulder replacement is a highly reliable surgery for pain relief (5).
  - A hemiarthroplasty replaces the humeral head; a total shoulder arthroplasty also replaces the glenoid.
  - Shoulder replacement should not be expected to restore normal shoulder motion (2).
  - For patients with primary osteoarthritis, total shoulder arthroplasty provides better results than hemiarthroplasty for pain, mobility, and activity.
  - It is an easy, economical, and dependable method of treating shoulders severely affected by rheumatoid arthritis.
- Arthrodesis can be functionally preferable to shoulder arthroplasty for the physical laborer with painful arthritis who is not required to perform overhead lifting.

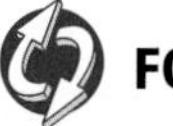

## FOLLOW-UP

### PROGNOSIS

- Osteoarthritis pain and progression vary widely among patients, but most patients are unlikely to improve with time.
- Shoulder arthroplasty has good long-term results.

### COMPLICATIONS

- Complications of arthroplasty include:
  - Loosening of the glenoid component
  - Infection
  - Dislocation
  - Nerve injury

### PATIENT MONITORING

Patients are treated nonoperatively until activities of daily living become compromised or pain becomes unmanageable.

### REFERENCES


1. Nakagawa Y, Hyakuna K, Otani S, et al. Epidemiologic study of glenohumeral osteoarthritis with plain radiography. *J Shoulder Elbow Surg* 1999;8:580–584.
2. Azar FM, Wright PE, II. Arthroplasty of shoulder and elbow. In: Canale ST, ed. *Campbell's Operative Orthopaedics*, 10th ed. St. Louis: Mosby, 2003:483–533.
3. Parsons IM, Weldon EJ, III, Titelman RM, et al. Glenohumeral arthritis and its management. *Phys Med Rehabil Clin North Am* 2004;15:447–474.
4. Bishop JY, Flatow EL. Management of glenohumeral arthritis: A role for arthroscopy? *Orthop Clin North Am* 2003;34:559–566.
5. Edwards TB, Kadakia NR, Boulahia A, et al. A comparison of hemiarthroplasty and total shoulder arthroplasty in the treatment of primary glenohumeral osteoarthritis: Results of a multicenter study. *J Shoulder Elbow Surg* 2003;12: 207–213.


### ADDITIONAL READING


Lehtinen JT, Kaarela K, Belt EA, et al. Incidence of glenohumeral joint involvement in seropositive rheumatoid arthritis. A 15-year endpoint study. *J Rheumatol* 2000;27:347–350.


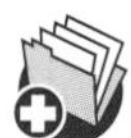

## MISCELLANEOUS

### CODES

#### *ICD9-CM*

716.91 Glenohumeral arthritis

### PATIENT TEACHING

- Shoulder arthroplasty can substantially improve symptoms of pain, but patients cannot be expected to regain normal motion.
- Physical therapy before and after surgery is beneficial to maximize strength and ROM.

### FAQ

- Q: What are the expectations for shoulder hemiarthroplasty or total arthroplasty for glenohumeral arthritis patients?
  - A: Patients can expect pain relief from shoulder arthroplasty with removal of osteophytes and repair of rotator cuff tendons. Patients can expect modest improvement in ROM, but it will not be full. Patients can expect improved function in activities of daily living.

S

# SHOULDER/PROXIMAL HUMERUS FRACTURE

Matthew D. Waites, AFRCS (Ed)
Barry Waldman, MD

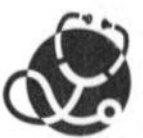

## BASICS

### DESCRIPTION

- The proximal humerus consists of the articular surface of the shoulder joint and the attachments of the rotator cuff to the greater and lesser tuberosities.
- Most of the blood supply to the humeral head comes from the anterior humeral circumflex branch of the axillary artery.
- >90% of proximal humeral fractures result from a low-energy fall directly onto the shoulder (1,2).
- Patients with osteoporotic bone are at the highest risk.
- In nonosteoporotic patients, fractures result from high-energy trauma.
- Classification:
  - Neer classification (3) divides the proximal humerus into 4 parts:
    - Articular surface
    - Greater tuberosity
    - Lesser tuberosity
    - Surgical neck (the border between the round proximal metaphysis and the diaphyseal portion of the bone)
    - Fractures are classified as having 1–4 parts, based on the number of fragments, with a fragment defined as a part if it is displaced >1 cm and/or angulated >45°.

### GENERAL PREVENTION

- Osteoporosis prevention
- Fall prevention

### EPIDEMIOLOGY

- Risk for a proximal humeral fracture increases with age, peaking in the 9th decade (4).
- The risk is closely related to the prevalence of osteoporosis.

#### *Incidence*

- 70 per 100,000 people (5).
- 3:1 Female:Male incidence (4).
- Proximal humerus fractures account for 10% of all fractures in patients >65 years old (6).

### RISK FACTORS

- Low bone mineral density
- Predisposition to falls:
  - Diabetes mellitus
  - Previous falls
  - Epilepsy and seizure medication (1)
  - Poor vision and balance
- Previous fractures after age 45 years (1)
- Reduced physical activity

#### *Genetics*

No known genetic association

### ETIOLOGY

- Mechanism of injury:
  - In elderly osteoporotic patients, 76% result from a fall that has a direct impact on the shoulder or upper arm (2).
  - In younger patients, high-energy injury such as a motor vehicle accident is primary cause.

### ASSOCIATED CONDITIONS

- Dislocation of the glenohumeral joint
- Complete rotator cuff tears occur in 20% of cases, particularly greater tuberosity fractures (7).
- Axillary and suprascapular nerve injury
- Vascular injury to axillary vessels or their branches, especially in the presence of atherosclerosis

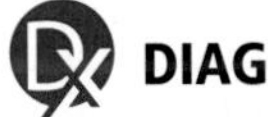

## DIAGNOSIS

### SIGNS AND SYMPTOMS

- Subcutaneous hematoma in 68% of patients sustaining fracture from a low-energy fall (2)
- Ecchymosis may extend to the elbow or chest wall and neck.
- Pain with ROM
- Patient supporting the affected arm

#### *History*

- Discover the mode of injury, low- versus high-energy fracture

#### *Physical Exam*

- Note loss of deltoid contour and limb posture, which may indicate an associated dislocation.
- Examine the skin to check its integrity.
- Palpate the humerus, clavicle, and scapula.
- Perform a neurovascular examination of the entire upper extremity to rule out an associated injury.
  - It is important to document sensation in the "regimental badge" area supplied by the axillary nerve's lateral circumflex branch.

### TESTS

#### *Lab*

No routine tests are indicated unless surgery is anticipated.

#### *Imaging*

- 3 views of the proximal humerus should be obtained for all fractures:
  - AP
  - Lateral
  - Axillary
- CT may be helpful in comminuted fractures when surgery is planned.

### DIFFERENTIAL DIAGNOSIS

- Acute rotator cuff tear or strain
- Anterior or posterior shoulder dislocation (similar presentation)
- Pain in the proximal shoulder (may be from AC joint dislocation or biceps tendon rupture)

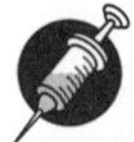

## TREATMENT

### GENERAL MEASURES

- Up to 85% of proximal humerus fractures are displaced minimally and can be treated nonoperatively (5).
  - A simple collar and cuff allows gravity to maintain alignment.
  - It is imperative that the patient maintains elbow and wrist movement.
- Dislocated shoulders require reduction with intra-articular block or sedation.

#### *Activity*

- Initially, the patient's arm is placed in a sling.
- The patient should begin gentle pendulum exercises of the shoulder.

#### *Nursing*

- Skin care under the axillary fold is important.
- A pad (changed daily) should be placed.
- The patient will require assistance with washing.

### SPECIAL THERAPY

#### *Physical Therapy*

- Patients with 2-part fractures have been shown to have less pain and better outcomes when treated with immediate physical therapy and pendular exercises than with delayed therapy (8).
- Early passive movement also is important in surgically repaired shoulders.
- Active motion should not begin until 4–6 weeks after surgery.

### MEDICATION (DRUGS)

#### *First Line*

Oral narcotic analgesics are appropriate in the acute setting.

### SURGERY

- Greater tuberosity fractures may need to be stabilized if they are displaced >5–10 mm.
- Displaced 2-part fractures in the young polytrauma victim should be treated surgically (plate, intramedullary nail, or multiple pins) to aid mobilization.
- Controversy exists over the best way to treat displaced osteoporotic 3- and 4-part fractures.
  - 2 studies have shown no benefit of surgical treatment over nonoperative treatment, although patients were not randomized to treatment groups and methods of fixation were not standardized (9,10).
- Because operative treatment of displaced 3- and 4-part fractures should preserve soft-tissue attachments and be mindful of the blood supply to the humeral head, treatment trends include minimal fixation with sutures, wires, or smooth pins.
- Displaced 4-part fractures have a high risk of osteonecrosis, and prosthetic replacement should be considered.

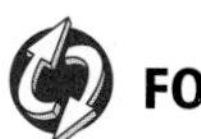

# FOLLOW-UP

## PROGNOSIS

- Most fractures unite without operative intervention.
- Some shoulder motion may be lost.

## COMPLICATIONS

- Osteonecrosis of the humeral head
- Nonunion
- Malunion
- Shoulder stiffness
- Axillary nerve injury in up to 58% of patients diagnosed with electromyography (11)
- Loss of fixation
- Axillary artery injury

## PATIENT MONITORING

Follow-up radiographs every 1–4 weeks to assess reduction of the fracture and bony healing.

## REFERENCES


1. Chu SP, Kelsey JL, Keegan THM, et al. Risk factors for proximal humerus fracture. *Am J Epidemiol* 2004;160:360–367.
2. Palvanen M, Kannus P, Parkkari J, et al. The injury mechanisms of osteoporotic upper extremity fractures among older adults: A controlled study of 287 consecutive patients and their 108 controls. *Osteoporos Int* 2000;11:822–831.
3. Neer CS, II. Displaced proximal humeral fractures. I. Classification and evaluation. *J Bone Joint Surg* 1970;52A:1077–1089.
4. Nguyen TV, Center JR, Sambrook PN, et al. Risk factors for proximal humerus, forearm, and wrist fractures in elderly men and women: The Dubbo Osteoporosis Epidemiology Study. *Am J Epidemiol* 2001;153:587–595.
5. Lyons RP, Lazarus MD. Shoulder and arm trauma: Bone. In: Vaccaro AR, ed. *Orthopaedic Knowledge Update 8*. Rosemont, IL: American Academy of Orthopaedic Surgeons, 2005: 267–281.
6. Baron JA, Karagas M, Barrett J, et al. Basic epidemiology of fractures of the upper and lower limb among Americans over 65 years of age. *Epidemiology* 1996;7:612–618.
7. Schai PA, Hintermann B, Koris MJ. Preoperative arthroscopic assessment of fractures about the shoulder. *Arthroscopy* 1999;15:827–835.
8. Hodgson SA, Mawson SJ, Stanley D. Rehabilitation after two-part fractures of the neck of the humerus. *J Bone Joint Surg* 2003;85B: 419–422.
9. Fjalestad T, Stromsoe K, Blucher J, et al. Fractures in the proximal humerus: Functional outcome and evaluation of 70 patients treated in hospital. *Arch Orthop Trauma Surg* 2005;125:310–316.
10. Ichmann T, Ochsner PE, Wingstrand H, et al. Non-operative treatment versus tension-band osteosynthesis in three- and four-part proximal humeral fractures. A retrospective study of 34 fractures from two different trauma centers. *Int Orthop* 1998;22:316–320.
11. Visser CPJ, Coene LNJEM, Brand R, et al. Nerve lesions in proximal humeral fractures. *J Shoulder Elbow Surg* 2001;10:421–427.


## ADDITIONAL READING


Sher JS, Lozman PR. Proximal humerus fractures and dislocations and traumatic soft tissue injuries of the glenohumeral joint. In: Brinker MR, ed. *Review of Orthopaedic Trauma*. Philadelphia: WB Saunders, 2001:239–254.


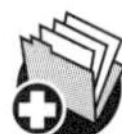

# MISCELLANEOUS

## CODES

### *ICD9-CM*

812.0 Fracture, upper end humerus, closed

## PATIENT TEACHING

- Emphasize importance of early passive exercises and active movements of the ipsilateral elbow and wrist.
- Explain that fractures may take 6–10 weeks to heal, and that some permanent shoulder stiffness is common.

### *Activity*

- As pain decreases, patients should increase their activity.
- For the first 3 months, the patient should not lift >10 pounds.
- After healing, the patient may resume normal activity gradually.

### *Prevention*

- Patients who have a fracture after the age of 50 years should be evaluated for osteoporosis with a DEXA scan.
- Osteoporosis prevention should be instituted.
- Elderly patients who fall should be evaluated to determine if falls can be prevented:
  - Physical therapist visit to the patient's home
  - Medical checkup for comorbidities that may cause falls, such as cataracts, dizziness, dementia, and polypharmacy

## FAQ

- Q: How are most fractures treated in the elderly patient?
  - A: Most proximal humerus fractures in the elderly can be treated without surgery.
- Q: How long should a sling be worn?
  - A: The sling is for comfort in the first 2–4 weeks after surgery. A sling prevents motion, and motion is desired after pain has resolved to prevent stiffness.

S

# SKELETAL SCINTIGRAPHY

*Heather A. Jacene, MD*

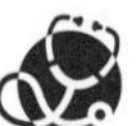

## BASICS

### DESCRIPTION

- Skeletal scintigraphy is a nuclear medicine imaging method for bone disease.
- Advantages:
  - High sensitivity for early detection of disease
  - Whole body survey
- Disadvantage:
  - Limited specificity

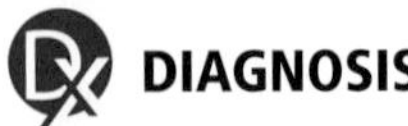

## DIAGNOSIS

### SIGNS AND SYMPTOMS

- Indications
  - Whole body skeletal scintigraphy:
    - Primary bone tumors
    - Osteomyelitis
    - Joint prosthesis pain
    - Occult fractures
    - Stress fractures and shin splints
    - Spondylosis
    - Reflex sympathetic dystrophy
    - Fracture nonunion
    - AVN
    - Musculoskeletal pain, etiology uncertain
    - Heterotopic bone formation
    - Metastases to bone
    - Paget disease and fibrous dysplasia
  - TPSS:
    - Osteomyelitis
    - Stress fracture
    - Reflex sympathetic dystrophy
    - Osteoid osteoma
- Radiopharmaceutical:
  - Technetium-99m-labeled phosphate and phosphonate compounds specifically localize in bone.
  - Regions of increased bone turnover (blastic response) have increased uptake.

### TESTS

- Technique
  - Whole body skeletal scintigraphy:
    - 20–30 mCi of technetium-99m-diphosphonate
    - Intravenous injection of radiopharmaceutical
    - Whole body imaging, 2–4 hours after radiopharmaceutical injection
  - TPSS (20–30 mCi of technetium-99m-diphosphonate):
    - Flow phase (phase 1): Bolus intravenous injection; 1–3-second images for 60 seconds, beginning at time of injection; spot imaging of area of interest for 1 minute to evaluate for the presence of altered regional blood flow
    - Extracellular (blood pool) phase (phase 2): High-count images immediately after the flow phase in various views
    - Delayed phase (phase 3): Whole body imaging 2–4 hours after radiopharmaceutical injection and special views of the region of interest
  - Optional imaging (phase 4):
    - 24-hour delayed imaging: More time for tracer localization in bone; for patients with poor blood flow (e.g., diabetes, peripheral vascular disease) and renal failure
    - SPECT: Improved contrast resolution and 3D cross-sectional images

#### *Pathological Findings*

- Primary malignant bone tumors:
  - Hyperemia on flow phase
  - Intense technetium-99m-diphosphonate in tumor on delayed images
- Primary benign bone tumors:
  - Uptake varies widely
  - Osteoid osteoma has high uptake.
    - Hyperemia on flow phase
    - Intense accumulation in the lesion on extracellular and delayed images
    - High sensitivity for lesion detection
    - Radionuclide-guided surgery can be performed.
- Osteomyelitis:
  - Findings ("3-phase positive"):
    - Focal arterial hyperemia
    - Extracellular phase: Increased focal bone accumulation
    - Delayed phase: Increased focal bone accumulation
  - Cellulitis without osteomyelitis: Increased regional flow and blood pool, but no delayed uptake
  - Cellulitis and osteomyelitis: Flow and extracellular phase may show diffuse uptake, but delayed images show focal bone uptake.
  - 90% accuracy in absence of complicating factors (e.g., hardware, recent fracture or surgery) (1), which may result in false-positives
  - Other conditions also result in similar findings that decrease the specificity of TPSS.
  - Clinical history and comparison with radiographs is essential.
  - Differential diagnosis of a 3-phase positive bone scan:
    - Fractures
    - Gout
    - Osteoarthritis
    - Charcot joint
    - Reflex sympathetic dystrophy
    - Healing phase osteonecrosis
    - Primary malignant bone tumors
    - Osteotomy
  - False-negatives:
    - Neonates
    - Elderly, particularly in setting of conditions that cause decreased blood flow (e.g., diabetes, peripheral vascular disease)
    - Antibiotics (Fig. 1)
- Septic joint:
  - 3-phase positive
  - Periarticular bone and joint space accumulation of radiopharmaceutical
- Complimentary nuclear medicine imaging
  - Radiolabeled leukocyte scintigraphy:
    - Leukocytes migrate to sites of infection.
    - Pitfall: Leukocytes also accumulate at sites of normal bone marrow.
    - Good accuracy, combined with bone scanning
    - Leukocyte/bone marrow scintigraphy: Accuracy of 89–98% (2); based on fact that only leukocytes but not bone marrow agents (sulfur colloid) will accumulate at a site of infection.
  - Sequential TPSS/gallium-67 scan:
    - Interpretative criteria are based on comparison of tracer localization and intensity of tracer uptake on the 2 scans (3).
    - Superior to bone scanning alone in the presence of incongruent image findings (4)
    - Large number of equivocal cases decreases the sensitivity and limits the utility of this combined study (3).

#### *Special Considerations*

- Vertebral osteomyelitis:
  - Intense uptake in adjacent vertebral bodies
  - Sensitivity of delayed bone imaging in 86–100% (5)
  - Combined bone/gallium scan increases specificity.
  - Radiolabeled leukocyte imaging of limited value: 40–50% false-negative rate (5)

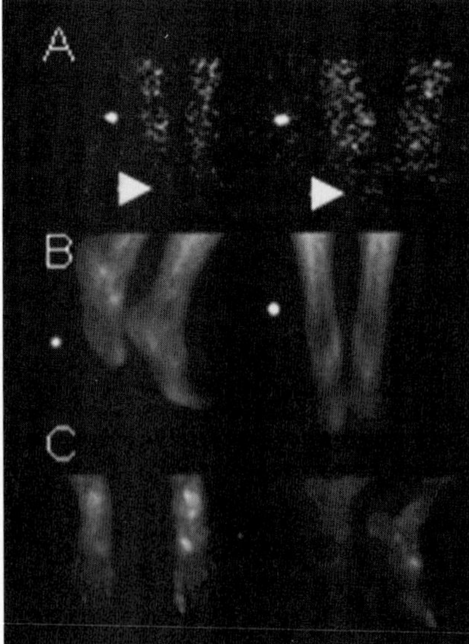


**Fig. 1.** 3-phase positive bone scan consistent with osteomyelitis of the right great toe. **A**: Flow phase with mildly increased flow to the right great toe. **B** and **C**: Increased tracer uptake in the right great toe on the extracellular and delayed phase images (**C**: Left image is plantar view).

- Diabetic foot:
  - TPSS: High negative predictive value for osteomyelitis
  - Forefoot:
    - Technetium-99m–exametazime-labeled leukocytes are the study of choice if the TPSS is positive or equivocal.
  - Mid- or hindfoot:
    - Neuropathic/Charcot joint can accumulate leukocytes in the absence of infection.
    - Study of choice: Combined indium-111-labeled leukocytes/technetium-99m-sulfur colloid
- Arthritis:
  - Diffuse periarticular increase of radiotracer
  - Focal osteoblastic activity in subchondral bone
- Occult fractures:
  - 3-phase positive
  - Visualization on skeletal scintigraphy:
    - 80% by 24 hours
    - 95% by 72 hours in those <65 years old
    - Maximum sensitivity to detect fractures is at 7 days in patients >65 years old
  - Skeletal scintigraphy returns to normal (6).
    - Nondisplaced fractures: 60–80% at 1 year; 95% at 3 years
    - Displaced fractures: Positive indefinitely
- Athletic injuries:
  - Stress fractures:
    - Positive 1–2 weeks before radiographic changes are visualized.
    - Intense, oval or fusiform uptake at fracture site
  - Shin splints:
    - Normal flow and extracellular phase
    - Mild to moderate, linear uptake on delayed imaging only
    - Most commonly, posteromedial aspects of bilateral tibias
- Painful prosthesis evaluation:
  - Skeletal scintigraphy is nonspecific for differentiating prosthesis loosening and infection.
  - Typical appearance shows loosening on bone scan:
    - Increased uptake in region of greater and lesser trochanters and at tip of the prosthesis
  - Increased uptake can be seen up to 1 year after cemented prosthesis placement and up to 2–3 years after noncemented prosthesis placement.
  - Study of choice is combined indium-111-labeled leukocytes/technetium-99m-sulfur colloid scan:
    - Sensitivity and specificities >90% (7)
    - False-positives (7): Displaced bone marrow (technetium-99m-sulfur colloid scan helps avoid this pitfall.)
- Bone grafts:
  - Technetium-99m-diphosphonate scan can detect early changes in vascular patency if used within 1 week after surgery.
    - Vascularized graft: Normal or diffusely increased tracer uptake and focally increased uptake at osteotomy site
    - Failed graft: Photopenic defect
  - Pitfalls:
    - New bone formation on a nonviable graft
    - Osteoradionecrosis
    - Postoperative changes
- Metastatic bone disease:
  - Metastatic bone disease from nonosseous tumors can present as several patterns on skeletal scintigraphy.
    - Multiple, randomly scattered lesions
    - Solitary lesion
    - Diffuse disease
    - Photopenic lesions
    - Reduced sensitivity and false-negatives with multiple myeloma, renal cell carcinoma, thyroid carcinoma, lymphoma
- Spinal surgery:
  - Normal: Diffuse uptake at surgical sites secondary to new bone formation
  - Nonunion/pseudarthroses:
    - Focal areas of intense uptake
    - SPECT improves sensitivity

### *Pediatric Considerations*

Young children may require sedation to remain still for the entire examination.

### *Pregnancy Considerations*

- Radiation exposure to a fetus from most studies using technetium-99m-labeled agent is <0.500 rad (8).
- Fetal risk is considered negligible at radiation exposures of <5 rad (8).
- However, the benefit of the single study should outweigh the risk of the exposure to the fetus and be given serious consideration.

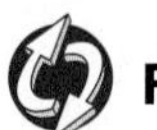

## FOLLOW-UP

- Follow-up skeletal scintigraphy can assess:
  - Stability of metastatic bone disease
  - Residual or recurrent primary bone tumors
  - Assessment of response to therapy
  - Malignancy
  - Infections
  - Persistent nonunion at fracture sites

### REFERENCES


1. Maurer AH, Chen DCP, Camargo EE, et al. Utility of three-phase skeletal scintigraphy in suspected osteomyelitis: Concise communication. *J Nucl Med* 1981;22:941–949.
2. Palestro CJ, Roumanas P, Swyer AJ, et al. Diagnosis of musculoskeletal infection using combined In-111 labeled leukocyte and Tc-99m SC marrow imaging. *Clin Nucl Med* 1992;17:269–273.
3. Palestro CJ, Torres MA. Radionuclide imaging in orthopaedic infections. *Semin Nucl Med* 1997;27: 334–345.
4. Rosenthall L, Lisbona R, Hernandez M, et al. $^{99m}$Tc-PP and $^{67}$Ga imaging following insertion of orthopaedic devices. *Radiology* 1979;133: 717–721.
5. Palestro CJ, Kim CK, Swyer AJ, et al. Radionuclide diagnosis of vertebral osteomyelitis: Indium-111-leukocyte and technetium-99m-methylene diphosphonate bone scintigraphy. *J Nucl Med* 1991;32:1861–1865.
6. Matin P. The appearance of bone scans following fractures, including immediate and long-term studies. *J Nucl Med* 1979;20:1227–1231.
7. Palestro CJ, Kim CK, Swyer AJ, et al. Total-hip arthroplasty: Periprosthetic indium-111-labeled leukocyte activity and complementary technetium-99m-sulfur colloid imaging in suspected infection. *J Nucl Med* 1990;31: 1950–1955.
8. Toppenberg KS, Hill DA, Miller DP. Safety of radiographic imaging during pregnancy. *Am Fam Physician* 1999;59:1813–1820.


### ADDITIONAL READING


- Holder L, ed. Orthopaedic nuclear medicine (part I). *Semin Nucl Med* 1997;27:309–400.
- Holder L, ed. Orthopaedic nuclear medicine (part II). *Semin Nucl Med* 1998;28:3–131.
- Palestro CJ. Radionuclide imaging after skeletal interventional procedures. *Semin Nucl Med* 1995;25:3–14.


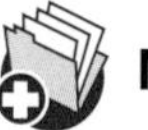

## MISCELLANEOUS

### PATIENT TEACHING

- Minimal preparation is required for patients undergoing skeletal scintigraphy.
- Patients should be advised of the following:
  - The total time of the test from the injection of radiotracer until completion of imaging is ~4 hours.
  - Patients will be required to lie flat and still for image acquisition.
  - If patients have severe pain that will not permit them to lie still, then pain medication should be considered.
  - After radiotracer injection, patients should drink plenty of fluids to reduce the radiation dose to the bladder and kidneys.

### FAQ

- Q: How long after a fracture occurs will the bone scan return to normal?
  - A: Most (60–90%) nondisplaced and uncomplicated fractures return to normal in 1 year; 95% return to normal in 3 years. Displaced and comminuted fractures and fractures around joints can have prolonged or indefinite positivity.
- Q: Which test should be ordered to distinguish between loosening and infection of a joint prosthesis?
  - A: In this setting, an indium-111-labeled- or technetium-99m-exametazime white blood cell study is the most accurate test. White blood cells accumulate in areas of infection but not in areas of bone remodeling (loosening). Because bone marrow may be displaced during surgery and normally accumulates labeled white cells, a technetium-99m-sulfur colloid study often is performed in conjunction with a white cell study. Infection is diagnosed in areas that accumulate white cells but not sulfur colloid.

# SLIPPED CAPITAL FEMORAL EPIPHYSIS

*Paul D. Sponseller, MD*

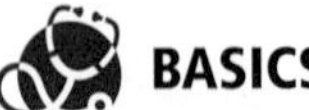

## BASICS

### DESCRIPTION

- SCFE is a disorder of the hips of adolescents or preadolescents in which the femoral head is displaced relative to the rest of the femur (Fig. 1).
  - The femoral head remains in the acetabulum.
  - Most notable features: The outward rotation of the lower femur and leg and a limp
- Classification:
  - Stable versus unstable (1):
    - Stable: Weightbearing without crutches is possible; 95% of patients have satisfactory results with proper treatment.
    - Unstable: Weightbearing without crutches is not possible; compared with stable type, this type has a higher rate of AVN and severe slip, so only 50% have satisfactory results with treatment.
  - Chronologic (1):
    - Acute (<3 weeks)
    - Chronic (>3 weeks)
  - Anatomic (1,2):
    - Grade 0 (preslip): Impending slip with no discernible displacement
    - Grade I (mild): 1–33% slip (Fig. 2)
    - Grade II (moderate): 33–50% slip (Fig. 3)
    - Grade III (severe): >50% slip

### EPIDEMIOLOGY

- 80% of cases occur during the growth phase of adolescence (boys, 10–16 years; girls, 10–14 years) (1).
- Male:Female ratio, 2.4:1 (3)

#### *Incidence*

- 2–10 per 100,000 in the general population per year (3)
- Substantial seasonal variation (3)
  - Highest in September, lowest in March
  - Variation is presumed to be secondary to late effects of vitamin D exposure or to activity.

### RISK FACTORS

- Adolescence
- Male gender
- Obesity: A weight:height ratio >90th percentile in 50–75% of patients (2)
- African American race (3)
- Contralateral SCFE: 50% of patients eventually have a bilateral slip (25% at initial presentation) (4).
- Delayed skeletal maturity

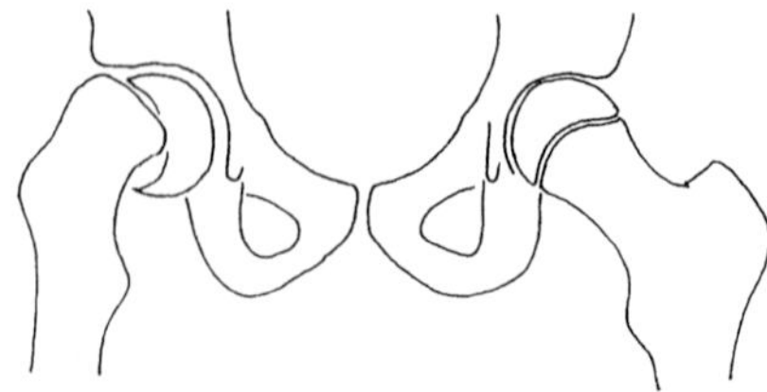

**Fig. 1.** SCFE occurs through the growth plate, as seen in the right hip here.

#### *Genetics*

A 5–7% incidence is noted in family members of patients who have SCFE compared with 2–10 per 100,000 in the general population (1).

### ETIOLOGY

- Likely multifactorial, resulting in a weakened growth plate (physis) with higher-than-normal stresses placed across it
- Endocrine factors such as hypothyroidism, panhypopituitarism, hypogonadal conditions, and renal osteodystrophy may weaken the physis, but such occurrences are rare (1).
- During the preadolescent or adolescent age, the growth plate is weakened by the process of rapid growth.
- Increased shear stress may be generated by obesity or trauma.

### ASSOCIATED CONDITIONS

- Hypothyroidism
- Hyperparathyroidism
- Chronic renal failure
- Radiation therapy to pelvis

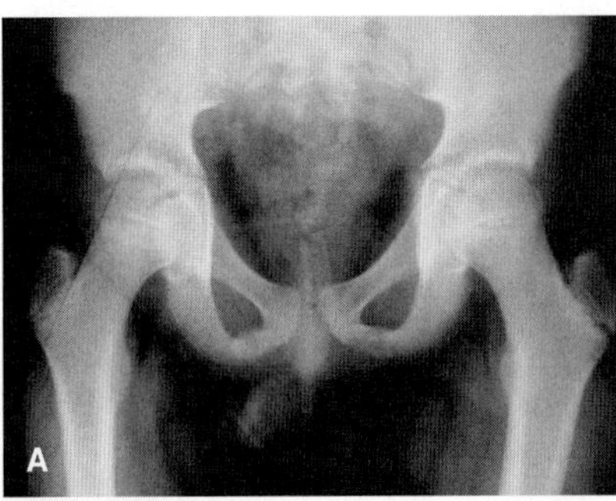


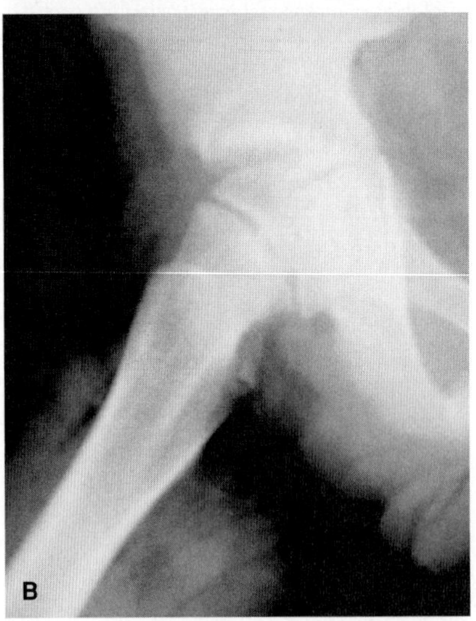


**Fig. 2.** Subtle (grade 1) SCFE. **A:** Note the subtle loss or epiphyseal height on the right hip and the greater lucency at the physis. **B:** Slip is more obvious on the lateral view.

## DIAGNOSIS

### SIGNS AND SYMPTOMS

- Symptom: Pain:
  - Acute (<3 weeks) or chronic (>3 weeks)
  - Occurs in the groin, medial thigh, or knee
- Signs:
  - Decreased internal rotation of the hip
  - Limp
  - Trendelenburg gait
  - Antalgic gait (patient bears the weight on the affected side for as little time as possible.)
  - Externally rotated gait
- Symptoms and signs of hypothyroidism or other endocrine disorder, including cold intolerance, delayed bone age, lethargy, coarse hair

#### *History*

- The problem usually develops spontaneously, with no major incident, although in some patients, an episode of trauma may exist.
- Often the pain is not severe, and the patient does not seek medical attention until late.
- Some patients simply feel more easily tired.
- Many patients present with a primary complaint of knee pain (a referral pattern), which often delays the proper diagnosis.

#### *Physical Exam*

- Pain (mild) on palpation of groin or proximal femur
- Pain greatest with internal rotation or abduction
- Hip external rotation >internal rotation
- The hip automatically goes into more external rotation as it is flexed.
- Most patients have little or no internal rotation of the hip.
- The affected limb rests in more external rotation than the contralateral limb.
- Rule out endocrine disorders, such as hypothyroidism, panhypopituitarism, hypogonadal conditions, and renal osteodystrophy by history.

### TESTS

#### *Lab*

An endocrine workup is indicated for patients with substantial delay in skeletal maturity or with symptoms suggesting an endocrine problem.

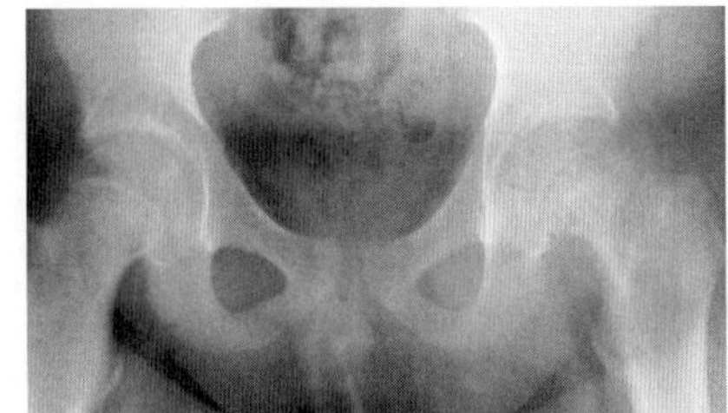

**Fig. 3.** This pelvic radiograph shows a grade-2 slip on the left hip and a grade-1 slip on the right.

### *Imaging*

- Radiography:
  - Plain AP and lateral views usually are adequate for diagnosis.
    - Findings are most pronounced on the lateral view.
  - Varus angulation of the epiphysis on the femoral neck may be apparent, and the appearance of the epiphysis has been likened to "ice cream falling off of its cone."
  - "Kline line" (loss of the intersection of the epiphysis by the lateral cortical line of the femoral neck) is best seen on a lateral view.
  - Widening and blurring of the physis
  - A relative decrease in the height of the epiphysis (compared with contralateral side)
  - "Pistol-grip deformity": In chronic stages, reactive bone forms along the inferomedial portions of the femoral neck.
- CT or MRI usually shows an impending slip (also called a *preslip*) if the diagnosis is suspected or radiographs do not show it.
  - In a preslip, MRI shows increased edema in the region of the physis.

### DIFFERENTIAL DIAGNOSIS

- Perthes disease: Usually presents as a painless limp at a young age (4–8 years) and distinguishable on radiographs
- Proximal femoral fractures: 90% with high-energy trauma (5)
- A stress fracture of proximal femur is more common after skeletal maturity (5).

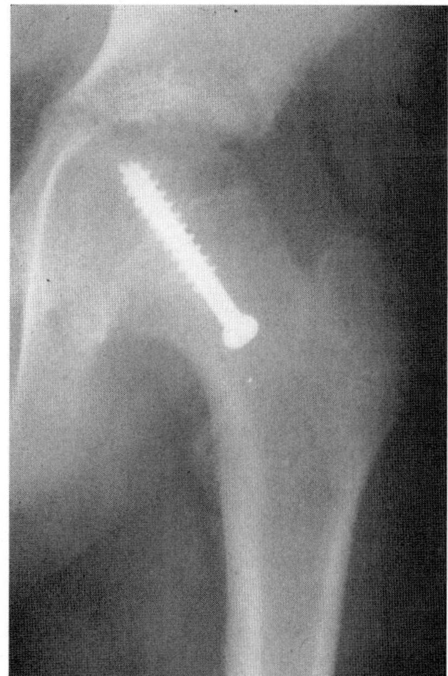

**Fig. 4.** *In situ* fixation of SCFE with 1 cannulated screw.

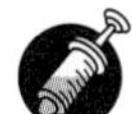

## TREATMENT

### GENERAL MEASURES

- Complete avoidance of weightbearing is needed until the slip is stabilized.
  - Prevention of additional slip is the cornerstone of therapy.
  - Place the child immediately on bed rest and admit for surgery.
    - Surgery usually is done with 1 percutaneously placed screw to close the physis (Fig. 4).

### SPECIAL THERAPY

#### *Physical Therapy*

Postoperative instruction in ambulation with crutches or a walker is indicated, with partial weightbearing if the slip is stable.

### SURGERY

- The goal is to prevent additional slippage by inducing closure of the physis.
- 1 guide pin is placed percutaneously from the anterior neck into the center of the femoral epiphysis.
- The starting point is on the anterior femoral neck rather than on the lateral cortex of the proximal femur.
- An appropriate-length 6.5- or 7.3-mm cannulated screw is placed over the guide wire.
- Care is taken to avoid leaving a screw that penetrates the chondral surface of the epiphysis because such penetration likely will lead to chondrolysis.
- In severe unstable slips, some surgeons attempt reduction of the slip by traction, gentle closed manipulation, or open reduction.
- Osteotomies for severe slips may be performed to correct severe deformity.
  - Although controversial, prophylactic fixation of the contralateral hip is justifiable in very young patients, patients with known metabolic or endocrine disorders, or patients in whom appropriate follow-up is unlikely.
- Removal of the screw is not recommended.
- For patients with degenerative joint disease in later life resulting from SCFE, options are hip fusion in the young patient and total hip replacement in the older patient.

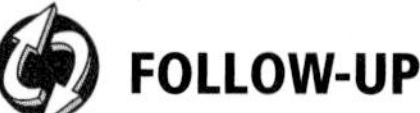

## FOLLOW-UP

### PROGNOSIS

- Prognosis depends on the severity of the slip and the presence of complications.
- Even without complications, a high incidence of degenerative joint disease still is possible (6).
- If the patient is able to lose weight, it will help decrease the risk of degeneration and increase the success of total hip replacement.

### COMPLICATIONS

- Osteonecrosis:
  - Blood supply to the femoral head is lost, leading to collapse and severe degenerative joint disease.
  - Most strongly associated with unstable slip: 40% risk (5% risk for stable slips) (5).
- Chondrolysis: Acute dissolution of articular cartilage with subsequent pain and stiffness
- Degenerative joint disease: Undiagnosed or untreated SCFE leading to degenerative joint disease is a common cause of total hip replacement in the United States (4).

### REFERENCES


1. Kay RM. Slipped capital femoral epiphysis. In: Morrissy RT, Weinstein SL, eds. *Lovell and Winter's Pediatric Orthopaedics*, 6th ed. Philadelphia: Lippincott Williams & Wilkins, 2006:1085–1124.
2. Mooney JF, III, Podeszwa DA. The management of slipped capital femoral epiphysis. *J Bone Joint Surg* 2005;87B:1024–1025.
3. Brown D. Seasonal variation of slipped capital femoral epiphysis in the United States. *J Pediatr Orthop* 2004;24:139–143.
4. Kocher MS, Bishop JA, Hresko MT, et al. Prophylactic pinning of the contralateral hip after unilateral slipped capital femoral epiphysis. *J Bone Joint Surg* 2004;86A:2658–2665.
5. Mullins MM, Sood M, Hashemi-Nejad A, et al. The management of avascular necrosis after slipped capital femoral epiphysis. *J Bone Joint Surg* 2005;87B:1669–1674.
6. Carney BT, Weinstein SL, Noble J. Long-term follow-up of slipped capital femoral epiphysis. *J Bone Joint Surg* 1991;73A:667–674.


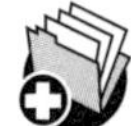

## MISCELLANEOUS

### CODES

#### *ICD9-CM*

732.2 Slipped capital femoral epiphysis

### PATIENT TEACHING

- The child and parent must understand the need for immediate nonweightbearing and early (usually the same day) surgery to prevent additional slip and the need for careful postoperative monitoring for osteonecrosis, chondrolysis, degenerative joint disease, and (most importantly) SCFE of the contralateral hip.
- Any pain in the contralateral thigh should be reported immediately.
- After surgery, the patient should maintain partial weightbearing to nonweightbearing for 6 weeks.
- Vigorous sports are not allowed until the physis has closed (usually ~6 months postoperatively).

#### *Prevention*

Although controversial, prophylactic pinning of the contralateral hip is recommended for patients in whom communication is impaired or appropriate follow-up is unlikely (4).

### FAQ

- Q: What causes the slip?
  - A: It is a combination of increased forces (weight and activity) on a physis that may be weakened by the growth spurt and other individual factors.
- Q: What is the risk of osteoarthritis?
  - A: It is increased to at least 25–50% at 30 years after the slip.

S

# SNAPPING HIP

*Paul D. Sponseller, MD*

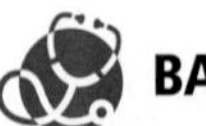

## BASICS

### DESCRIPTION

- Snapping of the hip is a sensation that is normally felt on an infrequent basis by many people.
  - If it becomes frequent or painful, patients may seek attention and treatment.
  - The causes may include structures outside or inside the joint.
- Synonyms: Popping hip; Tendinitis; Coxa saltans

### GENERAL PREVENTION

- Perform adequate stretching before and after sports.
- Avoid frequent intramuscular injections into the gluteal muscles.

### EPIDEMIOLOGY

- Snapping of the hip may occur at any age, including in the elderly.
- It is slightly more common in females than in males.

#### *Incidence*

- Uncommon clinical problem
- No statistics on frequency or prevalence

### RISK FACTORS (1–4)

- Coxa vara, or decreased angle of the femoral neck, renders the greater trochanter more prominent and increases the risk of snapping.
- Another risk factor is a history of multiple intramuscular injections into the buttock, which may cause fibrosis of the gluteus and, in turn, may predispose to snapping.
- Athletes who increase their training to an extreme degree may also develop this condition.

#### *Genetics*

No known genetic predisposition exists.

### ETIOLOGY

- Internal:
  - A structure in front of the joint, such as the psoas tendon, causes the snapping by riding over the front of the femoral head or the pubic ramus.
- External:
  - May be from snapping of the iliotibial band or the anterior fibers of the gluteus maximus riding over the greater trochanter.
  - May follow multiple intramuscular injections into the buttock, which render the gluteus and iliotibial band fibrotic and contracted.
- Intra-articular:
  - Includes loose bodies or a tear in the acetabular labrum, which may cause sensation of snapping or clicking.
  - Rarely, may occur after total hip arthroplasty secondary to malposition or loosening of the femoral component.

### ASSOCIATED CONDITIONS

Snapping hip usually occurs in isolation and is not related to any systemic conditions or other skeletal problems.

## DIAGNOSIS

### SIGNS AND SYMPTOMS

- The patient has a sensation of muscle jumping over the front or the side of the hip.
  - The patient may be able to point to the location of snapping, thus aiding in the diagnosis.
- The patient may have difficulty getting into or arising from a squat.
- The diagnosis may be confirmed by blocking the movement of the psoas or the iliotibial band during flexion and extension of the hip.

#### *History*

- Patients note the spontaneous onset of snapping or popping of the hip, usually in the absence of trauma.
- It is more common in athletes than in the general population, and typically begins in the juvenile or adolescent period (1,2).
- Ask the patient about what activity or position produces the snapping, and its frequency.

#### *Physical Exam*

- Ask the patient to point to the area where the snapping is felt.
  - This procedure is helpful in distinguishing snapping of the iliotibial band (lateral) from the psoas (anteriorly).
- Ask the patient if, he/she can reproduce the snapping.
- For psoas tendon snapping over the pectineal eminence, the "figure 4" test is helpful.
  - This test consists of the patient actively moving the affected hip from extension to a "figure 4" or flexed and abducted position while keeping the foot in the midline (Fig. 1) (1).
- To test for the snapping iliotibial band, the patient is placed in the lateral position on the opposite hip, and the hip in question is flexed and extended in progressively greater adduction.
  - Note the presence of abduction contracture, reproduction of symptoms, and actual snapping.

### TESTS

#### *Imaging*

- Plain radiography of the pelvis is indicated to rule out any bony abnormality of the pelvis or joint.
- CT scan may be helpful if a structural abnormality is found.
- Ultrasound has been reported to document dynamically the snapping and possibly to guide injection, but it requires experience (1,5).
- Iliopsoas bursography is done under fluoroscopy, with contrast medium injected anteriorly into the bursa.
  - If the psoas tendon is the cause, it may be seen to flip over the front of the hip corresponding with the symptoms.
  - Psoas tendon and bursa can be injected with steroid and lidocaine at this time.
  - If the injection relieves symptoms, it is additional confirmation of the diagnosis.

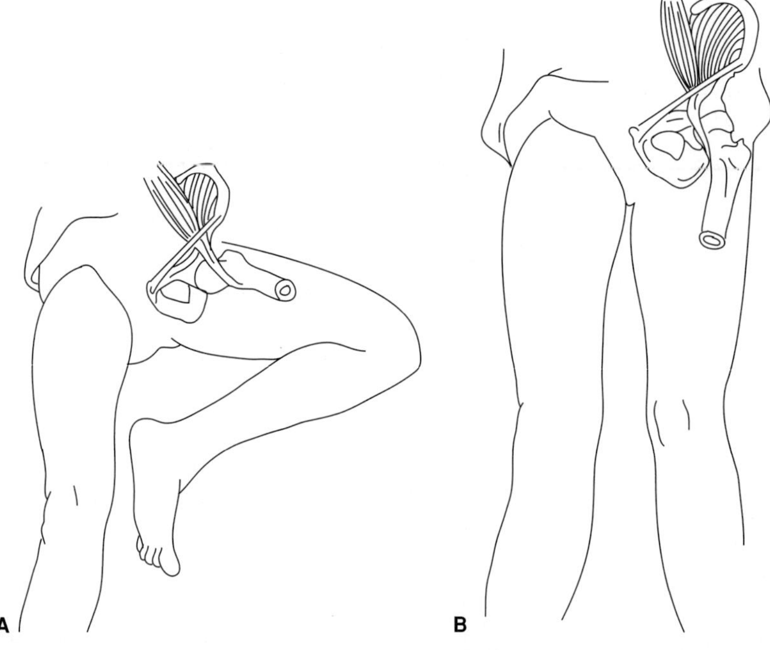


**Fig. 1.** Artist's sketch of movement of the iliopsoas tendon during snapping hip. **A**: The tendon is lateral to the pelvic brim with the hip in flexion and abduction. **B**: Snapping hip is reproduced as the tendon moves to a more medial position on the pelvic brim with extension and adduction of the hip. (Reprinted with permission of Dobbs MB, Gordon JE, Luhmann SJ, et al. Surgical correction of the snapping iliopsoas tendon in adolescents. *J Bone Joint Surg* 2002;84A:420–424.)

- Injection of the greater trochanteric bursa does not require imaging but is a helpful confirmatory test.
- A hip arthrogram, combined with CT scan may be helpful in diagnosing a torn acetabular labrum.
- MRI may be helpful to rule out other conditions or diagnose acetabular labral tears (5,6).

### *Diagnostic Procedures/Surgery*
Hip arthroscopy may be useful in confirming an intra-articular cause and treating a torn labrum or loose body.

### *Pathological Findings*
- Internal type of snapping hip:
  - The psoas and iliacus tendons ride in a shallow groove between the iliopectineal eminence and the anterior inferior iliac spine.
  - They may cause snapping by riding over each other, over the psoas bursa, or over the bone during flexion and extension.
- The iliotibial band attaches to the tensor fasciae latae and the gluteus maximus and minimus.
  - It remains taut during flexion and extension, and it rides over the trochanteric bursa.
  - Any thickening of this bursa, or increasing tension of the tendon, may contribute to the snapping.

## DIFFERENTIAL DIAGNOSIS
- Snapping of the meniscus may masquerade as snapping hip because the hip and knee usually flex together.
- Exostosis around the hip may contribute to snapping.
- Habitual hip subluxation in children and adolescents is an uncommon phenomenon, which may be confused with a snapping hip.

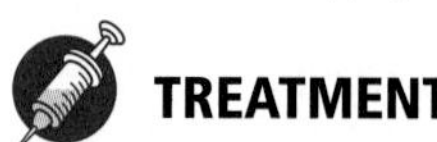

# TREATMENT

## GENERAL MEASURES
- Injection into the appropriate region is an intermittent step between physical therapy and surgery.
  - It may be done using a mixture of local anesthetics (e.g., lidocaine) to confirm the diagnosis and steroids to interrupt the inflammatory cycle and perhaps provide permanent relief.
- Make the diagnosis by physical examination and imaging.
- The extent of treatment depends on how much snapping bothers the patient.
  - If the snapping is severe, the following are advised:
    - Avoidance of provocative activities
    - Stretching exercises
    - Anti-inflammatory medications
    - Injection with steroids may be repeated every 6 months.
    - Surgery
- The patient should refrain from activities involving flexion and extension, or adduction (such as running on the side of an incline), which may predispose to snapping.

## SPECIAL THERAPY
### *Physical Therapy*
Stretching the iliotibial band or psoas tendon may alleviate the problem.

## MEDICATION (DRUGS)
### *First Line*
- NSAIDs:
  - Dosing schedules vary from quick-onset, short duration, to once-a-day agents, which are less effective for acute pain.
  - Gastrointestinal upset is a possible side effect, and these drugs are to be used cautiously in patients with a history of gastric ulcer disease.
- Narcotics should be avoided.

## SURGERY
- If other measures do not help, surgery may be offered, depending on the underlying cause.
  - If the cause is the iliotibial band, it can be incised over the greater trochanter to relieve the pressure.
  - If the cause is the psoas tendon, it may be lengthened at the pelvic brim.
- Surgery is reserved for the most recalcitrant cases because the results are unpredictable when no structural abnormalities have been identified.
- Intra-articular factors, such as a loose body or a torn acetabular labrum, may be dealt with appropriately.

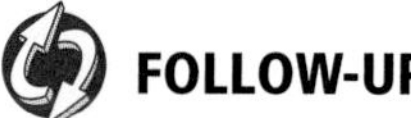

# FOLLOW-UP

## PROGNOSIS
- Usually not a long-standing problem
- Does not lead to arthritis

## COMPLICATIONS
- Failure to improve is the most common complication (1).
- Femoral neuropathy is another possible risk of psoas lengthening.

## PATIENT MONITORING
Because this condition is benign, patients may be allowed to self-monitor and return for follow-up if symptoms warrant.

## REFERENCES

1. Dobbs MB, Gordon JE, Luhmann SJ, et al. Surgical correction of the snapping iliopsoas tendon in adolescents. *J Bone Joint Surg* 2002;84A: 420–424.
2. Lyons JC, Peterson LFA. The snapping iliopsoas tendon. *Mayo Clin Proc* 1984;59:327–329.
3. Schaberg JE, Harper MC, Allen WC. The snapping hip syndrome. *Am J Sports Med* 1984;12: 361–365.
4. Wahl CJ, Warren RF, Adler RS, et al. Internal coxa saltans (snapping hip) as a result of overtraining. A report of 3 cases in professional athletes with a review of causes and the role of ultrasound in early diagnosis and management. *Am J Sports Med* 2004;32:1302–1309.
5. Shabshin N, Rosenberg ZS, Cavalcanti CFA. MR imaging of iliopsoas musculotendinous injuries. *Magn Reson Imaging Clin N Am* 2005;13: 705–716.
6. Tatu L, Parratte B, Vuillier F, et al. Descriptive anatomy of the femoral portion of the iliopsoas muscle. Anatomical basis of anterior snapping of the hip. *Surg Radiol Anat* 2001;23:371–374.


S

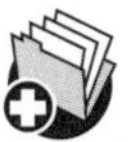

# MISCELLANEOUS

## CODES
### *ICD9-CM*
- 719.65 Snapping hip
- 726.0 Bursitis

## PATIENT TEACHING
The phenomenon of a snapping tendon or other structure, including the rationale for rest and stretching, should be explained to the patient.

## FAQ
- Q: Is snapping hip likely to lead to arthritis?
  - A: No. It does not normally lead to arthritis because most causes are outside the joint.

# SOFT-TISSUE TUMORS

*Constantine A. Demetracopoulos, BS*
*Frank J. Frassica, MD*

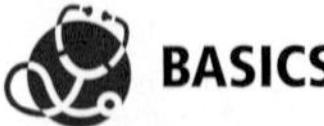

## BASICS

### DESCRIPTION
- Soft-tissue tumors may occur in any area of the skeleton and in individuals of any age.
- They may comprise fibrous tissue or tissue originating from muscle, fat, vessels, or nerves.
- Reactive lesions also cause soft-tissue tumors.
- Benign tumors far outnumber malignant ones.
- Differentiating the malignant from the benign can be difficult.
- Staging: The Musculoskeletal Tumor Society (called the "Enneking" system) (1,2) classifies benign and malignant tumors:
  - Benign lesions:
    - Stage 1: Inactive
    - Stage 2: Active
    - Stage 3: Aggressive
  - Malignant tumors:
    - Stage I: Low grade
    - Stage II: High grade
    - Stage III: Metastatic

### EPIDEMIOLOGY (3)
- Only 15% of sarcomas occur in children.
- >40% of sarcomas occur in patients >55 years old.
- Although soft-tissue tumors may occur at any age, types may vary.
- In childhood, the most common types include:
  - Popliteal cyst
  - Ganglion of wrist or ankle
  - Neuroblastoma
  - Neuroectodermal tumor
  - Rhabdomyosarcoma

#### *Incidence*
- Soft-tissue tumors in the aggregate are common.
- Although the ratio of benign to malignant types is 100:1 (3), vigilance must be maintained to avoid missing malignant tumors.

#### *Prevalence*
No difference in gender risk is noted overall, but sarcomas are more common in males.

### RISK FACTORS

#### *Genetics*
- Most soft-tissue tumors are not inherited.
- A notable exception is NF, which is associated with multiple soft-tissue tumors and is inherited in an autosomal-dominant manner.
- Genetic abnormalities (4):
  - Clear cell carcinoma: t(12;22)(q13;a12)
  - Extraskeletal myxoid chondrosarcoma: t(9;22)(q22;q12)
  - Synovial sarcoma: t(x;18)(p11;q11)
  - Alveolar rhabdomyosarcoma: t(2;13)(q35;q14)
  - Myxoid liposarcoma: t(12;16)(q13;p11)
  - Alveolar soft part sarcoma: t(x;17)(p11;q25)

### ETIOLOGY
- The cause is largely unknown.
- Myositis ossificans may occur with trauma.
- Reactive granuloma may occur with implantation or retention of a foreign body.

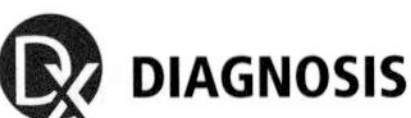

## DIAGNOSIS

### SIGNS AND SYMPTOMS
- Presence of a mass
- Possible loss of ROM of the adjacent joint
- Usually painless or minimally painful
- Absence of pain is not a reason to ignore the lesion.

#### *Physical Exam*
- Inspect the lesion for size, depth, and mobility.
- Obtain a history of recent growth.
- Note consistency and fixation to surrounding structures.
- It is more likely to be benign if it is small (<5 cm), soft, and superficial.
- It is more likely to be malignant if it is large (>5 cm), hard, and deep.
- Assess the effect on adjacent parts:
  - Presence of limp
  - Restricted joint motion
  - Palpation of lymph nodes
  - Examination of abdomen

### TESTS

#### *Lab*
Laboratory tests usually are not helpful, but screening tests may be helpful if a workup for malignant disease is undertaken.

#### *Imaging*
- Radiography:
  - Plain radiographs should be obtained first to look for phleboliths (indicating hemangioma) or rings and stipples (indicating chondroma).
  - A lesion may appear radiodense or radiolucent if it is sandwiched between 2 tissues of lower density, as in deep lipomas in which the fat is contrasted between bone and muscle.
  - Spotty calcifications occur in 20–30% of synovial sarcomas (3).
- Ultrasound is used to look for homogeneity and size, but it has largely been replaced by MRI.
- MRI (5):
  - Superior in its ability to provide excellent soft-tissue definition and to characterize some tissues
  - Many new signal combinations are available.
  - The technique may need to be discussed with the radiologist beforehand.

#### *Pathological Findings*
- Careful histologic evaluation is necessary, taking into account cell features, matrix production, and tissue organization.
- Incorrect histologic diagnosis is not uncommon.

### DIFFERENTIAL DIAGNOSIS
- Intramedullary bone tumor with soft-tissue extension
- Bone tumor arising from the surface of the bone

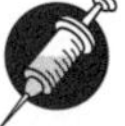

# TREATMENT

## GENERAL MEASURES
- Observation:
  - For inactive benign lesions (e.g., lipomas, ganglions) if they are not causing symptoms
- If the nature of a lesion is not clear, it is important not to fall into the trap of complacency.
- Initiate a diagnostic workup under the direction of an orthopaedist knowledgeable about the diagnoses.

### *Activity*
Activity may increase the symptoms of some tumor types, such as a popliteal cyst, ganglion, or myositis ossificans.

## SPECIAL THERAPY
### *Physical Therapy*
Physical therapy often is used postoperatively to restore function.

## MEDICATION (DRUGS)
- Chemotherapy is an effective adjuvant for a few of the malignant soft-tissue tumors (e.g., rhabdomyosarcoma and Ewing sarcoma).
- Protocols vary from type to type, and chemotherapy may be used before surgery in some types to shrink the tumor and to make resection more feasible.

## SURGERY
- The extent of surgery depends on the degree of malignancy.
  - Benign tumors may be excised at their margins.
  - Malignant tumors (sarcomas) should be excised with a layer of normal tissue around them.
    - ~95% of patients are treated with limb-sparing surgery.
- Attachment to nerves or major vessels may prevent effective resection of malignant tumors.
- If the lesion cannot be safely removed leaving a functional limb, amputation may be recommended.
- Radiation therapy often is used to decrease the risk of local recurrence.

# FOLLOW-UP

## PROGNOSIS
- Depends on the following:
  - Grade of malignancy
  - Anatomic extent
  - Treatment given
- Superficial sarcomas (located above the fascia) have an excellent prognosis (>80%), whereas deep, large, high-grade lesions have the worst prognosis (only 50–60% long-term survival) (3).

## COMPLICATIONS
- Infection
- Recurrence
- Misdiagnosis
- Injury to local nerves and vessels

## PATIENT MONITORING
- Follow the patient at suitable intervals with physical examination or, in some cases, serial MRI scans.
- After the resection of malignant tumors, patients are followed at 3-month intervals for 2 years to look for pulmonary metastases (CT scans) and then every 4–6 months for 5 more years.
- MRI scans are used to check for local recurrence 6 months after surgery and then once a year.

## REFERENCES

1. Enneking WF. A system of staging musculoskeletal neoplasms. *Clin Orthop Relat Res* 1986;204:9–24.
2. Frassica FJ, McCarthy EF, Bluemke DA. Soft-tissue masses: when and how to biopsy. *Instr Course Lect* 2000;49:437–442.
3. Weiss SW, Goldblum JR. General considerations. In: Weiss SW, Goldblum JR, eds. *Enzinger and Weiss's Soft Tissue Tumors*, 4th ed. St. Louis: Mosby, 2001:1–19.
4. Lin PP. Cellular and molecular biology of musculoskeletal tumors. In: Menendez LR, ed. *Orthopaedic Knowledge Update: Musculoskeletal Tumors*. Rosemont, IL: American Academy of Orthopaedic Surgeons, 2002:11–20.
5. Frassica FJ, Khanna JA, McCarthy EF. The role of MR imaging in soft tissue tumor evaluation: perspective of the orthopaedic oncologist and musculoskeletal pathologist. *Magn Reson Imaging Clin North Am* 2000;8:915–927.


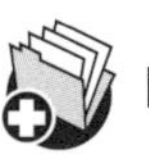

# MISCELLANEOUS

## CODES
### *ICD9-CM*
238.1 Neoplasm, connective tissue, uncertain behavior

## PATIENT TEACHING
- The patient should be given a general understanding of the behavior of the tumor type.
- Discuss the importance of follow-up and the risk of recurrence.

## FAQ
- Q: Should all patients with a soft-tissue mass have an MRI?
  - A: If the clinician is positive of the behavior of the mass, such as a subcutaneous lipoma or wrist ganglion, then an MRI is not necessary. In contrast, if the clinician does not know the nature of the mass, an MRI is necessary.
- Q: Is a biopsy necessary for all soft-tissue masses?
  - A: If the clinician does not know the nature of the mass, a biopsy is necessary.

# SPINA BIFIDA

*Paul D. Sponseller, MD*

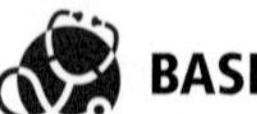

## BASICS

### DESCRIPTION

- Incomplete closure of the laminar arches of the spine (Fig. 1)
- Occurs at birth but may not be detected until later
- An unrelated variety, spina bifida occulta, is a small defect in the 5th lumbar or 1st sacral arches, a benign finding of no clinical consequence.
- May be a clinically significant problem if it is associated with congenital neurologic deficit at the open bony levels
- May occur at any level of the spine or at multiple levels, although it is most common at the caudal aspect of the spine
- In the presence of a neurologic deficit, secondary problems may develop in the genitourinary tract and lower limbs.
- Classification:
  - Spina bifida occulta: Skin-covered defect in the lower lumbar spine with no neurologic deficit, associated with slightly increased risk of spondylolisthesis
  - Myelomeningocele:
    - Combination of several absent laminae, with exposed meninges and usually neurologic deficit at the same level
    - High risk of hydrocephalus
  - Lipomeningocele:
    - Caudal fatty mass arising from the spinal canal, palpable under the skin, with an associated neurologic deficit but no substantial risk of hydrocephalus (1)
- All patients with spina bifida should be classified by motor level (i.e., the lowest level with antigravity strength).
- Synonyms: Spinal dysraphism; Neural tube defect; Myelomeningocele

### GENERAL PREVENTION

Folate, 0.4 mg daily, used in the 1st few months of pregnancy, may prevent spina bifida.

### EPIDEMIOLOGY

Males and females are affected equally.

#### *Incidence*

- The incidence of spina bifida occulta is 2–3% of the general population (2).
- The overall incidence of neural tube defects in the United States is ~1 per 1,000 births (2).
- The risk of occurrence in 1st-degree relatives is slightly higher than that in the general population (3.2%) (2).

#### *Prevalence*

- Slightly higher in Caucasians and lower in African Americans than in the general population (1,2).
- The rate varies from country to country.

### RISK FACTORS

- Affected 1st-degree relatives
- Poor perinatal nutrition

#### *Genetics*

- Not inherited in a Mendelian fashion
- Follows a polygenic pattern
- No known single genetic defect

### ETIOLOGY

- Failure of closure or late rupture of neural tube:
  - Mechanism of this failure is unknown.

### ASSOCIATED CONDITIONS

- Hydrocephalus
- Chiari malformation
- Syringomyelia
- Kyphosis
- Scoliosis
- Renal problems
- Latex allergies
- Sprengel deformity
- Pathologic fracture

## DIAGNOSIS

### SIGNS AND SYMPTOMS

- Local signs:
  - Abnormality in the skin of the back over site of lesion, ranging from a dimple to a hairy or vascular marking
  - Fatty mass (lipomeningocele)
  - Exposure of the meninges (myelomeningocele)
  - Spina bifida occulta has no physical signs.
- Generalized signs:
  - Motor weakness
  - Atrophy of the calf or thigh
  - Sensory defect corresponding to the motor defect
  - Neurogenic bladder
- Symptoms:
  - None are attributable directly to the spina bifida, except that it predisposes to an increased incidence of tethered cord and spondylolisthesis, which may cause backache.

#### *Physical Exam*

- Examine the patient for scoliosis and kyphosis.
- Note the quality of the skin covering because it predicts the late risk of breakdown.
- Record the motor level of the lesion on each limb as the lowest that has contraction against resistance.
- Record the strength in the major muscle groups for future comparison.
- Record the lowest level of sensation because it predicts pressure sores.
- Note the presence of contractures or deformities of each joint.
- Observe the patient's gait, if possible.
- Look for signs of hydrocephalus or Chiari malformation (Fig. 2).

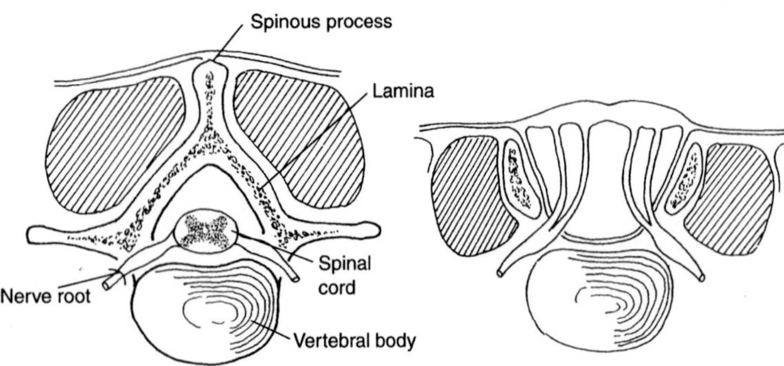


**Fig. 1.** Normal posterior spinal elements (*left*) are disrupted in spina bifida (*right*).

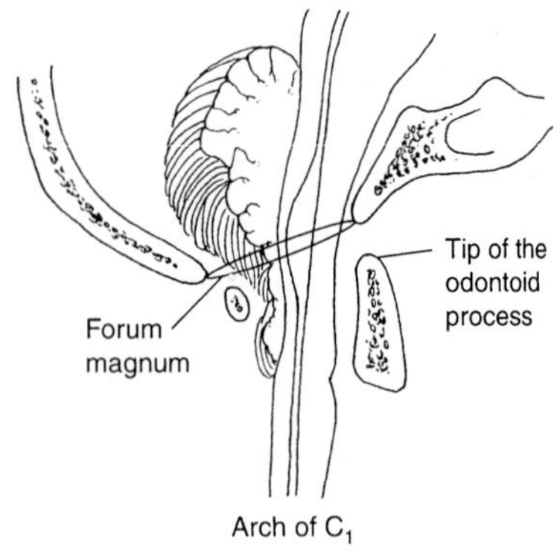


**Fig. 2.** Chiari malformation with cerebellar compression may cause brainstem symptoms in spina bifida.

## TESTS

### Lab

- Prenatal screening with amniocentesis and determination of $\alpha$-fetoprotein and acetylcholinesterase are available for those at increased risk of a neural tube defect.
- Ultrasound may be used as a prenatal imaging test.

### Imaging

- Radiography:
  - Baseline radiography of the spine early in infancy to rule out congenital anomalies such as hemivertebrae and fusion between vertebrae, which are present in up to 20% of children with true spina bifida (1,3)
  - Baseline AP pelvis radiograph
- MRI of the neuraxis, if needed, to determine the presence of a syrinx, Chiari malformation, or tether of the spinal cord

### Pathological Findings

- The pathologic features of a typical myelomeningocele include a flattened spinal cord with scarring and abnormal neural elements.
- Often present is associated hydrocephalus or Chiari malformation with herniation of the cerebellar tonsils through the foramen magnum.

## DIFFERENTIAL DIAGNOSIS

- Defect from previous laminectomy
- Radiographic delay in ossification of an intact arch

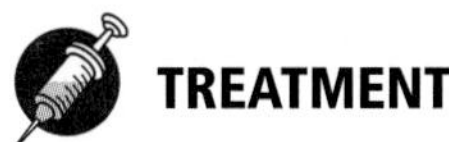

# TREATMENT

## GENERAL MEASURES

- An experienced neurologist, as well as a neurosurgeon, orthopaedic surgeon, and urologist, should see the child at birth.
- Avoid latex exposure (4).
- Offer genetic counseling to the family.
- Prescribe long-term, low-dose prophylactic antibiotic therapy for patients with recurrent urinary tract infections.
- Monitor motor strength and sensory level and record throughout the patient's life to detect tethering or other complications.
- Treat clubfoot deformities by casting initially.
- Treat other deformities by stretching, bracing, or surgery.
- Teach the family how to protect insensate skin.
- Involve the family in a support group such as the Spina Bifida Association of America.
- Some instances of hip subluxation do not need surgery, especially if the condition is high and bilateral in a nonambulatory patient.

### Activity

- Encourage patients to maximize activity by the most efficient means, either by using a wheelchair or by walking with braces.
- Offer wheelchair sports to those athletically inclined, as a means of building social skills and self-image.

## SPECIAL THERAPY

### Physical Therapy

- Patients should be followed throughout growth to maximize mobility, to monitor use of equipment (wheelchair or braces), and to monitor muscle strength.
- A therapist and a nutritionist may help the patient to prevent weight gain.

## SURGERY

- Clubfoot:
  - The 1st step is the Ponseti treatment (2,5) (casting), which may result in partial or total correction.
  - Surgery, if needed, to lengthen tendons and realign bones to create a foot that will be flat on the ground
- Other foot and leg correction may be offered as needed.
- Spine surgery is indicated for patients with scoliosis or kyphosis causing unbalanced sitting, to straighten and fuse the spine with implanted rods (3,6).

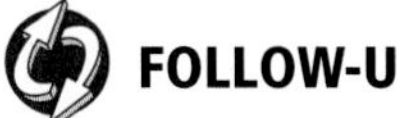

# FOLLOW-UP

## PROGNOSIS

- Currently, infant mortality is only slightly higher than that in the general population, especially for those with severe degrees of spina bifida cystica, because of excellent neonatal care.
- Long-term independence is not possible for some patients with central nervous system complications.

## COMPLICATIONS

- Shunt failure
- Cord tethering at the site of opening, causing weakness with growth
- Fracture: Higher risk with higher neurologic deficit
  - Signs of fracture in patient with spina bifida include:
    - Low-grade fever
    - Swelling
    - Warmth without pain
- Pressure sore over insensate skin, especially of the ischium, foot, or trochanter
- Renal failure secondary to poor self-care

## PATIENT MONITORING

- Follow patients with myelomeningocele every 4–6 months (5):
  - To detect new deformities
  - To monitor the fit of braces and equipment (6,7)
  - To monitor for signs of neurologic deterioration (1), which may be secondary to shunt failure, syrinx (cyst in the cord), tethering of the cord, or Chiari malformation

## REFERENCES


1. McLone DG, Herman JM, Gabrieli AP, et al. Tethered cord as a cause of scoliosis in children with a myelomeningocele. *Pediatr Neurosurg* 1990;16:8–13.
2. Lindseth RE. Myelomeningocele. In: Morrissy RT, Weinstein SL, eds. *Lovell and Winter's Pediatric Orthopaedics*, 5th ed. Philadelphia: Lippincott Williams & Wilkins, 2001:601–632.
3. Guille JT, Sarwark JF, Sherk HH, et al. Congenital and developmental deformities of the spine in children with myelomeningocele. *J Am Acad Orthop Surg* 2006;14:294–302.
4. Tosi LL, Slater JE, Shaer C, et al. Latex allergy in spina bifida patients: Prevalence and surgical implications. *J Pediatr Orthop* 1993;13:709–712.
5. Asher M, Olson J. Factors affecting the ambulatory status of patients with spina bifida cystica. *J Bone Joint Surg* 1983;65A:350–356.
6. Mazur JM, Kyle S. Efficacy of bracing the lower limbs and ambulation training in children with myelomeningocele. *Dev Med Child Neurol* 2004;46:352–356.
7. Mitchell LE, Adzick NS, Melchionne J, et al. Spina bifida. *Lancet* 2004;364:1885–1895.


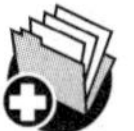

# MISCELLANEOUS

## CODES

### ICD9-CM

- 741.93 Lumbar spina bifida
- 756.17 Spina bifida occulta

## PATIENT TEACHING

- Teach which products contain latex and how to avoid them.
- Discuss signs and symptoms of shunt failure, if applicable.
- Teach prevention of skin pressure sores.
- Teach bowel and bladder continence.
- Encourage weight control early in childhood.

## PREVENTION

Folate, 0.4 mg daily, used periconceptually, may prevent spina bifida.

## FAQ

- Q: If my 1st child has spina bifida occulta, what are my chances that a subsequent child will have spina bifida cystica?
  - A: The risk is approximately the same as that of the general population. Spina bifida occulta does not increase appreciably the risk of neural tube defects.
- Q: Do patients with spina bifida have normal intelligence?
  - A: Intelligence varies widely. Hydrocephalus and its complications can take its toll. In general, the mean IQ is diminished somewhat in the population with spina bifida, but many patients can become independent and receive advanced degrees.
- Q: What are the chances that my child with spina bifida can walk?
  - A: They vary with the motor level of the child. Patients affected at a high lumbar level or above do little functional walking.

# SPINAL STENOSIS

*Dhruv B. Pateder, MD*

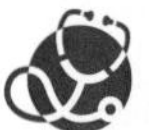

## BASICS

### DESCRIPTION
- Compression of neural elements secondary to osteoarthritic changes (bone spurs, hypertrophied ligamentum flavum, disc space narrowing) at intervertebral levels and facet joints
- Characterized by back and/or lower extremity pain, numbness, weakness, and possible bladder/bowel dysfunction.

### GENERAL PREVENTION
No known preventive measures

### EPIDEMIOLOGY
- Symptoms develop during the 5th and 6th decades.
- No gender predominance
- Degenerative spondylolisthesis with spinal stenosis is 4 times more common in females (1–3).

#### *Incidence*
1.7–8% (1–3)

### RISK FACTORS
Increasing age and spinal arthritis

#### *Genetics*
No definitive genetic links

### PATHOPHYSIOLOGY
- Disc dehydration leads to loss of height with bulging of the annulus and ligamentum flavum into the spinal canal, thus increasing joint loading of the facets.
- Increased joint loading leads to reactive sclerosis and osteophytic bone growth, which in turn leads to additional compression of the neural elements.

### ETIOLOGY
- Congenital:
  - Chondrodystrophy
  - Idiopathic
- Acquired:
  - Degenerative
  - Spondylolytic
  - Iatrogenic
  - Posttraumatic
  - Paget disease

## DIAGNOSIS
- Long-standing back pain that progresses to buttock and lower extremity pain
- Neurogenic claudication (pain, tightness, numbness, and subjective weakness of lower extremities)
- Symptoms worsen with standing, walking, and back extension.
- Symptoms improve with sitting or leaning forward.

#### *History*
- Insidious onset
- Progresses slowly
- Symptoms worse when walking "uphill" and improve with leaning forward (e.g., while pushing a cart in a grocery store)

#### *Physical Exam*
- Few physical findings may be present even in affected patients.
  - Gait alteration (Rule out cervical myelopathy or intracranial pathology.)
  - Loss of lumbar lordosis
  - Decreased ROM of the lumbar spine
  - Straight-leg-raise test may be positive if nerve root entrapment is present.
  - Muscle weakness, most commonly in the L5 distribution.
  - Consider rectal examination to rule out cauda equina syndrome in selected patients.

### TESTS
Spinal stenosis usually is diagnosed with a combination of history, physical examination, and imaging studies.

#### *Lab*
Complete blood cell count, C-reactive protein, and ESR usually are used if infection or cancer is in the differential diagnosis.

#### *Imaging*
- AP and lateral spine radiographs:
  - Show degenerative changes or spondylolisthesis
  - Rule out fractures, infection, or tumor
  - Flexion/extension views help evaluate instability.
- MRI shows compression of neural elements.
- CT-myelography:
  - Comparable to MRI in showing neural compression, but an invasive procedure (contrast injection associated with subsequent headache)
  - Often obtained in patients who have had previous spinal instrumentation or cannot tolerate an MRI examination (e.g., those with claustrophobia, pacemaker)

#### *Diagnostic Procedures/Surgery*
Selective injections can be used to localize the source of pain in patients with multiple sites of neural compression and unclear findings.

#### *Pathological Findings*
- Decreased disc height
- Facet hypertrophy
- Spinal canal and/or foraminal narrowing
- Disc herniation of bulging
- Possible intervertebral instability

### DIFFERENTIAL DIAGNOSIS
- Vascular claudication (symptoms do not improve with leaning forward)
- Cervical myelopathy
- Spinal stenosis in the thoracic spine

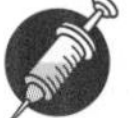

# TREATMENT

## GENERAL MEASURES

- Brace or corset may help for a short time, but it is not recommended for long term because it leads to paraspinal muscle weakness.
- Weight loss

### *Activity*

As tolerated, as long as no other pathology (e.g., fractures, gross instability, etc.) is present

## SPECIAL THERAPY

### *Physical Therapy*

- General conditioning (Patients can ride an exercise bicycle without many problems because they can lean forward and relieve symptoms.)
- Aquatic therapy
- Back extensor muscle strengthening
- Abdominal muscle strengthening
- Gait training

## MEDICATION (DRUGS)

No role for maintenance opiates

### *First Line*

- Anti-inflammatory medications (in absence of gastrointestinal side effects)
- Enteric-coated aspirin (fewer gastrointestinal side effects)
- Acetaminophen

### *Second Line*

- COX-2 inhibitors (Be aware of a changing side-effect profile.)
- Lumbar epidural steroids

## SURGERY

- Indicated when nonoperative treatment fails, and the patient cannot attain a tolerable quality of life.
  - Preoperative clearance by an internist, cardiologist, and/or anesthesiologist is necessary.
- Decompression of neural elements is a mainstay of treatment.
  - Generally includes a laminectomy, but foraminotomies and discectomy also should be performed if they are involved in neural compression
- Fusion is necessary in the presence of instability or if extensive decompression results in instability (with disruption of the pars interarticularis and/or >50% of articular facets)
- Instrumentation with pedicle screws commonly is used to achieve fusion.

# FOLLOW-UP

Routine follow-up is at 6 weeks, 3 months, 6 months, 1 year, 2 years, and then every 2 years.

## PROGNOSIS

- Spinal stenosis generally worsens with time.
- Surgery is successful in improving pain and symptoms in patients for whom nonoperative treatment fails.

## COMPLICATIONS

- Severe spinal stenosis can lead to bowel and/or bladder dysfunction.
- Surgical complications include infection, neurologic injury, pseudarthrosis, chronic pain, and disability.

## PATIENT MONITORING

Patients are monitored for resolution of symptoms, fusion (if arthrodesis was performed), and development of any complications.

## REFERENCES


1. Amundsen T, Weber H, Lilleas F, et al. Lumbar spinal stenosis. Clinical and radiologic features. *Spine* 1995;20:1178–1186.
2. Hilibrand AS, Rand N. Degenerative lumbar stenosis: Diagnosis and management. *J Am Acad Orthop Surg* 1999;7:239–249.
3. Zucherman JF, Hsu KY, Hartjen CA, et al. A multicenter, prospective, randomized trial evaluating the X STOP interspinous process decompression system for the treatment of neurogenic intermittent claudication: Two-year follow-up results. *Spine* 2005;30:1351–1358.


## ADDITIONAL READING


Yuan HA, Garfin SR, Dickman CA, et al. A historical cohort study of pedicle screw fixation in thoracic, lumbar, and sacral spinal fusions. *Spine* 1994;19:2279S–2296S.


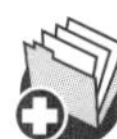

# MISCELLANEOUS

## CODES

### *ICD9-CM*

- 723.0 Cervical spinal stenosis
- 724.00 Spinal stenosis
- 724.02 Lumbar spinal stenosis

## PATIENT TEACHING

Patients should be educated about the natural history of the condition and about awareness of progressive motor weakness and bladder/bowel dysfunction.

## FAQ

- Q: What is the most common symptom of spinal stenosis?
  - A: Positional pain (worse with lumbar spine in extension and better with lumbar spine in flexion).
- Q: What is the best imaging modality to diagnose spinal stenosis?
  - A: MRI.

# SPINE FUSION

*David B. Cohen, MD*
*Andrew P. Manista, MD*

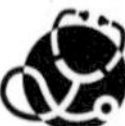

## BASICS

### DESCRIPTION

- Spine fusion is a surgical procedure that causes 2 or more vertebral levels to be joined with solid bony healing in the spine.
- It is performed to correct spinal instability from traumatic, degenerative, or iatrogenic causes and to prevent spinal deformity progression.

### EPIDEMIOLOGY

#### *Incidence*

Over the last 2 decades, the incidence of spinal fusion in the United States has more than doubled in the adult population (1).

### RISK FACTORS

- Diabetes mellitus leads to increased risk of infection in patients undergoing spine fusion.
- Diabetes mellitus or tobacco use (2) leads to high rates of pseudarthrosis (nonunion).

### ETIOLOGY

- Spinal fusions often are indicated for (3):
  - Congenital scoliosis
  - Idiopathic scoliosis
  - Spondylolisthesis
  - Degenerative scoliosis
  - Spinal fractures
  - Postsurgical instability

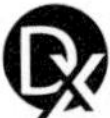

## DIAGNOSIS

### SIGNS AND SYMPTOMS

#### *Imaging*

- Plain radiographs are used to assess the adequacy and maturation of a spinal fusion (4).
  - The presence of continuous bridging bone over the fusion site is the best evidence of a well-healed fusion.
- When failure to heal (pseudarthrosis) is suspected, the following are indicated:
  - CT scan
  - 3D reconstructions of a CT scan
  - Conventional radiographs, often with flexion and extension views

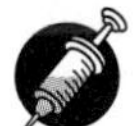

## TREATMENT

### GENERAL MEASURES

- Success of an individual fusion depends on:
  - Patient age
  - Surgical technique
  - Use of bone graft (5)
  - Patient's nutritional status
  - Patient's smoking status: Cigarette smoking can increase the rate of pseudarthrosis by up to 8-fold (2).

### SPECIAL THERAPY

#### *Physical Therapy*

- Physical therapy helps increase walking ability and improve aerobic conditioning.
- It is not required after spinal fusion.
- Individual surgeon preference

### SURGERY

- The choice of surgical approach (anterior or posterior) depends on the requirements of an individual case (e.g., the need for correction of rigid versus flexible deformities or the need to decompress neural elements) (6).
- Fusion can be facilitated by combining instrumentation techniques (e.g., pedicle screws, pedicle hooks, sublaminar wires) and various types of bone graft (e.g., local, iliac crest, rib, fibula, or allograft).

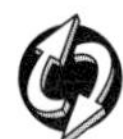

## FOLLOW-UP

- During the 1st year after spinal fusion surgery, patients require follow-up with the treating surgeon every 2–3 months for healing assessment.
- Once solidly healed, patients should be followed every few years to monitor for developing pseudarthrosis or problems related to early degenerative changes at levels adjacent to the fused levels.

### PROGNOSIS

- The prognosis varies greatly, depending on:
  - Diagnosis
  - Smoking status
  - Surgical technique
- Patients with impending litigation and those injured at work tend to have less favorable results than patients without these conditions (7).

## COMPLICATIONS (8)

- Depending on the indications for surgery:
  - Failure to return to normal function
  - Pseudarthrosis
- Depending on the surgical technique:
  - Pseudarthrosis rates of 10% are not uncommon in the literature, but not all pseudarthroses are painful or require treatment.
  - Spinal fusion increases load and stresses at levels adjacent to the fusion, a situation that can lead to an increased rate of early degeneration at the junctional levels (9).
  - Neurologic injury

## PATIENT MONITORING

- Activity:
  - For 6 weeks after surgery (during healing and maturation of the fusion), patients often have activity restrictions, which vary from surgeon to surgeon.
  - By 6 months after surgery, most patients are released to unlimited activities, but most physicians advise against high-impact activities such as running, downhill skiing, and lifting heavy weights.
- Follow-up care:
  - In general, bone is the slowest healing tissue in the human body, but it has the ability to heal completely without a scar.
  - Healing of the spinal fusion is similar to fracture healing.
    - Spinal instrumentation and appropriate immobilization limit the local motion, which allows a fusion to heal.
    - In adults, it takes up to 6 months for a fusion to become solid and up to 2 years for it to attain full strength.
    - In children, bone heals more rapidly, and full fusion strength can occur in 6–12 months.

## REFERENCES


1. Deyo RA, Gray DT, Kreuter W, et al. United States trends in lumbar fusion surgery for degenerative conditions. *Spine* 2005;30:1441–1445.
2. Glassman SD, Anagnost SC, Parker A, et al. The effect of cigarette smoking and smoking cessation on spinal fusion. *Spine* 2000;25:2608–2615.
3. Hanley EN, Jr, David SM. Who should be fused? Lumbar spine. In: Frymoyer JW, ed. *The Adult Spine: Principles and Practice*, 2nd ed. Philadelphia: Lippincott-Raven, 1997:2157–2174.
4. Hilibrand AS, Dina TS. The use of diagnostic imaging to assess spinal arthrodesis. *Orthop Clin North Am* 1998;29:591–601.
5. Louis-Ugbo J, Boden SD. Spinal fusion. In: Bono CM, Garfin SR, Tornetta P, et al., eds. *Spine*. Philadelphia: Lippincott Williams & Wilkins, 2004:297–324.
6. Liew SM, Simmons ED, Jr. Thoracic and lumbar deformity: Rationale for selecting the appropriate fusion technique (anterior, posterior, and 360°). *Orthop Clin North Am* 1998;29:843–858.
7. Atlas SJ, Chang Y, Kammann E, et al. Long-term disability and return to work among patients who have a herniated lumbar disc: The effect of disability compensation. *J Bone Joint Surg* 2000; 82A:4–15.
8. Brown CA, Eismont FJ. Complications in spinal fusion. *Orthop Clin North Am* 1998;29:679–699.
9. Hilibrand AS, Carlson GD, Palumbo MA, et al. Radiculopathy and myelopathy at segments adjacent to the site of a previous anterior cervical arthrodesis. *J Bone Joint Surg* 1999;81A:519–528.


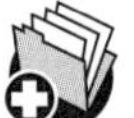

# MISCELLANEOUS

## PATIENT TEACHING

- Spinal fusion predisposes to additional spinal difficulties.
- Generalized total body fitness, avoiding smoking, and preventing osteoporosis are important factors for minimizing these problems.

## FAQ

- Q: How are spinal fusions obtained?
  - A: Spinal fusions occur as a result of the process of incorporating bone graft between adjacent spinal segments while maintaining a stable spinal segment, often with spinal instrumentation.
- Q: What are 2 factors that increase the rates of pseudarthrosis (nonunion) after a spine fusion.
  - A: Diabetes mellitus and smoking.

# SPONDYLOLISTHESIS

*Michael K. Shindle, MD*
*David B. Cohen, MD*
*A. Jay Khanna, MD*

## BASICS

### DESCRIPTION
- Spondylolisthesis is an abnormal AP translation of 2 vertebral bodies relative to each other (Fig. 1).
  – This translation is secondary to a defect in the pars interarticularis (spondylolysis) or the posterior ligamentous-bony restraints.
- Spondylolisthesis is classified by type (Table 1) and by the severity of the slip (Table 2) (1,2).

### GENERAL PREVENTION
- No preventive measures except long-term brace wear have been found to be effective in decreasing the progression of spondylolisthesis.
- Because major progression is rare, brace treatment commonly is not recommended.

### EPIDEMIOLOGY
- Isthmic spondylolisthesis usually begins in childhood, but a slight increase in incidence occurs in adolescence, up to 6% in males (3).
- Degenerative spondylolisthesis occurs mainly in older adults.
- Compared with males, females develop spondylolisthesis more often and develop more pronounced slips at a younger age (4).

#### *Incidence*
- 5% of the general population has spondylolysis or spondylolisthesis (3,4).
- It does not occur until 5–6 years of age, when the incidence is 3.3% (3,4).

#### *Prevalence*
- The prevalence is 0% at birth, 3–4% at 6 years, and 5–6% in adulthood (4).
- Spondylolysis occurs most often at L5.

### RISK FACTORS
- A family history of spondylolisthesis
- Particular physical activities in adolescence that involve hyperextension of the spine, such as playing the lineman position in football and participating in gymnastics, have been associated with a high incidence of isthmic spondylolisthesis (5,6).

#### *Genetics*
- An increased risk is associated with a positive family history.
- ~1/4 of affected patients have a positive family history of spondylolisthesis.

### ETIOLOGY
- The cause of isthmic spondylolisthesis is a stress fracture through a thin portion of the posterior elements (pars interarticularis).
- The causes of degenerative spondylolisthesis are degeneration and instability of the disc.

### ASSOCIATED CONDITIONS
- Most people with the condition are otherwise physically normal.
- However, an increased risk is present if one has a connective-tissue disorder, such as Marfan syndrome, or neuromuscular conditions, such as athetoid cerebral palsy.

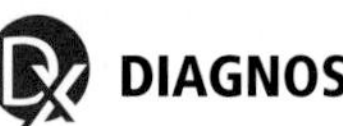

## DIAGNOSIS

### SIGNS AND SYMPTOMS
- Symptoms often can be insidious, but they may follow a relatively minor injury.
- Pain localized to the low back and thigh area may be seen in association with sciatica from an L5 radiculopathy.
- Back or leg pain
- Gait abnormality
- Abnormal posture (hyperlordotic)
- History of trauma: Acute or mild repetitive, often sports-related

#### *Physical Exam*
- Evaluate ambulation and forward bending.
- Perform a careful neurologic examination, including assessment of rectal sensation and function.
- Patients may present with a hypolordotic posture.
- Patients with a severe slip may show L5 radiculopathy.
- Perform the limited straight-leg-raise test: A patient with spondylolisthesis will have limited lumbar flexion with major hamstring tightness.

### TESTS

#### *Lab*
Perform electromyography and nerve conduction velocities to assess L5 root compression.

#### *Imaging*
- Conventional radiographs, including a spot lateral of L5–S1, allow assessment of the presence and degrees of spondylolisthesis.
  – Oblique views show the pars interarticularis (neck of the "Scotty dog") and visualize the pars defect.
  – Flexion and extension views can illustrate stability, particularly for degenerative and iatrogenic slips.

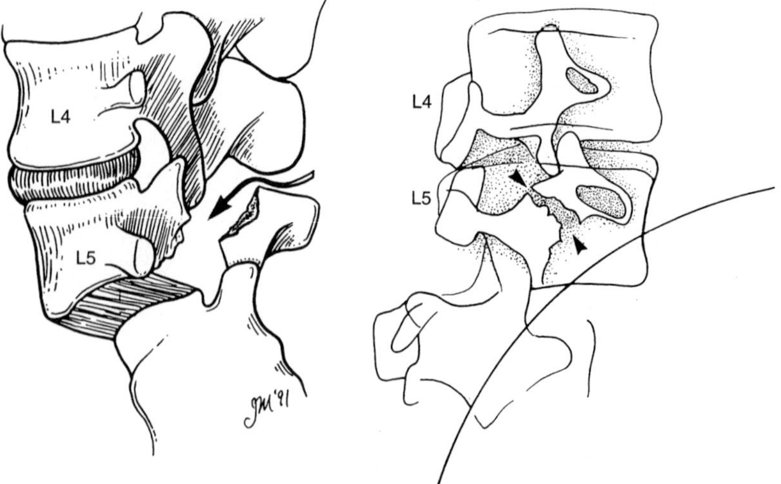


**Fig. 1.** Lateral **(A)** and oblique **(B)** views of spondylolytic spondylolisthesis. The *arrows* point to a defect in the pars interarticularis.

**Table 1. Classification of Spondylolisthesis**

| Class | Associated Risk Factors |
|---|---|
| Isthmic | Family history, gymnastics, football lineman |
| Congenital | Spina bifida occulta |
| Pathologic | Metastatic cancer or infection |
| Traumatic | Often associated with spinal cord injury |
| Degenerative | Seen in 6th and 7th decades of life at L4–L5 level |
| Iatrogenic | Removal of posterior restraints at prior surgery |

**Table 2. Grade of Spondylolisthesis**

| Spondylolisthesis Grade | Percentage of Slip |
|---|---|
| Grade 0 | 0 |
| Grade I | <25 |
| Grade II | 25–50 |
| Grade III | 51–75 |
| Grade IV | 76–100 |
| Grade V | Complete displacement |

- When a clear pars defect is not visualized, and early spondylosis is suspected in an adolescent, a technetium bone scan can be used.
  - For this study, a SPECT scan should be ordered.
- CT can aid in the diagnosis of occult pars interarticularis defects.
- MRI often is not useful for identifying spondylitic defects, but it can help in assessing the degrees of neural compression and the hydration status of the L4–L5 disc.
- Use discography or selective blocks to assess whether the L4–L5 disc or the pars defect is a patient's pain generator.

### *Pathological Findings*

- The most common finding is a defect in the pars interarticularis that resembles a fibrous union or pseudoarthrosis.
- The fibrous mass of the pars defect sometimes pins the L5 nerve root beneath it.

### DIFFERENTIAL DIAGNOSIS

- The differential diagnosis of spondylolisthesis is extremely important because the presence of a spondylitic defect is not necessarily the source of a patient's pain.
- A common cause of pain in a patient with a spondylolisthesis is an L4–L5 disc herniation.
  - The differential diagnosis of back pain should include tumor, infection, facet arthropathy, stenosis, or degenerative disc disease.

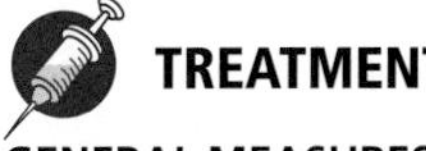

## TREATMENT

### GENERAL MEASURES

- Children and adolescents:
  - Lumbar bracing in lordosis may be used for up to 6 months to relieve pain.
  - Nonoperative treatment: Good to excellent results in up to 91% of patients (7,8)
  - Once the patient is asymptomatic without the brace, serial radiographs may be evaluated every 1–2 years until skeletal maturity.
  - Patients for whom a 12-month regimen of nonsurgical treatment fails or who have symptomatic high-grade slips may require posterolateral fusions.
- Adults:
  - Patients with grade 0 and grade I slips can be treated as for simple mechanical back pain.
  - Patients with more severe slips (grade II or higher) require posterior spine fusion and possible nerve root decompression.
  - Reduction of high-grade slips, the need for anterior spinal fusion, and the levels to be fused are all controversial topics.

### *Activity*

- Patients (any age) with asymptomatic grade 0 and grade I spondylolisthesis have no restrictions.
- Symptomatic patients (any age): Activity restriction until they regain painless lumbar flexion and rotation

### SPECIAL THERAPY

### *Physical Therapy*

Hamstring stretching and lumbar lordosis may relieve the discomfort in patients with symptomatic grade 0 or grade I spondylolisthesis.

### MEDICATION (DRUGS)

Medications used for children or adults should be those typically administered for the relief of back pain: An analgesic with or without muscle relaxant.

### SURGERY

- For high-grade slips and patients in whom nonoperative therapy fails, posterior spinal fusion is indicated.
- The most common procedure is a posterolateral 1-level L5–S1 fusion (9).
- If reduction of the spondylolisthesis is attempted or an L5 radiculopathy is present, the L5 nerve root should be widely decompressed.
- The addition of anterior spinal surgery:
  - Is reserved for the more severe grades
  - May increase the chance of fusion
  - May prevent postsurgical progression of the spondylolisthesis

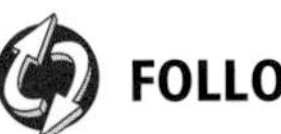

## FOLLOW-UP

### PROGNOSIS

- Spondylolisthesis slightly predisposes an individual to problems with chronic back pain.
- Most symptomatic low-grade slips in children and adolescents can be treated nonsurgically and lead to no long-term disability.

### COMPLICATIONS

- Greatly variable
- If the slip progresses to a high grade, compression of the cauda equina with loss of bowel and bladder function may occur occasionally.
- Many different reduction techniques have been described, including halo-femoral traction, cast reduction, and open reduction and internal fixation.
  - After reduction, radiculopathy secondary to L5 nerve root dysfunction can occur (10).

### REFERENCES


1. Meyerding HW. Spondylolisthesis. *Surg Gynecol Obstet* 1932;54:371–377.
2. Wiltse LL, Newman PH, Macnab I. Classification of spondylolysis and spondylolisthesis. *Clin Orthop Relat Res* 1976;117:23–29.
3. Fredrickson BE, Baker D, McHolick WJ, et al. The natural history of spondylolysis and spondylolisthesis. *J Bone Joint Surg* 1984;66A:699–707.
4. Baker D, McHollick W. Spondylolysis and spondylolisthesis in children. *J Bone Joint Surg* 1956;38A:933–934.
5. d'Hemecourt PA, Gerbino PG, Micheli LJ. Back injuries in the young athlete. *Clin Sports Med* 2000;19:663–679.
6. Eddy D, Congeni J, Loud K. A review of spine injuries and return to play. *Clin J Sport Med* 2005;15:453–458.
7. d'Hemecourt PA, Zurakowski D, Kriemler S, et al. Spondylolysis: returning the athlete to sports participation with brace treatment. *Orthopedics* 2002;25:653–657.
8. Rubery PT, Bradford DS. Athletic activity after spine surgery in children and adolescents: results of a survey. *Spine* 2002;27:423–427.
9. Smith MD, Bohlman HH. Spondylolisthesis treated by a single-stage operation combining decompression with in situ posterolateral and anterior fusion. An analysis of eleven patients who had long-term follow-up. *J Bone Joint Surg* 1990;72A:415–421.
10. Transfeldt EE, Dendrinos GK, Bradford DS. Paresis of proximal lumbar roots after reduction of L5-S1 spondylolisthesis. *Spine* 1989;14:884–887.


### ADDITIONAL READING


- King EC, Sarwark JF. Spondylolysis and spondylolisthesis. In: Sponseller PD, ed. *Orthopaedic Knowledge Update: Pediatrics 2*. Rosemont, IL: American Academy of Orthopaedic Surgeons, 2002:329–339.
- Puschak TJ, Sasso RC. Spondylolysis-spondylolisthesis. In: Vaccaro AR, ed. *Orthopaedic Knowledge Update 8*. Rosemont, IL: American Academy of Orthopaedic Surgeons, 2005:553–563.


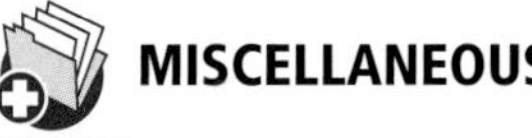

## MISCELLANEOUS

### CODES

### *ICD9-CM*

- 738.4 Isthmic spondylolisthesis, degenerative spondylolisthesis

### PATIENT TEACHING

- Educate patients with a high-grade slip about looking for progressive bladder dysfunction.
- After recovery from a symptomatic episode, new onset of bowel or bladder symptoms may indicate slip progression.

### FAQ

- Q: Which nerve root is most likely to be affected by a reduction and fusion of a high-grade L5–S1 spondylolisthesis?
  - A: The L5 nerve root. For this reason, the L5 nerve root should be decompressed carefully before an attempt at reduction. Also, neuromonitoring may be used during the surgical procedure.
- Q: What grade slip does a patient with 20% anterior translation of L4 on L5 have?
  - A: Grade I. (Table 2.)

# SPRAINS

*John H. Wilckens, MD*

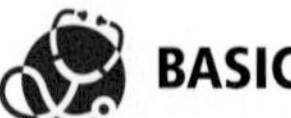

## BASICS

### DESCRIPTION

- Sprains refer to damaged ligaments, and they are the result of overstretching of the tissues.
- Injuries to the ligamentous structures of movable joints are among the most common complaints seen in primary care medicine, as well as in the subspecialty areas of orthopaedic surgery.
- Sprains can occur in any movable joint.
- Classification: 3 grades are recognized (1):
  - Grade I: Interstitial injury with no disruption of fiber continuity
  - Grade II: Partial tear of the ligament with mild laxity but no instability of the involved joint; preservation of the ligament's continuity
  - Grade III: Complete tear of injured ligament
- Synonym: Ligament injury

### GENERAL PREVENTION

Proper warm-up exercise is indicated before a workout or before participating in sports.

### EPIDEMIOLOGY

- No age-related factors.
- Both genders are affected equally.
- Sprains are common.

### RISK FACTORS

- "Weekend" athletes
- Running, throwing, or jumping sports
- Inadequate warm-up exercises
- Anabolic steroids (2)

### ETIOLOGY

Abrupt, overstretching of the ligament from an externally applied force or a force generated by the periarticular muscles can lead to various degrees of ligamentous injuries.

## DIAGNOSIS

### SIGNS AND SYMPTOMS

- Pain or swelling occurs in minor sprains.
- Patients with incomplete ligament tears may have mildly increased laxity on stress examination.
- Ecchymosis over the involved area or gross instability of the joint can be seen in cases of ligament disruption.

#### *Physical Exam*

- Ecchymosis or tenderness over the area of the ligament strongly suggests the diagnosis.
- Tenderness over the ligament occurs during testing for stability (stretching of the injured ligament).
- Gross instability of the involved joint is diagnostic.

### TESTS

#### *Lab*

No laboratory tests aid in the diagnosis.

#### *Imaging*

- Radiography:
  - Stress radiographs may show grade II and grade III injuries.
  - Obtain plain films to rule out associated fractures or dislocation.
- MRI is best for assessing soft-tissues injuries, but not always necessary.

#### *Pathological Findings*

- Grade I: Grossly intact ligament, but hemorrhages and tearing (seen microscopically) in small areas within the ligament
- Grade II: Partial ligament injury with increased joint laxity
- Grade III: Complete ligament disruption

### DIFFERENTIAL DIAGNOSIS

- Muscle strain
- Contusion
- Fracture

## TREATMENT

### GENERAL MEASURES

- Initial treatments consist of the RICE protocol.
  - Ice minimizes swelling through local vasoconstrictive effects, dulls pain receptors, and decreases spasm.
  - Compression and elevation further limit soft-tissue swelling.
- Grade I and grade II injuries:
  - Treat with initial immobilization and gradual, pain-free physical therapy to preserve ROM and to avoid disuse atrophy.
  - Normal activity can be resumed gradually once the pain and swelling subside.
- Grade III injuries require longer immobilization to allow the ligament to heal, especially in nonoperative cases (3).

### SPECIAL THERAPY

#### *Physical Therapy*

- Ice
- Contrast treatment with hot and cold compresses
- Massage
- Ultrasound
- Pain-free, protected, ROM exercises
- Muscle strengthening
- Proprioception training (4)

### SURGERY

- Most ligament injuries heal without surgical intervention.
  - Rupture of the ACL represents the notable exception and usually requires surgical reconstruction.
- Repairs may be done by direct suture of the torn ligament.

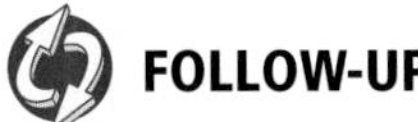

# FOLLOW-UP

## PROGNOSIS

Prognosis generally is excellent with nonoperative treatment in most patients with ankle and knee collateral ligament injuries.

## COMPLICATIONS

- Joint instability
- Chronic pain
- Stiffness

## PATIENT MONITORING

Patients are followed at 2–3-week intervals to assess ROM.

## REFERENCES


1. Davis PF, Trevino SG. Ankle injuries. In: Baxter DE, ed. *The Foot and Ankle in Sport*. St. Louis: Mosby-Year Book, 1995:147–169.
2. Freeman BJC, Rooker GD. Spontaneous rupture of the anterior cruciate ligament after anabolic steroids. *Br J Sports Med* 1995;29:274–275.
3. Frey C. Ankle sprains. *Instr Course Lect* 2001;50: 515–520.
4. Hewett TE, Paterno MV, Myer GD. Strategies for enhancing proprioception and neuromuscular control of the knee. *Clin Orthop Relat Res* 2002;402:76–94.


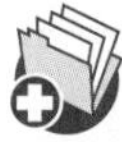

# MISCELLANEOUS

## CODES

### *ICD9-CM*

- 845.00 Ankle sprain
- 848.9 Sprain/strain, site unspecified

## PATIENT TEACHING

- Outline the treatment plan clearly.
- Patient compliance is important in achieving a good outcome.

### *Prevention*

Proper warm-up exercise is indicated before a workout or before participating in sports.

## FAQ

- Q: When can a patient with a grade I ankle sprain safely return to activity?
  - A: Patients with minor ankle sprains can return to activity when the ankle achieves full ROM, good muscle strength, and minimal pain. Until a patient has complete return of strength and proprioception, an ankle splint should be worn during activities to prevent reinjury.

S

# SPRENGEL DEFORMITY

*Paul D. Sponseller, MD*

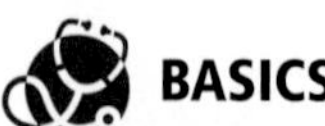

## BASICS

### DESCRIPTION

- Sprengel deformity:
  - Congenital elevation of the scapula (Fig. 1)
  - Small scapula with restricted ROM
  - Often, congenital anomalies coexist.
- This condition:
  - Is present from birth
  - May be discovered at birth or after the child starts to use the arms
  - Usually is diagnosed within the 1st few years of life
- Surgery is best performed in patients 2–8 years old, although satisfactory results have been reported as late as 14 years of age.
- Synonyms: Undescended scapula; Congenital high scapula

### EPIDEMIOLOGY

#### *Incidence*

Rare

#### *Prevalence*

- <1 per 10,000 (1)
- More common in girls than in boys, with a ratio of 3:1 (1)

### RISK FACTORS

- Myelomeningocele
- Congenital cervical fusion

#### *Genetics*

- It is almost always a sporadic condition.
- Only a small number of familial cases have been reported (1) in which the pattern was autosomal dominant.

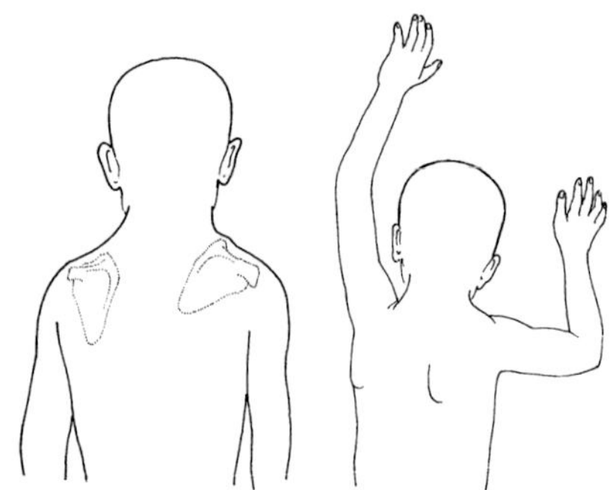

**Fig. 1.** Sprengel deformity is an elevated, downward-rotated scapula. This produces limitation of abduction (*right*).

### ETIOLOGY

- The normal scapula:
  - Appears in the 5th week of embryonic life, located in the neck, opposite the C5–T1 segments
  - Migrates distally to its position in the thoracic region
- Therefore, Sprengel deformity is a failure of descent of the scapula.
  - Its cause is unknown.
  - It may be secondary to defective formation or later contracture of musculature.
  - 1 theory is that abnormally located "blebs" of cerebrospinal fluid interfere with scapular descent (1,2).

### ASSOCIATED CONDITIONS

- Klippel-Feil (cervical fusions) syndrome
- Myelomeningocele
- Congenital scoliosis
- Syringomyelia
- Renal malformations
- Limb malformations may each occur sporadically with this condition, or Sprengel deformity may occur in isolation.

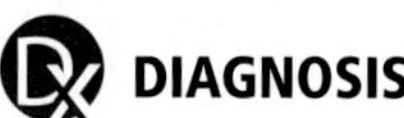

## DIAGNOSIS

### SIGNS AND SYMPTOMS

- Most commonly unilateral, but may be bilateral
- The scapula:
  - Small and elevated
  - Rotated so the glenoid faces more downward than normal, placing the inferomedial pole closer to the spine and the superomedial pole farther from it
  - The superomedial pole is prominent in the base of the neck.
- The angle of the neck on affected side may appear more blunted than that on the opposite side.
- Variation occurs in the degrees of severity, from obvious to barely noticeable deformity.
- Abduction of the arm is limited because the glenoid is turned downward and because the motion of the scapula is decreased.
  - Causes the patient to tilt the trunk when reaching upward; this motion often is the 1st to bring the diagnosis to light.

#### *Physical Exam*

- Note the prominence of the scapula in the angle of the neck from anterior and posterior aspects.
- Palpate the superomedial aspect of the scapula to check for a bony connection (omovertebral bar) to the spine.
- Measure the ROM, especially abduction (raising up to side).
- Check neck ROM.
- Perform the spine-bending test to look for scoliosis.
- If the patient has congenital cervical fusions, test the hearing because an increased risk of hearing abnormalities is possible.

### TESTS

#### *Lab*

Test results are normal.

#### *Imaging*

- Radiography:
  - On the cervical spine, look for associated congenital anomalies.
  - On the thoracolumbar spine, rule out scoliosis.
- In addition, ultrasound of the kidneys, ureter, and bladder is indicated because of the high incidence of associated anomalies.

#### *Pathological Findings*

- Scapula:
  - Smaller than normal
  - May be attached at its upper portion to the spinous processes of the lower cervical or upper thoracic spine by a bar of bone or cartilage known as an omovertebral bar
  - Upper portion is curved abnormally forward.
  - The muscles that normally attach the scapula are hypoplastic.
- Multiple other congenital malformations of other systems may be associated, in random fashion.

### DIFFERENTIAL DIAGNOSIS

- Congenital cervicothoracic scoliosis may distort the trunk and ribs, thus giving an appearance similar to that of Sprengel deformity.
- Birth palsy of the upper portion of the brachial plexus may cause an inability to abduct the extremity, so use of the arm resembles that of a patient with Sprengel deformity.
- Injury to the axillary nerve, such as after a shoulder dislocation, produces deltoid-muscle weakness, with inability to abduct the shoulder.
- Injury to the long thoracic nerve produces winging of the scapula.
- Fascioscapulohumeral dystrophy produces bilateral shoulder weakness.

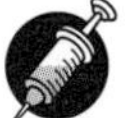

# TREATMENT

## GENERAL MEASURES

- Stretching and strengthening are recommended initially, but it is doubtful whether they make any major improvement.
- During these early years, the patient should be observed to determine the degrees of visibility of the deformity and its impact on the function of the arm.
- Problems in these areas are indications for surgery.

### *Activity*

- Parents or physicians should not restrict activity.
- Often, these children are surprisingly functional.

## SPECIAL THERAPY

### *Physical Therapy*

- Physical therapy is useful in nonoperative cases to improve the range of abduction.
  - Active and passive stretching exercises, to be maintained by the parents
- The family can assess whether the results over the first 2–4 years of the patient's life are satisfactory.

## SURGERY

- For patients who are unwilling to accept the degree of deformity or limitation of abduction that Sprengel deformity produces, surgical relocation of the scapula is the only option.
- Several techniques are used to accomplish this goal, all of which involve detaching the muscles from their origins or insertions (2,3).
- Results:
  - Noticeable improvement, but not restoration of appearance or function to normal
  - Improved range of abduction
  - The incision on the back may tend to spread and become wider than incisions in other areas.

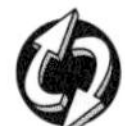

# FOLLOW-UP

## PROGNOSIS

- The deformity usually is static and does not improve or worsen with time.
- No evidence indicates that it causes arthritis of the shoulder, although the affected side may be weaker than the contralateral side.

## COMPLICATIONS

- The results of surgery usually are good, but complications include:
  - Brachial plexus stretch
  - Weaknesses of the shoulder muscles
  - Incomplete correction
  - A wide incision scar

## PATIENT MONITORING

- The family should bring the child in for several visits, ~6–12 months apart, when trying to decide about surgery.
- The best age for surgery is when the patient is 2–8 years old, although it has been successfully done on both older and younger patients.

## REFERENCES


1. Tsirikos AI, McMaster MJ. Congenital anomalies of the ribs and chest wall associated with congenital deformities of the spine. *J Bone Joint Surg* 2005;87A:2523–2536.
2. Cavendish ME. Congenital elevation of the scapula. *J Bone Joint Surg* 1972;54B:395–408.
3. Woodward JW. Congenital elevation of the scapula: Correction by release and transplantation of muscle origins. *J Bone Joint Surg* 1961;43A:219–228.


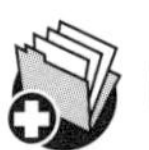

# MISCELLANEOUS

## CODES

### *ICD9-CM*

755.52 Sprengel deformity

## PATIENT TEACHING

- Parents should be:
  - Shown the normal and abnormal positions of the clavicle
  - Told that stretching results in slight improvement, and surgery results in a good deal more
  - Informed about the length of the surgical incision

## FAQ

- Q: Is surgery mandatory for Sprengel deformity?
  - A: It is not mandatory if the appearance of the shoulder and the degree of abduction are acceptable to the patient.

S

# STERNOCLAVICULAR JOINT DISLOCLATION

*Theodore T. Manson, MD*
*John H. Wilckens, MD*

## BASICS

### DESCRIPTION
- The medial end of the clavicle dislocates from its articulation with the sternum.
- Dislocations may be anterior or posterior.
  - Posterior dislocations:
    - May cause neurovascular or respiratory compromise.
  - Posterior reductions:
    - Must be reduced.
  - Anterior dislocations often are unstable, even if reduced, but few functional deficits occur with this instability.

### EPIDEMIOLOGY
- Rare injury (1):
  - 1% of all joint dislocations
  - 3% of all shoulder girdle injuries
  - 40% from vehicular trauma
  - 21% from sports-related injury
  - 63% of dislocations are anterior.

### PATHOPHYSIOLOGY
- The sternoclavicular joint is a diarthroidal connection between the clavicle and sternum.
- Strong ligaments bind the 2 bones together.
  - The capsular sternoclavicular ligaments are the primary restraints to AP movement.
  - Assisting the capsular ligaments are the costoclavicular and intra-articular disc ligaments.
- Several vital structures lie immediately posterior to the sternoclavicular joint (Fig. 1).
  - Innominate artery and vein
  - Trachea
  - Esophagus
  - Vagus and phrenic nerves
  - Anterior jugular vein
  - Posterior dislocation can cause compression of these structures.
- The medial clavicular physis is the last physis to fuse, usually at the age of 23–25 years.
  - A presumed sternoclavicular dislocation in a patient <25 years old may be a physeal fracture rather than a dislocation.
  - The prognosis for physeal fractures is better than that for dislocations.

### ETIOLOGY
- Often a result of motor vehicle collisions or sports
- 2 common mechanisms:
  - Direct blow to medial clavicle:
    - Usually causes posterior dislocation
  - Lateral compression of shoulder:
    - Football pile up
    - Side-impact motor vehicle collision

### ASSOCIATED CONDITIONS
High-energy injuries should have a full ATLS workup (2) to exclude additional thoracic, spinal, and extremity injury.

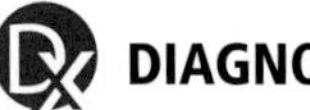

## DIAGNOSIS

### SIGNS AND SYMPTOMS
- Patients may report history of direct blow or lateral compression injury.
- Patients usually report pain with any movement of arm.
  - Worse with compressing shoulders together
  - Patient usually supports arm with the contralateral hand.

#### *History*
- Ask about numbness or weakness in arms.
- Ask about shortness of breath or difficulty with talking.
- Ask about difficulty with swallowing.

#### *Physical Exam*
- With anterior dislocations, the medial end of the clavicle will be more prominent than the contralateral side.
- With posterior dislocations, the medial clavicle may no longer be palpable and a sulcus may be present.
- The affected shoulder appears shortened and thrust forward.
- Perform a thorough neurologic examination of both arms.
- Compare pulses between arms.
- Look for venous congestion in the neck and arms.

### TESTS
#### *Imaging*
- Radiography:
  - The sternoclavicular joint is difficult to image on plain radiographs.
  - A chest radiograph may give some hint of deformity, and specialized views are difficult to obtain and interpret.
- CT:
  - Provides most information about a sternoclavicular dislocation
  - Shows the bony anatomy of the dislocation
  - Shows what, if any, structures are being compressed in a posterior dislocation
  - Is the study of choice if a sternoclavicular joint dislocation is suspected
  - If a posterior dislocation is suspected, consider using CT angiography.

### DIFFERENTIAL DIAGNOSIS
- The sternoclavicular joints also can be sprained, for which the treatment is symptomatic sling use.
- Other thoracic trauma, such as a pneumothorax, can cause shortness of breath, in which case the ATLS protocol should be followed.

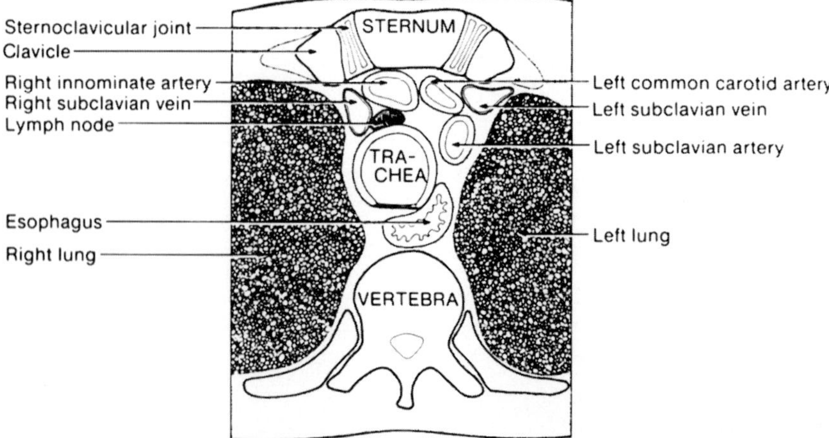


**Fig. 1.** Cross-sectional view of the anatomy of the vital structures posterior to the sternoclavicular joint. (Reprinted by permission from: Rockwood CA, Jr. Disorders of the sternoclavicular joint. In: Rockwood CA, Jr, Matsen FA, III, eds. *The Shoulder:* Philadelphia: WB Saunders, 1990;477–525.

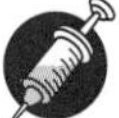

## TREATMENT

### INITIAL STABILIZATION

- In general, sternoclavicular dislocations should be reduced.
- Anterior dislocations often are unstable after reduction, but most orthopaedic surgeons prefer an attempt at reduction.
- Posterior dislocations always should be reduced and usually are stable thereafter.

### GENERAL MEASURES

- Reduction of a sternoclavicular joint dislocation often can be performed closed, but general anesthesia or deep sedation often is necessary secondary to pain and muscle spasm.
- Reduction of an anterior dislocation:
  - Position the patient supine with a 3–4-inch bolster between the scapulae.
    - A common error is to use too small a bolster.
    - Abduct the affected shoulder to 90°.
    - Extend the affected shoulder 15°.
    - Have the assistant apply traction to affected arm.
    - Apply direct posterior pressure to the medial clavicle.
    - Place the affected arm in a figure-8 bandage or sling and swath after reduction.
- Reduction of a posterior dislocation:
  - Position the patient supine with a 3–4-inch bolster between the scapulae.
  - A thoracic surgeon should be involved when reducing a posterior dislocation because a clavicle pulled from a punctured subclavian vessel or lung can lead to a catastrophic intrathoracic hemorrhage or pneumothorax.
  - 2 common techniques of closed reduction:
    - Abduction traction technique; apply traction to the abducted, extended arm; apply downward pressure to the shoulder over the glenohumeral joint; grasp the medial clavicle with fingers and attempt to pull the clavicle anteriorly; if closed manipulation fails, prepare the skin and use a sharp towel clamp to grasp the medial clavicle and pull it anteriorly; the clavicle usually reduces with an audible and palpable pop.
    - Adduction traction technique:
      - Adduct the arm; apply lateral traction to the adducted arm; push down on the shoulder over the glenohumeral joint; if needed, grasp the medial clavicle with fingers or a sterile towel clamp; after reduction, place the arm in a sling and swathe or figure-8 dressing.

#### *Activity*

- The affected arm should be immobilized for 4–6 weeks after reduction.
- Patients may benefit from sleeping upright (i.e., in a recliner) for pain relief and comfort.

#### *Nursing*

- Patients should have parenteral access and adequate pain relief.
- Patients may be more comfortable sitting upright with a sling until definitive treatment is rendered.

### SPECIAL THERAPY

#### *Physical Therapy*

- Hand and wrist exercises and elbow ROM exercises can begin immediately.
- Shoulder exercises usually should wait 4–6 weeks.

### MEDICATION (DRUGS)

- Medications for pain control are appropriate.
  - Parenteral and oral narcotics in the acute setting
- NSAIDs in the acute and chronic settings

### SURGERY

- Posterior dislocations for which closed reduction has failed should undergo open reduction in the operating room.
  - A thoracic surgeon should be present.
  - After open reduction, the stability of the joint is assessed (often, it is stable).
  - Unstable joints may be stabilized with one of many suture techniques and a graft reconstruction.
  - Kirschner wire or Steinmann pin fixation are contraindicated secondary to the disastrous sequelae of implant migration into the mediastinum.
- Posterior dislocations untreated for >7–10 days after injury often require open reduction because of retrosternal adhesions.
- In most cases, anterior dislocations with instability or residual deformity may be treated nonoperatively.
  - Residual anterior subluxation or dislocation usually causes few functional problems.
  - Symptomatic patients may be treated using open reduction and stabilization, much like patients with a posterior dislocation.

## FOLLOW-UP

- A patient with a sternoclavicular joint dislocation should be referred to an orthopaedic surgeon for follow-up.
- Shoulder ROM exercises usually can be started at 4–6 weeks.
- In stable reductions, a sling and swathe or figure-8 dressing usually is worn for 4–6 weeks.
- Unstable anterior dislocations can be treated symptomatically with a sling until symptoms resolve.

### PROGNOSIS

- Posterior dislocations usually are stable after reduction.
- Anterior dislocations often are unstable, but the instability causes few functional deficits.
  - An unstable anterior dislocation usually remains prominent with a cosmetic deformity.

### COMPLICATIONS

- The most disastrous complications occur with posterior sternoclavicular dislocations (3).
  - Compression or laceration of great vessels
  - Compression of trachea, resulting in respiratory compromise
  - Compression of esophagus, causing swallowing difficulties
  - Brachial plexopathy
  - TOS
- Anterior dislocations can have sequelae as well, but they are much more benign.
  - Cosmetic deformity (less than a surgical scar)
  - Degenerative changes
  - Recurrent instability and pain with activity

### PATIENT MONITORING

Patients should be followed until pain resolves and motion and function are restored.

### REFERENCES


1. Wirth MA, Rockwood CA, Jr. Injuries to the sternoclavicular joint. In: Bucholz RW, Heckman JD, eds. *Rockwood and Green's Fractures in Adults*, 5th ed. Philadelphia: Lippincott Williams & Wilkins, 2001:1245–1294.
2. American College of Surgeons Committee on Trauma. *Advanced Trauma Life Support Program for Doctors*, 6th ed. Chicago: American College of Surgeons, 1997.
3. Gove N, Ebraheim NA, Glass E. Posterior sternoclavicular dislocations: A review of management and complications. *Am J Orthop* 2006;35:132–136.


### ADDITIONAL READING


- Bicos J, Nicholson GP. Treatment and results of sternoclavicular joint injuries. *Clin Sports Med* 2003;22:359–370.
- Rudzki JR, Matava MJ, Paletta GA, Jr. Complications of treatment of AC and sternoclavicular joint injuries. *Clin Sports Med* 2003;22:387–405.
- Wirth MA, Rockwood CA, Jr. Acute and chronic traumatic injuries of the sternoclavicular joint. *J Am Acad Orthop Surg* 1996;4:268–278.


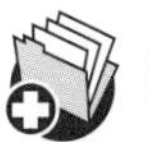

## MISCELLANEOUS

### CODES

#### *ICD9-CM*

839.61,839.71 Dislocation, sternoclavicular joint

### FAQ

- Q: If a patient has a posterior sternoclavicular joint dislocation and difficulty with swallowing, shortness of breath, difficulty with talking, or neck venous distention, how urgent is the condition?
  - A: In this scenario, the patient should be emergently transferred to a facility with a CT scanner and a thoracic or trauma surgeon. The medial clavicle has injured or compressed 1 of several important mediastinal structures: The trachea, esophagus, and/or the subclavian vessels.

# STRESS FRACTURE

*John H. Wilckens, MD*
*Simon C. Mears, MD, PhD*

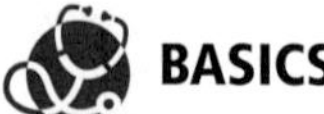

## BASICS

### DESCRIPTION

- A stress (microscopic) fracture occurs when:
  - Repetitive stresses are applied to a bone faster than it is able to remodel to withstand this challenge.
    - As the stressing force continues, the bone gradually fatigues and eventually breaks.
    - Remodeling occurs in response to the stress but does not happen quickly enough to prevent the break.
  - Suddenly increased forces are applied to a normal bone (e.g., a metatarsal stress fracture that occurs in a military recruit who marches 20 miles without adequate conditioning).
- Related to the stress fractures is the insufficiency fracture, in which normal forces cause a fracture of weakened bone (e.g., a femoral neck fracture in an osteopenic elderly woman).
- Weightbearing bones of the lower extremity are affected, most commonly:
  - Metatarsus (Fig. 1)
  - Calcaneus
  - Tibia (Fig. 2)
  - Fibula
  - Femoral neck
- Classification/radiographic grading (1):
  - Grade I: Normal radiograph, positive STIR
  - Grade II: Normal radiograph, positive STIR, positive T2-weighted MRI
  - Grade III: Periosteal reaction on radiograph, positive T1- and T2-weighted MRI, STIR without definite cortical break
  - Grade IV: Fracture line or periosteal reaction, fracture line on T1- and T2-weighted MRI
- Synonyms: March fracture; Fatigue fracture

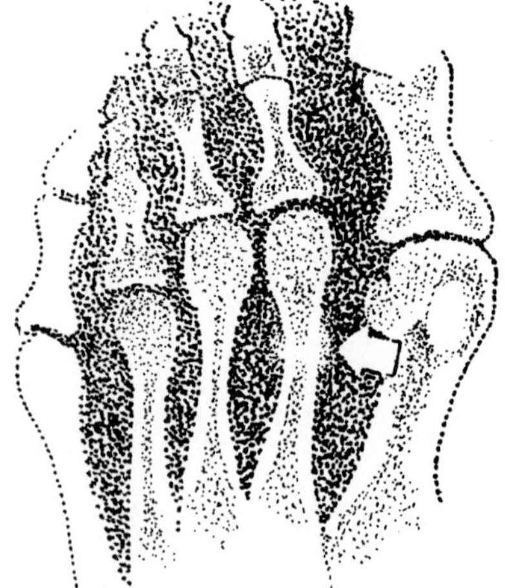

**Fig. 1.** Stress fracture of the foot most commonly involves the metatarsal shafts. It is signified by sclerosis or a periosteal reaction (*arrow*).

### GENERAL PREVENTION

- Avoid sudden increases in physical activity levels, especially when involving walking or running.
- Runners should be educated to reduce mileage and to rest when they have acute, new-onset pain with activity.

### EPIDEMIOLOGY

- Can occur at any age (2):
  - Typically, people ≤60 years old develop stress fractures after sustained or cyclic exertion.
  - Persons >60 years old develop stress fractures from normal stress to a weak bone.

#### *Incidence*

- Stress and insufficiency fractures occur more often in females than in males.
- Commonly occur in:
  - Running and jumping athletes
  - 5% of military recruits (3)
  - In a recent study, elite tennis players had a 12% rate of stress fracture (4).

#### *Prevalence*

Femoral stress fractures occur at a rate of 20 per 100,000 person-years; 1/2 are within the femoral neck (5).

### RISK FACTORS

- Female triad (eating disorder, amenorrhea, stress fracture [osteoporosis])
- Rapid change in conditioning program:
  - >10% increase in running mileage per week
  - Military recruit in boot camp
- Skeletal malalignment:
  - Pes cavus, pes planus
  - Excessive external rotation of the hip
- Muscle fatigue: As muscles fatigue, they absorb less shock, which is transmitted to the bone (e.g., marathon running).
- Low bone density
- Gender: Female recruits have higher rates of stress fracture than do male recruits (6).
- Low aerobic fitness is a predictor of stress fracture in recruits (7).

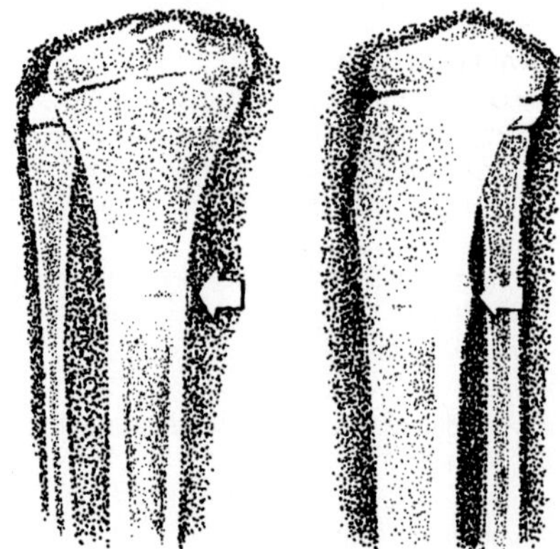

**Fig. 2.** Stress fracture of the tibia, with sclerosis and periosteal reaction.

### ETIOLOGY

- Sudden increase in strenuous activity in young people
- Minimal stress in people with weak or osteopenic bone

### ASSOCIATED CONDITIONS

- Osteopenia
- Metabolic bone disease
- Female triad

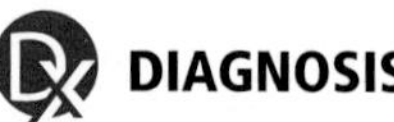

## DIAGNOSIS

### SIGNS AND SYMPTOMS

- The patient initially presents with a 2–3-week history of a vague, dull ache with exertion or impact loading.
- As the injury progresses, the pain becomes sharper and localized and begins earlier in training.
- If a stress fracture progresses to complete (macroscopic) fracture, pain occurs at rest.

#### *Physical Exam*

- Antalgic gait may be present.
- Point tenderness is noted in the affected bone.
- Observe swelling and thickening of the soft tissues over the affected bone.
- Pain in the hip with resisted active straight-leg raise (Stinchfield sign).

### TESTS

#### *Lab*

No serum laboratory tests

#### *Imaging*

- Radiography:
  - Plain radiographs (AP and lateral views) typically do not show findings until 2 weeks after the onset of symptoms.
  - What usually is observed is healing, periosteal callus, or sclerosis at the fracture site.
- Bone scan:
  - Very sensitive
  - Findings may be delayed 48–72 hours in elderly patients with insufficiency fractures.
- MRI:
  - Very sensitive
  - Allows for classification and prognosis
  - Can rule out other soft-tissue injuries in the differential diagnosis

### DIFFERENTIAL DIAGNOSIS

- Infection
- Fracture
- Soft-tissue injury
- Exertion or chronic compartment syndrome
- Tumor

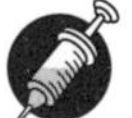

# TREATMENT

## GENERAL MEASURES

- In general, the patient must reduce activity below the threshold of pain.
  - If the patient has pain with walking, crutches should be used.
  - If the patient has pain with motion, or at rest, the injured part should be immobilized in a cast or fracture splint.

### *Activity*

- After initial treatment, activity should be increased gradually.
- Once the patient is pain free, low-impact training can be started and advanced as tolerated.
- Once running is resumed, mileage should be increased slowly.

## SPECIAL THERAPY

### *Physical Therapy*

- Identify training errors that led to the stress fracture.
- Identify and correct mechanics and muscle imbalance.
- Core strengthening

## MEDICATION (DRUGS)

NSAIDs can be given, but they have an inhibitory effect on bone healing, making them a controversial intervention.

### *First Line*

Acetaminophen

## SURGERY

- For high-risk stress fractures:
  - Fractures whose displacement would cause catastrophic complications:
    - Femoral neck fractures require emergent internal fixation because a complete, displaced femoral neck fracture is associated with a high incidence of AVN (8).
  - Fractures associated with a high rate of delayed union or nonunion (8): Patella, tarsal navicular, talus

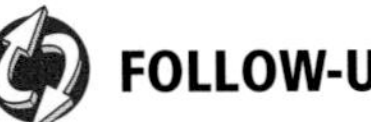

# FOLLOW-UP

## DISPOSITION

### *Issues for Referral*

High-risk fractures (see what has been determined previously)

## PROGNOSIS

- Stress fractures in young people have a good prognosis.
- Older patients or those with metabolic bone disease typically continue to develop insufficiency fractures in other bones.
- Time to return to full activity (1):
  - Grade I: 3+ weeks
  - Grade II: 5+ weeks
  - Grade III: 11+ weeks
  - Grade IV: 14+ weeks

## COMPLICATIONS

- Completion of fracture, the most common complication of stress fractures, substantially prolongs healing and may require internal fixation.
- Continued pain even after fracture healing may occur.

## PATIENT MONITORING

Radiographs are obtained every 4–6 weeks to monitor progress to healing.

## REFERENCES


1. Arendt E, Agel J, Heikes C, et al. Stress injuries to bone in college athletes: a retrospective review of experience at a single institution. *Am J Sports Med* 2003;31:959–968.
2. Bennell K, Grimston S. Risk factors for developing stress fractures. In: Burr DB, Milgrom C, eds. *Musculoskeletal Fatigue and Stress Fractures*. Boca Raton: CRC Press, 2001:35–54.
3. Armstrong DW, III, Rue JPH, Wilckens JH, et al. Stress fracture injury in young military male and females. *Bone* 2004;35:806–816.
4. Maquirriain J, Ghisi JP. The incidence and distribution of stress fractures in elite tennis players. *Br J Sports Med* 2006;40:454–459.
5. Niva MH, Kiuru MJ, Haataja R, et al. Fatigue injuries of the femur. *J Bone Joint Surg* 2005;87B: 1385–1390.
6. Gam A, Goldstein L, Karmon Y, et al. Comparison of stress fractures of male and female recruits during basic training in the Israeli anti-aircraft forces. *Mil Med* 2005;170:710–712.
7. Shaffer RA, Rauh MJ, Brodine SK, et al. Predictors of stress fracture susceptibility in young female recruits. *Am J Sports Med* 2006;34:108–115.
8. Boden BP, Osbahr DC. High-risk stress fractures: Evaluation and treatment. *J Am Acad Orthop Surg* 2000;8:344–353.


## ADDITIONAL READING


Brukner PD, Bennell KL. Stress fractures. In: O'Connor FG, Wilder RP, eds. *Textbook of Running Medicine*. New York: McGraw-Hill, 2001:227–256.


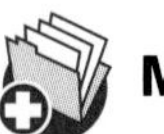

# MISCELLANEOUS

## CODES

### *ICD9-CM*

733.11 Stress fracture

## PATIENT TEACHING

Gradual increase in training intensity (e.g., <10% in running mileage per week)

### *Prevention*

- Patient education:
  - With new-onset pain with activity, the patient should rest and reduce training.
  - The patient should try to identify and correct any training errors.

## FAQ

- Q: Do all high-risk stress fractures require surgery?
  - A: No. These fractures can be treated with prolonged nonweightbearing and immobilization. However, they are associated with a high risk of nonunion. Surgical fixation allows earlier weightbearing, less immobilization, improved predictable healing, and earlier return to activity.
- Q: Can you get a stress fracture in nonweightbearing bone?
  - A: Any bone subjected to an increased mechanical load (including repetitive muscle use) can develop stress fractures. For example, overhead athletes, such as pitchers, can develop stress fractures in the humerus and olecranon, and rowers can develop stress fractures of the ribs.
- Q: When can an athlete return to activity?
  - A: Athletes with stress fractures can participate in "active rest," decreasing their activity below the threshold of pain. If an athlete has a stress fracture in a weightbearing bone, then core strengthening and balancing exercises and aquatic (or hydroaerobic) exercises can be done. Once pain-free, an athlete can begin low-impact aerobics, such as stationary cycling or elliptical training. If the athlete is pain free with these activities, jogging and sports-specific activities can be begun.

# SUBACROMIAL INJECTION

*Timothy S. Johnson, MD*

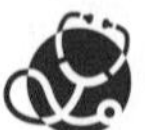

## BASICS

- Shoulder injection sites:
  - Subacromial area: Most common site
  - Other potential sites include:
    - Bicipital tendon sheath
    - Glenohumeral joint
    - Sternoclavicular joint
    - AC joint
- To avoid confusion:
  - Always refer to these injections by describing the anatomic location of the shot.
  - Avoid describing any of these injections as a "shoulder injection."
- Subacromial injection is reserved for pain that has been resistant to NSAIDs, activity modification, and physical therapy.
- The most common sources of pain include:
  - Subacromial bursitis
  - Shoulder impingement
  - Rotator cuff tendinitis
  - Partial-thickness rotator cuff tears

**Table 1. Impingement Test**

| Result upon Re-examination | Potential Explanations |
|---|---|
| 100% Pain relief | Rotator cuff disease: Subacromial bursitis, rotator cuff tendonitis, rotator cuff tear |
| Partial pain relief | Rotator cuff disease plus another source of shoulder pain. Re-examine thoroughly to define and treat the other source (e.g., cervical radiculitis, AC joint arthritis, labral tear, etc.). |
| No pain relief | Rotator cuff disease in not the source of pain. Re-examine thoroughly to define and treat the true source (e.g., cervical radiculitis, biceps tendonitis, labral tear, etc.). |
| | The medication did not go into the subacromial space. |

- Impingement test:
  - This test involves injection with local anesthetic only.
  - It is used to confirm subacromial disease/rotator cuff abnormality as the source of pain.
  - Because diagnosing shoulder abnormality is difficult to master, shoulders are injected diagnostically more often than any other joint.
  - Although rotator cuff disease is probably the most common shoulder ailment, the clinician should keep in mind that many other causes of shoulder pain exist.
  - Always re-examine the patient after the local anesthetic has taken effect.
    - If the subacromial space was injected correctly, the local anesthetic should alleviate the pain (Table 1).

## TREATMENT

- Therapeutic injection:
  - Repetitive corticosteroid injections into the subacromial space can lead to tendon rupture, atrophy, and retraction (1–3).
  - Always use a low dose (e.g., $<10$ mg of triamcinolone) of corticosteroid and re-examine the patient afterward (Table 1).
  - Inject local anesthetic with the corticosteroid.
    - Good pain relief shortly after the injection (5 minutes, with recurrence of pain at a later date usually bodes well for early surgical intervention; refer such patients for surgical evaluation).
  - Chronic, massive, retracted rotator cuff tears with atrophy are not repairable surgically.
- Several techniques are used for therapeutic injection of the shoulder, the easiest and most common of which follows (Fig. 1). (Right shoulder injection is explained for demonstration purposes. Switch hands when performing a left subacromial injection [2].)

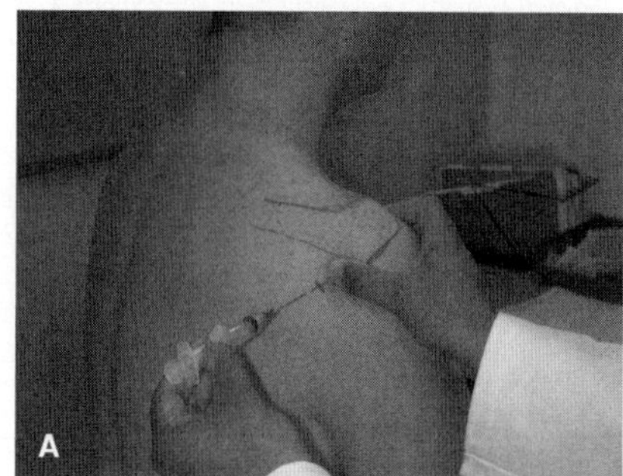


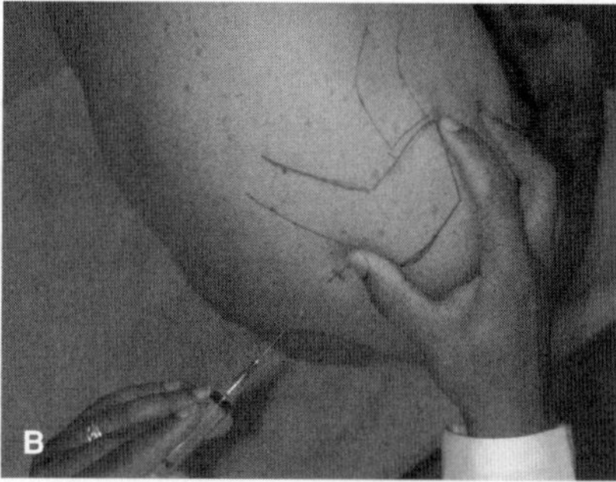


**Fig. 1.** Subacromial injection technique for the right shoulder. **A:** Posterior view. **B:** Superior view.

- Have the patient remove the shirt and expose the entire right shoulder girdle.
- Identify bony landmarks of the shoulder; it may be helpful to mark the landmarks with a pen.
  - Acromion
  - Spine of the scapula
  - Greater tuberosity
  - Clavicle
  - AC joint
- Perform a wide, standard sterile skin preparation of the posterior shoulder, and stand behind the patient.
- The clinician should place the ulnar border of the right thumb on the posterolateral border of the acromion with the right index finger on the leading edge of the anterolateral acromion.
- Insert the needle inferior to the acromion (below the examiner's right thumb), aiming anteriorly just below the tip of the index finger.

## REFERENCES

1. Akpinar S, Hersekli MA, Demirors H, et al. Effects of methylprednisolone and betamethasone injections on the rotator cuff: An experimental study in rats. *Adv Ther* 2002;19:194–201.
2. Mathews PV, Glousman RE. Accuracy of subacromial injection: Anterolateral versus posterior approach. *J Shoulder Elbow Surg* 2005;14:145–148.
3. Scutt N, Rolf CG, Scutt A. Glucocorticoids inhibit tenocyte proliferation and tendon progenitor cell recruitment. *J Orthop Res* 2006;24:173–182.

## ADDITIONAL READING

Ford LT, DeBender J. Tendon rupture after local steroid injection. *South Med J* 1979;72:827–830.

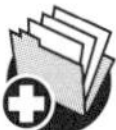

## MISCELLANEOUS

### FAQ

- Q: The subacromial injection is 1 of how many common locations injected in the shoulder?
  - A: 5: The subacromial bursa, bicipital tendon sheath, glenohumeral joint, sternoclavicular joint, and AC joint.
- Q: In addition to infection, what is 1 of the more common complications of repetitive corticosteroid injection of the subacromial space?
  - A: Rotator cuff rupture.

# SUBTROCHANTERIC FRACTURE

*Carl Wierks, MD*
*Emmanuel Hostin, MD*

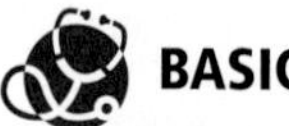

## BASICS

### DESCRIPTION

- By definition, subtrochanteric hip fractures (or, simply, subtrochanteric fractures) extend into the region between the lesser trochanter and a point 5 cm distally.
- Classification:
  - Multiple systems exist, but prognostically the most critical factor is fracture stability, which is based on the degrees of comminution of the medial and posteromedial cortex.
  - The Russell and Taylor classification (1):
    - Useful for guiding treatment because it differentiates fractures that extend into the piriformis fossa from those that do not.
    - This distinction is important because a cephalomedullary nail enters the femur at the piriformis fossa and therefore should not be used if the fossa is fractured (2).
- The medial and posteromedial cortices sustain the great compressive forces.
  - Comminution in this area renders the fracture unstable.

### GENERAL PREVENTION

- Fall precautions in the elderly
- Wearing safety belts in automobiles

### EPIDEMIOLOGY

- A bimodal age distribution:
  - 1/3 of these fractures occur in patients ≤50 years old (3).
- Young patients typically present after undergoing high-energy trauma, whereas low-energy trauma is the typical cause in the geriatric population (3).

#### *Incidence*

Subtrochanteric fractures account for ~10–34% of all hip fractures (3).

### RISK FACTORS

Any condition that generally (such as osteoporosis) or focally (such as metastatic disease) weakens the bone may predispose to such an injury with low-energy trauma or even without trauma.

### ETIOLOGY

- In young patients with normal bone, the mechanism of injury is high-energy trauma, as occurs in motor vehicle collisions, falls from substantial heights, or gunshot wounds.
- In the geriatric population with weakened bone, low-energy trauma (such as a minor fall) is a more common cause.
- Less commonly, the pathologic fracture occurs in which weakened bone stock (e.g., secondary to neoplasm or metabolic bone disease) is unable to withstand the mechanical stresses of normal ambulation or other low-impact activity.
- The mechanical stresses on the femur are highest in the subtrochanteric region.

### ASSOCIATED CONDITIONS

- When the fracture is associated with high-energy trauma, a high index of suspicion should exist for other injuries in the ipsilateral extremity or pelvis and elsewhere (e.g., cranial and vertebral injuries).
- These injuries can be associated with substantial hemorrhage; therefore, the patient should be monitored for hypovolemic shock.
- In addition, compartment syndrome of the thigh is possible, although rare.
- With any such fracture associated with previous symptoms of pain, a limp, or with minimal trauma, neoplasm should be ruled out by appropriate methods, including bone biopsy at the time of treatment.

## DIAGNOSIS

### SIGNS AND SYMPTOMS

- The clinical picture often is not subtle and resembles that in any patient with an intertrochanteric or a femoral shaft fracture.
- Pain and deformity are common, although nondisplaced fractures also are seen.

#### *History*

Trauma or fall

#### *Physical Exam*

- Generally, a shortened extremity with a swollen thigh is most evident on examination.
- A complete neurovascular examination of the extremity should be performed.
- An open injury should be ruled out.

### TESTS

#### *Lab*

- A complete blood count to evaluate the hematocrit is advisable in patients with any trauma.
  - Preoperative laboratory tests should be obtained in case operative treatment is necessary.
- Urine and serum electrophoresis may be obtained if pathologic fracture is suspected.

#### *Imaging*

- Radiography:
  - AP radiographs of the pelvis and AP and lateral films of the hip and femur should be obtained with particular attention being paid to including the femoral neck to rule out concurrent, ipsilateral injury and to help dictate treatment options.
  - The "cross-table lateral" hip view is advised rather than the "frog-leg" view.

### PATHOPHYSIOLOGY

- The proximal portion of the femur is pulled into abduction, external rotation, and flexion by the gluteus, external rotator, and iliopsoas muscles, respectively.
- The distal fragment is pulled proximally and into varus by the iliopsoas, producing a shortened femur with varus deformation.
- Recognition of these deformities is important and aids the surgeon in reducing the fracture.

### DIFFERENTIAL DIAGNOSIS

- Traumatic injury
- Pathologic fracture

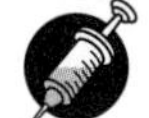

## TREATMENT

### GENERAL MEASURES

- Initial assessment after the trauma includes the ATLS (4) protocol when appropriate.
  - Treatment of any urgent concomitant injuries should be done while traction splinting is in place.
- Skeletal traction should be initiated if the patient is going to be treated nonoperatively or if surgical fixation will be delayed.
- Nonoperative treatment may be indicated for elderly patients who are poor operative candidates.
  - Skeletal traction or cast bracing may be used, although these treatments commonly result in shortening, rotational or varus deformity, malunion, or nonunion.
- After the immediate posttraumatic stabilization and workup, medical issues include intravascular volume, antithromboembolic prophylaxis (keeping in mind the timing of definitive surgical management), and treatment of pre-existing medical problems.

#### *Pediatric Considerations*

- Unless the bone is weakened by an inherent process such as a simple bone cyst, fibrous dysplasia, or osteoporosis, subtrochanteric femur fractures in children are secondary to high-energy trauma and much less common than more proximal femoral fractures.
- The vascular supply to the femoral head is not at risk as it is in femoral neck fractures.
- The potential for leg-length discrepancy is present even if no obvious damage to the physis is present.
  - Attention to leg length and rotational orientation should be a priority during treatment (5).
- Treatment can involve closed reduction and spica cast, external fixation, or internal fixation.

### *Activity*
- Patients should be nonweightbearing until definitive stabilization of the fracture.
- Postoperative weightbearing:
  - Toe-touch weightbearing with crutches or a walker should be initiated within the first 2–3 days.
  - Full weightbearing should be achieved gradually over a 3-month period, guided by radiographic healing.
- Elderly patients are allowed to bear weight as tolerated.

## SPECIAL THERAPY
### *Physical Therapy*
Patients may begin ROM and hip strengthening in the early postoperative period.

## MEDICATION (DRUGS)
Narcotic pain medicines are necessary after subtrochanteric fractures.

## SURGERY
- Open reduction and internal fixation comprise the treatment of choice for most fractures because this approach allows for early mobilization and better achieves near-normal anatomy than do nonoperative procedures.
- The goals of treatment are to restore femoral length and rotational alignment and to maintain the abductor muscle lever arm by preventing varus deformity.
- Because this area of the femur undergoes substantial compressive and tensile stresses with normal gait, implant failure is of concern, particularly with unstable fractures.
- The main operative treatment options include static interlocking nails, cephalomedullary reconstruction nails with locking screws placed into the femoral head, a sliding hip screw, and a 95° angled blade plate (6).
  - Static interlocking nails can be used if both trochanters are intact.
  - Cephalomedullary nails are indicated if loss of the posteromedial cortex is present.
  - A sliding hip screw can be used only for proximal fractures because the compression screw must cross the fracture and, for compression to occur, the plate cannot be fixed to the proximal fragment.
  - A device called the Medoff plate allows sliding along the head–neck axis and the shaft.
    - Results in a blinded study comparing the Medoff plate to an intramedullary nail favored the use of the nail (7).
    - A 95° angled blade plate has been shown to provide good results when a sliding hip screw cannot be used because of comminution in the trochanteric area and fracture extension into the lateral cortex (8).
    - Dynamic condylar screw plate fixation is not as reliable as intramedullary nail fixation (9).

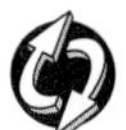

# FOLLOW-UP
- Patients should be seen within 1–2 weeks after surgical fixation to confirm fracture and implant stability.
- Subsequently, they should be seen monthly to assess healing radiographically and clinically.

## PROGNOSIS
- Most patients can return to near-prefracture activity level, given appropriate treatment (10).
- A recent review (11) of 302 patients with low-energy subtrochanteric fractures treated with a cephalomedullary nails found that:
  - At 1 year, 34.5% of the patients had died.
  - Survivors had an increased level of social dependence, an increased use of walking aids, and reduced mobility.
  - Of the 211 patients who were evaluated at 1 year after the injury, 42% had some degree of hip discomfort but only 2 described the pain as severe and disabling.
  - Reoperation was required in 8.9% of the patients, with a 1-year nail revision rate of 7.1%.
  - 2% of the patients had nonunion.

## COMPLICATIONS
- The most common complications of treatment of subtrochanteric fractures are nonunion, malunion, shortening, and implant failure.
- Stable, near-anatomic reduction and internal fixation of these injuries with attention paid to avoiding premature weightbearing help decrease the incidence of such complications.
- Loss of fixation in plate and screw devices usually is secondary to screw pullout from the femoral head in osteoporotic bone and should be managed with revision to an intramedullary nail (12).
- Failure of interlocking nails can be secondary to failure to lock the device statically, fracture at the entry site, or an undersized nail.
  - These complications can be treated with nail replacement using a larger-diameter nail.
- Penetration of the distal anterior femoral cortex also is a potential complication with an intramedullary nail (13).
- Nonunion is defined by pain or tenderness at the fracture site after 3–6 months.
- Symptoms of malunion include limp, rotational deformity, and leg-length discrepancy.
  - Treatment involves valgus osteotomy, revision internal fixation, and bone grafting.
- AVN of the femoral head may occur in children with open physes, if standard intramedullary nailing is performed through the piriformis fossa.

## REFERENCES

1. Russell TA, Taylor JC. Subtrochanteric fractures of the femur. In: Browner BD, Jupiter JB, Levine AM, et al., eds. *Skeletal Trauma. Fractures, Dislocations, Ligamentous Injuries*. Philadelphia: WB Saunders, 1992:1485–1524.
2. Sims SH. Subtrochanteric femur fractures. *Orthop Clin North Am* 2002;33:113–126.
3. Bedi A, Le TT. Subtrochanteric femur fractures. *Orthop Clin North Am* 2004;35:473–483.
4. American College of Surgeons Committee on Trauma. *Advanced Trauma Life Support Program for Doctors*, 6th ed. Chicago: American College of Surgeons, 1997.
5. Jarvis J, Davidson D, Letts M. Management of subtrochanteric fractures in skeletally immature adolescents. *J Trauma* 2006;60:613–619.
6. Kregor PJ, Obremskey WT, Kreder HJ, et al. Unstable pertrochanteric femoral fractures. *J Orthop Trauma* 2005;19:63–66.
7. Miedel R, Ponzer S, Tornkvist H, et al. The standard Gamma nail or the Medoff sliding plate for unstable trochanteric and subtrochanteric fractures. A randomised, controlled trial. *J Bone Joint Surg* 2005;87B:68–75.
8. Yoo MC, Cho YJ, Kim KI, et al. Treatment of unstable peritrochanteric femoral fractures using a 95 degrees angled blade plate. *J Orthop Trauma* 2005;19:687–692.
9. Kulkarni SS, Moran CG. Results of dynamic condylar screw for subtrochanteric fractures. *Injury* 2003;34:117–122.
10. Cheng MT, Chiu FY, Chuang TY, et al. Treatment of complex subtrochanteric fracture with the long gamma anteroposterior locking nail: A prospective evaluation of 64 cases. *J Trauma* 2005;58:304–311.
11. Robinson CM, Houshian S, Khan LA. Trochanteric-entry long cephalomedullary nailing of subtrochanteric fractures caused by low-energy trauma. *J Bone Joint Surg* 2005;87A:2217–2226.
12. Barquet A, Mayora G, Fregeiro J, et al. The treatment of subtrochanteric nonunions with the long gamma nail: Twenty-six patients with a minimum 2-year follow-up. *J Orthop Trauma* 2004;18:346–353.
13. Ostrum RF, Levy MS. Penetration of the distal femoral anterior cortex during intramedullary nailing for subtrochanteric fractures: A report of three cases. *J Orthop Trauma* 2005;19:656–660.


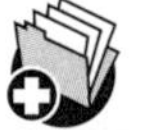

# MISCELLANEOUS

## CODES
### *ICD9-CM*
820.32 Subtrochanteric fracture

## PATIENT TEACHING
- Patients should be advised of the risk of malunion, nonunion, or implant failure, especially if they have osteoporotic bone.
- Protected weightbearing in the early postoperative period is essential to allow adequate reconstitution of this mechanically stressed area.

## FAQ
- Q: What is the best treatment for a subtrochanteric femur fracture?
  - A: Intramedullary nailing using a cephalomedullary device allows for stable fixation of subtrochanteric fractures. Reduction and anatomic fixation is paramount. The fracture must be reduced before nail insertion.

S

# SUBUNGUAL HEMATOMA

*Scott Berkenblit, MD, PhD*
*Dawn M. LaPorte, MD*

## BASICS

### DESCRIPTION

- Subungual hematoma is a localized collection of blood between the nail and nail bed of a finger or toe that results from an injury or laceration of the soft tissue of the nail bed under an intact nail.
- Pressure of the hematoma against the periosteum of the distal phalanx produces severe pain.
- Classification of the injury to the underlying nail bed tissue:
  - Simple laceration
  - Stellate laceration
  - Crush injury

### EPIDEMIOLOGY

- Older children and young adults are the most commonly affected individuals.
- One of the most common hand injuries seen in the office or emergency room
- The long finger is most frequently injured of all of the digits because of its prominence.

### ETIOLOGY

- Blunt trauma to the distal phalanx causes this condition.
- Injury in a door is the most common mechanism, followed by smashing between 2 objects and injury by a saw.

### ASSOCIATED CONDITIONS

Distal phalanx fracture

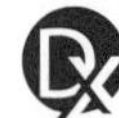

## DIAGNOSIS

### SIGNS AND SYMPTOMS

- Typically, in an acute injury, the patient complains of localized pain and gives a history of trauma to the finger or toe.
- Nail deformity is a late sign of a neglected nail bed injury.

#### *Physical Exam*

- On inspection, the hematoma is visible through the nail.
- If an underlying fracture of the distal phalanx is present, diffuse swelling of the digit tip is seen.

### TESTS

#### *Imaging*

Plain films of the affected digit should be obtained to rule out an associated fracture of the distal phalanx.

### DIFFERENTIAL DIAGNOSIS

- Contusion or fracture of the distal phalanx without hematoma formation
- Subungual melanoma, if history of injury is not clear
- Pyogenic granuloma at base of the nail, usually caused by perforation with cuticle scissors

## TREATMENT

### GENERAL MEASURES

- Treatment for a painful subungual hematoma involving <50% of the nail bed (1):
  - Prepare the nail in sterile fashion before the procedure (Fig. 1).
  - It is not necessary to anesthetize the finger.
  - Drain the hematoma by trephining 1–3 holes in the nail over the affected area with a battery-powered cautery such as an ophthalmic cautery (preferred method), a heated paper clip, or a 16-gauge needle, while the patient presses the pad of the finger firmly against a hard surface.
  - Drainage provides prompt relief of pain.
- Treatment for a hematoma involving >50% of the nail bed or with an underlying fracture:
  - Remove the nail to inspect and repair the underlying nail bed injury.
  - For an underlying fracture:
    - Splint the distal phalanx in addition to replacing the nail.
    - A displaced fracture may require reduction and fixation.

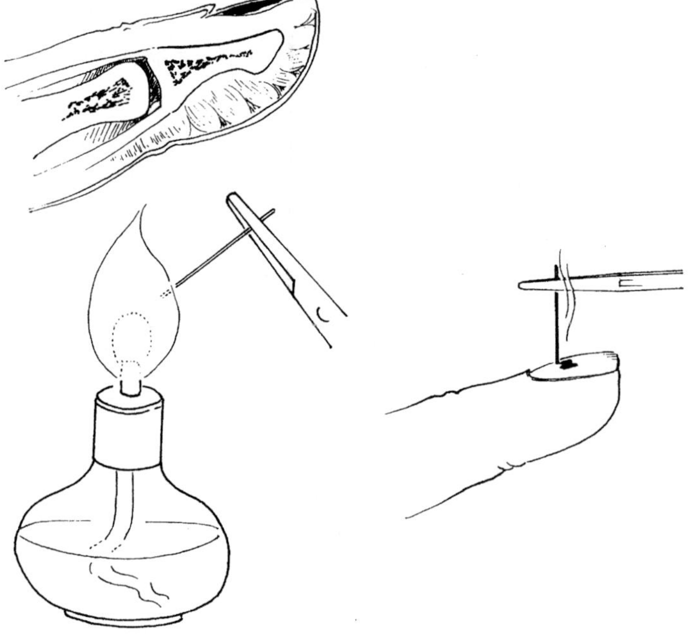

**Fig. 1.** A subungual hematoma may be decompressed with a cautery or hot needle for pain relief.

### *Activity*
The patient may continue activity as tolerated.

## SPECIAL THERAPY
### *Physical Therapy*
A hand therapist can fashion a tip protector to wear until the end of the finger is less sensitive.

## MEDICATION (DRUGS)
- Prescribe NSAIDs for pain relief.
- Prophylactic antibiotics should be given.

## SURGERY
- Surgical repair of a nail bed laceration requires nail removal.
  - Use a digital nerve block to obtain adequate regional anesthesia.
  - Grasp the distal edge of the nail with a clamp and bluntly dissect the nail from the nail bed and eponychium.
  - After irrigation, repair the laceration with fine absorbable sutures (e.g., 6-0 or 7-0 chromic).
  - Splint the eponychial fold to prevent formation of adhesions, which can result in deformity of the regrown nail.
    - Use the proximal part of the removed nail or a piece of heavy foil (suture wrapper) as a splint.
    - The replaced nail may be sutured to the eponychium with 5-0 nylon.
    - Cover the exposed nail bed with petrolatum gauze and apply a tubular gauze dressing.

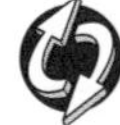

# FOLLOW-UP

## PROGNOSIS
The prognosis is excellent, if proper assessment and treatment are performed.

## COMPLICATIONS
- Nail deformity (i.e., fissured nail) if the eponychial fold is not properly splinted after removal of the nail or if a nail bed laceration is not repaired
- Split or nonadherent nail
- Osteomyelitis, a complication of unsterile drainage of the hematoma and improper wound dressing

## PATIENT MONITORING
The patient should be given a follow-up appointment within 1 week if nail bed repair has been performed.

## REFERENCE

1. Seaberg DC, Angelos WJ, Paris PM. Treatment of subungual hematomas with nail trephination: a prospective study. *Am J Emerg Med* 1991;9: 209–210.


## ADDITIONAL READING

- Batrick N, Hashemi K, Freij R. Treatment of uncomplicated subungual haematoma. *Emerg Med J* 2003;20:65.
- Roser SE, Gellman H. Comparison of nail bed repair versus nail trephination for subungual hematomas in children. *J Hand Surg* 1999;24A:1166–1170.
- Sommer NZ, Brown RE. The perionychium. In: Green DP, Hotchkiss RN, Pederson WC, et al., eds. *Green's Operative Hand Surgery*, 5th ed. Philadelphia: Elsevier Churchill Livingstone, 2005:389–416.


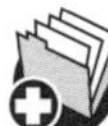

# MISCELLANEOUS

## PATIENT TEACHING
Patient should be counseled about signs of infection.

### *Prevention*
- Late deformity of the nail is difficult to reconstruct, and the results are unpredictable.
- Therefore, guidelines given earlier for inspecting and repairing nail bed injury should be followed to minimize the risk of late deformity.

## FAQ
- Q: How is the pain associated with subungual hematoma addressed?
  - A: The pain is secondary to the pressure of blood in this confined space, and evacuation of the hematoma is indicated to relieve the pain. The finger is prepped with Betadine, and a battery-powered microcautery tip is used to burn a hole through the nail.
- Q: Is nail removal and nail bed repair always indicated in subungual hematoma?
  - A: Nail removal and nail bed repair are considered if >50% of the nail is undermined by blood and the nail is broken or the nail edges are disrupted.

# SUPRACONDYLAR ELBOW FRACTURE

*Melanie Kinchen, MD*
*Simon C. Mears, MD, PhD*

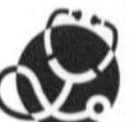

## BASICS

### DESCRIPTION

- Occurs at the metaphyseal–diaphyseal junction of the distal humerus
  - The fracture goes through the olecranon fossa of the distal humerus, which is a weak area.
- The mechanism (hyperextension) usually causes elbow dislocation in adults, supracondylar humerus fractures in children, and fractures through the growth plate of the distal humerus in toddlers.
- Classification:
  - By mechanism of injury:
    - Hyperextension type (95% of fractures)
    - Flexion type
  - The Gartland classification system is the most commonly used (1).
    - Type I: Nondisplaced
    - Type II: Displaced, but with an intact cortex; hinge or greenstick
    - Type III: Completely displaced, with no continuity between fragments; at highest risk for complications
- Synonym: Distal humerus fracture

### EPIDEMIOLOGY

- These fractures affect the distal humerus of children at a rate of 308 per 100,000, and 56% of those elbow fractures are supracondylar (2).
- Mean age of patients at time of injury is ~8 years (2).
- Distribution between genders is approximately even (2).
- This fracture is rare in adults, with rates of distal humerus fractures at 5.7 cases per 100,000 (3).

### RISK FACTORS

Fall on an outstretched arm

### ETIOLOGY

- A fall on an outstretched hand with the elbow hyperextended
- A fall onto a flexed elbow (extremely rare)

### ASSOCIATED CONDITIONS

- Ipsilateral distal forearm fractures
- Ipsilateral midshaft humeral fractures
- Nerve and artery damage (Fig. 1)

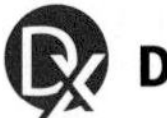

## DIAGNOSIS

### SIGNS AND SYMPTOMS

- Pain, swelling, and possibly instability occur after an acute traumatic event.
- After a few hours, typically ecchymosis occurs in the antecubital region.
- Nerve injuries are common with this fracture, signaled by lack of full active ROM.
- Arterial injuries also are possible and produce loss of pulse, color, temperature, and later, movement.

#### *Physical Exam*

- Swelling and tenderness are common.
- With type III fractures, an S-shaped deformity at the elbow is common and may be mistaken for a dislocation.
- Perform a thorough neurovascular examination of the involved extremity because a substantial risk of injury exists.
- Document full active flexion and extension of all digits at both MCP and IP joints.
- Substantial pain on passive stretch of the fingers may signal compartment syndrome.
- Check pulse, color, and temperature to assess vascular status.

### TESTS

#### *Imaging*

- AP and lateral radiographs usually are sufficient for diagnosing the injury.
- For nondisplaced fractures, a posterior fat pad sign may be the only radiographic finding.
- When ordering a radiograph of a suspected supracondylar fracture, specify the distal humerus as the part to be examined rather than the elbow because the patient may not be able to straighten the elbow fully.

### DIFFERENTIAL DIAGNOSIS

- Elbow dislocation
- Bicondylar humeral fracture
- Growth plate fracture (in toddlers)

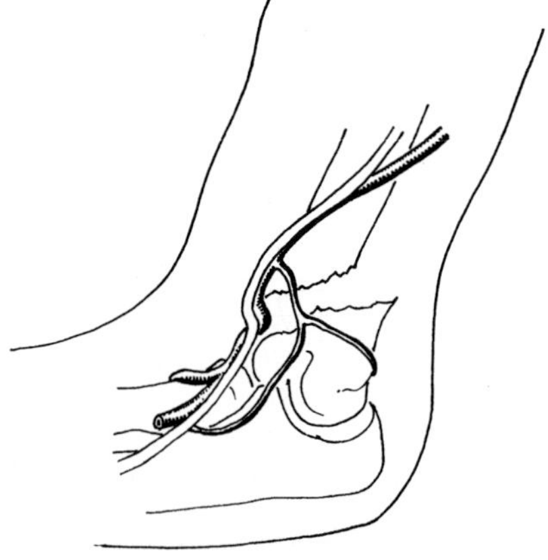

**Fig. 1.** A supracondylar fracture of the distal humerus may injure the brachial artery or the medial, radial, or ulnar nerve.

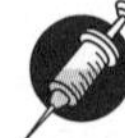

## TREATMENT

### INITIAL STABILIZATION

Initial treatment should involve immobilization of the injured elbow in 20–30° of flexion to prevent additional displacement or neurovascular damage until an orthopaedic surgeon can evaluate the patient.

### GENERAL MEASURES

- Type I injuries: Immobilization
- Type II injuries: Closed reduction and immobilization or operative intervention
- Type III injuries: Operative intervention
- Immobilization should be at <90° of flexion because flexion of >90° leads to increased compartment pressures and risk of compartment syndrome (4).

### SPECIAL THERAPY

#### *Physical Therapy*

- Physical therapy for children has not been shown to improve results (5).
- Physical therapy is useful in adult fractures.
  - Timing depends on healing and strength of internal fixation.
  - ROM is emphasized, followed by strength.

### MEDICATION (DRUGS)

Acetaminophen or acetaminophen with codeine for pain control

### SURGERY

- For type II fractures angulated >5–10° and for type III fractures, closed reduction should be attempted with the patient under adequate analgesia or anesthesia.
  - If anatomic reduction cannot be achieved by closed reduction, open reduction should be performed.
  - Fractures without vascular injury may be splinted and pinned on a delayed basis.
  - A delay of <24 hours does not seem to alter outcomes (6,7).
- An unstable fracture should be stabilized with percutaneous pin fixation.
  - 2 lateral pins and crossed medial and lateral pins give mechanical stability.
  - Use of only lateral pins prevents possible injury to the ulnar nerve (8).
  - Flexion injuries are treated with reduction and pinning (9).
  - After surgery, the elbow is immobilized at 90° of flexion for 3–4 weeks.
  - The pins are removed at 4–6 weeks.
- Compartment syndrome:
  - May be prevented by timely recognition of arterial injury
  - If ischemia time exceeds ~6 hours, fasciotomy of the forearm probably should be included in the treatment.

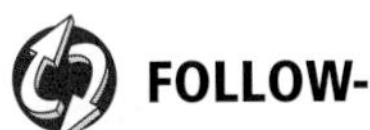

## FOLLOW-UP

### PROGNOSIS

- Prognosis is excellent with anatomic reduction (10).
- If malunion occurs, additional surgery may be needed to correct the deformity.

### COMPLICATIONS

- Nerve injuries: The median nerve is the most commonly injured, followed by the radial nerve.
- It may take several months to regain normal function (11).
- Arterial injuries: The brachial artery is the most commonly injured.
- Compartment syndrome may result in Volkmann ischemic contracture.
- Varus deformity of the elbow
- Elbow stiffness: Uncommon with anatomic reduction
- AVN of the trochlea, leading to a fishtail deformity

### PATIENT MONITORING

- Patients require radiographs and examinations at 1–2 weeks and ~6 weeks after fracture to ensure maintenance of the reduction during fracture healing.
- A small risk of malreduction exists.
- Patients should be seen after bone healing to document good alignment and ROM.

### REFERENCES


1. Gartland JJ. Management of supracondylar fractures of the humerus in children. *Surg Gynecol Obstet* 1959;109:145–154.
2. Houshian S, Mehdi B, Larsen MS. The epidemiology of elbow fracture in children: analysis of 355 fractures, with special reference to supracondylar humerus fractures. *J Orthop Sci* 2001;6:312–315.
3. Robinson CM, Hill RMF, Jacobs N, et al. Adult distal humeral metaphyseal fractures: epidemiology and results of treatment. *J Orthop Trauma* 2003;17:38–47.
4. Battaglia TC, Armstrong DG, Schwend RM. Factors affecting forearm compartment pressures in children with supracondylar fractures of the humerus. *J Pediatr Orthop* 2002;22:431–439.
5. Keppler P, Salem K, Schwarting B, et al. The effectiveness of physiotherapy after operative treatment of supracondylar humeral fractures in children. *J Pediatr Orthop* 2005;25:314–316.
6. Gupta N, Kay RM, Leitch K, et al. Effect of surgical delay on perioperative complications and need for open reduction in supracondylar humerus fractures in children. *J Pediatr Orthop* 2004;24:245–248.
7. Sibinski M, Sharma H, Bennet GC. Early versus delayed treatment of extension type-3 supracondylar fractures of the humerus in children. *J Bone Joint Surg* 2006;88B:380–381.
8. Skaggs DL, Hale JM, Bassett J, et al. Operative treatment of supracondylar fractures of the humerus in children. The consequences of pin placement. *J Bone Joint Surg* 2001;83A: 735–740.
9. De Boeck H. Flexion-type supracondylar elbow fractures in children. *J Pediatr Orthop* 2001;21: 460–463.
10. Mangwani J, Nadarajah R, Paterson JMH. Supracondylar humeral fractures in children: ten years' experience in a teaching hospital. *J Bone Joint Surg* 2006;88B:362–365.
11. Ramachandran M, Birch R, Eastwood DM. Clinical outcome of nerve injuries associated with supracondylar fractures of the humerus in children: the experience of a specialist referral centre. *J Bone Joint Surg* 2006;88B:90–94.


### ADDITIONAL READING


Storm SW, Williams DP, Khoury J, et al. Elbow deformities after fracture. *Hand Clin* 2006;22:121–129.


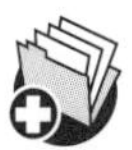

## MISCELLANEOUS

### CODES

#### *ICD9-CM*

- 812.41 Closed supracondylar fracture
- 812.51 Open supracondylar fracture

### PATIENT TEACHING

Adult patients and parents of injured children should be informed about the signs of ischemia and compartment syndrome (increasing pain, loss of finger motion, cold fingers, and loss of color) because compartment syndrome may (rarely) occur in the 1st few days after reduction secondary to tight dressings or intimal injury to the vessels.

#### *Activity*

To prevent refracture, rough play should be prohibited for a month after pin removal.

### FAQ

- Q: Which supracondylar fractures should be treated with surgery?
  - A: Type II fractures with an unsatisfactory reduction require reduction and pinning. Type III fractures require reduction and percutaneous pinning.

# SYNDACTYLY

*Dawn M. LaPorte, MD*
*John J. Hwang, MD*

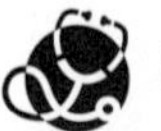

## BASICS

### DESCRIPTION

- Webbed fingers (or toes) (Fig. 1), usually detected at birth
- Classification:
  - Internal involvement: Simple (skin only) versus complex (bony involvement/fusion)
  - Extent of syndactyly: Complete (entire length of digits involved) versus incomplete (some part of fingers joined)
- Synonym: Webbed digits

### EPIDEMIOLOGY

More common in Caucasian males

#### *Incidence*

- Syndactyly occurs per ~1 per 2,000 births (1).
- It is seen bilaterally in 50% of cases (1).

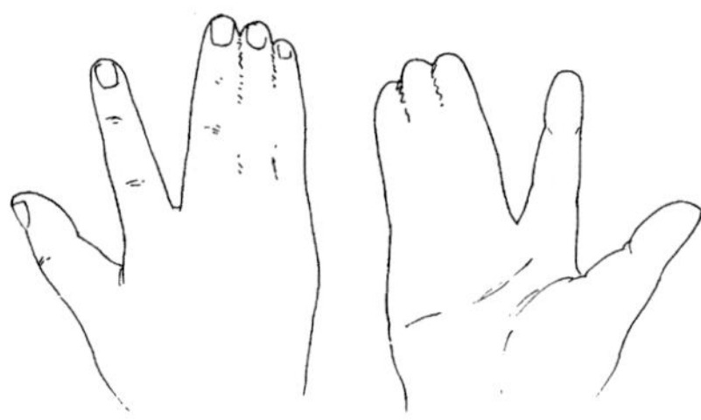

**Fig. 1.** Syndactyly, or webbing of the fingers, can be simple or complex.

### RISK FACTORS

The presence of other congenital abnormalities constitutes a risk factor for this condition.

#### *Genetics*

- 10–40% of the cases are familial (2).
- 80% of cases are sporadic (3).

### ETIOLOGY

- Syndactyly occurs secondary to a failure of separation of the digits in the 6th–8th weeks of intrauterine life.
- The specific cause is unknown.
- Although syndactyly may be associated in some cases with a positive family history or with a syndrome, in most cases it is an isolated finding.

### ASSOCIATED CONDITIONS

- Apert syndrome: Acrocephalosyndactyly
- Poland syndrome: Associated with chest wall anomalies and cardiac anomalies
- Congenital constriction band syndrome
- Fenestrated syndactyly (joined at the tips)
- Proteus syndrome
- NF: A slight increase in incidence

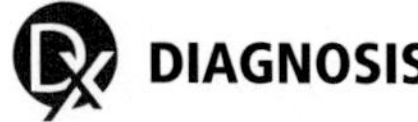

## DIAGNOSIS

### SIGNS AND SYMPTOMS

No pain is associated with this condition.

#### *Physical Exam*

- Observe joined fingers, which can be associated with many anomalies.
- Examine the joints for active and passive ROM.
- Test the 2 joined digits at each level for independent movement.
  - The ability to move separately indicates no bony or complex syndactyly.
- The amount of excess skin between the digits is a sign of the difficulty of reconstruction.
- Inspect the nails.
  - If they are joined, it is likely that the underlying bones are joined also.

### TESTS

#### *Imaging*

- Plain radiography is indicated to differentiate simple from complex syndactyly.
- Angiography or MRA may be needed in difficult cases of syndactyly to assess the structure of the underlying vascular supply of the 2 digits.
  - Vasculature branching distally instead of proximally may limit the extent of possible separation.

#### *Pathological Findings*

- Insufficient amount of skin present
- Abnormal fascial interconnections
- Abnormal interconnection between flexor and extensor tendons
- Various anomalies of bones and joints

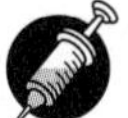

# TREATMENT

## GENERAL MEASURES

- Release of webbing:
  - Can improve cosmesis and function
  - Webs less than a few millimeters distally, or those causing minimum inhibition to spread of the fingers, do not need surgical intervention.
- Complex syndactyly, especially with only 1 branching neurovascular bundle, can be difficult to correct surgically.
- The timing of surgery is controversial, but usual recommendations are:
  - >6 months of age for border digits (thumb/index finger and ring/small finger)
  - >12 months for central digits

## SPECIAL THERAPY

### *Physical Therapy*

Physical therapy is not needed unless for postoperative scar management, web space splinting, and/or motion.

## SURGERY

- The degree of syndactyly dictates which of the many available release techniques is used.
- A large dorsal flap with a wider proximal base than the distal end is a good technique for simple and incomplete syndactyly.
- Skin grafting usually is necessary, depending on the amount of skin defect after release.
- Division of bones is needed in complex syndactyly.
- Postoperative dressing is an important part of treatment.
  - The dressing is extended above the elbow, and an above-the-elbow plaster cast can be beneficial.
  - The same dressing is continued until postoperative day 14.

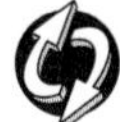

# FOLLOW-UP

## PROGNOSIS

The prognosis is good, although minor differences in width and appearance of the reconstructed digit are common.

## COMPLICATIONS

- Stiffness
- Wound dehiscence
- Scar contracture
- Partial web recurrence
- Circulatory deficit, resulting in loss of digit:
  - Rare
  - Can be minimized by operating on only 1 side of the digit at a time, so that a collateral vessel is preserved.

## PATIENT MONITORING

As children grow, they should be monitored for partial recurrence of the web or scar contracture.

## REFERENCES

1. Kay SP, McCombe D, Kozin SH. Deformities of the hand and fingers. In: Green DP, Hotchkiss RN, Pederson WC, et al., eds. *Green's Operative Hand Surgery*, 5th ed. Philadelphia: Elsevier Churchill Livingstone, 2005:1381–1444.
2. Ger E. Syndactyly. In: Buck-Gramcko D, ed. *Congenital Malformations of the Hand and Forearm*. London: Churchill Livingstone, 1998:131–140.
3. Trumble TE. Congenital hand deformities. In: Trumble TE, ed. *Principles of Hand Surgery and Therapy*. Philadelphia: WB Saunders, 2000:579–601.

## ADDITIONAL READING

Fearon JA. Treatment of the hands and feet in Apert syndrome: an evolution in management. *Plast Reconstr Surg* 2003;112:1–12.

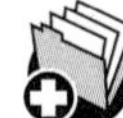

# MISCELLANEOUS

## CODES

### *ICD9-CM*

755.1 Syndactyly

## PATIENT TEACHING

- The patient or parents should be educated about the complexity of procedure, which they often underestimate.
- In particular, the need for obtaining soft-tissue coverage and the difficulty of increasing ROM of an abnormal joint should be explained.

## FAQ

- Q: Is syndactyly typically bilateral?
  - A: It occurs bilaterally 50% of the time.
- Q: What is the classification system for syndactyly?
  - A: Syndactyly is "complete" if the web space extends to include the fingertip and "incomplete" when the web space occurs anywhere between the normal web and the fingertips. "Simple" syndactyly has only skin/soft tissue connections, and "complex" syndactyly is marked by skeletal anomalies.
- Q: At what age should surgery be performed for syndactyly?
  - A: Syndactyly release usually is performed in patients ~12 months old. It is performed earlier for the border digits or with increasing angular deformity.

# TALUS FRACTURE

*Derek F. Papp, MD*

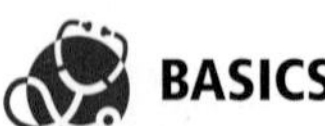

## BASICS

### DESCRIPTION

- The talus, a small bone in the hindfoot:
  - Articulates with the calcaneus and the remainder of the midfoot bones
  - Supports the body's weight and distributes the body's forces to the foot
  - Is critical to proper function of the foot
  - Is covered (~60%) with articular cartilage
  - Is vascularly supplied by vessels through a small area of the talar neck
- Because of its the tenuous blood supply, the talus is predisposed to posttraumatic osteonecrosis.
  - Fractures of the talus may be difficult to diagnose, and the clinician must understand the presenting features of this injury because of the high rate of osteonecrosis.
  - The talus may fracture in different anatomic locations, including the talar neck, the talar body, and the processes of the talus.
  - Another common talus fracture is the talar dome osteochondral fracture (see "Osteochondral Defect of the Talus" chapter).
- Classification of fracture patterns:
  - Talar neck fractures: Modified Hawkins system (1):
    - Type I: Nondisplaced vertical fracture of the talar neck
    - Type II: Displaced fracture of the talar neck with subluxation or dislocation of the subtalar joint; ankle joint is normal
    - Type III: Displaced fracture of the talar neck, associated with dislocation of the ankle and subtalar joints
    - Type IV: Extrusion of the talus
  - Talar body fractures:
    - Type I: Coronal or sagittal fractures
    - Type II: Horizontal fractures
  - Talar process fractures:
    - Posterior process fractures
    - Lateral process fractures

#### *Pediatric Considerations*

Because children have a higher cartilage-to-bone ratio than do adults, the pediatric talus is more prone to bend and thus better tolerates deforming forces.

### EPIDEMIOLOGY

No age- or gender-related associations

#### *Incidence*

- Talar fractures represent 3% of all foot fractures, and 50% are in the talar neck (2).
- Talar body fractures are less common, accounting for 7–38% of all tarsal fractures (2).

### RISK FACTORS

- Motor vehicle collisions
- High-energy falls
- Snowboarding

### PATHOPHYSIOLOGY

- Neck fractures occur with impaction of the neck of the talus against the distal anterior tibia during severe dorsiflexion of the foot.
- Among snowboarders, lateral process fractures are common, with external rotation forces applied to the booted, dorsiflexed foot.
- Body fractures occur from axial compression between the tibia and calcaneus.

### ETIOLOGY

The cause is high-energy trauma with forefoot hyperextension.

### ASSOCIATED CONDITIONS

Talar neck fractures commonly are associated with medial malleolar fractures.

## DIAGNOSIS

### SIGNS AND SYMPTOMS

- Extreme pain about the talus and hindfoot, associated with high-energy trauma
- Ecchymosis and swelling
- Deformity

#### *History*

- Commonly caused by motor vehicle accidents and falls from a height.
- Historically associated with pilots because they place their feet against the rudder controls (aviator's astragalus).

#### *Physical Exam*

- Check the ankle and hindfoot for:
  - Focal tenderness
  - Deformity
  - Ankle and subtalar motion
- Clinicians should carefully examine patients with mid- or hindfoot sprains and maintain a high index of suspicion for radiographic and CT findings.
- Talar process fractures may be missed easily.

### TESTS

#### *Imaging*

- Radiography:
  - AP and lateral radiographs of the ankle and foot are the baseline studies.
  - An oblique view of the talar neck can be helpful.
    - The foot is held in maximal equinus (plantarflexion) and 15° of pronation for this view.
- CT is required to delineate fracture displacement.

#### *Pathological Findings*

Occasionally, fractures occur through cysts or bone tumors.

### DIFFERENTIAL DIAGNOSIS

- Ankle fractures
- Ankle dislocation
- Talar dislocation
- Calcaneus fracture
- Navicular fracture

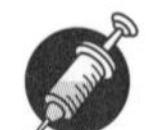

## TREATMENT

### INITIAL STABILIZATION

- Ice, immobilization, and elevation are indicated.
- Immediate reduction of displaced fragments is recommended to reduce risk of skin necrosis and secondary infection.

### GENERAL MEASURES

- Nondisplaced fractures may be treated with a below-the-knee cast for 12 weeks and nonweightbearing for 6 weeks.
- Type II talar neck fractures require reduction by closed or open (surgical) means.
- Type III talar neck fractures almost always require surgery to obtain an adequate reduction.
- Talar body fractures:
  - Have a higher incidence of osteonecrosis than do talar neck fractures
  - Should be treated surgically for the best reduction, if possible
- Established osteonecrosis of the talus is very difficult to treat, given the bone's minimal blood supply.
- Displaced fractures that cannot be reduced require open reduction and internal fixation.
- Displaced fractures are more predisposed to skin necrosis and infection because of the lack of protective subcutaneous tissue, especially dorsally.
  - Displaced fragments can distort surrounding tissues, which may lead to necrosis and secondary infection.
- A talar process fracture <1 cm in size and displaced <2 mm is treated with a nonweightbearing cast for 6 weeks (3).

#### *Pediatric Considerations*

- Nondisplaced fractures are treated in an above-the-knee plaster cast for 6–8 weeks.
- With the remodeling potential of pediatric patients, displacement of <5 mm and <5° of malalignment on an AP view are acceptable after reduction (4).

#### *Activity*

Nonweightbearing for at least 4–6 weeks

### SPECIAL THERAPY

#### *Physical Therapy*

ROM exercises are begun after removal of the cast.

### MEDICATION (DRUGS)
Pain can be controlled with opioid analgesics as appropriate, with transition to NSAIDs or acetaminophen as appropriate.

### SURGERY
- Open or closed reduction
- Open reduction of the talus and the talar neck is performed through incisions over the medial or lateral aspects of the hindfoot.
  - Incision placement depends on the precise fracture geometry.
  - Displaced fractures generally require 2 incisions to ensure precise reduction.
- Fractures are reduced using intraoperative fluoroscopy.
  - Cannulated screws are used for fixation and can be placed in an anterograde or retrograde manner.
  - Comminuted fractures of the talar neck have little support for screw fixation, and plate fixation may be preferred.
- Talar body fractures are more difficult to approach than are talar neck fractures.
  - A medial malleolar osteotomy often is required for visualization.
  - Screw heads should be buried into the articular surface.
- Process fractures >1 cm in size or displaced >2 mm are thought to have a better outcome with open reduction and internal fixation.
  - Either small cannulated screws or Kirschner wires may be used (5).
- After surgery, swelling should be monitored carefully for signs of compartment syndrome.
  - If necessary, compartment pressure should be measured in the foot.
  - Fasciotomies should be performed if compartment syndrome exists.
- Postoperatively, a well-modeled splint should be placed and then converted to a below-the-knee, nonweightbearing cast after swelling is reduced.

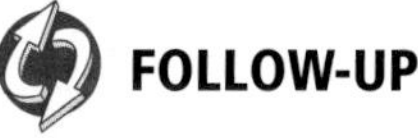

## FOLLOW-UP

### DISPOSITION
- Pain should be well controlled.
- Radiographic follow-up should continue for at least 18–24 months for nondisplaced fractures and for longer periods for displaced fractures and those complicated by posttraumatic osteonecrosis.

### PROGNOSIS
- Prognosis is directly related to the degree of initial injury, often regardless of anatomic reduction and fixation (6).
- Talar body fractures have a poor prognosis and often are associated with posttraumatic osteonecrosis and/or arthritis; 1 series reported that 88% of patients had 1 or both entities (7).

### COMPLICATIONS
- Osteonecrosis
- Skin necrosis and infection
- Delayed union is common, given the relatively poor blood supply.
- Nonunion leads to chronic pain and may require bone grafting or fusion procedures.
- Malunion can redistribute forces on the foot and cause chronic foot pain.
- Posttraumatic arthritis:
  - Can occur with or without associated osteonecrosis
  - Subtalar or pantalar fusion may be required as a salvage procedure.

### PATIENT MONITORING
- The integrity of the talar vascular supply can be confirmed with follow-up radiographs.
  - The Hawkins sign is a subchondral lucency (talar dome subchondral bone osteopenia) that results from bone resorption after a talus fracture with an intact blood supply.
  - The presence of a Hawkins sign excludes osteonecrosis of the talus.
- Diagnosis of osteonecrosis can be confirmed with MRI.

### REFERENCES

1. Canale ST, Kelly FB, Jr. Fractures of the neck of the talus. Long-term evaluation of seventy-one cases. *J Bone Joint Surg* 1978;60A:143–156.
2. Juliano PJ, Dabbah M, Harris TG. Talar neck fractures. *Foot Ankle Clin* 2004;9:723–736.
3. Valderrabano V, Perren T, Ryf C, et al. Snowboarder's talus fracture. Treatment outcome of 20 cases after 3.5 years. *Am J Sports Med* 2005;33:871–880.
4. Ribbans WJ, Natarajan R, Alavala S. Pediatric foot fractures. *Clin Orthop Relat Res* 2005;432: 107–115.
5. Berkowitz MJ, Kim DH. Process and tubercle fractures of the hindfoot. *J Am Acad Orthop Surg* 2005;13:492–502.
6. Lindvall E, Haidukewych G, DiPasquale T, et al. Open reduction and stable fixation of isolated, displaced talar neck and body fractures. *J Bone Joint Surg* 2004;86A:2229–2234.
7. Vallier HA, Nork SE, Benirschke SK, et al. Surgical treatment of talar body fractures. *J Bone Joint Surg* 2003;85A:1716–1724.


### ADDITIONAL READING

Kanlic EM, Pirela-Cruz MA. Fractures and injuries of the foot. In: Perry CR, Elstrom JA, eds. *Handbook of Fractures*, 3rd ed. New York: McGraw-Hill, 2006:386–409.


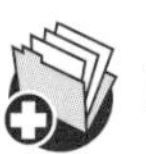

## MISCELLANEOUS

### CODES
#### *ICD9-CM*
825.21 Talus fracture

### PATIENT TEACHING
- Inform patients of the high incidence of talar osteonecrosis.
- Teach proper cast care and stress the importance of nonweightbearing during the healing period.
- Inform patients about the severity of the injury and the often poor long-term results.
- Review the potential need for later hindfoot fusion.

#### *Activity*
- Crutch walking and nonweightbearing until instructed otherwise.
- Physical therapy to increase ROM and strength after cast removal

### FAQ
- Q: How soon should a displaced talar fracture be reduced?
  - A: Talar fractures of the neck or body should be reduced as soon as possible to prevent soft-tissue complications. Some authors believe that emergent surgery is not necessary because the risk of posttraumatic arthritis is far greater than that of osteonecrosis.
- Q: How likely am I to return to full activities after a talar fracture?
  - A: After a displaced fracture, osteonecrosis may occur. The rate of osteonecrosis depends on the severity of the initial injury. If osteonecrosis occurs, a high likelihood exists that a fusion will be required. Hindfoot fusion results in ankle stiffness and difficulty in walking on uneven ground and in climbing. Most patients with displaced talar neck or body fractures have arthritis and chronic pain.

# TARSAL TUNNEL SYNDROME

*Marc D. Chodos, MD*

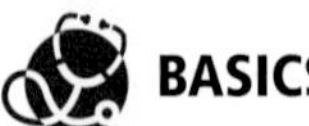

## BASICS

### DESCRIPTION

- Tarsal tunnel syndrome is entrapment of the tibial nerve or its distal branches caused by compression or traction as the nerve courses through the tarsal tunnel.
- Anatomy (1):
  - Proximal tarsal tunnel:
    - Fibro-osseous space that contains (from anterior to posterior) the PTT, flexor digitorum longus tendon, posterior tibial artery and vein, tibial nerve, and flexor hallucis longus tendon.
    - The tarsal tunnel is a continuation of the deep posterior compartment of the leg.
    - The floor is composed of the medial surface of talus, the sustentaculum tali, and the medial wall of the calcaneus.
    - The roof is composed of the flexor retinaculum, which begins up to 10 cm proximal to the medial malleolus; each tendon and the neurovascular bundle is contained by separate fibro-osseous compartments that connect with the retinaculum.
  - The tibial nerve gives rise to the MCN, MPN, and LPN; nerve anatomy can be variable.
    - MCN:
      - 69–90% of the time, arises directly from the tibial nerve
      - Also can arise from the LPN
      - Single nerve branch in 79%, but can be multiple branches
      - Provides sensation to medial heel
    - MPN and LPN:
      - Formed by terminal bifurcation of tibial nerve
      - 93–96% of the time, bifurcation takes place within the tarsal tunnel.
      - Remainder occurs proximal to tarsal tunnel, in the leg.
    - MPN:
      - Provides sensation to plantar foot, big toe, 2nd toe, 3rd toe, and medial border of the 4th toe
      - Provides motor innervation to the abductor hallucis, flexor digitorum brevis, flexor hallucis brevis, and 1st lumbrical
    - LPN:
      - Provides sensation to lateral border of the 4th toe and to the 5th toe
      - Provides motor innervation to the quadratus plantae, abductor digiti minimi, flexor digiti minimi brevis, lateral 3 lumbricals, adductor hallucis, and the interossei
      - Most common nerve involved in tarsal tunnel syndrome
      - The distal tarsal tunnel begins as the MPN and LPN pass through separate fibrous tunnels deep to abductor hallucis.
    - MPN may be trapped between the navicular and the abductor hallucis, or at the knot of Henry.
    - The 1st branch of the LPN may be trapped in fascia of abductor hallucis as it travels to abductor digiti quinti, causing heel pain.

#### *Pregnancy Considerations*

- Tarsal tunnel syndrome can occur during pregnancy, typically secondary to local compression caused by fluid retention and volume changes.
- Care usually is supportive until after delivery, because many cases resolve after pregnancy.

### EPIDEMIOLOGY

- In a literature review of 186 cases, patients ranged from 14–80 years old (2).
- Slightly more common in females (56%) than in males (2)

#### *Incidence*

Unknown

### RISK FACTORS

- No clear risk factors have been proven, but several authors have associated tarsal tunnel syndrome with certain occupations and activities.
  - Jogger's foot: Excessive hindfoot valgus is theorized to stretch the tibial nerve during repetitive activity such as running (1).
  - Activities that consist of repetitive squatting or crouching, such as in race jockeys (1,2)

### PATHOPHYSIOLOGY

- Tarsal tunnel syndrome is caused by compression or tension on the tibial nerve, resulting in damage (1).
- Unyielding structure of tarsal tunnel places nerve at risk for injury from local volume changes.
- Compressive etiologies: Sensory abnormalities are hypothesized to result from nerve ischemia, whereas late motor dysfunction may be the result of direct nerve compression injury.
- Chronic traction injuries produce fibrosis of the epineurium and stiffness, which makes the nerve less able to compensate for other insults.

### ETIOLOGY

- The specific cause is identifiable in only 60–80% of patients (1); causes can be grouped into 3 categories: Trauma, space-occupying lesion, and deformity.
- Most common causes (2):
  - Trauma: 17%
  - Varicosities: 13%
  - Hindfoot varus: 11%
  - Fibrosis: 9%
  - Hindfoot valgus: 8%
- Other causes of compression include ganglia, lipoma, neurilemmoma, inflammatory synovitis, PVNS, tarsal coalition, and accessory musculature.

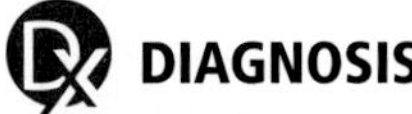

## DIAGNOSIS

### SIGNS AND SYMPTOMS

Frequently misdiagnosed because of poorly localized and variable symptoms

#### *History*

- Insidious/intermittent onset of pain and paresthesias
- Location of symptoms defined by the nerves involved
- Neurogenic pain (burning, paresthesias, numbness)
- Pain can radiate proximally up the medial leg (Valleix phenomenon) in 33% of patients with severe compression, or distally along path of involved nerves (1,2).
- Pain usually worse with standing or activity
- Some patients have substantial night pain, which may be related to venostasis.
- Symptoms improve with rest, loose shoe wear, and elevation.

#### *Physical Exam*

- Perform a complete foot and ankle examination.
- Foot alignment:
  - Examine for hindfoot varus or valgus abnormalities.
  - Exaggerating heel dorsiflexion, inversion, or eversion may reproduce symptoms by stretching or compressing the nerve.
- Palpate the tarsal tunnel and course of the tibial nerve for:
  - Tenderness
  - Swelling consistent with a space-occupying lesion
- Tinel sign: Percussion over the course of the tibial nerve may produce paresthesias and distal symptoms.
- Cuff test: Using a pneumatic cuff to create a venous tourniquet may cause engorgement of varicosities and reproduce symptoms.
- Compression test: Applying pressure to tarsal tunnel for 60 seconds may reproduce symptoms.
- Sensory examination:
  - The MCN usually is spared, but numbness and altered sensation may be present in the distribution of the MPN or LPN.
  - 2-point discrimination is decreased early in the disease process.
- Motor examination:
  - Intrinsic weakness is difficult to assess.
  - Rarely, weakness of toe plantarflexion may be noted.
  - Atrophy of the abductor hallucis or abductor digiti minimi may be seen late in the disease process.

### TESTS

#### *Lab*

Routine laboratory tests can be used to rule out other conditions that may mimic tarsal tunnel syndrome, including peripheral neuropathy caused by diabetes or other systemic illnesses.

#### *Imaging*

- Routine weightbearing radiographs to assess for fracture or exostoses
- MRI:
  - Can be helpful in assessing the tarsal tunnel for masses or other sources of nerve compression before surgery
  - In 1 study, a causative agent was identified in 88% of symptomatic feet (3).

#### *Pediatric Considerations*

MRI is recommended for evaluating pediatric tarsal tunnel syndrome because compression by a neoplastic mass is not uncommon (3).

#### *Diagnostic Procedures/Surgery*

- Electrodiagnostic studies (4):
  - Can evaluate for evidence of underlying peripheral neuropathy
  - Isolated motor latencies have a lower sensitivity than sensory or mixed action potentials.
  - Sensory action potentials are the most sensitive test (90.5%), but they also have the highest false-positive rate (8%).
  - Mixed motor and sensory conduction velocities are abnormal in 85.7%, with a very low false-positive rate.
  - It is important to evaluate for proximal nerve compression, including a lumbar radiculopathy or a double-crush phenomenon.

#### *Pathological Findings*

- At the time of surgical exploration, the following may be found:
  - Focal swelling, scarring, or nerve abnormalities
  - A pathologic source of compression

### DIFFERENTIAL DIAGNOSIS

- Peripheral neuropathy (diabetes)
- Peripheral neuritis
- Peripheral vascular disease
- Morton neuroma
- Metatarsalgia
- Subtalar joint arthritis
- Tibialis posterior tendinitis/dysfunction
- Plantar fasciitis
- Complex regional pain syndrome
- Proximal injury or compression of the tibial branch of the sciatic nerve
- Lumbar radiculopathy

## TREATMENT

### GENERAL MEASURES

- Initially, nonoperative management is recommended except for acute tarsal tunnel syndrome or in the setting of a known space-occupying lesion (excluding synovitis) (1).
  - Rest/immobilization
  - Orthotics
  - Anti-inflammatories, including steroid injections and nonsteroidal drugs
  - Medications that alter neurogenic pain (tricyclic antidepressants, antiepileptic drugs, nerve blocks)
  - Physical therapy (desensitization)
  - Compression stockings
  - Weight loss

### SURGERY

- Surgery is indicated (1,2):
  - If nonoperative measures fail after a 3–6-month trial
  - In the setting of acute tarsal tunnel syndrome
  - If the cause is a space-occupying lesion
- Use a curved posteromedial incision, following the course of the tibial nerve.
- Release the entire flexor retinaculum.
- Release the MPN and LPN distally as they pass deep to the abductor hallucis and into the plantar foot.
- Excise space-occupying lesions and address underlying pathology such as tendon dysfunction and tarsal coalition.
- Minimize surgical dissection to help limit scar formation.

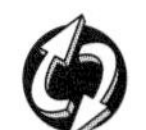

## FOLLOW-UP

- Postoperative management includes:
  - Nonweightbearing splint until incision heals (2–3 weeks), followed by progressively increased weightbearing and ROM exercises.
  - RICE protocol to limit swelling

### PROGNOSIS

- Best results are seen in young patients, when surgery is performed early in the disease process (before motor abnormalities occur) or when a discrete lesion is found.
- In a review of 25 articles, 91% of 110 patients had improvement or resolution of symptoms with surgery (1).
- A more recent study with longer patient follow-up and more stringent criteria has shown poorer outcomes, with deteriorating results over time (5).

### COMPLICATIONS

- The main adverse outcome is unsuccessful surgical intervention: No improvement, partial/incomplete improvement, or temporary improvement with recurrence of symptoms (6).
- 5 causes of failed tarsal tunnel release:
  - Incorrect diagnosis
  - Incomplete release
  - Adhesive neuritis (external scar formation)
  - Intraneural damage (systemic disease, direct nerve injury)
  - Failure to treat all sources of nerve compression in a double-crush phenomenon
- Examination of the incision length is the most important part of the physical examination in determining whether an adequate release was done initially.
- Electrodiagnostic studies are not helpful for diagnosing tarsal tunnel syndrome after a failed release.
- Repeat surgical release, combined with a barrier procedure (vein or synthetic graft wrapping around the nerve), is the operative treatment of choice for adhesive neuritis.
- Results for revision surgery are poorer than those for primary surgical release.

### REFERENCES


1. Lau JTC, Stavrou P. Posterior tibial nerve—primary. *Foot Ankle Clin* 2004;9:271–285.
2. Cimino WR. Tarsal tunnel syndrome: Review of the literature. *Foot Ankle* 1990;11:47–52.
3. Frey C, Kerr R. Magnetic resonance imaging and the evaluation of tarsal tunnel syndrome. *Foot Ankle* 1993;14:159–164.
4. Galardi G, Amadio S, Maderna L, et al. Electrophysiologic studies in tarsal tunnel syndrome. Diagnostic reliability of motor distal latency, mixed nerve and sensory nerve conduction studies. *Am J Phys Med Rehabil* 1994;73: 193–198.
5. Pfeiffer WH, Cracchiolo A, III. Clinical results after tarsal tunnel decompression. *J Bone Joint Surg* 1994;76A:1222–1230.
6. Raikin SM, Minnich JM. Failed tarsal tunnel syndrome surgery. *Foot Ankle Clin* 2003;8: 159–174.


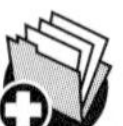

## MISCELLANEOUS

### CODES

#### *ICD9-CM*

355.5 Tarsal tunnel syndrome

### PATIENT TEACHING

The patient should be actively involved in the decision-making process, with a clear understanding of the risks and benefits of surgical and nonsurgical treatments.

### FAQ

- Q: Electrodiagnostic studies for tarsal tunnel syndrome can also rule out what important conditions included in the differential diagnosis?
  - A: Peripheral neuropathy and lumbar radiculopathy.
- Q: What is the recommended treatment for acute tarsal tunnel syndrome, such as occurs with calcaneal or talar fracture?
  - A: Acute tarsal tunnel syndrome from trauma is caused by displaced fracture fragments, tension on the nerve structures, or compression by hematoma. Acute surgical decompression of the tarsal tunnel is combined with fracture reduction and fixation to relieve pressure on the tibial nerve.

# TENNIS ELBOW

*Mark Clough, MD*

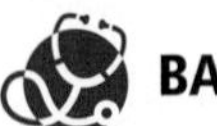

## BASICS

### DESCRIPTION

- Lateral epicondylitis (tennis elbow) is a tendinopathy of the origin of the ECRB tendon.
- The lateral epicondyle is the origin of the common wrist extensor tendon, including:
  - ECRL
  - ECRB
  - Extensor digitorum communis
  - Extensor carpi ulnaris
- The ECRB lies beneath the ECRL.
- These extensors stabilize the wrist and are used in sports (such as tennis) during a backhand stroke.
- Lateral epicondylitis typically occurs from overuse in the nonathlete's dominant arm during the 4th and 5th decades.

### GENERAL PREVENTION

Use of good form while playing tennis (i.e., proper grip size, backhand technique)

### EPIDEMIOLOGY

Occurs equally in males and females

#### *Incidence*

The peak incidence is in the 5th decade (1).

### RISK FACTORS

- Patients are susceptible with activities of repetitive supination and pronation of the forearm in which the elbow is near full extension (such as in tennis).
- Although tennis elbow is its common name, lateral epicondylitis can be seen in other racket sports, fencing, and certain occupations with repetitive actions (e.g., plumbing, painting, knitting, and dentistry).
- Associations have been made to poor stroke mechanics, improper racket grip size, racket weight, and racket stringing.
- Harder playing surfaces produce more force on the ball and therefore create greater transmitted forces to the lateral epicondyle.

### ETIOLOGY

- Initiated as a microtear within the origin of ECRB.
- The ECRL and extensor digitorum communis also are susceptible.
- Insufficient healing response leaves the ECRB origin vulnerable to secondary injury.

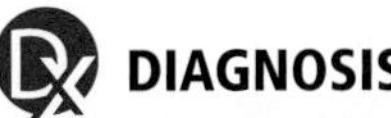

## DIAGNOSIS

### SIGNS AND SYMPTOMS

- Patients usually have a history of repetitive activity.
- Pain is present at the lateral epicondyle with resisted wrist extension that is made worse when the elbow is extended.
- Symptoms are exacerbated with activity and improve with rest.
- Patients report pain with grasping objects.
- Elbow ROM usually is not compromised.

#### *Physical Exam*

- Tenderness over the origin of the common wrist extensor tendons at the lateral epicondyle
- Tenderness may extend distally.
- Reproduction of pain with passive flexion of the wrist with the elbow extended
- The clinician should check for radial tunnel syndrome, in which pain is reproduced with active middle finger extension against resistance.
- A cervical spine examination is warranted for all patients, especially if symptoms are bilateral.

### TESTS

#### *Imaging*

- Radiographs:
  - AP and lateral radiographs of the elbow are obtained to rule out fractures or other lesions in the elbow.
  - AP and lateral plain radiographs usually are negative, but 23% of patients may show calcifications in the local soft tissue (2).
  - Consider cervical spine radiographs if symptoms possibly originate from the neck.
- CT may be warranted for detailed evaluation of the joint in cases of a loose body or arthritis.
- MRI usually is not necessary, but it may show tendon thickening with increased T1 and T2 signals.

#### *Diagnostic Procedures/Surgery*

Electromyography may be helpful in distinguishing radial tunnel syndrome from lateral epicondylitis (see "Differential Diagnosis").

#### *Pathological Findings*

- Microscopic tears within the substance of the ECRB
- Histology shows replacement of tendon collagen fibers with vascular granulation-like tissue and fibroblasts, termed "angioblastic proliferation."

### DIFFERENTIAL DIAGNOSIS

- Differential diagnosis includes cervical spine disease with radiculopathy.
- Radial tunnel syndrome (5% coexistence reported, compression of posterior interosseous nerve as it enters the supinator muscle) (3)
- Olecranon bursitis
- Medial epicondylitis
- UCL strain/sprain
- Intra-articular disease, such as arthritis, osteochondritis dissecans of the capitellum, or loose body

## TREATMENT

### GENERAL MEASURES

- Nonoperative treatment includes rest, counterforce straps, wrist splint, activity modification, cryotherapy, NSAIDs, and physical therapy initially.
- Athletes should improve technique and mechanics and modify equipment as detailed above.
- If results are poor with initial therapy, then consider corticosteroid injection.
  - Caution should be used, because multiple injections or incorrectly given injections increase the risk of tendon rupture.
- Nonoperative treatment is successful in 95% of patients (1).
- Newer treatments, including low-level laser and extracorporeal shock wave, have not shown substantial benefit when compared with placebo treatment in a recent meta-analysis (4).

#### *Activity*

Patients should be instructed to rest the affected extremity and that activity can be resumed in a graduated fashion as symptoms improve.

### SPECIAL THERAPY

#### *Physical Therapy*

- If pain continues, physical therapy (including ultrasound, iontophoresis, friction massage, and counterforce bracing [tennis elbow strap]) may be helpful.
- Once symptoms have diminished, a stretching and strengthening program directed at forearm extensors may help to prevent recurrence.

### SURGERY
- If nonoperative therapy fails over a 6-month period, operative treatment may be warranted.
- Traditional surgery consists of resection of the degenerated ECRB origin.
- The 5% coexistent radial tunnel syndrome also should be released (3).
- Arthroscopic débridement of the ECRB origin represents a promising surgical procedure with quicker return to activity (5).

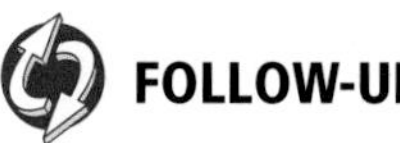

## FOLLOW-UP

- The splint is removed in 1 week, and ROM exercises are initiated.
- Once the wound is well healed, strengthening exercises are added to the therapy program and pain-limited activity can be started.
- Full activity usually is possible in ~3 months.

### PROGNOSIS
- Lateral epicondylitis has the potential to be a chronic problem with periods of exacerbation and relief.
- Patients usually (95%) have success with nonoperative treatment (1).

### COMPLICATIONS
- Few complications occur with nonoperative therapy.
- Potential surgical complications include tendon rupture (retear), infection, decreased ROM, and stiffness.

### PATIENT MONITORING
Repeat radiographs in 3 months if the pain persists.

### REFERENCES

1. Coonrad RW. Tennis elbow. *Instr Course Lect* 1986;35:94–101.
2. Nirschl RP. Muscle and tendon trauma: Tennis elbow. In: Morrey BF, ed. *The Elbow and Its Disorders*. Philadelphia: WB Saunders, 1985: 481–496.
3. Werner CO. Lateral elbow pain and posterior interosseous nerve entrapment. *Acta Orthop Scand Suppl* 1979;174:1–62.
4. Speed CA, Nichols D, Richards C, et al. Extracorporeal shock wave therapy for lateral epicondylitis—a double blind randomised controlled trial. *J Orthop Res* 2002;20:895–898.
5. Baker CL, Jr, Murphy KP, Gottlob CA, et al. Arthroscopic classification and treatment of lateral epicondylitis: Two-year clinical results. *J Shoulder Elbow Surg* 2000;9:475–482.


### ADDITIONAL READING

- Azar FM. Shoulder and elbow injuries. In: Canale ST, ed. *Campbell's Operative Orthopaedics*, 10th ed. St. Louis: Mosby, 2003:2339–2375.
- Bisset L, Paungmali A, Vicenzino B, et al. A systematic review and meta-analysis of clinical trials on physical interventions for lateral epicondylalgia. *Br J Sports Med* 2005;39:411–422.
- Brashear HR, Jr, Raney RB, Sr. Affectations of the elbow, wrist, and hand. In: Brashear HR, Jr, Raney RB, Sr, eds. *Handbook of Orthopaedic Surgery*, 10th ed. St. Louis: CV Mosby, 1986:476–497.
- Ilfeld FW. Can stroke modification relieve tennis elbow? *Clin Orthop Relat Res* 1992;276:182–186.
- Jobe FW, Ciccotti MG. Lateral and medial epicondylitis of the elbow. *J Am Acad Orthop Surg* 1994;2:1–8.
- Nirschl RP, Pettrone FA. Tennis elbow. The surgical treatment of lateral epicondylitis. *J Bone Joint Surg* 1979;61A:832–839.
- Porretta CA, Janes JM. Epicondylitis of the humerus. *Mayo Clin Proc* 1958;33:303–306.
- Tearse DS. Sports injuries. In: Clark CR, Bonfiglio M, eds. *Orthopaedics: Essentials of Diagnosis and Treatment*. New York: Churchill Livingstone, 1994:237–247.


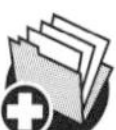

## MISCELLANEOUS

### CODES
#### *ICD9-CM*
726.32 Tennis elbow (lateral epicondylitis)

### PATIENT TEACHING
Lateral epicondylitis is typically a result of chronic overload of the wrist extensors.

#### *Activity*
Activity modification is an important element of treatment.

#### *Prevention*
- Proper technique and grip size for playing tennis
- 2-hand backhand eliminates strain on the ECRB.

### FAQ
- Q: What devices can one wear to relieve lateral epicondylitis?
  - A: Patients with lateral epicondylitis typically respond to counterforce strapping (placing a strap around the proximal forearm) and wrist splinting (immobilizing the wrist puts the wrist extensors at rest).
- Q: When would injecting lateral epicondylitis with cortisone be considered?
  - A: If symptoms persist after activity modification, physical therapy, and bracing.

# TENOSYNOVITIS

*Gregory Gebauer, MD, MS*

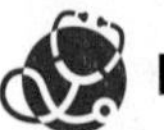

## BASICS

### DESCRIPTION

- Tenosynovitis is the painful inflammation of a tendon and its surrounding synovial sheath.
- It affects long tendons, most commonly in the fingers, wrist, or ankle.
- The inflammation may be related to an acute injury, chronic overuse, a systemic inflammatory disease (rheumatoid arthritis) or infection, or it may be idiopathic in origin.
- The condition is rare in children and is most common in early to middle adulthood.
- Classification:
  - By duration:
    - Acute: Few days' duration of symptoms; usually resolves promptly with rest and NSAIDs
    - Chronic: Duration of symptoms >2–3 weeks; may have more changes in tendon and its sheath; more difficult to cure
  - By common locations:
    - Posterior tibialis tenosynovitis (1)
    - Flexor tenosynovitis
    - Biceps tenosynovitis
    - de Quervain tenosynovitis (of the thumb extensor and abductor tendons) (2)
- Synonym: Tendinitis

### GENERAL PREVENTION

In general, it is difficult to predict who will be affected by tenosynovitis, making prevention in the general population difficult.

### EPIDEMIOLOGY

- 1 of the most common musculoskeletal problems affecting the general population
- Most people experience at least 1 episode of tenosynovitis in their lifetime.
- Females are affected slightly more frequently than are males.

### RISK FACTORS

- Systemic inflammatory diseases such as rheumatoid arthritis
- Previous episodes of tenosynovitis
- Unclear if repetitive motion is linked

### ETIOLOGY

- Excessive use or constriction of a tendon causes inflammation of the sheath (tenosynovium), which then becomes thickened.
- Females in the 30–50-year age group who are engaged in activity involving repetitive motion constitute most of the noninfectious, nonrheumatologic cases.
- Rheumatoid arthritis, lupus, or other inflammatory arthritides can manifest as tenosynovitis.
- Infectious causes of tenosynovitis are associated with a cut or break in the skin that extends deep into the flexor sheath.

#### *Pregnancy Considerations*

Pregnancy can precipitate tenosynovitis, especially de Quervain.

### ASSOCIATED CONDITIONS

- Rheumatoid arthritis
- Inflammatory arthropathies

## DIAGNOSIS

### SIGNS AND SYMPTOMS

- Pain over the affected tendon:
  - May be acute or insidious
  - Usually follows a period of unusual or new activity
  - Worse with continued use
- De Quervain tenosynovitis:
  - Tender on the radial side of the wrist
  - Worse with ulnar deviation
- Some patients may develop a trigger finger, in which inflammation and scarring of the long flexor tendons of the fingers causes a locking or snapping sensation as the tendon passes through the pulley systems along the palmar aspect of the fingers.

#### *Physical Exam*

- Tenderness in a longitudinal distribution, along the course of the involved tendon
- Tenderness can be mild, moderate, or severe.
- Possible associated swelling along the tendon sheath

### TESTS

#### *Lab*

- Laboratory studies may be useful to rule out infection, including complete blood count, sedimentation rate, and C-reactive protein.

#### *Imaging*

- Radiographs are needed:
  - If a history of penetrating trauma is present
  - To assess the presence of arthritis in adjacent joints or to exclude other possible causes of the patient's symptoms, such as fractures
- MRI and ultrasound may show inflammation in the tendon sheath and can be useful in confirming the diagnosis.

#### *Pathological Findings*

Localized inflammation and thickening of the tendon sheath are revealed microscopically by the presence of acute inflammatory cells (polymorphonuclear leukocytes).

### DIFFERENTIAL DIAGNOSIS

- Infection of the tendon sheath
- Trauma to tendon (e.g., strain or tear)

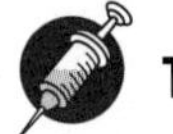

## TREATMENT

### GENERAL MEASURES

- Relative rest: Avoidance of offending activities and gentle ROM exercises
- Short-term splinting can be used for complete immobilization in extreme cases.

### SPECIAL THERAPY

#### *Physical Therapy*

- Physical and occupational therapists manage these problems, making use of:
  - Splints
  - Strengthening and stretching exercises
  - Job and activity modification

### MEDICATION (DRUGS)

- NSAIDs are the mainstay of treatment.
- Corticosteroid injection for de Quervain tenosynovitis (2)
- Tenosynovitis associated with systemic inflammatory diseases such as rheumatoid arthritis may respond to disease-modifying agents or to systemic anti-inflammatory medications.
- Infectious causes of tenosynovitis must be treated aggressively with antibiotics.

### SURGERY

- Indicated in patients for whom nonoperative measures have failed
- Release of the tendon sheath around the inflamed area, along with excision of tenosynovitis and tendon débridement
- de Quervain tenosynovitis may require complete release of the abductor pollicis longus, followed by splinting.
- For septic tenosynovitis: Release of the tendon sheath, decompression of purulence, and removal of inflamed/infected synovium

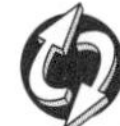

## FOLLOW-UP

### DISPOSITION

#### *Issues for Referral*

Patients with tenosynovitis secondary to a systemic inflammatory condition such as lupus or rheumatoid arthritis should be referred to a rheumatologist for medical management (including disease-modifying agents).

### PROGNOSIS

- Most cases resolve with nonoperative measures.
- The PTT and the Achilles tendon are especially prone to disease recurrence.

### COMPLICATIONS

Tenosynovitis may fail to resolve, usually because of chronic changes in the tendon.

### PATIENT MONITORING

Patients are followed at 4–6-week intervals to check ROM and healing of the tendon.

### REFERENCES


1. Bare AA, Haddad SL. Tenosynovitis of the posterior tibial tendon. *Foot Ankle Clin* 2001;6:37–66.
2. Weiss APC, Akelman E, Tabatabai M. Treatment of de Quervain's disease. *J Hand Surg* 1994;19A:595–598.


### ADDITIONAL READING


- Coughlin MJ. Disorders of tendons. In: Coughlin MJ, Mann RA, eds. *Surgery of the Foot and Ankle*, 7th ed. St. Louis: Mosby, 1999:786–861.
- Froimson AI. Tenosynovitis and tennis elbow. In: Green DP, ed. *Operative Hand Surgery*, 3rd ed. New York: Churchill Livingstone, 1993:1989–2006.


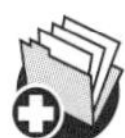

## MISCELLANEOUS

### CODES

#### *ICD9-CM*

727.0 Tenosynovitis

### PATIENT TEACHING

#### *Activity*

Patients should be instructed to avoid exacerbating activities.

#### *Prevention*

Patients should avoid repetitive manual activity or a sudden increase in activity.

### FAQ

- Q: What is tenosynovitis?
  - A: Tenosynovitis is an inflammation of the tendon and the tendon sheath. It can be caused by acute injury, overuse, systemic inflammatory diseases, or infection.
- Q: How do you treat tenosynovitis?
  - A: Treatment depends on the causes. Infections are treated with antibiotics and even surgical decompression. Overuse injuries are treated with anti-inflammatory medications and relative rest of the affected area. Systemic diseases leading to tenosynovitis may require a more aggressive medical regimen for treatment.
- Q: What is de Quervain tenosynovitis?
  - De Quervain tenosynovitis is an inflammation of the tendons of the 1st dorsal compartment of the wrist, namely the extensor pollicis brevis and abductor pollicis longus.

# THORACIC DISC HERNIATION

*Dhruv B. Pateder, MD*

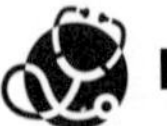

## BASICS

### DESCRIPTION

- Thoracic disc herniation is a difficult condition to diagnose and treat given its vague symptoms, which are often similar to those of other conditions.
- These difficulties are compounded by the fact that a high prevalence occurs of asymptomatic thoracic disc abnormalities and herniation.

### EPIDEMIOLOGY

- Symptomatic thoracic disc disease most commonly occurs in the 5th decade.
- A slight male predominance is noted.
- Up to 50% of patients report some traumatic event before the onset of symptoms (1–4).

#### Incidence

Symptomatic herniations occur in 1 per 1,00,000 patients per year (1–4).

#### Prevalence

- Up to 73% of patients have some thoracic disc abnormalities on MRI (4).
- 37% have asymptomatic disc herniations (4).

### RISK FACTORS

#### Genetics

No known genetic link

### PATHOPHYSIOLOGY

- Symptomatic disc herniations can lead to spinal cord or nerve root compression.
- Spinal cord compression can lead to signs of myelopathy without upper extremity involvement.

### ASSOCIATED CONDITIONS

Adolescents with Scheuermann disease often present with acute disc herniation.

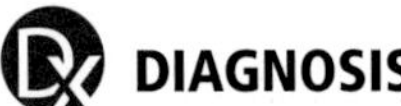

## DIAGNOSIS

### SIGNS AND SYMPTOMS

Patients may present with axial pain (localized from the middle to lower thoracic spine), radicular pain (T10 dermatomal is most common), or myelopathy (bowel and bladder dysfunction are seen in up to 20% of patients with symptomatic disc herniation) (1–6).

#### History

- This disorder has a very extensive differential diagnosis given the vague signs and symptoms, depending on the level of disc herniation.
- 2 separate clinical courses:
  - Young patients (usually <40 years old) with a soft disc herniation:
    - Usually present after a traumatic event
    - Usually have acute spinal cord compression
    - Respond well to nonoperative and operative treatment
  - Older patients (usually >40 years old) with long-standing symptoms and degenerative calcified discs:
    - Have no history of trauma
    - Have chronic cord or root compression

#### Physical Exam

- Neurologic examination:
  - Signs of myelopathy
  - Asymmetric contraction of rectus abdominus during sit-up
  - Superficial cremasteric reflex
  - Sensory levels:
    - T4: Nipple line
    - T7: Xiphoid process
    - T10: Umbilicus
    - T12: Inguinal crease
- Gait
- ROM

### TESTS

- Asymmetric contraction of rectus abdominus during sit-up
- Superficial cremasteric reflex

#### Lab

Complete blood cell count, ESR, and C-reactive protein usually are used if infection or cancer is in the differential.

#### Imaging

- Radiography:
  - AP and lateral radiographs of the spine show degenerative changes or spondylolisthesis and rule out fractures, infection, or tumor.
  - Radiographs should include the 1st rib, 12th rib, and sacrum to allow for appropriate localization of the level of abnormality.
- MRI:
  - Shows compression of neural elements
  - The sagittal and axial T1- and T2-weighted images should be used to evaluate the disc herniation.
  - Special attention should be given to confirming the level of the disc herniation.
  - A sagittal localizer pulse sequence should be used to count down from C2 and count up from the sacrum.
  - Correlation should be made with the conventional radiographs.
- CT-myelography is comparable to MRI in showing neural compression, but it is an invasive procedure (dye injection associated with subsequent headache).

#### Diagnostic Procedures/Surgery

Discography is controversial but often used to evaluate for axial back pain when multilevel disease or severe pain occurs in the presence of relatively normal imaging studies.

### DIFFERENTIAL DIAGNOSIS

- An extensive differential
- Intrathoracic abnormality
- Intra-abdominal abnormality
- Infectious
- Neoplastic
- Degenerative
- Metabolic
- Deformity
- Neurogenic

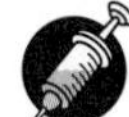

## TREATMENT

### GENERAL MEASURES

Acute thoracic disc herniations have a natural history similar to that of lumbar disc herniations and are managed similarly with nonoperative treatment in the absence of neurologic compromise.

#### Activity

As tolerated, as long as no other abnormality (e.g., fractures, gross instability, etc.) is present

### SPECIAL THERAPY

#### Physical Therapy

- Acute phase:
  - Passive modalities:
    - Heat
    - Ice
    - Ultrasound
- After overcoming the acute phase:
  - ROM
  - Flexibility
  - Strengthening exercises
  - Hyperextension exercises

### MEDICATION (DRUGS)

No role for maintenance opiates

#### First Line

- Anti-inflammatory medications (as long as no gastrointestinal side effects occur)
- Enteric-coated aspirin (fewer gastrointestinal side effects)
- Acetaminophen

#### Second Line

- COX-2 inhibitors (be aware of changing side-effect profile)
- Epidural or intercostals steroid injections

### SURGERY

- Indicated when nonoperative treatment fails and the patient cannot attain a tolerable quality of life
- Preoperative clearance by an internist, cardiologist, and/or anesthesiologist is necessary.
- Correct level of surgical excision is ensured by use of intraoperative radiographs.
- Anterior transthoracic approach is used most commonly.
- Posterior pediculofacetectomy is the only recommended posterior approach.
- Very high risk of neurologic injury with thoracic laminectomy (not recommended)
- Lateral extracavitary and costotransversectomy are the 2 lateral approaches.
- Video-assisted thoracoscopic surgery is a new, minimally invasive procedure.
- Thoracic fusion is controversial because some contend that the rib cage gives the thoracic spine inherent stability, whereas other surgeons cite the possibility of deformity and instability.

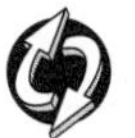

## FOLLOW-UP

Routine follow-up is at 6 weeks, 3 months, 6 months, 1 year, 2 years, and then every 2 years.

### DISPOSITION

#### *Issues for Referral*

Patients should be referred to appropriate specialists (thoracic or general surgeons, rheumatologists, etc.) if other conditions cannot be ruled out as part of the differential diagnosis.

### PROGNOSIS

Most patients who undergo disc excision have excellent or good long-term results (6).

### COMPLICATIONS

- The overall surgical complication rate after thoracic disc excision was 14.6% in a series of 82 patients (6).
- The most serious complication is paralysis or paraparesis.
- Myelopathy and/or neurologic compromise is also a potential complication of nonoperative treatment.

### PATIENT MONITORING

Patients are monitored for resolution of symptoms, fusion (if arthrodesis was performed), and development of any complications.

### REFERENCES


1. Brown CW, Deffer PA Jr, Akmakjian J, et al. The natural history of thoracic disc herniation. *Spine* 1992;17:S97–S102.
2. Carson J, Gumpert J, Jefferson A. Diagnosis and treatment of thoracic intervertebral disc protrusions. *J Neurol Neurosurg Psychiatry* 1971;34:68–77.
3. Vanichkachorn JS, Vaccaro AR. Thoracic disc disease: Diagnosis and treatment. *J Am Acad Orthop Surg* 2000;8:159–169.
4. Wood KB, Garvey TA, Gundry C, et al. Magnetic resonance imaging of the thoracic spine. Evaluation of asymptomatic individuals. *J Bone Joint Surg* 1995;77A:1631–1638.
5. Regan JJ. Percutaneous endoscopic thoracic discectomy. *Neurosurg Clin N Am* 1996;7:87–98.
6. Stillerman CB, Chen TC, Couldwell WT, et al. Experience in the surgical management of 82 symptomatic herniated thoracic discs and review of the literature. *J Neurosurg* 1998;88:623–633.


### ADDITIONAL READING


Simpson JM, Silveri CP, Simeone FA, et al. Thoracic disc herniation: Re-evaluation of the posterior approach using a modified costotransversectomy. *Spine* 1993;18:1872–1877.


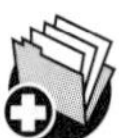

## MISCELLANEOUS

### CODES

#### *ICD9-CM*

- 722.11 Thoracic intervertebral disc without myelopathy
- 722.72 Intervertebral disc disorder with myelopathy, thoracic region

### PATIENT TEACHING

- Patients should be educated about:
  - Being aware of progressive motor weakness and bladder/bowel dysfunction
  - The natural history of the condition

### FAQ

- Q: What is the most common surgical approach to perform a thoracic discectomy?
  - A: Anterior approach.

# THORACIC OUTLET SYNDROME

*Chris Hutchins, MD*
*John H. Wilckens, MD*

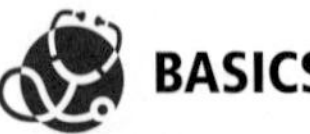

## BASICS

### DESCRIPTION

- TOS is a group of signs and symptoms that result from compression of the neurovascular supply to the upper limb in the supraclavicular area and shoulder girdle (1).
- Synonyms: Scalene anticus syndrome; Costoclavicular syndrome; Hyperabduction syndrome; Cervical rib syndrome; Droopy shoulder syndrome

### EPIDEMIOLOGY

#### *Incidence*

- Incidence unknown
- Condition not common

#### *Prevalence*

- Most common in young to middle-aged adults
- Occurs more often in females than males

### RISK FACTORS

- Cervical ribs
- Congenital fibrous bands
- Diabetes mellitus
- Thyroid disease
- Alcoholism
- Aggravating factors:
  - Obesity
  - Extremely large breasts in females
  - Emotional depression, causing patients to adopt a slumping posture
  - Repetitious overhead activity

### ETIOLOGY

- Frequently multifactorial and may be influenced by trauma, repetitious job activities, anatomic predisposing factors, and some systemic diseases (e.g., diabetes, thyroid disease)
- A job that requires continuous overhead activity (e.g., painting ceilings) may cause signs and symptoms of brachial plexus compression over a short period.
- A job that requires repetitive motions of the upper extremities, but in less extreme elevation (e.g., keyboard operator, truck driver), may cause similar symptoms, but over a period of years.

### ASSOCIATED CONDITIONS

- CTS and cubital tunnel syndrome complaints:
  - It is believed that a nerve that has some degrees of compression in the neck is more sensitive to nerve compression problems at other points along its course, such as at the elbow or the wrist.
  - Thus, patients with TOS are more susceptible to developing CTS and cubital tunnel syndromes, and vice versa.
  - This phenomenon has been termed the "double crush syndrome."
- Patients with arthritis, diabetes mellitus, thyroid disease, and alcoholism have nerves with increased susceptibility to the development of superimposed nerve compression.

## DIAGNOSIS

### SIGNS AND SYMPTOMS

- Neural compression:
  - Patients may complain of pain in the neck or shoulder, and numbness and tingling involving entire upper limb or forearm and hand (Fig. 1).
    - The ulnar side of the limb and the 2 ulnar digits are involved predominantly, although the middle finger also may be included.
    - Sensory findings often are subtle, are usually on the ulnar aspect of the hand, and may include the medial aspect of the forearm.
  - Nocturnal pain and paresthesias are common and must be differentiated from symptoms caused by CTS, which commonly affects the radial side of the hand.
  - Frequently, patients experience difficulty in using the limb in an elevated, overhead position, such as when holding a hair dryer.
  - Some patients show a decline in the strength or dexterity of the hand, even without obvious atrophy.
  - Headache and pain in the arm, shoulder, neck, and chest may accompany any of these other complaints.
- Arterial compression:
  - Coolness
  - Weakness
  - Easy fatigability of the arm
  - Diffuse pain
  - Occasionally, Raynaud-like symptoms
- Venous compression:
  - May be intermittent or, less frequently, constant
  - Results in limb swelling
  - Varying degrees of cyanosis

#### *Physical Exam*

- The diagnosis of TOS is a clinical one (2).
- Assess the neck and supraclavicular fossa on both sides.
  - The affected scapula may be held lower and more anteriorly than the opposite scapula.
  - The clavicle may appear more horizontal than normal.
  - Tenderness may be present over the brachial plexus.
- Tinel sign may be present (pain referred to the ulnar aspect of the hand).
- Examine the shoulder girdle for glenohumeral instability, which may produce symptoms similar to those of TOS.
- Perform a complete, bilateral, upper extremity motor and sensory examination.
- Test the intrinsic muscle strength in the hand.
- Document the vasomotor status of the limb and the presence or absence of swelling.
- "Stress tests" or provocative maneuvers used in the clinical diagnosis of TOS:
  - These tests must be interpreted carefully. (It is not clinically significant, for example, to be able merely to obliterate the pulse by some position of the arm, because doing so is possible in many asymptomatic people.)
  - A test is not positive unless, without prompting, the patient complains of reproduction of the symptoms when the arm is placed in the provocative position.
  - Conduct the Adson maneuver with the patient's arm at the side, the neck hyperextended, and the head turned toward the affected side.
  - Perform the Wright maneuver with the patient's arm abducted and externally rotated.
    - The test is more sensitive when the patient holds a deep breath.
    - The patient's elbow should be extended to limit the effects of possible ulnar neuropathy at the elbow (which would be exacerbated by elbow flexion).

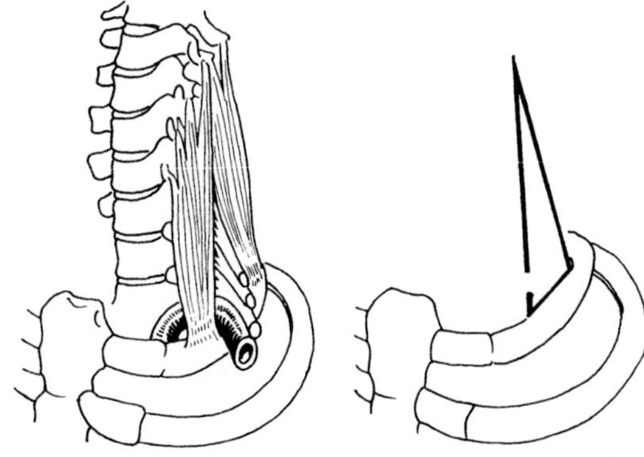

**Fig. 1.** In TOS, the brachial plexus or subclavian artery (*left*) may be compressed in the scalene triangle (*right*) or by an extra rib.

## TESTS

### Imaging

- Radiography
  - Obtain plain AP and lateral radiographs of the cervical spine to evaluate for discogenic disease, adventitious ribs, or overly long transverse processes.
  - Evaluate the chest radiograph for apical lung tumors, which may be responsible for neurovascular compression, especially in patients with a history of smoking.
  - MRI is useful if a strong suspicion exists of disc disease, but it does not help in the diagnosis of TOS.
- Electrodiagnostic studies may be helpful in identifying associated CTS and cubital tunnel syndrome.
- Vascular studies if compression of the subclavian artery or vein is suspected

### Pathological Findings

Compression of the neurovascular supply to the upper limb in the region of the suprascapular area and shoulder girdle is noted.

## DIFFERENTIAL DIAGNOSIS

- Lesions of the cervical spine:
  - Degenerative disc disease
  - Cervical spondylosis
- Lesions compressing the brachial plexus (e.g., tumors of the apex of the lung)
- Trauma
- Compression of the peripheral nerves:
  - CTS (entrapment neuropathy of the median nerve)
  - Ulnar nerve compression or dislocation at the elbow
  - Compression of the radial or suprascapular nerves
- Neuropathies of alcoholism, heavy metal intoxication, avitaminosis, or diabetes mellitus
- Complex regional pain syndromes
- Arterial lesions:
  - Peripheral or coronary atherosclerosis
  - Aneurysm
  - Occlusive changes
  - Embolism
  - Raynaud disease
  - Vasculitis
- Venous lesions:
  - Effort vein thrombosis
  - Thrombophlebitis

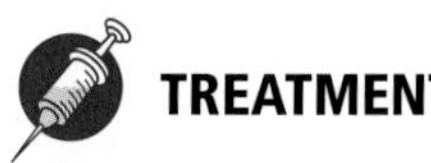

# TREATMENT

## GENERAL MEASURES

Nonoperative management should be tried initially for all patients with TOS (3).

## SPECIAL THERAPY

### Physical Therapy

- The cornerstone of nonoperative therapy is a carefully regulated program of muscle strengthening and postural re-education exercises.
- The trapezius, rhomboid, and levator scapulae muscles can be strengthened by the use of elastic bands or free weights with the arms elevated $<90^\circ$ and with avoidance of bracing of the scapulae to prevent provocative positions.
- Patients often do not experience symptomatic improvement before 2 months.
- Exercises must be continued until muscular atrophy and weakness is reversed and correct posture is developed.
- The preoperative exercise routine can be resumed 1 month postoperatively.

## MEDICATION (DRUGS)

- Nonoperative therapy is based on a stringent program of exercises to strengthen the muscles of the pectoral girdle.
- The goal is to augment the tone of the suspensory muscles of the AC joint so the costoclavicular space can remain wide.
- Patients must continue with the exercises until they have reversed the muscular atrophy and weakness and have developed an awareness of correct posture.
- If a carefully supervised exercise and postural program fails, and the patient has intractable pain, surgery may be indicated.
  - Surgery should be presented as an option only for those patients who believe that they cannot continue with the condition as it is and who understand the potential risks and benefits of the proposed procedure.
- Explanation of the pathologic process of TOS helps to alleviate a patient's concerns and makes the patient more receptive when instructed to avoid certain activities and postures.
  - Specific contributory factors, such as repetitive elevated positioning of the arms at work, should be identified and, when possible, addressed.

## SURGERY

- Scalenectomy or 1st rib resection, or some combination thereof, represents the most common surgical treatment for patients with TOS.
- A patient with an arterial or venous lesion may require vessel repair or grafting in addition to decompression.

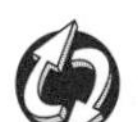

# FOLLOW-UP

## PROGNOSIS

- Nonoperative management is successful in most patients.
- With proper selection of patients for surgery, most improve.

## COMPLICATIONS

- Pneumothorax
- Infection
- Vascular injury
- Injury to brachial plexus
- Shoulder girdle instability

## PATIENT MONITORING

- Follow the patient's physical therapy progress.
- Postoperative disease recurrence is possible, secondary to scapular muscle weakness and an inability to support the shoulder girdle or inadequate release of the site of compression.

## REFERENCES


1. Fechter JD, Kuschner SH. The thoracic outlet syndrome. *Orthopaedics* 1993;16:1243–1251.
2. Abdollahi K, Wood VE. Shoulder. Section O. Thoracic outlet syndrome. In: DeLee JC, Drez D, Jr, Miller MD, eds. *DeLee & Drez's Orthopaedic Sports Medicine: Principles and Practice*, 2nd ed. Philadelphia: WB Saunders, 2003:1161–1169.
3. Roos DB. The thoracic outlet syndrome is underrated. *Arch Neurol* 1990;47:327–328.


## ADDITIONAL READING


Leffert RD. TOS. *J Am Acad Orthop Surg* 1994;2:317–325.


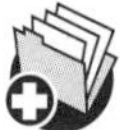

# MISCELLANEOUS

## CODES

### ICD9-CM

353.0 Thoracic outlet syndrome

## PATIENT TEACHING

- Explain the pathogenesis of TOS to patients, because an understanding of the mechanism helps the patient recognize the need for modifying activities and postures that would narrow the thoracic outlet, such as overhead movements, hyperabduction of the arm, use of shoulder straps, and carrying heavy handbags.
- Attempts to alter the ergonomic characteristics of the job should be made, or a new job should be considered.

### Prevention

- No known fully effective means of prevention
- The patient can diminish the risk by avoiding frequent overhead lifting or hyperabduction of the arm and by weight control.

## FAQ

- Q: What are the most common signs and symptoms of TOS?
  - A: Pain, weakness, fatigability, numbness, and tingling in the upper extremity. These symptoms may be intermittent and have inconsistent presentations. A high clinical suspicion is needed, and definitive diagnosis may require several studies.
- Q: Do all patients with TOS require surgery?
  - A: Although most patients respond to physical therapy and postural education, those with anatomic lesions and overhead occupations or recreations are best treated with surgery.

# THORACOLUMBAR SPINE FRACTURE AND DISLOCATION

*Dhruv B. Pateder, MD*

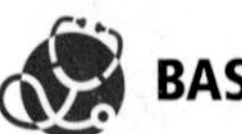

## BASICS

### DESCRIPTION
- Most spine fractures occur in the thoracolumbar region.
- T11–L1 is the most frequently injured area.
- Concomitant spine injuries are present in up to 15% of patients (1–5).
- Associated abdominal injuries are present in ~20% of patients (1–5).
- The Denis 3-column classification (1,2) is the system most commonly used to describe thoracolumbar fractures.
  - Divides the thoracolumbar spine into 3 columns:
    - Anterior column: Anterior 2/3 of the vertebral body/disc
    - Middle column: Posterior 1/3 of the vertebral body/disc and posterior longitudinal ligament
    - Posterior column: Pedicles, facets, lamina, transverse, and spinous processes
  - Divides fractures into minor and major injuries:
    - Minor injuries: Fractures of spinous and transverse processes, pars interarticularis, and facets
    - Major injuries: Compression fractures, burst fractures, distraction-flexion injuries, fracture-dislocations, and distraction-extension injuries

### EPIDEMIOLOGY
- Most injuries occur in males 15–30 years old (3–5).
- Motor vehicle accidents and other high-energy forces
- Elderly patients with osteopenic/osteoporotic bones sustain fractures with low-energy injuries.

### RISK FACTORS
- Age 15–30 years
- Motor vehicle accidents
- High-energy trauma
- Osteoporotic bone

### ASSOCIATED CONDITIONS
- Contiguous and noncontiguous spinal column injuries
- Neurologic injuries
- Spinal shock
- Abdominal injuries:
  - Splenic rupture
  - Liver lacerations
  - Bowel injuries

## DIAGNOSIS

### SIGNS AND SYMPTOMS
#### *History*
- For high-energy trauma, obtain history from patient and the emergency medical personnel on the scene.
- Question the patient about pertinent medical history (e.g., AS, previous spine surgery, etc.).

#### *Physical Exam*
- 1 of the most important components of caring for trauma patients, particularly patients with spine injuries
- Documentation of each examination is very important because deteriorating neurologic assessments often provide the 1st clue of an underlying injury.
- Document the initial examination and compare it to the results of the examination in the field.
- Inspect for any visible bruising, deformity, or step-offs around the spine.
- Inspect for associated injuries (e.g., seat-belt marks).
- Palpate the entire spine for areas of tenderness.
- Grade the motor examination on a 0–5-point scale.
  - 0: No motor activity
  - 1: Flicker of activity
  - 2: Full motion across a joint without gravity
  - 3: Full motion across a joint against gravity
  - 4: Motion across a joint against some external resistance
  - 5: Motion across a joint against full external resistance
- Assess the sensory levels.
  - T4: Nipple line
  - T7: Xiphoid process
  - T10: Umbilicus
  - T12: Inguinal crease
  - L1: Proximal 1/3 anterior thigh
  - L2: Middle 1/3 anterior thigh
  - L3: Over superior portion of patella
  - L4: Over medial malleolus
  - L5: Over dorsum of 3rd toe
  - S1: Over dorsum of small toe
- Assess the reflexes.
  - L4: Patellar reflex
  - L5: No reflex
  - S1: Gastrocnemius-soleus reflex
- Perform a rectal examination.
  - Tone
  - Volition
  - Perianal light touch and pinprick sensation (S2–S5)
  - Bulbocavernosus reflex
  - Anal wink reflex

### TESTS
#### *Lab*
All trauma patients routinely undergo metabolic panel, complete blood cell count, prothrombin time/INR, partial thromboplastin time, and urinalysis.

#### *Imaging*
- Radiography:
  - Trauma series:
    - Lateral cervical spine, chest, and pelvic radiographs
    - Radiographs of the spine are ordered if the patient is having back pain or an abnormality is noted on physical examination.
  - Thoracolumbar spine
- CT:
  - Ordered for additional evaluation of an injury or abnormality seen radiographically
  - Also can be very useful for preoperative planning
- MRI is ordered if soft-tissue injury (disc extrusion, ligamentous injury) is suspected because it cannot be visualized on CT.

### DIFFERENTIAL DIAGNOSIS
- In high-energy trauma, not much of a differential diagnosis exists, given the acute nature of the injury and the correlative findings on physical examination and imaging studies.
- Patients >50 years old who sustain thoracolumbar spine fractures after low-energy trauma must be evaluated for osteoporosis, and pathologic fractures must be ruled out.

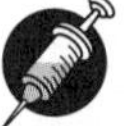

## TREATMENT

### INITIAL STABILIZATION
- Nonoperative fractures can be treated in a TLSO with a cervical extender if the fracture is above T7 and a unilateral thigh extender if necessary.
- Patients with fractures that may require surgical intervention can be on bed rest until they undergo definitive fixation.

## GENERAL MEASURES

- Compression fractures:
  - Nonoperative treatment with a TLSO (add cervical extension if fracture is above T7)
  - Vertebral augmentation procedures (kyphoplasty and vertebroplasty) are used more frequently to treat osteoporotic and osteolytic vertebral compression fractures.
  - Treatment of the underlying osteoporosis is of critical importance in avoiding additional fractures.
- Burst fractures:
  - Involve 2 of the 3 columns
  - Nonoperative treatment consists of progressive weightbearing in a TLSO
  - Surgery usually is indicated in the presence of:
    - Neurologic injury and/or kyphosis of >20°
    - Facet subluxation
    - Increased interspinous distance
    - >50% loss of anterior vertebral body height
    - >50% canal occlusion
  - However, all these parameters are relatively "soft," and the overall clinical scenario should be considered when deciding on nonoperative or surgical management.
- Distraction-flexion injuries:
  - Distraction of the posterior elements usually leads to ligamentous injury, and compression of the anterior column leads to a vertebral body fracture.
  - Nonoperative management rarely is indicated because ligamentous healing is unpredictable in these unstable injuries.
  - During surgery, care should be taken to avoid causing spinal canal narrowing (with bone fragments or disc material) during fracture reduction.
- Fracture-dislocations:
  - Findings include facet fracture-dislocation, rotational, or translational deformity.
  - Nonoperative management rarely is indicated because ligamentous healing is unpredictable in these unstable injuries.
  - Surgical intervention usually begins with a posterior reduction and stabilization before an anterior decompressive/fusion procedure can be considered.
- Distraction-extension injuries:
  - Very rare; tend to occur in patients with underlying metabolic bone disease
  - Nonsurgical treatment is not a good option because these injuries are very unstable.
  - Surgery generally begins with posterior instrumentation and fusion, with possible anterior correction.

### *Activity*

- Patients treated with a TLSO or operative fixation can advance to progressive weightbearing.
- Patients with neurologic injury need rehabilitation and can advance with activity, depending on the extent of injury.

### *Nursing*

A sequential neurologic examination with vital signs should be performed by a trained medical practitioner.

## SPECIAL THERAPY

Patients with neurologic injury often need counseling and benefit from peer support groups.

### *Radiotherapy*

Radiation therapy has a role for patients with pathologic thoracolumbar fractures to decrease tumor size and burden.

### *Physical Therapy*

Plays a very important role in mobilizing patients after spinal injury, particularly those with neurologic injury

## MEDICATION (DRUGS)

No role for maintenance opiates

### *First Line*

- Anti-inflammatory medications (as long as no gastrointestinal side effects occur)
- Enteric-coated aspirin (fewer gastrointestinal side effects)
- Acetaminophen

### *Second Line*

COX-2 inhibitors (Be aware of changing side-effect profile.)

## SURGERY

- The goal of surgery is to decompress the neural elements and achieve rigid spinal fixation.
- The surgical approach is surgeon- and injury-pattern-dependent.
  - With the advent of pedicle screws, posterior instrumentation usually is favored because it allows excellent fixation and alignment of the spine without the morbidity associated with the anterior approach.
  - The anterior approach also has an important role in decompression when bone fragment retropulsion is present in the spinal canal.

# FOLLOW-UP

Routine follow-up is at 2 weeks, 6 weeks, 3 months, 6 months, 1 year, 2 years, and then every 2 years thereafter.

## DISPOSITION

### *Issues for Referral*

- Patients with chronic pain issues should be referred to a pain medicine specialist.
- Patients with neurologic injury should be followed by a physical medicine and rehabilitation specialist.
  - Neurologic consultation may be obtained if the pattern of neurologic deficit does not correlate with the spinal injury.
- Physical and occupational therapists also play important roles in recovery.

## PROGNOSIS

- Prognosis depends on injury severity.
- Neurologically intact patients with low-energy injuries have excellent recovery.
- Patients with neurologic injury have major issues that may require alteration in their personal and professional lives.

## COMPLICATIONS

- Surgical complications include:
  - Infection
  - Neurologic injury
  - Pseudarthrosis
  - Spinal deformity
  - Junctional degeneration and stenosis
  - Chronic pain and disability
- Skin problems from pressure points on TLSO braces

## PATIENT MONITORING

Patients are monitored for resolution of symptoms, fusion (if arthodesis was performed), and development of any complications.

## REFERENCES


1. Denis F. The three column spine and its significance in the classification of acute thoracolumbar spinal injuries. *Spine* 1983;8:817–831.
2. Denis F. Spinal instability as defined by the three-column spine concept in acute spinal trauma. *Clin Orthop Relat Res* 1984;189:65–76.
3. Singh K, Vaccaro AR. Thoracic and lumbar trauma. In: Bono CM, Garfin SR, Tornetta P, et al., eds. *Spine*. Philadelphia: Lippincott Williams & Wilkins, 2004:45–57.
4. Spivak JM, Vaccaro AR, Cotler JM. Thoracolumbar spine trauma: II. Principles of management. *J Am Acad Orthop Surg* 1995;3:353–360.
5. Spivak JM, Vaccaro AR, Cotler JM. Thoracolumbar spine trauma: I. Evaluation and classification. *J Am Acad Orthop Surg* 1995;3:345–352.


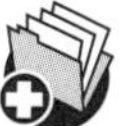

# MISCELLANEOUS

## CODES

### *ICD9-CM*

- 805.2 Dorsal [thoracic], closed
- 805.3 Dorsal [thoracic], open
- 805.4 Lumbar, closed
- 805.5 Lumbar, open
- 805.8 Unspecified, closed
- 805.9 Unspecified, open

## PATIENT TEACHING

- Patients should be educated about:
  - Being aware of progressive motor weakness and bladder/bowel dysfunction
  - The natural history of the condition

## FAQ

- Q. Who should care for patients with a thoracolumbar spine fracture dislocation and a major neurologic injury?
  - A. Patients benefit from a multidisciplinary team composed of orthopaedic surgeons, neurosurgeons, physiatrists, counselors, and others. Many complications may develop, requiring meticulous care.

T

# THUMB ARTHRITIS

*Darryl B. Thomas, MD*
*Dawn M. LaPorte, MD*

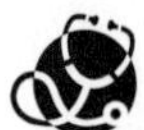

## BASICS

### DESCRIPTION

- Degenerative joint disease commonly presents in the hand and is associated with pain, swelling, loss of motion, and, later, deformity.
- Frequently, the thumb is the earliest site of involvement, with the CMC joint affected 1st, especially in osteoarthritis.
- The 1st CMC joint is considered the most important joint of the hand.
- Thumb arthritis, which may be unilateral or bilateral, occurs as commonly in the nondominant hand as in the dominant one.
- It generally affects more females than males (1).
- Various forms of arthritis affect the thumb, including:
  - Osteoarthritis
  - Rheumatoid arthritis
  - Gout

### EPIDEMIOLOGY

#### *Incidence*

The incidence is highest in persons ≥55 years old.

### RISK FACTORS

Increased body mass index (1)

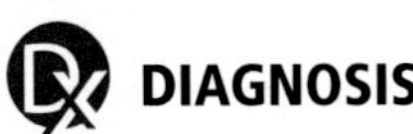

## DIAGNOSIS

### SIGNS AND SYMPTOMS

- Joint pain
- Warmth
- Swelling
- Stiffness
- Crepitus
- Triggering (catching of tendon, with snapping and locking), most noticeably during activities such as pinching and grabbing

#### *Physical Exam*

- Perform a careful and thorough examination of the hand and thumb, with attention to ROM of the joints (CMC, MCP, IP) and associated swelling, erythema, and soft-tissue masses.
- Test for "snuffbox" tenderness and tendinitis (Finkelstein test).

### TESTS

#### *Lab*

No serum laboratory tests are needed.

#### *Imaging*

Plain radiographs reveal a loss of joint space, sclerosis, spur formation, and subchondral cysts.

#### *Pathological Findings*

- Rheumatoid arthritis: Hypertrophic synovitis that eventually destroys joint cartilage, compresses or disrupts tendons, compresses adjacent nerves, and dislocates and erodes the joint
- Osteoarthritis: Loss of articular cartilage associated with spur formation and loss of motion, but not associated with tendon ruptures or triggering as frequently as in rheumatoid arthritis

### DIFFERENTIAL DIAGNOSIS

- Ligamentous injuries
- Tendon injuries (e.g., de Quervain tenosynovitis)
- Scaphoid fractures

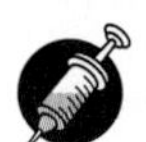

## TREATMENT

### GENERAL MEASURES

- Supportive measures include rest, heat, analgesics, splint immobilization, and NSAIDs.
- Intra-articular corticosteroid injections may be helpful during flare-ups.
- Activity limitation or modification
- Rheumatologic or orthopaedic consultation for those with symptoms refractory to nonoperative management

### SPECIAL THERAPY

#### *Physical Therapy*

- A hand therapist can fashion a splint to immobilize the thumb while preserving wrist ROM.
- Therapy often is helpful after surgery to reduce swelling and regain motion and function.

### MEDICATION (DRUGS)

- NSAIDs
- Intra-articular steroid injection, although not shown to be effective versus placebo in CMC arthritis (2)

### SURGERY

- MCP joint:
  - Early surgical treatment may involve synovectomy of the joint and tendon advancement or tendon transfer.
  - If the joint is grossly unstable, or the articular surface is destroyed, arthrodesis (fusion) may be indicated.
- CMC joint:
  - Treatment may involve arthroplasty, consisting of resection of the trapezium and replacement with the patient's own tendon.
  - If arthroplasty fails, arthrodesis may be performed.

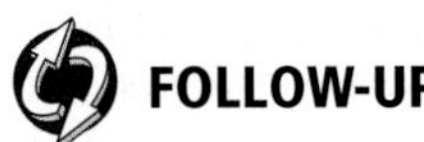

## FOLLOW-UP

### PROGNOSIS

- The prognosis is fairly good.
- Arthrodesis is the most reliable pain relief procedure, but it results in permanent limited motion.
- Interpositional tendon arthroplasty is the most common and overall most effective procedure for CMC arthritis.
  - Patients enjoy decreased pain and improved quality of life (3).

### COMPLICATIONS

- Surgery may be complicated by:
  - Damage to the radial sensory nerve
  - Wound infection
  - Nonunion
  - Chronic subluxation
  - An unstable joint

### PATIENT MONITORING

Patients must be followed at 4–12-week intervals for assessment of function and for detecting postoperative wound complications.

### REFERENCES

1. Haara MM, Heliovaara M, Kroger H, et al. Osteoarthritis in the carpometacarpal joint of the thumb. Prevalence and associations with disability and mortality. *J Bone Joint Surg* 2004;86A: 1452–1457.
2. Meenagh GK, Patton J, Kynes C, et al. A randomised controlled trial of intra-articular corticosteroid injection of the carpometacarpal joint of the thumb in osteoarthritis. *Ann Rheum Dis* 2004;63:1260–1263.
3. Angst F, John M, Goldhahn J, et al. Comprehensive assessment of clinical outcome and quality of life after resection interposition arthroplasty of the thumb saddle joint. *Arthritis Rheum* 2005;53:205–213.

### ADDITIONAL READING

- Siegel D, Jupiter JB. Osteoarthritis of the hand and wrist. In: Jupiter JB, ed. *Flynn's Hand Surgery*, 4th ed. Baltimore: Williams & Wilkins, 1991:407–417.
- Tomaino MM, King J, Leit M. Thumb basal joint arthritis. In: Green DP, Hotchkiss RN, Pederson WC, et al. eds. *Green's Operative Hand Surgery*, 5th ed. Philadelphia: Elsevier Churchill Livingstone, 2005: 461–485.

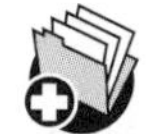

## MISCELLANEOUS

### CODES

#### *ICD9-CM*

716.95 Arthritic hand

### FAQ

- Q: How is thumb arthritis diagnosed?
  - A: Patients present with complaints of pain and possibly deformity. They are tender over the affected joint(s) and may have limited ROM and crepitus at the joint with motion. The diagnosis is confirmed with plain radiographs showing decreased joint space and possibly sclerosis, osteophyte formation, and/or cystic change.
- Q: How is thumb CMC arthritis treated?
  - A: The 1st line of treatment is with splint immobilization and anti-inflammatory medication. The splint used is a hand-based thumb-keeper splint and is to be worn as much as possible during daily activity. If symptoms persist, a corticosteroid injection may be helpful. For patients with persistent or recurrent severe pain, surgical treatment is warranted, using CMC arthroplasty and tendon interposition.

# THUMB LIGAMENT INJURIES

Dawn M. LaPorte, MD
Darryl B. Thomas, MD

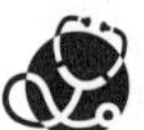

## BASICS

### DESCRIPTION

- Thumb ligament injuries most commonly involve an incomplete or complete rupture of the UCL resulting from a forced radial deviation (abduction).
- The RCL also can be injured, but it occurs less commonly.
- Thumb ligament injuries occur in males and females of all ages.
- Classification:
  - These injuries are complete or incomplete, based on the integrity of the ligament and its bony insertion.
- Synonyms: Gamekeeper's thumb; Skier's thumb

### GENERAL PREVENTION

Prevention involves knowing the mechanism associated with this injury.

### EPIDEMIOLOGY

#### *Incidence*

These injuries occur most commonly in skiers and ball-handling athletes.

### RISK FACTORS

- Skiing accidents involving ski poles or falls
- Athletic activities involving ball handling, such as baseball, football, or basketball

### ETIOLOGY

Forced radial deviation (abduction) of the thumb is the cause.

### ASSOCIATED CONDITIONS

- Avulsion fracture of the tendon insertion
- Capsular injuries or Stener lesions:
  - Complete rupture of the UCL with the adductor aponeurosis interposed between the distally avulsed ligament and its insertion into the base of the proximal phalanx
  - Important to recognize but not always readily apparent

## DIAGNOSIS

### SIGNS AND SYMPTOMS

- Pain
- Swelling
- Weakness
- Deformity localized to the ulnar base of the thumb
- Loss of pinch function

#### *Physical Exam*

- Ulnar swelling, weakness, or a local palpable mass from a rolled avulsed ligament or bone fragment may be present.
- The examiner often can radially deviate the patient's thumb passively to a marked angle, as compared with the opposite, uninjured thumb.
  - Absence of an "endpoint" to joint opening is diagnostic.
  - Radiographs should be reviewed before testing for joint stability to assess for a fracture (so as not to displace a fracture if present).
- Often a digital block is necessary to complete a full examination because of pain and swelling in the acute setting.
- Surgical repair often is necessary in the presence of joint opening.

### TESTS

#### *Imaging*

- Acute injuries:
  - Plain films are necessary to rule out fracture.
  - Stress testing usually is not needed.
- Chronic injuries:
  - Radiographs should be obtained to assess for degenerative changes.
  - Stress radiographs may be helpful.

#### *Pathological Findings*

Attenuation or rupture of the UCL of the thumb is noted.

### DIFFERENTIAL DIAGNOSIS

- 1st metacarpal or proximal phalanx fractures
- 1st CMC joint arthritis
- Volar plate injury

## TREATMENT

### GENERAL MEASURES

- A thumb spica splint or cast immobilization is indicated for 4 weeks for a partial rupture, or up to 6 weeks if an associated avulsion fracture is present (1).
- For acute injury:
  - Rest, elevation, ice
  - Immobilization in a thumb spica splint
  - Analgesics
  - Orthopaedic follow-up
- For chronic injury:
  - Thumb spica brace
  - Activity modification
  - Orthopaedic surgery consultation for elective ligament repair/reconstruction

### SPECIAL THERAPY

#### *Physical Therapy*

Physical therapy is helpful postoperatively to increase ROM and strength and to assist in resuming activities.

### MEDICATION (DRUGS)

- Commonly, proper rest is all that is needed for restoration of function, although pain and swelling may persist for several weeks.

### SURGERY

- Surgical treatment in the acute setting is by suture repair.
- For old injuries, tendon or fascial grafts may be necessary.
- When crepitus or pain is present on a grinding type of joint manipulation (development of arthritis), arthrodesis (fusion) may provide the best result (check radiographs to diagnose arthritis).
- If the ligament rupture is complete and acute, primary repair should be performed.
- When the diagnosis is delayed for ≥1 month, fibrosis makes identification and repair of the ligament more difficult.

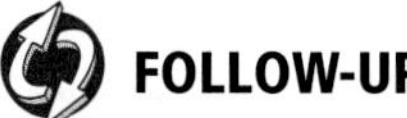

## FOLLOW-UP

### PROGNOSIS
Generally, the prognosis is good.

### COMPLICATIONS
- Chronic instability
- Nonunion of avulsed fragment
- Degenerative joint disease

### PATIENT MONITORING
- Monitoring is performed by the orthopaedic surgeon to assess proper restoration of function and stability.
- Patients are followed at 4–8-week intervals until healing is complete, with a full ROM and restoration of strength.

### REFERENCE
1. Campbell JD, Feagin JA, King P, et al. Ulnar collateral ligament injury of the thumb. Treatment with glove spica cast. *Am J Sports Med* 1992;20: 29–30.

### ADDITIONAL READING
- Glickel SZ, Barron OA, Catalano LW, III. Dislocations and ligament injuries in the digits. In: Green DP, Hotchkiss RN, Pederson WC, et al., eds. *Green's Operative Hand Surgery*, 5th ed. Philadelphia: Elsevier Churchill Livingstone, 2005:343–388.
- Trumble TE. Hand fractures. In: Trumble TE, ed. *Principles of Hand Surgery and Therapy*. Philadelphia: WB Saunders, 2000:41–89.

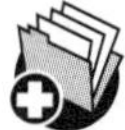

## MISCELLANEOUS

### CODES

#### *ICD9-CM*
842.10 Thumb ligament sprain

### PATIENT TEACHING
Patients should limit activities with immobilization to allow for healing, followed by removable splinting as needed while activities are resumed slowly.

### FAQ
- Q: How is a partial UCL tear treated?
  - A: Incomplete tears of the UCL are managed with immobilization of the thumb metacarpal joint for 4 weeks in neutral varus/valgus alignment and slight flexion. It can be immobilized with an Orthoplast splint or a cast.
- Q: How is the diagnosis of a complete UCL tear made?
  - A: Physical examination is usually adequate for diagnosis. The metacarpal joint is tested in 30° of flexion, and absence of an endpoint to joint opening with radial stress is key to the diagnosis. Plain radiographs should be obtained to assess for presence of an avulsion fracture, but avulsion fracture and complete tear of the UCL can occur in the same thumb.

T

# TIBIAL PLAFOND FRACTURE

*Jason W. Hammond, MD*
*Peter R. Jay, MD*

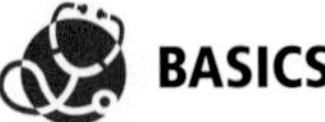

## BASICS

### DESCRIPTION

- Tibial plafond (or pilon) fractures, a subset of ankle fractures, are intra-articular fractures of the distal tibia involving varying degrees of articular and metaphyseal injury (Fig. 1).
  - The word "pilon" comes from the French root meaning "pestle" or "rammer," conveying the idea that the talus drives into the tibial articular surface.
  - The distal tibia also is known as the plafond (roof) over the talus; thus, these fractures also are called "plafond fractures."
- These high-energy, often-devastating injuries:
  - Often are associated with marked soft-tissue injury
  - Can be associated with substantial neurovascular compromise
  - Can be associated with other lower extremity, spinal, pelvic, abdominal, thoracic, or cranial injuries
  - Are associated with the population at risk for high-level trauma (i.e., young males)
- Practitioners should be even more vigilant about open injuries and vascular or tissue compromise in elderly or debilitated patients.
- Multiple classification systems exist, but the Ruedi and Allgower (1) system is the most commonly used:
  - Type I: Nondisplaced or minimally displaced intra-articular fracture
  - Type II: Displaced intra-articular fracture with minimal comminution
  - Type III: Displaced fracture with marked comminution
- The Ruedi and Allgower (1) classification system has clinical and prognostic implications:
  - Type I can be treated with splint or cast immobilization; good prognosis
  - Types II and III require surgical intervention; associated with a more guarded prognosis

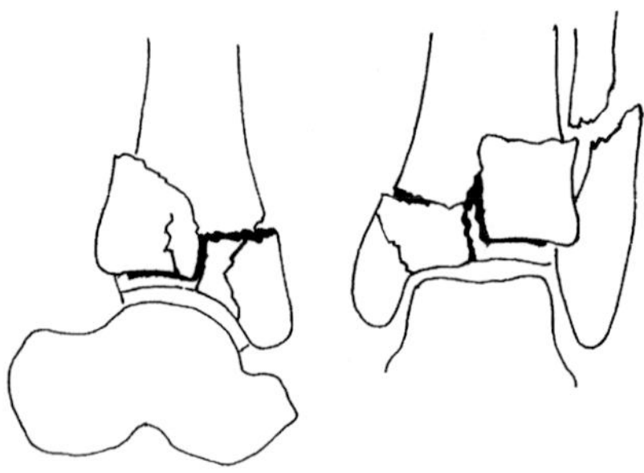

**Fig. 1.** Tibial plafond fracture.

### EPIDEMIOLOGY

#### *Incidence*

- These rare injuries are associated with high-energy trauma.
- Anecdotally, the incidence has been increasing with the advent of the automobile airbag.

### RISK FACTORS

- Individuals at risk for high-level trauma (e.g., young males, alcohol abuse, drug use)
- Individuals who work at heights

### ETIOLOGY

- High-energy injuries:
  - Motor vehicle accident
  - Fall from height
  - High-energy axial loading is the common denominator.
- Some low-energy (e.g., skiing) injuries

### ASSOCIATED CONDITIONS

Patients are at high risk for associated pelvic, spinal, abdominal, thoracic, or cranial injuries.

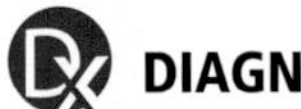

## DIAGNOSIS

### SIGNS AND SYMPTOMS

#### *History*

- Severe pain
- Swelling
- Inability to bear weight

#### *Physical Exam*

- 1st, perform a complete trauma assessment with a primary survey of airway, breathing, circulation and then a secondary survey of the head, neck, chest, abdomen, spine, pelvis, and all extremities per the ATLS protocol (2).
- Evaluate soft-tissue status, including swelling, fracture blisters, open fracture.
- Perform a careful neurovascular examination.
- Monitor for compartment syndrome.
- Use the wrinkle test: Swelling is decreased and ready for surgery when the skin wrinkles with pinching.

### TESTS

#### *Lab*

- Order appropriate tests for the level of injury:
  - Hematocrit
  - Type and cross-match
  - Urine and stool check for blood, as indicated
  - All preoperative laboratory tests necessary for age group, level of injury, and institution

#### *Imaging*

- Plain radiographs:
  - AP, lateral, and mortise views of the ankle
  - AP and lateral views of the foot
  - Tibia-fibula
  - Some surgeons find that radiographs of the opposite extremity assist in reconstruction in severe cases.
- If displacement or comminution is present, a CT scan can be helpful for surgical planning.

### DIFFERENTIAL DIAGNOSIS

- Ankle fracture
- Talus fracture
- Tibial shaft fracture
- Calcaneus fracture
- Midfoot fracture
- Forefoot fracture

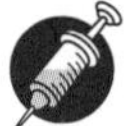

## TREATMENT

### GENERAL MEASURES

- The soft tissue often is the limiting factor, as well as the major cause for complications.
- Type I: Nondisplaced fracture:
  - Responds well to closed therapy, including a well-padded splint, ice, elevation, nonweightbearing
  - The splint can be converted to a cast when swelling begins to subside.
- Types II and III: Displaced fractures:
  - Require surgical intervention
  - Are associated with poor results and multiple complications
  - Debate continues on whether to perform open reduction with internal fixation or external fixation with or without limited internal fixation.
  - The current trend is toward external fixation with limited internal fixation because of its equivalent clinical results and lower complication rate.
  - Treatment may use a staged approach.
    - Initial treatment with an external fixator is important to prevent limb shortening.
    - Limited percutaneous fixation may provide some fracture fixation.
    - After soft-tissue swelling has decreased, the fixator may be removed, and the fracture may be plated.
  - With severe injuries, primary arthrodesis rarely has a role.

- Weightbearing is delayed until fracture union, no matter what mode of therapy is used.
- The time frame often is 3–4 months, but it can be shorter for type I fractures treated nonsurgically.

### *Activity*

Fractures should be splinted and the limb kept elevated.

### *Nursing*

- Always evaluate the neurovascular and soft-tissue status.
- Compartment syndrome checks

## SPECIAL THERAPY

### *Physical Therapy*

Physical therapy to address ankle ROM, leg strengthening, and gait after fracture healing

## MEDICATION (DRUGS)

Patients require pain medication in the acute setting.

## SURGERY

- In general, most plafond fractures are treated using a staged surgical protocol.
- Staged treatment using initial external fixation followed by later internal fixation has decreased complication rates, especially those related to soft-tissue healing (3).
- External fixation:
  - A spanning fixator is placed using calcaneal transfixion pins and tibial half-pins.
  - A ringed fixator may be used with thin wires.
  - The fibula must be brought out to length.
  - If the lateral skin is not too swollen, the fibula should be fixed with a plate.
  - The tibial articular surface should be aligned with traction and ligamentous taxis.
  - Limited percutaneous fixation should be considered to reduce the fracture further.
  - The external fixator allows the soft tissues to heal for later definitive plating and bone grafting.
- Open reduction and internal fixation:
  - Soft-tissue swelling must be resolved before an open approach to the distal tibia, which may require waiting several weeks.
  - An anterior approach often is necessary to expose the fracture and allow precise reduction.
  - Reconstruct the distal tibial articular surface with lag screws.
  - Bone graft the tibial metaphyseal defect.
  - Stabilize the distal articular surface to the proximal tibia.
  - Contoured plates are available that fit the medial or lateral surface of the tibia.
  - Modern plates allow for percutaneous subperiosteal placement and the use of locking technology.

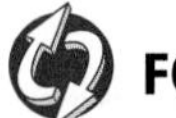

# FOLLOW-UP

## PROGNOSIS

- High-energy pilon fractures have a devastating effect on patients.
  - In 1 study at 3 years after injury, patients had decreased SF-36 scores, and 40% were not able to work (4).
  - Negative effects of the fracture can remain at the 5-year follow-up (5).

## COMPLICATIONS

- Chronic ankle pain
- Early ankle degenerative joint disease
- Need for revision operations or ankle arthrodesis
- Compartment syndrome
- Soft-tissue coverage issues
- Wound dehiscence
- Superficial wound infection
- Pin infection with external fixation
- Deep wound infection
- Osteomyelitis
- Posttraumatic arthrosis

## PATIENT MONITORING

- Patients are monitored for wound-healing problems, maintenance of fracture reduction, radiographic union of fracture, and advancement of weightbearing status.
- Patients should be treated with DVT prophylaxis after injury and while immobilized.

## REFERENCES

1. Ruedi TP, Allgower M. Fractures of the lower end of the tibia into the ankle-joint. *Injury* 1969;1:92–99.
2. American College of Surgeons Committee on Trauma. *Advanced Trauma Life Support Program for Doctors*, 6th ed. Chicago: American College of Surgeons, 1997.
3. Sirkin M, Sanders R, DiPasquale T, et al. A staged protocol for soft tissue management in the treatment of complex pilon fractures. *J Orthop Trauma* 2004;18:S32–S38.
4. Pollak AN, McCarthy ML, Bess RS, et al. Outcomes after treatment of high-energy tibial plafond fractures. *J Bone Joint Surg* 2003;85A:1893–1900.
5. Marsh JL, Weigel DP, Dirschl DR. Tibial plafond fractures. How do these ankles function over time? *J Bone Joint Surg* 2003;85A:287–295.

## ADDITIONAL READING

Borrelli J Jr, Ellis E. Pilon fractures: Assessment and treatment. *Orthop Clin North Am* 2002;33:231–245.

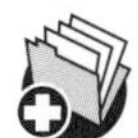

# MISCELLANEOUS

## CODES

### *ICD9-CM*

823.8 Tibial plafond fracture

## PATIENT TEACHING

Patients are counseled on the risk of posttraumatic arthritis and the risk of long-term pain and disability.

## FAQ

- Q: Is a pilon fracture more severe than an ankle fracture?
  - A: Yes. A pilon fracture is a high-energy fracture affecting the weightbearing articular surface of the ankle. Patients are at high risk for long-term ankle pain and dysfunction.
- Q: Should all pilon fractures be treated with open reduction and internal fixation?
  - A: No. Skin integrity is the overriding concern. If the ankle is very swollen, open reduction should be delayed and the ankle treated in a staged manner with external fixation and limited percutaneous fixation.

# TIBIAL PLATEAU FRACTURE

*Peter R. Jay, MD*
*Jason W. Hammond, MD*

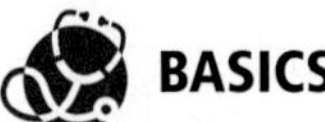

## BASICS

### DESCRIPTION

- The tibial plateau is the proximal weightbearing surface of the tibia.
  - Articulates with the femoral condyles to form the knee joint
  - Can be divided into medial and lateral components
- A tibial plateau fracture is any fracture involving the proximal articular surface of the tibia (Fig. 1).
- Classification by Schatzker et al. (1):
  - Type I: Lateral split fracture
  - Type II: Lateral split/depression fracture
  - Type III: Central depression fracture
  - Type IV:
    - Medial plateau fracture (with or without intercondylar spine involvement)
    - Represents a fracture dislocation and has the highest concurrence of vascular or neurologic injury
  - Type V: Combined medial and lateral plateau fracture
  - Type VI:
    - Fracture of the metaphysis separating the articular portion of the fracture from the tibial shaft
    - Often the result of high-impact trauma, so associated abdominal, thoracic, pelvic, spinal, skeletal, or cranial injury may be present.
- Neurovascular injury and compartment syndrome may occur with any tibial plateau fracture, but they are more common with high-energy injuries (type IV, V, and VI fractures).
- Associated soft-tissue injuries to the knee are likely.
  - Involvement of these structures may be as high as 77% for 1 or more cruciate or collateral ligaments, 91% for lateral meniscus abnormality, 44% for medial meniscus tears, and 68% for tears of 1 or more of the posterolateral corner structures of the knee (2).

### EPIDEMIOLOGY

#### *Incidence*

- Tibial plateau fractures comprise 1% of all fractures and 8% of fractures in elderly persons (3).
  - Fractures in the elderly usually result from a low-energy fall (4).
- Isolated medial plateau fractures comprise ~10–23% of these injuries (1,5).
- Isolated lateral plateau fractures comprise ~55–70% of these injuries (1,5).
- Combined medial and lateral plateau fractures comprise ~11–31% of these injuries (1).

### RISK FACTORS

- Those at risk for high-velocity trauma (e.g., young age, male gender, alcohol and drug abuse, urban environment)
- The elderly with poor bone quality are at risk for fractures from falls.

### ETIOLOGY

- Isolated varus, valgus, or axial force, or a combination thereof
- Most fractures are the result of motor vehicle accidents, pedestrian versus motor vehicle accidents, and falls from a height.
- Less frequently, fractures are caused by a skiing or bicycle accident, or other sports injury.

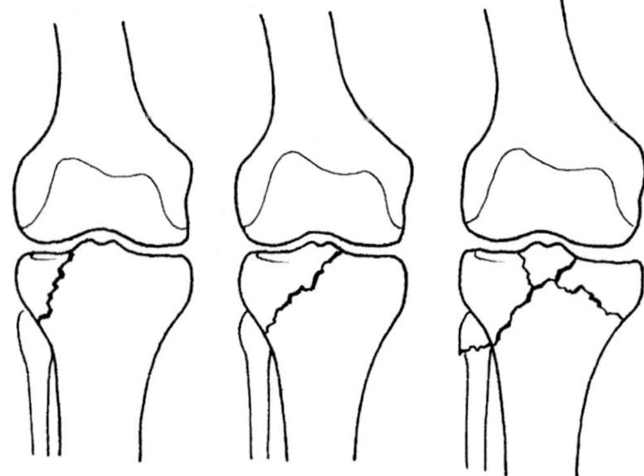

**Fig. 1.** Tibial plateau fracture may involve 1 or both sides of the joint.

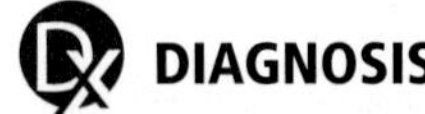

## DIAGNOSIS

### SIGNS AND SYMPTOMS

- Pain, swelling, and often deformity
- Inability to bear any or full weight
- Inability to move the knee partially or fully

#### *Physical Exam*

- The patient requires a complete trauma evaluation.
- Special care must be taken to evaluate the skin and subcutaneous tissue (open versus closed, and tissue quality).
- Perform a careful neurologic examination for nerve injury (most often peroneal).
- Perform a careful vascular examination.
  - If pulses are not equal, the arterial brachial index should be measured and, if abnormalities are found, a vascular surgeon should be consulted urgently.
  - Arteriogram and revascularization may be required.
- Patients must be examined for compartment syndrome.
- Varus and valgus stability can be assessed gently, and pseudolaxity may be determined.

### TESTS

#### *Imaging*

- Radiography:
  - High-quality AP and lateral radiographs are used to identify the fracture lines and estimate displacement.
  - Oblique radiographs may be helpful in assessing fracture lines.
- CT:
  - This important adjunctive study to plain radiographs influences decision-making.
  - Obtain scout views to ensure the images are tangent to the articular surface; cuts of ≤5 mm are recommended.
  - Helps plan surgery and assess the articular surface of the joint
- MRI:
  - Useful in identifying soft-tissue injury, including ligamentous and meniscal injury
  - Also useful for diagnosing nondisplaced fractures

### DIFFERENTIAL DIAGNOSIS

- Femur fracture
- Supracondylar fracture
- Femoral condylar fracture
- Tibia metaphyseal injury
- High tibial shaft injury
- Soft-tissue injuries, such as of the ACL, PCL, LCL, MCL, meniscus, or any combination thereof

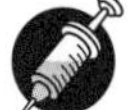

# TREATMENT

## GENERAL MEASURES

- Ice, elevation, and immobilization should be initiated as early as possible.
- A large, bulky dressing with plaster and splints or a well-padded knee immobilizer is used to prevent excessive swelling.
- Nondisplaced fractures may be treated without surgery, but they should be immobilized initially and then placed in a hinged knee brace.

### Activity

Regardless of treatment, patients should not bear weight until the fracture is healed.

## SPECIAL THERAPY

### Physical Therapy

ROM and quadriceps strengthening exercises are performed until full ROM is achieved.

## MEDICATION (DRUGS)

### First Line

Opioid analgesics usually are required for pain control.

## SURGERY

- Indications:
  - Open fracture
  - Intra-articular step-off of >3–5 mm or tilt of a condyle of >5°
  - Varus or valgus angulation of the extended knee
  - Floating knee (fracture of the tibia and femur, the knee floats in between)
- Types of fixation:
  - External fixation:
    - Bridging: The pins are placed in the distal femur and midtibia to immobilize the knee and stabilize the fracture while the soft tissues heal (temporary fixation).
    - Hybrid frame: The tensioned wires are placed just below the tibial articular surface and standard 5-mm pins are placed in the tibial diaphysis, providing stabilization of the fracture fragments (open definitive fixation).
  - Internal fixation:
    - Elevate depressed parts of the joint.
    - Use bone graft or bone substitutes to maintain elevation of articular surface.
  - Limited percutaneous fixation:
    - Use cannulated screws and fluoroscopy.
    - Can be combined with limited reduction and elevation of the joint surface
    - Can be combined with external fixation
    - Can be performed with arthroscopic assistance
  - Plating:
    - Buttress plating: Medial or lateral plates, depending on the type of fracture; use of a raft of subchondral screws to support the articular surface
    - Contoured locking plates: Available to fit the lateral side of the proximal tibia precisely; screws lock into the plate to add support; may be used to support bicondylar fractures
    - Double plating: Must be done carefully to prevent soft-tissue stripping, the "dead bone sandwich"
  - Combined external/internal fixation:
    - Initial bridging external fixation followed by delayed plating
    - Allows for rest and healing of the soft-tissue envelope
    - Favored in high-energy injuries
  - Arthroscopic-assisted fixation:
    - Allows for diagnosis of intra-articular abnormality
    - Direct visualization of joint step-off
    - Care must be taken to avoid fluid extravasation and compartment syndrome.
  - Weightbearing is delayed usually until fracture is healed clinically.
  - With adequate stabilization, surgically treated knees should start early ROM exercises.

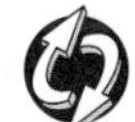

# FOLLOW-UP

## PROGNOSIS

- These fractures can be devastating injuries.
- The incidence of posttraumatic arthritis is related to the age of the patient, amount and location of initial displacement, and reduction of the fracture (6).
- In 1 series, high-energy fractures treated with a staged approach with initial external fixation had only a 5% incidence of wound problems (7).
- Patients with high-energy fractures of the tibial plateau treated with external fixation have been shown to have 5-year knee scores comparable to those of age-matched controls (8).

## COMPLICATIONS

- Skin compromise
- Infection
- Compartment syndrome may occur in as many as 10% of plateau fractures (9).
- Loss of fixation
- Malunion
- Nonunion
- Posttraumatic arthritis
- Stiffness
- Pain

## PATIENT MONITORING

After fracture fixation, patients should be monitored with monthly radiographs until fracture healing.

## REFERENCES


1. Schatzker J, McBroom R, Bruce D. The tibial plateau fracture. The Toronto experience, 1968–1975. *Clin Orthop Relat Res* 1979;138:94–104.
2. Gardner MJ, Yacoubian S, Geller D, et al. The incidence of soft tissue injury in operative tibial plateau fractures: A magnetic resonance imaging analysis of 103 patients. *J Orthop Trauma* 2005;19:79–84.
3. Singer BR, McLauchlan GJ, Robinson CM, et al. Epidemiology of fractures in 15,000 adults: The influence of age and gender. *J Bone Joint Surg* 1998;80B:243–248.
4. Keating JF. Tibial plateau fractures in the older patient. *Bull Hosp Jt Dis* 1999;58:19–23.
5. Berkson EM, Virkus WW. High-energy tibial plateau fractures. *J Am Acad Orthop Surg* 2006;14:20–31.
6. Gaston P, Will EM, Keating JF. Recovery of knee function following fracture of the tibial plateau. *J Bone Joint Surg* 2005;87B:1233–1236.
7. Egol KA, Tejwani NC, Capla EL, et al. Staged management of high-energy proximal tibia fractures (OTA types 41): The results of a prospective, standardized protocol. *J Orthop Trauma* 2005;19:448–455.
8. Weigel DP, Marsh JL. High-energy fractures of the tibial plateau. Knee function after longer follow-up. *J Bone Joint Surg* 2002;84A:1541–1551.
9. Chang YH, Tu YK, Yeh WL, et al. Tibial plateau fracture with compartment syndrome: a complication of higher incidence in Taiwan. *Chang Gung Med J* 2000;23:149–154.


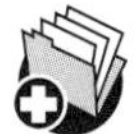

# MISCELLANEOUS

## CODES

### ICD9-CM

832.00 Tibial plateau fracture

## PATIENT TEACHING

Compliance with motion and weightbearing status is essential for a good outcome.

### Activity

- Patients should begin ROM exercises of the knee as soon as possible.
- Weightbearing should be delayed until the fracture is healed.

## FAQ

- Q: Which patients are at risk of compartment syndrome after tibial plateau fracture?
  - A: All patients are at risk. Patients with high-energy fractures and those with coagulopathies are at highest risk.
- Q: Which patients are at highest risk of vascular injury?
  - A: Patients with high-energy fractures and fractures of the medial condyle (type IV fractures) are at highest risk.

T

# TIBIAL SHAFT FRACTURE

*Simon C. Mears, MD, PhD*
*Michelle Cameron, MD*

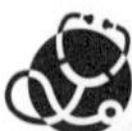

## BASICS

### DESCRIPTION

- A fracture of the diaphysis (usually midportion) of the tibia
- Classification:
  - Fractures are classified by the amount of comminution and the position of the fracture.
  - The AO system can be used to describe the fracture further (1).
  - Open fractures are classified by the system of Gustilo and Anderson (2).

### EPIDEMIOLOGY

- Can occur in any age group
- In 1 study, 76% of fractures were closed (3).

#### *Prevalence*

Fractures occur most commonly in people <40 years old (4).

### RISK FACTORS

- Motor vehicle accident
- High-impact sports
- Bumper injuries

### ETIOLOGY

- Low-energy falls
- Twisting mechanisms
- High-energy crush injuries
- High-impact injuries

### ASSOCIATED CONDITIONS

- Fibular fracture
- Knee ligament injuries
- Femur fractures
- Neurovascular injury
- Compartment syndrome

## DIAGNOSIS

### SIGNS AND SYMPTOMS

- Instability of the leg at the fracture site
- Swelling
- Ecchymosis
- Pain
- Tenderness

#### *Physical Exam*

- Evaluate the knee and ankle.
- Perform a skeletal screening examination.
- Scrutinize the leg closely for signs of skin penetration or open fracture.
- Carefully evaluate swelling for compartment syndrome.
- Examine the patient's neurologic and vascular status.

### TESTS

#### *Imaging*

Obtain AP and lateral radiographs of the tibia, which include the ankle joint distally and the knee joint proximally.

#### *Diagnostic Procedures/Surgery*

If concern exists for compartment syndrome, compartment pressures should be measured.

### DIFFERENTIAL DIAGNOSIS

- Compartment syndrome
- Fibular fracture
- Open versus closed fracture

## TREATMENT

### GENERAL MEASURES

- Closed fractures:
  - Fractures that are <50% displaced, are <1 cm shortened, and have <10% of angulation in any plane:
    - May be treated in an above-the-knee cast (5)
    - The cast is converted to a functional brace after 6–8 weeks (6).
  - Fractures with greater displacement, angulation, or comminution are treated with reduction and fixation using an intramedullary nail.
- Open fractures:
  - Treated with urgent and often repetitive irrigation and débridement
  - Intravenous antibiotics are given for 24–48 hours.
  - Definitive treatment is based on the nature of the fracture and involves external fixation or open reduction with an intramedullary nail, depending on fracture severity.
- Tibial shaft fractures often are associated with compartment syndrome and neurovascular injury.
  - Closely monitor compartment tension.
  - Evaluate the neurovascular status of the limb immediately on presentation and frequently thereafter.

#### *Activity*

Tibial shaft fractures often require 2–6 months of protected weightbearing on the affected extremity.

## SPECIAL THERAPY

### *Physical Therapy*

Gait training for nonweightbearing is indicated.

## MEDICATION (DRUGS)

Analgesics

## SURGERY

- Internal fixation:
  - Placement of an intramedullary nail starting at the knee and extending to the ankle or placement of a plate and screws
  - Nails may be inserted through the patellar tendon or with a lateral or medial parapatellar insertion.
    - The method of insertion does not seem to relate to later anterior knee pain (7).
  - Nails may be reamed or unreamed.
    - Reaming of the canal allows for a larger diameter nail to be placed.
    - Reamed nails have lower rates of hardware failure and nonunion (8).
    - The term "unreamed" is really a misnomer, because some amount of reaming must be done to place even the smallest nail.
  - Plate fixation often is necessary for fractures that involve the proximal or distal 1/3 of the tibia.
  - Pediatric fractures may be treated with multiple elastic nails that can be inserted without damage to the growth plate (9,10).
  - Open fractures have lower nonunion and infection rates when treated with recombinant BMP-2 in addition to intramedullary nailing (11).
- External fixation:
  - Placement of pins in the proximal and distal portions of the fracture and reduction of the fracture and maintenance of the reduction with the external frame
  - Indications:
    - Soft-tissue injury preventing intramedullary nail insertion
    - Damage control orthopaedics in the multiply injured patent
    - Pediatric tibia fractures

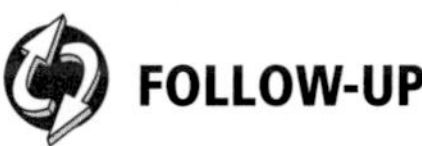

# FOLLOW-UP

## PROGNOSIS

- Low-energy injuries with displacement of <50% have a good prognosis (12).
- The incidence of complications increases and the prognosis worsens with high-energy, comminuted fractures.
- Distal fractures and those with a remaining fracture gap after fixation have been shown to have a high rate of nonunion (13).
- Open fractures have the worst prognosis and the highest incidence of complications (13).
- Severe tibia fractures with major soft-tissue injuries have a poor prognosis (14).
- Patients who smoke have a higher rate of nonunion than do nonsmokers (15).

## COMPLICATIONS

- Compartment syndrome
- Neurovascular injury
- Malunion
- Delayed union
- Nonunion
- Osteomyelitis
- Hardware pain
- Anterior knee pain

## PATIENT MONITORING

Closely monitor the patient's neurovascular status and look for compartment swelling.

## REFERENCES


1. Müller ME, Nazarian S, Koch P, et al. *The Comprehensive Classification of Fractures of Long Bones*. Berlin: Springer-Verlag, 1990.
2. Gustilo RB, Anderson JT. Prevention of infection in the treatment of one thousand and twenty-five open fractures of long bones: Retrospective and prospective analysis. *J Bone Joint Surg* 1976;58A:453–458.
3. Court-Brown CM, McBirnie J. The epidemiology of tibial fractures. *J Bone Joint Surg* 1995;77B:417–421.
4. Grutter R, Cordey J, Buhler M, et al. The epidemiology of diaphyseal fractures of the tibia. *Injury* 2000;31:C64–C67.
5. Schmidt AH, Finkemeier CG, Tornetta P, III. Treatment of closed tibial fractures. *Instr Course Lect* 2003;52:607–621.
6. Sarmiento A, Gersten LM, Sobol PA, et al. Tibial shaft fractures treated with functional braces. Experience with 780 fractures. *J Bone Joint Surg* 1989;71B:602–609.
7. Toivanen JAK, Vaisto O, Kannus P, et al. Anterior knee pain after intramedullary nailing of fractures of the tibial shaft. A prospective, randomized study comparing two different nail-insertion techniques. *J Bone Joint Surg* 2002;84A:580–585.
8. Larsen LB, Madsen JE, Hoiness PR, et al. Should insertion of intramedullary nails for tibial fractures be with or without reaming? A prospective, randomized study with 3.8 years' follow-up. *J Orthop Trauma* 2004;18:144–149.
9. Kubiak EN, Egol KA, Scher D, et al. Operative treatment of tibial fractures in children: Are elastic stable intramedullary nails an improvement over external fixation? *J Bone Joint Surg* 2005;87A:1761–1768.
10. Vallamshetla VRP, De Silva U, Bache CE, et al. Flexible intramedullary nails for unstable fractures of the tibia in children. An eight-year experience. *J Bone Joint Surg* 2006;88B:536–540.
11. Govender S, Csimma C, Genant HK, et al. Recombinant human bone morphogenetic protein-2 for treatment of open tibial fractures: A prospective, controlled, randomized study of four hundred and fifty patients. *J Bone Joint Surg* 2002;84A:2123–2134.
12. Milner SA, Davis TRC, Muir KR, et al. Long-term outcome after tibial shaft fracture: Is malunion important? *J Bone Joint Surg* 2002;84A:971–980.
13. Audige L, Griffin D, Bhandari M, et al. Path analysis of factors for delayed healing and nonunion in 416 operatively treated tibial shaft fractures. *Clin Orthop Relat Res* 2005;438:221–232.
14. MacKenzie EJ, Bosse MJ, Pollak AN, et al. Long-term persistence of disability following severe lower-limb trauma. Results of a seven-year follow-up. *J Bone Joint Surg* 2005;87A:1801–1809.
15. Harvey EJ, Agel J, Selznick HS, et al. Deleterious effect of smoking on healing of open tibia-shaft fractures. *Am J Orthop* 2002;31:518–521.


## ADDITIONAL READING


- Forster MC, Bruce ASW, Aster AS. Should the tibia be reamed when nailing? *Injury* 2005;36:439–444.
- Mashru RP, Herman MJ, Pizzutillo PD. Tibial shaft fractures in children and adolescents. *J Am Acad Orthop Surg* 2005;13:345–352.


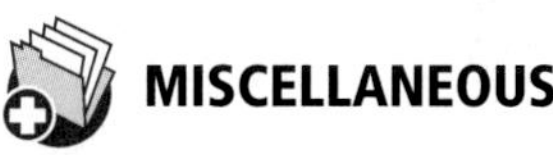

# MISCELLANEOUS

## CODES

### *ICD9-CM*

- 823.2 Closed tibial shaft fracture
- 823.3 Open tibial shaft fracture

## PATIENT TEACHING

- Patients should be:
  - Informed that tibial fractures are occasionally difficult to treat and may have a prolonged healing time
  - Encouraged to stop smoking

## FAQ

- Q: Does a closed tibial shaft fracture require surgery?
  - A: Surgery may allow for earlier weightbearing and return to function. Fractures that are well reduced have an excellent prognosis with nonoperative treatment (functional brace).
- Q: How should severe open tibial fractures be treated?
  - A: Severe open tibial fractures are treated with stabilization of fracture fragments followed by soft-tissue coverage. Amputation is sometimes necessary secondary to infection or soft-tissue injury.

T

# TIBIAL SPINE FRACTURE

*Jason W. Hammond, MD*
*Peter R. Jay, MD*

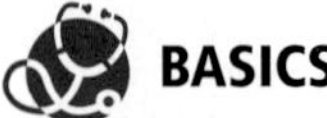

## BASICS

### DESCRIPTION

- A fracture of the tibial spine or intercondylar eminence of the proximal tibia (Figs. 1 and 2)
- Either the anterior tibial spine or, less commonly, the posterior tibial spine is affected; rarely are both involved.
- The anterior tibial spine supplies part of the insertion for the ACL.
- In the skeletally immature knee, the ACL is thought to be stronger than the incompletely ossified tibial spine to which it attaches.
  - Thus, an avulsion of the tibial spine occurs instead of a torn ACL.
  - Occasionally, midsubstance ACL tears do occur in children.
    - A narrow femoral notch predisposes to midsubstance ACL injuries rather than tibial spine fractures (1).
- Classification: The Meyers and McKeever classification (2) is based on the degrees of fracture displacement.
  - Type I: Minimally displaced
  - Type II: Displacement of the anterior portion of the fragment with a posterior hinge intact
  - Type III: Complete separation of the fragment with upward displacement and rotation

### EPIDEMIOLOGY

#### *Incidence*

In 1 study, 4 times as common in children as in adults (3)

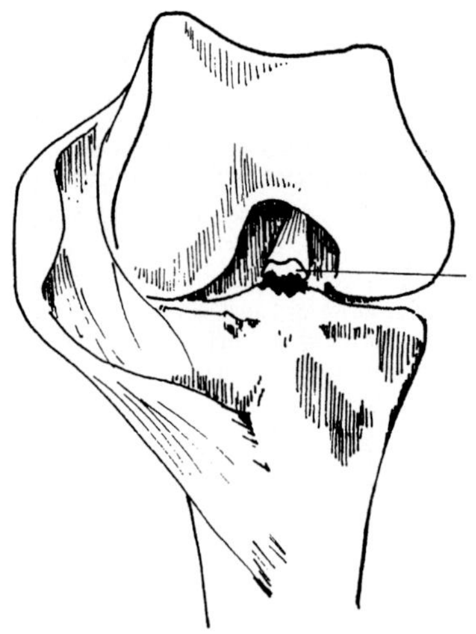

**Fig. 1.** Tibial spine fracture.

### ETIOLOGY

- Fractures of the tibial spine result from violent twisting, varus-valgus injuries, or hyperextension.
- Fractures may occur from direct contact with the adjacent femoral condyle.
- Fall from a bicycle, athletic injury, or motor vehicle accident

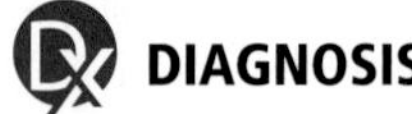

## DIAGNOSIS

### SIGNS AND SYMPTOMS

#### *History*

- History of trauma to the leg
- Ask patients about other injuries.

#### *Physical Exam*

- Pain, swelling, and effusion associated with hemarthrosis
- Reluctance to bear weight
- Lack of full extension secondary to bony block
- Gently assess for knee stability (anterior, posterior, varus, or valgus), which often is difficult to detect in the acute setting because of guarding.
- Anterior laxity may be present.

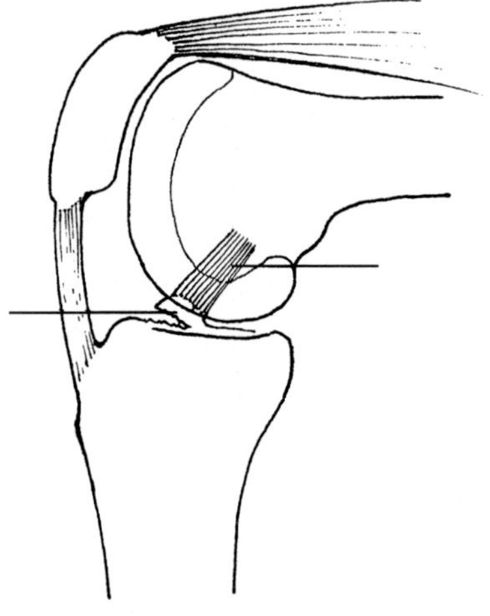

**Fig. 2.** A tibial spine fracture is best seen on the lateral radiograph and may involve only a small fragment of bone.

### TESTS

#### *Imaging*

- Plain radiographs:
  - AP and lateral views of the knee usually are adequate.
  - Findings on the lateral radiograph are the foundation of the classification system and help to guide appropriate therapy.
  - A tunnel view or a radiograph parallel to the slant of the tibia can be helpful sometimes.
- CT scanning may reveal other fracture lines or tibial plateau fracture.
- MRI: Compared with tibial spine fractures in children, those in adults have a higher incidence of concomitant injuries (such as meniscal tears) requiring surgical treatment, and MRI is recommended (4).

#### *Pathological Findings*

- An avulsion at the insertion of the ACL
- The ACL fans out and also inserts on the anterior horn of the medial meniscus, which can be pulled into the fracture site and can block reduction (5,6).

### DIFFERENTIAL DIAGNOSIS

- Isolated ligamentous injuries
- Coincidental ligamentous injuries (ACL, PCL, MCL, LCL)
- Patellar fracture
- Patellar tendon rupture
- Tibial tubercle fracture
- Tibial plateau fracture
- Isolated or coincidental meniscal injury

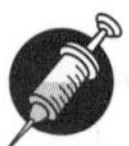

## TREATMENT

### GENERAL MEASURES

- Initial measures:
  - Ice, elevation, and immobilization should be initiated, even during evaluation.
  - If the hemarthrosis is causing severe pain, aspiration under sterile conditions helps relieve pressure in the knee.
- Type I and II fractures:
  - Treat with closed reduction and an above-the-knee cylinder cast.
    - Placing the leg in full extension or hyperextension reduces the fragment.
    - The leg should be immobilized in a position between full extension and 10° of flexion.
    - The length of immobilization is 4–6 weeks.
- Type III fractures:
  - Fractures should be reduced and immobilized.
  - Surgical treatment is recommended for most fractures to ensure reduction (7).

***Activity***
Patients may bear weight with the leg immobilized in extension.

**SPECIAL THERAPY**
***Physical Therapy***
Physical therapy should begin after immobilization to work at ROM and strengthening of the leg.

**MEDICATION (DRUGS)**
***First Line***
Pain medications should be given as needed after fracture.

**SURGERY**
- Indicated for fractures that are not reduced.
- Some clinicians have recommended surgical treatment for all type III tibial spine fractures.
- Surgery can be accomplished via an open or arthroscopic approach.
  - The arthroscopic approach has become more popular.
- Fractures should be reduced, and reduction should be maintained with internal fixation.
  - Sometimes reduction requires the removal of interfracture soft tissue.
- Fixation can be with a screw or heavy suture, depending on the size of the fracture.
- A recent biomechanical study has suggested that fixation with fiber wire is stronger than that with screws (8).
- In children, screws should not cross the physis unless the child is nearing skeletal maturity.

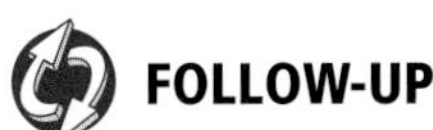

## FOLLOW-UP

**DISPOSITION**
***Issues for Referral***
Tibial spine fractures should be referred to an orthopaedic surgeon.

**PROGNOSIS**
- Functional results of both screw and suture fixation are excellent if the fracture is reduced (9,10).
- Measurement of ACL function with a KT-1000 arthrometer has shown excellent stability after fixation (11,12).
- Excessive or symptomatic knee laxity may require ACL reconstruction (13).

**COMPLICATIONS**
- Loose bodies
- ACL laxity
- Knee arthritis
- Knee stiffness
- Postoperative wound infection
- DVT

**PATIENT MONITORING**
- The patient should be followed closely to rule out fracture displacement.
- After healing, the knee should be examined for ACL laxity.

**REFERENCES**

1. Kocher MS, Mandiga R, Klingele K, et al. Anterior cruciate ligament injury versus tibial spine fracture in the skeletally immature knee: A comparison of skeletal maturation and notch width index. *J Pediatr Orthop* 2004;24:185–188.
2. Meyers MH, McKeever FM. Fracture of the intercondylar eminence of the tibia. *J Bone Joint Surg* 1959;41A:209–220; disc. 220–222.
3. Molander ML, Wallin G, Wikstad I. Fracture of the intercondylar eminence of the tibia: A review of 35 patients. *J Bone Joint Surg* 1981;63B:89–91.
4. Ishibashi Y, Tsuda E, Sasaki T, et al. Magnetic resonance imaging aids in detecting concomitant injuries in patients with tibial spine fractures. *Clin Orthop Relat Res* 2005;434:207–212.
5. Kocher MS, Micheli LJ, Gerbino P, et al. Tibial eminence fractures in children: Prevalence of meniscal entrapment. *Am J Sports Med* 2003;31:404–407.
6. Lowe J, Chaimsky G, Freedman A, et al. The anatomy of tibial eminence fractures: Arthroscopic observations following failed closed reduction. *J Bone Joint Surg* 2002;84A: 1933–1938.
7. Mulhall KJ, Dowdall J, Grannell M, et al. Tibial spine fractures: An analysis of outcome in surgically treated type III injuries. *Injury* 1999;30: 289–292.
8. Bong MR, Romero A, Kubiak E, et al. Suture versus screw fixation of displaced tibial eminence fractures: A biomechanical comparison. *Arthroscopy* 2005;21:1172–1176.
9. Ahn JH, Yoo JC. Clinical outcome of arthroscopic reduction and suture for displaced acute and chronic tibial spine fractures. *Knee Surg Sports Traumatol Arthrosc* 2005;13:116–121.
10. Hunter RE, Willis JA. Arthroscopic fixation of avulsion fractures of the tibial eminence: Technique and outcome. *Arthroscopy* 2004;20: 113–121.
11. Ahmad CS, Stein BE, Jeshuran W, et al. Anterior cruciate ligament function after tibial eminence fracture in skeletally mature patients. *Am J Sports Med* 2001;29:339–345.
12. Senekovic V, Veselko M. Anterograde arthroscopic fixation of avulsion fractures of the tibial eminence with a cannulated screw: Five-year results. *Arthroscopy* 2003;19:54–61.
13. Horibe S, Shi K, Mitsuoka T, et al. Nonunited avulsion fractures of the intercondylar eminence of the tibia. *Arthroscopy* 2000;16:757–762.


**ADDITIONAL READING**

- Accousti WK, Willis RB. Tibial eminence fractures. *Orthop Clin North Am* 2003;34:365–375.
- Lubowitz JH, Elson WS, Guttmann D. Part II: Arthroscopic treatment of tibial plateau fractures: intercondylar eminence avulsion fractures. *Arthroscopy* 2005;21:86–92.


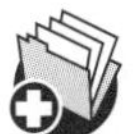

## MISCELLANEOUS

**CODES**
***ICD9-CM***
823.05 Avulsion of tibial spine

**PATIENT TEACHING**
***Activity***
- After injury, patients should be mobilized gradually.
- Nonoperative treatment requires the leg to be left in extension for 4–6 weeks, followed by a gradual increase in knee motion.
- Mobilization after surgery should be gradual and depends on the rigidity of fixation.
- Often, a knee brace is used and flexion is increased gradually over time.

**FAQ**
- Q: What is the risk of ACL laxity with need for ligament reconstruction?
  - A: With reduction of the fracture, the risk of ACL laxity is quite low. If the fracture is not reduced, the risk is much higher.

# TIBIAL TORSION

*Paul D. Sponseller, MD*

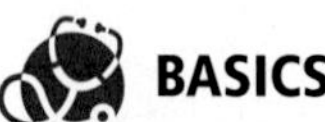

## BASICS

### DESCRIPTION

- A condition in which the tibia, along with the ankle and foot, is rotated internally or externally (i.e., inward or outward) on its axis (Fig. 1)
- This rotation is seen in the course of normal development, but on occasion it may represent a developmental abnormality.
- Abnormal values usually are described as >2 standard deviations from the mean for a given age.
- Classification:
  - Internal tibial torsion
  - External tibial torsion
  - Neuromuscular torsion: May be associated with cerebral palsy or spina bifida
- Synonyms: In-toeing (internal torsion or "pigeon toeing"); Out-toeing (external torsion)

### EPIDEMIOLOGY

- Abnormal internal or external tibial torsion as an isolated deformity is common (1,2).
  - Usually seen in infants and children <3 years old, after walking has developed
  - In general, younger children display more internal than external rotation.
  - No particular predilection for males or females has been noted.

#### *Incidence*

Persistent torsion that does not resolve is seen in <1% of children (2).

### RISK FACTORS

#### *Genetics*

- Internal tibial torsion is presumed to be caused by a combination of genetic factors and intrauterine position.
- A family history is important because the subdivision into hereditary and nonhereditary forms is of practical importance in the prognosis and treatment.

### ETIOLOGY

Caused by a combination of genetic factors and intrauterine position

### ASSOCIATED CONDITIONS

In infants, abnormal medial tibial torsion may coexist with congenital metatarsus varus or developmental genu varum.

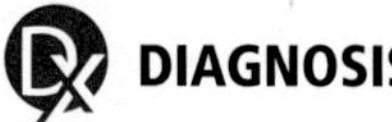

## DIAGNOSIS

### SIGNS AND SYMPTOMS

- Parents often are concerned about the difference between a child with tibial torsion and other siblings who do not have this condition.
- A parent who was treated for the same condition with an orthosis may believe that the child will require the same treatment.
- The primary concern often is the appearance of the child's legs while walking or running.
- Tripping and falling may be noticed by the parent.
- Pain is rare; parents may describe the child as having a limp, but no painful component to the gait is present.

#### *Physical Exam*

- Assess the child from the hips to the toes.
- 1st, if the child is ambulatory, observe the child's gait, which usually demonstrates the problem that concerns the parents.
  - Look for a heel-toe gait and a limp:
    - The absence of a heel-toe gait may be the initial sign of an underlying neurologic disorder (e.g., cerebral palsy).
    - A limp may explain the rotational position of the extremity because the child may be positioning the limb in a more comfortable position to avoid pain while walking.
    - Unilateral DDH of the hip may present as in-toeing associated with a limp.
  - Foot-progression angle:
    - Observe the angle between the long axis of the foot and the line of progression the child is moving along.
    - The normal foot-progression angle is slightly external, but has a range of ~15° in either direction.
- Then, the child should lie down for the rest of the examination.
  - Check the child's hips for stability in the supine position before specifically assessing for rotational malalignment.
  - Then place the child in a prone position to evaluate hip rotation and tibial torsion.
  - For proper measurement, the pelvis must remain level and stationary during the examination.
  - Note the clinical estimates of femoral anteversion and tibial torsion.
    - Femoral anteversion is estimated by the angle between the vertical axis and the long axis of the leg at the position in which the greater trochanter is the most prominent on internal and external rotation.
    - Tibial torsion can be assessed by comparing the bimalleolar axis with the position of the tibial tubercle.
  - Note the foot shape: Metatarsus adductus may be the primary cause of in-toeing, particularly in the infant.

### TESTS

#### *Imaging*

- Physical examination usually provides the information needed to form a treatment plan, but radiographs are indicated in some instances.
- Radiography:
  - If asymmetric limitation of hip abduction is present or if hip abduction in the toddler is <60°, an AP radiograph of the pelvis is needed to rule out hip dysplasia.
  - Radiographs of the feet may help to quantify clinically suspected metatarsus adductus.
  - Radiographs of the tibia are not helpful in assessing tibial torsion.
- CT is the most widespread imaging technique for evaluating femoral rotation, but this test often is unnecessary because these conditions usually can be evaluated clinically.

### DIFFERENTIAL DIAGNOSIS

- Blount disease (pathologic genus varum with internal tibial torsion)
- Abnormal femoral anteversion
- Metatarsus adductus
- Cerebral palsy
- Hip dysplasia

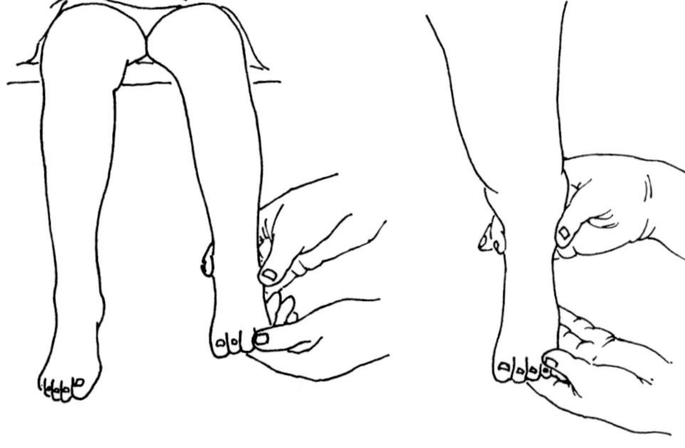

**Fig. 1.** Internal tibial torsion is characterized by inward rotation of the foot with respect to the knee.

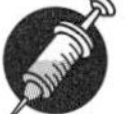

## TREATMENT

### GENERAL MEASURES

- Internal tibial torsion is the most common cause of in-toeing in children <3 years old (2).
- With increasing age and growth, tibial torsion tends toward a normal tibial position, with the lateral malleolus 20–30° posterior to the medial malleolus.
- Virtually all children born with internal tibial torsion have improvement by age 3–5 years.
- Most nonsurgical treatment consists of a careful explanation to the parents of the course of in-toeing or out-toeing in the examined child, because most rotational concerns normalize with time and growth.
- Because the use of night splints (i.e., Dennis Browne bars), braces, heel or sole wedges, or orthotics has not been proven to influence rotation of the tibia (2), most orthopaedic surgeons do not use these devices.
- In children born with excessive external tibial torsion, particularly if it is asymmetric, spontaneous correction is less common, and rotational osteotomy may be needed later (3).
- For children with excessive or asymmetric tibial torsion after age 7–10 years, derotational tibial osteotomy may be considered if the parents are concerned about the gait.
- Often, the persistence or worsening of in-toeing beyond 3–4 years of age is the result of the emergence of abnormal femoral anteversion.
- Children born with "normal" external tibial torsion usually do not undergo additional external rotation during the 1st few years of life, and the final tibial torsion stays within the normal range.

#### *Activity*

No particular modification is needed.

### SPECIAL THERAPY

#### *Physical Therapy*

- Formal physical therapy usually is not indicated or beneficial.
  - The time frame for improvement in torsion, which is measured in years, is not compatible with physical therapy.
- Some physicians advise parents to involve the children in activities for which foot position is important, such as ice skating, roller skating, track, or ballet.
  - Although little evidence suggests that these activities produce correction, such activities encourage parents to monitor the limbs and shows the child's functional potential.

### SURGERY

- Derotation osteotomy is the only surgical treatment to consider for children with rotational abnormalities.
  - However, surgery should be considered only after age ~7–10 years.
  - Before surgery, the clinician must be certain that the expected natural derotation will not correct the rotational abnormality sufficiently.
- In general, tibial rotational osteotomy seldom is needed in children <5 years old.
- In children with cerebral palsy, early surgery is more likely to be followed by recurrence of the torsion.
- Tibial derotation osteotomy may be appropriate if the thigh–foot angle remains internally rotated ≥20° or if the external tibial rotation is ≥35°.
  - However, this decision is an elective best left up to the family.
- Rotational osteotomy is performed most commonly just above the distal tibial growth cartilage and is immobilized with a cast with or without internal fixation for 6–8 weeks.

## FOLLOW-UP

### PROGNOSIS

- This condition usually is self-limiting and part of natural development.
- If the tibias of the parents and the adolescent siblings have normal alignment, the probability of spontaneous correction in the affected child by the age of 7–8 years is great (1).
- If a familial incidence of persistent abnormal internal tibial torsion exists, the prognosis for spontaneous correction is slightly lower (1).

### COMPLICATIONS

Potential surgical complications include growth-plate injuries, neurovascular injuries, nonunion, and implant problems.

### PATIENT MONITORING

Annual or biannual observation and examination are useful for documenting the expected rotational changes with growth, particularly if the parents need periodic reassurance.

### REFERENCES


1. Schoenecker PL, Rich MM. The lower extremity. In: Morrissy RT, Weinstein SL, eds. *Lovell and Winter's Pediatric Orthopaedics*, 6th ed. Philadelphia: Lippincott Williams & Wilkins, 2006:1157–1211.
2. Staheli LT, Corbett M, Wyss C, et al. Lower-extremity rotational problems in children. Normal values to guide management. *J Bone Joint Surg* 1985;67A:39–47.
3. Wedge JH, Munkacsi I, Loback D. Anteversion of the femur and idiopathic osteoarthrosis of the hip. *J Bone Joint Surg* 1989;71A:1040–1043.


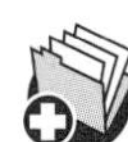

## MISCELLANEOUS

### CODES

#### *ICD9-CM*

736.89 Internal tibial torsion

### PATIENT TEACHING

- Education of the parents is of paramount importance in managing family concerns.
- Most patients with tibial torsion improve to a satisfactory degrees naturally.
- Showing a graph of the normal improvement with age may be helpful.

### FAQ

- Q: By what age should my child's torsion improve?
  - A: Every child is different. As long as improvement is seen, continued watching and waiting is appropriate. If no improvement is seen by age 8–10 years, surgery may be justified if the parents are interested.
- Q: Does internal or external tibial torsion pose a risk of arthritis of the knee, hip, or back?
  - A: No. Several studies suggest that no such risk exists.

# TOE FRACTURE

Mark Clough, MD

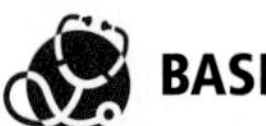

## BASICS

### DESCRIPTION

- Fracture of the proximal, middle, or distal phalanx:
  - The hallux, or great toe, has 2 phalanges.
  - The 2nd–5th toes each have 3 phalanges (1).
- Most common fracture of the forefoot (2)
- Hallucal or proximal phalanx fractures are seen with stubbing injuries, whereas distal phalanx fractures are seen in crush-type injuries (2).

#### *Pediatric Considerations*

- Often Salter-Harris injury of phalangeal growth plate
- Often a benign injury with good prognosis
- In rare cases of severe displacement or angulation, operative reduction may be indicated.

### GENERAL PREVENTION

Protective shoe wear, such as steel-toed shoes, should be worn as appropriate.

### EPIDEMIOLOGY

#### *Incidence*

Incidence is 140 per 100,000 population per year, and the Male:Female ratio is 1:6 (3).

### RISK FACTORS

- Heavy construction work
- Improper protective foot wear or walking barefoot
- Ambulating at night in the dark without proper footwear

### ETIOLOGY

- The mechanism of injury is usually in the form of direct trauma (a stubbing or crushing injury).
- The lesser toes are subject to abduction injuries such as the "night walker fracture" (3).

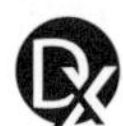

## DIAGNOSIS

### SIGNS AND SYMPTOMS

- Pain
- Swelling
- Ecchymosis
- Painful weightbearing
- Difficult ROM ambulation
- Difficulty with donning shoe wear

#### *Physical Exam*

- Tenderness to palpation
- Swelling and ecchymosis
- Limited ROM
- Angulation or deformity
- Subungual hematoma with crush injury of toe

### TESTS

#### *Imaging*

AP, lateral, and oblique radiographs of the toe (not foot) identify the fracture and help dictate necessary treatment.

### DIFFERENTIAL DIAGNOSIS

- Contusion
- DIP joint sprain
- PIP joint sprain
- Joint dislocation

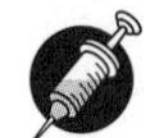

## TREATMENT

### GENERAL MEASURES

- Closed, nondisplaced fractures:
  - Buddy taping immobilization and a rigid-soled shoe for help with ambulation/protection (3)
  - Rest, cryotherapy, and elevation acutely
- Displaced fractures or dislocated toes:
  - Reduction and appropriate splinting before referral to an orthopaedic surgeon (2)
- Subungual hematomas can be decompressed with hot sterile needle or electrocautery (2).

#### *Activity*

- Buddy taping and weightbearing as tolerated in protective or hard-soled shoe
  - Children: 3–4 weeks usually is sufficient (3).
  - Adults: 4–6 weeks may be necessary.
- Swelling of toe and difficulty with tight-fitting shoe wear may last 2–3 months after fracture.

### SPECIAL THERAPY

#### *Physical Therapy*

Not generally applicable or necessary

### MEDICATION (DRUGS)

- NSAIDs
- Analgesics

### SURGERY
- Open fractures should be débrided and irrigated thoroughly in addition to antibiotic treatment for prevention of osteomyelitis (4).
- Open reduction and internal fixation is recommended for displaced, angulated, and intra-articular fractures.
  - In the hallux, screws, pins, and plating may be used (3).
  - In the lesser toes, Kirschner wires or miniscrews may be appropriate (3).

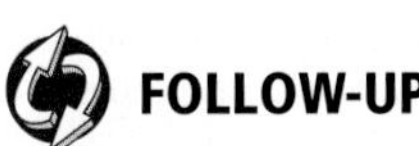

## FOLLOW-UP

### PROGNOSIS
The prognosis is good.

### COMPLICATIONS
- Malunion
- Nonunion
- Infection/osteomyelitis
- Nail bed deformity (3)

### PATIENT MONITORING
Serial radiographs are obtained.

### REFERENCES

1. Hatch RL, Hacking S. Evaluation and management of toe fractures. *Am Fam Physician* 2003;68: 2413–2418.
2. Armagan OE, Shereff MJ. Injuries to the toes and metatarsals. *Orthop Clin North Am* 2001;32:1–10.
3. Mittlmeier T, Haar P. Sesamoid and toe fractures. *Injury* 2004;35:S-B87–S-B97.
4. Ribbans WJ, Natarajan R, Alavala S. Pediatric foot fractures. *Clin Orthop Relat Res* 2005;432: 107–115.


### ADDITIONAL READING

- Sanders R. Fractures of the midfoot and forefoot. In: Coughlin M, Mann R, eds. *Surgery of the Foot and Ankle*, 7th ed. St. Louis: Mosby, 1999:1574–1605.
- Thordarson DB. Fractures of the midfoot and forefoot. In: Myerson MS, ed. *Foot and Ankle Disorders*. Philadelphia: WB Saunders, 2000: 1265–1296.


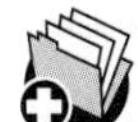

## MISCELLANEOUS

### CODES
#### *ICD9-CM*
826.0 Fracture of the phalanx

### PATIENT TEACHING
- Patients should be told to protect the injured foot with a rigid-soled shoe.
- Pain and swelling should be expected to last several weeks to months after successful fracture healing.

#### *Activity*
Typically, weightbearing as tolerated in hard-soled surgical postoperative shoe

### FAQ
- Q: What are 2 common mechanisms of injury producing toe fractures?
  - A: Jamming/stubbing trauma and crush injury.
- Q: What types of toe fractures typically require surgical treatment?
  - A: Open fractures require débridement, whereas displaced, angulated, or intra-articular fractures should be reduced and stabilized.

# TOE WALKING

*Paul D. Sponseller, MD*

## BASICS

### DESCRIPTION

- Idiopathic toe walking in toddlers is common.
- Most commonly caused by a shortened Achilles tendon
- Some of these children eventually adopt normal walking patterns with growth.
- Persistent and exclusive toe walking beyond 3 years of age should prompt an examination for underlying neuromuscular problems.
- However, most children have what is termed, by exclusion, "idiopathic toe walking."

### EPIDEMIOLOGY

Usually noted when a child begins to walk

#### *Incidence*

Common

#### *Prevalence*

Both genders equally affected

### RISK FACTORS

- Positive family history
- History of premature birth
- Low Apgar score

#### *Genetics*

Up to 50% of patients have a positive family history (1,2).

### ETIOLOGY

- Neuromotor patterning
- Shortened Achilles tendon

## DIAGNOSIS

- Idiopathic toe walking is diagnosed on the basis of the history and physical examination.
- A diagnosis of exclusion:
  - Neuromuscular abnormality must 1st be excluded.

### SIGNS AND SYMPTOMS

#### *Physical Exam*

- Examination should be made with the child wearing shorts.
- Note the position of the feet during all phases of walking and standing.
- Perform neurologic examination to detect spasticity or myopathy.
- Note the range of ankle dorsiflexion, with the knee both flexed and extended.
- Palpate the calf for any abnormal masses.
- Examine the hamstrings and adductors for tightness.
- Document passive and active ankle ROM.

### TESTS

- Additional testing is indicated only if the physical examination suggests a neurologic or myopathic cause.
- Computerized gait analysis may differentiate a child with mild cerebral palsy from an idiopathic toe walker.
  - An out-of-phase gastrocnemius complex on electromyographic analysis strongly suggests a neurologic abnormality in a toe walker.
- Creatinine phosphokinase, muscle biopsy, or mutation analysis may be useful if a dystrophic process is suspected.

#### *Imaging*

MRI of the spine may be performed if a suspected spinal abnormality is causing spasticity.

### DIFFERENTIAL DIAGNOSIS

- Arthrogryposis
- Cerebral palsy
- Familial spastic paraparesis
- Muscular dystrophy
- Tethered cord syndrome
- Charcot-Marie-Tooth disease

## TREATMENT

### GENERAL MEASURES

- Stretching and encouragement are the usual 1st-line means of treatment.
- Orthotics, by themselves, do not seem to be effective.
- Casting:
  - Increased ankle dorsiflexion can be achieved by stretching and serial casting, placing the foot in maximum dorsiflexion (i.e., at least 10° of ankle dorsiflexion, while allowing the normal heel–toe gait to develop).
  - The cast should be changed weekly until the desired ankle ROM is obtained.
- Initially, patients should be seen weekly for cast changes.
- Night braces with the ankle in maximal dorsiflexion may be helpful for maintaining the dorsiflexion achieved with casting or surgery.

### SPECIAL THERAPY

#### *Physical Therapy*

- Passive and active ROM exercise of the ankles may be used to treat patients with mild cases (3).
- If the ROM of the ankle allows some dorsiflexion, teaching children to practice walking on the heels may help to enforce a normal gait pattern (3).

### SURGERY

- If other methods fail, Z-lengthening of the Achilles tendon can improve ankle dorsiflexion.
  - May be done through percutaneous or open methods (1,3)
  - Usually performed if a child does not adopt a normal gait pattern by the start of school years

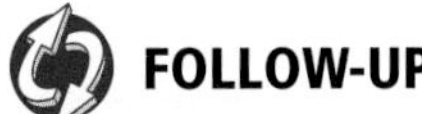

## FOLLOW-UP

### DISPOSITION

#### *Issues for Referral*

- Toe walking begins *de novo* after a period of normal heel–toe gait.
- A child does not improve by the start of kindergarten.
- Patients should be referred to a pediatric orthopaedic surgeon if possible.

### PROGNOSIS

- Many idiopathic toe walkers develop a normal gait by the age of 3 years.
- Persistent toe-strike gait into maturity may cause problems with metatarsal callous formation and impaired balance.

### COMPLICATIONS

- Undiagnosed neurologic abnormality
- Overlengthening of the heel cord
- Recurrence

### REFERENCES

1. Hemo Y, Macdessi SJ, Pierce RA, et al. Outcome of patients after Achilles tendon lengthening for treatment of idiopathic toe walking. *J Pediatr Orthop* 2006;26:336–340.
2. Kalen V, Adler N, Bleck EE. Electromyography of idiopathic toe walking. *J Pediatr Orthop* 1986;6:31–33.
3. Eiff MP, Steiner E, Judkins DZ. Clinical inquiries. What is the appropriate evaluation and treatment of children who are "toe walkers"? *J Fam Pract* 2006;55:447,450.

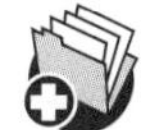

## MISCELLANEOUS

### CODES

#### *ICD9-CM*

727.81 Toe walking

### PATIENT TEACHING

- Patients and their families may be instructed to perform home heel-cord stretching exercises and heel walking at home.
- Some idiopathic toe walkers can assume a heel–toe gait with persistent persuasion.

### FAQ

- Q: What is the cause of toe walking if other usual causes are excluded?
  - A: It is likely that a subtle difference in central locomotor patterning is present.
- Q: Will a child grow out of the habit of toe-walking?
  - A: Many children will do so before the start of kindergarten. However, if the child does not, referral to a specialist is indicated.

T

# TORTICOLLIS

*Barry Waldman, MD*
*Andrew P. Manista, MD*

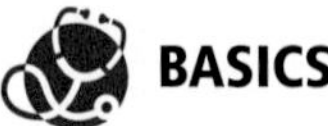

## BASICS

### DESCRIPTION
- A limitation of motion of the cervical spine that causes the head to be held in a tilted position
- May result from muscular, skeletal, or neurologic abnormalities (1) (Fig. 1)
- Classification (3):
  - Congenital abnormalities
  - Acquired abnormalities
- Synonyms: Skeletal wry neck; Congenital wry neck; Cock-robin deformity; Sandifer syndrome (torticollis resulting from gastroesophageal reflux disease and hiatal hernia) (2)

### GENERAL PREVENTION
The condition cannot be prevented, but prompt referral and treatment may preclude the need for surgery.

### EPIDEMIOLOGY
- The most common cause is rotatory subluxation of the atlantoaxial joint, an acquired condition.
- Congenital muscular torticollis usually is evident in the first 6–8 weeks of life.
- Other causes may appear throughout childhood or may become evident well into adulthood.
- Males and females are affected equally.

#### *Incidence*
- Because of the multiple causes, it is difficult to give a specific figure for incidence.
- It affects an estimated 1 per 100 to 1 per 1,000 patients (4).

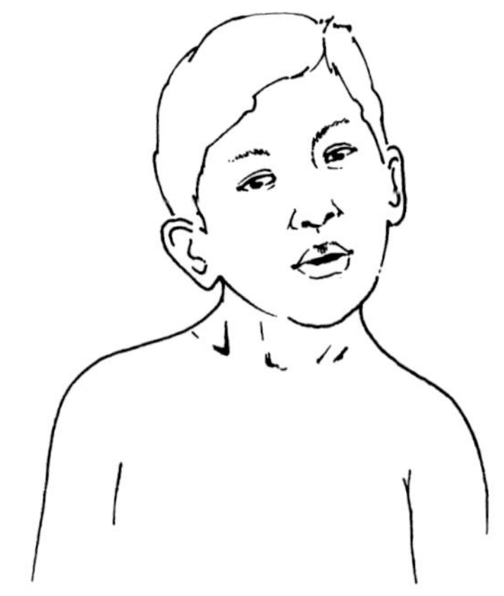

**Fig. 1.** Torticollis typically produces lateral flexion to 1 side and rotation to the other.

### RISK FACTORS
- Local trauma to the infant's neck during delivery, especially during a difficult delivery
- For atlantoaxial rotatory subluxation: Upper respiratory infection, pharyngitis, or trauma

#### *Genetics*
- Multiple congenital causes of torticollis exist, of which a few have a genetic predisposition.
- Skeletal dysplasias are the most common genetic syndromes associated with torticollis.

### ETIOLOGY
- Congenital muscular torticollis is caused by contracture of the sternocleidomastoid muscle.
- Congenital bony torticollis may be secondary to occipitocervical abnormalities.
- Acquired torticollis may result from neurogenic, traumatic, inflammatory, or idiopathic causes (see "Differential Diagnosis").
- Bony abnormalities: Atlanto-occipital synostosis, basilar impression, odontoid abnormalities, cervical hemivertebrae, or asymmetry of occipital condyles
- Atlantoaxial rotatory subluxation, the most common bony abnormality, is characterized by rotatory displacement of C1 on C2 and may be congenital or secondary to inflammation or trauma.

## DIAGNOSIS

### SIGNS AND SYMPTOMS
- Hallmark sign: Tilting of the head to 1 side with limitation of ROM
- Usually the patient rotates the head away from the neutral (straight) position, but not toward it.
- Patients may present with a neck mass (contracted sternocleidomastoid muscle).
- Neck pain is a common complaint, but it usually occurs in adults.
- Patients also may complain of occipital pain, vertigo, or dizziness aggravated by certain movements of the head.
- If torticollis persists beyond infancy, secondary asymmetry of the cranium (plagiocephaly) may remain.

#### *Physical Exam*
- The patient's head is tilted, with the ear toward the involved side and the chin rotated away, with limitation of ROM toward the corrected position.
- In some cases of muscular torticollis, a palpable mass may be present on the involved side (contracted sternocleidomastoid muscle).
- Remodeling of the head or face may result from pressure while sleeping.
- A short, broad neck with a low hairline may be seen in patients with bony abnormalities or Klippel-Feil syndrome.

### TESTS
#### *Lab*
- No specific laboratory tests, unless an inflammatory or neoplastic origin is being considered
- Ophthalmologic, audiologic, and gastroenterologic evaluations sometimes are needed if no obvious skeletal causes are seen.

#### *Imaging*
- AP and lateral radiographs of the cervical spine should be obtained for any patient with torticollis to identify bony abnormalities.
- CT is used to evaluate rotatory subluxation, dislocation, or fracture.
- MRI is used if a neurologic lesion of the brainstem or neck is suspected.

#### *Pathological Findings*
In congenital muscular torticollis, the sternocleidomastoid muscle is fibrotic, replaced by scar tissue in a nonspecific fashion.

### DIFFERENTIAL DIAGNOSIS
- Neurogenic causes:
  - Spinal cord tumors of the cervical spine
  - Cerebellar tumors
  - Syringomyelia
  - Ocular dysfunction
- Traumatic causes:
  - Subluxations
  - Fractures and dislocations of the occipitocervical junction
- Inflammatory causes:
  - Cervical adenitis
  - Rheumatoid arthritis
- Idiopathic causes:
  - Atlantoaxial rotatory subluxation or displacement

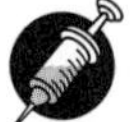

## TREATMENT

### GENERAL MEASURES
- Congenital muscular torticollis:
  - Responds to stretching exercises in nearly 100% of patients treated before 1 year of age (5,6)
  - Positioning of toys in the crib will encourage the child to stretch the involved side.
- Atlantoaxial rotatory subluxation (7):
  - Patients usually recover with physical therapy if the condition is detected within the 1st week of onset.
  - Use of a soft collar and analgesics is for patients with atlantoaxial rotatory subluxation patients.
  - Patients with recalcitrant cases may require muscle relaxants and a hard collar or brace.
  - If treatment is delayed, traction or even surgery is required.

### *Activity*

- Contact sports and vigorous athletics should be restricted until the condition has been treated.
- Specifics depend on the underlying cause.

### SPECIAL THERAPY

#### *Physical Therapy*

- Stretching exercises may be beneficial in patients with muscular torticollis or recent-onset rotatory subluxation.
- Specific instructions should be given to the therapist.

### MEDICATION (DRUGS)

Analgesics (acetaminophen, ibuprofen)

### SURGERY

- Congenital muscular torticollis that is refractory to stretching may require release of the sternocleidomastoid muscle.
- Severe atlantoaxial rotatory subluxation or other severe bony abnormality may require fusion of C1 and C2.

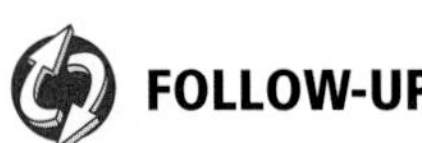

## FOLLOW-UP

### PROGNOSIS

Most cases resolve spontaneously or with treatment.

### COMPLICATIONS

- Fixed subluxation
- Plagiocephaly (in late-treated muscular torticollis)

### PATIENT MONITORING

- Neurologic status should be followed closely.
- Bony abnormalities, such as rotatory subluxation, may require repeated CT scans.

### REFERENCES


1. Nucci P, Kushner BJ, Serafino M, et al. A multi-disciplinary study of the ocular, orthopaedic, and neurologic causes of abnormal head postures in children. *Am J Ophthalmol* 2005;140:65–68.
2. Ramenofsky ML, Buyse M, Goldberg MJ, et al. Gastroesophageal reflux and torticollis. *J Bone Joint Surg* 1978;60A:1140–1141.
3. Cheng JCY, Tang SP. Outcome of surgical treatment of congenital muscular torticollis. *Clin Orthop Relat Res* 1999;362:190–200.
4. Cheng JCY, Au AWY. Infantile torticollis: A review of 624 cases. *J Pediatr Orthop* 1994;14:802–808.
5. Canale ST, Griffin DW, Hubbard CN. Congenital muscular torticollis. A long-term follow-up. *J Bone Joint Surg* 1982;64A:810–816.
6. Morrison DL, MacEwen GD. Congenital muscular torticollis: Observations regarding clinical findings, associated conditions, and results of treatment. *J Pediatr Orthop* 1982;2:500–505.
7. Phillips WA, Hensinger RN. The management of rotatory atlanto-axial subluxation in children. *J Bone Joint Surg* 1989;71A:664–668.


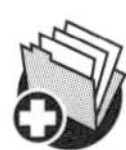

## MISCELLANEOUS

### CODES

#### *ICD9-CM*

- 754.1 Congenital torticollis
- 847.0 Traumatic torticollis

### PATIENT TEACHING

- Once the cause is known, anatomic models may be used to explain the cause of the torticollis to patients and families.
- Patients and families should be made aware of the usual course of the condition and the possible need for different methods of therapy.

### FAQ

- Q: When is congenital torticollis usually 1st evident clinically?
  - A: In the first 6–8 weeks of life.
- Q: What does a neck mass in a patient with torticollis often represent?
  - A: A contracted sternocleidomastoid muscle. However, additional evaluation may be required in some cases to rule out other causes.

# TRIANGULAR FIBROCARTILAGE COMPLEX TEAR

*Barry Waldman, MD*
*Dawn M. LaPorte, MD*

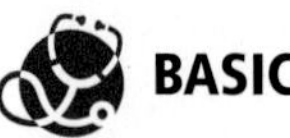

## BASICS

### DESCRIPTION
- The TFCC:
  - A group of ligaments and cartilaginous structures that stabilize the distal radioulnar joint during pronation and supination of the forearm
  - Extends from the ulnar styloid to the sigmoid notch of the distal radius
  - Central portion:
    - More cartilaginous than its periphery
    - Acts as a meniscal homolog, similar to the menisci of the knee joint
- Injury to the TFCC may result in acute or chronic wrist pain, often on the ulnar side.
- A few wrists contain a true meniscus with a free edge that can be seen arthroscopically.
- Synonym: Ulnar-sided wrist pain

### EPIDEMIOLOGY
#### *Incidence*
- Uncommon
- Peak incidence: 30–60 years of age

### RISK FACTORS
- Jobs that require:
  - Repeated, loaded pronation and supination of the wrist
  - Heavy lifting

### ETIOLOGY
- Hyperpronation or dorsiflexion of the wrist may result in a tear of the TFCC, equivalent to a distal dislocation of the ulna (Fig. 1).
- It may be associated with fracture of the distal radius or ulna or both.

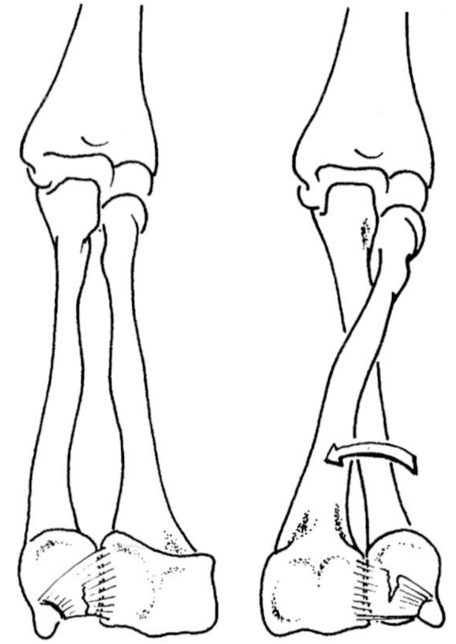

**Fig. 1.** TFCC tear may occur with forearm rotation.

## DIAGNOSIS

### SIGNS AND SYMPTOMS
- Most common complaint is ulnar-sided wrist pain, especially with repeated pronation and supination
- Clicking
- History of:
  - Hyperpronation or dorsiflexion injury to the wrist (acute cases)
  - Repeated pronation and supination (chronic cases)

#### *Physical Exam*
- Localize the area of pain carefully (e.g., use the tip of the index finger to isolate the area of tenderness precisely).
- Examine each joint of the wrist and hand for ROM and to detect crepitus, pain, or snaps.
- TFCC compression test:
  - Provocative maneuver, for which elicited pain is a positive test
  - Axially load while rotating the ulnar-deviated wrist.
  - A click may reproduce the patient's symptoms, causing pain.
- Palpate the extensor carpi ulnaris while flexing and extending and while pronosupinating the wrist to rule out subluxation.
- Assess the neurovascular status of the hand and forearm.

### TESTS
- Arthrography of the wrist may be indicated.
  - A tear of the TFCC allows dye to extrude into the radioulnar joint, which does not normally communicate with the radiocarpal joint.
- Some patients may require later injections of the distal radioulnar or midcarpal joint for full evaluation.

#### *Imaging*
- Radiography:
  - AP and lateral radiographs of the wrist
  - Radiographs of the wrist in pronation and supination may be helpful in assessing radioulnar joint instability.
  - Ulnar height should be assessed on "0 rotation" views.
    - In the normal wrist, the distal radial and ulnar joint surfaces should be at the same level on the AP radiograph.
    - Positive variance of the ulna may result from fracture or instability of the distal radioulnar joint.
- CT scan of both wrists in pronation and supination also can aid in diagnosis of instability.

### DIFFERENTIAL DIAGNOSIS
- Fracture of the radius, ulna, or any of the carpal bones
- Rupture or tendinitis of the extensor carpi ulnaris, flexor carpi ulnaris, or the carpal ligament
- Extensor carpi ulnaris subluxation
- Arthritis of the ulnocarpal, pisotriquetral, or distal radioulnar joint
- Lunotriquetral ligament injury
- Ulnar artery thrombosis
- Ulnar impaction syndrome

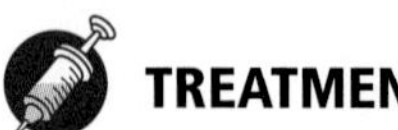

## TREATMENT

### GENERAL MEASURES
- Injury with fractures:
  - Reduce and immobilize the fracture.
  - Assess the distal radioulnar joint for reduction whenever distal forearm or wrist fractures are manipulated.
  - Acutely repair the TFCC when operative care of the fracture is indicated.
- Injuries without fracture:
  - Try nonoperative treatment with a below-the-elbow cast in neutral rotation and analgesics for 6 weeks.
  - Slowly reintroduce gentle ROM when the cast is removed.
  - Patients with continued pain and instability may require additional assessment and subsequent operative repair.

### SPECIAL THERAPY
#### *Physical Therapy*
Patients with reduced ROM after TFCC injury or fracture may benefit from stretching exercises.

### MEDICATION (DRUGS)
Analgesics are indicated.

### SURGERY
- Repair of the ruptured TFCC can be attempted arthroscopically or with an open procedure if sufficient tissue is present.
- Tears in the central area of the TFCC without instability may require arthroscopic débridement.
- Variance of the ulnar height may need to be addressed through shortening of the ulna.
- Reconstruction of the distal radioulnar joint with a tendon or band of fascia lata may be used to stabilize the joint.
- In severe cases, with advanced radioulnar arthritis, fusion of the joint (Sauve-Kapandji procedure) may be considered (1).

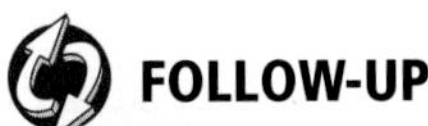

## FOLLOW-UP

### PROGNOSIS
- The prognosis is fair to good.
- Some persistent pain may occur even with adequate repair.

### COMPLICATIONS
Posttraumatic arthritis can occur, often delayed by years or even decades.

### REFERENCE

1. Carter PB, Stuart PR. The Sauve-Kapandji procedure for post-traumatic disorders of the distal radio-ulnar joint. *J Bone Joint Surg* 2000;82B:1013–1018.


### ADDITIONAL READING

- Aulicino PL, Siegel JL. Acute injuries of the distal radioulnar joint. *Hand Clin* 1991;7:283–293.
- Culp RW, Osterman AL, Kaufmann RA. Wrist arthroscopy: Operative procedures. In: Green DP, Hotchkiss RN, Pederson WC, et al., eds. *Green's Operative Hand Surgery*, 5th ed. Philadelphia: Elsevier Churchill Livingstone, 2005:781–803.
- Shih JT, Lee HM, Tan CM. Early isolated TFCC tears: Management by arthroscopic repair. *J Trauma* 2002;53:922–927.


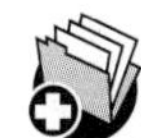

## MISCELLANEOUS

### CODES
#### *ICD9-CM*
842.00 Wrist pain

### FAQ
- Q: Do all TFCC tears need to be repaired?
  - A: Partial tears may respond well to splint immobilization and anti-inflammatory medicine or corticosteroid injection. Central tears of the TFCC can be treated with arthroscopic débridement. Complete TFCC tears and tears resulting in distal radial ulnar joint instability require repair.
- Q: How are TFCC tears repaired?
  - A: An open repair is performed for a complete peripheral tear. If the distal radial ulnar joint is stable, arthroscopic repair can be considered.

# TRIGGER FINGER

*Dawn M. LaPorte, MD*
*Chris Hutchins, MD*

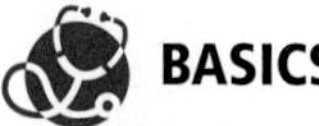

## BASICS

### DESCRIPTION

- A "trigger finger" is a manifestation of stenosing tenosynovitis that results in painful catching of the involved flexor tendon as the patient flexes and extends the digit.
- As the affected digit is slowly flexed, it snaps or triggers into a flexed position.
- Once the digit triggers, extension is difficult and, occasionally, must be obtained manually.

#### *Pregnancy Considerations*

- Incidence in pregnant females may be higher than that in the general population.
- Treat with corticosteroid injection for temporary triggering relief because it likely will resolve or not recur.

### EPIDEMIOLOGY

- Affected digits:
  - In the adult, all digits, but most commonly, the thumb, ring, and middle fingers
  - In the child, primarily the thumb
- Children (congenital type) and middle-aged patients predominate.
- The adult variety of trigger finger is more common in females than in males.

#### *Incidence*

The lifetime incidence in nondiabetic adults >30 years old is reported to be 2.2% and that in adults with insulin-dependent diabetes mellitus is up to 10% (1).

### RISK FACTORS

- Rheumatoid arthritis
- Increased age
- Diabetes mellitus

### ETIOLOGY

- A nodule usually develops on the flexor tendon, most likely in response to abrasion of the tendon in the tendon sheath.
- The nodule then impinges on one of the rings of fibrous tissue encircling the flexor tendon sheath known as the A1 pulley; the result is "triggering" when the digit is extended (Fig. 1).
- This problem is self-perpetuating because the irritation from triggering prevents a decrease in the swelling.
- In the pediatric population (<2 years old), a congenital narrowing of the tendon sheath or a nodular thickening in the tendon (Notta node) may be present, resulting in congenital trigger digit, most commonly the thumb.

### ASSOCIATED CONDITIONS

- In congenital trigger digit, an association with trisomy 13 exists.
- In the adult patient, other disorders related to tenosynovitis, such as de Quervain tenosynovitis and CTS, may be present.
- Systemic disorders that cause connective tissue abnormalities, such as diabetes, gout, and rheumatoid arthritis, also may be present.

## DIAGNOSIS

### SIGNS AND SYMPTOMS

- Sign: A nodule in the palm of the hand, just distal to the distal palmar crease
- Symptom: Painful locking or snapping of the digit into a flexed position with flexion

#### *Physical Exam*

- By gently palpating the flexor tendon sheath of the affected digit in the region of the distal palmar crease and then having the patient flex the digit, the offending nodule and/or triggering sometimes may be palpated.
- In children <2 years old, 30% have bilateral involvement (2–4).

### TESTS

#### *Lab*

No serum laboratory tests aid in this diagnosis.

#### *Imaging*

Imaging studies usually are not necessary because trigger finger is a clinical diagnosis.

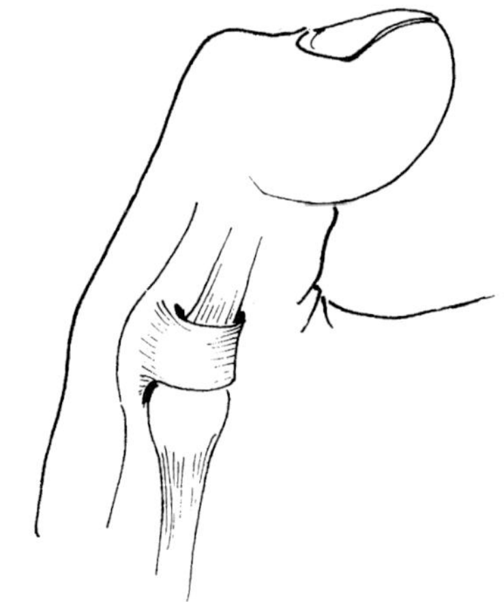

**Fig. 1.** In trigger finger, a nodule in the tendon sheath prevents it from sliding under the pulley. The finger does not extend.

### DIFFERENTIAL DIAGNOSIS

- Tendon rupture
- Contracted (ankylosed) joints
- Congenital clasped thumb
- Absent extensor
- Tumor of tendon sheath
- Loose body in the MCP joint

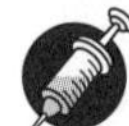

## TREATMENT

### GENERAL MEASURES

- Triggering may unlock with rest.
- In children:
  - <6 months old: 30% resolve spontaneously (2).
  - 6–30 months old: Only 12% resolve spontaneously (2).
  - Many require surgical intervention, which is recommended before 4 years of age to prevent permanent contracture of the IP joint (5)
- In adults: Corticosteroid injection is 1st line of treatment.
- When nonoperative therapy fails, surgical incision of the A1 pulley has a 98% cure rate.
- No restrictions are placed on activity after injection.

### SPECIAL THERAPY

#### *Physical Therapy*

None is needed.

### MEDICATION (DRUGS)

#### *First Line*

- In adults, treatment commences with injection of the tendon sheath (but not the tendon) with lidocaine and cortisone in the region of the A1 pulley.
  - A single injection results in a 44–93% success rate (6–8).
  - The use of >3 injections has a 77–88% success rate (6–8).

### SURGERY

- A small transverse or oblique incision is made in the region of the A1 pulley (just distal to the distal transverse palmar crease) and overlying the affected flexor tendon.
- The A1 pulley is incised.
- After surgical release, the hand is bandaged for several days.
- Activity is resumed gradually.

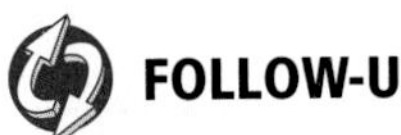

## FOLLOW-UP

### PROGNOSIS
The prognosis is good.

### COMPLICATIONS
- Errant injections may result in damage to the tendon or digital nerves and vasculature, but these complications are rare.
- Surgical risks include digital nerve laceration, tendon rupture, infection, and reflex sympathetic dystrophy.

### PATIENT MONITORING
None is necessary after surgical release.

### REFERENCES

1. Stahl S, Kanter Y, Karnielli E. Outcome of trigger finger treatment in diabetes. *J Diabet Complications* 1997;11:287–290.
2. Dinham JM, Meggitt BF. Trigger thumbs in children. A review of the natural history and indications for treatment in 105 patients. *J Bone Joint Surg* 1974;56B:153–155.
3. Ger E, Kupcha P, Ger D. The management of trigger thumb in children. *J Hand Surg* 1991;16A:944–947.
4. Wood VE, Sicilia M. Congenital trigger digit. *Clin Orthop Relat Res* 1992;285:205–209.
5. Wolfe SW. Tenosynovitis. In: Green DP, Hotchkiss RN, Pederson WC, et al, eds. *Green's Operative Hand Surgery*, 5th ed. Philadelphia: Elsevier Churchill Livingstone, 2005:2137–2159.
6. Freiberg A, Mulholland RS, Levine R. Nonoperative treatment of trigger fingers and thumbs. *J Hand Surg* 1989;14A:553–558.
7. Griggs SM, Weiss APC, Lane LB, et al. Treatment of trigger finger in patients with diabetes mellitus. *J Hand Surg* 1995;20A:787–789.
8. Rhoades CE, Gelberman RH, Manjarris JF. Stenosing tenosynovitis of the fingers and thumb. Results of a prospective trial of steroid injection and splinting. *Clin Orthop Relat Res* 1984;190: 236–238.


### ADDITIONAL READING

Lister G. Inflammation. In: *The Hand: Diagnosis and Treatment,* 3rd ed. New York: Churchill Livingstone; 1993:323–353.


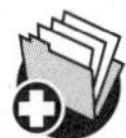

## MISCELLANEOUS

### CODES
***ICD9-CM***
- 727.03 Trigger finger, acquired
- 756.89 Congenital

### PATIENT TEACHING
Patients are advised to have surgical release for recurrent symptoms.

### FAQ
- Q: What is the initial treatment for a trigger digit?
  - A: Most trigger digits in adults can be treated successfully with corticosteroid injection.
- Q: Is trigger digit associated with any medical comorbidities, and does this affect prognosis?
  - A: "Secondary" trigger digit can be associated with diabetes mellitus, gout, renal disease, rheumatoid arthritis, and other rheumatic diseases. It is associated with a worse prognosis after nonoperative or operative management.

T

# TUMOR

*Constantine A. Demetracopoulos, BS*
*Kristy L. Weber, MD*
*Frank J. Frassica, MD*

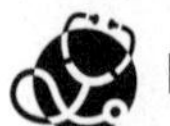

## BASICS

### DESCRIPTION

- Bone tumors can be divided into 4 categories:
  - Benign primary:
    - Common, usually in young patients
    - Most common forms: Osteochondromas, osteoid osteoma, and giant cell tumors
  - Malignant primary:
    - Rare, but more common in the 2nd and 3rd decades than at other ages
    - Responsible for <1% of deaths from cancer (1)
    - Most common forms in patients 10–25 years old: Osteosarcoma and Ewing tumor
    - Most common forms in older patients: Chondrosarcoma and MFH
  - Metastatic:
    - The most common destructive tumors encountered in adults, usually in the 4th–8th decades
  - Lesions that simulate bone tumors:
    - Uncommon
    - In children: Infection, EOG, and stress fracture
    - In adults: Paget disease, hyperparathyroidism
    - Myeloma and lymphoma are common malignancies that occur in bone but are not of mesenchymal origin.
    - Soft-tissue tumors are benign or malignant and rarely metastasize to bone.
    - Although primary soft-tissue sarcomas are twice as common as all bone sarcomas combined, together they constitute <1% of all cancer deaths (1).

### EPIDEMIOLOGY

#### *Incidence*

- 3,000 bone sarcomas per year (1)
- 9,000 soft-tissue sarcomas per year (1)

### RISK FACTORS

#### *Genetics*

Ewing tumor is associated with translocation t(11;22)(q24;q12) (2).

### ASSOCIATED CONDITIONS

- Conditions in which bone malignancies may develop:
  - Multiple hereditary exostoses
  - Solitary osteochondroma
  - Paget disease
  - Bone infarcts

## DIAGNOSIS

### SIGNS AND SYMPTOMS

- Pain:
  - Most patients with bone tumors present with musculoskeletal pain.
  - Typically, it is described as dull, deep, aching pain.
  - It often becomes constant and occurs at night.
- Swelling
- Loss of function at the involved site
- Weight loss occurs with metastatic disease.
- Acute symptoms of a pathologic fracture: In up to 5–10% of patients, pathologic fracture is the 1st evidence of the underlying disease (2).
- Soft-tissue tumors:
  - More common than bone tumors
  - Patients may present with a small lump or a large mass.
  - The lesion often enlarges and may be painful or painless.

#### *Physical Exam*

- Perform a complete musculoskeletal examination.
- Inspect the affected site for soft-tissue masses, overlying skin changes, and adenopathy.
- When metastatic disease is suspected, examine the thyroid gland, lungs, abdomen, prostate, and breasts.

### TESTS

#### *Lab*

- These tests often are nonspecific, but routine studies should be obtained in any patient with a suspected tumor.
  - Patients 5–30 years old:
    - Complete blood count with differential
    - Peripheral blood smear
    - ESR
  - Patients >40 years old:
    - Complete blood count with differential
    - Peripheral blood smear
    - ESR
    - Serum calcium and phosphate
    - Serum or urine protein electrophoresis
    - Urinalysis
  - Biopsy:
    - Key to diagnosis
    - It is beneficial to the pathologist and surgeon to have a narrow working diagnosis at the time of the biopsy.
    - The biopsy should be done at the center where the treatment is to be given.

#### *Imaging*

- Plain radiographs in 2 planes of the affected area are the 1st imaging examinations indicated.
  - Determine the matrix characteristics (bone, cartilage, or amorphous).
  - Determine the anatomic location within the bone (epiphyseal, metaphyseal, or diaphyseal).
  - Determine the number of lesions.
  - Determine the effect of the lesion on bone.
  - Determine the bone's response to the lesion.
- A chest view also should be obtained when malignancy is suspected.
- Technetium bone scanning is indicated for clinical suspicion of malignancy in the presence of normal plain radiographs.
- A skeletal survey is indicated for patients with myeloma for whom the bone scan may be negative.
  - AP and lateral views of the cervical spine, thoracic spine, and lumbosacral spine
  - AP views of the pelvis, femora, tibiae, fibulae, humeri, radii, and ulnae
- MRI:
  - Preferred modality for screening the spine for occult metastases, myeloma, or lymphoma
  - For soft-tissue tumors, best imaging modality for defining anatomy and precisely depicting lesion

### DIFFERENTIAL DIAGNOSIS

- Based on clinical and radiographic findings
- Patient age:
  - Young patients (10–25 years old)
    - Benign: Infection, EOG, enchondromatosis
    - Malignant: Osteosarcoma, Ewing sarcoma, leukemia, or lymphoma
  - Older adults (>25 years old):
    - Benign: Paget disease, hyperparathyroidism, enchondroma
    - Malignant: Metastatic bone disease, multiple myeloma, lymphoma, primary mesenchymal tumors, chondrosarcoma, MFH
- Matrix characteristics:
  - Cartilage calcification may appear stippled with apparent rings, whereas bone may be cloudlike and may show trabeculae.
  - Cartilage-forming tumors include enchondroma, osteochondroma, chondromyxoid fibroma, chondroblastoma, and chondrosarcoma.
  - Bone-forming tumors include osteoid osteoma, osteoblastoma, and osteosarcoma.

- Number of bone lesions:
  - Indicates whether the process is monostotic or polyostotic
  - Multiple destructive lesions in patients >40 years old are most likely metastatic bone disease, multiple myeloma, or lymphoma.
  - In younger adults, multiple lytic lesions are most likely a vascular tumor, multiple enchondromatosis, or LCH (EOG).
  - In children <5 years old, multiple destructive lesions may represent metastatic neuroblastoma, Wilms tumor, or LCH.
- Anatomic location:
  - Chondroblastoma most commonly occurs in the epiphysis of long bones.
  - Ewing tumor often involves the diaphysis.
  - Osteosarcoma most commonly is seen at the metaphysis of the distal femur and the proximal tibia.
- Effect of the lesion on bone:
  - A lytic (radiolucent) lesion is less dense than surrounding bone.
  - An osteoblastic (radiopaque) lesion is more dense than surrounding bone.
- High-grade malignant lesions:
  - Usually spread rapidly through the medullary canal
  - Cortical bone is destroyed early, and the tumor may spread to the soft tissues.
  - Often, the host bone has little ability to contain the process, and it may appear diffuse or permeative.
- Low-grade malignant lesions:
  - Tend to spread slowly
  - Host bone often can contain the lesion with a thickened cortex or rim of periosteal bone, to give a well-circumscribed appearance.
  - Reactive new bone formation with periosteal elevation into an "onion skin" pattern may suggest Ewing sarcoma, osteosarcoma, or osteomyelitis.

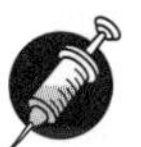

## TREATMENT

### GENERAL MEASURES

- Immediately after diagnosis:
  - Referral should be made to a musculoskeletal oncologist for proper staging, biopsy, and treatment as appropriate.
  - An improperly placed biopsy needle or biopsy incision can have a severely adverse affect on the patient's clinical course, and thus patients should be referred only to orthopaedists who specialize in tumor management.
  - A team approach to treatment includes an orthopaedic tumor surgeon, pathologist, medical or pediatric oncologist, radiation oncologist, social worker, and physical therapist.
  - For diagnosis of a malignant primary sarcoma, a pulmonary CT scan is performed to evaluate for metastases, which helps complete the staging and determine the treatment plan and prognosis.
- Treatment:
  - The diagnosis, histologic grade, and the size of the tumor:
    - Essential for determining treatment and prognosis
    - Helpful for determining whether adjunctive treatment (chemotherapy or radiation therapy) is to be given before surgical treatment
  - Options:
    - Neoadjuvant (preoperative) chemotherapy has a substantial impact on the efficacy of limb salvage and disease-free survival for patients with osteosarcoma and Ewing tumor.
    - External-beam irradiation is used for local control (Ewing tumor, lymphoma, myeloma, and metastatic bone disease) and adjunctively (in combination with surgery, for the treatment of soft-tissue sarcomas); the ionizing irradiation can be delivered preoperatively, perioperatively with brachytherapy after loading tubes, or postoperatively.

### SPECIAL THERAPY

#### *Radiotherapy*

- Used to destroy any cells that may have escaped surgical treatment
- In some cases, used to shrink the tumor preoperatively in locations where it is difficult to determine tumor margins clearly

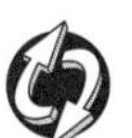

## FOLLOW-UP

### PROGNOSIS

- Depends on the specific lesions (in general, 5-year survival [2]):
  - Low grade: >90%
  - High grade: 40–60%

### COMPLICATIONS

- Cauda equina syndrome:
  - True orthopaedic emergency that can occur with metastatic tumors
  - Massive, central lumbar disc herniation with saddle anesthesia (S2–S4)
  - Bowel and bladder paralysis (unable to void, rectal incontinence)
  - Emergency MRI and discectomy or decompression needed

### PATIENT MONITORING

- The pulmonary system is monitored closely after treatment of primary sarcomas:
  - First 2 years: Every 3–4 months
  - From 2–5 years: Every 4–6 months
  - From 5–10 years: Every 6 months

### REFERENCES


1. American Cancer Society. *Cancer Facts & Figures 2006*. Atlanta, GA: American Cancer Society, 2006.
2. McCarthy EF, Frassica FJ. Primary bone tumors. *In: Pathology of Bone and Joint Disorders: With Clinical and Radiographic Correlation*. Philadelphia, WB Saunders, 1998;195–255.


### ADDITIONAL READING


- Frassica FJ, Frassica DA, McCarthy EF, Jr. Orthopaedic pathology. In: Miller MD, ed. *Review of Orthopaedics*, 3rd ed. Philadelphia: WB Saunders, 2000:379–441.
- Pommersheim WJ, Chew FS. Imaging, diagnosis, and staging of bone tumors: A primer. *Semin Roentgenol* 2004;39:361–372.
- Simon MA, Finn HA. Diagnostic strategy for bone and soft-tissue tumors. *J Bone Joint Surg* 1993;75A:622–631.


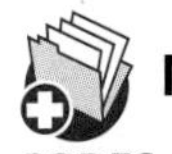

## MISCELLANEOUS

### CODES

#### *ICD9-CM*

238.0 neoplasm of uncertain behavior of other and unspecified sites and tissues (bone and articular cartilage)

### PATIENT TEACHING

Patients are apprised of the staging strategy and the treatment based on the diagnosis.

### FAQ

- Q: What are the most important presenting symptoms of a malignant bone tumor?
  - A: Bone pain at rest and at night are the most common symptoms. The pain often progresses from intermittent to constant and is not relieved by NSAIDs or weak narcotics.
- Q: What is the prognosis for the common malignant bone tumors in young patients?
  - A: Multiagent chemotherapy in both osteosarcoma and Ewing tumor has improved the 5-year disease-free survival to 60–70%.
- Q: Is a biopsy necessary to confirm the diagnosis of a malignant bone tumor?
  - A: In general, a needle or open biopsy is necessary to establish the diagnosis and to plan treatment.

# UNICAMERAL BONE CYST

*Constantine A. Demetracopoulos, BS*
*Frank J. Frassica, MD*

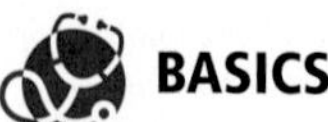

## BASICS

### DESCRIPTION

- A benign membrane-lined, fluid-filled lesion of bone that develops in childhood and fills in by maturity
- Location:
  - 80% occur in the proximal humerus and proximal femur (1).
  - Other, less common, areas are the proximal tibia, distal tibia, distal femur, calcaneus, distal humerus, radius, fibula, ilium, ulna, and rib.
  - Usually centrally located adjacent to the physeal plate or in the metaphyseal or diaphyseal region
  - Rarely, it crosses the physis into the epiphysis.
  - May also occur in flat bones
- Rarely seen in adults
- Classification:
  - Active:
    - Usually seen in children <10 years old
    - A lytic or lucent area abuts the physis and may fill the entire metaphyseal region.
    - Typically, it has a thinner cortical wall, which makes the lesion more prone to fracture and recurrence (~50%) (2).
  - Inactive:
    - Usually seen in children >10 years old
    - A lytic area is separated from the physeal plate by normal cancellous bone.
    - Typically, it has a thicker cortical wall, which makes it less prone to fracture and recurrence (2.)
- Synonyms: Simple bone cyst; Solitary bone cyst

### EPIDEMIOLOGY

All lesions are diagnosed in patients <20 years old (3).

#### *Incidence*

Male:Female ratio is 2:1 (4).

### RISK FACTORS

#### *Genetics*

No known relationship exists.

### PATHOPHYSIOLOGY

#### *Pathological Findings*

- Gross:
  - Examination reveals a cystic cavity with a membrane lining of variable thickness (2–10 mm) usually containing yellowish fluid that may be blood-tinged or frankly bloody if the fracture is recent or has been previously aspirated and injected.
  - Septa may be present with loculations of fluid, particularly with a history of fracture.
- Microscopic:
  - A membrane containing fibrous tissue and occasional spicules of bone is seen along with occasional osteoclasts, chronic inflammatory cells, and giant cells.

### ASSOCIATED CONDITIONS

None are known.

### ETIOLOGY

The origin is unknown, but suggested causes include an intraosseous hematoma, a necrotic lipoma, lymphatic or venous obstruction, or an intraosseous synovial rest.

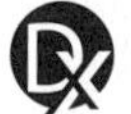

## DIAGNOSIS

### SIGNS AND SYMPTOMS

- The patient usually is asymptomatic unless fracture occurs as a result of a thinned-out cortex.
- Most cysts are discovered as a result of a fracture, which typically occurs with minimal trauma, such as throwing a ball.
- The remaining lesions usually are found incidentally.
- If symptomatic, the patient presents with localized pain and with swelling or stiffness of the adjacent joint.

#### *Physical Exam*

- Usually, nothing is detectable on examination unless the patient is symptomatic.
- With respect to recurrent fractures resulting from a unicameral bone cyst, patients must be examined for angular deformities resulting from malunion and for limb-length discrepancies secondary to growth arrest.

### TESTS

#### *Imaging*

- Radiography:
  - The typical appearance is a centrally located, expansile, radiolucent lesion with a well-marginated border in the metaphyseal region, causing thinning of the adjacent cortex.
  - The "fallen fragment" or "fallen leaf" sign indicates the presence of a fracture with movement of a cortical piece of bone to a dependant portion of the fluid-filled cyst and suggests the presence of a cavity instead of a solid tumor.
  - The cyst moves away from the epiphysis as the lesion becomes inactive (1).
- MRI:
  - May be performed if a question of a solid lesion remains
  - A bright uniform signal in the T2-weighted image is consistent with a high water content, suggesting a cyst.
  - An extraosseous soft-tissue mass never will be present.

### DIFFERENTIAL DIAGNOSIS

- Aneurysmal bone cyst
- Fibrous dysplasia
- Enchondroma
- Giant cell tumor
- EOG

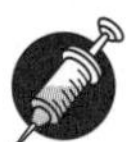

## TREATMENT

### GENERAL MEASURES

- If found incidentally, a unicameral bone cyst may be treated with observation or with dual-needle aspiration of the cyst followed by injection of methylprednisolone, bone marrow, or other substance.
- If it is discovered as a result of a pathologic fracture, the bone may be allowed to heal.
  - ~15% of fractures are followed by spontaneous healing of the cyst (5).
  - The remainder usually are offered injections.
  - Curettage and grafting rarely are necessary.

### SURGERY

- Needle aspiration may be performed by inserting 2 needles with stylets into the lesion under fluoroscopic guidance.
- Removal of the stylets and attempted aspiration will prove whether the lesion is fluid-filled.
- Proper needle placement may be confirmed with radiographic contrast agent.
- If the contrast agent cannot be injected or no fluid appears on aspiration, then an open biopsy should be performed, assuming the possibility of a solid lesion.
- If the lesion is fluid-filled: Injection:
  - It is thought that the injection may stimulate the cyst to heal.
  - If necessary, the injection may be repeated at 2-month intervals up to 3 times.
  - ~50% of patients require multiple injections (5).
  - Usually, 40–200 mg of methylprednisolone
  - Newer protocols include injecting other substances, such as marrow or bone-grafting substitutes.
- Persistent or recurrent cysts may require open curettage and bone grafting with autograft (cortical, cancellous, and bone marrow aspirate), allograft (cortical and cancellous), or injectable demineralized bone matrix.
- In critical, high-stress regions such as the base of the femoral neck and femoral head, internal fixation with a plate may be indicated.

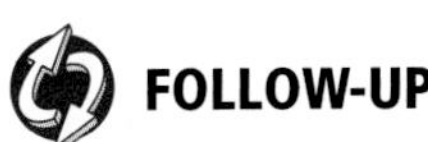

## FOLLOW-UP

### PROGNOSIS

- The unicameral bone cyst eventually heals spontaneously and fills in with bone, but it may involve recurrent fractures, injections, or curettage and bone grafting before resolution.
- Results of treatment vary with the location or size of a cyst and the age of the patient.
- Recurrence:
  - The rate of recurrence is higher when the cyst occurs in the proximal humerus than in the femur or tibia.
  - When a cyst is present in flat bones, recurrence is rare.
  - Smaller cysts have a lower rate of recurrence than do larger cysts.
  - Cysts presenting in patients in the 1st decade have a higher recurrence rate.
- Malignant degeneration of the unicameral bone cyst never occurs.

### COMPLICATIONS

- Growth arrest may occur, giving rise to limb-length discrepancies and malunions that cause angular deformities.
- AVN may occur as a result of fracture through proximal femoral lesions.

### REFERENCES


1. McCarthy EF, Frassica FJ. Bone cysts. In: *Pathology of Bone and Joint Disorders: With Clinical and Radiographic Correlation*. Philadelphia: WB Saunders, 1998:277–289.
2. Makley JT, Joyce MJ. Unicameral bone cyst (simple bone cyst). *Orthop Clin North Am* 1989;20:407–415.
3. Dahlin DC. Conditions that commonly simulate primary neoplasms of bone. In: *Bone Tumors: General Aspects and Data on 6,221 Cases*, 3rd ed. Springfield, IL: Thomas, 1978:356–419.
4. Campanacci M, Capanna R, Picci P. Unicameral and aneurysmal bone cysts. *Clin Orthop Relat Res* 1986;204:25–36.
5. Chang CH, Stanton RP, Glutting J. Unicameral bone cysts treated by injection of bone marrow or methylprednisolone. *J Bone Joint Surg* 2002;84B:407–412.


### ADDITIONAL READING


- Ahn JI, Park JS. Pathological fractures secondary to unicameral bone cysts. *Int Orthop* 1994;18:20–22.
- Rougraff BT, Kling TJ. Treatment of active unicameral bone cysts with percutaneous injection of demineralized bone matrix and autogenous bone marrow. *J Bone Joint Surg* 2002;84A:921–929.


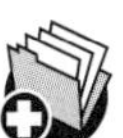

## MISCELLANEOUS

### CODES

#### *ICD9-CM*

733.21 Unicameral bone cyst

### PATIENT TEACHING

- Patients must be advised that the persistence rate is ~85% in cysts treated with observation after a fracture (5).
- The risk of refracture remains as long as the cyst is present.
  - Activity modification may greatly reduce the risk of refracture, but it may not be practical for this specific age group, depending on the patient.

#### *Activity*

- Children with unicameral bone cysts are allowed to participate in sports without restriction after partial or complete healing of the cyst.
- A risk exists for repeat fracture with heavy activities or even activities of daily living.

#### *Prevention*

- Prevention of fractures is difficult and often unpredictable.
- The clinician and parents can restrict sports activities in patients with large cysts.

### FAQ

- Q: Do unicameral bone cysts have any malignant potential?
  - A: Unicameral bone cysts can be very troublesome because of recurrent fractures, but they never become malignant.
- Q: Do unicameral bone cysts of the hip always need surgery?
  - A: Most children with unicameral bone cysts of the proximal femur require curettage, internal fixation, and bone grafting to prevent fracture and the associated risk of AVN of the femoral head.
- Q: Is a biopsy necessary to confirm the diagnosis of unicameral bone cysts?
  - A: Unicameral bone cysts have such characteristic radiographic findings that a biopsy is not necessary to establish the diagnosis.

# VERTEBRAL OSTEOMYELITIS

*Henry Boateng, MD*
*Damien Doute, MD*
*A. Jay Khanna, MD*

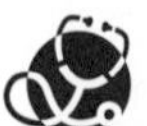

## BASICS

### DESCRIPTION
Infection of the vertebral bony elements, not including the disc space

### GENERAL PREVENTION
- Prevention of HIV and hepatitis
- Early treatment of hematogenous infection
- Postoperative wound care, including dressing changes and prophylactic postsurgical antibiotics

### EPIDEMIOLOGY
- Bimodal distribution:
  - Small peak in youth (10–20 years old)
  - Largest peak in adults >50 years old
- Increasing rates in young adults with HIV or other immunocompromise
- Males affected more than females (60–80% of cases) (1,2)

#### *Incidence*
Rare: 1 per 250,000 (1)

#### *Prevalence*
2–8% of all osteomyelitis cases (1)

### RISK FACTORS
- HIV
- Diabetes
- Organ transplant recipient
- Spine surgery
- Intravenous drug use
- Immunosuppression
- Alcoholism (3)

#### *Genetics*
No known Mendelian genetic association

### PATHOPHYSIOLOGY
- Thought to be primarily secondary to vascular spread of pathogens:
  - Most spinal infections originate from a hematogenous source.
  - The spine's large venous and arterial circulation at both endplates and body facilitates hematogenous spread (3).
- In postoperative patients with hardware, bacteria may adhere to instrumentation via glycocalyx and develop into osteomyelitis.

### ETIOLOGY
- *Staphylococcus aureus*: Most common pathogen
- *Pseudomonas*: Seen in immunocompromised patients and those with a history of intravenous drug use
- *Klebsiella*, *Escherichia coli*, and *Proteus* may be seen in patients with previous genitourinary infection and subsequent vertebral osteomyelitis.
- Postoperative infections usually are caused by *S. aureus* and have a higher rate of antibiotic resistance than do infections from other organisms (3).
- Mycobacterium tuberculosis (Potts disease) is now rare, but it can occur in developing countries and in immunocompromised patients.

### ASSOCIATED CONDITIONS
- Epidural abscess
- HIV
- Intravenous drug abuse
- Discitis
- Paravertebral abscess
- Meningitis
- Myelitis
- Sepsis

## DIAGNOSIS

### SIGNS AND SYMPTOMS
- Back pain is the most common presenting symptom.
- Constitutional symptoms of infection, including fever, anorexia, night sweats, chills
- Spinal deformity in late cases secondary to bony destruction
- Postoperative infections may show discharge and purulence from incision.

#### *History*
- Back pain: Insidious but may be acute
- Fever
- Chills, night sweats
- Irritability and fussiness in children
- Neurologic deficits may occur in rare cases.

#### *Physical Exam*
- Paraspinal tenderness and muscle spasm
- Torticollis
- Generalized weakness
- Kernig sign and symptoms of meningitis
- Hamstring spasm
- Many clinical findings of infection may be reduced or absent in immunocompromised patients.

### TESTS

#### *Lab*
- Complete blood count with differential may be elevated in 50% of patients (1).
- ESR is the most sensitive marker for infection.
  - Normal rate is 0–20
  - Elevated in 90% of patients with infection, but also elevated postoperatively and thus lacks the specificity on its own for confident diagnosis
- C-reactive protein is a more specific marker of acute infection.
  - Returns to normal 6–10 days postoperatively
  - Thus, an elevated rate for >10 days is suspicious for infection.
- Blood cultures
- Fungal cultures
- History-driven specific labs such as exposure to tuberculosis

#### *Imaging*
- Conventional radiography:
  - Changes on radiographs occur late, and initial radiographs may be normal.
  - If clinically suspicious, obtain MRI.
- MRI:
  - Best study: Low on T1-weighted scans, high on T2-weighted scans
  - Post-gadolinium images show ring-enhanced areas of signal intensity.
- CT scan: Osteolysis (3)

### *Diagnostic Procedures/Surgery*
- Nuclear medicine studies are useful in MRI-contraindicated patients (e.g., those with pacemakers)
- Bone scan
- Indium-labeled white blood cell count:
  - High false-negative rate
  - Do not use as stand-alone test.
- Biopsy: Percutaneous or open at the time of surgery (1)

### *Pathological Findings*
- Biopsy material may contain organisms:
  - Inflammatory cells
  - Caseating necrotic granulomas in patients with tuberculosis

## DIFFERENTIAL DIAGNOSIS
- Fracture
- Tumor
- Disc herniation
- Infections:
  - Typically cross the endplate
  - Tumor usually spares the endplate (per MRI).

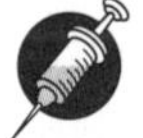

# TREATMENT

## INITIAL STABILIZATION
- Intravenous antibiotics:
  - Initially, broad spectrum until organism sensitivities are obtained, and the specific antibiotics can be administered.
- Spine immobilization

## GENERAL MEASURES
- Obtain cultures of blood and, if possible, bone before starting antibiotics.
- Biopsy is critical for treatment: Should attempt percutaneously if possible.
- Immobilize spine.

### *Activity*
- Bed rest
- Thoracolumbosacral orthotic for immobilization, if needed

### *Nursing*
- Patients may be critically ill and may require intensive care.
- Patients should be hospitalized for intravenous administration of antibiotics and for observation and management of medical comorbidities.

## SPECIAL THERAPY
### *Physical Therapy*
- No role for physical therapy in acute infection
- Increased pain postoperatively with physical therapy may be a signal of infection.

## MEDICATION (DRUGS)
### *First Line*
Broad-spectrum antibiotics

### *Second Line*
- After biopsy, culture-specific antibiotics:
  - Vancomycin for methicillin-resistant organisms
- Zosyn (piperacillin and tazobactam) for *Pseudomonas* and Gram-negative organisms

## SURGERY
- Indications for surgical management (4):
  - Failure of nonoperative treatment
  - Need for open biopsy
  - Presence of spinal abscess
  - Sepsis
  - Progressive spinal deformity
  - Refractory pain
  - Spinal Instability
  - Neurologic deficit
- Surgical treatment principles in infection are (1):
  - Adequate débridement
  - Neurologic decompression if needed
  - Rigid fixation

# FOLLOW-UP

- Continue intravenous antibiotics for 6–8 weeks.
- Follow-up with infectious-disease specialist.
- Early and progressive mobilization

## COMPLICATIONS
- Abscess formation
- Vertebral collapse
- Neurologic compromise
- Paralysis
- Cauda equina syndrome
- Untreated infections may lead to sepsis and possible death.

## PATIENT MONITORING
- Repeat radiographs every 4–8 weeks until radiographically and clinically stable.
- Follow-up ESR and C-reactive protein
- Repeat MRI if pain or fever continues.

## REFERENCES

1. Carragee EJ. Pyogenic vertebral osteomyelitis. *J Bone Joint Surg* 1997;79A:874–880.
2. Sapico FL, Montgomerie JZ. Vertebral osteomyelitis. *Infect Dis Clin North Am* 1990;4: 539–550.
3. Eastlack RK, Kauffman CP. Pyogenic infections. In: Bono CM, Garfin SR, Tornetta P, et al., eds. *Spine*. Philadelphia: Lippincott Williams & Wilkins, 2004:73–80.
4. Emery SE, Chan DPK, Woodward HR. Treatment of hematogenous pyogenic vertebral osteomyelitis with anterior debridement and primary bone grafting. *Spine* 1989;14:284–291.


## ADDITIONAL READING

Stone DB, Bonfiglio M. Pyogenic vertebral osteomyelitis: a diagnostic pitfall for the internist. *Arch Intern Med* 1963;112:491–500.


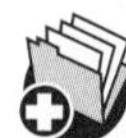

# MISCELLANEOUS

## CODES
### *ICD9-CM*
730.28 Vertebral osteomyelitis

## PATIENT TEACHING
- Early treatment of infectious processes, especially in immunocompromised patients.
- It is essential that patients complete the course of intravenous antibiotics.

### *Activity*
- Immobilization in acute phase with brace
- Early mobilization after surgical stabilization

## FAQ
- Q: Is emergent surgery indicated once the diagnosis of vertebral osteomyelitis is suspected?
  - A: The 1st-line treatment for this condition is intravenous antibiotics and immobilization. Surgery is indicated in the presence of neurologic deficit, worsening pain, deformity, or the presence of an epidural abscess.
- Q: Is neurologic compromise the most common presenting symptom in patients with vertebral osteomyelitis?
  - A: No. Neurologic compromise actually is quite rare. One should suspect possible vertebral osteomyelitis in immunocompromised or postsurgical patients with worsening back and spine pain. Appropriate imaging and laboratory studies should be obtained.

# VERTICAL TALUS

*Paul D. Sponseller, MD*

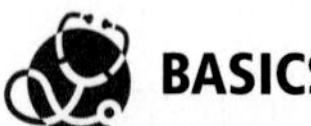

## BASICS

### DESCRIPTION

- Congenital vertical talus is an uncommon disorder, a rigid flatfoot that requires early identification and treatment.
- Its essence is a dislocation of the talonavicular joint with associated adaptive changes.
- It may be unilateral or bilateral.
- > 1/2 of affected patients have other neurologic, genetic, or connective tissue disorders.
- The deformity occurs *in utero*, but it may be 1st identified any time from infancy to adulthood.
- Classification:
  - Isolated
  - Syndrome-related
- Synonyms: Congenital convex pes planus; Congenital rigid rocker-bottom foot

### EPIDEMIOLOGY

#### *Incidence*

- Rare, but a high association with other disorders and anomalies:
  - 10% of children with myelodysplasia have congenital vertical talus (1).
  - It also can be associated with trisomy 13, 15, and 18 and with arthrogryposis or Larsen syndrome.
- In 20–40% of cases, congenital vertical talus occurs as an isolated anomaly (1,2).
- It affects males and females equally.

### RISK FACTORS

- Myelodysplasia
- Ligamentous laxity
- Arthrogryposis multiplex

#### *Genetics*

- Unknown, but probably variable
- In some cases, vertical transmission as an autosomal dominant trait with incomplete penetrance has been described.

### ETIOLOGY

- Muscle imbalance between the dorsiflexor muscles of the forefoot and plantarflexor muscles of the hindfoot cause disruption in the middle of the foot (talonavicular joint).
- Ligamentous laxity and *in utero* malposition may be causative factors in some cases.

### ASSOCIATED CONDITIONS

- Arthrogryposis
- Larsen syndrome
- Myelomeningocele
- Trisomy 13, 15, 18

## DIAGNOSIS

### SIGNS AND SYMPTOMS

- Signs: Moderate reversal of the arch and a crease on the dorsum of the foot near the sinus torsi
- Symptoms: Lack of push-off strength, painful callus under the head of the talus possible if untreated by walking age

#### *Physical Exam*

- Check the other extremities, as well as the spine, for anomalies.
- Measure strength in both lower extremities.
- Observe the foot in stance and gait if the child is walking.
- It is easily distinguishable from the more common calcaneovalgus and flexible flatfoot.
- The sole of the foot is convex, has a rocker bottom, and is rigid.
- The heel is in a fixed equinus with a tight Achilles tendon.
- The head of the talus is prominent and palpable medially in the sole of the foot.
- The hindfoot is in valgus.
- The forefoot is abducted and in dorsiflexion at the midtarsal joint (Fig. 1).
- As the patient becomes older, the appearance of the foot becomes more distinctive.

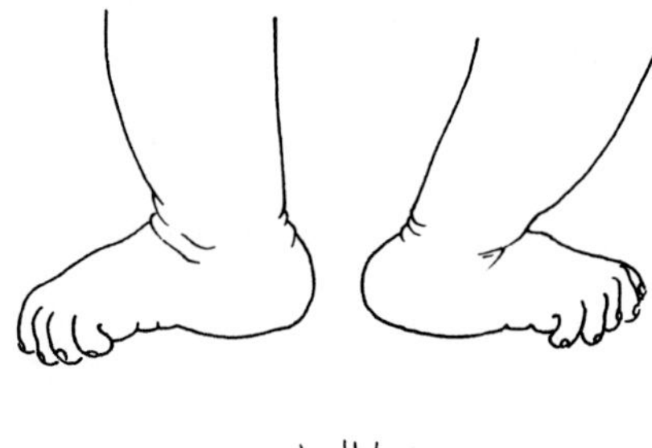

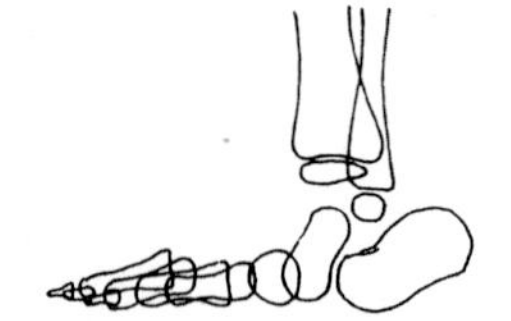

**Fig. 1.** Vertical talus produces a dorsal crease and a plantar prominence.

### TESTS

#### *Imaging*

- Obtain radiographs.
- The talus is plantarflexed (on lateral films) and angled medially (on AP films).
- The navicular is dislocated dorsally and is perched on the neck of the talus.
- The forefoot is displaced dorsally and abducted.
- The calcaneus is in a fixed equinus.
- Only the most posterior aspect of the talus articulates with the tibia and, in extreme cases, the talus is parallel to the tibia.
- The diagnosis is confirmed in extreme plantarflexed views, when the navicular will not reduce, and the line through the talar axis passes plantar to the metatarsal axis.
  - Normal is dorsal to the cuboid and in line with the metatarsal axis.
  - However, the navicular does not ossify until ~3 years of age, in the normal foot or the foot with congenital vertical talus.
  - The position of the navicular may be inferred from the orientation of the first metatarsal.

#### *Pathologic Findings*

- The calcaneus is in equinus and laterally displaced.
- The talus is hypoplastic, angled medially, and plantarflexed.
- Fixed dorsal dislocation of the navicular is noted.
- Contracture of the Achilles tendon (posteriorly) is evident.
- Contracture of the toe extensor and the tibialis anterior (anteriorly) is seen.
- Specially positioned plantar flexion lateral radiograph is helpful (see later).

### DIFFERENTIAL DIAGNOSIS

- Calcaneovalgus foot
- Flexible flatfoot

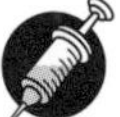

# TREATMENT

## GENERAL MEASURES

- Stretching
- Surgery
- If the condition is recognized, surgical intervention is preferred before the patient is 2 years old.
- Casting and manipulation alone usually are not effective, although they should be used preoperatively to stretch soft tissue.

### *Activity*

Unrestricted

## SURGERY

- The essential features are reduction (open or closed) and pinning of the talonavicular joint.
  - Although open surgery previously was the norm (1,3), reduction and percutaneous pin fixation with an Achilles tenotomy recently has become an accepted technique (4).
  - The associated contracted tendons (Achilles and, if needed, anterior tibialis) also should be lengthened.
  - The medial joint capsules may be stabilized, or, in children ≥3 years old, the talonavicular joint may be fused.
  - Children >5 years old may require triple arthrodesis.
- Postoperative percutaneous pins of the talonavicular joint usually are removed at 6 weeks.
- Postoperative bracing often is used for a number of months.
  - Late treatment requires subtalar fusion.
  - Recurrent deformity is treated with soft-tissue reconstruction and subtalar fusion.
- In adolescents and adults, salvage is performed by triple arthrodesis and often requires removal of a large portion of the talus.

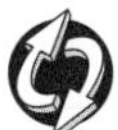

# FOLLOW-UP

Patients should be followed throughout childhood to monitor the growth of the foot.

## PROGNOSIS

If untreated, the condition produces progressive disability.

## COMPLICATIONS

- Complications of nontreatment: Callus, skin breakdown, poor push-off
- Complications of treatment: Stiffness, residual varus or valgus, need for additional surgery

## PATIENT MONITORING

Even after surgery, the patient should be followed periodically to verify normal growth.

## REFERENCES


1. Morrissy RT, Giavedoni BJ, Coulter-O'Berry C. The child with a limb deficiency. In: Morrissy RT, Weinstein SL, eds. *Lovell and Winter's Pediatric Orthopaedics*, 6th ed. Philadelphia: Lippincott Williams & Wilkins, 2006:1329–1381.
2. Ogata K, Schoenecker PL, Sheridan J. Congenital vertical talus and its familial occurrence: An analysis of 36 patients. *Clin Orthop Relat Res* 1979;139:128–132.
3. Seimon LP. Surgical correction of congenital vertical talus under the age of 2 years. *J Pediatr Orthop* 1987;7:405–411.
4. Dobbs MB, Purcell DB, Nunley R, et al. Early results of a new method of treatment for idiopathic congenital vertical talus. *J Bone Joint Surg* 2006;88A:1192–1200.


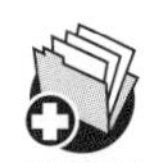

# MISCELLANEOUS

## CODES

### *ICD9-CM*

754.69 Congenital vertical talus

## PATIENT TEACHING

- Patients should be informed of the chances of inheritance in future children.
- The natural history of this condition, if left untreated, which is severe callus formation, skin breakdown, and poor push-off, also should be discussed.
- The risk of hip dysplasia should be mentioned and excluded.
- The possible need for additional surgery should be mentioned.

## FAQ

- Q: How is vertical talus commonly recognized?
  - A: By the deep crease in the sinus tarsi and the plantar convexity.
- Q: Does it resolve spontaneously?
  - A: No, it does not.

V

# WRIST ANATOMY AND EXAMINATION

*Marc W. Hungerford, MD*
*Dawn M. LaPorte, MD*

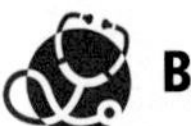

## BASICS

### DESCRIPTION

- Bones: The wrist is composed of 8 carpal bones in 2 rows (proximal and distal); from radial to ulnar:
  - Proximal row:
    - Scaphoid (or navicular)
    - Lunate
    - Triquetrum
    - Pisiform
  - Distal row:
    - Trapezium
    - Trapezoid
    - Capitate
    - Hamate
- Tunnels: The wrist has 6 dorsal and 2 volar (or palmar) compartments (or tunnels) that transport tendons to the hand.
  - Compartment I:
    - The 1st (most radial) tunnel transports the abductor pollicis longus and the extensor pollicis brevis tendons.
    - These tendons represent the radial border of the "anatomic snuffbox."
    - This compartment is a site for stenosing tenosynovitis (de Quervain tenosynovitis), characterized by inflammation of the synovial lining of the tunnel that narrows the opening and results in pain when the tendons move.
  - Compartment II:
    - On the radial side of the radial tubercle, it houses the extensor carpi radialis longus and brevis.
  - Compartment III:
    - On the ulnar side of the radial tubercle, it contains the extensor pollicis longus.
    - This compartment defines the ulnar border of the snuffbox.
    - Palpates along the length of this tendon to feel for signs of rupture.
    - It is not uncommon to find this tendon ruptured in association with rheumatoid arthritis.
  - Compartment IV:
    - Lies just ulnar to compartment III and just radial to the radioulnar articulation
    - Contains the extensor digitorum communis and the independent extensor indicis
  - Compartment V:
    - Overlies the distal ends of the radioulnar joint on the dorsum of the wrist
    - Contains the extensor digiti minimi tendon
  - Compartment VI:
    - Contains the extensor carpi ulnaris tendon and lies between the apex of the ulnar styloid process and the ulnar head
    - In rheumatoid arthritis, this tendon may become displaced in an ulnar direction or may rupture.

## DIAGNOSIS

### SIGNS AND SYMPTOMS

- Symptoms can be referred to the wrist from the elbow, shoulder, and the cervical spine, and causes include the following:
  - Herniated cervical discs
  - Osteoarthritis
  - Brachial plexus outlet syndromes
  - Elbow and shoulder entrapment syndromes

#### *History*

- Demographics: Age, handedness, occupation, avocational activities
- Previous wrist injury or surgery
- Chief complaint
- Symptoms: Onset, relation to activities, exacerbating/improving factors, frequency, duration, night/day
- Work status
- Workers' compensation status

#### *Physical Exam*

- Inspection:
  - Bilateral comparison is a useful, quick way to identify the presence of pathologic signs.
  - Because symptoms can be referred from other areas of the body, wrist examination requires exposure of the entire upper extremity, including the cervical spine.
  - The examiner may observe the patient's wrist movements as he or she undresses and determine whether motion is smooth and natural or stiff and jerky.
- Palpation of skin:
  - Evaluate for any unusually warm or dry areas.
  - Extensive localized warmth may indicate infection, whereas notable dryness (anhidrosis) may suggest nerve damage.
  - Give attention to any lesions, swellings, or scars observed during inspection.
- Palpation of bones:
  - Radial styloid process:
    - Lies lateral when the palm faces anteriorly
    - Its most prominent point lies just proximal to the wrist joint.
  - Anatomic snuffbox:
    - This small depression is located immediately distal and slightly dorsal to the radial styloid process (1).
    - Palpable and easy to visualize when the patient extends the thumb laterally away from the fingers
  - Scaphoid:
    - Lies on the radial aspect of the wrist and forms the floor of the snuffbox
    - The most commonly fractured of all the carpal bones
    - Tenderness to palpation over the snuffbox suggests a fracture of the scaphoid.
  - Trapezium:
    - Located on the radial side of the wrist and articulates with the 1st metacarpal.
    - The palpable saddle-like trapezium–1st metacarpal joint is most commonly involved in degenerative joint disease.
    - Grind test:
      - This test evaluates for 1st CMC joint degenerative joint disease.
      - The examiner stabilizes the CMC joint with 1 hand and, with the other, axially loads the patient's hand.
      - The examiner's 1st hand then moves the metacarpal base laterally in several directions, to exacerbate symptoms.
      - Reproduction of the patient's symptoms (a positive result) supports the presence of 1st CMC arthritis.
  - Capitate:
    - Largest of all the carpal bones
    - Palpable immediately proximal to the base of the 3rd metacarpal (the largest and most prominent of the metacarpal bases).
  - Lunate:
    - Lies just proximal to the capitate, in the proximal carpal row, and articulates proximally with the radius and distally with the capitate.
    - The most frequently dislocated and the 2nd most often fractured wrist bone.
    - The lunate, capitate, and base of the 3rd metacarpal are in line with each other and are covered by the ECRB tendon, which inserts into the base of the 3rd metacarpal.
  - Ulnar styloid process:
    - Can be palpated at the distal aspect of the ulna medially and posteriorly
    - A groove on its distal tip houses the extensor carpi ulnaris tendon.
  - Triquetrum:
    - Lies just distal to the ulnar styloid process
  - Pisiform:
    - This small sesamoid bone lies anterolateral to the triquetrum and sits within the flexor carpi ulnaris tendon.
  - Hook of the hamate:
    - Located slightly dorsal and radial to the pisiform
    - Forms the lateral (radial) border of the tunnel of Guyon, which encompasses the ulnar nerve and artery; the medial border of the tunnel of Guyon is the pisiform.
  - Finkelstein test:
    - This test evaluates specifically for stenosing tenosynovitis in compartment I tendons.
    - The patient is instructed to make a fist with the thumb tucked inside the other fingers.
    - Then the examiner stabilizes the patient's forearm with 1 hand and deviates the patient's wrist in an ulnar direction with the other hand.
    - Sharp pain felt in the tunnel region strongly supports a diagnosis of stenosing tenosynovitis.

- Palpation of the palmar aspect of the wrist:
  - Palmaris longus:
    - Bisects the anterior aspect of the wrist; its distal end also is the anterior surface of the carpal tunnel.
    - To palpate the palmaris longus, have the patient flex the wrist and touch the tips of the thumb and small finger together in apposition; the palmaris longus becomes prominent along the midline of the anterior aspect of the wrist.
  - Carpal tunnel:
    - Lies deep to the palmaris longus and is defined proximally by the pisiform and the tubercle of the scaphoid and distally by the hook of the hamate and the tubercle of the trapezium
    - The transverse carpal ligament, part of the volar carpal ligament, runs between those bony prominences and forms a fibrous sheath containing the carpal tunnel anteriorly within a fibro-osseous tunnel.
    - Posteriorly, the carpal tunnel is bordered by the carpal bones.
    - The compartment transports the median nerve and the finger flexor tendons from the forearm to the hand.
    - Clinical significance:
      - Compression of the median nerve (CTS) can restrict motor function and sensation along the median nerve distribution of the hand.
      - Patients note discomfort over the wrist and numbness of the thumb and the index and middle fingers.
      - Patients often have paresthesias at night.
    - To support a diagnosis of CTS, reproduce:
      - Pain in the median nerve distribution by tapping over the volar carpal ligament (Tinel sign) (1)
      - Symptoms by flexing the patient's wrist to its maximal degrees and holding for at least 1 minute (Phalen test) (1)
  - Flexor carpi radialis:
    - Flexor carpi radialis tendinitis can cause pain over the flexor aspect of the wrist.
    - On examination, pain is noted with palpation over the flexor carpi radialis tunnel (from 3 cm proximal to the wrist to the main insertion of the flexor carpi radialis on the base of the second metacarpal).
    - Examination also usually produces increased pain with resisted wrist flexion and resisted radial deviation of the wrist.
  - Vascular anatomy:
    - The radial artery can be palpated just radial to the flexor carpi radialis tendon.
    - The pulse of the ulnar artery may be palpated proximal to the pisiform bone just before it crosses the wrist on the anterior aspect of the ulna.
    - Most patients have both arteries, with the ulnar artery usually providing the dominant blood supply (2).
- ROM (use bilateral comparison to evaluate the patient's restrictions):
  - Flexion (normal, 70–80°)
  - Extension (normal, 70–80°)
  - Radial deviation (normal, up to ~20°)
  - Ulnar deviation (normal, up to ~30°)
  - Supination (normal, 90°)
  - Pronation (normal, 90°)
- Neurologic examination (the focus is on muscular assessment and sensation testing).
- Motor testing:
  - Wrist extension (C6)
  - Flexion (C7)
  - Supination (C5, C6)
  - Pronation (C6, C8, T1)
- Sensation testing (test volar and dorsal aspects of the wrist and compared results with those of the contralateral wrist)
- Peripheral nerve innervation (test sensation in the median, ulnar, and radial nerve distributions in the hand)

## TESTS

### *Imaging*

- Radiographs should include at least 3 views of the wrist (posteroanterior, lateral, and oblique).
  - A "scaphoid view" (wrist in ulnar deviation) can be helpful in assessing for a scaphoid fracture.
  - A "clenched fist" view can suggest a possible scapholunate ligament tear (3).
- Scaphoid fractures may not be evident on initial radiographs and may be seen on repeat radiographs 7–10 days later.

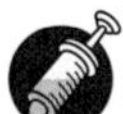

# TREATMENT

## GENERAL MEASURES

### *Pregnancy Considerations*

- If the pregnant patient has symptoms of numbness and tingling in her fingers, the clinician should have a high index of suspicion for CTS (median neuropathy at the wrist).
- An increased incidence of de Quervain tenosynovitis also occurs in new mothers. (The clinician should check for this condition by using the Finkelstein test.)

## REFERENCES


1. Hoppenfeld S. Physical examination of the wrist and hand. *In: Physical Examination of the Spine and Extremities.* Norwalk, CT: Appleton-Century-Crofts, 1976;59–104.
2. American Society for Surgery of the Hand. Examination of specific systems. In: *The Hand: Examination and Diagnosis.* New York: Churchill Livingstone, 1990:13–56.
3. Garcia-Elias M, Geissler WB. Carpal instability. In: Green DP, Hotchkiss RN, Pederson WC, et al., eds. *Green's Operative Hand Surgery*, 5th ed. Philadelphia: Elsevier Churchill Livingstone, 2005: 535–604.


## ADDITIONAL READING


Watson HK, Weinzweig J. Physical examination of the wrist. *Hand Clin* 1997;1:17–34.


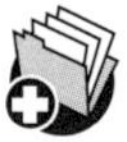

# MISCELLANEOUS

## FAQ

- Q: How can you differentiate between de Quervain tenosynovitis and thumb CMC arthritis on examination?
  - A: In de Quervain tenosynovitis, the patient is tender to palpation over the 1st dorsal compartment tendons over the radial styloid versus tenderness over the CMC joint in CMC arthritis. In de Quervain tenosynovitis, the patient has pain with ulnar deviation of the wrist with the thumb tucked into a fist, whereas with CMC arthritis, the patient has a positive grind test.
- Q: What is the anatomic landmark for the scaphoid?
  - A: The "anatomic snuffbox" is a small depression just distal and dorsal to the radial styloid process. It is easy to visualize when the patient extends the thumb laterally away from the fingers. Tenderness to palpation in this area after trauma suggests possible scaphoid fracture.

# WRIST PAIN

*Dawn M. LaPorte, MD*
*John J. Hwang, MD*

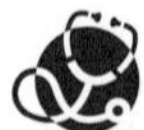

## BASICS

### DESCRIPTION

- Wrist pain, a common symptom, may be caused by different conditions, including trauma, overuse, and infection.
  - It is important to obtain a detailed history to make the correct diagnosis and to provide appropriate treatment.
  - The history should include onset, duration, frequency, and location of the pain.
  - Information regarding swelling, erythema, abnormal clicks, aggravating activities, ROM, sensory changes, motor strength, and general health conditions is essential.
- Classification:
  - Traumatic
  - Inflammatory
  - Degenerative
  - Infectious
  - Neurologic

#### *Pregnancy Considerations*

If numbness is present as well, it is most likely CTS.

### ASSOCIATED CONDITIONS

- Rheumatoid arthritis
- History of trauma
- Osteoarthritis
- Gout

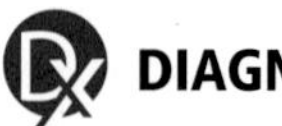

## DIAGNOSIS

### SIGNS AND SYMPTOMS

- The location of wrist pain is indicative of the cause.
- Patients may present with swelling and pain localized as radial wrist pain, dorsal wrist pain, ulnar wrist pain, palmar wrist pain, or general wrist pain.

#### *Physical Exam*

- Radial wrist pain:
  - De Quervain tenosynovitis:
    - Caused by inflammation of the 1st dorsal compartment (extensor pollicis brevis and abductor pollicis longus)
    - The patient may provide a history of repetitive wrist activities.
    - Finkelstein test (with thumb flexed into palm, pain is reproduced by ulnar deviation of the wrist) usually is positive.
  - Scaphoid fracture:
    - Patients usually have a history of trauma, most often a fall on an outstretched arm.
    - Tender to palpation over anatomic snuffbox
- Dorsal wrist pain:
  - Tenosynovitis of extensor tendons:
    - The patient usually presents complaining of pain in the dorsum of the wrist that may radiate proximally and distally.
    - Usually, the patient has a history of repetitive activities and overuse.
    - Pain occurs on flexion and extension.
    - Pain with resisted extension
    - Sometimes, a sharply demarcated scalloped edge of the extensor synovial sheath can be palpated with wrist motion.
  - Ganglion cyst:
    - This cyst is the most common mass on the dorsal surface of the wrist.
    - Most arise from the scapholunate ligament.
    - Generally, they are movable and transilluminate light.
    - The size of a cyst may vary with time.
  - Extensor carpi ulnaris tendinitis:
    - Pain over this tendon with combined supination and ulnar deviation against resistance
- Ulnar wrist pain:
  - Distal radioulnar joint instability:
    - Usually history of trauma to the wrist
    - Pain is located at the distal radioulnar joint, especially with pronation and supination.
    - Instability can be palpated or visualized with stress loading.
    - Radiographs may show increased space between the distal radius and ulna; if radiography is inconclusive, CT may be helpful.
  - Flexor carpi ulnaris tendinitis:
    - Pain at the flexor carpi ulnar usually is detected on resisted wrist flexion and ulnar deviation.
  - Fracture of the hook of the hamate:
    - Patients (especially golfers and tennis players) have a history of direct impact to the ulnar palm.
    - Pain occurs on palpation of hamate and resisted flexion of 4th and 5th fingers (1)
    - Radiographs of the wrist in the carpal tunnel view show the fracture.
  - TFCC tear:
    - Ulnar-sided wrist pain, often with clicking
    - Pain with axial load while rotating the ulnar-deviated wrist
- Palmar wrist pain:
  - Flexor tenosynovitis:
    - Similar to extensor tenosynovitis
    - The patient usually presents with a history of overuse of the wrist.
    - Pain, located on the palmar aspect of the wrist, is aggravated with wrist motion and with resisted wrist flexion; it may radiate proximally or distally.
  - CTS (2):
    - Most common compression neuropathy in the upper extremity.
    - Patients often complain of pain around the wrist, numbness and tingling in the radial 3 digits, clumsiness, and weakness.
    - Patients frequently wake up at night with numbness in the fingers.
    - Tinel test of the carpal tunnel and Phalen test may be positive.
    - Decreased sensibility in median nerve distribution and thenar atrophy are late signs.
- General wrist pain:
  - Arthritis:
    - Patients with inflammatory arthritis and osteoarthritis involving the radiocarpal, intercarpal, and CMC joints present with pain in the wrist.
    - Patients with osteoarthritis may have a history of trauma.
    - Swelling, stiffness, and decreased ROM usually are present.
    - Patients with inflammatory arthritis, especially rheumatoid arthritis, have swelling of tendon sheaths and synovial thickening.
    - Deformity of joints is a sign of advanced disease.
    - Radiographs of patients with osteoarthritis generally show narrowing of joint space, subchondral sclerosis, and osteophytes.
    - Radiographs of patients with inflammatory arthritis show narrowing of joint space, osteopenia, bone erosion, and deformity.
  - Wrist infection:
    - Immunocompromised patients or those with a history of intravenous drug use are at higher risk than the general population.
    - Pain, swelling, erythema, decreased ROM, and other cardinal signs of infection may be present.
    - Increased pain with ROM is characteristic.
    - Elevated leukocyte count, ESR, and C-reactive protein are signs of infection.
    - Joint fluid analysis: Findings of >80,000 white blood cells and >75% polymorphs strongly suggest a septic joint. (Absolute white blood cell counts may vary and overlap with other conditions.)

## TESTS

### *Lab*

White blood cell count, ESR, and C-reactive protein are indicated to assess for infection.

### *Imaging*

- Radiography:
  - Plain AP, lateral, and oblique radiographs are obtained to look for fracture, with a carpal tunnel view for fracture of the hook of the hamate.
  - A scaphoid view is used to assess scaphoid fracture (3).
- MRI may be useful in the diagnosis of TFCC tear (1).

## DIFFERENTIAL DIAGNOSIS

- Radial wrist pain:
  - De Quervain tenosynovitis
  - Scaphoid fracture or nonunion
  - Thumb CMC arthritis
  - Radiocarpal arthritis
- Dorsal wrist pain:
  - Tenosynovitis of extensor tendons
  - Ganglion cyst
  - Extensor carpi ulnaris tendinitis
- Ulnar wrist pain:
  - Distal radioulnar joint instability
  - Flexor carpi ulnaris tendinitis
  - Fracture of the hook of the hamate
  - TFCC tear
- Palmar wrist pain:
  - Flexor tenosynovitis
  - CTS
  - Palmar ganglion
- General wrist pain:
  - Arthritis
  - Infection

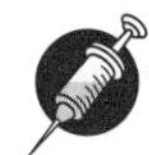

# TREATMENT

## GENERAL MEASURES

- Tendinitis and tenosynovitis can be treated with rest, modification of activity, ice, immobilization, NSAIDs, and local injection of steroid if warranted.
- Nondisplaced fractures should be treated with immobilization and NSAIDs.
- Rheumatoid arthritis of the wrist should be treated by a rheumatologist as a component of general systemic condition.
- Ganglion cysts may be aspirated (if dorsal) or excised.
- Patients with mild to moderate CTS symptoms can be treated nonoperatively (oral anti-inflammatory medicine, wrist splint, and activity modification).
  - Nonoperative interventions are unlikely to cure the condition but they may alleviate the symptoms enough to obviate the need for surgical intervention.
  - Injection of cortisone to the carpal tunnel may be indicated for persistent CTS before considering surgical management.
- Patients with wrist infections should be admitted to a hospital.
  - After joint fluid is sent for culture and sensitivity, intravenous antibiotics should be started as soon as possible.
  - Open irrigation usually is indicated, but serial aspiration of the joint is also an acceptable means of treatment.
  - After hospital discharge, antibiotics usually are continued for several weeks; early ROM is paramount in preserving long-term joint function.

## MEDICATION (DRUGS)

### *First Line*

- NSAIDs
- Local steroid injection for tenosynovitis and tendinitis in persistent case
- Intravenous antibiotics for wrist infection

## SURGERY

- De Quervain tenosynovitis: A few patients require surgical release of the 1st dorsal compartment.
- Displaced scaphoid fracture: Internal fixation
- Distal radioulnar joint instability:
  - If the TFCC is involved, treatment is controversial.
  - Patients who cannot be treated by immobilization may require arthroscopy and open repair of the TFCC tear.
  - If accompanied by intra-articular and extra-articular fracture of the distal radius or ulna, fixation of fracture and Kirschner wire pinning of the distal radioulnar joint instability are indicated.
- Fracture of the hook of the hamate:
  - This fracture tends to be displaced, and the incidence of nonunion is high if it is left untreated.
  - If the fragment is small, its surgical excision is recommended.
  - For a fracture at the hook's base, open reduction and internal fixation are recommended.
- Flexor tenosynovitis:
  - Surgical tenolysis is indicated for chronic recalcitrant tendinitis.
- CTS:
  - Surgical release (considered definitive treatment) is indicated when nonoperative treatment has failed or when signs of advanced CTS (including decreased sensibility, muscle atrophy, and substantial nerve conduction study and electromyographic changes) exist.
- Arthritis:
  - Surgical intervention (e.g., arthroplasty, resection, fusion) is reserved for patients with severe symptoms in whom nonoperative treatment has failed.

# FOLLOW-UP

## PROGNOSIS

Most cases can be largely alleviated by 1 of the forementioned methods.

## REFERENCES


1. Cooney WP, Bishop AT, Linscheid RL. Physical examination of the wrist. In: Cooney WP, Linscheid RL, Dobyns RL, eds. *The Wrist: Diagnosis and Operative Treatment*. St. Louis: Mosby, 1998:236–261.
2. Gelberman RH, Rydevik BL, Pess GM, et al. Carpal tunnel syndrome. A scientific basis for clinical care. *Orthop Clin North Am* 1988;19:115–124.
3. Amadio PC, Moran SL. Fractures of the carpal bones. In: Green DP, Hotchkiss RN, Pederson WC, et al., eds. *Green's Operative Hand Surgery*, 5th ed. Philadelphia: Elsevier Churchill Livingstone, 2005:711–768.


## ADDITIONAL READING


- Aulicino PL, Siegel JL. Acute injuries of the distal radioulnar joint. *Hand Clin* 1991;7:283–293.
- Donatto KC. Orthopaedic management of septic arthritis. *Rheum Dis Clin North Am* 1998;24: 275–286.
- Gelberman RH, Wolock BS, Siegel DB. Fractures and non-unions of the carpal scaphoid. *J Bone Joint Surg* 1989;71A:1560–1565.
- Harvey FJ, Harvey PM, Horsley MW. De Quervain's disease: Surgical or nonsurgical treatment. *J Hand Surg* 1990;15A:83–87.


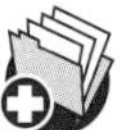

# MISCELLANEOUS

## CODES

### *ICD9-CM*

- 714.0 Rheumatoid arthritis
- 727.04 De Quervain tenosynovitis
- 727.41 Ganglion of joint
- 814.01 Scaphoid fracture

## PATIENT TEACHING

Patients with work-related CTS may alleviate the condition by job modification.

## FAQ

- Q: What causes radial-side wrist pain?
  - A: The most common cause is de Quervain tenosynovitis (inflammation of the 1st dorsal compartment tendons characterized by tenderness and a positive Finkelstein test). The 2nd most common cause is thumb CMC arthritis (tender at CMC joint and positive "grind test"). The 3rd is radiocarpal arthritis (characterized by pain with radial deviation of the wrist). With a history of trauma, one also should consider a scaphoid fracture as a possible diagnosis.
- Q: What must be considered in ulnar-side wrist pain?
  - A: The differential diagnosis includes TFCC, distal radioulnar joint instability, flexor carpi ulnaris tendinitis, and fracture of the hook of the hamate.

# WRIST SPRAIN

*Peter R. Jay, MD*
*Dawn M. LaPorte, MD*

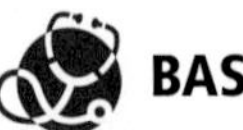

## BASICS

### DESCRIPTION
- A wrist sprain is an injury to the bones and ligaments of the wrist that results in pain from an incomplete ligament tear.
  - No associated long-term disability
  - Because many serious injuries are easily confused with wrist sprains, the patient with substantial swelling or persistent pain should be suspected of having a more serious injury.
- Classification:
  - Grade I: No ligament damage (stretch of the ligament without tearing)
  - Grade II: Partial tear
  - Grade III: Complete tear

### EPIDEMIOLOGY
- Wrist sprain occurs most commonly in adults; it is rare in children.
- Suspect an injury to the growth plate if swelling and tenderness are seen.
- Elderly persons are more likely to suffer a fracture.
- Males and females are affected equally.

#### *Incidence*
This is a common injury because the wrist is part of the 1st reflexive defense against injury.

### RISK FACTORS
- Frequent falls
- Overuse

### PATHOPHYSIOLOGY
#### *Pathological Findings*
- A sprain of the wrist involves partial stretching or disruption of the ligaments holding the radius and the carpal bones in alignment.
- No major interosseous ligament injury or fracture should be seen.

### ETIOLOGY
- This injury usually occurs from a fall on an outstretched hand.
- It also may occur from a twisting injury as the hand is grasping an object.
- Overuse or unusually heavy activity with wrist

### ASSOCIATED CONDITIONS
- A fall on an outstretched hand produces a continuum of injury from stretching and mild tearing of the ligament to fracture of the bones and dislocation of the articulation, such as the following:
  - Scaphoid fracture
  - Radial styloid fracture
  - Perilunate dislocation

## DIAGNOSIS

### SIGNS AND SYMPTOMS
- Signs: Swelling over the wrist joint
- Symptoms:
  - Pain on ROM
  - Stiffness
  - Decreased grip strength
  - Little pain on axial loading

#### *Physical Exam*
- Inspect the wrist for amount of swelling.
- Carefully perform ROM.
  - It should be possible to achieve a complete range if done slowly.
  - Check pronation and supination of the wrist.
- Palpate the structures on the dorsum of the wrist individually for tenderness and to focus the subsequent radiographic examination.
- Palpate the volar part of the wrist; tenderness increases the likelihood of a serious injury.
- Inspect the snuffbox for tenderness.
- Palpate the wrist extensor tendons, both over and away from the wrist.

### TESTS
#### *Lab*
No serum tests

#### *Imaging*
- Radiography:
  - Obtain AP, lateral, and oblique films of the wrist.
    - The oblique film (also termed the "navicular view") is most useful to rule out an occult injury to this bone.
  - Order a clenched-fist view if scapholunate instability is suspected.
    - A positive view shows >3 mm of space between the scaphoid and lunate (1).
  - A coned (specially focused) lateral view of the wrist may be needed to rule out avulsion fractures of the triquetrum or of the lunate.
- MRI or fluoroscopy may be used by the orthopaedist or hand surgeon in cases of an unclear diagnosis or to search for an occult injury.
- If plain radiographs are normal, a bone scan may be ordered to rule out occult fracture (2).

### DIFFERENTIAL DIAGNOSIS
- The diagnosis of a wrist sprain is clinical and made primarily by palpation over the ligaments and by the exclusion of more serious injuries.
  - Navicular or scaphoid fracture:
    - This serious injury may progress to a painful nonunion if it is not immobilized.
    - Signaled by pain in the "snuffbox" area of the hand, between the extensor and abductor tendons to the thumb
    - A scaphoid radiographic view usually shows it.
    - If not, a bone scan may be ordered, or the wrist may be immobilized in a thumb spica cast for 2 weeks and then rechecked (2).
- Scapholunate interosseous ligament injury:
  - This tear of the ligament that joins the lunate and scaphoid bones may result in late wrist instability, clicking, and degeneration.
  - The signs are a gap >3 mm between the scaphoid and lunate on plain posteroanterior radiograph or an angle of >60° between these bones on the lateral radiograph (1).
- Avulsion or "chip" fracture of the lunate or triquetrum:
  - This injury, which may simulate a sprain, is best seen on coned or detailed lateral films of the wrist.
  - Longer immobilization is required.
- De Quervain tenosynovitis:
  - This overuse injury of the extensor-abductor tendons of the thumb results in aching on the radial side of the wrist and a positive Finkelstein test (3).
- TFCC tear:
  - This tear involves the distal radioulnocarpal joint and causes ulnar-sided wrist pain.
- Distal radioulnar joint subluxation:
  - This injury is noted by a dorsal prominence over the distal ulna, especially in pronation (4).
- Subluxation of the extensor carpi ulnaris tendon:
  - This injury usually occurs with pronation and supination of the wrist and causes pain that is frequently associated with "snapping."
- Lunate dislocations:
  - These serious injuries occur after falls and high-energy trauma to the wrist.
  - The lunate is completely dislocated on the radiographs.
  - This injury frequently is overlooked on initial plain radiographs.

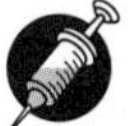

## TREATMENT

### GENERAL MEASURES
- Immobilization for comfort
- Counseling to return to activity when symptoms subside
- Specialist referral if symptoms persist
- If a scaphoid fracture is suspected, the wrist should be immobilized in a thumb spica cast and re-examined in 2 weeks.
- If carpal instability is suspected, refer patient to a specialist.
- If a sprain is suspected, ice, immobilization, and analgesics are appropriate.
- A wrist splint may be made of padded plaster or fiberglass or may be ready-made for easy removal and reapplication.
- Remove the wrist splint when the pain subsides, usually in 5 days, at the most.
- If pain persists >5 days and is not improving, referral to a specialist may be indicated.

### Activity

- When pain subsides, early return to activity should be encouraged.
- If clicking or pain develops, the wrist should be re-evaluated.

## SPECIAL THERAPY

### Physical Therapy

- The patient may perform therapy at home with an exercise program or directly under the supervision of a therapist.
- The goals of rehabilitation are return to preinjury ROM, strength, and dexterity.

## MEDICATION (DRUGS)

### First Line

NSAIDs are useful for patients with pain.

## SURGERY

- Surgery is not indicated for simple wrist sprains.
- Major ligament tears that result in instability often necessitate surgical repair (ligament reconstruction, or partial or complete wrist fusion) (1).

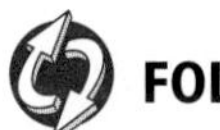

# FOLLOW-UP

## PROGNOSIS

- Full recovery is expected after a wrist sprain.
- If it is not achieved, evaluate the patient for other conditions.

## COMPLICATIONS

- Reflex sympathetic dystrophy, a syndrome of sympathetically maintained pain resulting in exaggeration of the injury response
- Ankylosis

## PATIENT MONITORING

- The patient should be seen 7–14 days after the injury.
- If the pain has resolved, no additional evaluation is necessary.
- If substantial pain is still present, radiographs and consultation with an orthopaedic or hand surgeon should be obtained.

## REFERENCES


1. Garcia-Elias M, Geissler WB. Carpal instability. In: Green DP, Hotchkiss RN, Pederson WC, et al., eds. *Green's Operative Hand Surgery*, 5th ed. Philadelphia: Elsevier Churchill Livingstone, 2005:535–604.
2. Amadio PC, Moran SL. Fractures of the carpal bones. In: Green DP, Hotchkiss RN, Pederson WC, et al., eds. *Green's Operative Hand Surgery*, 5th ed. Philadelphia: Elsevier Churchill Livingstone, 2005:711–768.
3. Wolfe SW. Tenosynovitis. In: Green DP, Hotchkiss RN, Pederson WC, et al., eds. *Green's Operative Hand Surgery*, 5th ed. Philadelphia: Elsevier Churchill Livingstone, 2005:2137–2159.
4. Adams BD. Distal radioulnar joint instability. In: Green DP, Hotchkiss RN, Pederson WC, et al., ed. *Green's Operative Hand Surgery*, 5th ed. Philadelphia: Elsevier Churchill Livingstone, 2005:605–644.


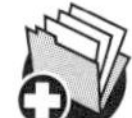

# MISCELLANEOUS

## CODES

### ICD9-CM

842.00 Wrist pain

## PATIENT TEACHING

Instruct the patient to remove the splint in 5 days and to begin ROM and activities of daily living.

### Prevention

If feasible, patients should avoid falling on the outstretched hand.

## FAQ

- Q: How is the diagnosis of wrist sprain made?
  - A: The diagnosis is based on clinical examination and careful exclusion of more serious injuries. The patient is tender to palpation over the wrist ligaments.
- Q: How should a wrist sprain be treated?
  - A: The wrist should be immobilized in a splint for patient comfort. Anti-inflammatory medication may be helpful initially. If the patient is tender over the anatomic snuffbox, but no scaphoid fracture is seen, the splint should be a below-the-elbow thumb spica, and the patient should have a follow-up examination in 7–14 days for repeat radiographic evaluation.

W

# GLOSSARY

| Abbreviation | Definition | Abbreviation | Definition |
|---|---|---|---|
| 3D | three-dimensional | MDI | multidirectional instability |
| AC | acromioclavicular | MFH | malignant fibrous histiocytoma |
| ACL | anterior cruciate ligament | MPN | medial plantar nerve |
| AO/ASIF | Arbeitsgemeinschaft fur Osteosyntheses/Association for the Study of Internal Fixation | MRA | magnetic resonance arthrography |
| | | MRI | magnetic resonance imaging |
| AP | anteroposterior | MTP | metatarsophalangeal |
| AS | ankylosing spondylitis | NF | neurofibromatosis |
| ATFL | anterior talofibular ligament | NOF | nonossifying fibroma |
| ATLS | Advanced Trauma Life Support | NSAIDs | nonsteroidal anti-inflammatory drugs |
| AVN | avascular necrosis | OATS | osteochondral autogenous transplantation (proprietary term) |
| CFL | calcaneofibular ligament | | |
| CMC | carpometacarpal | OCD | osteochondral defect |
| CR | computed radiography | OI | osteogenesis imperfecta |
| CT | computed tomography | OSD | Osgood-Schlatter disease |
| CTS | carpal tunnel syndrome | PCL | posterior cruciate ligament |
| DDH | developmental dysplasia (or dislocation) of the hip | PE | pulmonary embolism |
| DEXA | dual-energy x-ray absorptiometry | PINS | posterior interosseous nerve syndrome |
| DIP | distal interphalangeal | PIP | proximal interphalangeal |
| DR | direct radiography | PTFL | posterior talofibular ligament |
| DVT | deep venous thrombosis | PTT | posterior tibial tendon |
| ECRB | extensor carpi radialis brevis | PVNS | pigmented villonodular synovitis |
| ECRL | extensor carpi radialis longus | RCL | radial collateral ligament |
| EOG | eosinophilic granuloma | RICE | rest, ice, compression, elevation |
| ESR | erythrocyte sedimentation rate | ROM | range of motion |
| HIV | human immunodeficiency virus | SCFE | slipped capital femoral epiphysis |
| HMPAO | $^{99m}$Tc-exametazime | SCIWORA | spinal cord injury without radiographic abnormality |
| INR | international normalized ratio | | |
| IP | interphalangeal | SI | sacroiliac |
| ITBS | iliotibial band syndrome | SLAP | superior labral anterior and posterior |
| JIA | juvenile idiopathic arthritis | SPECT | single-photon emission tomography |
| LCH | Langerhans cell histiocytosis | STIR | short T1 inversion recovery |
| LCL | lateral collateral ligament | TFCC | triangular fibrocartilage complex |
| LPN | lateral plantar nerve | TLSO | thoracolumbosacral orthosis |
| MCL | medial collateral ligament | TNF | tumor necrosis factor |
| MCN | medial collateral nerve | TOS | thoracic outlet syndrome |
| MCP | metacarpophalangeal | TPSS | three-phase skeletal scintigraphy |
| MFA | malignant fibrous histiocytoma | UCL | ulnar collateral ligament |

# INDEX

Note: Page numbers followed by f indicate figures; t indicate tabular material.